Principles of

Clinical Laboratory Utilization and Consultation

Principles of

Clinical Laboratory Utilization and Consultation

Brenta G. Davis, EdD, CLS, MT(ASCP)

Professor and Chair
Department of Clinical Laboratory Sciences
College of Allied Health Sciences
University of Tennessee—Memphis
Memphis, Tennessee

Diana Mass, MA, CLS, MT(ASCP)

Clinical Professor and Director
Clinical Laboratory Sciences Program
Department of Microbiology
College of Liberal Arts and Sciences
Arizona State University
Tempe, Arizona

Michael L. Bishop, MS, CLS, MT(ASCP)

Training, Application, and Support Specialist
Sales Training Department
Organon Teknika Corporation
Durham, North Carolina

W.B. SAUNDERS COMPANY
A Division of Harcourt Brace & Company
Philadelphia London Toronto Montreal Sydney Tokyo

W.B. SAUNDERS COMPANY
A Division of Harcourt Brace & Company

The Curtis Center
Independence Square West
Philadelphia, Pennsylvania 19106

Library of Congress Cataloging-in-Publication Data

Principles of clinical laboratory utilization and consultation / [edited by] Brenta G. Davis, Diana Mass, Michael L. Bishop—1st ed.

p.   cm.

ISBN 0–7216–6934–4

1. Diagnosis, Laboratory.   2. Medical laboratories.   I. Davis, Brenta G.
II. Mass, Diana.   III. Bishop, Michael L.
[DNLM: 1. Laboratory Techniques and Procedures—utilization.   2. Referral and
Consultation.   QY 4 P957 1999]

RB37.P715 1999   616.07′56—dc21

DNLM/DLC   98–13149

PRINCIPLES OF CLINICAL LABORATORY UTILIZATION AND CONSULTATION   ISBN 0–7216–6934–4

Printed in the United States of America.

Last digit is the print number: 9   8   7   6   5   4   3   2   1

To all who value our profession and welcome the challenge of its transformation, and to my family for the pleasure they bring to everything in my life.

B. G. D.

To my mother and father, Ella and Joseph Rotman, for their guidance; to my husband, Monty, for his encouragement; and to my daughter, Jacquelyn, for enriching our lives.

D. M.

To Sheila, Chris, and Carson for their support and patience.

M. L. B.

Contributors

Shauna C. Anderson, PhD

Chair, Microbiology Department and Director, Clinical Laboratory Science Program, Brigham Young University, Provo, Utah

Thyroid Disorders; Disorders of the Parathyroid Glands; Disorders of the Adrenal Cortex; Male Reproductive Disorders

Brian D. Andresen, MS, PhD

Director, Forensic Science Center, Lawrence Livermore National Laboratory, Livermore, California

Hypertensive Disorders; Toxicology and Drug Monitoring

Judith T. Barr, ScD

Director, National Education and Research Center For Outcomes Assessment, Northeastern University, Boston, Massachusetts

Clinical Laboratory Utilization: Rationale

Vickie S. Baselski, PhD

Professor, Department of Pathology, University of Tennessee; Director, Clinical Microbiology, Regional Medical Center, and Baptist Regional Laboratories, Memphis, Tennessee

Septic Shock; Antimicrobial Therapy and Sensitivity Testing

Michael L. Bishop, MS, CLS, MT(ASCP)

Training, Application, and Support Specialist, Sales Training Department, Organon Teknika Corporation, Durham, North Carolina

Laboratory Results in the Newborn

Karen Brown, MS

Instructor in Hematology, Hemostasis, Phlebotomy, Department of Pathology, University of Utah, and Salt Lake Community College; Assistant Professor and Medical Laboratory Technician Program Director, University of Utah, School of Medicine, Salt Lake City, Utah

Leukocyte Abnormalities and Hematologic Malignancies

Eileen Carreiro-Lewandowski, MS

Professor, Department of Medical Laboratory Science, University of Massachusetts, North Dartmouth, Massachusetts

Pancreatitis

Louis B. Caruana, MS, PhD

Professor of Clinical Laboratory Science, Clinical Laboratory Science Program, Health Science Center, Southwest Texas State University, San Marcos, Texas

Osteomyelitis

Susan Cockayne, PhD

Associate Professor, Brigham Young University, Provo, Utah

Impaired Glucose Metabolism; Pituitary Disorders

Kozy Corsaut, MEd, MT(ASCP), CLS(NCA)

Associate Professor, Clinical Coordinator, Medical Laboratory Technician Program, Stark State College, Canton, Ohio

Degenerative Processes

Felicia A. Czekaj, MS

Assistant Professor of Clinical Laboratory Sciences, Medical Laboratory Technician and Medical Technology Programs, School of Health Related Professions, University of Medicine and Dentistry of New Jersey, Newark, New Jersey

Major Aminoaciduria

Brenta G. Davis, EdD, CLS, MT(ASCP)

Professor and Chair, Department of Clinical Laboratory Sciences, College of Allied Health Sciences, University of Tennessee, Memphis, Tennessee

Clinical Laboratory Utilization: Implementation

Catherine Downs, MA, CLS, MT(ASCP)

Clinical Professor, Clinical Laboratory Sciences Program, Department of Microbiology, College of Liberal Arts and Sciences, Arizona State University, Tempe, Arizona

Urinary Obstructive Disorders

Sharon S. Ehrmeyer, PhD

Professor, Pathology and Laboratory Medicine, University of Wisconsin, Madison, Wisconsin

Acute Respiratory Failure; Chronic Obstructive Pulmonary Disease; Pulmonary Thromboembolism; Lung Cancer

Gordon E. Ens, MT(ASCP)

President, Colorado Coagulation Consultants, Denver, Colorado; Associate Editor, Clinical Hemostasis Review, Tucson, Arizona

Hemostatic Disorders

Douglas W. Estry, PhD

Associate Professor, Medical Technology Program, Michigan State University, East Lansing, Michigan

Ulcers; Malignancies and Bleeding of the Gastrointestinal Tract

Kevin D. Fallon, PhD

Director of Scientific Affairs, Instrumentation Laboratory, Lexington, Massachusetts

Acute Respiratory Failure; Chronic Obstructive Pulmonary Disease; Pulmonary Thromboembolism

Deborah T. Firestone, MA, MT(ASCP), SBB

Chair, Clinical Laboratory Science Department, School of Health Technology and Management, State University of New York, Stony Brook, New York

Malnutrition, Eating Disorders, and Starvation

Maribeth L. Flaws, PhD, SM(ASCP)

Assistant Professor, Rush University, Chicago, Illinois

Infectious Processes (Neurologic)

H. Elise Galloway, MS, PhD

Professor Emeritus, Medical Laboratory Sciences, College of Health Professions, Medical University of South Carolina, Charleston, South Carolina

Disorders of Carbohydrate Metabolism

Lynn S. Garcia, MS, MT(ASCP), CLS(NCA), F(AAM)

Manager, Brentwood Annex (Microbiology, Special Manual Chemistry); and Clinical Laboratory, Santa Monica–UCLA Hospital, UCLA Medical Center, Department of Pathology and Laboratory Medicine, Los Angeles, California

Parasitic Infections

Jesse Guiles, EdD

Associate Professor of Clinical Laboratory Sciences, Department of Clinical Laboratory Sciences, School of Health Related Professions, University of Medicine and Dentistry of New Jersey, Newark, New Jersey

Major Aminoaciduria

Bethany W. Hurtuk, MS, PhD

Professional Laboratory Consultant, Cleveland, Ohio

Myocardial Infarction and Atherosclerotic Heart Disease

Lynn Ingram, MS

Associate Professor, University of Tennessee, Memphis, Tennessee

Heart Failure; Liver Disease: Jaundice, Cirrhosis; Hepatitis; Hepatic Failure

James A. Jackson, MS, PhD, MT (ASCP), CLS

Professor, Department of Medical Technology, Wichita State University, Wichita, Kansas

Cholestasis

Karen James, MS, PhD

Adjunct Assistant Professor, Department of Biology, Appalachian State University, Boone, North Carolina; Consultant, Health Care Development Services, Northbrook, Illinois

Acquired Immunodeficiency Syndrome (AIDS); Tumor Immunology and Tumor Markers

Rebecca Jensen, MT (ASCP)

Editor, Clinical Hemostasis Review, Hemostasis Resources, Tucson, Arizona

Hemostatic Disorders

Hal S. Larsen, PhD, MT (ASCP), CLS (NCA)

Associate Dean and Chair, Department of Diagnostic and Primary Care, Texas Tech University Health Sciences Center, Lubbock, Texas

Primary Immunodeficiencies; Allergies

Craig A. Lehmann, PhD

Associate Dean, Associate Professor and Chair, Division of Diagnostic and Therapeutic Sciences, School of Health Technology and Management, Health Sciences Center, State University of New York, Stony Brook, New York

Malnutrition, Eating Disorders, and Starvation; Hyperlipoproteinemias

Linda Luckey, MEd

Assistant Professor, Clinical Laboratory Sciences, University of Tennessee; Director, Clinical Laboratory, Baptist Memorial Hospital, Memphis, Tennessee

Clinical Laboratory Utilization: Implementation

Peggy Prinz Luebbert, MS, MT (ASCP), CIC

Instructor, University of Nebraska Medical Center, Risk Management Specialist, Alegent Health, Omaha, Nebraska

Nosocomial Infections

Connie R. Mahon, MS

Associate Professor and Undergraduate Program Director, Department of Clinical Laboratory Sciences, The University of Texas Health Science Center, San Antonio, Texas

Bowel Disorders; Skin and Soft Tissue Infections

Diana Mass, MA, CLS, MT (ASCP)

Clinical Professor and Director, Clinical Laboratory Sciences Program, Department of Microbiology, College of Liberal Arts and Sciences, Arizona State University, Tempe, Arizona

Consulting as a Professional Role for the Clinical Laboratory Scientist

Timothy G. McManamon, PhD, DABCC

Lecturer, Mercy School of Medical Technology and Clinical Laboratory Science; Clinical Chemist, Mercy Hospital Medical Center, Des Moines, Iowa

Fetal Monitoring

Elia Mears, MS, MT (ASCP) SM

Instructor, Department of Medical Technology, School of Allied Health Professions, Louisiana State University Medical Center, New Orleans; Laboratory Manager, Leonard Chabert Medical Center, Houma, Louisiana

Nutrition in the Hospitalized Patient

Herb Miller, PhD, MT (ASCP), CLS (NCA)

Acting Chairman, Director, and Associate Professor, Department of Medical Technology, Rush University, Chicago, Illinois

Pleural Effusions

Sharon M. Miller, PhC, MT (ASCP), CLS (NCA)

Professor and Associate Dean, College of Health and Human Sciences, Northern Illinois University, De Kalb, Illinois

Geriatric Changes in Laboratory Results

Theodore H. Morton, PharmD

Assistant Professor of Clinical Pharmacy and Clinical Laboratory Sciences, University of Tennessee; Clinical Pharmacy Specialist, Baptist Memorial Health Care, Memphis, Tennessee; Assistant Professor of Clinical Pharmacy Practice, University of Mississippi, Jackson, Mississippi

Antimicrobial Therapy and Sensitivity Testing

Martha Savage Payne, MPA

Associate Professor, Clinical Laboratory Science, University of Tennessee, Memphis, Tennessee

Renal Failure; Glomerulonephritis; Nephrotic Syndrome

Lucy J. Randles, MA, CLS/CLDir

President and Owner, Health Care Advantage, Copley, Ohio

Screening for Congenital Disorders

Lauren Roberts, MS, CLS, MT (ASCP)

Associate Clinical Professor, Clinical Laboratory Sciences Program, Arizona State University, Tempe, Arizona

Infectious Cardiomyopathy; Respiratory Tract Infections; Urinary Tract Infections; Sexually Transmitted Diseases

Linda L. Ross, MS

Assistant Professor, University of Tennessee, Memphis, Tennessee

Septic Shock; Infections in the Immunocompromised Host

Larry Schoeff, MS, MT (ASCP)

Director, Medical Technology Program, and Associate Professor, Department of Pathology, School of Medicine, University of Utah, Salt Lake City, Utah

Malabsorption

Marian Schwabbauer, PhD

Professor of Clinical Pathology, Department of Pathology, University of Iowa, Iowa City, Iowa

The Anemias

David L. Smalley, PhD, MT (ASCP), BCLD

Professor of Pathology and Associate Professor of Clinical Laboratory Sciences, University of Tennessee; Director, Diagnostic Immunology Laboratory and Profiling Laboratory, Baptist Regional Laboratories, Memphis, Tennessee

Autoimmune Diseases; Transplantation Immunology

Donna Spannaus-Martin, MS, PhD, MT(ASCP)

Assistant Professor, Department of Clinical Laboratory Sciences, University of Tennessee, Memphis, Tennessee

Osteoporosis

Thomas Spillman, PhD

Senior Technical Director, Laboratory Corporation of America, San Diego, California

Toxicology and Drug Monitoring

David P. Thorne, PhD

Assistant Professor, Michigan State University, Medical Technology Program, East Lansing, Michigan

Ulcers; Malignancies and Bleeding of the Gastrointestinal Tract

Denise Uettwiller-Geiger, MS, DLM

Administrative Director and Clinical Chemist, John T. Mather Memorial Hospital, Port Jefferson, New York

Pregnancy; Female Reproductive Disorders

Alexander von Laufen, MA

Clinical Neuropsychological Examiner, Department of Psychiatry and Behavioral Medicine, Bon Secours Venice Hospital, Venice, Florida

Cerebrovascular Accidents; Seizure Disorders, Epilepsy, and Other Convulsive States

Diane Wyatt, MS

Associate Professor, Department of Clinical Laboratory Sciences, University of Tennessee, Memphis, Tennessee

Hemolytic Disease of the Fetus and Newborn

Foreword

Over the past two decades the effect of laboratory science and technology on the day-to-day practice of medicine has changed dramatically. Laboratory analyses, which once required test tubes, beakers, and hot water baths in the 1960s and the monstrous sequential analyzers of the 1970s, are now commonly performed on desktop or handheld analyzers in a fraction of the time and with significantly better accuracy and reliability. Rather than a wait of 2 or 3 days for culture results, we frequently can know within hours the identity of an offending pathogen causing a sore throat, bacteremia, or meningitis. The sheer number of analytes that can be evaluated has dramatically increased. For example, in addition to testing for hepatitis antibodies and antigens, viral particles can now be quantitated; to evaluate myocardial injury, there are now analyses for Troponin I and T in addition to the old standbys of CPK, CK-MB and LDH. These changes have, to some extent, made the practice of medicine more exacting and definitely more complicated. Similarly, the field of laboratory science has evolved from one of complicated analytic procedures to one complicated by "black boxes," containing sophisticated electronics and an almost overwhelming array of test choices.

These advances have also created significant challenges for those at the interface between laboratory and clinical medicine. In additon to pathologists, others at this interface frequently include clinical laboratory supervisors, technical supervisors and consultants, and nonpathologist directors of physicians' office laboratories. Physicians read or hear about a new test and want its supposed benefits for their patients right away. Not infrequently, however, such tests are found to be less useful than initially predicted or advertised. Because of the pressures to achieve cost-effective outcomes resulting from the advance of managed care, to be successful in this new world, we must learn to use the most effective means, in terms of both cost and outcome, to diagnose and treat our patients. This requires those in the medical field, clinician and laboratory scientist alike, to work as a team, now more than ever before. We must respect and accept one another's areas of expertise to maximize the quality and effectiveness of the services we provide. To do so requires that we also understand, to some degree at least, one another's expertise. The clinician must become acquainted with such concepts as sensitivity, specificity, and positive and negative predictive values, in order to most cost-effectively use a test and apply the result to patient care. The laboratorian must understand the pathophysiology of disease, the concept of differential diagnosis, other nonlaboratory diagnostic tests and how test results contribute, or an accurate and timely diagnosis of a patient's malady.

This book was written with these needs in mind. It can and will serve as an excellent resource for the laboratory scientist and the busy clinician, and probably, most importantly, for those at the interface between the two fields of laboratory and clinical medicine. As director of a large physicians' office laboratory I expect this book to assist me greatly in answering the questions of my colleagues about laboratory testing and how it is best used in their practice of medicine. Undoubtedly it will serve similar needs wherever cost-effective diagnosis and treatment can be enhanced by appropriate and effective use of the clinical laboratory.

VERLIN K. JANZEN, MD, MT(ASCP)

Hutchinson Clinic
Hutchinson, Kansas

Preface

The clinical laboratory is changing and clinical laboratory scientists are changing with it. Even before the advent of managed care, medical necessity, and capitation, technological advances were creating new and different roles for us. Because of these changes, the skills that are valued now in the clinical laboratory are quite different from those that were necessary for success in the past. Quality has been, and will always be, the *sine qua non* of the clinical laboratory but an important new dimension has been added to considerations of quality: proper utilization of the laboratory for efficient and cost-effective diagnosis and treatment of the patient.

This book is based on the premise that the demands on the clinical laboratory have become so complex that merely reporting raw data without insight and understanding of the physician's needs can be counterproductive for the patient and for the fiscal health of the institution. Today it is no longer sufficient for laboratory results to be merely accurate and precise; they must also be useful in that they do not confuse the issue for the physician or add unnecessarily to costs because the results contribute nothing toward a diagnosis. Laboratory skills today often have less to do with performing a test than with determining whether the test should be done at all; with ensuring that follow-up testing is appropriate; and with assisting the clinician in asking the right laboratory question rather than using a "shotgun" approach to diagnostic testing. More is no longer better.

If we are to meet these needs and participate fully in this expanded view of clinical laboratory practice, we must understand clearly the bases on which clinical questions are formulated and acted upon by clinicians. We must know how to use our scientific and technical expertise to assist the clinician in choosing the right tests for a given patient to reach an accurate, timely, and cost-effective diagnosis. In doing this, we are in a unique position to integrate data from all of the laboratory disciplines in a relevant way. It is in this context—as we help the clinician to choose wisely from among the great variety of tests available—that laboratory data become the *means,* not the end, of clinical laboratory science practice.

Principles of Clinical Laboratory Utilization and Consultation approaches the profession from this standpoint. We have assumed that our readers are familiar with normal physiology and can address laboratory test methodology and related technical considerations elsewhere. This book does not address the "how to" of methodology; there are many excellent texts that do so. Instead, it addresses the "why" and the "when" of laboratory testing by means of a disease-oriented organization and content based on the perspective of the user of laboratory findings. Thus, the book begins with a chapter that describes why clinicians choose laboratory tests and the process by which test results are used to evaluate differential diagnoses, derived from the patient's presenting symptoms, history, and physical findings, so that a final diagnosis evolves from laboratory data. The next chapter provides practical guidelines for laboratory practitioners in the implementation of a laboratory utilization program and examples of the significant resultant cost savings for the institution and the patient. The latter represent powerful arguments that laboratorians can use in persuading administrators of the wisdom of implementing such programs. The disease-oriented sequence of chapters dealing with organ systems is generally ordered by acuity; for example, disorders of the heart or lungs can have an immediate and grave outcome for the patient who is not treated properly or promptly. Further, chapters are organized to facilitate the clinical laboratory scientist's understanding of the circumstances under which one particular test or method might be valuable and another less so. Accordingly, there is great emphasis on the characteristics of laboratory analyses and the pathophysiology of various disease processes that result in significant abnormal laboratory findings. At the same time, the clinical manifestations that also derive from the pathophysiologic process are discussed so that the laboratory scientist can interact meaningfully with clinicians making test choices in a given clinical situation. Similarly, brief discussions of treatment are provided, particularly as it affects specific laboratory findings, so that the assistance and contribution of the clinical laboratory scientist can continue beyond the initial diagnosis.

Laboratory practitioners and educators who find these concepts of clinical laboratory science practice to be innovative or unusual would do well to read the foreword of this text, the two chapters described above, and the chapter on the development of consultation skills. These initial chapters, together with this preface, are designed to provide a foundation and rationale for the remainder of the text. Except for a few chapters in which a different organization seemed more logical, the reader will find discussions of etiology and pathophysiology leading to a description of clinical manifestations, which in turn lead to discussion of effective and efficient laboratory approaches to the clinical questions involved. In many cases, algorithms and flow charts are provided to aid in test choices, interpretation, and follow-up. The concluding sections of most chapters include a brief discussion of treatment and one or more case studies that illustrate the topics addressed therein.

Several conventions are followed throughout the text.

One such convention is that the term *clinical laboratory scientist* as used is equivalent to a term that is, perhaps, more familiar: *medical technologist.*

Although this text is designed primarily for clinical laboratory science practitioners and students, it is hoped that other healthcare professionals who have an interest in better utilization of the clinical laboratory might also find it helpful. The clinical laboratory is a powerful tool in quality patient care if it is properly used, and to that end this book has been written.

BRENTA G. DAVIS
DIANA MASS
MICHAEL L. BISHOP

Acknowledgments

The authors wish to acknowledge the original contributions by the following individuals on which portions of this text are based: Joan E. Aldrich, Holly Alexander, Benjamin Andrusaitis, Michael Boroch, Peggy L. Bottjen, Linda H. Brooks, Scot C. Buessow, JoLynne Campbell, V. Michelle Chenault, R. Lyle Christensen, Patricia Collins, Suzanne W. Conner, Julia R. Crowley, Madeline J. Ducate, Paul G. Engelkirk, Mary J. R. Gilchrist, Linda Gorman, Bethany W. Hurtuk, Sharon Jackson, Cynthia Karr, Consuelo M. Kazan, Janice M. Klaasen, Robin Gaynor Krefetz, Bernhard Ludvigsen, Peggy Luebbert, Shirley MacManigal, Kathleen Becan-McBride, Mary Ann McLane, Sharon M. Miller, Barbara J. Minard, Maria Luisa J. Morsi, Jon O. Nilsestuen, Jane Sydney Oliver, Marie Pezzlo, Laura Martin Rahlfs, Michael Sealfon, Robert M. Shoemaker, Linda A. Smith, Michael W. Sullivan, Cheryl Swinehart, Jacqueline Swoyer, Kerry A. Upton, and Patricia Walsh.

The authors also wish to gratefully acknowledge Verlin K. Janzen, MD, MT(ASCP) for his contributions as medical consultant and content reviewer.

Contents

Section Three
Renal Disorders

Section Four
Gastrointestinal Disorders

Contents xix

Contents

Part I

Principles of Laboratory Utilization and Consultation

Chapter 1

Clinical Laboratory Utilization: Rationale

Judith T. Barr

In 1995, the United States spent more than $1 trillion on health care services, more than $3,400 for every man, woman, and child in this country, and more per person than any other country on earth. Growing health care costs, from 5% of the gross domestic product (GDP) in 1965 to 15% in 1995, are now diverting monies from other segments of the economy. Rather than improving educational systems, replacing deteriorating transportation infrastructures, or modernizing industrial production systems, a large proportion of the GDP is going toward the nation's health care industry.

Perhaps if the United States had the best health in the world, the expenditure could be justified, but this is not the case. Compared with 20 other industrialized countries, the United States ranks near the top in infant mortality and low birth-weight rates expressed as a percent of live births and only ranking in the middle as measured by years of life expectancy.[1] We are investing more in health care than any other country on earth, yet we are not receiving the maximal return on our investment.

Laboratory professionals should be concerned with these national health care issues because they affect us. They affect take-home salaries, the international competitiveness of American products and companies, and the daily role of the laboratorian. The health care system is being squeezed to become more efficient, to use as few human and consumable resources as possible, and, thus, to reduce costs.

All sectors of the health care industry are being examined for methods to increase efficiency and reduce health care spending. The clinical laboratory will be a prime target because over the last generation major expansions in health care technology and its associated expenses have come from the diagnostic side, with a rapid growth in the costs of laboratory tests and imaging procedures.[2] The challenge is to achieve the benefits of increased efficiency without compromising essential quality of services.

In October 1993, the Health Care Financing Administration (HCFA) reported that 154,403 laboratories had registered for regulatory oversight under the Clinical Laboratory Improvement Amendments of 1988. However, the HCFA estimated that there may be as many as 50,000 additional laboratories that have not yet registered. A large number of laboratories (67,000) perform only tests that are not technically or clinically complex and therefore are exempt from regulation.[3] More than half of the nation's laboratories are based in physician offices (58.7%), 7.7% are in nursing facilities, and 5.8% in hospitals. The remaining 27.6% of laboratories exist in such facilities as community clinics (4.6%), as independent laboratories (4.1%), and in home health agencies (3.3%), although the majority of laboratory procedures are performed in hospitals and independent laboratories. Collectively these laboratories produced over 9 billion tests in 1993,[4] more than double the estimated 4 billion tests performed in 1982.[5]

Clinical laboratories have begun to implement cost reduction efforts such as the substitution of less costly or generalist personnel, for costly and specialized professionals, the adoption of cost efficient testing methods, and the elimination of tests that are antiquated or provide no clinical value. For example, not too long ago, laboratory testing for hospital admission included a complete blood count (CBC) with differential cell count and a complete urinalysis with microscopic examination. No longer is this practiced because the labor-intensive differential and microscopic examination of urine sediment does not provide information of clinical value for the average patient being admitted. Now a white blood cell count, hematocrit, and a chemical screening of the urine are performed before admission, and only if any abnormalities are detected are the more expensive and labor-intensive tests performed. This testing strategy provides laboratory test results in a more cost-effective manner. Although there is a very low probability that some clinical information of value may be lost in this streamlined testing policy, policy makers have concluded that the cost of comprehensive admission testing is not worth the small amount of additional information that would be obtained.

These examples are only the beginning. As more health care is delivered through managed care organizations (MCOs) and as more health care providers are paid under a capitation system, the value received for our health care dollars will be more closely scrutinized. Health care services, including laboratory tests, will have to have value. In other words, laboratory tests will have to provide information that is meaningful and useful in the management of a patient's clinical course. Systems must be developed to prevent the performance of tests with no value, for example, duplicate testing, inappropriate timing, and "shotgun" ordering. Other systems must be implemented to assist clinicians in the appropriate and cost efficient utilization of laboratory services.

Laboratories and clinicians now have economic incentives to implement these changes. Clinical laboratories are now contracting with MCOs to provide laboratory services for members of their plan on a capitated basis. Under a capitation method of payment, a laboratory receives a set fee per member–per month to provide all laboratory services for that MCO. If the clinicians in the MCO collectively order more tests than the laboratory had estimated, the laboratory will lose money; if they order fewer tests, the laboratory makes a profit. Under capitation, clinical laboratories have an incentive to ensure that tests ordered by the managed care plan's clinicians are really necessary and that they contribute to the health of the plan's members. The introduction of administrative system changes such as utilization screens and laboratory testing guidelines are among the methods that laboratories are using to minimize the financial risk of a deficit operation. Other strategies include the utilization of clinical laboratory scientists in new and expanded roles within the institution to assist clinicians in using the laboratory efficiently and cost-effectively (see Chapter 2).

Physicians contract with MCOs and receive capitated payments to provide patient services such as office visits, referrals to specialists and therapists, and diagnostic testing. Just as the capitated method of payment provided an economic incentive for laboratories to implement administrative systems changes, capitation also provides an economic incentive for physicians to modify their test-ordering behavior. Because all services associated with their patients' care must be paid from the same pool of money that contains their income, physicians receiving capitated payments now realize that the more laboratory tests they order, the less take-home pay they will have at the end of the month. Because capitation does have the potential to lead to underutilization of services, MCOs must develop systems that monitor clinicians' behavior to ensure that the economic incentives of capitation lead to optimal use of laboratory and other health care services rather than suboptimal use, which can lead to poor patient outcomes and reduced income for the MCO.

Regardless of opinions about capitation as a method of payment, capitation has awakened the laboratory community to the need to understand and appreciate their role in the delivery of health care services, as well as their broader contribution to the nation's health care economy. Laboratorians now need to ask not only how they can best perform their traditional role of producing high-quality laboratory tests as efficiently as possible, but also how they can improve the utilization of the laboratory and the application of test results. Ultimately, laboratorians need to ask how their services can contribute to the broader societal aim of maximizing the number of years of healthy life gained as a result of the investment in laboratory services.

Although some of these concepts are new for the laboratory community, they are concepts that must be mastered for survival and success in a managed care environment. In the sections that follow, a comparison of the "traditional" vs. the "interactive" new role for the clinical laboratory in the changing health care environment is introduced. Then these new concepts are developed within the 11 steps of the "Total Testing Process," the organizing framework that provides the blueprint for the interactive laboratory to intervene and improve the efficiency and effectiveness of all phases of clinical laboratory testing. This new direction will challenge clinical laboratory scientists to apply their knowledge to new responsibilities, which require them to extend beyond the process of producing an analytic test result and to interact with clinicians in a collaborative effort to improve both the laboratory's input and its output. Improving the utilization of the clinical laboratory will improve the cost efficiency of the laboratory and the value of laboratory information. Improving the interpretation and application of test results will increase the clinical effectiveness of laboratory services and reinforce their value to those who make resource allocation decisions. Chapter 2 discusses these concepts in detail as they apply to clinical laboratory scientists.

Mastery of all three phases—the input (preanalytic), the process (analytic), and the output (postanalytic)—is critical. Each phase seeks to answer specific questions. First, the input—is the test appropriate for the clinical condition and is the specimen and its time of collection correct? Next, the process—within clinically relevant guidelines is the test result accurate and precise, and is the process responsive to the turn-around time (TAT) needs of clinicians? And third, the output—are the results being properly interpreted and integrated into proper patient care or is data overload confusing or misleading physicians? An optimal integration of all three phases will produce the most efficient and effective test. Otherwise, an accurate and precise laboratory result will be of no value if the test was not clinically indicated, if the laboratory's precision was beyond that needed for clinical judgments, or if the result was misinterpreted. Such tests are of little value because they unnecessarily consume limited health care resources and can potentially lead to patient harm.

THE TRADITIONAL VS. THE INTERACTIVE LABORATORY

Different incentives underlie the direction and operation of the traditional vs. the interactive laboratory and determine the roles and responsibilities of clinical laboratory scientists. The traditional laboratory is driven by the economic incentives inherent in the fee-for-service payment

The Traditional Laboratory

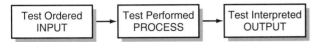

Figure 1–1. The traditional laboratory is isolated from what tests are ordered (input) and how their results are interpreted (output).

system, in which the more tests that are performed, the more the laboratory is paid. The interactive laboratory is shaped by a prospective or capitated method of payment. Under this system, the laboratory or physician receives a budget that must cover all services; therefore, the more that is done, the more that will be drained from the budgeted amount. These different economic incentives set the stage for the very different functionings of the traditional and interactive laboratory.

The Traditional Laboratory

The traditional role of the clinical laboratory has been to perform tests—to specialize in the process of producing names and numbers (raw data). Specimens are received, requested analyses are performed, and results are released. As depicted in the traditional laboratory model (Fig. 1–1), little laboratory input or communications occurred prior to the test being received or after the result was released. Within this model, the major emphasis was on the quality of the test performance and the internal organization and production features of the laboratory. Neither clinical appropriateness of test requests nor interpretation of test results were considered major concerns of the clinical laboratory. The laboratory performed the tests and billed for services under a fee-for-service payment system. The more tests the laboratory performed, the more money the laboratory made. By adopting quality control and automation principles from industry, traditional laboratories produced large quantities of high-quality data at low unit cost. Clinicians had unlimited access to laboratory testing, leading one laboratory observer to comment that "a significant proportion of the clinical laboratory tests ordered in the United States are not really needed for effective diagnosis and treatment," and that "the most important factor underlying the overuse of laboratory tests is physician behavior."[6]

Recently, economic incentives have changed under prospective payment systems, such as diagnosis-related groups (DRGs) and managed care. No longer is the laboratory viewed as a revenue-generating profit center: it is now a consumer of limited resources, a cost center. In response to these new economic forces, the traditional laboratory focused on reducing costs by increasing its internal efficiency of producing test results instead of improving appropriate utilization of its services. More structured cost-accounting methods were introduced, work flow patterns analyzed, automation increased, staffing and scheduling improved, and better volume discounts and leasing agreements negotiated. Discrete analyzers and other methodologies, using smaller reagent volumes, yielded additional savings and lowered unit cost. These strategies have limits that are often reached early in the cost-containment

process, however, and, from a cost-containment standpoint, there is a much greater payoff in attempting to reduce the numbers of unnecessary tests ordered than in attempting to further reduce the unit cost or charge per test.[6] Moreover, such internal restructuring, although necessary, did not enable clinical laboratory scientists to better integrate the process of laboratory testing into the total care of the patient for better patient outcomes, nor did these efficiencies enable the traditional laboratory to better control the use of services.

To respond to the pressures of prospective payment systems and to increase the clinical relevance of their services, clinical laboratory scientists found that they had to expand their views of the role and function of the clinical laboratory. Rather than focusing only on its internal *efficiency*, they believed that the laboratory must also examine its *effectiveness*. This involves not only the internal process of producing results (analytic process), but also outreach efforts to increase appropriate laboratory utilization (preanalytic input) and to assist clinicians by providing additional information to accompany test results (postanalytic output). Laboratories must now assume some measure of responsibility for the input and output components of their services. To achieve these goals, a new model of the clinical laboratory was developed, that of the "interactive" laboratory.

The Interactive Laboratory

Central to the current changes in the delivery of clinical laboratory services is the adoption of an expanded role for the clinical laboratory scientist, assisting the clinician in the appropriate utilization of laboratory services and the interpretation of its results. To implement this new role, we must understand why clinicians order laboratory tests, the cognitive process involved in ordering, why such variation occurs in test ordering patterns, and how the clinical laboratory scientist can assist in the effective and efficient use of the clinical laboratory.

The interactive laboratory broadens the mission of the traditional laboratory. In this model, clinical laboratory scientists expand beyond their traditional role as generators of test data to integrate themselves into all phases of the production of laboratory information and to influence the utilization of the department's resources and services. As depicted in Figure 1–2, clinical laboratory scientists in the interactive laboratory interact and collaborate with clinicians to improve the clinical appropriateness of test re-

The Interactive Laboratory

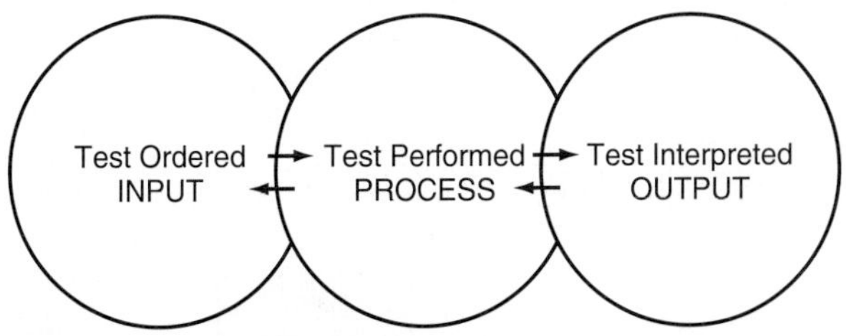

Figure 1–2. In the interactive laboratory, laboratorians and clinicians interact to improve how tests are ordered, how tests are performed, and how results are interpreted.

quests (preanalytic input), to improve the clinical relevance of the laboratory's offerings and procedures (analytic process), and to assist the clinician in the proper interpretation of laboratory information (postanalytic output).

To improve laboratory utilization, clinical laboratory scientists in the interactive laboratory must influence the test-ordering behavior and data interpretation of clinicians. To develop strategies to affect clinician behavior, laboratory scientists must examine why tests are ordered, what influences and cognitive steps are part of the laboratory utilization process, and how variation in test utilization patterns can be reduced. Then, in collaboration with clinicians, laboratory-based strategies, targeted to areas of weakness in the test-ordering process, can be developed to improve appropriate utilization and reduce unnecessary testing.

THE TOTAL TESTING PROCESS

A model of laboratory utilization must capture the interrelationship between the primary variables associated with laboratory test ordering and the sequential cognitive, organizational/environmental, and action processes leading from a clinical assessment, through the selection and ordering of a test, to the laboratory's performance of the test, and ultimately to the clinician's integration of the result into patient care. Institutional, laboratory, and medical staff characteristics and policies are known to affect the utilization pattern within a hospital. Also important are the characteristics of individual clinicians and the type and severity of each patient's illness.

Set in the context of regulatory, public health, insurance, and institutional policies, Figure 1–3 expands the earlier input-process-output model by graphically displaying a 10-step sequence of the total testing process. Although many feedback loops exist between various steps in the process, a simplified sequential model is presented. It incorporates all aspects of laboratory testing beginning with a clinical question that is prompted by the patient-clinician encounter and concluding with the impact of the test result on patient care.

This broad view of laboratory testing has evolved through a series of invitational institutes sponsored by the Centers for Disease Control and Prevention.[7, 8] At these institutes, laboratorians, clinicians, equipment and supply manufacturers, and laboratory regulators were challenged to examine laboratory quality from a broad, patient-centered perspective rather than a narrow, discipline-specific frame of reference. Multidisciplinary group discussions sensitized participants to the complexity and interrelationship of the multiple steps required to convert a test request into a test result that has an impact on patient care.

As seen in Figure 1–3, the total testing process begins and ends with patient care and consists of four major components: preanalytic (input), analytic (process), postanalytic (output), and regulatory environment within which the test is performed. The *preanalytic or input component* begins with a clinician-patient encounter that raises a clinical question that could be answered by a test (step 1). The clinician considers what tests might be appropriate to answer the clinical question and then selects a test (step 2). The selection is translated into a test order either directly by the clinician placing an electronic order or indirectly by a ward or office secretary transferring the written order to a laboratory request form (step 3). The preanalytic component concludes with specimen collection and the transport of the speciment to the clinical laboratory (step 4).

The *analytic or process component* involves the intra-laboratory processing (step 5) and testing of specimens (step 6) and the verification of test results (step 7). Because

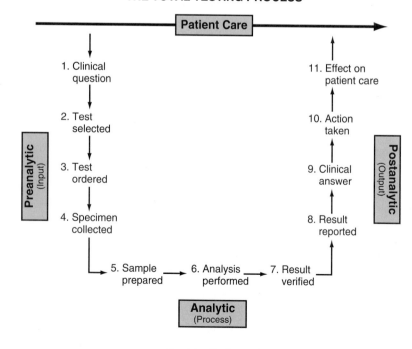

THE TOTAL TESTING PROCESS

Figure 1–3. The total testing process, grounded in what is of value to patient care, requires interaction between the clinician and laboratorian throughout the 11 steps of the process. From Barr JT, Schumacher GE: The total testing process applied to therapeutic drug monitoring. *In* Schumacher GE (ed): Therapeutic Drug Monitoring. Norwalk, Conn., Appleton & Lange, 1995

the ability to process and accurately analyze the specimen is dependent on the characteristics of the analytic system, considerations involving the selection of test methodology and quality control procedures would be included in this section.

The *postanalytic or output component* comprises the reporting of the test results (step 8), the interpretation of the result in light of the original clinical question (step 9), the actions taken in response to the result (step 10), and the result of these actions on patient care and ultimate patient outcomes.

The entire test ordering model is set within the context of "environmental" policies that are external to the specific patient and clinician but influence the use or nonuse of laboratory tests. Mandatory federal, state, and local laws as well as voluntary accreditation standards from the Joint Commission on the Accreditation of Healthcare Organizations (JCAHO) and the College of American Pathologists (CAP) influence the structure and process, and perhaps the outcomes, of laboratory testing. Several other examples of these "environmental" factors are an institution's standard operating procedures for admission and preoperative testing, an insurance company's or federal agency's denial of coverage if certain tests are used inappropriately or cannot be determined to be medically necessary, or the establishment of clinical management protocols.

This model explicitly identifies the "clinician" rather than the physician during the laboratory utilization process. Recognizing that patient assessment and test ordering are now performed, officially and unofficially, by a variety of practitioners (nurse practitioners, physician assistants, dentists, nurse midwives, clinical pharmacists, and nurses), the model suggests that strategies to improve laboratory utilization must be addressed to more than the physician population, and that different practitioner populations may require alternative types of interventions to improve the process.

Preanalytic Component

Why do clinicians order laboratory tests? When physicians at a major medical center were asked why they had ordered 1 or more of the 11 most frequently requested tests or panels, they indicated that 37% of their requests were for diagnostic purposes, 33% for monitoring, and 32% for screening. Only 1% of the tests were said to be ordered for medicolegal protection, 1% were for repeated testing because a previous result was not available, and none were for presentation to senior staff.[9] In addition to diagnosis, screening, and monitoring of disease, laboratory tests are also recognized to be useful in the determination of the severity of disease, the determination of the appropriate management of patients, the monitoring of therapy, and the prediction of response to treatment.[10]

Others have identified "the need to be complete" as a major impetus for test ordering. This compulsion to rule out or document every possibility, no matter how remote, creates much unnecessary testing.[11–15] Medical school faculty and hospital attending staff often reinforce this mentality by criticizing the omission of one laboratory test rather than rewarding restraint and thoughtful use of diagnostic tests.[12]

Last, physicians also use laboratory tests as a form of communication with patients, colleagues, and potential referral specialists.[16–20] Laboratory tests can be used to show the patient and other physicians that something is being done and can be used to reassure and please patients. Patients expect tests to be ordered, and physicians can both please the patient and signal the end of an office visit by ordering a test.

In a more cost efficient health care system, the clinical laboratory has a major role to play in improving the utilization of laboratory services. In an ideal world, clinicians would order only those tests that provide useful information for patient care or for epidemiologic purposes. In this ideal world, all clinicians facing the same clinical signs and symptoms would order the same tests that have proven to provide useful clinical information in the past. All practice guidelines or testing algorithms would be well developed, validated, and communicated to and accepted by clinicians.

Experience confirms, however, that this is not the case. Large variations exist in what clinicians order for laboratory tests.[21–26] Variations as large as 17-fold have been documented among physicians treating the same patient population.[22] Different clinicians will treat the same patient differently,[25] and the same clinician will treat patients with the same clinical presentation differently.[20] Although more efficient ordering strategies may improve this situation, great variation may remain in how a clinician approaches a case and progresses through each step in the total testing process. A number of factors can explain this variation—type and severity of illness, clinicians' educational preparation and personal characteristics, clinician-patient relationship, social and economic considerations, institutional and regional norms, and colleague expectations. Underlying them all, however, is a lack of standardization, or even consensus, in many of the steps in the total testing process, especially in the preanalytic or laboratory utilization phase. It is the responsibility of the laboratory to assist in the standardization of this process and to improve the appropriate utilization of the laboratory.

Step 1: Clinical Question

During the clinician-patient encounter, questions arise when the clinician detects certain signs and symptoms or needs additional data to guide therapy. Based on the condition of the patient, the clinician formulates clinical questions concerning diagnostic possibilities or changes in clinical status.[27, 28] All clinicians go through this question-posing step; whether or not they consciously analyze this step is largely dependent on their educational preparation. The more focused the clinical questions, the more likely that targeted, rather than "shotgun," test ordering will occur. The quality of the framing and focusing of the questions is dependent on individual clinician characteristics as well as prior education.[29, 30]

Before tests are ordered, clinicians should not only raise questions, but should accompany each question with a patient-specific probability assessment of how likely the patient is to have the condition under consideration. This probability estimate, taken before a test is ordered, is called a *prior probability*. It can be based on the patient's history or the clinician's previous experience with patients with similar clinical signs. Later in the total testing process, prior probability can be combined with information obtained from results of the test to yield a revised or *posterior probability* specific for the patient. Prior probability estimation has the potential to expand and personalize information contained in a laboratory result.[27]

Step 2: Test Selected

Given a clinical presentation and the resultant framed question, the clinician considers the array of tests that can be ordered to answer the question. Tests considered in this step are dependent on such factors as the clinician's ability to link the pathophysiology of the clinical question with possible tests to answer the question,[29] the clinician's experience with patients with similar clinical findings,[31] an understanding of the information content of each test and its ability to separate diseased from nondiseased populations,[27] knowledge of the laboratory's test offerings, and the algorithms or practice guidelines that the clinician must follow.

The clinical laboratory has a responsibility in this stage to ensure that its test offerings provide clinical value and that they are used appropriately.[32, 33] Laboratorians need to collaborate with clinicians to determine what tests the laboratory should offer for selection, for what patient populations they are appropriate, and when during the clinical course they should be selected. Such collaboration often occurs in the context of care management teams of which the clinical laboratory scientist is a member. New tests should be evaluated for both their economic impact and their ability to improve diagnostic accuracy. If a new test provides additional clinical information that is judged to be worth the additional cost, it should be added to the testing menu. At the same time, older tests providing less information for patient management and having the potential for incurring duplicative costs should be removed. With capitated budgets, laboratories now have an economic incentive to assist in test selection and improve the utilization of the laboratory. Methods to improve utilization are further discussed in a later section. At this point it is useful to consider a fundamental question: when should a test be selected? A laboratory test should meet three criteria. First, it should provide useful information for the diagnosis of disease, and treatment and monitoring of patients. Second, it should produce more benefit than harm to the tested population. And third, as a result of economic considerations, the test should be produced at a reasonable cost.

For example, consider population-based disease screening. Should all people be screened for a disease just because a screening test is available? Two recent studies indicate that the answer is no. General population screening for prostate-specific antigen (PSA) in asymptomatic men between 50 and 75 years resulted in greatly increased costs and poor health outcomes primarily associated with the aggressive follow-up for high numbers of false-negative results.[34] In a general population of nearly 55,000 pregnant women, prenatal screening for hemoglobinopathies identified 81 at-risk couples, but only 35% of them underwent amniocentesis.[35] In both cases untargeted, general screening increased costs, provided little patient management information, and, in one case, led to increased harm. Clinical

laboratory scientists need to improve test selection by developing screening guidelines based on disease prevalence in general and targeted populations, assessing test sensitivity and specificity, and reducing the cost of false positives and negatives.

From the possible tests being considered and whatever guidelines and algorithms are in place, the clinician now must select specific tests. The factors influencing this step include: the trade-off between the "need to be complete" vs. the need to contain costs,[15] the degree of uncertainty the clinician can tolerate (the more uncertain the clinician, the more tests ordered to reduce that uncertainty),[31, 36, 37] malpractice issues (tests are used to document that everything, no matter how remote, has been considered),[14] and the need to use the test to communicate to other clinicians or the patient.[20] Other factors influencing selection of tests include the style and expectation of attending staff and chief of service (the ordering pattern of those in power is emulated by others),[21, 22, 37–39] the type of medical specialty,[40–42] the teaching status of a hospital or floor,[43–47] and the payment mechanism for the laboratory charges.[9, 21, 39, 48–50]

At this step, the clinician should ask whether any results of each test considered would change the course of action. Generally, if the answer is no, the test should not be selected.

Step 3: Test Ordered

The tests selected by the clinician are converted into a test order. Depending on the sophistication of the institution's computer capabilities, clinicians can order the test through a computerized request system that transmits the order directly to the laboratory. In less integrated computer systems, the clinician places the order in the floor-based computer that does not communicate with the laboratory's computer, and a transcription step is required. In this instance, the clinician's order in the chart or the order book is transcribed to a test order form by the floor secretary or other support personnel.

Errors can occur within the ordering process procedure. In a recent survey of test ordering accuracy,[51] 577 institutions reported that 97.1% of physician test orders were completed by the laboratory. Of the ones that were not processed by the laboratory, 42% were incorrectly entered into the hospital computer and 13% of the test requisitions were incorrectly filled out. Although 2.9% may appear to be a low error rate, in this study population it represented 6,538 tests that were selected by the physician but not completed by the laboratory.

The organization and structure of laboratory test order forms can influence the number and types of tests that are ordered. Clinicians order more tests when the request forms are organized in bundled, multitest panels rather than by single laboratory test.[52, 53] According to a recent survey of laboratory practices, however, only 50% to 74% of clinical laboratories monitor the appropriate ordering of laboratory tests.[54]

Step 4: Specimen Collected

Patient identification, collection timing, patient preparation, and specimen quality are all important features of this step. Although it is obvious that proper patient identification is central to the total testing process, a nationwide survey indicated that 2.2% of patients' wristbands were missing or had errors.[55]

Sampling time criteria are critical for a number of laboratory analyses such as monitoring levels of glucose, some therapeutic drugs, and cardiac isoenzymes. A new concern has been raised about the timing of metabolic screening in newborns. With many MCOs providing incentives for mothers and their newborns to leave the hospital in less than 24 hours from delivery, the shortened hospital stay provides insufficient time for the infant to achieve a homeostatic balance that permits valid metabolic screening. Metabolic screening should not be performed before 24 hours of age; therefore, testing will have to be done after discharge, and a percentage of infants will be missed.[56]

Other critical areas require that specimen quality be assured (e.g., prevention of oxygen exposure to anaerobic cultures, hemolysis in venipuncture process) and that the specimen be labeled properly. Proper specimen collection is dependent primarily on the knowledge base of those collecting the specimen and the ability of a laboratory to evaluate specimen quality and to block samples determined to be unacceptable.

More than 75% of laboratories have a quality improvement program to monitor the frequency of unacceptable specimens, but only 50% to 75% of laboratories monitor the timeliness of specimen collection, the TAT to perform a phlebotomy, the frequency of redraws in phlebotomy, or the satisfaction of the outpatient population with the phlebotomy process.[54]

Analytic Component

Step 5: Specimen Prepared

For most forms of testing, step 5 involves the logging of the specimen into the laboratory computer system, the assignment of a laboratory acquisition number, preparation of the specimen for testing, and the storage of the sample if testing is not performed immediately. When specimens reach the laboratory, the time of receipt is noted and the specimens are logged in. Acquisition numbers or codes are assigned, and the number for each coded sample is placed on the laboratory worksheet. This phase of testing is labor intensive, with many possibilities for transcription and other human errors. Laboratory computer systems are being used to reduce the number of unit processes by having the computer generate worksheets from its centralized log-in record. Also, consolidation of testing with restructuring of laboratory boundaries and centralization of processing functions have led to lower costs and increased efficiencies.[57]

Bar codes, bar scanning computer equipment, and computerized data entry are being used to reduce errors in this step. Some hospitals have total hospital information systems that use patient-specific bar codes, assigned at admission, that are placed on all order forms and patient specimens. On receipt in the laboratory, the bar codes are scanned and worksheets generated. This and other technologies under development will simplify the log-in process, minimize transcription steps, and reduce associated errors.

Step 6: Analysis Performed

In step 6, the laboratory performs the analysis. In the selection of a testing system, five major points must be considered:

1. Analytic performance, including accuracy, reliability, specificity of reaction, and methodologic sensitivity within the expected range of possible values
2. Practicality, including ease of performance, time of analysis, volume of sample required, equipment calibration, and computer compatibility
3. Availability of laboratory equipment and supplies and personnel with appropriate skill levels
4. Economic aspects, including the initial purchase of equipment and reagents, quality control, and personnel costs
5. Location of the testing, including bedside, satellite, centralized, physician office, or other ambulatory environment

Whether the specimen received by the laboratory is actually tested depends on specimen quality and the appropriateness of the test given the screening or "gatekeeper" policies of the laboratory and institution. The laboratory may receive a specimen, but if the specimen does not meet specimen quality criteria such as timing requirements or specimen integrity, the test should not be performed. The analytic testing process may be correct if the test is performed; however, the test result will be faulty because the specimen will not reflect the physiologic status of the patient. In this case a correct analysis will produce an unrepresentative result that may lead to patient harm.

Other laboratory policies in this step can block the performance of a test order, even if the specimen quality is acceptable. Such policies involve the establishment of "reasonableness" or gatekeeper criteria. Examples include the following laboratory policies: a limit on the frequency of repeat urine cultures, the deletion of the white blood cell (WBC) differential count when the WBC count is normal, and not performing a lactate dehydrogenase (LD) isoenzyme assay when the LD level is normal.

The TAT for the analysis involves both clinical and economic considerations. For urgent situations, certain tests require a rapid TAT. This has led many clinicians to advocate point-of-care testing such as blood gas analyses and electrolytes in the operating room and bedside glucose testing on the units. Although there have been few comprehensive clinical and economic comparisons of well-organized, central laboratory testing vs. point-of-care testing, one glucose testing report indicated that the TAT with bedside testing was only 1 to 2 minutes shorter than central laboratory testing, no significant adverse medical outcomes were associated with the TAT difference, but that the cost of bedside testing was approximately twice that of central laboratory testing.[58]

Economic and clinical considerations are driving another aspect of reduced TAT. Automated systems within the clinical microbiology laboratory permit rapid in vitro susceptibility testing and bacterial identification. In one study, same-day antimicrobial susceptibility results reduced mortality related to infection in patients with infections of unknown antimicrobial susceptibility from 12.7% to 7%

and were projected to save the institution more than $2.4 million in charges over a year.[59] Patients with infections of unknown antimicrobial susceptibility are frequently started on multiple antibiotic therapy. Same day reporting identifies an effective antibiotic sooner, thus reducing the number of days patients are given expensive multiple antibiotics.[60]

Step 7: Results Verified

Results are verified before being released to patient care areas. Verification can involve both quality control (QC) and intrapatient checks. Routine QC samples of known values, performed in parallel with patient samples, are checked to determine if they are within their acceptable ranges. If the QC results are within range, the results are released. Given that these quality control samples are analyzed with the same procedure as the patients' samples, any defect in analytic processing should be detected by out-of-range values for the QC specimens.

Intrapatient checks are also used to detect results that vary significantly from a specific patient's previous results. Many automated computer systems perform "delta checks" by comparing the patient's current result with previous test values maintained in the laboratory's data bank. If the current results are similar to past values, the results are released; if they deviate, the testing station is notified and repeat testing may be necessary if the deviation cannot be accounted for by a change in the patient's status.

Postanalytic Component

Step 8: Result Reported

In step 8, the test result is released to the clinician. With integrated computer systems, laboratory results can be reported directly to the floor or clinician's office. The laboratory has a variety of methods by which it can communicate test results to the clinician. In order of increasing sophistication, the laboratory can release the results as a straight numeric value, as a value with accompanying referent ranges for a comparable population, as a value with out-of-referent values highlighted, as a predictive value with probabilistic estimates of disease/nondisease, or as an annotated report with recommendations for additional testing or treatment.[61, 62] Most laboratories have established "panic values"; when results occur outside these values, the laboratory immediately notifies the clinician or the patient's floor.

Little research has been conducted on the value of different reporting formats, their impact on clinician comprehension, or their effect on patient outcome. Applying the principles of total quality management strategies and determining what customers prefer, Peddecord and colleagues went to the main component of the laboratory's "customers," the clinicians, and asked them to identify opportunities for improvement in laboratory processing and reporting, especially as they relate to HIV and hepatitis B testing.[63] Their findings will be further evaluated in future prospective research.

Selective reporting has been used by the microbiology laboratory to help control the economic consequences of antibiotic selection. Some laboratories have listed the antibiotic susceptibility in rank order with respect to increasing cost. In this case, the least expensive antibiotic is listed first, followed by the increasing cost of the other susceptible antibiotic. In another laboratory, the computer issues a selective report of susceptible antibiotics. For example, if an organism is susceptible to a less costly first- or second-generation cephalosporin, the more expensive third generation cephalosporin is not reported.[60]

Overall, at least 75% of laboratories monitor the TAT from request to report for their urgent and nonurgent tests. Also at least 75% of laboratories notify clinicians of "panic results," results significantly outside referent range. Between 50% to 75% of laboratories monitor the overall timeliness of their reporting process.[54]

Step 9: Clinical Answer

In this step, information from laboratory results is used to answer the clinical question raised in step 1. Correct interpretation of laboratory results depends not only on the test results, but also on information about the quality of all preceding steps and characteristics of the individual patients and interpretative guidelines.

Concerning the quality of the preceding steps of the total testing process, interpretation of laboratory tests can be improved by explicitly recognizing the magnitude of variation and sources of error that are inherent in the total testing process. Both normal analytic and physiologic variation occur even though there is no real physiologic change in the patient. The magnitude of this variation needs to be qualified and combined with an assessment of the total "error" that is present in the testing methodology.[64] Only after that estimate is made can the clinician determine whether the change in a patient's test result is related to real physiologic change or to random error and variation within the testing system.

In step 1, clinicians used the clinical features of each patient to estimate the prior or pretest probability that a specific patient has a disease or clinical condition. Now in step 9 the information contained in the test result can be combined with the pretest probability from step 1 to produce a posttest probability of disease.[27, 65] This yields a patient-specific predictive value that can be used to help the clinician interpret a laboratory value in light of the patient's specific clinical condition. If laboratories required clinicians to submit prior probability information with each laboratory request, computer programs could combine the prior probability with the patient's results and issue an interpretative result based on the revised probability.

Last, clinicians frequently rely on diagnostic criteria as they interpret laboratory results; however, it is critical that these diagnostic criteria be frequently reviewed and updated as changes occur in testing methodology and understanding of the pathophysiology of the clinical condition. For example, the National Diabetes Data Group criteria for the diagnosis of gestational diabetes was compared to a modified, more inclusive, set of guidelines. Fifty percent more cases of gestational diabetes were identified using the more inclusive criteria. These additional cases had as high an incidence of maternal diabetes risk factors, infant macrosomia, and cord hyperinsulinemia as those cases identified by the earlier criteria.[66] If the criteria had not been reexamined, the cases would likely have been missed.

Steps 10 and 11: Action Taken and Impact on Patient Care

In these steps the clinician takes action based on the interpretation of the laboratory value, which has a direct impact on patient care. The laboratory has little influence in these steps, but it can monitor the outcomes of the clinician's action as well as other steps in the total testing process. For example, Medicare claims data have been used to follow patients with prothrombin and digoxin tests to determine if hospitalizations, related to the analyte being measured, occurred within a critical period after the test.[67–69] Models to link variations in patient outcomes with the variation in the structure and process of laboratory testing are needed in both the inpatient and ambulatory populations.[70]

METHODS TO IMPROVE LABORATORY UTILIZATION

All steps in the total testing process are worthy of efforts to improve the quality of the factors affecting that step; however, the remainder of this chapter examines efforts to improve the steps in the preanalytic stage, particularly targeted at improving the utilization of the clinical laboratory. This approach has been selected because research indicates that much improvement is possible in this stage, and improved laboratory utilization has both clinical and economic benefits. Clinically, increased targeting of laboratory testing increases the information content of the test results and avoids confusing and contradictory results. Economically, improved utilization generally leads to reductions in laboratory testing and lower laboratory and patient care expenses. By improving laboratory utilization, the clinical laboratory can add value and medical relevance to its services.[33, 71] Traditionally, the laboratory community has given more attention to advances in the analytic stage and has avoided interventions to modify clinician behavior and improve the appropriateness of laboratory utilization. However, success in a managed care environment will require laboratorians to abandon an avoidance strategy in favor of the more interactive strategies described in this book.

Many attempts have been made to modify the test-ordering behavior of physicians. Educational programs to improve test selection, cost awareness, and decision-making ability have been introduced into medical school curricula and sponsored by hospitals for their residents and attending staff. Other strategies have included rationing of laboratory tests, incentives to reduce utilization, and relative feedback programs. The strategies that have met with most success, however, achieve their effectiveness by changing policies and procedures, thereby establishing new clinical and administrative guidelines by which tests are ordered. Rather than relying solely on largely ineffective educational programs to modify laboratory utilization, these new strategies directly intervene in the test-ordering process by redefining previous "routine" procedures (e.g., eliminating microscopic examination for both routine urinalysis and complete blood counts), identifying "gatekeeper" tests (e.g., requiring abnormal creatine kinase [CK] level before CK isoenzyme assays are performed),

and creating barriers between steps (e.g., requiring additional forms or other types of justification for test selection).

Still, numerous medical educators have argued that the answer to inappropriate laboratory utilization lies not in the latter types of restricted access to testing, but rather in changing the ordering behavior of physicians by systematic instruction in clinical decision making,[72–74] appropriate use of clinical testing,[29] and the development of sequentially logical testing patterns based on priorities of cost-effectiveness.[75] To determine which strategy, or combination of strategies, would be most effective and efficient to improve laboratory utilization within an institution, therefore, the clinical laboratory scientist should be familiar with the variety of both non–laboratory- and laboratory-based interventions.

Three types of methods to improve laboratory utilization are highlighted: educational efforts, including feedback strategies; implementation of system changes; and the introduction of clinical appropriateness criteria, practice guidelines, and algorithms.

Educational Efforts

Laboratory utilization educational programs in medical schools are designed primarily to influence steps 2 and 3—the clinical question and test selection. Medical students are guided to convert a clinical assessment into a set of questions, link those questions to a group of tests, and then select the best test in the group to answer the question. Educational programs in hospitals include such varied interventions as simple passive distribution of information through lectures, newsletters, and booklets covering clinical appropriateness of certain tests or ordering strategies; feedback to physicians of patient-specific cost information or individual physician's ordering intensity relative to others in a group; and clinical appropriateness chart reviews with the house staff conducted by the attending staff. In this context, passive and active audits and other forms of feedback are considered informational inputs and, as such, are part of the educational process. This type of intervention is aimed primarily at improving step 2—selection of the specific test based on its ability to answer a clinical question.

The results of studies that have examined the effect on physician test-ordering behavior by educational efforts are mixed. These studies, primarily conducted in a retrospective reimbursement environment and targeted at step 2, suggest the following: (1) "single dose" educational programs have limited effect; (2) feedback to the requesting clinician about laboratory charges per hospital stay is relatively inexpensive and appears to have some effect; (3) relative rank feedback information concerning how physicians stand relative to their peers in the intensity of laboratory testing has no association with a reduction in unnecessary test orders and no effect on laboratory utilization; (4) interactive chart audits focused on clinical appropriateness are costly but are successful; and (5) the attending physician's attitude is a major contributing factor to the success of any intervention.[22, 29, 49, 76–89]

The conclusions concerning educational efforts directed at improving test utilization is that they are necessary but not sufficient unto themselves to achieve consistent improvement in the appropriateness of laboratory utilization.

System Changes

Rather than relying on the individual clinician to voluntarily modify test-ordering behavior, physician organizations, third-party payers, and hospital and laboratory administrators are reassessing what laboratory services and standard operating procedures can be modified or eliminated. Based on these and independent investigators' evaluations, the following four administrative or system changes that have been recommended are described: (1) modification or elimination of routine and preoperative testing (steps 2 and 3); (2) elimination of standing orders (steps 2 and 3); (3) modification of test request forms and the process by which tests are ordered (steps 3 and 4); and (4) development of "smart" computer ordering programs that will suggest tests, screen the appropriateness of the laboratory request, and block redundant, mistimed, or clinically inappropriate tests (steps 2 through 4).

Routine Testing

As mentioned earlier, there is clear evidence that routine admission and preoperative testing are unnecessary and expensive.[90–96] One study calculated that admission testing added 5% to the total cost of hospital care and was not associated with any evidence of benefit to the patient.[93] Routine preoperative testing also did not contribute to patient outcome; some recommended that it be eliminated for asymptomatic and clinically normal patients who are undergoing elective minor surgery,[93] whereas others question whether any unindicated, routine preoperative testing should be performed at all.[95–96] Unless clinical conditions suggest an atypical situation, routine admission and preoperative laboratory tests presently have been reduced to the minimum.

Standing Orders

The elimination of standing orders is another method used to increase appropriate laboratory utilization. The logic behind this administrative change is that physicians should formulate a diagnostic or monitoring strategy each day and not rely on repetitive daily orders. With more thought given to the value of each test, the logic continues, the physician should order only the needed and appropriate tests while eliminating the unnecessary ones. Although appearing to be a logical test reduction action,[97] few studies have evaluated its effectiveness, and in these, results are mixed.

Test Request Forms and Computer Request Screens

Unlike many other strategies, modifications involving the design and use of test request forms and computer request screens can be under the control of the laboratory. The laboratory can use the laboratory order form or computer screen to provide information as well as guide the clinician in the test selection process. At least two types of modifications have been evaluated: redesign of test presentation on the ordering form and the use of the request form as a type of "barrier" intervention.

In the first case, it has been suggested that the organization of the typical laboratory request forms encourages unfocused ordering and should be improved.[48, 98] In response to this problem, Wong and colleagues[53] created a problem-oriented form to be used for thyroid testing. The old form with four boxes to indicate if assays of triiodothyronine (T_3) uptake, thyroxine, T_3, and thyroid stimulating hormone were ordered was replaced with a form offering a thyroid function screen, hyperthyroid panel, hypothyroid panel, or "other" thyroid test. This problem-oriented test form eliminated the problematic test selection phase by having the clinician select the clinical problem directly, rather than choose individual laboratory tests. As a result, T_3 test requests declined 38% and thyrotropin by 68%. In commenting on this study, Lundberg[98] suggested that "the simplest, easiest, and cheapest, and probably most effective way to guide physicians to use a laboratory correctly is by designing test request forms properly."

Durnad-Zaleski and colleagues[99] redesigned the test request form for tumor markers and achieved a reduction of 25% in the ordering of these tests. Rather than simply listing the types of tumor markers that were available for testing, these investigators used the request form to provide information to clinicians in a form that would be useful at the time of test ordering. They created a matrix of boxes, rows being individual markers and columns indicating body systems. Each box at the intersection of a row and column was color coded to indicate whether or not a specific tumor marker was appropriate for the affected organ. This form guided the ordering of the tumor markers, reduced the number of inappropriate tests ordered, and reduced the costs associated with tumor marker testing.

Using a computer ordering system, Tierney and colleagues[100] had the computer screen display the charges for laboratory tests as tests were ordered on ambulatory patients. The addition of financial information as the test was ordered led to a reduction in the utilization of laboratory testing.

Other modifications of test request forms have included the alphabetical, rather than organ-clustered, listing of tests; the replacement of a chemistry panel or profile with the individual listing of its constituent tests; and the elimination of highly specialized, and overutilized, tests from the routine test request slips. These types of forms are used to stimulate the ordering of a specific test to answer a specific question, rather than the unfocused ordering induced by poorly designed forms.

Another use of the test request form is to make the process of ordering a test more difficult. This blocks the conversion of a test selected in step 2 to a test ordered in step 3. By increasing the "price" the clinician must "pay" to have the test performed, it is suggested that only those tests that are highly valued will be advanced through the barrier. Several of these "barrier" interventions include writing the order in a laboratory order book rather than simply checking off the test on the form; requesting approval to order restricted tests,[101] and justifying the test order by indicating a clinical condition on an additional test form.[102, 103] The effect of the first two has not been determined; several evaluations of the latter method offer important lessons for laboratory-based interventions.

The use of an additional or supplemental form has been reported to be successful in achieving test reductions of 25% to 44%.[102, 103] The decrease in testing was also associated with an improvement in the clinical appropriateness of the tests that rose from only 50% of the tests being clinically indicated prior to the supplemental form to an appropriateness level of 80% after the form was introduced.[103]

The laboratory request form can also be used to impose a form of rationing or limitation in the range of tests that can be ordered. Based on the sensitivity and specificity of laboratory tests in a population with a low prior probability of disease, Zaat and colleagues[104] in the Netherlands identified 15 "useful" tests for a general practice population. They modified their traditional laboratory test form by reducing the number of listed tests from 178 to these 15 hematologic and chemical tests plus several urine and feces tests. Space was allowed for "others" to be ordered. The new form was associated with an 18% decrease in laboratory testing, but when the traditional form was reintroduced, the testing returned to its former level.

The modifications of test order forms and computer order screens are some of the first that permit the laboratory to directly control one of the input variables into the laboratory. Hard copy forms are only the first examples. In institutions with computer-assisted test ordering, interactive programs have been developed that require clinicians to justify test selection. This will not only enable the laboratory to further manage test ordering, but also to provide assistance during the process.

Clinical Appropriateness Criteria, Practice Guidelines, and Algorithms

Clinical Appropriateness Criteria

Laboratories are beginning to implement guidelines that place restrictions on the performance of selected tests. As mentioned earlier, the once common complete blood count with differential cell count and routine urinalysis with microscopic examination are no longer performed routinely. Both types of microscopic examinations were labor intensive but contributed little additional clinical information when the white cell count was normal,[105–108] or the chemical screening of the urine was negative;[109, 110] therefore, laboratories have limited these follow-up tests to specimens with out-of-range cell counts or positive chemical screens. It is interesting to note that a Canadian hospital removed the differential white blood cell count from its requisition slips as early as 1973.[101] The development of criteria to judge the clinical appropriateness of test requests should be a collaborative effort between clinicians and laboratory scientists and is likely to improve all aspects of laboratory utilization.

Algorithms and Practice Guidelines

Algorithms and practice guidelines have been developed to guide clinicians in the sequence and selection of diagnostic tests. Previously published algorithms have emphasized diagnostic accuracy (hematuria[111, 112] and hypercalcemia[113, 114]) and cost-effectiveness. Others have focused on a reduction in unnecessary test requests.[115–118] More recent guidelines have emphasized testing within a managed care environment.[119, 120] Automated clinical practice guidelines and "smart" computer systems can guide the clinician at the point of order entry.[121]

Efficiencies achieved by algorithms and practice guidelines are expected to increase in a managed care environment. This text is an important contribution to improved testing and cost reduction in this regard because it includes a number of these tools. Not only can this information be used to assist clinicians in their test ordering, but it can also be used to develop triggered algorithms. When a primary result is abnormal, these algorithms could automatically initiate a properly structured sequence of clinically informative testing (triggered automatic test sequence).[32] Preventing batch or untargeted ordering would improve the appropriateness of testing and decrease the diagnostic time involved in the regular physician-initiated sequential testing.

Within the laboratory, multistage protocols have been implemented to structure the laboratory processing of requests. In these algorithms, certain screening or primary tests must be abnormal before further diagnostic study is performed. The less expensive primary tests serve as "gatekeepers" to the more expensive follow-up tests. For example, an algorithm was developed to differentiate between pleural effusions that were transudates and those that were exudates. Only those specimens meeting the exudate criteria would then have additional testing.[122] Similar staged strategies have been developed for immunoelectrophoretic analyses[123] and thyroid testing.[124]

Although algorithms and practice guidelines are methods to reduce variation and increase clinical utility of laboratory testing, they must be not be followed blindly, particularly during the early phase of their introduction. Process failures, built into the practice guidelines, have been detected by management information systems monitoring the process of care.[125] On balance, however, algorithms and practice guidelines communicate optimal quality and decrease testing costs while facilitating a more valid measurement of clinical processes and outcomes.[126]

THE ROLE OF THE CLINICAL LABORATORY SCIENTIST

In extending the role of the clinical laboratory scientist to assist clinicians in the proper utilization of the laboratory, much attention will be centered on the use of clinical appropriateness criteria and algorithms ensuring the most effective and efficient selection of tests and their useful interpretation. In order to function at this consultative level of collaboration with other professionals, clinical laboratory scientists must acquire the content (knowledge of subject matter) relevant to a disease-oriented, clinical approach to laboratory testing and the interactive skills necessary to establish themselves as the appropriate providers of this important service. Clinical laboratory scientists have for some time acquired the necessary content, although they must now view it from a somewhat different perspective—through the eyes of the consumer of laboratory services. Consultative skills necessary to become recognized as a useful resource in issues concerning laboratory utilization are new components of the laboratory scientist's body of knowledge. Chapter 2 addresses these issues in detail and offers useful suggestions for laboratory managers, practitioners, and educators in developing and meeting these opportunities in their own institutions. Patience and persistence in providing the unique expertise that integrates the right clinical question with the proper scientific and technical means to answer the question will benefit the patient, the clinician, and the profession of clinical laboratory science.

References

1. Schieber J, Poullier J, Greenwald L: Health system performance in OECD countries, 1980–1992. Health Aff 13:100–112, 1994.
2. Gold MR, Russell LB, Siegel JE, Weinstein MC: Cost-effectiveness in Health and Medicine. New York, Oxford University Press, 1996.
3. Health Care Financing Administration: Cholesterol Measurement: Test accuracy and factors that influence cholesterol levels, 1995. Washington, DC, Government Accounting Office, United States Government Printing Office, 1995.
4. Health Care Financing Administration: Statistics of CLIAC meeting, September 1994. Washington, DC, Division of Laboratory Standards and Performance, 1994.
5. MediTrends: The Hospital Research and Educational Trust. Chicago, American Hospital Association, 1986.
6. Sheinbach J: The clinical laboratories: Problems of cost containment as a challenge. *In* Benson ES, Rubin M (eds): Logic and Economics of Clinical Laboratory Use. New York, Elsevier North-Holland Biomedical Press, 1978.
7. Inhorm SL, Addison BV (eds): Proceedings of the 1986 Institute on Critical Issues in Health Practices: Managing the quality of laboratory test results in a changing health care environment. Wilmington, DuPont, 1987.
8. Martin ML, Addison BV, Eagner WM, Essien JDK: Proceedings of the 1989 Institute on Critical Issues in Health Laboratory Practice: Improving the quality of health management through clinician and laboratorian teamwork. Wilmington, DuPont, 1991.
9. Wertman BG, Sostrin SV, Pavlova Z, Lundberg GD: Why do physicians order laboratory tests? JAMA 243:2080–2082, 1980.
10. Young DS: The role of the laboratory in clinical decision making. *In* Connolly DP, Benson ES, Burke MD, Fenderson D (eds): Clinical Decisions and Laboratory Use. Minneapolis, University of Minnesota Press, 1982, pp 69–79.
11. Krieg AF, Gambino R, Galen RS: Why are clinical laboratory tests performed? When are they valid? JAMA 233:76–78, 1975.
12. Landau RL: Professors of medicine, stand up! Arch Intern Med 143:212–213, 1983.
13. Hardison JE: To be complete. N Engl J Med 300:193–194, 1979.
14. Feinstein AR: The "chagrin factor" and qualitative decision analysis. Arch Intern Med 145:1257–1259, 1985.
15. Reuben DB: Learning from diagnostic restraint. N Engl J Med 310:591–593, 1984.
16. Epstein AM, Martley RM, Charlton JR, et al: A comparison of ambulatory ordering for hypertensive patients in the United States and England. JAMA 252:1723–1726, 1984.
17. Sox HC, Marguiles I, Soc CH: Psychologically mediated effects of diagnostic tests. Ann Intern Med 95:680–685, 1981.
18. Woo B, Woo B, Cook EF, Weisberg M, et al: Screening procedures in the asymptomatic adult: Comparison of physicians' recommendations, patients' desires, published guidelines, and actual practice. JAMA 254:1480–1484, 1985.
19. Mills KA, Reilly PM: Laboratory and radiological investigations in general practice: II. Expectation and outcome. Br J Med 287:1111–1113, 1983.
20. Holmes MM, Rovner DR, Elstein AS, et al: Factors affecting laboratory utilization in clinical practice. Med Decis Making 2:471–482, 1982.
21. Freeborn DK, Baer D, Greenlick MR, Bailey JW: Determinations of medical care utilization: Physicians' use of laboratory services. Am J Public Health 62:846–853, 1972.
22. Schroeder SA, Kenders K, Cooper JK, Piemme TE: Use of laboratory tests and pharmaceuticals: Variation among physicians and effect of cost audit on subsequent use. JAMA 225:969–973, 1973.
23. Fineberg HV, Funkhouser AR, Marks H: Variation in medical practice: A review of the literature. *In* Egdahl R, Walsh DC (eds): Industry and Health Care: vol 1. Health Cost Management and Medical Practice Patterns. Cambridge, Mass, Ballinger, 1985, pp 143–168.
24. Schroeder SA, Schliftman A, Piemme TE: Variation among physicians in use of laboratory tests: Relation to quality of care. Med Care 12:709–713, 1974.
25. Hlatky MA, Lee KL, Botvinick EH, Brundage BH: Diagnostic test use in different practice settings. Arch Intern Med 143:1886–1889, 1983.
26. Johnson RE, Freeborn DK, Mullooly JP: Physicians' use of laboratory, radiology, and drugs in a prepaid group practice HMO. Health Serv Res 20:525–547, 1985.
27. Weinstein MT, Fineberg HV: Clinical Decision Analysis. Philadelphia, WB Saunders, 1980.
28. Johnson PE: Cognitive models of problem solvers. *In* Connelly DP, Benson ES, Burke MD, Fenderson D (eds): Clinical Decisions and Laboratory Use. Minneapolis, University of Minnesota Press, 1982.
29. Burke MD, Connelly DP: Systematic instruction in laboratory medicine. Hum Pathol 12:134–144, 1981.
30. Epstein AM, Begg CB, McNeil BJ: The effects of physicians' training and personality on test ordering for ambulatory patients. Am J Public Health 74:1271–1273, 1984.
31. Tversky A, Kahneman D: Judgment under uncertainty: Heuristics and biases. Science 185:1124–1131, 1974.
32. Barr JT: Improved laboratory utilization and information production: The administrator's new role. J Med Tech 3:511–521, 1986.
33. Hammond HC: Applying the value-of-information paradigm to laboratory management. Clin Lab Manage Rev 20:98–106, 1996.
34. Krahns MD, Mahoney JE, Eckman MH, et al: Screening for prostate cancer: A decision analytic view. JAMA 272:773–780, 1994.
35. Schoen EJ, Marks SM, Clemons MM, Bachman RP: Comparing prenatal and neonatal diagnosis of hemoglobinopathies. Pediatrics 92:354–357, 1993.
36. Greenland P, Mushlin AI, Griner PF: Discrepancies between knowledge and use of diagnostic studies in asymptomatic patients. J Med Educ 54:863–869, 1979.
37. Eisenberg J: Sociologic influences on decision-making by clinicians. Ann Intern Med 90:957–964, 1979.
38. Epstein AM, Begg CB, McNeil BJ: The effects of group size on test ordering for hypertensive patients. N Engl J Med 309:464–468, 1983.
39. Pineault R: The effect of prepaid group practice on physicians' utilization behavior. Med Care 14:121–136, 1976.
40. Noren J, Frazier T, Altman I, DeLozier J: Ambulatory medical care: A comparison of internists and family-general practitioners. N Engl J Med 302:11–16, 1980.
41. Everett GD, Chang P, deBlois CS, Holets TD: A comparative study of laboratory utilization behavior of "on-service" and "off-service" housestaff physicians. Med Care 21:1187–1191, 1983.
42. Garg ML, Mulligan JL, McNamara MJ, Skipper JK, et al: Teaching students the relationship between quality and cost of medical care. J Med Educ 50:1085–1091, 1975.
43. Jones KR: The influence of the attending physician on indirect graduate medical education costs. J Med Educ 59:789–798, 1984.
44. Busby DD, Leming JC, Olson MI: Unidentified educational costs in a university teaching hospital: An initial study. J Med Educ 47:243–253, 1972.
45. Schroeder SA, O'Leary DS: Differences in laboratory use and length of stay between university and community hospitals. J Med Educ 52:418–420, 1977.
46. Williams BT, Dixon RA: Biochemical testing for acute medical emergencies in four district general hospitals. Br Med J 1:1313–1315, 1979.
47. Martz EW, Ptakowski R: Educational costs to hospitalized patients. J Med Educ 53:383–386, 1978.
48. Epstein AM, Krock SJ, McNeil BJ: Office laboratory tests: Perceptions of profitability. Med Care 22:160–166, 1984.
49. Schroeder SA, Stowstack JA: Financial incentives to perform medical procedures and laboratory tests. Med Care 16:289–298, 1978.

50. Rice TH: The impact of changing Medicare reimbursement rates on physician-induced demand. Med Care 21:803–815, 1983.

51. Valenstein PN, Howanitz PJ: Ordering accuracy: A College of American Pathologists Q-probe study of 577 institutions. Arch Pathol Lab Med 119:117–122, 1995.

52. Tarpey A, Neithercut WD: Use of multichannel discrete analyser to reduce unnecessary biochemical tests. J Clin Pathol 46:459–461, 1993.

53. Wong ET, McCarron MM, Shaw ST: Ordering of laboratory tests in a teaching hospital: Can it be improved? JAMA 249:3078–3080, 1983.

54. Bachner P, Howanitz PJ, Lent RW: Quality improvement practices in clinical and anatomic pathology services: A College of American Pathologists Q-probe study of the program characteristics and performance in 580 institutions. Am J Clin Pathol 102:567–571, 1994.

55. Renner SW, Howanitz PJ, Bachner P: Wristband identification error reporting in 712 hospitals: A College of American Pathologists' Q-probe study of quality issues in transfusion practice. Arch Pathol Lab Med 117:573–577, 1993.

56. Coody D, Yelman RJ, Montgomery D, van Eys J: Early hospital discharge and the timing of newborn metabolic screening. Clin Pediatr (Phila) 32:463–466, 1993.

57. Staneck JL: Impact of technological developments and organizational strategies on clinical laboratory cost reduction. Diagn Microbiol Infect Dis 23:61–73, 1995.

58. Winkelman JW, Wybenga DR, Tanasijevic MJ: The fiscal consequences of central vs. distributed testing of glucose. Clin Chem 40:1628–1630, 1994.

59. Doern GV, Vautour R, Gaydet M, Levy B: Clinical impact of rapid in vitro susceptibility testing and bacterial identification. J Clin Microbiol 32:1757–1762, 1994.

60. Granato PA: The impact of same-day versus traditional overnight testing. Diagn Microbiol Infect Dis 16:237–243, 1993.

61. Hobbie RK, Reece RL: Interpretative reporting by computer. Hum Pathol 12:127–134, 1981.

62. Young DS: Interpretation of clinical chemical data with the aid of automatic data processing. Clin Chem 22:1555–1559, 1986.

63. Peddecord KM, Hofherr LK, Benenson AS, et al: Use of physician survey to identify opportunities for quality improvement. Clin Lab Sci 6:110–115, 1993.

64. Miller WG: Total error assessment of five methods for cholesterol screening. Clin Chem 39:297–304, 1993.

65. Barr JT, Schumacher GE: "The Total Testing Process" *In* Schumacher GE (ed): Therapeutic Drug Monitoring. Hartford CT, Appleton & Lange, 1995.

66. Magee MS, Walden CE, Benedetti TJ, Knopp RH: Influence of diagnostic criteria on the incidence of gestational diabetes and perinatal morbidity. JAMA 269:609–615, 1993.

67. Mennemeyer ST, Winkelman JW: Downstream outcomes: Using insurance claims data to screen for errors in clinical laboratory testing. QRB Qual Rev Bull 17:194–199, 1991.

68. Mennemeyer ST, Winkelman JW: Searching for inaccuracies in clinical laboratory testing using Medicare data: Evidence for prothrombin time. JAMA 269:1030–1033, 1993.

69. Winkelman JW, Mennemeyer ST: Screening for clinical laboratory errors with Medicare claims data: results for digoxin. Am J Med Qual 11:1–8, 1996.

70. Barr JT, Otto C: Is Variation in the Structure and Process of Bedside Glucose Testing Associated With Variations in Patient Outcomes? Denver, Clinical Laboratory Management Association, Annual Meeting Abstract, August 1996.

71. McDonald JM, Smith JA: Value-added laboratory medicine in an era of managed care. Clin Chem 41:1256–1262, 1995.

72. Connelly C, Steele B: Laboratory utilization: Problems and solutions. Arch Pathol Lab Med 104:59–62, 1980.

73. Kassirer JP, Pauker SG: Should diagnostic testing be regulated? N Engl J Med 299:947–949, 1978.

74. Davidoff F, Goodspeed R, Clive J: Changing test ordering behavior—A randomized controlled trial comparing probabilistic reasoning with cost containment education. Med Care 27:45–58, 1989.

75. Kassebaum DG: Teaching laboratory test use. J Med Educ 60:420–421, 1985.

76. Garland MJ: Integrating cost awareness with ethics in the undergraduate medical curriculum. J Med Educ 60:44–52, 1985.

77. Freeman RA: Cost containment. J Med Educ 51:157–158, 1976.

78. Spiegel CT, Knapp BA, Newman MA, et al: Modification of decision-making behavior of third-year medical students. J Med Educ 57:769–777, 1982.

79. Garg ML, Gliebe WA, Kleinberg WM: Student peer review of diagnostic tests at the Medical College of Ohio. J Med Educ 54:852–855, 1979.

80. Williams SV, Eisenberg JM, Kitz DS, Carroll JG, et al: Teaching cost-effective diagnostic test use to medical students. Med Care 22:535–542, 1984.

81. Rhyne RL, Gehlbach SH: Effects of an educational feedback strategy on physician utilization of thyroid function panels. J Fam Pract 8:1003–1007, 1979.

82. Karas S: Cost containment in emergency medicine. JAMA 243:1356–1359, 1980.

83. Martin AR, Wolf MA, Thibodeau LA, Dzau V: A trial of two strategies to modify the test-ordering behavior of medical residents. N Engl J Med 300:1330–1336, 1980.

84. Eisenberg JM: An educational program to modify laboratory use by house staff. J Med Educ 52:578–581, 1979.

85. Schroeder SA, Myers LP, McPhee SJ, et al: The failure of physician education as a cost containment strategy. JAMA 252:225–230, 1984.

86. Wones RG: Failure of low cost audits with feedback to reduce laboratory test utilization. Med Care 25:78–82, 1987.

87. Everett GD, deBlois CS, Chang P, Holets T: Effect of cost education, cost audits and faculty chart review on the use of laboratory services. Arch Intern Med 143:942–944, 1983.

88. Gortmaker S, Bickford A, Mathewson H, et al: A successful experiment to reduce unnecessary laboratory use in a community hospital. Med Care 26:631–642, 1988.

89. Berwick DM, Coltin KL: Feedback reduces test use in a health maintenance organization. JAMA 255:1450–1454, 1986.

90. Korvin CC, Pearce RH, Stanley J: Admissions screening: Clinical benefits. Ann Intern Med 83:197–203, 1975.

91. Hampton JR, Harrison MJG, Mitchell JRA, et al: Relative contributions of history-taking, physical examination, and laboratory investigations to diagnosis and management of medical outpatients. Brit Med J 2:486–489, 1975.

92. Sandler G: Costs of unnecessary tests. Brit Med J 2:21–24, 1979.

93. Durbridge TC, Edwards F, Edwards RG, Atkinson M: Evaluation of benefits of screening tests done immediately on admission to hospital. Clin Chem 22:968–971, 1976.

94. Delahunt B, Turnbull PRG: How cost effective are routine preoperative investigations? N Z Med J 92:431–432, 1980.

95. Kaplan EB, Sheiner LB, Boeckmann AJ, et al: The usefulness of preoperative laboratory screening. JAMA 253:3576–3581, 1985.

96. Lundberg GD: Is there a need for routine preoperative laboratory tests? JAMA 253:3589, 1985.

97. Sussman E, Goodwin P, Rosen H: Administrative change and diagnostic test use: The effect of eliminating standing orders. Med Care 22:569–572, 1984.

98. Lundberg GD: Laboratory request forms (menus) that guide and teach. JAMA 249:3075, 1983.

99. Durnad-Zaleski I, Rymer JC, Roudot-Thoraval F, et al: Reducing unnecessary laboratory use with new test request form: Example of tumour markers. Lancet 342:150–153, 1993.

100. Tierney WM, Miller ME, McDonald CJ: The effect of test ordering on informing physicians of the charges for outpatient diagnostic tests. N Engl J Med 322:1499–1504, 1990.

101. Gray G, Marton R: Utilization of a hematology laboratory in a teaching hospital. Am J Clin Pathol 59:877–882, 1973.

102. Novich M, Gillis L, Tauber AI: The laboratory test justified: An effective means to reduce routine laboratory testing. Am J Clin Pathol 84:756–759, 1985.

103. Barr JT: Design and analysis of interventions to modify utilization of therapeutic drug monitoring. Doctoral dissertation. Cambridge, MA: Harvard University, 1987.

104. Zaat JOM, van Eijk JTM, Bonte HA: Laboratory test form design influences test ordering by general practitioners in the Netherlands. Med Care 30:189–198, 1992.

105. Rich EC, Crowson TW, Connelly DP: Effectiveness of differential leukocyte count in case finding in the ambulatory care setting. JAMA 249:633–636, 1983.

106. Rock WA, Grogan JE: Demand versus need versus physician prerogatives in the use of the WBC differential. JAMA 249:613–616, 1983.

107. Shapiro MF, Hatch RL, Greenfield S: Cost containment and labor-intensive tests: The case of the leukocyte differential count. JAMA 252:231–234, 1984.

108. Wesson SK, Mercado T, Austin M, Schumacher HR: Differential counts and overuse of the laboratory. Lancet 1:552, 1980.

109. Shaw ST, Poon SY, Wong ET: "Routine urinalysis": Is the dipstick enough? JAMA 253:1596–1600, 1985.

110. Valenstein P: New roles for the urine dipstick. Medical Laboratory Observer 18:63–66, 1986.

111. Brewer ED, Benson GS: Hematuria: Algorithms for diagnosis: 1. Hematuria in the child. JAMA 246:877–880, 1981.

112. Benson GS, Brewer ED: Hematuria: Algorithms for diagnosis: 2. Hematuria in the adult and hematuria secondary to trauma. JAMA 246:993–995, 1981.

113. Wong ET, Freier EF: The differential diagnosis of hypercalcemia. An algorithm for more effective use of laboratory tests. JAMA 247:75–80, 1982.

114. Lum G, Deshotels SJ: The clinical usefulness of an algorithm for the interpretation of biochemical profiles with hypercalcemia. Am J Clin Pathol 78:479–484, 1982.

115. Orient JM, Kettel LJ, Sox HC, et al: The effect of algorithms on the cost and quality of patient care. Med Care 21:157–167, 1983.

116. Wachtel T, Moulton AW, Pezzullo J, Hamolsky M: Inpatient management protocols to reduce health care costs. Med Decis Making 6:101–109, 1986.

117. Young DW: An aid to reducing unnecessary investigations. Br Med J 281:1610–1611, 1980.

118. Taylor TR, Shields S, Black R: Study of cost-conscious computer-assisted diagnosis in thyroid disease. Lancet 2:79–83, 1972.

119. Scott DR: Influence of managed care and health maintenance organizations on the clinical microbiology laboratory. Diagn Microbiol Infect Dis 23:17–21, 1995.

120. Feldkamp CS, Carey JL: An algorithmic approach to thyroid function testing in a managed care setting. Am J Clin Pathol 105:11–16, 1996.

121. Friedberg RC, Moser SA, Jamieson PW, et al: Automating clinical practice guidelines: A corporate-academic partnership. Clin Lab Managem Review 10:120–123, 1996.

122. Peterman TA, Speicher CE: Evaluating pleural effusions: A two-stage laboratory approach. JAMA 252:1051–1053, 1984.

123. Rao KMK, Bordine SL, Keren DF: Decision making by pathologists: A strategy for curtailing the number of inappropriate tests. Arch Pathol Lab Med 106:55–56, 1982.

124. Hardwick DF, Morrison JI, Tydeman J, Cassidy PA, et al: Structuring complexity of testing: A process oriented approach to limiting unnecessary laboratory use. Am J Med Tech 48:605–608, 1982.

125. Banks NJ, Palmer RH, Berwick DM, Pisek P: Variability in clinical systems: Applying modern quality control methods to health care. Jt Comm J Qual Improv 21:407–419, 1995.

126. Gottlieb LK, Margolis CZ, Schoenbaum SC: Clinical practice guidelines at an HMO: Development and implementation in a quality improvement model. QRB Qual Rev Bull 16:80–86, 1990.

Chapter 2

Clinical Laboratory Utilization: Implementation

Linda Luckey and Brenta G. Davis

Old Laboratory vs. New Laboratory
Emerging Roles for Clinical Laboratory Scientists
Implementing New Roles in the Laboratory
New Roles and Expected Outcomes

For many years the services provided by clinical laboratory scientists (CLSs) have been essential in the diagnosis and treatment of patients. Their scientific and technical expertise has provided the information that clinicians find essential in carrying out patient care responsibilities. The clinician's reliance on the clinical laboratory has not changed; however, external forces, most notably in the form of managed care and capitation, are bringing about a major change in the way health care is delivered in the United States. The change is occurring rapidly, according to the Pew Health Professions Commission Report, transforming more traditional health care practice into "emerging systems of integrated care that combine primary, specialty, and hospital services" and requiring extraordinary collaboration skills across all levels and types of health care professions.[1] Nowhere is the change more evident than in the clinical laboratory, where the imperative exists to facilitate the wise and cost-effective use of laboratory services while maintaining, or even enhancing, the quality of the diagnostic and therapeutic decisions made by clinicians. Moreover, this transformation must take place in an environment that must use fewer resources more effectively to achieve "value added" outcomes (see Chapter 1).[2-7] Thus, for nonphysician laboratory managers and administrators, a unique set of challenges has emerged that require management expertise as never before. Also required is a cadre of practitioners who possess the knowledge and skills to assist in integrating management, fiscal, and laboratory utilization needs into an efficient and cost-effective system of providing the clinical laboratory services that are so essential to diagnosis and treatment.[8] It is no longer sufficient for laboratory results to be accurate and precise; they must also be useful in the sense that they contribute directly to timely and cost-effective diagnostic and therapeutic decisions.[9, 10] Changes in health care represent significant challenges, not only because of their magnitude, but also because of the speed at which they are occurring. Neverthe-less, they also represent extraordinary opportunities for clinical laboratory scientists who possess the knowledge of effective laboratory utilization and the willingness to use it.

OLD LABORATORY VS. NEW LABORATORY

To fully appreciate the new interactive laboratory described in Chapter 1 and the new roles required for CLSs, it is useful to review the comparison between the new laboratory and the old, or traditional, laboratory (see Figs. 1–1 and 1–2 in Chapter 1). In the traditional laboratory, in focus, almost to the exclusion of everything else, is the *process*, in which the actual performance of the test occurred, producing as accurate a number or a microbial identification as possible with all of the quality control accouterments, controls, and standards that accompany this phase. The input phase—that is, whether the right test had been used to answer a particular clinical question or to confirm a diagnosis—was not emphasized. If a test was ordered, it was performed, and the insurance company or the government (in the case of Medicare, for example), paid for it. Likewise, there was little focus in what happened after the laboratory result was reported. There was concern, of course, about the patient, but not much thought was given to the fact that a "good" result might not be put to good use. The exclusive focus and almost all of the effort was on the science, technology, and skill of testing, usually from within a very discipline-specific context. For example, the chemistry laboratory did chemical analyses and the hematology laboratory did hematologic analyses, and very little interaction between the two laboratories regarding the whole patient ever took place. If a result to two decimal places was good, a result to four decimal places was better. More was better, no matter what the cost and no matter if clinical need did not require that degree of accuracy or even that particular test.[11] In fact, the health care reimbursement system, in place for many years, encouraged overutilization: delivery of more services, including laboratory services, meant receipt of more income to providers and laboratories.[12]

Now, however, circumstances are very different. Current health care funding strategies punish rather than reward overutilization of services. Moreover, the complexity of the laboratory makes available what sometimes seems like an infinite array of test choices that have varying characteristics of sensitivity, specificity, and predictive value, depending on the clinical circumstances. This complexity makes it impossible for any physician to know everything; in addition, cost and technology must be considered. Now the potential exists, as never before, for laboratory results to make things worse, in terms of getting an accurate and cost-effective diagnosis. In the traditional laboratory, human technical skill was a highly prized and unique resource; now the technology is such that extensive technical skills are often irrelevant, and a different set of skills is valued. These skills have less to do with performing a test than with determining whether the test should be done at all, to help clinicians use the laboratory appropriately and more cost-effectively.[8] In the ideal new laboratory, only tests that actually contribute to an effective and efficient diagnosis are performed. Tests that contribute nothing to the diagnosis, or even confuse the issue because they address the wrong clinical question, would not be done. More is no longer better. Better is better. The legitimate concern of the laboratory is more than test performance. Process certainly is still very important, but now concern for input and output is added to the scope of the laboratory. The CLS is not the primary responsible party in the latter phases (input and output), because that is certainly still the physician, yet the CLS is an important participant/consultant in proper laboratory utilization that reaches the overall objective of accurate, efficient, and cost-effective diagnosis and treatment. All this is based on the premise that unless the right laboratory test has been ordered and interpreted properly, it does not matter how accurate and precise the result is. In the new laboratory the focus is on the patient and on an integrated view of laboratory data as a means to an end, rather than an end in itself.

EMERGING ROLES FOR CLINICAL LABORATORY SCIENTISTS

CLSs in laboratory management roles have become commonplace, and although their responsibilities have increased, the resources at their disposal have not. Many clinical laboratories, regardless of setting, are multimillion dollar enterprises, and they must be managed even more carefully, requiring professionals with enhanced management skills. Such skills also include the ability to advocate and to implement improved laboratory utilization, which is a major tool in delivering cost-effective, quality health care. In this context, appropriate laboratory utilization means that the "right test at the right time" is ordered, performed, and reported in a timely manner.

Providing advice about laboratory utilization issues is a new role for laboratory professionals, although it is emerging as an essential one.[1, 7, 9, 13–18] These roles may seem unusual or unrealistic, especially the suggestions that CLSs are developing collaborative, consultative relationships with clinicians who listen to them. However, these developments are occurring in environments where CLSs have sought opportunities to advance their reputations with physicians for credibility, competence, and the willingness to view the laboratory from the perspective that the laboratory is a means to an end, rather than an end in itself. The

---

Box 2–1. Laboratory Resource Management Consultant: Position Functions

Monitors utilization reports of high-volume test-usage patients

Communicates opportunities for improved utilization to case managers, physicians, and service line administrators

Assesses need for involvement of pathologists/administrators in utilization issues

Reviews care paths to affirm appropriate laboratory utilization

Consults with physicians, nurses, and laboratory professionals on current guidelines and protocols for proper test ordering

Educates physicians and nursing groups on current policies and procedures regarding laboratory utilization

Consults with laboratory administrators and practitioners about current laboratory utilization practices

---

development of this expanded role has occurred in environments where CLSs have felt confident enough about themselves and what they know (or can know) to attempt these interpersonal encounters and have done so skillfully enough to be successful. This new role is encompassed by a variety of titles, one of which is laboratory resource management consultant.[19] The stated purpose of this position is to facilitate and direct "proper utilization of laboratory services through testing protocols, case (care) management collaboration, physician education, and assessment of current health care goals and reimbursement plans." Box 2–1 lists the functions of this position and Box 2–2 outlines the requisite knowledge and skills. As this position has evolved and has become more integral to achieving the utilization goals of the laboratory, the title has been changed to laboratory resource manager. The consultation aspect is now so well understood that it is no longer necessary to emphasize it in the position title.[19]

Box 2–2. Laboratory Resource Management Consultant: Knowledge and Skills

Knowledge of data base, available information, and health care reimbursement

Knowledge of disease processes and the relationship to and/or need for laboratory tests

Understanding of sensitive customer needs and expectations

Knowledge of principles of total quality assurance

Clinical knowledge and critical thinking ability, independent judgment

Effective communication and motivational skills, knowledge of subject matter

Knowledge of educational methods and techniques

It is well documented that physician utilization of the laboratory can vary considerably in quality and quantity (see Chapter 1). Given the complexities of test choice described earlier, it is impossible for physicians to know everything about test characteristics, for example, the ability of the test to yield maximum information in a given clinical condition, the cost of procedures ordered vs. the cost of others that might yield as much information at less cost, and a host of considerations that include, but are not limited to, the accuracy of the clinical questions. Figure 2–1 depicts these relationships, including considerations that only CLSs can appropriately address because of their education, background, and experience.

If CLSs are to assume this function, they must be able to understand and participate in the sequence of events leading to the proper utilization of the laboratory, including how the physician arrives at the right clinical question (see Chapter 1 and Fig. 1–3). Figure 2–2 shows components of this process and suggests that CLSs have important roles to play in helping clincians at several points in the model, expanding their roles beyond test performance only. CLSs have the expertise to factor in all of the key elements, including the right clinical question in consideration of the right laboratory test.

Improving the quality of laboratory utilization has been a major goal of a number of groups for many years, because, in the final analysis, only by controlling the inappropriate and excessive use of laboratory testing can costs be managed. What is also emerging is the discovery that as laboratory utilization improves, quality and cost-effectiveness also improves.[9, 10, 20]

Use of clinical appropriateness criteria, algorithms, reflex testing, and other strategies discussed in Chapter 1 clearly cannot be initiated by the laboratory alone. Such tools must be the result of a collaborative effort between clinicians, CLSs, and others who understand enough about the parameters of the relevant clinical need to link it with the technical/scientific and economic characteristics of tests as diagrammed in Figure 2–1. There must also be room for flexibility. At times, the clinical need may require overriding the general rule, and CLSs must be able to understand and know when such deviations from the usual procedure by the physician are warranted.[20] Recent surveys of laboratory practitioners in a southeastern state[21] and of CLS educators nationally[8] found that many CLSs are already providing this type of expertise. A subsequent survey among laboratory managers in the southeast, determining their present need for individuals with these skills, found a growing demand for such expertise.[22] Other nonphysician health professionals have implemented such measures in their own fields, and CLSs that serve on care management and critical path teams are similarly involved.[23]

Other nonphysician health professionals, particularly pharmacists, who have faced similar changes and similar opportunities provide role models for CLSs, to some extent. As technology has advanced in the pharmacy field and began to have an impact on the traditional role and function of the pharmacist, the profession transformed itself and became as successful (or more) in expanded roles as they had been traditionally. Similarly, the roles of CLSs are changing in four directions, represented in Box 2–3.

These four general directions represent opportunities for CLSs in the new laboratory and in roles that may look unusual but that actually exist now in many institutions. Figure 2–3 depicts a decision-making flowchart of laboratory utilization at a large Midwestern hospital; other, similar, protocols exist across the country.[25]

As laboratory resources have been used more wisely, cost savings have resulted in millions of dollars, and quality of health care has not only been preserved, but overall patient care quality has improved.[25, 26] For expanded CLS roles to become more prevalent, CLSs must certainly ac-

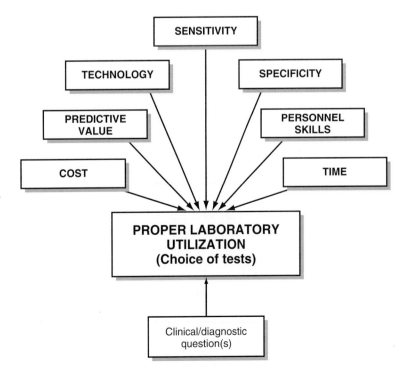

Figure 2–1. Laboratory utilization factors.

MODEL OF LABORATORY UTILIZATION

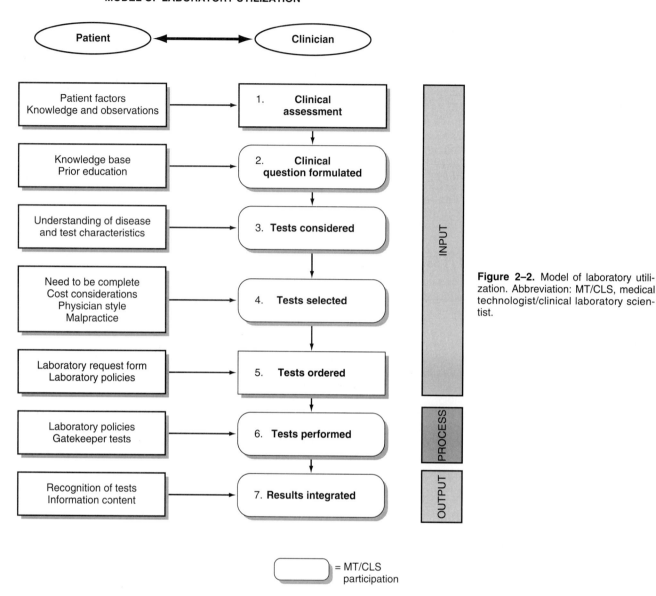

Figure 2–2. Model of laboratory utilization. Abbreviation: MT/CLS, medical technologist/clinical laboratory scientist.

quire a set of skills that may not seem traditional but are nonetheless essential for success in the new laboratory in an era of managed care. These are depicted in Box 2–4 and are discussed in depth in Chapter 3. Being successful in meeting new expectations and in fulfilling responsibilities in the "new laboratory" depends, in great part, not

only on the competence of CLSs but also on whether they seek opportunities to convey the professionalism they possess and whether they acquire the personal and interpersonal skills that make it possible. It is important to recognize, therefore, the affective, or attitude, component of the ability required to function in the new interactive laboratory. No matter how expert individuals may be, if they lack the confidence and empowerment to eagerly take on these new roles, success may be elusive. Figure 2–4 suggests that both knowledge and the inner power of knowing are essential components of being able to fill these new professional roles. It also suggests that the affective element is as important in the preparation and continuing education of CLSs as the traditional laboratory sciences.

IMPLEMENTING NEW ROLES IN THE LABORATORY

Changes of the magnitude now faced by the health care system in the United States are so profound and far-reach-

---

Box 2–3. Changing Roles and Future Opportunities

Increasing involvement in diagnosis and monitoring
Increasing use of laboratory staff at highest level of
   capability
Increasing emphasis on clinical problem orientation
   vs. narrow specialty
Increasing variety in practice sites outside the laboratory (e.g., bedside, home)

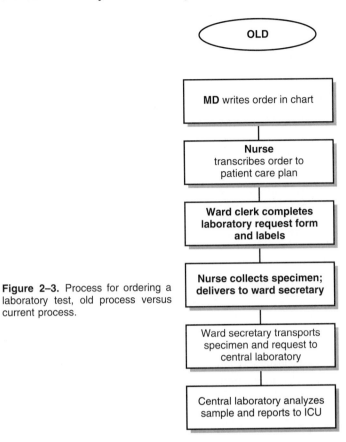

Figure 2–3. Process for ordering a laboratory test, old process versus current process.

ing that any element within the system that does not respond appropriately and quickly is at a great disadvantage competitively and is even likely to fail. Box 2–5 illustrates some of the specific changes that are occurring, which emphasize the need to adopt very different conceptual approaches in providing quality laboratory services in a managed care environment. This is particularly challenging in view of the perspective of hospital administrators who consider managing costs a greater challenge than maintaining quality.[27] It is vital to remember that the achievement of cost containment goals, to the exclusion of quality

goals, may permit survival in the short term; however, the additional achievement of quality goals will, in the longer term, determine the "winners."[9, 27] This will occur because eventually all of the players left in the game will be offering services at essentially the same price; only those who preserved quality during the cost containment process will survive from that point. A number of challenges are

---

Box 2–4. Skills Needed in the New Laboratory

Ability to adapt to change
Critical thinking abilities
Problem solving and troubleshooting skills
Communication skills
Attributes of a professional
THESE ARE ALSO CONSULTATION SKILLS

Box 2–5. How Has the Marketplace Changed?

Past	Present
Provider competition	Community delivery system
Fragmented care	Continuity of care
Sick care	Managed care
Reactive utilization review	Proactive practice guidelines
Cost per test	Length of stay
Test price	Test appropriateness

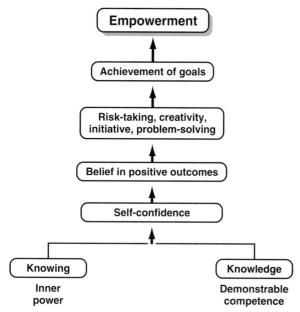

Figure 2–4. Empowerment.

the highest levels. The fact that the results of these strategies are the same as those desired by hospital administrators, and can be documented accordingly, is a great help in achieving the levels of administrative commitment and, ultimately, the physician support necessary for success.[20] Physicians and nurses generally have little understanding of the internal workings of the laboratory, the backgrounds of laboratory personnel, or the commitment of CLSs to the same patient care goals. The actions of the laboratory staff, which seem so logical to laboratorians, may seem arbitrary, unnecessary, or even uncaring to nonlaboratory professionals. Thus, the effort to promote wise use of the laboratory becomes a long-term effort of laboratorians to develop credibility with physicians and others and to provide them with information about the effects of their use of laboratory

facing clinical laboratories and laboratory managers, which are outlined in Box 2–6. One key element in achieving the goals of cost-effective laboratory services while maintaining quality is the availability of CLSs who have the skills and the knowledge to promote prudent utilization of the laboratory by individuals who depend on the laboratory for vital information. Such individuals include not only physicians and nurses but also pharmacists, service line managers, and social workers—anyone whose patient care efforts are affected by the need for timely diagnosis and treatment through reliable, accurate, and appropriate laboratory results.[20] Box 2–7 illustrates this concept as it is implemented by one of many service line (care management) teams in one large community hospital in the southeast.[28]

A growing number of health care institutions throughout the country rely on the expertise of laboratory managers and laboratory utilization advisors/consultants to achieve enhanced quality while achieving cost effectiveness.[29] The economic benefits of these management and utilization approaches to patients and health care institutions are significant in a health care system that spent $1 trillion in 1995, of which $130 billion was spent on laboratory services alone.[29] Among the increasing number of reported cost savings are such examples as 17% to 26% reductions in laboratory charges per patient case for selected medical conditions,[18, 29] and an almost 40% reduction in overall hospital costs for patients monitored by proactive and appropriate laboratory testing.[2, 18, 29] These and other specific examples represent multimillion dollar savings,[25, 26] and the potential for even greater cost savings, as well as patient satisfaction and outcomes, increases as the approaches are increasingly utilized by individuals trained in their application.[2, 18, 29]

As worthwhile as these goals and strategies are, no single laboratory professional can effect change without significant commitment by laboratory administrators, who in turn must be supported by institutional administrators at

---

Box 2–6. Hospital Rules for Success in Managed Care Arena

Maintain or Improve Quality Levels

1. Fulfill all requirements for regulatory agencies
2. Empower employees to do the right thing
3. Reward employees for quality performance
4. Implement quality indicators and monitor for compliance
5. Employ satisfaction surveys for employees

Improve Service Levels

1. Become more patient focused
2. Become more customer focused
3. Determine service levels required and work to meet these levels by employee involvement
4. Establish acceptable TAT with other departments, such as emergency department
5. Monitor TAT and share with customers
6. Ask for feedback
7. Develop customer designed panels
8. Reexamine traditional approaches

Reduce Cost of Service

1. Eliminate redundant and duplicate testing
2. Review testing menu—reduce number of profiles or numbers of tests included in profile
3. Reduce utilization (tests and blood products)
4. Review DRG data
5. Consolidate and cross-train
6. Develop appropriate ratio of MT/MLT
7. Reduce FTEs
8. Improve teamwork
9. Become involved with case management in order to

   - Reduce length of stay
   - Improve efficiency
   - Employ appropriate testing
   - Improve laboratory visibility

Abbreviations: TAT, turn around time; DRG, diagnosis-related groups; MT/MLT, medical technologist/medical laboratory technician; FTE, full-time equivalent.

Box 2–7. **Cardiovascular Services Medical Center: Service Line Team Meetings**

Purpose

To provide a forum for the members of the cardio-vascular team to discuss issues and develop action plans related to the delivery of care for cardiovascular patients at Baptist Memorial Hospital—Medical Center. Each team member is accountable for contributing to a seamless delivery of quality and efficient care as it relates to the cardiovascular patient population.

Functions

1. Development of operational goals and objectives that support the strategic initiatives of Baptist Memorial Hospital and The Baptist Heart Center.
2. Identification and resolution of operational issues that impair our ability to deliver a quality and efficient product consistently for the cardiovascular patient.
3. Joint development of quality improvement activities as they relate to cardiovascular services.

Membership

Respiratory therapy
Case managers
Patient care unit managers
Manager—invasive services
Manager—noninvasive services
Social services
Transplant services
Clinical laboratory services
Radiology
Service line educators
Surgery
Emergency department
Pharmacy
Infection control
House supervisor

---

services. It includes forming effective working relationships with a great variety of health professionals, and it certainly involves the exercise of patience and persistence on the part of the CLS.[31] Changing old habits is difficult, at best, and is fraught with resistance, confusion, and, often, misunderstanding. Despite these difficulties, the rewards, in terms of dollars saved and of quality improvement gained, are great and can provide the incentive for administrators, laboratorians, and other professionals to persist.[28] Persons

who serve as laboratory resource managers/consultants must have the knowledge and skills outlined in Boxes 2–1 and 2–2, and they must also be able to educate and lead their own laboratory colleagues as they reform their own approaches to providing laboratory services. For example, CLSs must learn to accommodate the concept of "clinical accuracy and precision" as opposed to the laboratory view of these parameters from an analytic perspective. The importance of accuracy and precision to the clinician depends

---

```
*****************************************************************
CLINICAL LABORATORY UPDATE               CLINICAL LABORATORY UPDATE
*****************************************************************


                    Patient _____ Admission Date _____
                    Diagnosis_____

FROM: _____
OFFICE NUMBER: _____
BEEPER NUMBER: _____
DATE: _____
TIME: _____

Clinical laboratory charges on this patient are at _____ for the following period: previous
week / previous month / since admission

Utilization during this period included: _____
_____
_____
_____
_____

This update is being provided to help make you aware of laboratory utilization. We hope this information
will help you in determining the most appropriate laboratory requests for your patient.

THIS UPDATE IS NOT A PERMANENT PART OF THE PATIENT'S MEDICAL RECORD
```

Figure 2–5. Laboratory test utilization review.

CLINICAL LABORATORY ORDERS AND TESTS

CH12	CH7	ELEC	LIVER A	MAG
				Magnesium
				POT
Sodium	Sodium	Sodium		Potassium
Potassium	Potassium	Potassium		**SOD**
Chloride	Chloride	Chloride		Sodium
Glucose	Glucose			
BUN	BUN			
Creatinine	Creatinine			
	CO₂	CO₂		
Calcium				
Protein				
Albumin			Albumin	
Alkaline Phosphatase			Alkaline Phosphatase	**MYOG**
AST			AST	Myoglobin
			ALT	**TROP**
Bilirubin, Total			Bilirubin, Total	Troponin 1
			Bilirubin, Direct	

MI1	MI2	MI3	MI4	CKMB
CK, Total		CK, Total	CK, Total	CK, Total
CK-MB		CK-MB	CK-MB	CK-MB
Myoglobin	Myoglobin	Myoglobin		
Troponin 1	Troponin 1	Troponon 1	Troponin 1	

CBCI	CBC	PLT	HGB	HCT
RBC	RBC			
Hemoglobin	Hemoglobin		Hemoglobin	
Hematocrit	Hematocrit			Hematocrit
RBC INDICES	RBC INDICES			
RDW	RDW			
Platelets	Platelets	Platelets		
MPV	MPV	MPV		
WBC	WBC			
Differential				
RBC Morphology				

Figure 2–6. Clinical laboratory test: chemistry and hematology. Abbreviations: BUN, blood urea nitrogen; AST, aspartate transaminase; CO₂, carbon dioxide; ALT, alanine transaminase; CK, creatine kinase; CK-MB, creatine kinase isoenzyme; RBC, red blood cell count; RDW, red-cell distribution width; MPV, mean platelet volume; WBC, white blood cell count.

entirely on the clinical context in which the result is to be used, and may well have to be sacrificed for another dimension of quality that is non–laboratory related.[32] For example, immediate information that covers a broad clinical range (normal/abnormal; elevated/decreased) may be more important in the emergency department, when faced with an unconscious diabetic patient, than are the more precise and accurate glucose measurements that will be necessary later to reestablish therapeutic stability in such a patient.

Documentation and tracking of problems is essential, and having the right tools to accomplish this is equally important. One way to focus the attention of the physician on the financial impact of the use of the laboratory is illustrated by the form shown in Figure 2–5. Note that a prominent notice indicates that this document will not become part of the patient's record.[28] An action as simple as providing convenient reminders to physicians and nurses

as to what combinations of tests are represented by specific laboratory orders can eliminate inadvertent and unnecessary testing. Figures 2–6, 2–7, and 2–8 are examples of three such efforts to inform "customers" about laboratory services. Figure 2–9 represents an internal tool in the laboratory that guides the laboratory staff in documenting, analyzing, and solving problems related to specimen collection, for example. Note that an area of the form is used to identify the negative effects of the identified problems on overall patient care. Figure 2–10 is a more general form suitable for internal laboratory use in identifying, analyzing, and solving a variety of problems. To truly provide patient-focused, high-quality "customer service," laboratory staff must be empowered to create and apply novel solutions to patient care problems. Examples of two reports documenting such actions can be found as Figures 2–11 and 2–12. It should be noted that the problems identified

CLINICAL LABORATORY ORDERS AND TESTS

APX	CLA	ACAG	ACAM
Prothrombin time INR value APTT	Prothrombin time INR value APTT Circulating lupus anticoagulant component ACAG Pathologist consultation	Anticardiolipin antibody, IgG Pathologist consultation	Anticardiolipin antibody, IgM Pathologist consultation

HEPA	PAD	PAB	PA
Heparin sensitive platelet aggregation Platelet antibody Platelet antibody to heparin Platelet count MPV Pathologist consultation	Platelet antibody Platelet antibody to a drug (specify drug)	Platelet antibody	Platelet aggregation Platelet count MPV Wu & Hoak Pathologist consultation

HP	PROC	PROS
Platelet factor 4 Prothrombin fragment 1.2 Antithrombin III level Protein C assay Protein S assay Factor VII assay D-Dimer assay by ELISA CLA panel Pathologist consultation	Protein C assay Factor VII assay Pathologist consultation	Protein S assay Factor VII assay Pathologist consultation

TSRT	RBC Order
ABO Rh Antibody screen	ABO Rh Antibody screen Crossmatch IS (each unit ordered)

Figure 2–7. Clinical laboratory test: coagulation and blood bank. Abbreviations: INR, International Normalized Ratio; APTT, activated partial thromboplastin time; ACAG, anticardiolipin antibody IgG; Ig, Immunoglobulin; MPV, mean platelet volume; CLA, cyclic lysine anhydride; ABO, blood group system; Rh, Rhesus factor; IS, immediate spin.

and solved in these two examples were quite different, yet both materially affected patient care and the institution's ability to provide cost-effective care and "customer satisfaction." "Customers" of the laboratory can be quite diverse, as in these examples, ranging from patients to nursing staff and physicians. Figure 2–13 is an example of a survey used to assess satisfaction about laboratory services on the part of professional staff in an emergency department. The data captured as a result of these efforts can be very valuable in developing inservice education for nursing staff, correcting and improving a variety of processes within the institution, and even revisiting decisions about such issues as job redesign. Figure 2–14 represents one way in which such data can be organized and reported to appropriate administrators, along with recommendations

for solutions. Similarly, other problems and their solutions, particularly if cost savings can be demonstrated, are important to report. In addition to Figures 2–11 and 2–12, Figures 2–15 and 2–16 are examples of reports that provide opportunities for the laboratory to demonstrate its value to the institution on an ongoing basis.

The opportunity to have a significant impact on care management is important to CLSs, not only from the point of view of quality of care but also as a professional opportunity. Figures 2–17 and 2–18 represent guidelines developed by care management teams that included CLSs and others (see Box 2–7). The unique expertise of CLSs can be a very valuable resource to such care efforts, in addition to expertise provided by physicians. These activities are particularly important as mechanisms to capture correct

Text continued on page 36

Are Coagulation Test Orders Confusing You?????

TEST	CODE	COMMENTS
Heparin sensitive platelet aggregation Includes: Platelet aggregation to heparin Platelet antibody Platelet antibody to a drug (heparin)	*HEPA*	Common ordering methods: Platelet-induced heparin aggregation and antibody. Assay for platelet sensitivity to heparin to include platelet aggregation, antiplatelet antibody to a drug (heparin) Platelet-induced antibody and aggregation for sensitivity to heparin Assay for aggregation and antibody for platelet sensitivity to heparin (HEPA-PAD heparin)
Platelet antibody	*PAB*	Antibody without drug
Platelet antibody to a drug Includes: PAB	*PAD*	Please put name of drug in the comment line *Each* drug must be set up individually Proper spelling of the drug is important
Platelet aggregation study	*PA*	Aggregation to ADP, collagen, and epinephrine
Protein C (functional)	*PROC*	Antigenic protein C (PCAG) requires pathologist's approval
Protein S (functional)	*PROS*	Antigenic protein S (PSAG) requires pathologist's approval
Circulating lupus anticoagulant	*CLA*	Includes antiphospholipid antibody (APA)
APX	*APX*	Includes APTT, PT ** and INR Putting the *anticoagulant* in the comment line will save you a telephone call from the laboratory
Activated clotting time	*ACT*	Notify laboratory, set up and performed by the laboratory

Figure 2–8. Specialty assays are available from the coagulation laboratory. Abbreviations: PAB, performance assessment battery; ADP, adenosine diphosphate; APTT, activated partial thromboplastin time; PT, prothrombin time; INR, International Normalized Ratio. ** All PTs include INRs.

```
                    CLINICAL LABORATORY
                       CQI MONITOR
                     PROBLEM SOLVING


                                             Date: _____
                                             Reported by: _____

Type of problem
        ☐ Misidentified specimen
        ☐ Adulterated specimen: IV _____ hyperal _____ other _____
        ☐ Unacceptable specimen _____
        ☐ Redundant order _____
        ☐ Incorrect order _____
        ☐ After tests are completed; Credits requested _____
        ☐ Volume of blood (inadequate/excessive) _____

Details
        Room no. and patient ID _____
        Lab number _____
        Collector code _____
        Date and time of problem _____
        Original result _____
        Recollect reported result _____

Laboratory action
        ☐ Recollected specimen; Repeated tests
        ☐ Recollected all tests; Repeated all tests
        ☐ Called correct report to nurse/MD
        ☐ Reported results via computer (Date: _____ Time: _____)

Effects
        ☐ Delay in reporting results
        ☐ Delay in surgery
        ☐ Cost of duplication/additional work
        ☐ Additional phlebotomies for patient
        ☐ Increased blood loss for patient

Supervisor action
```

Figure 2–9. Clinical laboratory CQI monitor problem solving. Abbreviations: CQI, continuous quality improvement; IV, intravenous.

DEPARTMENT OF PATHOLOGY
SERVICE RECOVERY

Date: ____________ Time: ____________

Reported by: ______________________

(Name and Title)

Details of problem:

____

____

____

____

____

Immediate action:

____

____

____

____

____

Problem resolved

Date and time: ______________

Name: ______________

Supervisor action:

____

____

____

____

Closure to customer's satisfaction

Date and time: ______________

Name: ______________

Figure 2–10. Service recovery form.

MEMORIAL HOSPITAL
Pathology and Clinical Laboratory Services
July 1998

Quality Measurement and Assessment

Issue: Pre-admission laboratory reports not printing to the most appropriate locations.

Key function: Care of patients: planning and providing care, assessment of patients, continuum of care, information management, improving organizational performance.

Contributing departments/ services: Pathology, information systems, nursing

Findings/trends: In January 1998, 4 months post–computer conversion, it was brought to the attention of laboratory personnel that pre-admission patient test results were not "expedite printing" to the most appropriate locations at East and Medical Center. The reports were being manually extracted from the system on a daily basis, which was costly in time and inherently inefficient. Having had experience with result reporting, laboratory personnel assessed the specific needs of pre-admission patients reporting at both East and Medical Centers. Distinct differences between the two locations were identified and proposed solutions discussed with nursing supervisors and computer support personnel. At East and Medical Center expedite printers needed to be defined for the appropriate pre-admission patient locations. A chart distribution was also created for the Medical Center due to differences in physical location of patient at time of pre-admission workup vs. actual day of admission to 12 Madison.

Conclusions: Due to the collaborative effort of laboratory, nursing, and information systems personnel, pre-admission laboratory results now expedite print to more efficient and effective areas, thus eliminating the need to manually print the results.

Recommendations/actions: No action at this time.

Figure 2–11. Example of an assessment report.

MEMORIAL HOSPITAL
Department of Clinical Laboratory Services
July 1998

Performance Assessment/Improvement Abstract

Issue: Effective communication regarding the appropriate collection container for a patient with platelets that clump in EDTA.

Key function: Care of patients: planning and providing care (TX), environment of care (EC), improving organizational performance (PI).

Contributing departments/ services: Pathology, phlebotomy, nursing

Findings/trends: A patient presented with the phenomenon of platelets that clump in EDTA. Upon confirmation of this situation by the laboratory, the hematology technologist notified nursing and phlebotomy that all platelet counts collected on this patient must be drawn in a blue-top tube rather than purple (EDTA) tube. Notification of special collection was placed in the patient's chart. Due to the fact that this was a somewhat isolated need and could not be addressed through the computer for this specific patient, the laboratory was dependent on verbal communication between nursing shifts and numerous phlebotomists.

The patient continued to have daily platelet counts collected in the wrong collection tube. A breakdown in communication between the patient's chart and the collection process was apparent. The hematology technologist readily identified the need for clear, concise communication of the special collection at the patient's bedside prior to the venipuncture. The technologist printed and laminated a small card indicating that all platelet counts were to be drawn in a blue-top tube. The technologist calmly, and with reassurance, explained to the patient that the card should be presented to anyone drawing blood to ensure proper collection and to prevent additional phlebotomies due to re-collections.

Conclusions: The laboratory is aware that communication of an isolated situation in a large institution can be frustrating as well as challenging. The hematology technologist quickly identified a problem and effectively developed a solution. The patient's platelet counts were collected properly once the bedside care was in place.

Recommendations/actions: All departments must be open to effective, efficient means of communication to better serve our customers. It is often necessary to seek means that challenge the norm and force us to ask, "Why not?"

Evaluation/follow-up:

Figure 2–12. Example of an assessment report. Abbreviation: EDTA, ethylenediaminetetraacetic acid.

Department of Pathology
Clinical Laboratory*—Medical Center

CUSTOMER SATISFACTION SURVEY
Emergency Department - Medical Center

	Strongly agree	Agree	No opinion	Disagree	Strongly disagree
Please circle the appropriate response					
TIMELINESS OF SERVICE					
1. Laboratory results are faxed or called in in a timely manner.	5	4	3	2	1
2. I am informed of critical values in a timely manner.	5	4	3	2	1
3. I am notified of recollects or problem specimens in a timely manner.	5	4	3	2	1
CUSTOMER SERVICE					
1. Laboratory personnel consistently use proper telephone etiquette.	5	4	3	2	1
2. When needed, an employee with technical knowledge is available to help resolve problems.	5	4	3	2	1
3. I am satisfied with the level of customer service provided by the clinical laboratory staff on all shifts.	5	4	3	2	1
RESULT REPORTING					
1. I receive my laboratory reports in a timely manner	5	4	3	2	1
2. Result reports are easy to read and designed so I can readily identify the patient results.	5	4	3	2	1
3. It is beneficial for laboratory reports to be faxed to the ED during computer down time.	5	4	3	2	1
REPUTATION					
1. The clinical laboratory provides quality service.	5	4	3	2	1
2. Errors are identified and corrected promptly.	5	4	3	2	1
3. Problems are resolved swiftly and effectively with adequate follow up.	5	4	3	2	1

SUGGESTIONS FOR IMPROVEMENT:

Your position is MD, RN, unit co-ordinator, other.

Thank you for taking time to provide honest feedback. We sincerely want to know your views regarding the strengths of the Clinical Laboratory—Medical Center and opportunities for improvement.

*Survey does not include Blood Bank Services

Figure 2–13. Example of a customer satisfaction survey. Abbreviation: ED, emergency department.

PERFORMANCE IMPROVEMENT MINUTES/REPORTING
Pathology and Clinical Laboratory/Resource Management
(Department/Service/Unit)

Key Function(s): CC, TX, Planning/Providing Care, PI

Dimension(s) Efficacy, Appropriateness, Effectiveness, Continuity, Safety, Efficiency, Respect, Caring

Measure/Issue: Monitor quality of blood specimen collections from redesign areas

In what way does your activity impact cost (quantity if possible)? Cost impact reflected in repeat venipunctures and repeat/redo laboratory work

Sample size   Total # reviewed 11,521   Denominator_____

Patient/Customer: All blood specimen collections performed by staff other than pathology phlebotomy team

Departments/Services/Disciplines: Redesign areas and pathology/medical center

DATE	FINDINGS/TRENDS/EVALUATIONS OF PREVIOUS ACTION	CONCLUSIONS	RECOMMENDATIONS/ACTION ASSIGN RESPONSIBILITY	FOLLOW-UP DATE
DEC. 1995	In December 1995, 11,521 blood specimen collections were performed by nonlaboratory personnel. During this period 473 specimen recollects were identified for reasons included in the weekly reports. The 4 major reasons flagged for recollects were 1) Hemolysis 2) Clotted 3) Underfilled 4) Verify Please note that the number of misidentified specimens (unlabeled and mislabeled) is significant. Issues continue to be addressed with the unit supervisors by Laboratory Resource Management Committee, through the use of CQI monitors.	In December 1995, recollect specimen collections were at 4.11% of total collections exceeding the goal of less than or equal to 3%. This reflects a decrease from 4.43% in November 1995. Please note that 1 day of recollect data was incomplete. This would be reflected in the number of recollects but would not affect the total number of collections.	Nursing services has hired additional phlebotomy support for early AM collections at East and Medical Center.	

Figure 2–14. Example of performance improvement minutes. Abbreviations: CC, continuum of care; Tx, care of patients; EC, entrance complaint; PI, improvement of organization performance.

PERFORMANCE IMPROVEMENT MINUTES/REPORTING
Pathology and Clinical Laboratory/Resource Management
(Department/Service/Unit)

Key Function(s): CC, TX, Planning/Providing Care, IM, PI   Dimension(s) Appropriateness, Efficacy, Effectiveness, Continuity, Timeliness,

Measure/Issue: Identification and intervention of redundant orders and incorrect test orders

In what way does your activity impact cost (quantity if possible)? Approximate savings of $25,000–30,000/month

Sample size   Total # reviewed_____   Denominator_____

Patient/Customer: All MC/Inpatients/ED/OPD/OBSV

Departments/Services/Disciplines: Clinical Laboratory — Medical Center

DATE	FINDINGS/TRENDS/EVALUATIONS OF PREVIOUS ACTION	CONCLUSIONS	RECOMMENDATIONS/ACTION ASSIGN RESPONSIBILITY	FOLLOW-UP DATE
DEC. 1995	Identification and intervention of redundant orders and incorrect test orders has always been an expectation of laboratorians. Intervention in overutilization and inappropriate test orders are warranting better documentation, increased staff awareness, and proactive action. This PIP aids in identifying problem areas with redundant orders, commonly misordered or inappropriate laboratory orders, and education opportunities.	In reviewing the Specimen Change Audit Report for the clinical laboratory in December 1995, **laboratorians intervened in saving $35,546.70 on redundant orders and duplicate orders.** This amount reflects a slight decrease compared to November, 1995. It is encouraging that the clinical laboratory is able to intervene in saving this amount of money. Opportunities continue to be available to educate physicians, nurses and unit coordinators on proper test codes/orders. Please note that 2 days of intervention data were incomplete. This would reflect an even greater amount for December 1995.	This continues to broaden the awareness of proactive intervention in all areas of the clinical laboratory.	

Figure 2–15. Example of performance improvement minutes. Abbreviations: CC, continuum of care; Tx, care of patients; IM, internal monitor; PI, improvement of organization performance; MC, medical center; ED, emergency department; OPD, outpatient department, OBSV, observation patients.

PERFORMANCE IMPROVEMENT MINUTES/REPORTING
Pathology and Clinical Laboratory/Resource Management
(Department/Service/Unit)

Key Function(s): CC, TX_____   Dimension(s)_Appropriateness, Efficiency, Effectiveness, Continuity,_
                                                            Timeliness, Efficacy

Measure/Issue:_Identification and intervention of unnecessary urine cultures_____

In what way does your activity impact cost (quantity if possible)?_Approximate savings of $1700-2,000/month_____

Sample size   Total # reviewed_2 week review____   Denominator_____

Patient/Customer:_All MC/Inpatients/ED/OPD/OBSV_____

Departments/Services/Disciplines: Clinical Laboratory - Medical Center/All Service Lines_____

DATE	FINDINGS/TRENDS/EVALUATIONS OF PREVIOUS ACTION	CONCLUSIONS	RECOMMENDATIONS/ACTION ASSIGN RESPONSIBILITY	FOLLOW-UP DATE
DEC. 1995	During the periods of 7/29/95–12/3/95, 2677 urine culture and sensitivities (UR) were ordered. Of that number 584 (21.8%) were screened negative for blood, nitrate, and/or leukocyte esterase and urine cultures were not performed. Four physicians requested cultures be performed regardless of the result of the urine screening. Three cultures showed no growth or non-significant urogenital flora. One culture grew coag negative staphylococcus. No specimens collected in surgery or the Myelosuppression Unit were included in this evaluation. Also, no bloody specimens were included.	Monitoring the urine cultures ordered and the number which were deemed unnecessary based on the screening procedure for blood, nitrate, and/or leukocyte esterase from 7/29–12/3/95 has shown **savings in cost to the laboratory of $10,512.00 and a savings in charges to patients of approximately $42,048.00.** Three of the 4 cultures showed no growth, questioning the necessity of these orders.	Based on the attached data, urine culture orders do not seem to be consistently increasing or decreasing. The laboratory will continue to monitor the ability of screening urines for culture to reliably identify those specimens which require culture, while effectively reducing costs to the laboratory and to patients.	

Figure 2–16. Example of performance improvement minutes. Abbreviations: CC, continuum of care; Tx, care of patients; MC, medical center; ED, emergency department; OPD, outpatient department, OBSV, observation patients.

AAA Repair/Aortic Graft

DRG 110/111   ICD/9 ___

PATIENT CARE GUIDE
Page 1 of 3

Target D/C Date _____

LOS: Expected _____

LOS: HCFA ___ 9.5 days ___

Verified→					
Date or time→					
Time frame→	Pre-Op	OR	POD1 ICU	POD2 Tel	POD3 Tel
ASSESSMENTS & EVALUATIONS	VS Laboratory data Knowledge base Medical history & existing problems	As needed	As needed	As needed Assess bowel function	As needed
CONSULTS	Anesthesia Social work RT	RT	PT	PT RT	PT RT
DIAGNOSTICS	CBC, SMAC, PX, APTT, T&C UA EKG CXR	CBC CCBP	CBC, K^+, creatinine	K^+	K^+
DIET/FLUID BALANCE	Reg. NPO-2400	NPO	NPO	NPO	NPO
ACTIVITY/ SAFETY	Up ad lib	Dangle	Dangle OOB & chair ×3	OOB & chair ×3 Ambulate	OOB & chair Ambulate
EDUCATION	Pre-Op educ. Review critical path				
TREATMENT MODALITIES	Body prep	Monitor ········· AFM (12 hr)·······> Pulse oximetry ······· Salem sump ····>Lo PA line········· Foley········· I&O········· IV fluid as prescribed···· Wound care as directed	BNC Incentive spirometry · Suction ·········	·······>D/C (per MD order) ········· ·······> ······> D/C ······> D/C (per MD order)	·················> ·················> Pulse oximetry spot check PRN ················>D/C ·················> ·················> ·················>
DISCHARGE PLANNING	Assess home eviron. Co-morbidities Formulate D/C plan	Update D/C plan	Update	Update	Update

CRITICAL PATHS DO NOT REPRESENT A STANDARD OF CARE. THEY ARE GUIDELINES FOR CONSIDERATION THAT MAY BE MODIFIED ACCORDING TO THE INDIVIDUAL PATIENT'S NEEDS.

Figure 2–17. Example of patient care guide.

Patient Care Guide

CORONARY STENT

DRG 112   Target LOS   3 days

Date/Init.	*Patient Problem List*	Res./Init.

DISCHARGE PLANNING

CONSULTS Case Mgr. ___ C. Rehab.___	**PHASE I** Entry Criteria: permit signed for PTCA, stent, Rotoblator, atherectomy.	**PHASE II** Entry Criteria: post-angioplasty with stent placement.	**PHASE III** Entry Criteria: sheath removed, bedrest completed, chest pain free (if applicable).	
	Pre-procedure	**Post-procedure—24 hr**	**24–48 hr**	**48–72 hr**
Date & Time >>				
ACTIVITIES	Pre-procedure sedation _____ d/c anticoagulant as ordered _____ Give pt. care teach guide to pt._____ Pre-procedure Coumadin _____ mg	Anticoag d/c'd (target in lab) time_____ initials_____ Sheath out when ACT < 175_____ time_____ initials_____ Extremity S & R D_____ E_____ N_____ d/c tele mon 4 hr post-sheath removal_____ Resume Hep drip 6 h after sheath removal time_____ initials_____ Bed alarms on D_____ E_____ N_____ O$_2$ d/c'd _____ Progress to short stay unit _____ Post-procedure Coumadin_____ mg APTT at therapeutic level D_____ , E _____ , N _____	Amb in room_____ ft. _____ft. _____ft. O$_2$ d/c'd _____ INR value:_____ Post-proc. Coumadin _____ mg	Amb in room_____ ft. _____ft. _____ft. O$_2$ d/c'd _____ INR value:_____ Heparin d/c'd _____ Post-proc. Coumadin _____ mg
MISC.				
OUTCOMES	Stabilization of V/S _____ Absence or relief of: 1. CP_____ 2. SOB_____ 3. Anxiety_____	Stabilization of V/S _____ Absence or relief of: 1. CP_____ 2. SOB_____ 3. Anxiety_____ Hemostasis at sheath site_____ Bedrest for (_____) hr_____ APTT at therapeutic level _____	Stable V/S_____ Performs ADLs w/o CP/SOB _____ Amb. in halls w/o CP/SOB _____ Hemostasis at sheath site_____ APTT at therapeutic level_____	Stable V/S_____ Performs ADLs w/o CP/SOB _____ Amb. in halls w/o CP/SOB _____ Hemostasis at sheath site_____ INR at therapeutic level_____
EDUCATION	Date & Initial: _____ _____ Pt Care Teach Guide P F O 1 2 3 4 _____ _____ Pre-procedure instruct. P F O 1 2 3 4 _____ _____ Disease process P F O 1 2 3 4 _____ _____ Risk factor prevention P F O 1 2 3 4 _____ _____ Diet instruction P F O 1 2 3 4 _____ _____ Report S&S to nurse P F O 1 2 3 4		_____ _____ Site care P F O 1 2 3 4 _____ _____ Medication instruct. P F O 1 2 3 4 _____ _____ D/C instruction P F O 1 2 3 4 _____ _____ Activity prescription P F O 1 2 3 4 _____ _____ Coum teach bk/diary P F O 1 2 3 4 _____ _____ P F O 1 2 3 4	

CRITICAL PATHS DO NOT REPRESENT A STANDARD OF CARE. THEY ARE GUIDELINES FOR CONSIDERATION THAT MAY BE MODIFIED ACCORDING TO THE INDIVIDUAL PATIENT'S NEEDS.

Figure 2–18. Example of patient care guide.

information about patient outcomes and the processes that contributed to them.[26] Because the laboratory is the largest single source of objective data about health status, it is an essential participant in analyzing the effect of process on outcomes.[10]

NEW ROLES AND EXPECTED OUTCOMES

For the institution and the laboratory, the major outcome is improved patient care without unnecessary or wasteful use of scarce resources. More appropriate laboratory testing reduces unnecessary or wasteful uses of laboratory staff, equipment, and supplies, while improving quality. For the CLS, benefits of new roles include an increased awareness of total patient care and a better understanding of the role of the laboratory in reaching cost-effective, high-quality outcomes. On a more personal level, CLSs enjoy the opportunities for increased interest in their work, recognition of their professional expertise and commitment, and, thereby, increased appreciation on the part of administrators and providers of the contribution by CLSs to the value-added patient outcomes so important in the continuing era of managed care.

References

1. Pew Health Professions Commission: Critical challenges: Revitalizing the health professions for the twenty-first century, report 3. San Francisco, UCSF Center for the Health Professions, 1995.
2. Landauer P: Moving toward managed care. Abbott Park, IL, Abbott Diagnostics, 1995.
3. Mennemeyer S, Windelman J: Searching for inaccuracy in laboratory testing using medicare data. JAMA 269:1030–1033, 1993.
4. Wilson I, Cleary P: Linking clinical variables with health related quality of life. JAMA 273:59–65, 1995.
5. Johnson E: Optimizing laboratory systems through reengineering. Adv Med Lab Professionals 7:10–13, 1995.
6. Bernstein L: Outcome management: a key factor that can "make or break" a lab. Adv Med Lab Professionals 8:16–18, 1996.
7. McDonald J, Smith J: Value-added laboratory medicine in an era of managed care. Clin Chem 41:1256–1262, 1995.
8. Harmening D, Castleberry B, Lunz M: Defining roles of MTs and MLTs. Lab Med 26:175–178, 1995.
9. Auxter S: Preserving quality through outcomes assessment. Clin Lab News 22:11, 1996.
10. Guterl G: Managed care seen as a "positive" for American public and the lab. Adv Med Lab Professionals 8:5, 17, 1996.
11. Rabbits D: Delivering diagnostic lab services in rapidly changing times: A commentary. Clin Lab Sci 10:102–105, 1997.
12. Wilde M: Competition force behind managed care. Adv Med Lab Professionals 8:5, 34, 1996.
13. Chapman B: Reducing lab test use. CAP Today 9:20–28, 1995.
14. Wong E: Improving laboratory testing: Can we get physicians to focus on outcome? Clin Chem 41:1241–1247, 1995.
15. Heacock D, Broust RA: A multidisciplinary approach to critical path development: A valuable CQI tool. J Nurs Care Qual 8:38–41, 1994.
16. Lumsdon K: Disease management. Hosp Health Netw 69:34–36, 38, 40–42, 1995.
17. Clare M, Sargent D, Moxley R, et al: Reducing health care delivery costs using clinical paths: A case study on improving hospital profitability. J Health Care Finance 21:48–58, 1995.
18. Wachtel T, O'Sullivan P: Practice guidelines to reduce testing in the hospital. J Gen Intern Med 5:335–341, 1990.
19. Pathology Department, Baptist Memorial Hospital: Position description, laboratory resource management consultant. Memphis, BMH, 1995.
20. Chapman B: Case pathways' "pluses" adding up. CAP Today 10:1,12–22, 1996.
21. Wyatt D, Davis B: 1995 Tennessee laboratory practitioner survey: Report of results and discussion. Memphis, University of Tennessee, Dept. of CLS, 1996.
22. Wyatt D, Davis B: 1994 Report of laboratory manpower survey. Memphis, University of Tennessee, Dept. of CLS, 1994.
23. Luckey L: Personal communication, Oct 15, 1996.
24. Karni K: Personal communication, Feb 20, 1995.
25. Bowie L: Implementing appropriate testing practices: The role of the laboratory in critical pathways. Clin Lab News 23:10–11, 1997.
26. Sokoll L, Li D, Dawson P, et al: Critical pathways: The laboratory's role in coronary artery bypass surgery. Clin Lab News 23:6–7, 1997.
27. Luckey L: The case for new roles: What they are, why they're needed and how everybody wins. Presentation at ASCLS Clinical Laboratory Educators' Conference, Atlanta, February 1996.
28. Scott S: Implementing new roles: Exactly what's involved and what the CLS needs to know and do. Presentation at ASCLS Clinical Laboratory Educators' Conference, Atlanta, February 1996.
29. Weissman D: Roadmaps to improved patient management. Labor Ind Rep IV:10–11, 1995.
30. Hamilton J: Baptist expands cost-control effort. Memphis Commercial Appeal (Business Section). May 11, 1993.
31. Lyon A, Greenway D, Hindmarsh J: A strategy to promote rational clinical chemistry test utilization. Am J Clin Pathol 103:718–724, 1995.
32. Watts N: Reproducibility (precision) in alternate site testing: A clinician's perspective. Arch Pathol Lab Med 119:914–917, 1995.

Consulting as a Professional Role for the Clinical Laboratory Scientist

Diana Mass

The emergence of clinical laboratory scientists as consultants represents a natural evolutionary growth of the clinical laboratory profession adapting to a changing environment. This emerging role is being fostered by two major developments (1) the need to improve laboratory test utilization[1-3] and (2) the extraordinary growth of decentralized testing.[4-6]

The first development is due to the increasing complexity of clinical laboratory science. Many physicians are seeking information and interpretive guidelines necessary to make optimal and cost-effective use of the laboratory. Similarly, rapid advances in clinical laboratory technology and diagnostic methods have made it nearly impossible for physicians and other health care providers to stay abreast of available tests and their implications for diagnosis and treatment. Laboratory consultants are needed to communicate to health care providers about appropriate laboratory utilization, which promotes a better integration of laboratory services into the patient care process.

Fueling this process are the medical necessity guidelines released by the Health Care Financing Administration (HCFA), which prohibits Medicare and Medicaid reimbursement for Part B services not medically necessary or reasonable for the diagnosis and treatment of disease. These requirements are part of an effort by this agency to control laboratory test utilization and thus reduce expenditures.[7] The clinical laboratory scientist is a natural link between the clinical laboratory and other providers or patients on matters of test selection, specimen collection, interpretation of test results in light of specimen quality and sources of interference, and patient education. Laboratory professionals are expected to provide information, solve problems, analyze situations, and implement decisions related to laboratory testing. Chapters 1 and 2 elaborate on this topic.

The second development, the growth of decentralized testing, is primarily the result of various incentives that have caused a shift of a great proportion of diagnostic testing to alternate sites outside of hospitals and private laboratories. Although this testing is often referred to as decentralized testing, a variety of terms—point-of-care, bedside ancillary, near patient testing—have emerged to describe this process within the hospital environment. The decentralized testing phenomenon also refers to the proliferation of physician office laboratories (POLs). Decentralized testing continues to grow in types and numbers of tests because technology has developed less labor-intensive, more compact, and less expensive equipment as well as reliable diagnostic kits that offer a wide range of testing. At these sites physicians and other health care providers require advice and instruction on clinical laboratory practice and management.[8, 9]

Accelerating the acceptance and legitimization of clinical laboratory consultants in decentralized sites is the federal regulatory authority of the Clinical Laboratories Improvement Act of 1988 (CLIA '88). CLIA '88 specifies the position of a "technical consultant" who is responsible for the technical and scientific oversight of laboratory testing in CLIA-defined moderate complexity laboratories. The specific responsibilities and qualifications of a technical consultant are listed in Box 3–1 and 3–2.[10] Many clinical laboratory scientists have the appropriate education and experience to fulfill these duties; however, if the evolutionary step toward consultation practice is to succeed, new concepts and new roles must be developed.

CONSULTATION PROCESS AND ROLES

Consultants are individuals with recognized expertise who are asked by a client to apply their knowledge and

---

Box 3–1. CLIA '88 Technical Consultant Responsibilities for Moderate Complexity Laboratory

- Selecting test methods
- Verifying test procedures (precision and accuracy)
- Enrolling and participating in a Department of Health and Human Services approved proficiency testing program
- Establishing a quality control program
- Resolving technical problems and ensuring that remedial actions are taken
- Ensuring that patient test results are not reported until all corrective actions have been taken
- Identifying training needs and ensuring that all testing personnel receive training appropriate for services performed
- Evaluating and ensuring the maintenance of staff competency
- Evaluating and documenting the performance of individuals responsible for moderate complexity

---

skills to a given situation. The consultation process involves the following general functions: evaluation of the problem, research, advising, planning, implementation, supervising, training, and evaluation of the result.

Consultants are hired to perform a specific function agreed on in advance. The expectations of both consultant and client are outlined in an initial letter of agreement or contract. After the consultant delivers a final report, which includes recommendations, the relationship usually terminates. However, in many instances, the consultant is retained to implement a plan of action.[11]

Consulting is aimed at helping a person or a group deal with confrontation of problems and efforts to change.

Box 3–2. CLIA '88 Technical Consultant Qualifications for Moderate Complexity Laboratory

- MD, DO, or DPM degree, and certified in anatomic or clinical pathology by ABP, AOBP, or equivalent qualifications
- MD, DO, or DPM degree, and 1 yr laboratory training/experience in the designated specialty/subspecialty of responsibility
- Doctorate in medical technology or chemical, physical, biologic, or clinical laboratory science and 1 yr laboratory training/experience in the designated specialty/subspecialty of responsibility
- Master's degree in medical technology or chemical, physical, biologic, or clinical laboratory science and 1 yr laboratory training/experience in the designated specialty/subspecialty of responsibility
- Bachelor's degree in medical technology or chemical, physical, biologic, or clinical laboratory science and 2 yr laboratory training/experience in the designated specialty/subspecialty of responsibility

---

Change is the operative word, because consultants deal primarily with the effect of change on an organization and on its personnel. Effective consultation requires that change occur. In this capacity, consultants act as change agents and must consciously create an environment where change choices occur.[12] For change to occur, the consultation service undertakes the following three major tasks:

- Assessing the environment, including the setting, the personnel, and the customers it serves
- Evaluating the individuals who will perform the job so that the required tools can be made available to them
- Teaching the individuals how to use the tools effectively

Consulting involves people dealing with people, as opposed to people dealing with machines or mathematical solutions. Successful consultants understand organizational dynamics and the unique functions and boundaries of the consultant role. They are aware of the effects and conflicts of using new technologies. They understand change processes and the powerful influence of individual and organizational resistance. They are clear about the boundaries of their role and they do not become involved in unproductive conflicts over authority and responsibility. They avoid using a narrow set of techniques without evaluating their relevance to a particular situation. The inability to understand these concepts and to apply these skills can produce barriers to positive outcomes, resulting in consultant services that are ineffectual.[13]

A consultant is also a facilitator and a specialist in diagnosing needs and identifying resources. During the consultation process, consultants are confronted with a series of decisions and possible alternatives. The primary value of a consultant lies in the expertise to accurately identify, analyze, and resolve the problems and needs of the client. It is not unusual for the initial problem identified by the client to be overshadowed by a more significant and complex one. Thus, the consultant must thoroughly explore and identify all facets of the problem before attempting to suggest a solution.[14, 15] The following are typical consultative roles that are correlated to problem-solving activities:

- The *fact finder* gathers data and stimulates thinking.
- The *informational expert* provides policy and practice decisions.
- The *advocate* proposes guidelines and persuades, or directs the problem-solving process.
- The *objective observer* raises questions for reflection.
- The *process counselor* observes the problem-solving process and raises issues.
- The *joint problem solver* offers alternatives and participates in decisions.
- The *trainer/educator* trains the client.

A consultant's proper diagnosis of the client's needs and problems determines the appropriate role for a given situation.[16]

CONSULTANT CHARACTERISTICS AND COMPETENCIES

Typically, the health care provider's perception of laboratory testing is very different than that of a clinical laboratory science consultant. Disparities occur in the need for detail, training, and documentation. To achieve compliance, the consultant must display certain personal characteristics. In addition to planning, communicating, and making decisions, successful consultants are innovative, creative, and flexible; able to deal with conflict, confrontation, and ambiguity; able to adapt to unfamiliar circumstances; and capable of high tolerance.[17, 18] In the decentralized testing environment, the consultative process is a personal relationship among people trying to solve a problem. Thus, these personal characteristics are vitally important.

The consultant's potential success to affect the quality of laboratory testing depends on the effectiveness of the consulting practice. A combination of interactive skills make a successful consultant. A consultant must excel in the area of technical knowledge and skill. The successful consultant translates expert knowledge into useful application. The consultant's knowledge must encompass the leading edge of the client's technology; he or she should be aware of emerging technologies and should evaluate their application. If consultants have the best information and

approach, or the most effective solution to a problem, but they do not have the ability to work with the client, then the result is negative and failure is inevitable. Therefore, a consultant must excel in interpersonal skills, the second area, which includes skills in leadership, communication, understanding value structures, conflict resolution, and teamwork.

Good conceptual skills are another important requirement. A consultant must be able to see beyond the immediate problem, relate all of the pieces, and integrate them into a conceptual working whole. Immediate problems are usually symptoms of another, larger problem. All changes in an organization have a ripple effect. If a recommendation is implemented that solves an immediate problem without regard for any other problems, then negative consequences may result, which exceed any potential gain to the client's organization.[13]

Consultative competencies have been identified and grouped according to the knowledge, skills, and attitudes necessary for success. These competencies are identified in Box 3–3.[16] If we examine these competencies and relate

---

Box 3–3. Consultant Competencies

Knowledge Areas

- Thorough grounding in the behavioral sciences
- Thorough foundation in administrative philosophies, policies, and practices of organizational systems and larger social systems
- Knowledge of educational and training methods, especially laboratory methods, problem-solving exercises, and role playing
- Understanding stages in the growth of individuals, groups, organizations, and communities and how social systems function at different stages
- Knowledge of how to design and help a change process
- Knowledge and understanding of human personality, attitude formation, and change
- Knowledge of personal motivations, strengths, weaknesses, and biases
- Understanding the leading philosophical systems as a framework for thought and a foundation for value system

Skill Areas

- Communication skills including listening, observing, identifying, and reporting
- Teaching and persuasive skills including the ability to effectively impart new ideas and insights and to design learning experiences that contribute to growth and change
- Counseling skills to help others reach meaningful decisions on their own
- Ability to form relationships based on trust and to work with a great variety of persons of different backgrounds and personalities; sensitivity to the feelings of others; ability to develop and share charisma

- Ability to work with groups and teams in planning and implementing change; skill in using group dynamics techniques and laboratory training methods
- Ability to utilize a variety of intervention methods and to determine which intervention is most appropriate at a given time
- Skill in designing surveys, interviewing, and other data-collecting methods
- Ability to diagnose problems with a client, to locate sources of help, power, and influence, to understand a client's values and culture, and to determine readiness for change
- Ability to be flexible in dealing with all types of situations
- Skill in using problem-solving techniques and in assisting others in problem solving

Attitude Areas

- Professional: competence, integrity, feeling of responsibility for helping clients cope with their problems
- Maturity: self-confidence, courage to stand by one's views, willingness to take necessary risks, ability to cope with rejection, hostility, and suspicion
- Open-mindedness: honesty, intelligence
- Possession of a humanistic value system: belief in the importance of the individual, belief in technology and efficiency as means and not ends, and trust in people and the democratic process in economic activities

them to a similar set for clinical laboratory sciences, we will find a great disparity. Since the traditional role and environment of the clinical laboratory scientist is remarkably different than that of a consultant, this should be expected. Consulting is based on the behavioral sciences, an area that is not stressed in the highly technical education of the clinical laboratory scientist.[13]

In response to a growing need to recognize qualified CLIA technical consultants, the American Society for Clinical Laboratory Science (formerly known as the American Society for Medical Technology) and the American Society of Clinical Pathologists-Associate Member Section (ASCP-AMS) jointly developed qualifications and competencies for this CLIA personnel position.[19] Refer to Box 3–4.

THE INTERNAL VS. THE EXTERNAL CONSULTANT

Consultants can be categorized as either internal or external. *Internal consultants* are employees of the organization for which they consult, and many clinical laboratory scientists have been serving in this capacity without being formally identified as such. *External consultants* are proprietors of private consulting businesses. These individuals have total responsibility, authority, and accountability for their professional practices.

The Internal Consultant

Internal consultant roles include laboratory scientists who attend patient rounds in teaching hospitals and advise

---

Box 3–4. Competency Statements for Personnel, Financial, Operations, and Quality Management Functions of the Laboratory

- Prepare job descriptions
- Recruit, interview, and select new employees
- Develop a wage and salary administration program
- Develop a system to evaluate and document competency of testing personnel and ensure that the staff maintain their competency to perform test procedures and report test results promptly, accurately, and proficiently
- Develop and present a program to identify training needs and ensure that each individual performing tests receives appropriate training for the type and complexity of the laboratory services performed
- Evaluate and counsel employees
- Develop a test request and reporting system that ensures that patient test results are not reported until all corrective actions have been taken and the test system is functioning properly
- Develop procedures for patient idenitification, specimen collection, handling, and processing
- Prepare work schedules
- Prepare and update procedure manuals
- Develop procedures for calibration, operation, and preventive maintenance of laboratory instruments
- Design and maintain an inventory control system for the laboratory
- Develop system for labeling, handling, and storing reagents and materials
- Evaluate and recommend reference laboratory services
- Design a billing and procedure coding system to obtain appropriate reimbursement
- Evaluate and recommend appropriate test methods, including reagents, supplies, and equipment, that are cost-effective and appropriate for the clinical use of the test results
- Establish reference ranges for tests
- Resolve technical problems and ensure that remedial actions are taken whenever test systems deviate from the laboratory's established performance specifications

- Verify the test procedures performed and establish laboratory test performance characteristics, including the precision and accuracy of each test and test system
- Evaluate and recommend an HHS approved proficiency testing program that is commensurate with the services offered
- Establish a comprehensive laboratory safety program to comply with federal, state, and local regulations
- Develop, implement, and monitor a quality control program that is appropriate for the testing performed and establishes the parameters for acceptable levels of analytic performance and ensures that these levels are maintained throughout the entire testing process, from the initial receipt of the specimen through sample analysis and reporting of test results
- Monitor and evaluate compliance with federal, state, and local regulations
- Establish procedures to evaluate the validity of the test results in terms of reference intervals (normal ranges), reportable ranges, quality control data, analytical system performance, correlations and interpretations with other test data, and clinical significance relative to patient status
- Develop a test priority list that ensures that work load is arranged to optimize patient care
- Evaluate and organize workflow to ensure maximum efficiency
- Design a system to constantly monitor process improvement using continuous quality improvement or total quality improvement or total quality management techniques

physicians on the selection of laboratory tests, or those who work for reference laboratories as sales or client representatives and advise physicians on proper screening methods with appropriate reflex (follow-up) testing. The internal consultant role is one that usually does not require the establishment of a formal consultant-client relationship each time service is provided. When clinical laboratory scientists who are internal consultants earn the respect of their colleagues in the organization, they often become essential participants on the health care team.

The consultant within the hospital environment can function in a variety of ways to improve patient care and to enhance the efficiency of the facility. One important activity that should be increased is the clinical laboratory scientist's involvement in interpreting and integrating laboratory data in the management of the patient's condition. Too often the role of the laboratory has been perceived to begin with receipt of a specimen and end with reporting of a result. Refer to Box 3–5 for an example of a position description for an internal consultant.

Laboratory professionals should be involved in ordering tests. What test will provide the most information? What type of specimen should be obtained? Under what conditions, when, and how often should the specimen be collected? Involvement in discussions with physicians about the patient's situation could avoid delays and inadequate or inappropriate samples, reduce patient trauma from unnecessary venipunctures, and improve the cost-effectiveness of patient care.

The laboratory's responsibility does not end when an accurate test value is obtained. The clinical laboratory scientist must ensure that the physician, nurse, therapist, pharmacist, or other health care provider understands the *meaning* of the results. The care these persons give depends on such understanding. Whether the test results are inconclusive or appropriate, subsequent steps are indicated; the laboratory scientist should discuss these steps with the physician or follow-up with institutionally sanctioned protocols. Refer to Chapter 2 for a detailed discussion of consultation activities of clinical laboratory scientists within an institutional setting.

The laboratory professional is qualified to serve as a consultant to a variety of departments within the institution, such as risk management, infection control, patient relations, respiratory care, and nuclear medicine. Assuming this consultative role, however, means leaving the laboratory and becoming involved in general institutional affairs. It means volunteering for additional responsibility. A role that has given many laboratory scientists new opportunities for professional growth has been as the CLIA designated technical consultant in hospital decentralized testing.

The External Consultant

An external consultant has a private consulting business or at least does not work in the client's organization. External consultants are hired to perform a specific function agreed on in advance. An example is a clinical laboratory consultant who has a contract to advise a physician group on the selection of an instrument or the Current Procedural Terminology (CPT) code for reimbursement. Generally,

---

Box 3–5. Sample Position Description: Internal Consultant

Position title: Clinical Laboratory Consultant

Qualifications: Bachelor's degree in clinical laboratory science, certification plus appropriate advanced degree

Skills and Experience: Good communication and interpersonal skills, 3 years of experience in clinical laboratory science

General Responsibilities

The individual fulfilling this role will be responsible for providing information concerning the laboratory service to physicians, nurses, therapists, other health care providers, and patients. This information may include ordering specific tests, interpreting test results, correlating test data from various sections of the laboratory, preparing patients for testing, performing appropriate follow-up procedures, and describing expected results following therapy. Information will also be technical, such as the time needed to perform specific tests and the nature of the specimens required. The position also carries responsibility for follow-up of problems associated with venipuncture and other specimen collection techniques.

Specific Duties

1. Daily patient rounds to respond to questions raised during phlebotomy
2. Participation in grand rounds
3. Responding to telephone inquiries about laboratory services
4. Monitoring ordering patterns for efficiency and cost-effectiveness
5. Working with human resources department to provide educational programs for patients and other health care professionals
6. Working with risk management department to identify, prevent, or solve problems related to the laboratory
7. Communicating with the originating site when inappropriate specimens are received in the laboratory
8. Providing information to laboratory personnel on changes in practice, trends, and new methods
9. Other communication as necessary to ensure maximally efficient use of the laboratory service

---

when the consultation has been completed, the consultant has no further ties to the client or the client's organization.

The clinical laboratory scientist who becomes an external consultant has, in effect, started a business. Just as in any other business venture, the consultant must recognize legal limits of liability and function competently within those limits. The possibility of incorporation should be investigated. Some amount of capital will be needed to purchase liability (malpractice) insurance, business cards, marketing materials, office equipment and supplies, and a telephone answering machine or service. The clinical laboratory scientist starting a consulting business might find it helpful to take advantage of some of the many books and workshops available to assist individuals who wish to start a small business.

Consultation outside of the hospital or decentralized laboratory is a growing opportunity for laboratory practitioners. Many institutions, organizations, industrial firms, and insurance companies require the information that can be provided by a laboratory scientist.

DECENTRALIZED TESTING

The Physician Office Laboratory

During the 1980s, economic and regulatory incentives as well as technological innovation in instrumentation and test methodology significantly changed the delivery of laboratory services. The diagnosis-related group (DRG) payment plan for Medicare patients altered the financial position of hospital-based clinical laboratories from an income center to a cost center. Capital for new laboratory instrumentation became a rare commodity, and the laboratory manufacturing industry was forced to look elsewhere for financial gain. At the same time, Congress passed direct billing laws that eliminated the customary practice of a physician's markup of laboratory charges for Medicare patients. If physicians were to profit from Medicare patient laboratory testing, the testing would have to be performed within the physician's practice site.[20, 21] Thus, new incentives were created for the laboratory manufacturing industry to develop instrumentation and less complicated testing methods for a new market—POL. In the ensuing 10 years, these two regulatory changes would forever alter the history and practice of laboratory services and would also play a major role in the development and transformation of the CLIA '88 regulations.

Just as physicians have guarded their role, so has the clinical laboratory community done so with respect to ownership of laboratory testing. Laboratory testing in the physician's office practice has always been a concern; however, there is a good case to be made for testing in this environment—the need for timely, effective, and efficient patient care. The medical evaluation of a patient is expedited when test results are available on-site, allowing for the prompt establishment of treatment plans. Physicians can order further diagnostic studies, if needed, while the specimen is still available. In addition, office testing is convenient for patients. In cases in which patients present with acute symptoms they can be evaluated in the office rather than being referred to a hospital emergency room, which generally results in higher cost and delay in alleviating pain. Also, many patients are anxious as they await the results of laboratory work, and having test results while the patient is in the office, or shortly thereafter, significantly reduces their anxiety. In this light, the consultative role of the laboratory scientist can make a major and positive impact, not only on the patient, but for the total health care delivery system.[8, 22] The growth of POL testing and implementation of CLIA '88, has provided consultants with opportunities to advise physicians on quality assurance measures to meet the standards for laboratory accreditation.

According to 1997 HCFA data,[23] 90,000 out of 160,000 CLIA certified laboratories, or 56%, are located in POLs. Categorized by type of complexity, these POLs are identified as follows:

- Waived provider   39%
- Provider performed microscopy (PPM)   30%
- Moderate   30%
- High   1%

It is predicted that the influx of managed care contracts, which limits in-office laboratory testing, will have a negative impact on these numbers unless physicians are able to negotiate more in-house testing.

CLIA '88 requires the POL to maintain quality control and quality assurance programs, to keep appropriate records, to employ personnel who meet Department of Health and Human Services (DHHS) qualifications, and to participate in DHHS approved proficiency programs.[10] The CLIA technical consultant does not have to be on-site at all times while testing is performed; however, the consultant must be available on-site, by telephone, or by electronic means. Although the laboratory's medical director can qualify for this technical and scientific oversight role, it is unlikely that he or she has been trained to fulfill the role. If POLs are to successfully comply with the CLIA standards, they will require assistance from clinical laboratory consultants.

Clinical laboratory consultants can advise physicians in several ways. First, consultants can help the physician develop specific policies and procedures to ensure accurate results. A consultant's technical expertise can prove invaluable in developing procedure and safety manuals and in designing appropriate documentation for patient results, quality control, instrument maintenance, and problem solving. In addition, evaluations of instruments and test kits may be more cost-effective and better focused under the direction of consultants familiar with the physician's test menu needs and volume, and with the education and skills of the personnel who will perform the testing. Consultants can also play a major role in selecting, evaluating, and training these personnel. Moreover, with continuous changes in clinical laboratory technology, consultants can assist physicians with new methods, reimbursement practices, and regulatory changes. The federal government has emphasized the importance of proficiency testing to ensure quality, and consultants can provide any support needed to perform follow-up assessments, corrective procedures, and training.[8, 22] Clinical laboratory scientists can provide a variety of services for physicians. The range of services usually available and needed is outlined in Box 3–6.[11] Individuals with knowledge and experience in these areas can perform an invaluable service. Another important role and contribution that laboratory consultants can provide is by improving test utilization, which is discussed in Chapters 1 and 2.

Management of Hospital Point-of-Care Testing

Historically, various diagnostic tests have been performed in hospitals by nonlaboratory personnel. Typically, nurses have performed urine dip stick analysis, hematocrit measurements, and blood glucose tests. Perfusionists have

---

Box 3–6. Services Typically Provided by Clinical Laboratory Consultants

LABORATORY DEVELOPMENT

- Evaluate laboratory facility
    Space and design
    Staff needs
- Evaluate product availability
    Instruments
    Reagents/controls/calibrators
    Test/kit systems
    Information systems
- Perform cost analysis
- Implement cost-effective purchasing/leasing
- Perform workflow analysis

TEST SELECTION AND PERFORMANCE

- Advise on in-house test menu
- Analyze test results
- Correlate results with clinical data
- Evaluate discrepancies
- Advise on test utilization and interpretation

PERSONNEL MANAGEMENT

- Write job descriptions
- Evaluate/supervise personnel
- Design/deliver in-service training
- Monitor safety policies

QUALITY ASSURANCE

- Develop/implement procedure manual
- Develop/implement quality control procedures
- Design/implement laboratory record system
- Monitor calibration, maintenance, problem-solving, and repair of instruments
- Evaluate proficiency testing
- Advise on procedure/system changes

REGULATION AND REIMBURSEMENT

- Advise on state/federal regulatory requirements
- Monitor and report on reimbursement policies
- Coordinate inspection/regulatory compliance

CONSULTANT ACTIVITIES AND RESPONSIBILITIES

The wide variety of potential consultant roles for the clinical laboratory scientist makes it difficult to describe a set of activities and responsibilities that apply to all situations; however, the following general areas provide insight into the process of consulting.

Providing Information

The most common responsibility of a consultant is to provide information to clients, and information is often all a client wants. The consultant must understand exactly why certain information is important to the client and how the client wishes to use that information.

Consultants must clearly identify their clients' needs. This exploration may result in the asking of questions that appear impertinent or irrelevant, but they are often neces-

---

Box 3–7. Implementing a Point-of-Care Testing Program

Elements of a Successful Point-of-Care Testing Program

- Designation of an individual, from the laboratory, who is responsible for administering the program
- Establishment of a point-of-care committee representing all affected parties
- Establishment of written policies and procedures
- Establishment of organized training and authorization program
- Implementation of a quality assurance program

Evaluation of Point-of-Care Testing

- Feasibility study (test volume anticipated, personnel number for training, procedure/instrument requirements, compliance expectations, and recommendation by point-of-care committee)
- Administrative approval

Training and Implementation

- Development of trainer(s)
- Development of training program
- Implementation of training program and authorization policies
- Establishment of competency program

Quality Assurance Program

- Written procedure following CLIA '88 requirements
- Quality control program
- Internal proficiency testing by correlation with central laboratory results
- Participation in an approved external proficiency testing (PT) program
- Periodic retraining and reauthorization
- Periodic quality assurance review by the laboratory

---

performed blood gas analyses and potassium measurements; cardiac surgical technicians have performed coagulation tests. Primarily to avoid turf wars, decentralized testing and its quality was often ignored by the hospital's laboratory administration. However, CLIA has forced hospital administrators to address this issue and treat decentralized testing with the same attention to quality that is typical in the clinical laboratory. Hospitals that include all diagnostic testing under one CLIA certificate have put the clinical laboratory in charge of all testing regardless of where it is performed or by whom. Refer to Box 3–7 for a description of the various activities needed to implement a successful point-of-care testing program.

sary to elicit information to meet underlying needs and integrate data for actual problem identification.

Providing information to clients may require surveys, cost studies, feasibility studies, or just using one's expertise and background in the field to provide up-to-date information. Sometimes, however, the actual information the client needs to address differs from the information the consultant is asked to provide. For example, an owner of a POL asked a consultant to solve an instrument problem that was resulting in incorrect laboratory findings. Upon investigation, the consultant found that the problem was a lack of proper personnel training, not technical difficulties with the equipment or reagents.

Often clients only need to make better use of available data to answer questions and solve problems. A consultant who wishes to develop an ongoing relationship with a client will find that helping a client to use available information to solve problems quickly and inexpensively can establish a high level of confidence and trust in the consultant's abilities.

Consultants must remember that they function at the client's pleasure, although not as his or her subordinate. Health care professionals who are consultants often have difficulty stopping work on a problem before an acceptable solution is reached. Although that characteristic is laudable, it is not always appropriate in a consultation. Information gathered and shared may never be used by the client, no matter how accurate and appropriate it may be for solving the problem. The client may determine that the consultation is over just as the consultant is on the verge of acquiring the requested information. The consultant may regard the client as applying the information inappropriately. The consultant has no control over client actions and no responsibility for the consequences. Consultants are responsible for keeping accurate and complete records of their activities and presenting a written report of results and recommendations.

Identifying and Solving Problems

Clients will sometimes approach consultants with a problem they want solved. For example, a laboratory manager may ask a consultant how to restructure the laboratory to adapt to changes in technology, or what are the best ways to decrease staff levels in response to a hospital administration's demand to cut costs. A group of physicians wishing to set up a laboratory in their private practice may engage a laboratory scientist as a consultant to determine what tests would be most effective for them to perform in-house, what space and equipment they will need, and what staff will be necessary to perform the testing.

Seeking solutions to such problems is certainly an appropriate function for a clinical laboratory science consultant; however, it is the consultant's responsibility to determine the overall extent of the problem before attempting to solve it. Relevant questions to ask include the following:

- What attempts have been made to solve the problem? With what results?
- Does the client have a solution in mind that has not been tried?
- Are any related aspects of the client's business not going well?

- Who besides the client must accept the solution to the problem for it to be implemented?
- Does the client have any predetermined limitations, such as space use or amount of money available?
- Do solutions exist that you know will not be implemented?

At the beginning of the consultation process it is wise to work with the problem as it has been defined by the client. At the same time, the consultant should look for underlying issues that might shed light on related factors or subjects that may be uncomfortable for the client to discuss openly. For example, the need for a group practice to set up its own laboratory may be a desire of one or two of the physicians in the group, whereas the others are satisfied with the service they have been receiving from another laboratory. In this case, any solution recommended by the consultant that addresses the original question of setting up a laboratory will meet opposition from some of the physicians in the practice. A feasibility study of the costs and benefits of developing an in-house clinical laboratory might be a more appropriate activity for initially addressing the problem. Depending on the results of the feasibility study and their acceptance, the consultation may continue or end. This reshaping can emerge gracefully if the consultant is sensitive to underlying issues and skillful in communicating with the client.

The most valuable consultant is one who can determine the exact nature of a client's problem while being sensitive to the client's comfort. The process of having an "outsider" come into the organization to diagnose the nature of a problem can often create stress between the consultant, including the consultant's staff and the client, even though the client has requested the consultation. Including the client and the client's staff in the exploration of the complexities of the problem is helpful, since a client who is actively involved in the process is more likely to discuss personal involvement with issues bearing on the problem and to accept suggestions.

Making Recommendations

A formal consultation usually concludes with a written report summarizing the situation and recommending action. The consultant may also be asked to present an oral report. Written and oral reports should be accurate and concise representations of the information gathered and the analysis of the problem. Recommendations may include alternative plans for action with an explanation of each alternative in terms of projected outcomes, costs, and benefits. In situations in which a consultation consists of only a short discussion with a client and the provision of information without research, the consultant should follow-up with a written report to the client. Written reports protect the consultant from potential misuse of the recommendations and provide the client with a written record for business and tax purposes. Even when consultations are provided informally and no charge is made for the service, good business practice dictates that a written report be prepared for the client.

If the consultant's recommendations are to be viewed as being credible and having much chance of being implemented, the recommendations must be stated in such a way as to demonstrate an in-depth knowledge of the problem and a sensitivity to the client's environment and constraints. All recommendations must be tailored to the client's specific ability to carry them out. A consistent, logical sequence of steps to solve a problem in one environment may not work in another. Situations occur in which strong and unpopular recommendations must be made to ensure quality performance and improved patient care. Consultants should not skirt around the issue when these situations arise, or they will jeopardize any credibility that has been established with the client. If the client has been actively involved in the consulting process, the resulting recommendations are more likely to be implemented. Clients should not receive a surprise at the final report, particularly if it is a surprise they are not going to like.

Assisting With Implementation

A consultant may be asked to assist a client in implementing the recommended changes. Participation in the implementation of change represents a modification of the relationship between the client and the consultant. Considerable debate surrounds the appropriateness of a management role for the consultant, and if there already is a manager in the organization, the potential for real conflict exists.

The extent of collaboration between client and consultant during consultation may set the tone for the continuation of the engagement into the implementation phase. If there was not a collaborative relationship during the consultation, then the client may only want to use the consultant's findings to implement unpopular decisions. However, if active collaboration was part of the consultation, then continuation into the implementation phase may be a natural progression for the consultant. The consultant knows better than anyone else how the recommendations were meant to be implemented and may bring new ways of problem-solving and innovation into the work setting.

CONSULTING WITHIN ETHICAL AND LEGAL BOUNDARIES

One of the major dangers inherent in the consultative process is the possibility of going beyond one's abilities or the limit of one's legal and ethical boundaries. Care must be taken to ensure that no harm is caused through advice provided by a consultant. At the same time, the consultant should not be limited by tradition and past practice or constrained by fear.

The scope of practice for some health care professionals is embodied within legal practice acts established by state governments. In the absence of such acts for laboratory personnel in most states, the practitioner must rely on a code of ethics[24] and the generally acknowledged scope of practice. The body of knowledge that has been delineated for the profession also represents an acceptable basis for establishing professional boundaries. Establishing the boundaries of one's expertise without infringing on the professional rights and responsibilities of others is perhaps one of the most difficult tasks of the consultant. In this arena there is no substitute for experience.

References

1. Barr JT: Clinical laboratory utilization: The role of the clinical laboratory scientist. *In* Davis BG, Bishop ML, Mass D (eds): Clinical Laboratory Science: Strategies for Practice. Philadelphia, JB Lippincott, 1989.
2. Finn AF Jr, Valenstein PN, Burk MD: Alteration of physician's orders by non-physicians. JAMA 259:2549, 1988.
3. Mass D: CLIA '88: Look for silver lining. Adv Med Lab Prof 4:4(1), 1992.
4. Check WA: How point-of-care is playing out. Coll Am Pathol 7:1(5), 1993.
5. Krienitz D, James L: How accelerated regulation will affect point-of-care testing. Med Lab Obs (special issue) 23:47–51, 1991.
6. Rock RC: Why testing is being moved to the site of patient care. Med Lab Obs (special issue) 23:2–5.
7. Auxter S: What to expect from HCFA's medical necessity policy. Clin Lab News 22:1–3, 1966.
8. Mass D: Laboratorians as consultants to physicians and POLs. Test Trends, vol 4, no. 2, 1990.
9. Mass D: Medical technologists of the future: New practice, new service, new functions. Lab Med 24:402–406, 1993.
10. Final regulations: Clinical Laboratory Improvement Amendments of 1988. Federal Register February 1992.
11. Mass D: Consulting in physician office laboratories. *In* Snyder JR, Wilkinson DS (eds): Management in Laboratory Medicine. ed 3. Philadelphia, JB Lippincott, 1997.
12. Ellis J, Helbig S: The Health Care Consultant as a Change Agent. Chicago, American Medical Record Association, 1981.
13. Mass D: The clinical laboratory scientist's transition to consulting. *In* Crowley JR (ed): A Manual for the Clinical Laboratory Scientist Consultant. The American Society for Medical Technology, 1988, pp 1–16.
14. Gallessich J: The Profession and Practice of Consultation. San Francisco, Jossey-Bass, 1982, pp 1–85.
15. Turner A: Consulting is more than giving advice. Harvard Bus Rev. Sept/Oct:120–129, 1982.
16. Lippitt G, Lippitt R: The Consulting Process in Action. La Jolla, University Associates, 1978.
17. Kelley RE: Consulting. New York, Charles Scribner & Sons, 1986, pp 1–40.
18. Meredith GG, Nelson RE, Neck PA: The Practice of Entrepreneurship. Geneva, Switzerland, International Labour Organization, 1982, pp 1–36.
19. Headley D: POL Forum: CLIA '88 regulations provide a new opportunity for technologists, Lab Med 24:46–48, 1993.
20. Prospective Payment for Inpatient Hospital Services; Social Security Amendments of 1983. Pub L No. 98–369, Title VI, Section 1886(d), April 1983.
21. Deficit Reduction Act of 1984: The Medicare and Medicaid Budget Reconciliation Amendments of 1984. Pub L No. 98–369, Title III, Division B, July 1984.
22. Crowley JR, Oliver JS: The physician office laboratory. *In* Davis BG, Bishop ML, Mass D (eds): Clinical Laboratory Science: Strategies for Practice. Philadelphia, JB Lippincott, 1989.
23. Health Care Financing Administration: Update on CLIA, Clinical Laboratory Improvement Amendment Advisory Committee Meeting, January 29, 1998. Atlanta, Centers for Disease Control and Prevention, 1998.
24. ASCLS House of Delegates: Consultant code of ethics. Clin Lab Sci 10:61, 1997.

Part II

Clinical Disorders

Chapter 4

Myocardial Infarction and Atherosclerotic Heart Disease

Bethany W. Hurtuk

ETIOLOGY AND PATHOPHYSIOLOGY

According to statistics available from the Centers for Disease Control and Prevention, about 500,000 Americans die from acute myocardial infarction (AMI) each year.[1] An infarct is a permanently damaged area of tissue, and in the majority of cases an AMI is the result of reduced blood supply, caused by atherosclerosis, to some area of myocardial tissue. Atherosclerosis is the deposition of lipids in blood vessels that results in narrowing of the lumina. It is believed to be a lifelong process beginning with the "fatty streak" found in the aorta of all infants by the age of 1 year and the coronary arteries by age 10 years. The fatty streak is a lipid-rich lesion that can enlarge into an atheroma or plaque. Many atheromas eventually undergo calcification, ulceration, thrombus formation, and aneurysmal dilation.

The aorta is the most common site for atherosclerotic plaque, followed by other major arteries. Elderly populations have more fibrous material in plaques, with marked calcification of vessels. Plaque formation is a complex process involving circulating lipoproteins, smooth muscle, macrophages (predominant cell found in the early fatty streaks), cellular enzyme systems, platelets, and endothelium. Hypercholesterolemia leads to changes in the endothelial lining of the vessels and in increased monocyte adherence, increased subendothelial migration, accumulation of lipids to form foam cells, and gradual accumulation of smooth muscle to form fatty streaks. At some sites, endothelial cells may separate, exposing foam cells, which in some cases may interact with platelets to form mural thrombi. Such interactions appear to lead to relatively rapid smooth-muscle proliferation.

Biochemically, the atherosclerotic plaques are associated with a predominant lipid fraction, the low-density lipoprotein (LDL). The cholesterol in the LDL fraction is blocked from reesterification, and localized cellular removal does not occur. The lipids deposited in the atherogenic lesions are not easily removable by normal cellular clearing mechanisms, and they begin to accumulate. By some unknown mechanism, the high-density lipoprotein (HDL) appears to retard this atherosclerotic process.

In addition to AMI caused by atherosclerosis alone, some sudden event, such as coronary thrombosis, may unfavorably alter the already precarious balance between myocardial oxygen demand and need in the atherosclerotic

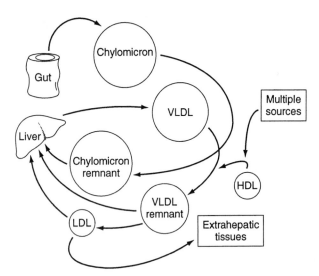

Figure 4–1. Pathways for lipoprotein metabolism.

(Fig. 4–1). Dietary cholesterol combined with chylomicrons enters the body. Chylomicron triglycerides are hydrolyzed, and residual particles, called *chylomicron remnants*, are rapidly removed by the liver. The liver also secretes triglyceride-rich lipoproteins called *very-low-density lipoproteins* (VLDLs), which are degraded into smaller VLDL remnants. The latter can be removed by the liver or converted to LDL. The LDLs are the major cholesterol-carrying lipoproteins in plasma. The major pathway for removal of LDLs is by way of LDL receptors on liver cells. To a lesser extent, LDLs can be cleared by extrahepatic tissues. HDLs may accept cholesterol from extrahepatic tissues and other sources and transfer it to VLDLs and LDLs.

Hypercholesterolemia has been linked to three processes: (1) the synthesis of LDL receptors, which is under feedback regulation responsive to the concentration of cholesterol in hepatic tissue; (2) the ability of hepatocytes to transport LDL receptors to the cell surface; and (3) the increased conversion of VLDLs to LDL, which appears to be modulated by diet.

Diet appears to be a significant factor for a large segment of the population. Certain individuals may be overly sensitive to excess dietary cholesterol, saturated fatty acids, or total calories, and may respond with an unusually marked increase in their LDL values. The sensitivity is the result of a genetic defect in the LDL receptor mechanism, resulting in increased levels of circulating LDL and cholesterol.

CLINICAL MANIFESTATIONS

A patient who experiences AMI may have a history of angina or substernal chest pain or pressure that begins during exposure to cold or a period of exertion and subsides when the activity is stopped. The pain usually lasts a few minutes. As narrowing of the arteries becomes more severe, the pain may occur at rest. Eventually blood supply ceases, resulting in myocardial infarction.

An individual may suffer from AMI and feel nothing or mistake the symptoms for indigestion. About 25% of all AMIs are asymptomatic or associated with atypical symptoms.[3] Most commonly, however, a deep heavy pain in the center of the chest is the presenting complaint of individuals suffering from AMI. The pain may begin when the patient is resting, but if it begins during activity, stopping the activity does not relieve the pain. Pain may also commonly radiate from the chest to the left shoulder and arm, back, or jaw, but rarely to the right arm or shoulder, back, or the face. Difficult breathing, sweating, nausea, vomiting, and a feeling of faintness usually accompany the pain.

A patient suffering from AMI may lose consciousness and stop breathing, requiring cardiopulmonary resuscitation (CPR), or the acute symptoms may pass but leave the patient sweaty and pale. Fifteen percent of AMI victims die within 1 hour of the onset of symptoms,[2] so prompt attention to an individual suspected of AMI is essential.

LABORATORY ANALYSES AND DIAGNOSIS
Lipids as Predictors of Risk

Total cholesterol measurement is the single most important laboratory test for assessing the risk of cardiovascu-

patient. Alternatively, the myocardial supply of oxygen in a patient with insignificant atherosclerosis may be suddenly reduced by a superimposed occlusive thrombosis or vasospasm. Whatever the sequence of events, as the blood flow decreases, the myocardium becomes ischemic and, eventually, necrotic.

At the cellular level, biochemical changes occur when blood flow to the myocardium decreases, and aerobic glucose metabolism is replaced by the Embden-Meyerhoff pathway. Pyruvate, the end product of anaerobic glucose metabolism, is reduced to lactate, which begins to accumulate. To provide the energy needed, myocardial uptake of glucose increases, resulting in increased glycogenolysis, which leads to more pyruvate, which is converted to lactic acid. The result is intracellular acidosis, which decreases glycolysis. Also, free fatty acids cannot be oxidized and, instead, tend to accumulate in the cells.

Loss of the energy necessary to maintain ionic equilibrium of the myocardial cell membrane results in ionic changes within the cell that cause loss of cellular integrity. Potassium is lost and sodium accumulates. With the increased sodium, an influx of chloride occurs, and the cell begins to swell.

Hence, as ischemia progresses, anatomic changes are observable at the cellular level. The mitochondria swell, the myofibrils become stretched, and areas of separation appear in the sarcolemma. The cell membrane is damaged. Ultimately, the infarction occurs, the myocardial cells are no longer intact, and cellular contents appear in general circulation.

The course of atherosclerosis and AMI can be affected by certain risk factors, some of which can be controlled individually. Advanced age definitely increases the chance for atherosclerosis to occur. Women, until the age of about 50 years, are less susceptible than men because of the protective effects of estrogen.[2] Diabetes, high blood pressure, smoking, obesity, and an inactive lifestyle result in increased atherosclerosis.

A significantly increased risk of atherosclerosis can be correlated with high total serum cholesterol values. The relationship between high cholesterol and coronary artery disease can best be understood by the lipoprotein system

Table 4–1. Cholesterol Risk Ranges for Cardiovascular Disease

Risk	Cholesterol (mg/dL)
Normal	<200
Moderate	200–239
High	>239

Data from Expert Panel Report on the National Cholesterol Education Program: Expert Panel on detection, evaluation and treatment of high cholesterol in adults. Arch Intern Med 148:36, 1988.

lar disease (see also Chapter 63). By monitoring total cholesterol levels and minimizing the factors that tend to elevate cholesterol, an individual may reduce his or her risk of cardiovascular disease. Hence, cholesterol screening has recently gained wide popularity.[4] The National Cholesterol Education Program (NCEP), under the auspices of the National Institutes of Health (NIH), has established risk ranges of cholesterol levels for cardiovascular disease (Table 4–1).[5]

Because of the preanalytical factors that affect cholesterol levels (i.e., weight and diet), a single test result is not a sufficient indication of risk.[3] Also, reference values for cholesterol vary with age and sex, so these variables, along with other risk factors, need to be considered when interpreting results.[6]

In addition to total serum level or plasma cholesterol level, several other lipid measurements have been recommended to assess risk associated with premature coronary artery disease. Most clinical laboratories now offer analysis of total cholesterol, total triglycerides, and HDL cholesterol as routine studies, and many can offer LDL measurement with the advent of a direct test. Although maintaining lower cholesterol and triglyceride levels is preferred, individuals with higher HDL cholesterol levels have less atherosclerosis.[7]

Enzymes

Enzymes and other proteins that are present at high concentrations in cardiac cells and are released into general circulation with cellular necrosis are the primary laboratory analytes used to identify AMI. Following AMI, each enzyme that appears in the serum in increased amounts does so for a certain period, depending on the size of the enzyme and its half-life in the blood stream. As the integrity of the cellular membrane deteriorates, smaller enzymes enter the general circulation sooner than larger enzymes. The pattern of serum enzyme elevation aids in both diagnosis and monitoring of the infarction (Fig. 4–2). The serum enzyme levels roughly depend on the extent of the cellular damage. Once the damage has occurred, the rise and eventual decrease in enzyme levels are helpful in monitoring patient recovery and ensuring that another infarction has not occurred. Successful treatment aids recovery and prevents further infarction but does not quicken return of enzyme levels to normal. The specific enzymes that may elevate and at which time intervals they may elevate are outlined in the following discussion.

Creatine Kinase

Creatine kinase (CK) is the first enzyme to show a serum elevation following AMI, with elevation onset 4 to 8 hours after infarction, a peak 12 to 24 hours following infarction, and a duration of 3 to 4 days (see Fig. 4–2). The enzyme may be elevated from 5 to 10 times the normal level. An elevation of more than 8 times the normal level is usually related to a serious infarct with a risk of mortality.

Because CK is present in body tissues other than the heart, several other abnormalities or conditions may have caused the elevation in the level of total CK; therefore, measurement of total CK is not as sensitive an indicator of AMI as is the measurement of the isoenzyme of CK with muscle and brain subunits (CK-MB or CK_2). CK_2 is found primarily in the heart and is responsible for the majority of the increase in total CK level from AMI (see Fig. 5–2). A CK_2 increase of at least 6%, together with other enzyme level increases, is a reliable indication that AMI has occurred. It is believed that the extent of necrosis can be estimated by analyzing the CK_2 time curve.[3] CK_2 is also

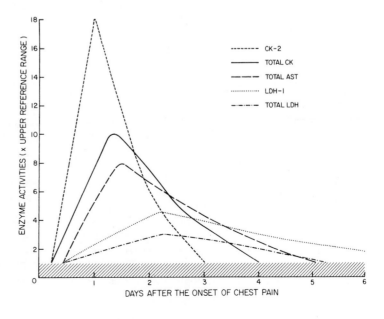

Figure 4–2. Typical pattern of changes in serum enzyme activities following an uncomplicated myocardial infarction. Depending on the location of the infarct and the enzyme assay method in use, these patterns and the magnitude of the peaks can vary quite markedly among patients. The *hatched area* indicates the reference interval of all enzymes. (From Burtis CA, Ashwood ER (eds): Tietz Textbook of Clinical Chemistry, ed 2. Philadelphia, WB Saunders, 1994, p 822.)

the most important enzyme used to assess the progress of thrombolytic therapy following AMI.[8]

Other instances occur in which the level of CK_2 is elevated, but the patient has not suffered AMI. Angina pectoris, coronary insufficiency, coronary bypass surgery, and electrical cardioversion result in elevated CK_2 with no occurrence of AMI.

Aspartate Aminotransferase

The second enzyme to show a serum elevation following AMI is aspartate aminotransferase (AST), which begins to elevate at 8 to 12 hours and peaks at 24 hours following the infarction (see Fig. 4–2). AST is usually elevated 2 to 3 times the reference range at its peak and remains elevated for about 5 days. An AST level more than 5 times the reference range indicates increased risk of mortality.

AST levels should not be used to aid in the diagnosis of myocardial infarction without the other enzyme levels discussed in this chapter, because several other pathologic conditions result in AST elevations, particularly diseases of liver, lung, and skeletal muscle. For this reason AST is less frequently used in diagnostic workups for AMI at the present time.

Lactate Dehydrogenase

Following AMI, lactate dehydrogenase (LD) is the last enzyme to show serum elevation. LD also remains elevated longer than either CK or AST (see Fig. 4–2). The elevation begins 12 to 24 hours after the infarction, peaks at 72 hours at 2 to 3 times the reference range, and remains elevated for about 10 days. Hence, LD measurements are useful for detecting an infarction that occurs more than 4 days before enzyme analysis, after CK and AST levels have already returned to normal. However, because LD is present in several different parts of the body, an increase in total LD is not indicative of AMI.

To aid in the diagnosis of AMI, LD isoenzyme analysis may be performed. After AMI the LD_1 isoenzyme increases, often to a level higher than that of the LD_2 isoenzyme (LD_2 level is usually higher than LD_1), a situation commonly called a "flipped" LD pattern. LD_1 may be elevated with no increase in the total LD concentration. Especially in conjunction with increased CK_2 levels, the "flipped" LD is indicative of AMI. The LD pattern may also be "flipped" in cases of renal cortex infarct, megaloblastic anemia, and intravascular hemolysis, but the CK_2 level is not elevated in these instances.

Because each enzyme elevation occurs within its own characteristic time frame, it is recommended that laboratory analyses for diagnosis of AMI be performed as a cardiac profile. Blood samples should be collected initially and then at specific intervals, usually every 12 hours for the next 48-hour period, and the enzymes that may increase in AMI should be quantitated on each sample. The enzyme analyses that may be performed without delay will depend on the services available in the laboratory. Total AST, CK, and LD levels are usually considered adequate for making immediate decisions regarding patient care. However, the CK_2 level, and later the LD_1 level and LD_1/LD_2 level, provide more sensitive information to confirm or rule out the diagnosis of AMI.

OTHER AMI MARKERS

Myoglobin

Myoglobin, a protein found in muscles, is elevated briefly before CK_2 elevation after myocardial infarction. Hence, myoglobin levels are helpful for early detection of AMI.[9] However, because there are significant amounts of myoglobin in skeletal muscle, the specificity of the analyte is low. If the clinical history is known, the cause of increased myoglobin may be more easily identified.

Troponin

Another marker that is useful within hours after the onset of symptoms is troponin. Both troponin-T and troponin-I have been found to be more specific for cardiac injury than CK_2. Both are present as early in the course of the disease but remain elevated longer. Adams and colleagues[10] found 100% diagnostic sensitivity for troponin-I and 99% diagnostic specificity in 108 patients who underwent either vascular or spinal surgery, 8 of whom had perioperative AMI. Because troponin-T appears to have prognostic value in unstable angina, both markers may be useful in rapidly assessing patient status.[11] This possibility has particular significance in the emergency department as an aid in making hospital admissions decisions and in initiating effective reperfusion therapy.

OTHER RELATED LABORATORY FINDINGS

Even though the analytes discussed in this chapter are the primary laboratory analytes that aid the physician in diagnosing atherosclerosis and AMI, several other laboratory findings are notable. Interest in the correlation between atherosclerosis and plasma concentrations of other analytes has grown. Apolipoprotein A_1, the major HDL protein, and apolipoprotein, the major LDL protein, have been studied. However, according to recent evaluations, measurements of fasting cholesterol, HDL cholesterol, and triglyceride provide as much information as measurement of the apolipoproteins.[13]

Lp(a) lipoprotein, an (a) apolipoprotein attached to an LDL particle, is considered a major risk factor that adds information unobtainable in any other way regarding the effectiveness of cholesterol-lowering medications.[13, 14] Routine Lp(a) measurements are not recommended because of lack of standardization.[13]

Arterial blood gas analyses may also appear abnormal following AMI. *Hypoxemia*, a deficiency of oxygen, is the condition usually found and is caused by poor aeration of the lung bases. Hence, oxygen therapy is provided to minimize myocardial damage at the location of the infarct, and arterial blood gases are frequently analyzed to verify adequate oxygenation.

TREATMENT

Several possible treatments for patients suffering from angina because of atherosclerosis are available. Cessation of smoking and changes in diet and exercise habits can be helpful. Medications are available that either reduce the oxygen demand of the heart or increase the blood supply. Available medications include nitrates, β-blockers, calcium-channel blockers, and aspirin, and may be given individually or in combination.

Two invasive techniques are also used to treat angina. In balloon angioplasty, a deflated balloon is inserted through a major artery to the coronary arteries via a catheter. The balloon is then inflated near a blockage to break it and stretch the artery, thereby increasing blood flow. Coronary artery bypass surgery, an operation in which obstructed or narrowed areas of coronary arteries are bypassed via new conduits, is common and successful. Such surgery provides complete relief from angina in about 70% of patients.[1]

When AMI is suspected, prompt and effective treatment is necessary to minimize the size of the infarct. An electrocardiogram (ECG) is performed to look for changes that are characteristic of AMI. Usual early treatments include intravenous administration of thrombolytic agents or emergency angioplasty to reestablish blood flow to the ischemic myocardium.

One important goal of treatment for AMI is to save the infarcted area by maintaining a balance between supply and demand of oxygen to the myocardium. Appropriate therapy includes relief of pain, rest, sedation, and a quiet atmosphere to lower the heart rate and thus reduce oxygen consumption. In addition, oxygen is usually given to raise the arterial partial pressure of oxygen. Morphine for relief from pain and benzodiazepines for sedation are commonly prescribed. If arrhythmias are present, additional medication such as procainamide, lidocaine, or quinidine is prescribed. In the presence of heart failure diuretics and angiotensin-converting enzyme (ACE) inhibitors are usually administered. For infarcts caused by any occlusive thrombus near an atherosclerotic plaque in a coronary artery, reperfusion therapy as early in the course of the disease as possible, using a thrombolytic agent, such as streptokinase or tissue plasminogen activator (t-PA) is indicated. Successful reperfusion therapy often results in CK_2 and myoglobin levels that are increased above the elevations that result from AMI.[9, 15]

Case Study

A 58-year-old, heavy-set man had been shoveling snow in his driveway. A neighbor noticed the man lying on the ground as though he had fainted or fallen and hit his head. The neighbor called for help and began CPR. The patient was taken to the hospital and admitted.

Questions

1. What is one of the most common disorders that the patient might have suffered, besides a blow to the head?

2. What laboratory test might be done initially to help diagnose the patient's condition?

3. What should the physician do if the laboratory test referred to in question 2 is normal?

Discussion

1. The patient may have suffered a myocardial infarction. Shoveling snow is one of the most strenuous tasks that can be undertaken by someone who is susceptible to a myocardial infarction, because of the cold temperatures as well as the physical exertion. A middle-aged overweight man may have a tendency for atherosclerosis.

2. A CK isoenzyme analysis would be very helpful. Evidence of a cerebral accident might show as an increase in the isoenzyme of creatine kinase with brain subunits (CK-BB), whereas evidence of a myocardial infarction might show as an increase in CK-MB.

3. A cardiac profile should be ordered a few hours after the patient has arrived at the hospital and again 24 hours later. From the repeated testing the physician may observe the typical increases and decreases in enzyme levels following a myocardial infarction.

References

1. Deckelbaum L: Heart attacks and coronary artery disease. *In* Zaret BL, Noser M, Cohen LS (eds): Yale University School of Medicine Heart Book. New York, Hearst Books, 1992, p 133.
2. McGoon MD (ed): Mayo Clinic Heart Book, New York, William Morrow & Co, 1993, p 19.
3. Burtis CA, Ashwood ER (eds): Tietz Textbook of Clinical Chemistry, ed 2. Philadelphia, WB Saunders, 1994, pp 820, 1056.
4. Ng R, Sparks K, Statland B: Performance of the CLA/200 ChemPro lipid analyzer for the measurements of cholesterol, HDL, and triglycerides. Lab Med 22:23, 1991.
5. Expert Panel Report on the National Cholesterol Education Program: Expert panel on detection, evaluation and treatment of high cholesterol in adults. Arch Intern Med 148:36, 1988.
6. Shaikh A: Patterns of cholesterol distribution in the participants of a screening project. Lab Med 22:258, 1991.
7. Waller K, Ward K, Rudmann S: Serum lipids, lipoproteins, and apoliproteins in the healthy elderly. Lab Med 23:109, 1992.
8. Guasco G, Hathorn G: Evaluation of preliminary screening methods for CK-MB isoenzymes used in the diagnosis of acute myocardial infarction. Clin Lab Sci 6:245, 1993.
9. Vaidya H: Myoglobin. Lab Med 23:306, 1992.
10. Adams JE, Sicard G, Allen B, et al: Diagnosis of perioperative myocardial infarction with measurement of cardiac troponin-I. N Engl J Med 330:670–674, 1994.
11. Hamm C, Ravkilde J, Gerhardt W, et al: The prognostic value of serum troponin T in unstable angina. N Engl J Med 327:146–150, 1992.
12. Wu A, Lan D: Metaanalysis in clinical chemistry: Validation of cardiac troponin T as a marker for ischemic heart disease. Clin Chem 41:1228–1233, 1995.
13. Schaefer E, McNamara J: Practice chemistry: Routine diagnostic testing for Apo A-I, Apo-B, Lp(a), and LDL cholesterol in clinical laboratories. Clin Lab Sci 7:205, 1994.
14. Naito H, Kwak Y: Practice chemistry: Lipoprotein(a) as a new biochemical marker for assessment of coronary heart disease risk. Clin Lab Sci 3:308, 1990.
15. Apple F: Creatine kinase-MB. Lab Med 23:298, 1992.

Chapter 5

Infectious Cardiomyopathy

Lauren Roberts

Infectious processes of the heart and the host inflammatory response to the infectious agent can be life-threatening. Infection of the heart results in cardiomyopathy with temporary or permanent effects on the anatomic structure or physiologic function of the heart. Infectious cardiomyopathy can involve the myocardium, pericardium, and/or endocardium. It may be difficult to differentiate one disorder from another because processes are often caused by the same infectious agent and can occur singly or in combination.

The pericardium is a double membranous, fibroserous sac that surrounds the heart and adjacent blood vessels. The inner layer, or *visceral pericardium*, is composed of a single layer of mesothelial cells, and the outer layer, or *parietal pericardium*, is a fibrous sac. The pericardial space lies between these layers and contains a small amount (15 to 50 mL) of fluid. The pericardium has several functions, including maintaining the heart in its fixed anatomic position and optimal shape and minimizing friction between the heart and surrounding tissues.[1] The term *pericarditis*

refers to inflammation of the pericardium. The middle and the thickest layer of the heart, composed of cardiac muscle, is the myocardium. The term *myocarditis* refers to inflammation of the myocardium. In some cardiomyopathies, both the pericardium and myocardium are affected simultaneously, resulting in myopericarditis. The endocardium is a thin, serous lining membrane of the inner surface of the heart. Inflammation of this region is referred to as *endocarditis*.

ETIOLOGY AND PATHOPHYSIOLOGY
Pericarditis

Pericarditis may present as the primary illness, or it may occur in the course of many other syndromes. This inflammatory process can result from many infectious agents, as well as some noninfectious conditions, including therapeutic agents, uremia, malignant diseases, or autoimmune diseases. Pericarditis can be classified both clinically and etiologically. Acute pericarditis is the most common form, and although it occurs in all ages, it occurs most frequently in young adults. It is often associated with pneumonitis and pleural effusions and usually lasts a few weeks. Acute pericarditis can be further classified as serofibrinous or purulent. Serofibrinous pericarditis is usually viral in origin, whereas purulent pericarditis is most often bacterial. Chronic pericarditis lasts for 6 months or longer and is associated with chronic granulomatous infections such as tuberculosis, or with noninfectious causes including trauma, irradiation, or autoimmune diseases.[1, 2] Table 5–1 identifies the infectious and noninfectious causes of pericarditis.

Virtually any microorganism that reaches the myocardium or pericardium is capable of causing pericarditis. Microbial agents can reach the pericardium as an extension of a pulmonary or myocardial infection, through blood stream or lymph dissemination, or through direct implant during surgery or trauma. Individuals with underlying noninfectious pericarditis have an increased susceptibility to hematogenous bacterial pericarditis. The pathogenesis of the disease involves a host inflammatory response to the etiologic agent, resulting in a buildup of serous fluid and an accumulation of cells. The intensity of the inflammatory process is related to the pathogenicity of the microorganism and varies from a small amount of serous fluid with mononuclear cells and fibrinogen to a large bloody effusion containing neutrophils. The inflammatory process interferes

Table 5–1. Infectious and Noninfectious Causes of Pericarditis

Infectious Causes

VIRUSES	BACTERIA
Coxsackievirus	*Staphylococcus aureus*
Echovirus	*Streptococcus pneumoniae*
Influenza virus	*Streptococcus pyogenes*
Adenovirus	*Haemophilus influenzae*
Mumps virus	*Neisseria gonorrhoeae*
Rubeola virus	*Neisseria meningitidis*
Cytomegalovirus	*Salmonella* spp.
Rubella virus	Other enteric gram-negative bacilli
Varicella-zoster virus	Anaerobic bacteria
Epstein-Barr virus	*Nocardia* spp.
	Mycobacterium tuberculosis

FUNGI	PARASITES
Histoplasma capsulatum	*Entamoeba histolytica*
Coccidioides immitis	*Toxoplasma gondii*
Cryptococcus neoformans	*Echinococcus granulosus*
Blastomyces dermatitidis	*Trichinella spiralis*
Candida spp.	*Plasmodium* spp.
Aspergillus spp.	*Trypanosoma cruzi*

CHLAMYDIA	OTHERS
Chlamydia trachomatis	*Rickettsia* spp.
Chlamydia psittaci	*Mycoplasma pneumoniae*

Noninfectious Causes

Acute myocardial infarction	Uremia
Neoplasia	Trauma
Aortic aneurysm	Radiation therapy
Familial Mediterranean fever	Acute rheumatic fever
Collagen vascular diseases	Drug-induced

with blood and lymphatic drainage, and the subsequent outpouring of fluid into the pericardial space results in pericardial effusion. If a sufficient amount of fluid accumulates, blood flow obstruction to the ventricles may result, and cardiac tamponade can occur. This is a serious complication and can be fatal if not treated promptly.[3]

The most common infectious cause of acute serofibrinous pericarditis is a virus, particularly the enteroviruses echovirus and coxsackievirus. Several other viruses have been associated with pericarditis (see Table 5–1). In some cases the viral agent is successfully isolated from the pericardial fluid, or antibody titers become elevated, enabling identification of the etiologic agent. In many situations acute pericarditis has followed another viral illness and is presumed to be caused by the same agent. Under appropriate conditions, pericarditis can follow an upper respiratory tract infection. Predisposing factors for pericarditis include alcohol use, trauma, age, hypertension, fatigue, and other viral infections. If a viral cause cannot be firmly established or excluded, the term *acute idiopathic pericarditis* is applied. Occasionally, nonviral agents cause this infection, including *Mycoplasma pneumoniae* and *Chlamydia* and *Rickettsia* species.

Acute purulent pericarditis is most often bacterial in nature. The pericardium thickens, and a viscid purulent fluid accumulates. The most common organisms responsible for this disease are *Staphylococcus aureus*, *Streptococcus pneumoniae*, *Haemophilus influenzae*, and *Neisseria meningitidis*. The incidence of bacterial pericarditis has decreased in the era of antibiotics, yet the mortality remains high. A large spectrum of bacteria is involved, including gram-negative bacilli and other hospital-acquired organisms. Even with antibiotic therapy, purulent pericarditis has a poor prognosis because it is usually indicative of an extensive infection of the mediastinum and lung. Fungal infections can also produce purulent pericarditis. An increasing number of cases of *Candida* or *Aspergillus* species infections have been reported in the United States, particularly in the immunosuppressed population. Parasitic infections of the pericardium are rare; however, when a hepatic abscess of *Entamoeba histolytica* ruptures through the diaphragm into the pericardium, amebic pericarditis can result. The pericardial fluid in amebic pericarditis is classically described as "anchovy sauce" pus.[4]

Chronic pericarditis is a granulomatous process and is often caused by *Mycobacterium tuberculosis* or by systemic fungi, such as *Coccidioides immitis* or *Histoplasma capsulatum*. In tuberculous pericarditis, the pericardium is infected through lymphatic spread. Tuberculous pericarditis is rare in the United States, but it must be considered as a possible etiologic agent, especially in patients with acquired immunodeficiency syndrome (AIDS). Chronic fungal pericarditis has increased in frequency over the years, particularly in the immunosuppressed population. Systemic fungal infections can complicate cancer chemotherapy. Infection can be widespread, invading the heart as well as the lungs, kidney, brain, and liver. In addition, infections that are typically slowly progressive and chronic in the immunocompetent host can develop in an acute fashion in the immunodeficient host.

Chronic constrictive pericarditis results when the healing of acute or chronic pericarditis is followed by pericardial thickening and fibrosis. The pericardial cavity becomes obliterated with the formation of granular scar tissue, which encases the heart and results in abnormal diastolic filling. Over time, atrophy to the myocardial tissue may decrease systolic function. Chronic constrictive pericarditis can follow tuberculous, bacterial, viral, or fungal pericarditis. It can also occur in noninfectious pericarditis because of neoplastic disease, autoimmune disorders, uremia, and chronic renal failure.[5]

Myocarditis

Myocarditis is defined pathologically as inflammation of the heart. This disease is most often caused by infectious agents, but it may also develop as a hypersensitivity reaction in acute rheumatic fever or as a result of radiation, chemicals, or drugs. The mechanism of pathogenesis involves direct toxicity of the microbe for myocardial cells, indirect toxicity through production of a microbial toxin, or inflammation due to autoimmunity following an infection. The infectious agents involved in myocarditis include the viruses, bacteria (including *Rickettsia*), fungi, and parasites described earlier for pericarditis.

Viruses are the most common infectious cause of myocarditis. In the United States, it is estimated that as many as 50% of cases can be attributed to infection with coxsackie B viruses.[6] Other picornaviruses are also important etiologic agents, and they have been isolated from inflamed myocardium. Laboratory studies demonstrate a strong tropism of these viruses for myocardial cells. Other viral agents implicated in myocarditis include influenza, Epstein-Barr, hepatitis, rubella virus, mumps virus, and cytomegalovirus. Myocarditis is a frequent condition in AIDS patients, and although it can be caused by organisms associated with immunodeficiency, it can also be directly attributed to human immunodeficiency virus.

Bacterial infections of the myocardium are rare, but they can occur during bacteremia. *N. meningitidis, S. aureus, Salmonella* species, and other bacteria have been responsible for this condition. These pathogens are directly toxic to the myocardium and produce lesions similar to those found in other tissues. A complication of endocarditis with *S. aureus* may result in myocardial abscesses. Infection with *Corynebacterium diphtheriae* represents the best example of a toxin-mediated myocarditis. The toxin produces cardiac damage by inhibiting protein synthesis, which leads to a dilated, flabby heart. This is the most common cause of death in diphtheria patients.[7] Lyme carditis occurs in about 10% of patients with *Borrelia burgdorferi* infection.

Disseminated fungal infections have also been involved in myocarditis. Systemic fungi, such as *C. immitis* and *H. capsulatum*, can produce diffuse or focal abscesses in normal hosts. In immunosuppressed patients, opportunistic fungi including *Aspergillus* species, *Candida* species, and *Cryptococcus neoformans* may result in myocarditis.

Chagas' disease, caused by the protozoan parasite *Trypanosoma cruzi*, is the major cause of myocarditis in the endemic areas of Central and South America. Although this infection is not common in the United States, in recent years the number of cases has increased as a result of immigration from endemic areas. *T. cruzi* has a particular tropism for the heart and is found in myocardial cells during the acute phase of illness. The chronic form of this illness results in extensive myocardial fibrosis and chronic inflammation. The inflammatory process is thought to be caused by cellular and humoral immune responses.[8] Other parasitic agents that have resulted in myocarditis include *Toxoplasma gondii, Trichinella spiralis, Schistosoma* species, and *Echinococcus granulosus*.

Endocarditis

Infective endocarditis is caused by microbial invasion of the endothelial lining of the heart. The infection produces vegetative lesions that usually occur on a heart valve. The descriptive terms for this disease, *acute* and *subacute bacterial endocarditis*, are based on the clinical course established in the era before antibiotics. Acute bacterial endocarditis (ABE) has an abrupt onset, and the infection has been present for less than 2 weeks when the diagnosis is made. Subacute bacterial endocarditis (SBE) has an insidious onset, with symptoms evolving over weeks to months. In addition to the duration of illness, these disease types have further important distinctions. ABE is often caused by more virulent pathogens that can attack normal healthy valves, whereas SBE is usually caused by less virulent organisms and occurs on previously damaged valves. Although these classifications are still useful terms for this disease, the most current classification is based on the anatomic site of infection and the infected population. Hence, infective endocarditis is now classified into native

valve endocarditis, prosthetic valve endocarditis (PVE), and endocarditis in intravenous (IV) drug abusers.[9]

The pathophysiology of infective endocarditis involves the presence of sterile thrombotic vegetations consisting of platelets and fibrin on the endocardium. These sterile thrombotic lesions usually form over areas of trauma to the endothelium and are known as nonbacterial thrombotic endocarditis (NBTE). Aggregates of platelets can occur on normal valves but are most often found on surfaces of valves damaged by congenital or rheumatic disease. Infective endocarditis develops when bacteremia allows microorganisms to attach to the sticky platelet-fibrin surface of the sterile vegetation and begin to multiply. The vegetation provides an ideal growth surface for the organism because essential nutrients can diffuse from the blood. The presence of the bacteria enhances further thrombosis, and as additional layers of fibrin deposit around the bacteria, the vegetations begin to enlarge, and phagocytes are not able to penetrate. The organisms gain entrance to the blood during transient bacteremias that occur during dental extraction, periodontal treatment, or invasive gastrointestinal, urologic, or gynecologic procedures.

Although endocarditis can occur in all valves, it most often occurs in high-pressure areas, on the downstream side of blood flow. Thus the left side of the heart is involved more often than the right side. In drug users, however, the incidence of right-sided valvular infection is much higher than in other patients with endocarditis. This may be due to an unusually high inoculum of organisms and prior damage to the tricuspid valve from the injected drugs or the impurities in the drugs.

Although the range of bacteria that can cause infectious endocarditis is wide, the majority of cases are caused by a few species (Table 5–2). The causative agents in non–drug abuser native valve endocarditis include streptococci (50% to 75%), staphylococci (25%), and enterococci (10%). The majority of the streptococci are α-hemolytic or viridans streptococci, which are normal inhabitants of the oropharynx. These organisms gain access to the blood during dental manipulations, and in most hosts they have a very low virulence; however, they are capable of settling on damaged valves. Enterococci are normal inhabitants of the

Table 5–2. **Etiologic Agents of Endocarditis**

Category of Endocarditis	Common Agents
Native valve	Viridans streptococci
	Streptococcus bovis
	Enterococcus faecalis
	Staphylococcus aureus
Prosthetic valve	*Staphylococcus epidermidis*
	Staphylococcus aureus
	Enterobacteriaceae
	Pseudomonas aeruginosa
	Candida spp.
	Diphtheroid bacilli
Intravenous drug abuse	*Staphylococcus aureus*
	Streptococcus spp.
	Enterococcus spp.
	Pseudomonas aeruginosa
	Enterobacteriaceae
	Candida spp.
	Other fungi

gastrointestinal tract, and they can attack normal or damaged valves. Enterococcal endocarditis is usually associated with patients who have had recent genitourinary tract manipulation or trauma. It is more common in men older than 60 years, or women younger than 40 years. *S. aureus* can attack normal or damaged valves and produce acute endocarditis with fulminant bacteremia. *S. epidermidis* is less common, and it usually infects abnormal valves. Almost any other species of bacteria can also be involved in native valve endocarditis. Spirochetes, rickettsiae, and chlamydiae are rarely involved. Fungi are not usually seen in native valve endocarditis unless the patient is an IV drug abuser. Other predisposing factors for fungemia can produce endocarditis in patients with IV catheters.

Approximately 10 to 20% of infective endocarditis cases involve prosthetic valves. PVE is categorized as early onset, when the symptoms develop within 60 days of surgery, or late onset, when they occur after 60 days. Early PVE indicates contamination during the perioperative period, and *S. epidermidis* is the most common organism involved. Late PVE is thought to reflect seeding of the valve by transient bacteremia, and viridans streptococci are the most common organisms involved.

IV drug users are at increased risk of infective endocarditis. Bacteremia develops either from direct injection of the organism or from a local infection at the injection site. The skin of the addict is the most frequent source of the organism, and thus *S. aureus* accounts for 60% of cases. Streptococci and enterococci account for 20% of cases, and gram-negative bacilli, primarily *Pseudomonas* species and *Serratia* species, constitute 10% of cases. The remaining 10% are due to fungi, primarily *Candida* species.[10]

Rheumatic Heart Disease

Acute rheumatic fever is one of the leading causes of cardiovascular disease in the world. Rheumatic fever is an inflammatory disease that can occur as a sequela to group A streptococcal pharyngitis and can affect the heart, joints, central nervous system, skin, and subcutaneous tissues. Damage to the heart results in rheumatic valvular heart disease (RVHD), the most serious manifestation of rheumatic fever. All layers of the heart may be involved in RVHD. The term *pancarditis* is used to describe inflammation involving the pericardium, myocardium, and endocardium. The classic inflammatory lesion that is pathognomonic for rheumatic fever is known as the myocardial Aschoff's body, a submiliary granuloma.[11]

Rheumatic fever most commonly occurs in children between the ages of 5 to 15 years. This reflects the age group with the greatest incidence of streptococcal throat infection. Epidemiologic studies reveal that environmental factors play a role in the development of this disease. Outbreaks of rheumatic fever are usually more prevalent in populations with crowded living conditions, poor nutrition, and limited medical care. The incidence of rheumatic fever in the United States decreased significantly following World War II, because of antimicrobial therapy availability and improved economic living conditions. In developing countries, however, rheumatic fever is still a major cause of death. In the mid-1980s the United States experienced a resurgence of rheumatic fever in separate geographic locations among children of high socioeconomic status who have ready access to medical care. These outbreaks were not typical of previous disease patterns, resulting in a renewed interest in this disease.

A clear relationship is evident between throat infections with group A streptococci and rheumatic fever, yet the exact pathogenic mechanism is still unclear. Numerous hypotheses have been proposed, but the lack of an experimental animal model for this disease has made laboratory studies difficult. The most widely accepted theory involves an abnormal host immunologic response to the antigens of group A streptococci. The group-specific carbohydrate of the bacterial cell wall is similar to glycoprotein found in human heart valves. On exposure to group A streptococci during infection, the host develops antibodies against the organism, which also react against the host's own tissue in an autoimmune-like response. Eventually this results in inflammation of the heart valves and leads to RVHD.[11, 12] Immunologic tests demonstrate that patients with rheumatic fever produce higher titers of streptococcal antibodies than patients with streptococcal infections who do not develop rheumatic fever. Genetic variables may also be an important component in the development of this disease. Rheumatic fever tends to be found in multiple members of some families, but this genetic predisposition is not fully understood. Recent studies have revealed a lymphocytic surface marker shown to be present in the majority of patients with rheumatic fever when compared to controls.[12] Further research needs to be performed to determine if this marker can be useful to detect susceptible individuals.

CLINICAL MANIFESTATIONS

Pericarditis

The signs and symptoms of infectious pericarditis are similar regardless of the etiologic agent. Purulent pericarditis, however, is usually a more dramatic presentation. The most frequent complaint in acute pericarditis is chest pain, although the quality and location varies. The pain is usually in the precordial area and radiates to the trapezius ridge and the neck, but it can be in the epigastric area and resemble an acute abdomen. The pain is described as sharp, dull, aching, and increases during inspiration and recumbency, but the pain improves when the patient is sitting up and leaning forward. Other symptoms in acute viral pericarditis include fever, dyspnea, nonproductive cough, fatigue, and malaise. Some patients report a recent respiratory or gastrointestinal illness. Fever, chills, and night sweats are more prominent in bacterial pericarditis.[13] Although chest pain is the primary complaint in pericarditis, it may be mild or absent in up to 50% of patients, especially in uremic and tuberculous pericarditis.[14]

If the patient experiences a rapid accumulation of pericardial fluid, cardiac tamponade may occur. Because of restricted cardiac filling, the patient will experience severe dyspnea with coughing and distended neck veins. A large quantity of fluid will produce a sensation of fullness or heaviness in the chest. Edema in the feet or ankles may appear if congestive heart failure or cardiac tamponade develop.

One of the most helpful signs in diagnosing pericarditis

is the pericardial friction rub. This is a scratching, sandpaper-like sound detected with the stethoscope that originates from the grating of the epicardial and pericardial surfaces. The sound has been described as the squeak of leather on a new saddle under a rider.[13]

Myocarditis

The clinical manifestations of myocarditis are variable and range from asymptomatic, in focal inflammation, to fulminant congestive heart failure, in diffuse myocarditis. In many cases the clinical manifestations are vague and nonspecific, and the condition is detected because of electrocardiographic abnormalities. Infants and young children have a more fulminant course beginning with fever, tachycardia, and difficulty feeding. Rapid progression and cardiac failure may ensue within a few days of the illness. Adults have a slower progression with an initial viral infection in the upper respiratory tract. Myocardial involvement begins 1 to 2 weeks after the initial infection, and the patient experiences fever, malaise, fatigue, dyspnea, and tachycardia.[15] Chest pain may appear in some patients, especially if pericarditis is also present. Some patients present with symptoms similar to those of a myocardial infarction.

Endocarditis

Symptoms of infectious endocarditis usually occur 2 weeks following the initiating bacteremia. Nonspecific symptoms include malaise, fatigue, night sweats, loss of appetite, and weight loss. Fever is a prominent feature of this disease and is low grade, except in acute disease. Many patients experience musculoskeletal symptoms of arthritis and arthralgia. Patients with acute endocarditis experience more rapid and severe symptoms of high fevers, chills, and prostration, often leading to hospitalization within a few days. In subacute endocarditis, the symptoms develop gradually. Patients often do not seek medical attention immediately because they believe they have the flu.

Numerous physical findings are associated with infectious endocarditis. Heart murmurs are present in almost all patients, thus infective endocarditis should be suspected in all patients with fever, anemia, and heart murmur. Splenomegaly is another common feature and is found in about one third of patients. Intravascular lesions are demonstrated by petechiae on the skin, conjunctiva, and oral mucosa and splinter hemorrhages under the nails. Septic emboli can result in Janeway's lesions, small, flat red spots that develop on the palms of the hands and soles of the feet.

Systemic emboli may affect the spleen, kidney, gastrointestinal tract, or heart. Neurologic manifestations can include cerebral emboli, aneurysms, brain abscesses, and meningitis. Renal disease may be present due to abscesses, an infarction, or glomerulonephritis. The most common complication is congestive heart failure caused by to valvular destruction, myocarditis, coronary artery emboli, or myocardial abscesses.[16]

Rheumatic Heart Disease

Carditis is the most important clinical manifestation of acute rheumatic fever because it can lead to acute heart failure and death. Rheumatic carditis usually does not cause symptoms and is often discovered on examination of a patient with suspected rheumatic fever, who presents with arthritis or chorea (irregular movements of the facial muscles or limbs). This prompts the examination of the heart, and murmurs are detected, which are caused by mitral and aortic regurgitation from valvular inflammation. If other symptoms of rheumatic fever are not apparent, and if the carditis is not severe enough to cause heart failure, the carditis may not be detected. A clinical diagnosis of carditis can be made if any one of the following is demonstrated in a patient with active rheumatic fever: organic heart murmur or murmurs not previously present, definite enlargement of the heart, congestive heart failure, or a pericardial friction rub or effusion.[11, 17]

LABORATORY ANALYSES AND DIAGNOSIS

Pericarditis

The diagnosis of acute pericarditis is confirmed by an electrocardiogram. Electrocardiographic changes can be detected within hours after the onset of pericardial pain. Chest radiographs do not usually provide diagnostic information unless the pericarditis is associated with tuberculosis or malignancy. Detecting the presence of pericardial effusion using the echocardiogram is necessary to provide material that can be analyzed to identify the etiologic agent.

A definitive diagnosis can be established by aspiration and laboratory analysis of pericardial fluid or a pericardial biopsy. However, these invasive techniques carry a significant risk and are not always indicated. In uncomplicated cases, those consistent with viral pericarditis, rheumatic fever, or uremia, pericardial aspiration does not usually provide a substantial diagnostic yield.[2, 13] Pericardiocentesis is indicated in complicated cases, when bacterial pericarditis is suspected, or when cardiac tamponade develops. In cases of tuberculosis, histoplasmosis, or coccidioidomycosis, pericardial tissue obtained through biopsy will provide a better yield of these organisms than pericardial fluid. If pericardial aspiration or biopsy is indicated, the laboratory should be notified in advance so that appropriate media, tissue culture media, or stains will be available. The pericardial fluid should be examined by Gram stain and acid-fast stains and cultured for aerobes, anaerobes, and mycobacteria. Depending on the results obtained from these tests, additional microbiologic studies, including viral and fungal cultures, may be ordered.

Additional laboratory findings in pericarditis include nonspecific indicators of inflammation. The white blood cell (WBC) count may be mildly elevated, and the erythrocyte sedimentation rate (ESR) may be increased. Cardiac enzyme levels are usually normal, but in some patients with epicardial inflammation the MB fraction of the isoenzyme of creatine kinase (CK_2) may be elevated. Other laboratory studies may be warranted depending on the clinical presentation. Blood cultures should be collected on febrile patients to detect possible infective endocarditis and bacteremia. Viral cultures or acute and convalescent serologic studies can be performed to establish a specific viral agent. Fungal serologic testing is indicated in patients that reside in or have traveled to an endemic area, or in immunocompromised patients. Antinuclear antibody (ANA) titers and tests for rheumatoid factor can be helpful in differentiating autoimmune pericarditis from infectious pericarditis. In children with suspected rheumatic fever, an anti–streptolysin O (ASO) titer may be ordered.

Myocarditis

Myocarditis is often a clinically silent disease and may be detected when electrocardiographic abnormalities are discovered. Because the cardiovascular signs and symptoms of myocarditis are often nonspecific, the identification of the specific etiologic agent responsible is usually dependent on extracardiac findings. When patients develop myocarditis following a viral illness, cultures can be performed from stool, throat washings, blood, myocardium, or pericardial fluid. Unfortunately, viral cultures are not always successful in yielding the organism. By the time the cultures are collected, the patient may no longer be actively shedding the virus. Serologic tests demonstrating a four-fold rise in antibody titer to a specific viral agent can also be used to determine the etiology. These tests may reveal a recent infection, but they are not specific for the diagnosis of viral myocarditis. Other laboratory findings in myocarditis include elevated WBC count and ESR. Some individuals experience elevated levels of myocardial enzymes, and it may be difficult to distinguish myocarditis from an acute myocardial infarction.

Endocarditis

The most important diagnostic test for the confirmation of infective endocarditis is the blood culture. Blood cultures are positive in more than 95% of patients who have not had antimicrobial therapy. The bacteremia is continuous, so if any culture becomes positive, all are likely to be positive. In patients with subacute disease who have not had prior antimicrobial therapy, three blood cultures should be collected at least 1 hour apart and then therapy initiated. Blood should be collected from separate venipuncture sites and cultured for aerobes and anaerobes. In acute disease, therapy should not be delayed, and cultures should be collected 30 minutes apart.[16, 18] When a patient has had antimicrobial therapy 1 to 2 weeks before admission, two separate blood cultures on 3 successive days are recommended.[19]

In some cases of infectious endocarditis the results of blood cultures are negative, and the diagnosis is based on clinical information and the use of echocardiography. Negative blood cultures are often a result of previous antimicrobial therapy, but they can also result from infection with fastidious organisms that are more difficult to cultivate. In fungal endocarditis, the organisms often become entrapped in emboli or in capillary beds and are more difficult to isolate. Culture-negative endocarditis must be differentiated from other fever-causing illnesses.

There are several hematologic findings noted in patients with infective endocarditis. A normochromic, normocytic anemia develops in most cases. In subacute disease the WBC count is normal, but the differential cell count reveals a slight shift to the left. In acute disease, leukocytosis and thrombocytopenia are present, but anemia is not as common. The ESR is almost always elevated.

Additional laboratory findings include the presence of circulating immune complexes. Rheumatoid factor is found in 50% of patients who have endocarditis for 3 to 6 weeks.[10, 16] Urinalysis results are usually abnormal and reveal proteinuria or microscopic hematuria. In patients with abnormal renal function, especially diffuse glomerulonephritis, serum complement levels are reduced. Other cardiologic procedures are used to detect the nature of the lesion and the size of the vegetations.

Rheumatic Heart Disease

Establishing the diagnosis of rheumatic heart disease is contingent on the diagnosis of rheumatic fever. No specific tests for the diagnosis of rheumatic fever exist, but certain laboratory results are supportive of clinical findings. Documenting a previous group A streptococcal infection and detecting the presence of a persistent inflammatory process provides supporting evidence for this disease.[17]

Detection of a recent streptococcal infection can be made by throat culture or antibody determinations. Throat cultures may no longer be positive by the time rheumatic fever is detected. If they are positive, it is not certain whether the patient is harboring the same organism or has been reinfected with a new strain. Streptococcal antibody tests are more useful because a rising titer is indicative of a recent infection. The serologic tests available include the ASO titer antideoxyribonuclease B (anti–DNase B), and antihyaluronidase. The ASO is the most widely used test and is considered significant when a rise in titer of 2 dilution units or more between an acute and convalescent serum sample occurs. If only a single serum is tested, the upper limits of normal are 85 Todd units for preschool-age children; 170 Todd units for school-age children; and 85 Todd units for adults.[20] If normal or borderline ASO results are demonstrated, the anti–DNase B assay can be performed. The Streptozyme test is another laboratory test that detects antibodies against several streptococcal antigens. Because this test measures antibodies against multiple streptococcal antigens, it may detect more positive specimens than tests like the ASO that measure a single streptococcal antibody. Therefore, it is possible for a patient to have a negative ASO test and a positive Streptozyme test. Clinicians must be advised of the type of test being performed when they request a streptococcal antibody titer.

Inflammation is detected by the presence of acute phase reactants. The most common tests include measurements of C-reactive protein (CRP) and the ESR. These tests are not specific for rheumatic fever, but they are almost always abnormal in this disease. Other laboratory findings include leukocytosis, increases in serum complement, mucoproteins, and α_2- and γ-globulins. A normocytic normochromic anemia due to the chronic inflammatory process may also be demonstrated.

TREATMENT
Pericarditis

The management of acute pericarditis first requires establishing whether the pericarditis is related to an underlying disorder that requires specific therapy. General supportive measures include bedrest until fever and pain disappear and analgesics for pain. Nonsteroidal anti-inflammatory agents are usually effective in managing the pain. If the pain does not respond to this treatment, corticosteroids may be administered. Anticoagulants should not be administered because they may precipitate bleeding into the pericardial space.

Viral pericarditis is usually self-limited with clinical and laboratory signs of inflammation disappearing within 2 to 6 weeks; however, some patients experience one or more recurrences after the inital episode.[13] No specific treatment is available for the viral agent, but supportive care is extremely valuable.

Acute bacterial pericarditis is a more serious illness, with a mortality of 50% to 70%. Successful therapy requires isolation of the organism through pericardial effusion. Specific antimicrobial therapy can be administered for 4 to 6 weeks, and surgical intervention is sometimes necessary. Antituberculous or antifungal agents may be appropriate if these organisms are responsible.

Myocarditis

The treatment of myocarditis includes supportive measures and therapy directed at the etiologic agent. Viral myocarditis is treated with bedrest, corticosteroids, and monitoring the patient for complications. Nonsteroidal anti-inflammatory agents are not recommended during the acute stages of illness because they can increase myocardial damage. Congestive heart failure is managed with short-acting digitalis, diuresis, and controlled salt intake. When myocarditis is due to other infectious agents (bacteria, fungi, parasites), more specific therapy is administered.

Endocarditis

Infective endocarditis is always fatal if untreated. In order to cure endocarditis, all microorganisms must be eradicated from the vegetation.[18] Surgery for valve replacement may be required in addition to antimicrobial therapy. The goal of antimicrobial therapy is to achieve a high enough concentration of the drug for a long enough time to sterilize the vegetation. The antimicrobial agents must be bactericidal rather than bacteriostatic. The appropriate treatment depends on the isolation of the causative agent and accurate determination of its susceptibility.

Antimicrobial susceptibility testing should include the determination of the minimal inhibitory concentration (MIC) and the minimal bactericidal concentration (MBC). The MIC test demonstrates the minimal amount of antimicrobial agent that inhibits visible in vitro growth of the bacteria. The MBC test reveals the minimal concentration that results in a 99.9% kill of the bacteria. These concentrations may be different, which is critical in achieving effective kill of the bacteria in the patient. Schlicter's test or the serum bactericidal activity test can be helpful in determining the effectiveness of treatment, although there is controversy over its use as a prognostic indicator. These tests measure the highest dilution of the patient's serum that kills a standard inoculum of the organism in vitro. A peak serum bactericidal titer of 1:8 or greater usually indicates an adequate therapeutic effect.

To prevent infectious endocarditis in high-risk patients, antimicrobial prophylaxis is recommended during procedures that cause transient bacteremia. High-risk patients are those with known congenital or valvular heart disease, with an intracardiac prostheses, or with a previous episode of endocarditis. The American Heart Association determines which procedures require prophylaxis through consideration of the frequency with which the procedure is associated with endocarditis; the frequency with which the procedure is associated with producing bacteremia; and whether the organisms that enter the blood during the procedure are associated with endocarditis.[21] Box 5–1 lists the procedures for which prophylaxis is recommended.

Rheumatic Heart Disease

Rheumatic fever is best prevented by ensuring early treatment of pharyngeal infection with group A streptococcus.[11] No specific cure for rheumatic fever is available, but supportive therapy can reduce the mortality and morbidity. The goal of therapy is to eradicate the group A streptococ-

---

Box 5–1. Recommendations for Endocarditis Prophylaxis

Dental Procedures

All procedures known to cause gingival or mucosal bleeding
Extraction
Professional cleaning
Periodontal surgery

Respiratory Tract Procedures

Tonsillectomy
Adenoidectomy
Surgery involving respiratory mucosa
Bronchoscopy using a rigid bronchoscope

Gastrointestinal Procedures

Gall bladder surgery
Esophageal dilation
Surgery involving the intestine

Genitourinary Procedures

Cystoscopy
Urethral dilation
Prostate surgery
Surgery of the urinary tract (in the presence of infection)
Urethral catheterization (in the presence of infection)

Gynecologic and Obstetric Procedures

Vaginal hysterectomy
Vaginal delivery in the presence of infection

Surgery Involving Contaminated Tissues

Incision and drainage of infected tissue

cal infection, to reduce inflammation, and to treat congestive heart failure, if present. When rheumatic fever is first diagnosed, the patient should be treated with a course of penicillin to eliminate group A streptococcus, even if the organism cannot be cultured at this time. Additionally, long-term prophylaxis is recommended by the American Heart Association. This secondary prophylaxis involves an intramuscular injection of penicillin every 4 weeks. Because the injection is quite painful, oral secondary prophylaxis is used in the United States, and penicillin V or oral sulfadiazine is administered daily. The duration of the prophylaxis may be continued indefinitely, especially in patients with increased exposure to group A streptococcus.[22] Patients who have valvular heart disease also require endocarditis prophylaxis as discussed previously.

Inflammation is reduced with the use of salicylates in patients with arthritis or with corticosteroids in patients with carditis. If congestive heart failure develops, measures are taken to eliminate the congestion. Bedrest is necessary to reduce the cardiac work. The mortality and morbidity of this disease can be reduced with early diagnosis, careful monitoring, and prevention of recurring episodes.

Case Study

A 37-year-old man presented to the emergency department complaining of fever, malaise, fatigue, night sweats, arthralgia, and loss of appetite. He had been experiencing this flulike illness for about 2 weeks and symptoms were worsening. Further questioning revealed that approximately 1 week before symptoms began he broke a tooth during lunch, and it was later extracted. He had no previous history of heart disease, but his mother had told him that he had rheumatic fever at 6 years of age. On physical examination, a diastolic murmur was audible, and splenomegaly was noted.

The following laboratory results were noted on admission:

Hemoglobin	(Hgb) 10.9 g/dL
Hematocrit	(Hct) 33%
WBC 12.0 × 10⁹/L	(differential cell count revealed a shift to the left)
ESR	Elevated
CRP	Positive
Urinalysis	Proteinuria and hematuria

Three sets of blood cultures were collected 1 hour apart from separate sites. On the second day of incubation the blood cultures were positive for viridans streptococci.

Questions

1. What is this patient's disorder?
2. What is the best treatment for this disorder?
3. What other tests or procedures could help assess the severity of the damage to the cardiac tissue?
4. What is the prognosis?
5. Should prophylactic antibiotics be used with this patient?

Discussion

1. The disorder is infectious endocarditis, resulting from viridans streptococci organisms that have settled on a previously damaged valve from childhood rheumatic fever. The organisms gained access to the blood stream from the oral mucosa.

2. A regimen of penicillin for 4 weeks along with gentamicin or vancomycin has been shown to be very effective in preventing relapses.

3. An echocardiogram would demonstrate vegetations larger than 3 mm and lesions of the valves. Surgical intervention may be necessary to remove infected tissue, correct defects, or restore valvular function.

4. Untreated, the prognosis is poor. Mortality can be reduced by early diagnosis, appropriate antibiotic therapy, and prevention of recurring infections.

5. Antimicrobial prophylaxis should be used in this patient for any future surgery on any infected or contaminated tissue; surgery of the genitourinary tract, respiratory mucosa, or gastrointestinal tract; and all dental procedures.

References

1. Braunwald E: Pericardial disease. *In* Isselbacher KJ, Braunwald E, Wilson JD, et al (eds): Harrison's Principles of Internal Medicine, ed 13. New York, McGraw-Hill, 1994, p 1094.
2. Smith CB: Pericarditis. *In* Hoeprich PD, Jordan MC, Ronald AR (eds): Infectious Diseases, ed 5. Philadelphia, JB Lippincott, 1994, pp 1222–1228.
3. Spodick DH: The Pericardium: Structure, function, and disease spectrum: *In* Spodick DH (ed): Pericardial Diseases. Philadelphia, FA Davis, 1976, p 7.
4. Roberts WC, Spray TL: Pericardial heart disease. *In* Spodick DH (ed): Pericardial Diseases. Philadelphia, FA Davis, 1976, p 32.
5. Andreoli TE, Carpenter CC, Plum F, et al: Cecil Essentials of Medicine, ed 2. Philadelphia, WB Saunders, 1990, p 111.
6. Ray CG: Enteroviruses. *In* Ryan KJ (ed): Sherris Medical Microbiology, ed 3. Norwalk, Conn. Appleton & Lange, 1994, p 489.
7. Wynne J, Braunwald E: The Cardiomyopathies and myocarditides. *In* Isselbacher KJ, Braunwald E, Wilson JD, et al (eds): Harrison's Principles of Internal Medicine, ed 13. New York City, McGraw-Hill, 1994, p 1093.
8. Markell EK, Voge M, John DT: Medical Parasitology, ed 7. Philadelphia, WB Saunders, 1992, pp 143–145.
9. Durack DT: Infective and noninfective endocarditis. *In* Schlant RC, Alexander RW (eds): Hurst's The Heart, ed 8. New York, McGraw-Hill, 1994, p 1681.
10. Korzeniowski OM, Kaye D: Endocarditis. *In* Gorbach SL, Bartlett JG, Blacklow NR (eds): Infectious Diseases. Philadelphia, WB Saunders, 1992, pp 548–552.
11. Stollerman GH: Rheumatic fever. *In* Isselbacher KJ, Braunwald E, Wilson JD, et al (eds): Harrison's Principles of Internal Medicine, ed 13. New York, McGraw-Hill, 1994, pp 1047–1052.
12. Kaplan EL: Acute rheumatic fever. *In* Schlant RC, Alexander RW (eds): Hurst's The Heart, ed 8. New York, McGraw-Hill, 1994, p 1452.
13. Lorell BH, Braunwald E: Pericardial disease. *In* Braunwald E (ed): Heart Disease: A Textbook of Cardiovascular Medicine, ed 4. Philadelphia, WB Saunders, 1992, pp 1469–1472.
14. Dunn M, Rinkenberger RL: Clinical aspects of acute pericarditis. *In* Spodick DH (ed): Pericardial Diseases, Philadelphia, FA Davis, 1976, p 134.
15. Smith CB: Myocarditis. *In* Hoeprich PD, Jordan MC, Ronald AR (eds): Infectious Diseases, ed 5. Philadelphia, JB Lippincott, 1994, p 1231.
16. Korzeniowski OM, Kaye D: Infectious endocarditis. *In* Braunwald E (ed): Heart Disease: A Textbook of Cardiovascular Medicine, ed 4. Philadelphia, WB Saunders, 1992, p 1085–1089.

17. Stollerman GH: Rheumatic fever and other rheumatic diseases of the heart. *In* Braunwald E (ed): Heart Disease: A Textbook of Cardiovascular Medicine, ed 4. Philadelphia, WB Saunders, 1992, pp 1727–1728.

18. Kaye D: Infective endocarditis. *In* Isselbacher KJ, Braunwald E, Wilson JD, et al (eds): Harrison's Principles of Internal Medicine, ed 13. New York City, McGraw-Hill, 1994, p 523.

19. Shea YR: Specimen collection and transport. *In* Isenberg HD (ed): Clinical Microbiology Procedures Handbook. Washington, DC, American Society for Microbiology, 1992, p 1.1.10.

20. Powell C, Parks D: Anti-Streptolysin O Microtitration. *In* Isenberg HD (ed): Clinical Microbiology Procedures Handbook. Washington, DC, American Society for Microbiology, 1992, p 9.4.3.

21. Molavi A: Endocarditis: Recognition, management, and prophylaxis. *In* Frankl WS, Brest AN (eds): Valvular Heart Disease: Comprehensive Evaluation and Treatment, ed 2. Philadelphia, FA Davis, 1993, p 164.

22. Burge DJ, DeHoratius RJ: Acute rheumatic fever. *In* Frankl WS, Brest AN (eds): Valvular Heart Disease: Comprehensive Evaluation and Treatment, ed 2. Philadelphia, FA Davis, 1993, pp 17–19.

Hypertensive Disorders

Brian D. Andresen

In 1731, English pastor Stephen Hales performed the first blood pressure measurements with a live mare. Although his experiments were most crude, Hales's observations were remarkably accurate and laid the foundation for modern blood pressure measurements. In 1896, an Italian physician, Riva-Rocci, built and used a prototype sphygmomanometer, incorporating the first pressure cuff, an ascending mercury column, and a pressure scale to make measurements. Today, blood pressure is now most easily measured and is generally the first indicator that a patient has hypertension. Nevertheless, statistics indicate that only one-half of all Americans who suffer from hypertension are ever aware of their illness. Of those who are diagnosed, only 50% receive adequate treatment.

ETIOLOGY AND PATHOPHYSIOLOGY

Hypertensive disorders are characterized by systolic and diastolic blood pressures exceeding 140 and 90 mm Hg, respectively (140/90). A blood pressure that consistently exceeds a diastolic value greater than 90 mm Hg is observed in approximately 15% to 25% of the U.S. adult population. For reasons that are not entirely clear, the reported incidence of hypertension in black persons is more than twice that in whites.

Repeated measurements of blood pressures over 200/140 mm Hg are very serious. Untreated, this "malignant" form of hypertension can quickly lead to death. "Benign"

forms of hypertension typically reveal no apparent symptoms until the advanced stages. Unaware of the disorder, the patient is at risk for heart, eye, kidney, and brain injury, and early death as a result of long-term physiologic damage. Subtle arteriosclerotic changes are also present in the patient with benign hypertension that can lead to a severely compromised blood flow in the extremities and brain. High blood pressure forces the heart to pump harder than normal because of increased vascular resistance. Over time, the overworked heart may fail.

Hypertension is most common in adults older than 65 years. Approximately 35% to 50% of the elderly have blood pressures in excess of 160/90 mm Hg. Many of these persons suffer from congestive heart failure, heart disease, ventricular hypertrophy, and vascular complications. In addition, strokes and other cardiovascular complications can occur as a result of sustained high blood pressure. Thus, the identification and management of hypertension are most important.

Children have substantially lower blood pressures than adults. Blood pressure gradually increases with age through puberty. Only 1% to 2% of children younger than 14 years have pressures in excess of 140/90 mm Hg. It has been suggested that children with slightly elevated blood pressures have greater risk of developing hypertension as adults. The parents of hypertensive offspring often have demonstrated elevated blood pressures as well, suggesting a hereditary component.

Hypertensive patients can be classified using two different approaches.[1,2] One method is by the *degree of hypertension*, which is important prognostically. The second method is to classify the hypertensive patient according to the *underlying etiology*. The latter approach is most important for selecting the appropriate therapy.

Degree of Hypertension

Patients can be categorized according to the degree of their hypertension. Hypertension that is immediately life threatening is termed *malignant*. Hypertension that is not immediately life-threatening is termed *benign*, although long-term benign hypertension can also be life threatening eventually; it may persist for decades, leading to physiologic complications and a shorter life span for affected patients than for average, age-matched, nonhypertensive patients.

Patients with malignant hypertension have a very poor

prognosis. If the disease is untreated, 60% die in 6 months, and 80% die within 1 year.[3] Untreated, malignant hypertension leads to inflammation and necrosis of the arterioles. This arteriolophathy can be visualized on physical examination as changes in the ocular fundus, which reveals hemorrhages, exudates, and papilledema. Papilledema under these circumstances usually results from ischemia of the optic nerve as a consequence of a damaged vasa nervorum and does not imply increased pressure of the cerebrospinal fluid. Similar vascular lesions can be found in the kidneys, where the severity of the disease is reflected by proteinuria, hematuria, red blood cell casts, and progressive renal failure.

Primary Hypertension

Although hypertension can be caused by a number of conditions, more than 90% of patients have "primary," "idiopathic," or "essential" hypertension, for which the etiology is unknown.[4] There is typically no common profile for patients with primary hypertension, and it is believed that a mosaic of many interacting factors causes the disease. Generally, all hypertension is considered primary until discovery of a distinct etiology that may respond to a specific therapy.

The mosaic of factors leading to primary hypertension includes age, race, posture, salt intake, emotional state, hormonal balance, and medication, all of which can interact to influence blood pressure. An initial consideration in primary hypertension is a defect in the transport of sodium in the renal tubules. In theory, the renal retention of sodium would lead to expanded intravascular volume and increased vascular resistance, and would signal the release of angiotensin. As a result, cardiac output would be elevated and blood pressure would increase. The increase in pressure and fluid exchange should promote sodium excretion; however, this might not be the case if a faulty autoregulatory mechanism prevents adequate tissue perfusion.

Ingestion of sodium appears to be very important in the etiology of primary hypertension.[5] Various studies have shown that populations consuming relatively small amounts of sodium (less than 60–80 mEq/day) have little hypertension and minimal or no increase in blood pressure with age.

It has also been suggested that most sodium-associated hypertension is caused by an imbalance of the interaction of sodium and the blood pressure regulatory mechanisms, which are sympathetic function, angiotensin, vasopressin, and vascular reactivity. Various abnormalities in sodium and calcium transport in the red cell and leukocyte membranes of patients with primary hypertension have also been reported. These findings lead to further speculations that membrane defects in vascular smooth muscles may be involved in the pathogenesis of high blood pressure.

Primary hypertension can be further subdivided into two groups according to whether the abnormalities are in the *hemodynamic* or in the *renin-angiotensin* system.[6] Hemodynamic abnormalities are often most associated with *labile hypertension*. This subclassification of primary hypertension is generally applied when cardiac output increases but vascular resistance remains unchanged or is considered "inappropriate" to match cardiac output. If the sympathetic nervous system function is altered in a patient with essen-

tial hypertension by increased visual or emotional stress, extremes of heat or cold, or heavy or mild forms of exercise, an exaggerated response can be evoked in the heart rate, cardiac output, renal renin release, and blood pressure. In the patient with labile hypertension, the imbalance in hemodynamics is accentuated and may evolve into fixed or established hypertension. Unfortunately, the mechanisms involved in labile hypertension are not yet well enough understood to enable the development of an adequate drug regimen or other treatment.

The status and possible role of the renin-angiotensin system in patients with primary hypertension has been thoroughly investigated, and studies point to a variety of causative factors. Renin is a proteolytic enzyme that catalyzes the conversion of a tetradecapeptide substrate to angiotensin I, which is later converted by a variety of tissues to angiotensin II (Fig. 6–1). False substrates, diminished receptor sites, and poor conversion owing to a variety of biochemical factors may lead to altered levels of angiotensin II and essential hypertension. In comparison with normotensive control patients, almost 70% of the patients with essential hypertension have normal plasma renin activity (PRA) levels, 20% to 25% have abnormally low PRA, and 5% to 10% have high PRA levels.[1]

Some research findings point to inappropriate levels of renal vasodilator substances in primary hypertension.[7] For example, researchers have reported that reduced levels of renal kallikrein, the enzyme which catalyzes the formation

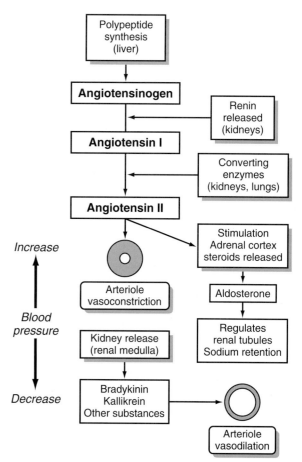

Figure 6–1. Renin-angiotensin system.

of the vasodilator bradykinin, are observed in the urine of the hypertensive patient.

Prostaglandins, particularly of the E series, are also able to cause renal vasodilatation, natriuresis, and renin release. However, the role of prostaglandins in hypertension is not well understood.

Calcium ions are directly linked with the contraction of vascular smooth muscles, and free intercellular Ca^{2+} levels can greatly influence blood pressure. Fixed hypertension can result from increased peripheral vascular resistance. Inhibition of Ca^{2+} across the cellular membranes through calcium channels can result in decreased peripheral vascular resistance. Therefore, Ca^{2+}-channel blocker drugs that inhibit transmembrane calcium transport have a significant impact on the control of hypertension. All therapeutic Ca^{2+}-channel blockers approved for clinical use also decrease coronary vascular resistance and increase coronary blood flow. It is interesting to note that an older treatment for *toxemia of pregnancy*, which can involve dangerously high blood pressures, was controlled by infusions of magnesium sulfate. Magnesium ions apparently competed for Ca^{2+} channels and disrupted peripheral vascular smooth muscle contraction.

Secondary Hypertension

Hypertensive Emergencies

Secondary hypertension is identified with a distinct disease state that is responsible for the elevated blood pressure.[3] Only 5% to 10% of the cases of hypertension in the United States are secondary. Although this form of hypertension is much less prevalent than primary hypertension, it is important to identify the etiology of secondary hypertension, because the underlying problem, even when relatively serious, may often be cured if identified.[8] The patient with secondary hypertension can be further classified either as a candidate for diagnostic procedures or as an individual in hypertensive crisis. The former state is not considered life threatening, and there is time for thorough laboratory studies. The latter state, however, requires immediate emergency care to prevent irreversible or lethal complications of the disease.[1, 9] Box 6–1 highlights those situations in which immediate or emergency treatment for hypertensive crisis is mandated.

Box 6–1. Hypertensive Emergencies

Malignant Hypertension

- Rapid funduscopic changes with necrotizing arteriolitis
- Hypertensive encephalopathy

Hypertension Associated With:

- Acute left ventricular failure
- Coronary insufficiency
- Aortic dissection or a leaking aneurysm
- Intracranial hemorrhage
- Postoperative bleeding

Box 6–2. Disorders Responsible for Secondary Hypertension

- Renal (parenchymal and vascular)
- Adrenal (cortical and medullary)
- Neurogenic
- Parathyroid or thyroid (hyperthyroid and myxedema)
- Coarctation of aorta (thoracic and abdominal)
- Toxemia of pregnancy (preeclampsia and eclampsia)
- Drug-induced (therapeutic and abusive)
- Increased left ventricle stroke volume
- Decreased aortic distensibility (arteriosclerosis and coarctation)

Clinically Demonstrable Hypertension

Although they are eventually life-threatening, other forms of secondary hypertension are more subtle in their initial stages. If left untreated, however, these disease states may also develop to a crisis level. Box 6–2 lists several disorders clearly responsible for secondary hypertension that can typically be associated with a certain target tissues.[4]

RENAL HYPERTENSION (see also Chapter 17)

Parenchymal Hypertension. Mild and severe diseases of the vascular and parenchymal tissues of the kidney are associated with hypertension.[6, 10, 11] Several important disease states associated with parenchymal deterioration are highlighted in Box 6–3.

Hypertension is observed in both acute and chronic glomerulonephritis. In the acute disease, volume overload is usually the most prominent feature. In the chronic disease, the hypertension usually is not severe unless associated with high levels of urea, creatinine, and other nonprotein nitrogen substances in the serum.

Pyelonephritis may also induce hypertension by causing

Box 6–3. Disease States Associated with Parenchymal Deterioration

Glomerulonephritis
Chronic pyelonephritis
Diabetic nephropathy
Interstitial nephritis
Polycystic kidney
Connective tissue disease
Hydronephrosis
Hypernephroma
JG cell tumor
Wilms' tumor
Solitary renal cyst
Perinephritis
Renal hematoma
Fibrous constriction (Ask-Upmark kidney)

renal failure or by interfering with intrarenal circulation. The severity of the hypertension does not parallel the severity of the disease, and renin concentrations may remain normal.[12]

The type of hypertension that commonly develops in patients with diabetic nephropathy is related to impairment of renal function often generated from intercapillary glomerulosclerosis or from chronic pyelonephritis. Plasma renin activity measurements in diabetics are often lowered owing to volume expansion, sympathetic neuropathy, or both.

Hypertension associated with polycystic kidney disease has not been correlated to renin concentrations. In contrast, renal compression caused by hematomas, perinephritis, and renal scars or obstructions may cause renin-dependent hypertension.[11]

Severe hypertension is often associated with connective tissue disorders such as scleroderma and systemic lupus erythematosus. The resultant hypertension may in turn accelerate the development of renal insufficiency, further accelerating the underlying disease state.

Abnormal parenchymal growths, such as renal cell carcinomas and cysts or other large intrarenal masses, occasionally cause hypertension, presumably by interfering with renal circulation and subsequent stimulation of renin release.[12] Hyperreninemia is also observed with many other types of renal tumors or compression lesions that cause hypertension.[13] Juxtaglomerular (JG) cell tumors and hemangiopericytomas of the kidney may produce severe hypertension, with hyperreninemia, secondary hyperaldosteronism, and marked hypokalemia. These tumors, which are more common in the young, tend to be small and may be missed radiologically unless selective renal angiography is performed. Wilms' tumor and some rare forms of extrarenal malignancies also may produce renin-like material and cause severe hypertension.

Renal Vascular Disease. Box 6–4 lists various disease states associated with renovascular diseases.[11, 13, 14] All are associated with abnormalities of the blood flow and perfusion of the kidney. One or both kidneys may be involved.

Hypertension is secondary to these renovascular diseases in only 1% to 2% of patients.[15, 16] Although almost half of patients with secondary hypertension have some type of renovascular lesion, only a few of these lesions actually cause the hypertension. Generally, atherosclerosis is more common in men and involves the proximal portion of the renal artery. Fibrous dysplasia, from either infection or congenital abnormalities, is more often diagnosed in women and affects the middle and distal portion of the renal vessels. Fibromuscular hyperplasia may also involve

---

Box 6–4. **Disorders Associated with Renovascular Disease**

Atherosclerotic, thrombotic, or embolic obstructions
Fibromuscular hyperplasia
Aneurysm or dissecting aneurysm
Inflammation (infection)
Hypoplasia

---

arteries elsewhere in the body, leading to ischemia of other organs and additional blood pressure elevations.

ADRENAL HYPERTENSION

Abnormalities of the adrenals can broadly be classified as mineralocorticoid excess syndromes.[6–8] Steroids that are important in hypertension are those involved in the biosynthesis of corticosteroids from cholesterol. Steroid production abnormalities can be grouped into aldosterone-producing adenoma, adrenocortical hyperplasia, Cushing's syndrome, and metabolic errors of steroid hydroxylation (hydroxylase deficiencies). Hypertension is secondary to primary hyperaldosteronism in approximately 1% of hypertensive patients. Of these, approximately 75% have an isolated primary, aldosterone-producing adenoma. The remaining 25% have *idiopathic hypotension* and typically have hyperplastic, nodular masses on one or both adrenal glands. Patients with primary hyperaldosteronism have spontaneous hypokalemia, an inability to concentrate urine, tetany, glucose intolerance, and overall depressed muscle strength. Abnormally low plasma renin activity (PRA) values are another important feature of hyperaldosteronism. In fact, the triad of *hypertension, hypokalemia,* and *low plasma renin levels* is highly suggestive of mineralocorticoid excess.

Cushing's Syndrome. The abnormal overproduction of cortisol or related corticosteroids, Cushing's syndrome results in a constellation of clinical signs and symptoms.[17] One of these is hypertension. However, the hypertension in most patients with Cushing's syndrome is not directly related to mineralocorticoid excess and is of unknown etiology. In addition, there is a group of patients with essential hypertension who have some similarities to patients with mineralocorticoid excess but have normal aldosterone secretions (morning cortisol plasma levels of 5–23 μg/dL).

Genetic Defects. Genetic defects involving enzymatic reactions that hydroxylate at the 11, 17, 18, or 19 carbon position of cortisol have also been identified as contributing to hypertension. Most of these enzyme deficiencies result in an excess production of deoxycorticosterone (DOC). Hydroxylation at carbon 18 or 19 generates 18-hydroxy-DOC or 19-hydroxy-DOC, respectively, both of which are associated with hypertension.

Pheochromocytoma. Usually derived from the adrenal medulla, pheochromocytoma is a rare chromaffin tissue tumor that causes excess secretion of catecholamines, resulting in hypertension.[18] Catecholamines are biosynthesized from phenylalanine and are very important in a variety of regulatory processes. Interest in pheochromocytoma arises because the tumor can cause a dramatic and potentially lethal elevation of blood pressure. The tumors are found in only 0.1% to 0.3% of the hypertension population and originate in the adrenal medulla in approximately 90% of these patients. In the remaining 10%, the catecholamine-generating tumors originate from the Zuckerkandl's organs, paraganglionic cells of the sympathetic nervous system, bladder, aorta, or carotid.

Pheochromocytoma is easily diagnosed[18] and is surgically correctable. Most signs and symptoms can be directly related to an overproduction of catecholamines secreted by the tumor. However, patients can be misdiagnosed as having disorders such as thyrotoxicosis, severe anxiety, diabetes mellitus, or hyperventilation. Onset at an early age is often characteristic of pheochromocytoma. There is also a familial association, and family members should be screened to identify asymptomatic individuals. Familial pheochromocytoma may be associated with other neural crest tissue tumors. These include tumors of the pituitary and pancreas and medullary carcinoma of the thyroid and parathyroid gland. Other associated disorders are cerebellar hemangioblastoma and retinal angioma. Approximately 10% of patients with pheochromocytoma have malignant diseases. When the metastatic lesions are slow growing, death usually results from hypertension rather than from the malignancy.

NEUROGENIC HYPERTENSION

Many types of neurologic conditions may cause hypertension. They include intracranial lesions, tumors, hematomas, subdural hygromas, carotid sinus denervation, familial dysautonomia, and spinal cord transection. In addition, various peripheral neuropathies, such as those seen with infectious polyneuritis, tabes dorsalis, porphyria, and lead poisoning, may cause hypertension.[19]

THYROID AND PARATHYROID DISEASES

Myxedematous patients all tend to have hypertension that, when correctly diagnosed, can be corrected by the administration of thyroid hormone.[20] Approximately one-third of the patients with hyperparathyroidism have hypertension,[2] which can often be attributed to renal parenchymal damage due to nephrolithiases (stones) and nephrocalcinosis (salt deposits). The observed hypertension usually disappears when the hypercalcemia is corrected. Elevated angiotensin levels, which are also common with hyperthyroidism, may play a role in the hypertension.

COARCTATION OF THE AORTA

Hypertension is often associated with a congenital defect leading to a constriction in the aorta.[1, 21] The constriction is usually located distal to the insertion of the ductus arteriosus and near the subclavian artery, but it can be in any portion of the aorta. It occurs most commonly in males and is associated with Turner's syndrome and other cardiac abnormalities, such as bicuspid aortic valve, ventricular septal defect, patent ductus arteriosus, mitral valve abnormalities, and berry aneurysms of the carotid circulation.[22] The hypertension may be caused by the constriction itself or may result from a form of renal arterial hypertension. The diagnosis is most evident from clinical and routine radiographic findings.[23, 24]

TOXEMIA OF PREGNANCY

In the United States, approximately one-fifth of all maternal deaths and 25,000 stillbirths and neonatal deaths are a direct result of hypertension during pregnancy.[25] A sustained increase in pressure of 30/15 mm Hg or any level exceeding 140/90 mm Hg is considered hypertensive. Hypertension during pregnancy can be defined by four different forms of pregnancy-related elevations of blood pressure; these are: (1) acute hypertension in pregnancy, preeclampsia-eclampsia (pregnancy-induced hypertension [PIH]); (2) chronic hypertension during pregnancy; (3) chronic hypertension during pregnancy with superimposed acute hypertension (preeclampsia), and (4) transient hypertension in pregnancy that occurs during labor or immediately postpartum and then subsides.

Acute hypertension during pregnancy is a condition that is most often associated with toxemia of pregnancy and preeclampsia-eclampsia.[2] *PIH* is the most current terminology for this form of hypertension. Typically, after the 24th week of gestation, a mildly preeclamptic patient develops overt edema of the face, hands, or feet, blood pressures in excess of 140/90 mm Hg, and proteinuria. There are no other typical clinical signs. In 90% of the patients, the sequential development of *edema, hypertension*, and *proteinuria* clearly identifies mild preeclampsia. The mild forms of pregnancy-induced hypertension are treatable but not preventable. The development of PIH consists of mild preeclampsia progressing to severe preeclampsia and then to eclampsia. The patient with severe preeclampsia is seriously ill; she must be hospitalized and her blood pressure continuously monitored and controlled. The severe forms of hypertension have a maternal mortality of 10% and a perinatal mortality of greater than 30%. The cause of preeclampsia is unknown, and extensive research is in progress to identify a "factor" or group of chemicals that may be responsible for the disease.[8] The incidence is increased in daughters of mothers who have had preeclampsia and in women with hydatidform mole, diabetes, Rh incompatibility, alpha-thalassesmia, preexisting renal disease, and chronic hypertension.

Chronic hypertension during pregnancy is defined as hypertension usually recorded *before* the pregnancy or *before the 24th week* of gestation. It appears that pregnancy often unmasks hypertension, which is seen most often in multigravida women. Chronic hypertension of pregnancy is divided into primary and secondary types. The former is not related to any specific disease state and accounts for 95% of cases. Like other forms of hypertension, secondary hypertension can be associated with an underlying disease process.

DRUG- AND DIET-INDUCED HYPERTENSION

Many types of drugs can precipitate abnormally high blood pressure, leading to stroke and cardiac arrest. For example, numerous deaths associated with high blood pressure and arrythmias have been reported by the national news media among athletes using illicit drugs (e.g., cocaine). The most commonly reported drug-induced hypertension, however, is associated with oral contraceptives in young and middle-aged women.

Oral Contraceptives. Thorough studies of large populations of women show that, with prolonged use, hypertension develops in approximately 5% of women taking oral contraceptives. In addition, there appears to be a threefold risk of developing hypertension when oral contraceptives are used for more than 5 years. Over a period of months, the systolic pressure increases 8 to 10 mm Hg, at which time some women may develop severe hypertension. Studies of large populations of women show that an association can be made between the development of hypertension with previous toxemia of pregnancy, familial hypertension, obesity, use of contraceptives, age, or preexisting borderline hypertension. The use of oral contraceptives appears to increase renin production, angiotensin II, aldosterone secretion, and salt and water retention. The increase in angiotensin II may raise vasoconstriction, leading to hypertension.

The hypertension morbidity reported with oral contraceptives appears to be associated with cardiovascular effects, including thromboembolism, stroke, and myocardial infarction. Myocardial infarctions appear to be most closely correlated with cigarette smoking.[25] In addition, oral contraceptives seem to increase serum levels of very-low-density lipoproteins, blood glucose, and platelet aggregation factors (prostaglandins). Estrogen-related steroids, used to treat postmenopausal women, have also been associated with elevated blood pressures.

Other Pharmacologic Agents. An adverse reaction leading to hypertensive crisis can be observed in patients who receive monoamine oxidase inhibitors (drugs prescribed for depression) and whose diet is high in tyramine from such sources as cheese, wines, herring, and liver.[1, 8] These drugs prevent the degradation of tyramine and tyrosine (biologic precursors for catecholamines), alter the chemical balance of catecholamines in tissues, and markedly enhance their physiologic effects. Other drugs that mimic catecholamines (e.g., amphetamine, cocaine) have been reported to elevate blood pressure significantly. Finally, drugs used to combat inflammation (e.g., indomethacin and other prostaglandin synthesis inhibitors) have been associated with hypertension. The actual mechanism for these effects is not clearly known; however, these agents may alter the correct balance between prostacyclins, thromboxanes, and prostaglandins in blood vessels. Box 6–5 lists drugs known to cause hypertension.

Foods. Interestingly, excessive licorice ingestion (50 to 100 g/day) can produce hypertension and hypokalemia,

owing to the compound glycyrrhizic acid, which exhibits mineralocorticoid action.

CLINICAL MANIFESTATIONS
Blood Pressure and History

Any blood pressure reading with a value greater than 140/90 mm Hg suggests possible hypertension.[24] A family history of hypertension and reported episodes of labile hypertension usually point to primary hypertension. Newly elevated blood pressure readings in a patient younger than 35 years or older than 50 years is usually associated with secondary hypertension. A history of repeated urinary tract infections (UTIs) with proteinuria, kidney stones, significant side pains, or use of steroids or oral contraceptives is very suggestive of a possible diagnosis of secondary hypertension.[8, 12] Nocturia and polydipsia with hypertension usually indicate endocrine disease.

A history of significant weight loss points to pheochromocytoma. Patients with hypertension secondary to pheochromocytoma manifest cyclic hypertension and the absence of obesity. Hypertension with obesity is most often associated with Cushing's syndrome. It is also observed that greater than 95% of pheochromocytomas are located in the abdomen, and 90% are in one or both adrenals. Multiple pheochromocytomas are more common in children.

In contrast, weight gain associated with a round face reflects Cushing's syndrome. Inappropriate development of muscle strength or weakness in the extremities, along with differences in pulse pressures, suggests coarctation of the aorta. Detailed examination of the ocular fundi identifies the duration and prognosis of the hypertension.

Detailed examination of the heart and lungs is also essential to identify unique sounds pointing to ventricular hypertrophy, cardiac decompensation, murmurs, rales, and bruits in the cardiovascular system. Palpitation of the abdomen may reveal aneurysms or enlarged kidneys. Neurologic examination points to cerebrovascular accidents (CVAs) or other pathologic events.

Symptomatology

In the majority of cases of primary hypertension, patients are unaware of their elevated blood pressure. The hypertension can persist for decades with no apparent symptoms to warn of future difficulties. Some persons may complain of fatigue, nervousness, dizziness, palpitation, insomnia, weakness, and headaches. When hypertension is left untreated, strokes, myocardial infarctions, and chronic renal failure are the major problems. Only with malignant hypertension is a patient possibly aware of some underlying problem.[1] Severe throbbing headaches, vomiting, visual disturbances (including blindness), paralysis, angina pectoris, convulsions, stupor, and blackout periods are typical symptoms of malignant hypertension.[26] Clinical findings in secondary hypertension are related to the underlying disease process responsible for the hypertensive state.

LABORATORY ANALYSES AND DIAGNOSIS

After a review of the various disease states, it is important to consider diagnostic methods to identify the un-

---

Box 6–5. **Drugs Known to Cause Hypertension**

- Corticosteroids
- Oral contraceptives
- Sympathomimetic amines or combinations:
    Phenylpropanolamine
    Guanethidine
- Vasopressin (Pitressin)
- Oxytocin
- Pentazocine (Talwin)
- Carbenoxolone
- Drugs of abuse (e.g., nicotine, PCP, cocaine)

derlying causes of hypertension. The evaluation of the patient should have two objectives: (1) to identify secondary forms of hypertension and (2) to determine the presence and extent of hypertensive vascular disease. Because primary hypertension has no clearly identifiable etiology, most of the diagnostic procedures performed in the clinical laboratory center on secondary hypertension. Generally, diagnostic procedures consist of history, routine laboratory studies, common ancillary tests, and special tests (Figs. 6–2 and 6–3; Box 6–6). A variety of laboratory tests aid in determining the degree and type of hypertension.[4, 6, 8, 10, 12, 27, 28]

Evaluation of Renal Status

Evaluation of renal status is carried out using a series of tests, including urinalysis, a urine culture, determinations of the serum creatinine level, renal ultrasound, and captopril renogram. This approach identifies the majority of patients with renal disease and differentiates renal arterial and parenchymal lesions. If parenchymal lesions are found, it may be difficult to ascertain whether the disease is causing or results from the hypertension.

Evaluation of the Renin-Angiotensin System

It is well established that assessment of renin production by each kidney is a most useful diagnostic test.[1] The test

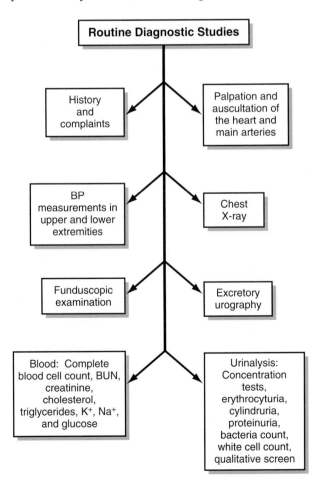

Figure 6–2. General approach to the hypertensive patient. Abbreviations: BP, blood pressure; BUN, blood urea nitrogen.

can be performed on peripheral blood or differentially on renal vein plasma obtained by direct catheterization of the two renal veins under fluoroscopic control.

PLASMA RENIN ACTIVITY

Renin activity is measured indirectly by the ability of the patient's plasma to generate angiotensin I from angiotensinogen by renin (see Fig. 6–1). The value obtained is expressed as nanograms of angiotensin I produced per milliliter of plasma per hour (ng/L/hr). Radioimmunoassay techniques are used, and normal values depend on the particular methodology used. These values are subject to the patient's sodium and potassium levels, posture, and exposure to drugs.[28] Box 6–7 lists the normal values for plasma renin activity. Typically, the values decrease with age and are slightly lower in women than in men. Several sample collection and processing precautions are necessary to ensure an accurate assay.

For PRA assay, blood should be drawn into a tube containing Na-EDTA (ethylene diaminetetra-acetic acid) (1 mg/mL), not K-EDTA. The Na-EDTA specifically inhibits converting enzymes that stop renin reaction at angiotensin I, and inactivates enzymes that may destroy renin. The sample should be centrifuged quickly, and the plasma frozen at −20°C to impede the activation of prorenin or the abnormal release of angiotensin. Small amounts of these compounds are always present; therefore, split sample measurements are made before and after incubation. Neomycin, sulfonyl fluoride, 8-hydroxyquinoline sulfate, and dimethcaprol are added to inhibit bacterial growth and help retard proteolysis. To obtain the maximum rate of renin activity, sufficient amounts of angiotensinogen should be added. A standard, competitive binding radioimmunoassay is performed with ^{125}I-angiotensin I. Box 6–8 indicates how renin activity is related to various disease states.[4]

Drugs can affect the PRA levels.[1] Drugs that tend to elevate renin include chlorthalidone, diazoxide, ethacrynic acid, oral contraceptives, estrogens, furosemide, guanethidine in sodium-depleted patients, hydralazine, spironolactone, and thiazide diuretics. Drugs that tend to lower PRA values are carbenoxolone, clonidine, deoxycorticosterone, glycyrrhiza, guanethidine in patients with normal sodium levels, methyldopa, prazosin, and propanolol. Patients should not receive drugs that affect renin for 1 week before a PRA assay.[29] Box 6–9 displays other factors leading to either high or low plasma renin values.

FUROSEMIDE STIMULATION TEST

Plasma renin activity varies significantly according to a patient's hydration and sodium intake.[30] The administration of furosemide, an effective diuretic, can be used to ascertain the response to dehydration and production of plasma renin. The patient is given furosemide orally and remains upright until blood is drawn several hours later; the renin levels are measured. Patients with renovascular disease have renin values 5 times (10–20 ng/mL/hr) normal values. Patients with primary hyporeninemic hypoaldosteronism usually have low levels of plasma renin (0.5–1.0 ng/mL/hr) and low aldosterone levels (5–10 ng/dL). Patients with suppressed renin values should be considered for possible

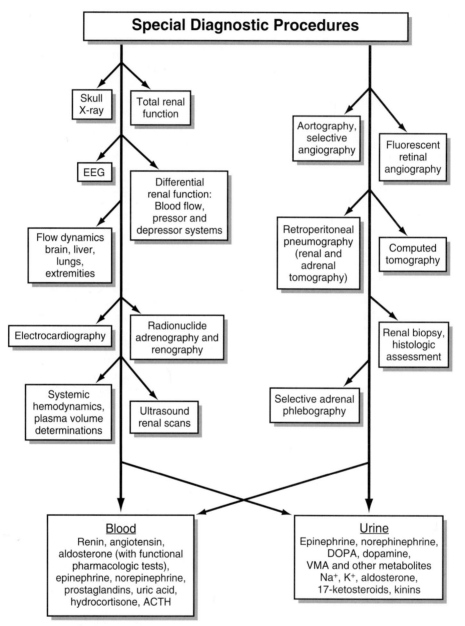

Figure 6–3. Special diagnostic procedures. Abbreviations: EEG, electroencephalography; ACTH, adrenocorticotropic hormone; DOPA, dihydroxyphenylalanine; VMA, vanillylmandelic acid.

Box 6–6. Tests, Special Studies, and Reference Ranges Expected for the Evaluation of Hypertension

History and Physical Examination

Duration, severity, previous response to drug therapy; family history, habits, emotional status and attitude; diet, medications, gastric ulcers, and general health; blood pressure in each arm and leg while standing, seated, and recumbent; arm-to-leg pulse delay time, flank bruits; ocular fundi and changes.

Urinalysis

- Glucose (<0.5 g/day, 1–15 mg/dL)
- Protein (1–14 mg/dL/24 hr)
- Sediment:
  Red blood cells (1 or 2 cells by high power, may indicate renal disease, RBC casts point to glomerular pathology)
  White blood cells (1 to 5 cells by high power, indicates all renal diseases, WBC casts reflect pyelonephritis)
- Urine culture—negative
- 24-hour urine for catecholamines, metanephrine, or vanillylmandelic acid

Blood

- Hemoglobin (12–17 g/dL, adult)
- Urea nitrogen (7–21 mg/dL, plasma)
- Creatinine (<1.3 mg/dL, serum or plasma)
- Uric acid (3–8 mg/dL, serum)
- Fasting sugar and 2–hour postprandial sugar (<120 mg/dL)
- Sodium (136–146 mEq/L, serum or heparinized plasma)
- Potassium (3.5–5.1 mEq/L, serum)
- Calcium (8.4–10.0 mg/dL, total, serum, fasting)
- Triglycerides (M: 40–160 mg/L; F: 35–135 mg/dL; serum)
- Thyroxin (serum, total T_4: 5–10 μg/dL)
- Carbon dioxide (32–48 mm/Hg $PaCO_2$, arterial)

Other Tests

- Electrocardiogram (ECG)
- Posteroanterior chest x-ray
- Rapid-sequence intravenous pyelogram

Special Tests

- When Cushing's syndrome is suspected:
  Plasma cortisol (A.M.: 5–23 μg/dL; P.M.: 3–15 μg/dL)
  24-hour urine 17-hydroxysteroid or 17-ketosteroid measurements (3–10 mg/day)
  Dexamethasone suppression test
- When renal artery stenosis is suspected:
  Radioisotope renogram (adrenoscintigraphy, CT scan, ultrasound, split renal function tests)
  Renal arteriogram
  Renal vein plasma vein activity
  Ureteral catheterization studies
- When hypokalemia points to aldosteronism:
  Plasma renin activity with sodium restriction
  Plasma aldosterone measurements
  24-hour urine aldosterone with sodium loading
  Adrenal venography
- Adrenal vein aldosterone
- Angiotensin II antagonist test: blood pressure measurements during the rapid infusion of saralasin (polypeptide)

---

primary aldosteronism and should be studied further. Patients with very high renin values may have renal artery stenosis or pheochromocytoma.

DIFFERENTIAL RENAL VEIN RENIN TEST

In patients with renovascular hypertension, the plasma renin activities are higher on the involved side. A differential renal vein renin test can be performed on patients who initially have been on a low-sodium, high-potassium diet and on diuretic medications 3 to 4 days prior to the test.[2, 18] During percutaneous catheterization under fluoroscopic guidance, blood is obtained from both renal veins and the inferior vena cava for later determinations of renin activities. Ratios of renin activity (affected side compared with unaffected side) greater than 1.5 indicate significant renovascular disease.

Pharmacologic Diagnostic Tests

A pharmacologic procedure useful for identifying defects in angiotensin II production is based on the infusion of the antagonist, saralasin, 1-(N-methylglycine)-5-valine-8-alanineangiotensin II. A reduction of 7 to 10 mm Hg in diastolic pressure in response to a rapid infusion of saralasin is a positive response. This test result correlates well with renovascular hypertension.[4, 8]

Another pharmacologic diagnostic test is the infusion of angiotensin II. In theory, hypertensive patients with renovascular hypertension show very little response from preexisting high levels of endogenous circulating angiotensin II.[1] Owing to many variables, however, this test often generates inconsistent results.

Angiotensin Assay

In normal patients, the plasma concentration of angiotensin II is 10 to 60 pg/mL. The plasma concentration of angiotensin I is less than 25 pg/mL.[28] Both polypeptides are measured with radioimmunoassay. As with any immunoassay procedure, the antisera used for angiotensin determinations often lack specificity, and reagents cross-react with many types of polypeptides. The lower limit of sensi-

Box 6–7. Plasma Renin Activities— Formation of Angiotensin I

Age (yr)	ng/mL/hr
2–4	2.37 ± 0.57
5–6	1.48 ± 0.17
7–9	2.13 ± 0.44
10–11	1.96 ± 0.36
14–15	1.18 ± 0.28
16–17	1.08 ± 0.25
Normal sodium diet	
Supine	1.6 ± 1.5
Standing	4.5 ± 2.9
Low sodium diet	
Supine	3.2 ± 1.1
Standing	9.9 ± 4.3

Box 6–8. Laboratory Renin Activity

Elevated

- Secondary aldosteronism
- Malignant or severe hypertension
- Bilateral renal disease
- Renal parenchymal disease
- Renin-secreting tumors
- Oral contraceptive induced
- Edematous normotensive states:
  Cirrhosis of the liver
  Nephrosis
  Congestive heart failure
- Hypokalemic normotensive states:
  Bartter's syndrome (JG cell)
  Kidney disease (Na and K release)
  Electrolyte loss (alimentary route)

Depressed

- Adrenal cortical disease:
  Primary aldosteronism
  Adrenal carcinoma
  Adrenal enzyme defects
  Steroid excess
- Without cortical disease:
  Liddle's syndrome
  Licorice ingestion
  Mineralocorticoids
- Normotensive patients:
  Renal parenchymal
  Autonomic disorders
  Postural hypertension
  Uninephrectomized patients
  Adrenergic blockers
  Hyperkalemia

tivity is 10 pg per sample using commercial antisera. Active proteinases may destroy angiotensin following a phlebotomy, although it has been found that Fuller's earth is capable of minimizing this problem. This agent's protective capability is probably due to the attraction and denaturing of specific enzymes on its surface that otherwise would degrade angiotensin. Drugs such as captopril or saralasin, which influence plasma renin activity, also affect the levels of angiotensin.

Evaluation of Adrenal Hypertension

Because of the biologic activity of steroids with respect to sex characteristics, many clinical symptoms are apparent in individuals with hypertension associated with mineralocorticoid abnormalities due to enzyme deficiencies and adrenal hyperplasia.[17] Depending on which hydroxylase is missing, various deficiencies and excesses are also noted in the hypertensive individual. Table 6–1 outlines these effects.

Diagnosis of excess mineralocorticoid production is based not only on the levels of steroids in the urine and blood, but also on how the secretion rates change with increases or decreases in volume. These tests can be performed following salt restriction or the ingestion of large amounts of salt over several days. Table 6–2 shows how a diagnosis can be made.

Steroid Measurements

The literature concerning the analysis of steroids in body fluids is extensive.[7, 14, 17] An approach for the analysis is based on the choice of specimen, levels encountered, accuracy needed, and method of analysis. Until the advent of sensitive analytical methods, most assay procedures focused only on urine analysis. More than 40 steroids are produced by the adrenals. Urinary and plasma cortisol determinations appear to be useful for the assessment of adrenal cortical function and have found application in clinical practice. Although other steroids and metabolites can be measured, cortisol measurements are the key to evaluating suspected abnormalities of glucocorticoid production.

The differential diagnosis of primary aldosteronism (adenoma or hyperplasia of the adrenals) from the secondary form can also be made following the administration of spironolactone.[8] Primary aldosteronism is controlled within 3 to 5 weeks, whereas the hypertension of the secondary form of aldosteronism is not. Spironolactone probably displaces aldosterone competitively from specific receptors and interferes with the normal reabsorption of sodium. Patients with adenomas can be distinguished from those with hyperplasia because the former appear to have higher aldosterone secretion rates, higher sodium and bicarbonate levels, and lower potassium levels and plasma renin activities.[7]

Diagnosis of Errors in Steroid Metabolism

METYRAPONE TEST

The rationale of this test is that 11 β-hydroxylase, the last enzyme in the biosynthesis of cortisol, is inhibited by metyrapone. As the blood level of cortisol falls, adrenocorticotropic hormone (ACTH) is released from the pituitary to stimulate the adrenal cortex to release more 11-deoxy-

---

Box 6–9. **Factors that Raise or Lower PRA Levels**

High Plasma Renin Activity

- Primary hypertension (5%–10%)
- High salt intake
- Adrenergic hypertension:
  Pheochromocytoma
  Hyperthyroidism
- Renal hypoperfusion:
  Renovascular disease
  Heart failure
  Malignant hypertension
- Renal compression:
  Tumors (JG cell or Wilms' tumor, hypernephroma, hematoma, cysts)
  Scars, bands, (Ask-Upmark kidney, perinephritis,
  radiation nephritis)
- Miscellaneous:
  Renal failure
  Glomerulonephritis
  Hydronephrosis

Low Plasma Renin Activity

- No mineralocorticoid excess:
  Essential hypertension (20%–25%)
  Race (40%–45% black persons are hypertensive)
  Reduced renal mass or responsiveness
  Reduced sympathetic activity:
    Idiopathic
    Adrenergic inhibitors (beta blockers, methyldopa, clonidine, rauwolfia derivatives)
- Mineralocorticoid excess:
  Aldosterone excess:
    Primary hyperaldosteronism
    Idiopathic hyperaldosteronism
    Congenital hyperaldosteronism
    Adrenal carcinoma
  Deoxycorticosterone (DOC) excess:
    Adrenal adenoma
    Ectopic ACTH-producing tumor
    17-α-hydroxylase deficiency
    11-β-hydroxylase deficiency
    18-Hydroxy-DOC excess

---

cortisol. Normal 11-deoxycortisol rises to more than 7 μg/dL after the metyrapone dose. Failure to respond reveals pituitary hypothalamic disease or the extraneous production of excess amounts of cortisol.

SINGLE-DOSE DEXAMETHASONE SUPPRESSION TEST

Dexamethasone suppresses the nocturnal rise in ACTH and resultant morning cortisol production in normal subjects (<3μg/dL). Patients with Cushing's syndrome, however, demonstrate cortisol levels in excess of 10 μg/dL. Patients who take phenytoin or phenobarbital may generate more cortisol because of enhanced metabolism of dexamethasone.

DIFFERENTIAL DIAGNOSIS OF CUSHING'S SYNDROME

In patients with documented elevations of cortisol, additional testing must be performed in order to identify the cause. Most cases can be attributed to a pituitary adenoma that produces excess ACTH; this is called "pituitary" Cushing's syndrome or simply Cushing's syndrome. However, adrenal adenomas, adrenocortical carcinomas, and ectopic ACTH syndromes (nonmalignant tissues that produce excess ACTH) must also be considered. Table 6–3 shows a differential diagnosis of Cushing's syndrome. The differential diagnosis of pituitary Cushing's syndrome from other causes is clearly made with the dexamethasone suppression test.

SALINE SUPPRESSION TEST

The rapid infusion of normal saline should suppress plasma aldosterone levels in normal patients, but not in individuals with primary aldosteronism, which is characterized by hypertension and hypokalemia. After the patient has been in an upright position for 2 hours, blood is drawn to determine the baseline aldosterone values. Next, while

---

Table 6–1. **Types of Metabolic Blocks In Adrenal Hyperplasia**

Missing Enzyme	Deficient	Excess	Phenotype
Desmolase	All steroids	Lipids in adrenals	Adrenal insufficiency
3β-ol-Dehydrogenase	Corticoids Andosterone	Dehydroepiandosterone	Salt-loser; male, hypospadias; female, mild virilism
17-hydroxylase	Androgens Estrogens Cortisol Andosterone	Corticosterone, 11-deoxycorticosterone	Immature female Hypertension Low potassium Alkalosis
21-hydroxylase	Aldosterone Corticoids	Androgens	Masculinization
11-hydroxylase	Corticoids Aldosterone	Androgens, 11-deoxycorticosterone	Masculinization Hypertension
18-hydroxylase	Aldosterone	Corticosterone	Salt-loser

Table 6–2. Renin-Aldosterone and Blood Volume Correlations in Diagnosis of Adrenal Hypertension

Stimulus	Secretion of Renin			Secretion of Aldosterone		
	Essential Hypertension	Renovascular Hypertension	Aldosterone	Essential Hypertension	Renovascular Hypertension	Aldosterone
Increased circulating volume (high salt intake, >100 mEq/day)	Down	Down	Down	Down	Varies	Up
Decreased circulating volume (low salt intake, only 10 mEq/day or acute diuresis and upright posture)	Varies	Up	Down	Up	Up	Up

the patient is in a supine position, 2 L of saline (0.9g/dL) is infused over 4 hours. Subsequent aldosterone determination in normal patients yield values less than 5 ng/dL, whereas patients with primary aldosteronism have plasma aldosterone levels in excess of 5 ng/dL.

FLUDROCORTISONE SUPPRESSION TEST

Fludrocortisone, a cortisone acetate that is fluorinated at the 9 position, suppresses the production of aldosterone in normal subjects, yet not in subjects with primary aldosteronism. In this test, the drug is administered at intervals over a period of 3 days. Twenty-four-hour urine collections are obtained for the measurements of aldosterone 1 day prior to and on the third (last) day after exposure to fludrocortisone. Normal subjects have urine aldosterone values less than 20 µg/day. Primary aldosterone patients have values greater than 20 µg/day.

Evaluation for Pheochromocytoma

The definitive diagnosis of pheochromocytoma is made through measurements of urinary catecholamines and their metabolites. Urinary excretion of catecholamines is elevated in more than 95% of patients with pheochromocytoma, regardless of the extent of the blood pressure. Any stress may exacerbate the excretion of catecholamines in normotensive individuals and may lead to false-positive results. The reference ranges of catecholamines are shown in Box 6–10. If the excreted catecholamines contain less than 20% epinephrine, the tumor is still in the adrenals.[28]

CATECHOLAMINE MEASUREMENT

Plasma. Because blood catecholamines are present at very low concentrations (pg/mL),[2, 28] specific methods that also possess high sensitivity and good selectivity must be

employed. Currently, the method of choice for fractionated catecholamine determination is high-pressure liquid chromatography (HPLC) with electrochemical detection.

In order to obtain valid laboratory results, an indwelling intravenous (IV) line is required for the collection of blood samples. This procedure eliminates patient stress, which may cause transitory increases in circulating catecholamines. The posture of the patient must be correctly maintained to obtain accurate catecholamine baseline values. Finally, cooled blood samples must be centrifuged immediately, and the plasma quickly separated, to obtain accurate catecholamine levels that otherwise may be depressed owing to red blood cell metabolism. Patients with pheochromocytoma generally have markedly elevated levels compared with those of normal patients.

Urine. Because measurement of plasma catecholamines presents a number of difficulties, urinary measuremets are preferred. Urine catecholamines and their metabolites can be quantitatively measured by means of chemical reactions that generate fluorescent products,[17, 18] although this approach possesses many analytical problems. Drugs that can be made to be or are fluorescent (e.g., ampicillin, methyldopa, promethazine, protamine, aspirin, sulfonamides, vitamin B complex), as well as certain beverages (containing cocoa, coffee, tea, etc.) and foods (i.e., bananas, vanilla extract, citrus fruits) often can interfere with the fluorometric assays. In addition, laboratory lighting can photochemically degrade catecholamines and their fluorescent products, fluorophors. Brown or red glassware or subdued laboratory lighting can be employed to reduce analytical variability.

Greater sensitivity can be achieved in urine assays by the hydrolysis of glucuronide and sulfate conjugates. Significant amounts of catecholamine-related compounds are excreted as conjugates. Many urine assay methods have been published; however, most employ enzymatic hydroly-

Table 6–3. Differential Diagnosis of Cushing's Syndrome

Underlying Disease State	Plasma ACTH	Dexamethasone Suppression Test	Metyrapone Test
Pituitary Cushing's syndrome (bilateral adrenal hyperplasia)	Normal to slight elevation	Positive	Positive
Ectopic ACTH production	Very high	Negative	Negative
Adrenal adenoma	Low	Negative	Variable
Adrenal carcinoma	Low	Negative	Negative

Box 6–10.	Reference (Abnormal) Ranges of Catecholamine and Metabolites

Urine

Norepinephrine: 10–70 μg/24 hr
Epinephrine: 0–20 μg/24 hr
(Total catecholamines: >250 μg/24 hr)
Normetanephrine plus metanephrine:
   <1.3 mg/24 hr
Vanillylmandelic acid: 1.8–9.0 mg/24 hr
(Metabolite: >10 mg/24 hr)
Dopamine: <200 μg/24 hr

Blood (Plasma)

Catecholamines: <1000 pg/mL
Norepinephrine: 104–548 pg/mL
Epinephrine: <88 p/mL

Adrenal medulla

Norepinephrine: 0.04–0.16 mg/g of tissue
Epinephrine: 0.22–0.84 mg/g of tissue

sis, followed by organic solvent extractions, concentration of a residue, acetylation with an appropriate derivatization reagent (e.g., perfluorobutyrate), and gas chromatographic analysis with an electron capture detector. This approach enables a complete chemical profile of all catecholamines and metabolites in a 24-hour urine sample to be obtained.

Metanephrine. Most authorities recommend the measurement of urinary metanephrine as the first test for pheochromocytoma.[28] Very few false-negative results are observed, and only rarely are false-positive results encountered. False-positive results are most often seen in severely stressed patients. In these individuals, false-positive results are ruled out when catecholamines are measured at a later time, when the patient is relaxed. The urinary values of metanephrine are expressed in relation to creatinine. A normal value (metanephrine-creatinine ratio) is less than 1.2 μg metanephrine/mg creatinine.

Clonidine Suppression Test. Clonidine significantly suppresses the production of catecholamines in normal subjects but not in patients with pheochromocytoma.[31] Clonidine is given orally to a recumbent patient. From an indwelling IV line, blood samples are then taken for the determination of plasma catecholamine levels before and after a 3-hour period. Plasma norepinephrine levels that remain constant or elevated at 3 hours strongly point to pheochromocytoma.

Vanillylmandelic Acid and Other Metabolites. In certain patients with pheochromocytoma, the production and metabolism of catecholamines may be intermittent, or the uptake and degradation of catecholamines (half-life approximately 2 minutes) may be so great that normal or near-normal levels of catecholamines are observed in the blood or urine. In these patients, however, metabolites of cate-

cholamines are elevated, pointing to the underlying disease state. The principal end product of norepinephrine and epinephrine is vanillylmandelic acid (VMA). This metabolite reflects total catecholamines rather than the specific catecholamines.[28] In addition, although urinary VMA measurements are more specific, they are less sensitive and more subject to diet and drugs than metanephrine-creatinine determinations.

The urinary excretion of norepinephrine precursors, dopa, dopamine, and metabolites (homovanillic acid and 3-methoxytyramine), are more commonly identified with neuroblastomas. Malignant pheochromocytomas also often secrete dopa, dopamine, and their metabolites. Benign tumors in adults do not secrete these compounds.

PHARMACOLOGIC APPROACHES

A pharmacologic approach can also be applied to the diagnosis of phenochromocytoma. This approach is somewhat dangerous because it either temporarily blocks the action of circulating catecholamines or enhances the release of catecholamines from tissue reserve.[8] One example, phentolamine, an alpha-adrenergic blocking drug, is given intravenously to reduce blood pressure. A very small dose (1 mg) produces a profound effect in patients with pheochromocytoma. A blood pressure drop of 35/25 mm Hg lasting 4 minutes or longer is considered a positive phentolamine test result. A simultaneous fall in blood glucose and rise in insulin are also noted as a positive response.

Another pharmacologic approach is the administration of histamine, which releases catecholamines from nerve endings, or glucagon, which stimulates glycogenolysis in tissue stores. A blood pressure rise of 50/25 mm Hg is highly indicative of pheochromocytoma. Urinalyses to determine the ratio of epinephrine and norepinephrine are very useful to ascertain tumor location. If norepinephrine accounts for greater than 80% of the two, the tumor is not on the adrenals. Urinary vanillylmandelic acid–catecholamine ratios are also valuable to ascertain the size of catecholamine-secreting tumors. If the ratio favors epinephrine and norepinephrine, the tumor is newly active and typically less than 50 grams. Large tumors are able to metabolize more of the catecholamines and generate more metabolite, so the ratio of products favors vanillylmandelic acid.

TREATMENT AND PROGNOSIS
Primary Hypertension

The prognosis of patients with primary hypertension is quite good if the disease does not progress to the malignant form. No known therapy can correct and reverse the course of the disease. Long-term reduction of the blood pressure does appear beneficial. It is now well established that exercise, meditation, avoidance of emotional stress, and control of overeating or intemperate drinking can lower blood pressures of many individuals with primary hypertension.[1, 14, 32] Restriction of sodium chloride intake to less than 1 gram per day significantly lowers the blood pressure in more than one-third of patients with primary hypertension.

The number of drugs and drug combinations used to

treat primary hypertension has dramatically increased. Not only has the number of drugs in each treatment category risen, but the number of categories has increased. Successful hypertensive treatment does not merely lower elevated blood pressure; it should also reduce the cardiovascular risk factors (which promote stroke, heart attacks, congestive heart failure, renal dysfunction) while maintaining the patient's remaining health assets. A drug regimen may occasionally reduce blood pressure at the expense of other body functions, which may be intolerable for some patients (e.g., tachycardia, impotence, increased lipids, decreased HDL cholesterol, muted response to hypothyroidism or hypoglycemia, or dry cough). There is much discussion in the medical literature about the application of hypertensive treatment research data to clinical situations. Differences of opinions do exist. Clinical observation and judgment cannot be overemphasized in the treatment of chronic conditions such as hypertension.

Useful drugs included in the treatment of primary hypertension are as follows:

β-Adrenergic Blockers

β-Adrenergic blocking agents are effective for the treatment of hypertension, but the mechanisms of action are unclear. Reduced cardiac output, decreased norepinephrine release at postganglionic sympathetic nerve endings, reduced renin secretion, and suppressed central sympathetic outflow are regarded as possible mechanisms.[32, 33] β-blockers have been shown in controlled trials to decrease mortality in patients with hypertension and in patients who have suffered myocardial infarction.[34]

β-Adrenergic blockers may be less effective in black patients. However, the β-blocker Labetalol (Normodyne) combines nonselective β-blockade with α-adrenergic receptor blockade. It appears equally effective in black and in white patients, and does not affect serum triglycerides as do some other β-blockers. Orthostatic hypotension is more of a concern than with other β-blockers.[35]

Diuretics

Like β-blockers, diuretics have been shown to decrease mortality in patients with hypertension.[32] Hydrochlorothiazide (HCTZ) and chlorthalidone are two of the thiazide-type diuretics that continue to be widely used to treat hypertension. Research has shown that single-drug regimens using doses as low as 12.5 mg daily and combinations with other drugs as low as 6.25 mg daily are effective hypertension therapy with reduced magnitudes of side effects, compared with previous regimens, especially for elderly patients.[36, 37] Diuretics and calcium channel blockers are more effective than β-blockers and ACE inhibitors for hypertension control in blacks.[38]

Potassium-sparing diuretics are often combined with potassium-losing diuretics to correct or prevent hypokalemia. Caution is urged to prevent hyperkalemia with these diuretic drugs as well as with the potassium-sparing single agents.

Calcium Channel Blocking Agents

Calcium channel blockers are excellent hypertensive medications, are well tolerated, but have become the subject of considerable debate in the current medical literature.[39–41] Calcium channel blockers cause vasodilatation, which decreases peripheral resistance and induces variable cardiac response. The class of short-acting dihydropyridines are chemically diverse and have been shown in some clinical settings to be associated with great mortality from myocardial infarction.

Side effects of calcium channel blockers vary but are generally mild. These agents do not affect serum lipids as do the diuretics and β-blockers, but they should be used with caution with β-blockers.[42]

Angiotensin-Converting Enzyme (ACE) Inhibitors

ACE inhibitors are very well tolerated by hypertensive patients, but apparently are less effective in blacks than in whites.[42] They have no effect on plasma lipid concentrations or glucose tolerance.[43, 44] They appear to preserve renal function in diabetics.[45, 46] The most common side effect of ACE inhibitors is a dry cough,[47] which cromolyn (Intal) may relieve.[48] Potential for hyperkalemia is reported with ACE inhibitors, particularly in patients taking potassium-sparing diuretics or those with decreased renal function. Some patients with high levels of plasma renin activity may be too sensitive (large hypotensive response) to ACE inhibitors, including volume-depleted and diuretic patients. Angioedema occurs in 0.1% to 0.2% of patients taking this antihypertensive drug class, and may be serious to life threatening.[42] ACE inhibitors are not to be used in pregnant women because of the risk of fetal injury and death.[49]

Angiotensin Receptor Antagonist

A new anti-hypertensive is entering the marketplace. An angiotensin receptor antagonist interferes with the attachment of angiotensin II to angiotensin I receptors. This agent for blood pressure treatment may prove as effective as the ACE inhibitors, without the dry cough. It may also prove less effective in black patients.[42]

Secondary Hypertension

The successful treatment of secondary hypertension is based on the identification and treatment of the underlying disease,[2] as discussed in the following section.

Renovascular Hypertension

The prognosis of the disease depends upon the age of the patient, extent of renovascular disease, duration of the hypertension, and selection of the appropriate surgical approach. Surgery is usually employed for endarterectomy, bypass grafts utilizing synthetic grafts or the patient's own veins, and complete revascularization of the affected areas. Nephrectomy is the treatment of choice only in advanced parenchymal disease secondary to vascular problems. In one study, long-term observations of a large group of patients who underwent unilateral nephrectomy in connection with arterial hypertension revealed a 73% remission of arterial hypertension and a return to normal or an improvement in the course of the disease. Arterial hypertension continued in 18% of the cases, and death occurred in 9%, in the first 6 years following nephrectomy. Partial nephrectomy is also beneficial in partially cystic and infarcted kidneys.

Acute Glomerulonephritis

Most cases of acute glomerulonephritis are related to infections (typically, β-hemolytic group A streptococci). Penicillin is the drug of choice. Some patients may take 2 months to 2 years to show normal urinalysis and return to normal hypertensive values.

Chronic Glomerulonephritis

Most patients who have chronic glomerulonephritis had, at one time, episodes of acute glomerulonephritis. No specific treatment is known, and in the asymptomatic phase, no therapy appears to be needed. Only when hypertension is apparent and sustained is drug therapy warranted.

Nephrotic Syndrome

Patients with edema, heavy albuminuria, hyperlipidemia, low blood albumin, and hypertension are candidates for nephrotic syndrome. Children generally recover. Adults who progress to glomerulosclerosis generally have a poor prognosis. Treatment with prednisone helps with remission. Steroids do not help with infection-induced nephrotic disease. Azathioprine and cyclophosphamide have been used successfully in patients with no response to steroids. Diuretics, low-sodium diet, and correction of potassium depletion significantly aid in the control of nephrotic syndrome.

Arteriolar Nephrosclerosis

Kidney lesions involving the small glomerular arterioles are often associated with hypertension. Although the kidney is affected, the patient is usually asymptomatic.[13] Death usually results from cardiac failure or cerebral hemorrhage with uremia.

Benign nephrosclerosis is usually seen in adults from 35 to 55 years of age. In these individuals, hypertension is recorded prior to any urinalysis changes. This contrasts with the diagnosis of glomerulonephritis, in which the urinalysis changes are observed before any hypertension is noted. Typically, treatment is similar to that of primary hypertension. Normal renal function is desired to aid in the repair of the sclerotic tissue. No treatment is required other than the control of the hypertension.

Chronic Pyelonephritis

A bacterial infection is most often associated with pyelonephritis. However, the prolonged abuse of analgesics containing phenacetin or other nephrotoxins can also lead to tissue destruction. The treatment of the underlying infection is most important in controlling pyelonephritis. No known treatment is known to stop the progressive deterioration of the renal function, and secondary hypertension is a final outcome.

Pheochromocytoma

When catecholamines are indicated as the underlying cause of the hypertension, surgical procedures are utilized (except in cases of malignant disorders).

Hyperparathyroidism

Often associated with kidney stones, hyperparathyroidism can be treated surgically. A successful cure depends on the removal of the excess functioning tissue and reversal of the renal damage. Typically, after surgery, the urine calcium phosphate falls to near zero. Vitamin D therapy may be needed for 1 to 2 months to stimulate a rise in circulating calcium.

Cushing's Syndrome

The successful therapy for Cushing's syndrome is based on correcting the hyperfunction of the adrenal cortex. Initially, heavy particle irradiation of the pituitary has been used to decrease tissue mass and hormone synthesis. This approach is successful in about 20% of the patients. If this approach fails, bilateral adrenalectomy has been used if the hypertension cannot be controlled and the clinical course demands a surgical intervention. Most steroid- or ACTH-producing neoplasms are surgically removed. Metastatic forms of the disease have a poor prognosis. Metyrapone can be administered as an adrenal inhibitor and to control any hypokalemia resulting from a hyperfunction of the adrenal cortex.

Case Study 1

A 43-year-old man presented to the hospital emergency room in a confused state. He was unable to move the left side of his body, his skin was cold and moist, and the blood pressure in both arms was 240/195 mm Hg. The pulse was 140 beats/min and regular. His temperature was 101.6 °F. Funduscopic examination revealed grade 2 hypertensive retinopathy that changed rapidly with the development of necrotizing arteriolitis.

The hematocrit was 60%, and the white cell count was 20.0×10^9L, with 85% neutrophils. The specific gravity of the urine was 1.020, with a + + + test for albumin and with a few coarse and finely granular casts per high-power field in the sediment. The blood urea nitrogen level was 60 mg, the creatinine 4.4 mg, and fasting blood sugar 114 mg/dL. The serum sodium value was 145 mEq/L, the potassium 3.7 mEq/L, and the chloride 110 mEq/L. Plasma renin and cortisol values were all normal.

The patient was treated initially with reserpine. After the second 1-mg injection, however, the blood pressure dropped to zero. He remained cold and clammy; the output of urine was negligible, and the venous pressure was also low. An infusion of 500 mL of dextran restored the blood pressure to 160/110 mm Hg.

On the second day of admission, the blood pressure varied from 180/120 to 240/140 mm Hg and was unresponsive to IV injections of reserpine. An IV injection of 5 mg of phentolamine lowered the pressure to 98/60 mm Hg. Dibenzyline was administered by mouth, but it did not control the blood pressure. With intermittent phentolamine injections, the blood pressure was controlled, and on the third day, the neurologic symptoms cleared.

Urinary excretion of VMA and catecholamines was not increased. A renal arteriogram was normal. The patient was discharged with a blood pressure of 140/100 mm Hg. His medications consisted of hydrochlorothiazide and hydralazine daily. The patient returned to the hospital frequently with acute hypertension. One minute after his hands and wrists were immersed in ice water, the blood pressure would rise dramatically. He would go into shock following small doses of pharmacologic agents or when a minimum of blood was removed. Clinical laboratory results could not support a diagnosis of pheochromocytoma. This patient was finally diagnosed as having sudden (paroxysmal) hypertension,[30] with clinical, hemodynamic, and metabolic hypersensitivity and possible signs of sympathoadrenal discharge. His condition was finally controlled with guanethidine and a diuretic.

Questions

1. Do the laboratory findings support the diagnosis of primary hypertension with an underlying hemodynamic etiology?
2. Why were the laboratory studies apparently not ordered immediately when the patient presented to the emergency department?

Discussion

1. The laboratory findings do not indicate primary or secondary hypertension of renal origin, nor do the cortisol catecholamine and VMA results indicate adrenal hypertension or pheochromocytoma.
2. The clinical findings in this patient indicated a hypertensive emergency: malignant hypertension with rapid funduscopic changes. In this situation, the patient must be stabilized before differential diagnostic studies can be performed.

Case Study 2

A 49-year-old man entered the hospital with an 18-month history of "lightheadedness." Blood pressure determinations on multiple occasions over 10 days were between 190/110 and 220/136 mm Hg. Readings were the same in both arms. Examination of the blood showed a hemoglobin of 15.1 g/dL, a hematocrit of 45% and a white blood cell count of 10.0×10^9/L. The specific gravity of the urine was 1.015 with a normal sediment. The blood urea nitrogen level was 21 mg, and the creatinine 1.6 mg/dL. Electrolytes and fasting blood sugar results were normal.

A renal arteriogram substantiated the history of the patient's right kidney removal 13 years earlier and showed that his left kidney was functioning normally. However, there was a clear sign of left renal artery narrowing. Before surgical opening of the renal artery, the blood pressure was 55/40 mm Hg distal to the stenosis. It was 140/90 immediately following repair.

The patient's blood pressure 3 years after surgery was 130/90 mm Hg, and his dizzy spells had been eliminated.

Question

The serum creatinine was just out of the reference range (0.6–1.3 mg/dL). Would this value have given any indication of renal compromise?

Discussions

Creatinine values alone are not a sensitive indicator of early renal disease. However, in this patient, slightly elevated creatinine values pointed to chronic renal functional impairment and would tend to make one suspect renal involvement.

References

1. Conn R (ed): Current Diagnosis 7. Philadelphia, WB Saunders, 1985.
2. Nies AS: Hypertension. *In* Melmon K, Morrelli HF (eds): Clinical Pharmacology, ed 2. New York, Macmillan, 1978.
3. Hypertension in the USA and USSR: Basic, Clinical and Population Research. Second USA-USSR Joint Symposium, Williamsburg, VA, May 14–16, 1979, NIH Publication No. 80-2016. Bethesda, Md, National Institutes of Health, 1980.
4. Chobanian AV: Hypertension. Clin Symp 34:3–32, 1982.
5. Heymans C (ed): The Pathogenesis of Essential Hypertension—Proceedings of the Prague Symposium. New York, Macmillan, 1962.
6. Philips T, Distler A: Hypertension: Mechanism and Management. New York, Springer-Verlag, 1980.
7. Whitley RJ, Meikle AW, Watts NB: Endocrinology. *In* Burtis CA, Ashwood ER (eds): Textbook of Clinical Chemistry, ed 2. Philadelphia, WB Saunders, 1994.
8. Bauer J: Differential Diagnosis of Internal Diseases. New York, Grune & Stratton, 1967.
9. Nies AS: Shock. *In* Melmon K, Morrelli HF (eds): Clinical Pharmacology, ed 2. New York, Macmillan, 1978.
10. Smith L, Wyngaarden, J (eds): Review of General Internal Medicine: A Self-Assessment Manual. Philadelphia, WB Saunders, 1980.
11. Muehrcke RC, Kark RM, Pirani CH, et al: Biopsy of the kidney in the diagnosis and management of renal disease. N Engl J Med 253:537–546, 1955.
12. Krupp MA: Physician's Handbook, ed 21. Los Altos, Cal, Lange Medical Products, 1982.
13. Imber I, Clymer RH: Obstruction of the renal artery producing malignant hypertension. N Engl J Med 252:301–304, 1955.
14. Marable SA, Moore FT, Schieve JF, et al: Treatment of hypertension associated with the solitary ischemic kidney. N Engl J Med 275:1278–1282, 1966.
15. Fruchtman M, Caldwell JR: Hypertension due to renal infarction. N Engl J Med 263:907–909, 1960.
16. Margolin EG, Merrill JP, Harrison JH: Diagnosis of hypertension due to occlusions of the renal artery. N Engl J Med 256:581–588, 1957.
17. Henry JB, Alexander DR, Eng CD, et al: Evaluation of endocrine function. *In* Henry JB (ed): Clinical Diagnosis and Management of Laboratory Methods, ed 19. Philadelphia, WB Saunders. 1996.
18. Brunjes S: Catecholamine metabolism in essential hypertension. N Engl J Med 271:120–124, 1964.

19. Masland RP, Heald FP, Goodale WT, et al: Hypertensive vascular disease in adolescence. N Engl J Med 255:894–897, 1956.
20. Epstein FH, Freedman LR, Levitan H, et al: Hypercalcemia, nephrocalcinosis and reversible renal insufficiency associated with hyperthyroidism. N Engl J Med 258:782–785, 1958.
21. Shaw RS: Acute dissecting aortic aneurysm. N Engl J Med 253:331–333, 1955.
22. Agress C, Estrin HM: Biochemical Diagnosis of Heart Disease. Springfield, IL, Charles C Thomas, 1963.
23. Silver EN, Katz LN: Heart Disease. New York, Macmillan, 1975.
24. Hurst JW, Schlant RC, Alexander RW (eds): The Heart, New York, McGraw-Hill, 1994.
25. Rayburn W, Zuspan F (eds): Drug Therapy in Obstetrics and Gynecology, ed 2. St Louis, Mosby, 1992.
26. Ewald CA, McKenzie CR: Manual of Medical Therapeutics, ed 28. Boston, Little, Brown, 1995.
27. Collins RD: Illustrated Manual of Laboratory Diagnosis. Philadelphia, JB Lippincott, 1968.
28. Pruden EL, McPherson RA (eds): Clinical Guide to Laboratory Tests. Philadelphia, WB Saunders, 1995.
29. Hoffman WS: The Biochemistry of Clinical Medicine, ed 4. Chicago, Yearbook Medical, 1973.
30. Cohn JN: Paroxysmal hypertension and hypovolemia. N Engl J Med 275:643–646, 1966.
31. Krupp K, Chatton MJ, Werdegard D: Current Medical Treatment. Los Altos, CA, Lange Medical, 1985.
32. Landsberg L, Young JB: Physiology and pharmacology of the autonomic nervous system. *In* Isselbacher KJ, Braunwald E, Wilson JD, et al (eds): Harrison's Principles of Internal Medicine, ed 12. New York, McGraw–Hill, 1994.
33. Williams GH: Hypertensive vascular disease. *In* Isselbacher KJ, Braunwald E, Wilson JD, et al (eds): Harrison's Principles of Internal Medicine, ed 12. New York, McGraw–Hill, 1994.
34. Drugs for Hypertension. Med Lett Drugs Ther 37:926, 1995.
35. Materson BJ, et al: Single-drug therapy for hypertension in men. N Engl J Med 328:914–921, 1993.
36. Siscovick DS, Raghunathau TE, Psaty BM, et al: Diuretic therapy for hypertension and the risk of primary cardiac arrest. N Engl J Med 330:1852–1857, 1994.
37. Is indapamid (Lozol) safer than a thiazide? Med Lett Drugs Ther 31:103, 1989.
38. Drugs for hypertension. Med Lett Drugs Ther 31:50, 1995.
39. Fagan TC: Calcium antagonists and mortality [editorial]. Arch Intern Med 155:2145, 1995.
40. Epstein M: Calcium antagonists should continue to be used for first-line treatment of hypertension [commentary]. Arch Intern Med 155:2150, 1995.
41. Furberg CD: Should dihydropyridines be used, as first-line treatment of hypertension?—the con side [commentary]. Arch Intern Med 155:2157, 1995.
42. Drugs for hypertension. Med Lett Drugs Ther 37:948–949, 1995.
43. Drugs for chronic heart failure. Med Lett Drugs Ther 35:41, 1993.
44. An ACE inhibitor after a myocardial infarction. Med Lett Drugs Ther 36:69, 1994.
45. Lewis EJ, Huntsicker LG, Bain RP, et al: The effect of angiotensin-converting enzyme inhibition on diabetic nephropathy. N Engl J Med 329:1456–1462, 1993.
46. Ravid M, Savin H, Jutrin I, et al: Long-term stabilizing effect of angiotensin-converting enzyme inhibition on plasma creatinine and on proteinuria in normotensive type II diabetic patients. Ann Intern Med 118:577–581, 1993.
47. Ravid D: Angiotensin-converting enzyme inhibitors and cough: A prospective evaluation in hypertension and in congestive heart failure. J Clin Pharmacol 34:1116–1120, 1994.
48. Hargreaves MR, Benson MK: Inhaled sodium cromoglycate in angiotensin-converting enzyme inhibition cough. Lanced 345:13–16, 1995.
49. Shotan A, Wilderhorn J, Hurst A, et al: Risk of angiotensin-converting enzyme inhibition during pregnancy: Experimental and clinical evidence, potential mechanisms, and recommendations for use. Am J Med 96:451–456, 1994.

Heart Failure

Lynn Ingram

Heart failure is a clinical condition that results from failure of the heart to pump blood effectively. Often used interchangeably with heart failure, the term *congestive heart failure* (CHF) refers to a group of symptoms resulting from fluid accumulation in the lungs, throughout the body, or both. The National Heart, Lung, and Blood Institute describes the condition as follows:

> Heart failure occurs when an abnormality of cardiac function causes the heart to fail to pump blood at a rate required by the metabolizing tissues or when the heart can do so only with an elevated filling pressure. The heart's inability to pump a sufficient amount of blood to meet the needs of the body tissues may be due to insufficient or defective cardiac filling and/or impaired contraction and emptying. Compensatory mechanisms increase blood volume and raise cardiac filling pressures, heart rate, and cardiac muscle mass to maintain the heart's pumping function and cause redistribution of blood flow. Eventually, however, despite these compensatory mechanisms, the ability of the heart to contract and relax declines progressively, and the heart failure worsens.[1]

CHF affects approximately 1 of every 100 people in the United States, and it is estimated that 2 million people are being treated for heart failure.[2] More than 400,000 people are diagnosed annually with CHF, and the Framingham Study estimates that the prevalence of CHF increases progressively with age from about 1% prevalence in those aged 50 to 59 years to a prevalence of about 10% in persons aged 80 to 89 years.[3]

ETIOLOGY AND PATHOPHYSIOLOGY

The causes of CHF are diverse (Box 7–1). CHF may result if the heart muscle is weakened, as occurs with cardiomyopathies, myocardial ischemia, myocardial infarction, or myocarditis. Heart failure may also result if the heart is stressed beyond its ability to respond, which might occur with a severe infection, profound anemia, or pulmonary embolism. In addition, an inefficient pumping action that develops with arrhythmias or valvular heart disease frequently leads to CHF.

For whatever reason, if the heart is unable to pump efficiently, then a diminished cardiac output occurs. If the left side of the heart fails, excess fluid accumulates in the lungs, leading to pulmonary edema and diminishing the output to the systemic circulation. The kidneys respond to this decreased blood flow with excessive fluid retention that actually makes the heart failure worse. If the right side of the heart fails, excess fluid accumulates in the systemic venous circulatory system, and generalized edema results. Diminished blood flow to the lungs and to the left side of the heart also occurs, resulting in decreased cardiac output to systemic arterial circulation.

Coronary Artery Disease

Coronary artery disease (CAD) is the most common cause of heart failure in the United States. Management

---

Box 7–1. Causes of Congestive Heart Failure

Ischemic heart disease
Cardiomyopathies
Valvular heart disease
Hypertension
Alcoholism
Myocarditis
Infiltrative disorders
Congenital heart disease
Idiopathy

---

and prognosis for CHF caused by CAD are poor, with an average annual mortality of 30% to 40%.[4]

Atherosclerosis of myocardial blood vessels leads to *ischemia*, a process causing active cardiac muscle to be replaced with fibrous material that does not function as cardiac muscle. The occlusion of cardiac vessels reduces blood flow and forces the heart to use anaerobic metabolism, the products of which can quickly damage the tissue cells. Necrosis occurs, leading to loss of cardiac muscle mass. A decrease in cardiac mass increases the load carried by the remaining viable tissue, resulting in increased cardiac stress and damage. See Chapter 4 for further discussion of coronary artery disease.

Cardiomyopathies

Cardiomyopathy is a term used to describe a group of cardiac conditions resulting from abnormalities of the heart muscle or myocardium in contrast to those that occur as a result of hypertension, valvular disease, coronary artery disease, or congenital heart defects. The three anatomic and physiologic categories of cardiomyopathies are dilated cardiomyopathy, restrictive cardiomyopathy, and hypertrophic cardiomyopathy.

The primary defect in all dilated cardiomyopathies is an abnormality in heart muscle contraction. When the heart is unable to contract efficiently, the heart dilates out of proportion, resulting in an enlarged heart with relatively thin cardiac walls. This increases the stress on the cardiac walls and restricts blood flow to the heart muscle itself, leading to further cardiac dysfunction. In most cases, the originating myocardial insult is unknown, but the result is a replacement of myocardial cells with fibrous connective tissue. Dilated cardiomyopathy may be the result of an autoimmune response, small blood vessel disease, or direct myocardial toxicity, as appears in alcohol-induced cardiomyopathy and anthracycline cardiotoxicity. Alcohol is harmful to cardiac tissue and is a significant factor in the development of dilated cardiomyopathy in 20% to 30% of patients.[5] A multitude of biochemical changes associated with excessive alcohol intake weaken the heart muscle and adversely affect blood flow, pumping pressures, and tissue tone. Arteriolar constriction caused by ethanol results in peripheral edema and pulmonary problems that complicate the cardiomyopathy.

Patients with restrictive cardiomyopathy exhibit an abnormal increase in diastolic pressure, resulting in reduced ventricular filling and distribution of reduced ventricular blood volume to the body. This condition can be caused by an intrinsically abnormal myocardium, infiltration of the myocardium with collagen or other abnormal proteins, endomyocardial disease, or space-occupying lesions (thrombi or tumors).[5]

Amyloidosis is a condition causing the deposit of fibrous proteins in various tissues. As a factor in the development of restrictive cardiomyopathy, it is second only to idiopathic causes. Patients with restrictive cardiomyopathy as a result of amyloidosis have a very poor prognosis. *Hemochromatosis*, an infiltration of iron into tissues, can adversely affect heart muscle and lead to loss of contractility and muscle function. Iron is probably the best known metal infiltrate, but other metals such as arsenic, lead,

or magnesium have also been implicated in restrictive cardiomyopathy.

Hypertrophic cardiomyopathy is characterized by hypertrophy of the ventricular septum, which is out of proportion to the other ventricular walls, and is often called asymmetric septal hypertrophy (ASH). ASH appears to be inherited as an autosomal dominant trait in 50% to 75% of cases, but the etiology of many abnormal hypertrophy cases remains unknown.

Inflammatory Heart Disease

Inflammation and immune-mediated mechanisms can be responsible for cardiac injury, although most cases of inflammatory heart disease resolve spontaneously without serious long-term sequelae. Viral myocarditis is the most common cause of inflammatory heart disease, but it can also be a result of bacterial and parasitic infections, an immunologic injury to the tissues, or an idiopathic cause. Numerous types of organisms adversely affect the normal heart tissue (Table 7–1).

The immunologic injury seen in rheumatic fever is an example of the type of myocarditis that occurs with many infections. In rheumatic fever, the bacterial antigens cross-react with circulating antibodies to form complexes that deposit in the myocardium, resulting in destruction of tissue leading to myocardial weakness and loss of cardiac wall tone. The patient often has symptoms of weakness, fever, and/or joint pain that mask the myocardial involvement. Inflammation of the pericardium causes fluid to accumulate in the pericardial space, constricting the heart and altering stroke volumes. Resolution of the inflammatory process may leave adhesions between the visceral and parietal membranes of the pericardium that restrict the contraction of the heart muscle and interfere with pumping function.

The restrictive characteristics of myocarditis are also seen in idiopathic states. Most common is the development of pericarditis after myocardial infarction involving areas adjacent to the pericardium. A fibrous buildup occurs with correction of the pericarditis that complicates the recovery from myocardial infarctions and may lead to CHF.

Valvular Heart Disease

CHF is an extremely serious complication of valvular heart disease. It indicates that the valve lesion is severe, and it is often closely related to a deterioration in the

Table 7–1. Organisms Known to Cause Myocarditis

Bacterial	Protozoal	Viral
Corynebacterium diphtheriae	*Trypanosoma cruzi*	Coxsackie B enterovirus
Treponema pallidum	*Toxoplasma gondii*	Echovirus
Borrelia recurrentis	*Taenia echinococcus*	Cytomegalovirus
Rickettsia		Influenza virus
Chlamydia		Infectious mononucleosis
Coxiella		Poliovirus
Mycoplasma pneumoniae		Measles
		Hepatitis
		Psittacosis

patient's clinical course. Valvular malfunctions alter the blood volume that the heart must regulate. Valves that remain only partially open cause inefficient pumping action and backup of blood into heart and lung circulation. Valves that remain partially closed throughout pumping result in inappropriate ventricular filling and emptying. Valvular disorders may be congenital or the result of infection. The endocarditis of rheumatic fever and the stenosis of other infections have been discussed in Chapter 5. Valvular damage in a patient with myocardial infarction can be precipitated by rupture of the papillary muscles, which causes the valve to retain partial function, although it no longer closes completely or opens sufficiently. Such patients will progress to cardiac failure as the blood volume changes alter blood load for ventricles and atria. The progression to CHF in these patients depends on the severity of valvular damage. Factors such as hypertension, total area of ischemia, or increase in immunologic complexes may cause the development of thrombi, which can either remain within the ventricle or pass through, posing a risk for reducing blood output and increasing back pressure. Thrombi that obstruct valve openings prevent blood flow and increase the risk of heart failure.

Congenital Heart Disease

Unlike many of the disorders in adults with acquired heart disease for which the development of CHF necessitates the risk of surgery, most congenital heart defects are corrected or palliated before the development of CHF.[6] Prevention of CHF through early intervention, usually by surgery, is the most effective management of heart failure in these patients. Adults with a congenital heart defect are an increasing patient population because correction of the defect early in life increases patient survival.[6] Moreover, they have the opportunity to develop other risk factors for coronary disease. The combination of the congenital defect repair and concurrent heart disease increases patient risk for CHF and results in a more difficult disease process to manage effectively.

Cardiac Conduction Dysfunctions

Arrhythmias, or malfunctions of the cardiac conduction system, may be caused by ischemia, infarction, infiltrates, electrolyte imbalances, or chemical toxins. Tachycardia of more than 160 beats per minute often results in inadequate ventricular filling and reduced diastolic volume, stroke volume, and cardiac output. Paroxysmal tachycardia can lead to a vicious cycle of increased oxygen need, followed by electrical instability and increased contraction with further oxygen demands. Recognition of the ischemia and initiation of corrective measures are necessary to alleviate tachycardia. Arrhythmias directly involving loss of sinoatrial (S-A) node control or atrioventricular (A-V) node conduction present problems involving heart failure. The irregular cardiac rhythms, seen when the S-A node is not controlling cardiac muscle depolarization,[7] precipitate heart congestion and alteration of heart chamber filling capacities. These changes can increase pressure problems as well as create inefficiencies of blood flow. Arrhythmias involving the A-V node often cause a slow or unresponsive

depolarization of the ventricles to the S-A stimulus. Without A-V node response an uncoordinated contraction occurs between the atrial and ventricular chambers. This inefficiency of heart pumping can also be caused by fibrous deposits that isolate the A-V node from the heart conduction system.

Other Causes of CHF

The disease states discussed below are seldom solely responsible for heart failure, but when they develop in the presence of underlying heart disease, heart failure may be precipitated. A healthy individual could compensate for the additional stress on the heart caused by these conditions, but this may not be true of patients with a diseased or damaged heart.

Hypertension is a frequent cause of CHF in the United States, and cardiac problems are 6 times more likely in hypertensive patients than in normotensive patients.[8] Hypertension leads to CHF primarily as a result of its chronic effects, especially the hypertrophy of heart muscle, which eventually leads to decreased efficiency of cardiac function when severe enough. Hypertension does not cause CHF from the increase in blood pressure, but the added pressure on the heart may lead to heart failure. The increase in blood pressure increases the resistance that the left ventricle must overcome to maintain cardiac volumes.[7]

The association of hypertension with myocardial infarction gives rise to an even higher risk of CHF by accelerating the progression of atherosclerosis. Existing hypertension has an adverse prognostic impact on the outcome of a myocardial infarction. The onset of hypertension after a myocardial infarction also increases the risk of recurrent infarction.[9] Antihypertensive therapy reduces the risk of development of CHF. Recent studies have reported a 52% reduction of CHF in patients who undergo successful treatment of hypertension compared with untreated control subjects.[9]

The very nature of connective tissue diseases eventually affects cardiac function. Deposition of abnormal materials into the heart results in vasculitis and a deterioration of cardiac function. Cardiac involvement is common in systemic lupus erythematosus, scleroderma, and polymyositis but rare in other connective tissue diseases such as rheumatoid arthritis. Pericarditis, cardiomyopathy, conduction system defects, and vascular abnormalities are the most common cardiac complications leading to CHF.

Sickle cell anemia, polycythemia, and vitamin B_1 deficiencies can also result in CHF. Strict control of these primary conditions will significantly reduce the likelihood of CHF development.

Heart function may be adversely affected by various endocrine disorders. Hyperthyroidism, with its unrestrained activity of thyroxine (T_4) and triiodothyronine (T_3), can cause the heart to pump vigorously without restraint. The adrenal hormones such as cortisol, cortisone, and aldosterone play an integral part in heart function by controlling metabolism, catabolism, and electrolyte balance. The effects of catecholamines and their part in the development of systemic hypertension are discussed in Chapter 6.

Good nutrition, including proper fluid and electrolyte balance, has had a significant role in maintaining adequate cardiac function. Vitamin B_6 deficiencies have been implicated in cardiomyopathies in which cardiac muscle fibers deteriorate and are replaced with fibrous strands. Toxic doses of vitamins can significantly alter the biochemistry of body cells, including myocardial cells.

Toxicity from substances that upset the biochemical functions of myocardial cells leads to myocardial weakness. Drug toxic effects can lead to loss of heart muscle contraction, increased volume loads, and relaxation of muscle tone. Cocaine is particularly harmful to cardiac muscle.[10] Poisons that inhibit sodium-potassium adenosine triphosphatase (ATPase) activity or the movement of calcium to and from muscle fibers will adversely affect the contraction and relaxation of heart muscle.

Contributing Factors to CHF

When cardiac function is already diminished, any additional stress placed on the heart may cause further damage to the cardiac muscle and worsening of the patient's symptoms. The patient may be able to compensate for the primary heart failure but unable to maintain adequate cardiac function when one or more of the following factors is added to the patient's condition. Box 7–2 lists the major contributing factors to CHF.

Anemia is a major contributing factor to CHF because it lowers blood viscosity and produces arteriolar dilatation as a result of hypoxia. Arterial pressure decreases, and the left ventricle undergoes hypertrophy because of increased venous return. Also, anemia reduces the oxygen-carrying capacity of the blood, which magnifies the pulmonary symptoms associated with CHF. Fever increases cellular metabolism and oxygen demand, and the body rids itself of excess heat through vasodilatation and increased blood flow to the skin surface. These mechanisms increase the demand for blood, significantly increasing the workload for the heart.

Chronic supraventricular tachycardia can induce cardiomyopathy and lead to cardiac dysfunction, though the exact mechanism has not been identified.[8] Poor diet or anorexia, often seen in ill cardiac patients, and abnormalities in water and electrolyte balance will affect heart dysfunction. Reduced renal blood flow as a result of CHF diminishes renal control of plasma electrolyte concentrations, which in turn have a direct effect on cardiac function.

Severe electrolyte abnormalities can cause either ventricular arrhythmias or decreased muscle contractility. Potassium and magnesium concentrations are particularly important in maintaining proper cardiac pumping rhythm; calcium is the primary cation responsible for controlling cardiac contractility. Regular monitoring of these electrolytes is required to ensure proper cardiac function, especially when diuretics are a part of the patient's treatment plan.

Obesity can contribute to CHF because cardiac output must increase to meet the oxygen demand of the excess adipose tissue. Increasing the stroke volume while the resting heart remains unchanged generally achieves the necessary output.[11]

Pulmonary disease increases stress on the heart, which struggles to meet the increased work of breathing and to overcome the hypoxia, hypercapnia, and metabolic and electrolyte imbalances caused by the pulmonary problems.

Environmental factors such as extremes of heat, humidity, and cold also stress the cardiac system. Well-documented cases of patients with significant myocardial dysfunction show that controlled climates are required to minimize undue stress on the heart.[12]

Effects of CHF on Other Organs

CHF produces a diverse pattern of symptoms and abnormalities, primarily because of impaired blood flow to the entire body. Patients with CHF experience diminished function of other organ systems as well as heart function, but the two organs most affected are the lungs and kidneys.

Left-sided heart failure causes pulmonary congestion and edema. The edema leads to stiffening of lung tissues and, if unchecked, reduces the surface area available for exchange of oxygen and carbon dioxide. The accompanying dyspnea may first present as paroxysmal nocturnal dyspnea (in which fluid collects in the spaces only at night) or orthopnea (in which fluid collects in the spaces when the patient is lying down).[7]

Increases in blood pressure may cause rupture of small pulmonary blood vessels, resulting in areas of hemorrhage and secondary infarction in the patient with CHF. The decrease in left ventricular function increases the demand on the right ventricle to handle excessive volumes of blood. Pooling of blood in the circulation causes systemic congestion and edema, especially in the lower extremities. The increased systemic congestion and pressure lead to hepatic congestion and hepatomegaly. This congestion causes hemorrhagic damage to liver cells, resulting in fibrotic changes and loss of liver function.

Chronic lung disease may cause a secondary form of heart failure commonly referred to as *cor pulmonale*. Two mechanisms are thought to be associated with the development of cor pulmonale: (1) respiratory disease causing increased pulmonary vascular resistance and pulmonary hypertension, which increases the right heart load; and (2) hypoxemia or respiratory acidosis, which leads to respiratory malfunction and a reduction in the ability of the myocardium to cope with normal blood volumes.[7]

The first mechanism of cor pulmonale can increase the blood volume load on the right ventricle, resulting in right ventricular hypertrophy and failure. Often there is a lack of pulmonary congestion or dyspnea until the left ventricle also becomes involved.[7] The lack of respiratory gas ex-

---

> ┌─────────────────────────────────────┐
> **Box 7–2. Factors Contributing to Congestive Heart Failure**
>
> Anemia
> Chronic supraventricular tachycardia
> Poor diet or anorexia
> Electrolyte imbalances
> Reduced renal blood flow
> Drugs
> Obesity
> Pulmonary disease
> Environment (heat, humidity, cold)

Box 7–3. Signs and Symptoms of Congestive Heart Failure

Dyspnea
Orthostatic dyspnea
Cough
Angina
Pulmonary infection
Confusion
Fatigue
Weight gain
Nocturia
Sinus tachycardia
Pulmonary rales
Mitral insufficiency
Paroxysmal nocturnal dyspnea
Edema
Shortness of breath
Pulmonary congestion
Exercise intolerance
Insomnia
Weakness
Abdominal discomfort/nausea/vomiting
Ascites
Increased jugular venous pressure
3rd or 4th heart sound
Hepatic congestion

---

rate at which the cardiac performance becomes impaired, and the ventricle initially involved in the disease process.[2] Vigilant attention to patient history, a thorough physical examination, radiologic examinations, and laboratory testing can facilitate early detection of CHF. CHF is readily detectable if it involves a patient with myocardial infarction, angina, pulmonary problems, or arrhythmias, but CHF is most commonly investigated because of dyspnea, edema, cough, and/or angina. Many patients have already experienced pulmonary congestion and have had frequent bouts with pulmonary infection. Other symptoms such as exercise intolerance, fatigue, and weakness are common. The signs and symptoms associated with CHF are listed in Box 7–3.

Left-sided heart failure results in dyspnea on exertion, orthopnea, paroxysmal nocturnal dyspnea, and, finally, dyspnea at rest. Right-sided heart failure leads to dependent edema, abdominal discomfort due to congestion of the liver and spleen, and, occasionally, ascites. If the CHF continues to progress, then angina and arrhythmias may develop. Criteria for cardiac failure are listed in Box 7–4.

Presenting symptoms of dilated cardiomyopathy are dyspnea on exertion, orthopnea, paroxysmal nocturnal dyspnea, and chest discomfort similar to angina. Physical findings include sinus tachycardia, elevated jugular venous pressure, pulmonary rales, a third and/or fourth heart sound, mitral insufficiency, and, in severe cases, hepatic congestion and peripheral edema.

change in the second mechanism of cor pulmonale quickly increases the level of toxic metabolites. Normal blood volumes high in lactic acid and carbon dioxide hinder myocardial respiration, and toxic metabolites increase heart workload and reduce myocardial effectiveness.

Alterations in blood flow also affect kidney function and contribute to the edema common in CHF. The increase in renal sympathetic nerve discharge, caused by a decrease in renal blood flow, causes kidney release of renin and stimulates the renin-angiotension system to increase blood volume and peripheral vasoconstriction, resulting in increased blood pressure.[10] The kidneys, trying to improve renal blood flow, contribute to fluid retention and edema in the pulmonary and/or systemic circulations in the patient with CHF.

An atrial natriuretic factor (ANF), released from secretory granules of the heart atria, helps regulate blood volume and blood pressure by providing negative feedback for release of antidiuretic hormone.[13] The action of ANF suggests that it is released to counteract many of the fluid problems that may develop in a CHF patient.

Other organs and organ systems affected by CHF are the liver, pancreas, and musculoskeletal and hematologic systems.

CLINICAL MANIFESTATIONS

Clinical indications of CHF range from very mild symptoms, which appear only on exertion, to the most advanced conditions, in which the heart is unable to function without external support. The clinical manifestations of CHF vary widely and depend on the age of the patient, the extent and

---

Box 7–4. Criteria for Cardiac Failure*

Major Criteria

Paroxysmal nocturnal dyspnea
Neck vein distention
Rales
Cardiomegaly
Acute pulmonary edema
S3 gallop
Increased venous pressure
Hepatojugular reflux

Minor Criteria

Ankle edema
Night cough
Dyspnea on exertion
Hepatomegaly
Pleural effusion
Vital capacity reduced ⅓ from maximum
Tachycardia

Major or Minor Criteria

Weight loss of 4.5 kg over 5 days in response to treatment

---

*Patients with two of the major criteria or one of the major and two of the minor criteria are prime candidates for a diagnosis of cardiac failure.

Data from Breast AN (ed): Congestive Heart Failure. New York, Medcom Press, 1975.

LABORATORY ANALYSES AND DIAGNOSIS

Radiologic Testing

Radiologic testing, such as chest radiography, is the primary means for diagnosing heart failure. Common findings on x-ray film are prominent pulmonary vessels, pulmonary infiltrates, and effusions. Echography, angiography, and fluoroscopy are definitive techniques for pinpointing heart problems. Echocardiography is used to detect valvular or structural abnormalities and damaged or poorly functioning heart muscle. Although an echocardiogram may be nonspecific, it provides a baseline for future comparison and can determine the extent of ischemia, the presence of hypertrophy, and rhythm disturbances. Angiography of coronary vessels is used to assess coronary artery disease.

Computed tomography and magnetic resonance imaging gated to the cardiac cycle may soon be more widely available and can provide information on systolic and diastolic function in patients undergoing these studies for other indications, such as pericardial disease, cardiac tumors, aortic disease, or pulmonary vascular disease.[14]

Clinical Laboratory Analyses

Laboratory involvement in heart failure primarily involves measuring the effects of heart failure on other organs, such as lung congestion and kidney failure. The laboratory is also invaluable for monitoring drug therapy following the diagnosis of heart failure.

Clinical laboratory assessment of heart failure may be helpful in early detection of the disease in patients with pulmonary congestion or edema. Blood gas analyses aid in determining the acid-base and oxygen status of the patient. Respiratory acidosis with elevated arterial carbon dioxide tension ($PaCO_2$) levels is often seen in these patients. The patient with edema develops electrolyte and osmolality changes as a result of fluid buildup and ionic redistribution. An increased excretion of potassium and a decrease in urinary sodium may be early indicators of these imbalances. Decreased cardiac output results in renal sodium retention, which also causes increased fluid retention; therefore, the serum sodium level generally stays within the reference ranges or is slightly decreased. Serum electrolyte determinations (including sodium, potassium, chloride, and calcium) are important to monitor diuretic and drug therapy in patients being treated for heart failure.[13]

The laboratory's role in detecting secondary causes of heart failure is also valuable. The patient who has secondary heart failure due to thyroid dysfunction can be identified by a highly sensitive thyroid-stimulating hormone assay. The presence of chest pain may suggest a need for performing cardiac enzyme profiles to eliminate the possibility of myocardial infarction.[13]

A patient suspected of having CHF should also be screened for kidney and liver involvement. Blood urea nitrogen (BUN) and creatinine levels are useful in assessing kidney function. The patient with heart failure who has an elevated creatinine level probably has already developed some kidney complication, and an elevated BUN level is an early indicator of uremia. Aspartate aminotransferase (AST), alanine aminotransferase (ALT), and alkaline phosphatase (ALP) measurements usually show elevations in patients with chronic right ventricular failure.[13] In addition, the γ-glutamyl-transferase (GGT) value is usually twice the value of the upper limit of the normal range, suggesting progressive liver congestion.

The routine complete blood cell count (CBC) is important for detecting anemias and infections. Hemolysis may indicate additional testing for hemoglobinuria and myoglobinuria, indicators of cardiovascular damage and myocardial disease. An increase in the number of white blood cells may indicate pericarditis, endocarditis, or valvular infections. If kidney dysfunction has occurred, anemia caused by decreased production of renal erythropoeitin may develop.

The infections associated with pericarditis, endocarditis, and valvular problems should be identified by blood cultures as described in Chapter 5. Microbiologic cultures of

---

Box 7–5. Drugs Used in Treatment of Congestive Heart Failure

Diuretics: Relieve Circulatory Congestion and Pulmonary and Peripheral Edema

Thiazide diuretics
  Hydrochlorothiazide
  Chlorthalidone
Loop diuretics
  Furosemide
  Bumetanide
  Ethacrynic acid
  Torsemide
Potassium-sparing diuretics
  Triamterene
  Amiloride
  Spironolactone

Inotropic Support: Increase Cardiac Pumping Ability

Digitalis glycosides
Phosphodiesterase inhibitors
Dobutamine

Vasodilators: Increase Stroke Volume, Reduce Ventricular Filling Pressure, and Improve Tolerance for Exercise

Angiotensin-converting enzyme (ACE) inhibitors
  Captopril
  Enalapril
  Lisinopril
  Ramipril
Hydralazine
Minoxidil
Organic nitrates

Anticoagulants: Prevent Thromboembolic Episodes

Aspirin
Warfarin

material from the pericardium and endocardium may also be performed if a pericardial infection is suspected.

The laboratory's role during the treatment of heart failure may extend to the provision of blood components, particularly when surgical intervention is needed. Bypass grafting, correcting valvular defects, and other surgical procedures to correct heart failure will involve the use of blood components during the surgery and the recovery period.

TREATMENT

The optimal treatment for heart failure is prevention. A sensible diet, weight control, and regular exercise are important. Treatment of hypertension and the avoidance of smoking, excessive alcohol intake, and illicit drug use are also critical preventive measures.[10]

When a patient is diagnosed with heart failure, dietary sodium is restricted and medications are prescribed. Diuretics are given to help the kidneys clear excess water and sodium to reduce blood volume and the workload placed on the heart. Digitalis strengthens the pumping action of the heart, and hydralazine, or other angiotensin-converting enzyme (ACE) inhibitors, such as captopril, dilate the peripheral arteries, decreasing the amount of effort that the heart expends pumping blood. Calcium-channel blockers dilate blood vessels and β-blockers slow the heart rate.[10] Antiarrhythmic agents may be given for regulation of any arrhythmias that may be present.

Cardiac glycosides, particularly digoxin, are used to increase the contractility of the heart and slow the conduction impulses. When monitoring patients on digoxin, attention must be paid to the drug level and the BUN/creatinine ratios because digoxin has a narrow therapeutic range, is strongly bound to protein, and is dependent on adequate kidney function for elimination. The potassium level must also be closely monitored if the patient is taking diuretics.

Box 7–5 lists medications currently used for the treatment of CHF and describes their effects.

PROGNOSIS

CHF is a lethal condition even when treated vigorously. In the Framingham Study, 37% of men and 38% of women died within 2 years of CHF diagnosis, and after 6 years of follow-up, 82% mortality in men and 67% mortality in women was seen. Sudden death, common in CHF, occurs at 5 times the rate for the general population. Substantial morbidity is also associated with CHF, with a significant increase in the risk of stroke and myocardial infarction.[3] Symptoms of overt CHF limit a patient's ability to perform even the most basic of daily activities. Patients with CHF consistently describe a poor quality of life because of physical symptoms, functional disability, emotional and economic burdens, frequent hospitalizations, and poor prognosis.[15] Advances in medical and surgical treatments during the past 40 years have not significantly improved the dismal prognosis for CHF.

Case Study

A 55-year-old man with a history of alcohol abuse was admitted to the hospital with shortness of breath and hyperventilation. His history revealed a chronic cough and fatigue. The physical examination revealed edema of the feet and legs, moderate respiratory distress, a blood pressure of 160/90 mm Hg, pulse rate of 70 per minute, and hepatomegaly. Laboratory assessment revealed changes from normal reference ranges as follows:

Laboratory Findings

Electrolytes

Sodium	132 mmol/L
Potassium	5.5 mmol/L
Chloride	106 mmol/L
Total CO_2	32 mmol/L

Blood Gases

pH	7.46
$Paco_2$	22 mm Hg
Pao_2	76 mm Hg
$\%O_2$ sat	91%

Liver Enzymes

AST	48 IU/L
ALT	52 IU/L
ALP	145 IU/L
GGT	90 IU/L

Other Values

BUN	40 mg/dL
Creatinine	2.1 mg/dL
Bilirubin	1.3 mg/dL
Hematocrit	12.6%
CBC	Normal
Microbiology cultures	Negative

Questions

1. What physiologic condition do the blood gas analyses and the patient's symptoms suggest?
2. What kind of heart failure is probably involved?
3. What are the implications of the other abnormal laboratory values?

Discussion

1. The physiologic condition indicated is respiratory alkalosis due to hyperventilation.
2. CHF due to alcohol cardiomyopathy is probably involved. Increased blood pressure indicates hypertension, which is most likely as much an etiologic factor as the alcohol.
3. Elevated liver enzyme levels and hepatomegaly suggest liver congestion, probably a result of right ventricular failure and damage due to alcohol abuse. BUN and creatinine values suggest poor renal perfusion from decreased cardiac output.

References

1. Report of the Task Force on Research in Heart Failure. National Heart, Lung, and Blood Institute. Washington, DC, 1994.
2. Braunwald E, Colucci WS, Grossman W: Clinical aspects of heart failure: High-output heart failure; pulmonary edema. *In* Braunwald E (ed): Heart Disease: A Textbook of Cardiovascular Medicine, vol 1, ed 5. Philadelphia, WB Saunders, 1997, pp 445–470.
3. Kannel WB, Belanger AJ: Epidemiology of heart failure. Am Heart J 121:951–957, 1991.
4. Smith WM: Epidemiology of congestive heart failure. Am J Cardiol 55:3A–8A, 1985.
5. Hosenpud JD: The cardiomyopathies. *In* Hosenpud JD, Greenberg BH (eds): Congestive Heart Failure: Pathophysiology, Diagnosis, and Comprehensive Approach to Management. New York, Springer-Verlag, 1994, pp 196–222.
6. Morton MJ: Heart failure secondary to congenital heart disease. *In* Hosenpud JD, Greenberg BH (eds): Congestive Heart Failure: Pathophysiology, Diagnosis, and Comprehensive Approach to Management. New York, Springer-Verlag, 1994, pp 246–257.
7. Emes JH, Nowak T: Introduction to Pathophysiology—Basic Principles of the Disease Process. Baltimore, University Park Press, 1983.
8. Hassapoyannes CA, Nelson WP, Hoopkins CB: Other causes and contributing factors to congestive heart failure. *In* Hosenpud JD, Greenberg BH (eds): Congestive Heart Failure: Pathophysiology, Diagnosis, and Comprehensive Approach to Management. New York, Springer-Verlag, 1994, pp 281–300.
9. Vasan RS, Levy D: The role of hypertension in the pathogenesis of heart failure: A clinical mechanistic overview. Arch Intern Med 156:1789–1796, 1996.
10. Soufer R: Heart Failure. *In* Zaret BL, Noser M, Cohen LS (eds): Yale University School of Medicine Heart Book, Hearst Books, New York, 1992, pp 177–214.
11. Messerli FH, Sundgaard-Riise K, et al: Dimorphic cardiac adaptation to obesity and arterial hypertension. Ann Intern Med 99:757–761, 1983.
12. Spann JF, Mason DT, Zelis RC: Recent advances in the understanding of congestive heart failure. Mod Concepts Cardiovasc Dis 39:115–120, 1970.
13. Burtis CA, Ashwood ER (ed): Teitz Textbook of Clinical Chemistry, ed 2. Philadelphia, WB Saunders, 1994.
14. Redfield MA: Evaluation of congestive heart failure. *In* Giuliani ER, Gersh BJ, McGoon MD, et al (eds): Mayo Clinic Practice of Cardiology. St. Louis, Mosby–Year Book, 1994, pp 569–587.
15. English MA, Mastrean MB: Congestive heart failure: Public and private burden. Crit Care Nurs Q 18:1–6, 1995.

Pulmonary Disorders

Chapter 8

Acute Respiratory Failure

Kevin D. Fallon and Sharon S. Ehrmeyer

ETIOLOGY AND PATHOPHYSIOLOGY

Respiratory failure, or acute respiratory insufficiency, is a term applied to a variety of problems in which the pulmonary system fails to provide the body with adequate oxygen for tissue metabolism and fails to remove an appropriate amount of the carbon dioxide produced as an end product. A condition results in which the arterial oxygen tension (PaO_2) is below the predicted normal range for the patient's age in the absence of another defined cause, such as left-to-right shunt; and the arterial carbon dioxide tension ($PaCO_2$) is above 50 mm Hg, in the absence of compensation for metabolic alkalosis.

Many types of disorders, some which are respiratory in origin, can lead to respiratory failure. The generic causes of respiratory failure are as follows:

Brain	Drugs or injury that affect the respiratory center
Spinal cord	Trauma or degenerative disease
Neuromuscular	Drugs, starvation, muscular atrophy
Thorax	Fatigue, rib damage
Airways	Obstructions
Cardiovascular	Cardiac disease

Box 8–1 lists some examples of specific nonrespiratory causes of failure.[1]

Among the respiratory failure mechanisms that can lead to insufficiency is hypoventilation, which is characterized by movement of an inadequate amount of air into and out of the alveoli. One cause might be partial or total blockage of the airway due to foreign material, such as mucus, or by constriction of the muscles of the bronchial tree. A decrease in mechanical action, resulting in movement of inadequate volumes of air, is associated frequently with trauma, fractured ribs, abdominal pain, and fatigue. Another significant cause of hypoventilation is neurologic in nature, resulting from brain injury, changes in neuromuscular transmission, or drugs. Drugs can also affect brain sensitivity to carbon dioxide (CO_2), which controls signals to the respiratory muscle and signal transmission at the neuromuscular junction.

Inadequate diffusion is another cause of respiratory failure and results in the impairment of gas exchange at the alveolocapillary interface. This is most frequently due to pulmonary edema, which has a variety of causes but is most commonly associated with infections, particularly pneumonia.

Shunting, or ventilation-to-perfusion inequality, is characterized by a percentage of the cardiac output that does not participate in gas exchange in the alveoli. Anatomic connection between the venous and arterial circulation, other than in the lungs, is an example of a shunt. However, in the acute care patient, the more usual cause of a shunt is obstruction (mucus plugs) in the lower bronchi.

Perfusion-to-ventilation inequality results in increased dead space, that is, volumes of air in the lung that do not exchange with the blood because large areas of the lung that are ventilated adequately are not perfused with blood.

Box 8–1. **Examples of Causes of Respiratory Failure: Nonpulmonary in Origin**

Ventilation	Respiratory	Injury	Cardiac
Drugs	Trauma	Lung trauma	Fluid overload
Anesthesia	Hemorrhage	Smoke	Congestive heart failure
CNS	Shock	Aspiration pneumonia	Acute heart failure
(central nervous system)			
Spinal cord injury	Pulmonary embolism	Pulmonary disease	
	Pneumonia		

Data from Shoemaker WC: Pathophysiology and fluid management of postoperative and post-traumatic ARDS. *In* Shoemaker WC, Thompson W, Holbrook P, et al: Textbook of Critical Care, ed 2. Philadelphia, WB Saunders, 1989, p 615–636.

The principal cause of the decrease in perfusion is emboli in the pulmonary circulation that block the flow of blood to sections of the lung. Another major problem arises when the pulmonary arterial pressure is inadequate to overcome the resistance provided by the pulmonary microcirculation. Two different physiologic conditions can cause this: (1) a severe drop in arterial pressure caused by heart failure, or (2) an increase in resistance to blood flow caused by fluid buildup in lung areas when mechanical ventilation pressure is too high. Infections are a frequent cause of this increased resistance, but the condition can also result from immobility. Proper nursing care calls for frequent turning of the patient who has pain or is receiving medication to prevent hypoventilation in some areas of the lung that could result in mucus plugging, pneumonia, and respiratory failure. The weakened patient has to expend considerable energy by increasing both the rate and the volume of breathing to ventilate the lungs. Patients frequently are paralyzed and put on mechanical ventilators to conserve energy for healing processes.

The adult respiratory distress syndrome (ARDS) is a form of severe respiratory failure that continues to be one of the more lethal conditions that can threaten a patient. In one multihospital study, 633 of 1,426 patients (44.4%) with acute respiratory failure (ARF) did not survive hospitalization.[2] Other studies have shown the mortality rate of ARDS to be between 50% and 70%.[3]

ARDS is ARF caused by diffuse alveolar injury and is considered the end stage of multiple insults such as accidental and surgical trauma, hemorrhage, sepsis, atelectasis, smoke inhalation, and many other conditions that result in direct damage to the alveolocapillary interface. ARDS affects large numbers of patients and prognosis is usually poor if prolonged supplemental high concentrations of oxygen (>50%) are required to achieve adequate PaO$_2$.

ARDS is characterized by severe hypoxemia refractory to high inspired oxygen concentrations, with diffuse interstitial or alveolar infiltrates that are generally bilateral on chest radiography. Edema and the presence of abnormal airways results in a decrease in thoracic compliance (loss of elasticity). The alveolar-arterial difference in partial pressure of oxygen (PA-aO$_2$) is generally less than 0.3, and pulmonary microvascular permeability is increased. Proper management and monitoring of respiratory failure is necessary to prevent high morbidity and mortality rates. Although ARDS is often impossible to prevent, it is easier to prevent than to cure.

The physiologic response to ARDS is extremely complicated. It can be characterized by ventilation-to-perfusion mismatches, reduced functional residual capacity (usable lung volume), and diminished compliance that leads to hypoxemia. A massive response in the release of hormones and other agents leads to cellular and functional changes in the lung. ARDS involves diffuse lung injury, leading to pulmonary edema. This is not to be confused with cardiogenic pulmonary edema, although respiratory failure can result from both. Frequently, the use of a pulmonary artery catheter with a thermistor for determining cardiac output by thermal dilution is required to ascertain the status of the heart and to distinguish between pulmonary and cardiogenic pulmonary edema.

Before 1950, respiratory failure was not diagnosed as frequently as it is now because necessary laboratory analyses were not available. Determination of arterial oxygenation was performed by volumetric analysis (Van Slyke's method), which required more than 30 minutes for a single determination and, therefore, could not be of more than academic benefit to the patient.

Fewer people actually die from respiratory failure now because of rapid diagnosis and relatively effective treatment. One study reported that only 15% of patients in an ARDS group died from respiratory failure.[4] However, large numbers of people survive the ventilation crisis only to succumb to other complications associated with long-term illness, such as sepsis, stress ulcers with hemorrhage, and heart or renal failure (Box 8–2). Sepsis is the major cause of death in ARDS patients who survive the initial trauma. If the infection precedes the development of ARDS, the source is usually in the abdomen, whereas infection occurring after ARDS develops is usually pulmonary in origin.[5]

Respiratory arrest can be transient and, if properly managed, can be resolved within a short time. ARDS is usually preceded by a catastrophic event, such as multiple trauma, occurring in an otherwise healthy individual.

Among the causes of transient respiratory insufficiency is ingestion of drugs, both controlled and uncontrolled. Narcotics affect the opiate receptors in the brain stem and can cause respiratory depression. Morphine has been linked to delayed respiratory suppression when injected into the epidural space for local anesthesia. Almost any of the arsenal of drugs used by anesthesiologists, in sufficient dose, cause respiratory depression through any one of several mechanisms (e.g., impairment in chemoreceptor func-

Box 8–2. **Some Nonpulmonary Complications Associated with ARDS**

Medical Complications	**Therapy Complications**	**Ventilator Complications**
Disseminated intravascular coagulation	Fluid overload	Barotrauma
Sepsis	Shock	Bacterial pneumonia
Malnutrition	Overmedication	Pneumothorax
Stress ulcers	Gastric distention	Subcutaneous emphysema
Atelectasis		Reduced cardiac output

Modified from Lake KB: Adult respiratory distress syndrome: High permeability pulmonary edema. *In* Hodgkin JE, Burton GC (eds): Respiratory Care: A Guide to Clinical Practice. Philadelphia, JB Lippincott, 1984, p 873.

tion, interference with neuromuscular transmission, or changes in metabolism). Properly managed, these situations are resolved by short-term ventilation support. Delays in treatment, frequently associated with overdoses of street drugs, can cause a patient's condition to deteriorate to the point at which more aggressive therapy may be required. Pain caused by abdominal incisions, broken ribs, and similar trauma can elicit shallow breathing (hypoventilation). The deep breath, or sigh, becomes too painful, and periodic inflation of the alveoli stops.

Obesity is another cause of hypoventilation. Excessive weight creates pressure and a need for increased ventilation to support the metabolism of the added tissue mass. As a result, respiratory mechanics are altered so that the work of breathing increases significantly. Morbidly obese people often underventilate and are actually prone to apnea.

CLINICAL MANIFESTATIONS

The symptoms of respiratory failure include tachypnea, dyspnea, an ashen-gray appearance, cyanosis, agitation, and anxiety. Two types of failure may occur. One exhibits hypoxemia (low oxygen levels with either eucapnia [normal CO_2 levels] or hypocapnia [low CO_2 levels]), whereas the second exhibits hypoxemia with hypercapnia (high CO_2 levels). The first is usually associated in adults with ARDS resulting from acute lung injury. Stiff or noncompliant lungs are generally observed in these cases, along with sepsis. In the second type of respiratory failure, patients generally have chronic problems superimposed on an acute episode. Some patients exhibit both types of problems during an illness, and in many instances it is necessary to use a pulmonary artery catheter to determine whether the edema is caused by a cardiogenic or fluid overload problem or is pulmonary in origin.

LABORATORY ANALYSES AND DIAGNOSIS

Respiratory Failure

The primary concern in the support of the patient with ARF is maintenance of respiration. Adequate ventilation of the lung and maintenance of cardiac output is required for adequate oxygen delivery to the tissues. For proper management, arterial blood gas analyses must be available at all times. These provide the following crucial information:

Pao_2

Arterial oxygen tension indicates respiratory failure when the Pao_2 falls below 50 mm Hg. Oxygenation of the tissues is inadequate. Alveolar ventilation is determined by $Paco_2$. An elevated $Paco_2$ indicates hypoventilation and respiratory failure.

ACID-BASE STATUS

This is determined by the $Paco_2$, pH, and bicarbonate concentration.

A combination of ventilation-to-perfusion mismatching, alveolar hypoventilation, and, occasionally, abnormalities in respiratory drive will produce significant hypoxemia (Pao_2 >50 mm Hg). In previously healthy patients, the $Paco_2$ may be low initially as the patient hyperventilates to compensate. However, as the respiratory muscles tire, hypercapnia ($Paco_2$ >50 mm Hg) and acidemia (pH <7.35) occur. In patients with chronic hypoventilation, the $Paco_2$ may be high initially. In any case, as the concentration of CO_2 rises, acidemia results. Blood gas values frequently change very rapidly and without warning, so the analysis must be available at all times (Table 8–1).

Acid-base disorders result in compensatory responses of the lungs and kidneys; as a result, clinical assessment of patients' laboratory findings is initially difficult because the physician does not know if the findings represent an initial or a compensated situation. Frequent blood gas values must be obtained, therefore, and aggressive ventilatory

Table 8–1. **Laboratory Results in Acute Respiratory Failure**

Cause	Pao_2	$Paco_2$	pH
Nervous system	↓	↑	↓
Neuromuscular	↓	↑	↓
Thorax	↓	↑	↓
Cardiovascular	↓	↓	N or ↑
ARDS			
Early	↓	N ↓	N or ↑
Late	↓	↑	↓

Abbreviation: N, normal.

Data from Lake KB: Adult respiratory distress syndrome: High permeability pulmonary edema. *In* Hodgkin JE, Burton GC (eds): Respiratory Care: A Guide to Clinical Practice. Philadelphia, JB Lippincott, 1984, p 873 and Bone R: Acute respiratory failure and chronic obstructive lung disease: Recent advances. Med Clin North Am 65:563, 1981.

support provided. Because the goal is always to remove the patient from the ventilator as quickly as possible, laboratory data are consulted carefully to determine the most aggressive course possible for weaning the patient from the ventilator. The precision and timeliness of the laboratory analyses, starting with obtaining the sample and continuing through the analysis, are critical to this process. Small changes, if reliable, can confirm a trend and accelerate further modifications in therapy.

ARDS

In ARDS the PaO_2 falls despite oxygen enrichment of inspired gas. It is possible that some time (days) can elapse after the insult before frank ARDS develops. Because ARDS is such a complicated condition and is usually compounded by other serious conditions in the patient, it is necessary to assess a large number of biochemical variables in ARDS patients.

Fluid and electrolyte management is a high priority. Even small changes in serum electrolyte concentrations may represent fluid-electrolyte shifts that can delay or prevent recovery. Resuscitation of trauma victims often requires large amounts of blood and other fluids. Hormonal changes or kidney or cardiac problems associated with the trauma may prevent the excretion of the excess fluid. Proper management of fluid-electrolyte problems involves a consideration of the following three dimensions: (1) the total amount of the electrolyte (concentration and volume of distribution), (2) body balance (rate of movement into and out of the body), and (3) body composition (movement into and out of body compartments). These require serum electrolyte determinations.

Coagulation problems, particularly disseminated intravascular coagulation (DIC), have been found to be common in patients with ARDS, and evaluation of the patient's coagulation status is often indicated. Coagulation tests such as fibrinogen, platelet count, activated partial thromboplastin time, ethanol gelation test, and fibrin degradation products are less predictive than antithrombin III, plasminogen (low values), or factor VIII (higher values) in assessing coagulation disorders in these patients. The platelet count seems to be the most sensitive indicator and should be considered when transfusions are part of the overall therapy. A plasma complement profile has been proposed as an early warning of impending coagulopathy. Sepsis syndrome is specifically defined by clinical signs and laboratory tests, and can be a warning of impending ARDS.

A low serum protein concentration, disturbed renal function, and a low PaO_2/FiO_2 (O_2 concentration of inspired air) in drowning victims indicate a greater risk for development of ARDS. Aggressive therapy is required from the start.

The white blood cell (WBC) count has a potential predictive value for patients who have a high risk for developing ARDS. Counts below $5.0 \times 10^9/L$ associated with respiratory failure indicate the onset of ARDS.

A strong correlation between immunoreactive trypsin and both ARDS and sepsis has been found, suggesting that proteinases are implicated in the development of ARDS. Because of the variety of pathologic conditions that result from trauma and other conditions that lead to or result from ARDS, the involvement of the laboratory in the treatment of these patients is very extensive. Very aggressive management of pulmonary function, involving blood gas analyses, carbon monoxide (CO) oximetry (including total hemoglobin), and related calculated parameters is necessary. Cardiac output is correlated with these values to ensure that adequate oxygen is being carried to the tissues. Hemoglobin concentrations must be adequate, and the affinity of hemoglobin for oxygen must provide for adequate oxygen delivery.

Fluid volumes must be maintained so that cardiac output is adequate. Dilution of all electrolytes is a potential hazard, so constant monitoring of these concentrations is required.

Kidney failure is not uncommon, and therefore constant evaluation of creatinine, urea nitrogen, and other renal function indicators is routine.

Liver function is carefully monitored using serum enzymes and other analytes that may indicate any changes in this organ. As discussed earlier, infections are the most common problem in these patients; therefore, proper identification of the causative agent, so that specific antibiotic selection can be made, is crucial for survival. Nutritional status is determined by a variety of methods, many of which are of marginal value. Twenty-four-hour urine nitrogen, albumin, and transferrin tests are used by clinicians to follow the patient's nutritional status.

TREATMENT

Treatment for respiratory distress is centered on achieving adequate oxygenation of the tissues. Oxygen therapy is necessary but must be administered carefully and monitored because toxicity or depression of the ventilatory response can occur in some patients. Moreover, decisions to intubate are always made with care because a number of complications can ensue. Alteration of the rate and volume of ventilation and diuresis are mechanisms used to improve the respiratory status of the patient. ARDS is particularly difficult to treat because it represents a complicated mix of syndromes that are not well understood at this time. Blood gas analyses are essential in monitoring the effectiveness of treatment. The responsibility of the laboratory is to produce useful, accurate information in a timely manner.

Case Study

A 22-year-old man involved in a motor vehicle accident was brought to the emergency room and admitted to the surgical intensive care unit with multiple traumatic injuries. The patient was conscious and breathing spontaneously. The next day the patient became tachypneic and complained of difficulty in breathing (dyspnea).

Two days after admission, the chest radiograph showed diffuse infiltrates. Laboratory findings during the course of the hospital stay were as follows:

Day 2

PaO_2=75 mm Hg $PaCO_2$=60 mm Hg

pH=7.301 FiO_2=.21

(fraction of inspired oxygen)

Day 3

PaO_2=70 mm Hg   PaCO_2=70 mm Hg

pH=7.295   FIO_2=.40

Day 4

PaO_2=73 mm Hg   PaCO_2=76 mm Hg

pH=7.288   FIO_2=.50

On day 3, x-ray films showed increased pulmonary edema. On day 5, the patient developed a fever (39.2 °C).

Questions

1. Given the laboratory results, how do you explain the development of the patient's condition by day 3, and what steps should be taken?

2. What would you predict the blood and tracheal aspirate cultures taken on day 5 will show?

3. What analyses would the laboratory be performing on a frequent basis?

4. Given the laboratory findings later in the hospital stay, what is the prognosis for this patient?

Discussion

1. The patient developed respiratory failure subsequent to trauma. Given that the PaO_2 has fallen even though the FIO_2 had increased, ARDS is likely unless aggressive treatment is undertaken. In this case the patient was intubated and was ventilated with positive end expiratory pressure (PEEP). A pulmonary artery catheter was placed for determining cardiac output by thermal dilution and for obtaining blood for frequent blood gas analyses.

2. Because sepsis is a frequent complication of respiratory failure, especially ARDS, the cultures would be expected to be positive. The presence of fever and the high WBC count with a shift to the left support the suspicion of infection. In this case the blood culture and tracheal aspirate grew *Staphylococcus aureus*. Appropriate antibiotic therapy was instituted.

3. Blood gases and CO-oximeter panels were determined 4 or more times per day to guide aggressive respiratory management. Electrolytes were also carefully monitored.

4. Because oxygen concentration and FIO_2 increased, the prognosis is good. Once weaned from the respirator, the patient will probably do well breathing on his own.

References

1. Shoemaker WC: Pathophysiology and fluid management of postoperative and post-traumatic ARDS. *In* Shoemaker WC, Thompson W, Holbrook P, et al (eds): Textbook of Critical Care, ed 2. Philadelphia, WB Saunders, 1989, pp. 615–636.

2. Vasilyev S, Schaap RN, Mortensen JD: Hospital survival rates of patients with acute respiratory failure in modern respiratory intensive care units: An international, multicenter, prospective survey. Chest 107:1083, 1995.

3. Seidenfeld JJ, Pohl DF, Bell RC, et al: Incidence, site, and outcome of infections in patients with the adult respiratory distress syndrome. Am Rev Respir Dis 134:12, 1986.

4. Montgomery BR, Stager MA, Carrico CJ, et al: Causes of mortality in patients with adult respiratory distress syndrome. Ann Intern Med 99:293, 1983.

5. Lake KB: Adult respiratory distress syndrome: High permeability pulmonary edema. *In* Burton GC, Hodgkin JE (eds): Respiratory Care: A Guide to Clinical Practice. Philadelphia, JB Lippincott, 1984, p 873.

6. Bone R: Acute respiratory failure and chronic obstructive lung disease: Recent advances. Med Clin North Am 65:563, 1981.

Chapter 9

Chronic Obstructive Pulmonary Disease

Sharon S. Ehrmeyer and Kevin D. Fallon

The umbrella term, *chronic obstructive pulmonary disease* (COPD), is used to describe a group of pulmonary diseases characterized by the chronic or recurrent limitation to air flow within the lungs. The air flow is obstructed either by reduction in outflow pressure or by increased airway resistance due to a narrowing of the passages. In emphysema, the septal walls are damaged and collapse, causing a loss of elastic recoil of the lung and a reduction of expiratory airflow. Asthma, usually more spasmodic than chronic, narrows the airways.

ETIOLOGY AND PATHOPHYSIOLOGY

Emphysema

Emphysema is defined as the abnormal, permanent enlargement of the acinar air spaces distal to the terminal bronchiole caused by the destruction of the interalveolar walls.[1] With the destruction, adjacent capillaries also break down, causing the alveoli to coalesce into enlarged structures called *bullae* that contain less surface area for gas exchange. The small airways that were once held open by the elastic fibers of the surrounding alveoli collapse, resulting in air trapping or wasted ventilation.

Emphysema may occur by itself or in conjunction with chronic bronchitis. Most patients do not present with full-blown, disabling symptoms until between the fourth and

sixth decades of life; however, ventilatory deficits may appear much earlier.

Emphysema is classified according to the portion of the acini involved. As emphysema becomes more severe, classification becomes difficult, and more than one pattern may be present. The two most common types, centriacinar and panacinar, are shown in Figure 9–1. With centriacinar emphysema, the distention and destruction usually affects the proximal part of the acinus, the respiratory bronchioles, and the alveolar ducts. The respiratory bronchioles merge, and the more distal alveolar ducts and sacs remain unaffected. Panacinar emphysema involves the entire acinus, including the respiratory bronchiole, alveolar duct, alveolar sac, and alveoli, and all segments of the respiratory tree distal to the respiratory bronchiole are distended.

Localized emphysema destroys alveoli in only one or few locations within the lung. It often predisposes patients to pneumothorax, and progression can result in more extensive destruction of lung tissue. Irregular emphysema usually is associated with scars from an inflammation. Typically, patients with these last two types are asymptomatic, and the affected area, as long as it is an isolated finding, is not associated with COPD.

Although there is an incomplete understanding of the pathogenesis and etiology of emphysema, the single most recognized cause is cigarette smoking. The severity of emphysema caused by cigarette smoking is dose-related. Nonsmokers usually have infrequent and low-grade emphysema, whereas heavy smokers develop a more severe and extensive disease. Smoking also adds to the effects of other contributory factors, such as occupational and environmental air pollutants and any familial or genetic predisposition.

The dominant hypothesis to account for alveolar wall destruction is the proteolysis-antiproteolysis theory.[2] Alveolar wall destruction occurs when there is an imbalance between the release and destruction of proteases (mainly elastase). Inhalation of smoke causes neutrophils to accumulate and to release proteolytic enzymes. In addition, smoke increases the release of elastase, and the oxidants in cigarette smoke decrease antielastase activity.[3]

α_1-Antitrypsin (AAT), a serum glycoprotein synthesized and secreted by the liver, is a major inhibitor of a variety of proteolytic enzymes, including elastase. AAT deficiency may be congenital or acquired. With the congenital defi-

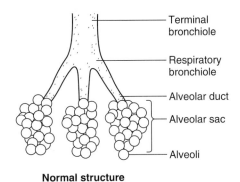

Normal structure

Figure 9–1. The effect of the centrilobular emphysema and panlobular emphysema upon the respiratory tract. Note that in CLE the respiratory bronchioles merge, whereas the more distal alveolar ducts and sacs remain unaffected. In PLE, however, all segments of the respiratory tree distal to the respiratory bronchiole are distended. (From Davis BG, Bishop ML, Mass D (eds): Clinical Laboratory Science: Strategies for Practice. Philadelphia, JB Lippincott, 1989, p 128.)

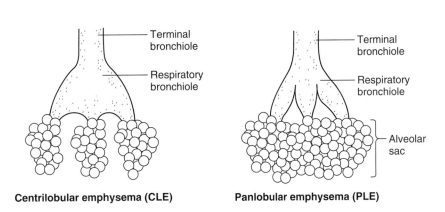

Centrilobular emphysema (CLE)   **Panlobular emphysema (PLE)**

ciency, the normal antiproteolytic activity of serum globulins is lacking, and individuals are likely to develop early and severe emphysema. Nearly 70% to 80% of individuals homozygous for the protease inhibitor gene type ZZ (PiZZ) develop COPD; however, as few as 1% of patients with emphysema have AAT deficiency.[4]

Recurrent respiratory infections and inhalation of irritants have been indirectly linked to permanent airway damage and the development of COPD in later life.

Asthma

Asthma is classified as COPD because the disease interferes with air flow through the lung. Asthma is characterized by bronchial hyperactivity of the airways.[5, 6] This leads to episodic bronchoconstriction due to increased responsiveness of the tracheobronchial tree to a variety of stimuli that normally would not affect nonasthmatics. Asthmatic episodes cause swelling of the bronchial mucosa, excessive secretion of viscous mucus, and secondary pulmonary hyperinflation. Hyperinflation occurs because of the constriction of small airways and the resultant air trapping. Although severe during asthmatic episodes, these characteristics may completely disappear following a remission of the attack (Fig. 9–2). Asthma's principal clinical characteristic is reversible airway obstruction. This feature is useful for differentiating asthma from other forms of obstructive lung disease.

Asthma is a common disease, occurring in 5% of the general population, although incidence among children is higher (10%). In adults, asthma affects both sexes equally, but in children it is twice as common in boys. About half the cases in children develop before they reach the age of 10 years. Asthma is classified into two major categories based on the factors that trigger the episodes. Extrinsic asthma is an allergic condition, and immunologic, antigen-antibody mechanisms trigger bronchospasm. With intrinsic or idiosyncratic asthma, irritants or other factors cause airway reactivity in the absence of an immune reaction. The distinction between the two types of asthma is important when instituting preventive measures against future attacks, but the differences have little value in the acute treatment of the disease because both forms require very similar therapy. Tables 9–1 and 9–2 list common features and stimuli that provoke acute episodes for both categories of asthma.

Asthma can also be classified according to the mechanism or principal stimulus that causes bronchial hyperactivity. Several mechanisms are postulated, although the mechanisms are probably interrelated. In extrinsic asthma, on exposure to aerosolized antigens, immunoglobulin E (IgE) antibodies are formed that are capable of binding to mast cells, basophils, and eosinophils.[7] Once the patient is sensitized to a specific antigen, on reexposure, the antigen reacts with the antibody on the activated cells, causing the release of inflammatory mediators and chemotactic factors. Bronchoconstriction results, in conjunction with increased capillary permeability, inflammatory cell entry, increased mucus secretion, and mucosal edema. Inflammatory cells contribute to airway inflammation and subsequent chronic bronchial obstruction and hyperirritability.

Many mechanisms for intrinsic asthma, triggered by

Bronchiole obstructed
on expiration by:

1. Muscle spasm
2. Swelling of mucosa
3. Thick secretions

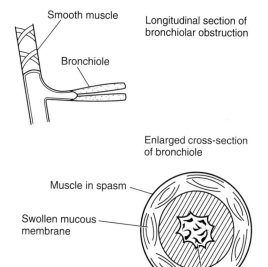

Smooth muscle

Longitudinal section of
bronchiolar obstruction

Bronchiole

Enlarged cross-section
of bronchiole

Muscle in spasm

Swollen mucous
membrane

Thick secretions

Figure 9–2. Mechanism of bronchial asthma.

Table 9–1. Extrinsic Asthma

Synonyms	Stimuli That Provoke Acute Episodes of Asthma	Common Features

IgE-mediated asthma
Allergic asthma
Atopic asthma
Reagin-mediated asthma
	Exposure to external or environmental antigens (allergens) that cause an immunologic response.
	Common offenders include
	  Pollens (grass, trees, flowers, etc.)
	  Feathers
	  House dust
	  Dander from cats, dogs, and horses
	  Dermatophagoides
	  Mold spores (e.g., *Aspergillus*)
	  Ingested materials such as dairy products, chocolate, fish, and alcohol (less common)
		Best understood form of asthma
		Personal and/or family history of allergic diseases
		Asthmatic attacks less frequent with time, and may disappear in adulthood
		Most often observed in children and young adults (<35 years old)
		Frequently seasonal unless antigens are present in environment continuously
		Increased serum levels of IgE

Table 9–2. Intrinsic Asthma

Synonyms	Stimuli That Provoke Acute Episodes of Asthma	Common Features
Nonallergic asthma Nonatopic asthma Idiosyncratic asthma	Infections—most often respiratory tract Exercise Emotional stress Air pollution Drugs	Negative personal and/or family history of allergic diseases Disease usually more severe than extrinsic and may become worse with time Typically appears later in life (>35 years old) Normal serum levels of IgE

several factors, have been postulated. Stimuli may activate sensory fibers of the vagus nerve in the lining of the upper and lower airways, which increase in airway resistance and bronchial secretions. Other mechanisms include immunoglobulin E (IgE)- and G (IgG)-mediated reactions, direct liberation of bronchoconstrictors, and hypersensitivity of unknown origin.[3, 8]

CLINICAL MANIFESTATIONS

Emphysema

Symptoms associated with emphysema are generally nonspecific and variable; however, symptoms occur with increasing frequency as the disease state progresses. Patients usually present with unremitting dyspnea that is often described as insidious in onset and steadily progressive. One of the characteristic observations is a pattern of breathing with a very slow, forced expiration that is laborious and may sometimes be associated with the use of pursed-lip breathing. Another sign associated with this pattern of breathing is the distention of the neck veins during the expiratory period and their immediate collapse on inspiration. The chest is frequently overexpanded because of the loss of elastic recoil in the lung, resulting in the characteristic barrel chest.

Tachypnea is common, often resulting in increased use of accessory muscles during the inspiratory cycle. With the rapid breathing, the arterial oxygen tension (PaO_2) is usually sufficient to saturate hemoglobin. Coughing may be minimal, with expectoration of only a scant amount of mucoid sputum. The chest is hyperresonant to percussion because of the general overexpansion, and breath sounds are usually diminished and faint. High-pitched wheezes are sometimes heard toward the end of expiration when the airways are beginning to close.

Cardiovascular signs are indicative of the body's attempt to compensate for the hypoxemia and include increased cardiac output, heart rate, and blood pressure and abnormal heart sounds. Cyanosis of the lips, earlobes, skin, and fingernail beds is seen in advanced stages of emphysema and is associated with the developing hypoxemia. Other observations during the advanced state include clubbing of the fingertips and, possibly, weakness and weight loss.

Asthma

The clinical spectrum of asthma ranges from intermittent mild forms of bronchospasm to very severe, unremitting, and life-threatening asthmatic episodes. Changes in the severity of asthma may occur spontaneously or as a result of therapy. The most severe and acute form, *status asthmaticus*, compromises ventilatory function to a life-threatening degree.

The clinical symptoms of bronchial asthma include wheezing; dyspnea; cough productive of thick, tenacious mucus; chest tightness; night attacks; agitation; fatigue; and, in more severe stages, inability to talk. The more common symptoms are caused by increased airway resistance and air trapping, which result in a decreased PaO_2 and hypoxemia. The hypoxemia causes tachypnea through stimulation of the peripheral chemoreceptors.

The cardiovascular consequences of hypoxemia include increased heart rate, cardiac output, and blood pressure. In more severe stages, in which the work of breathing is greatly increased, associated cyclic changes in blood pressure follow respiration. During inspiration, the pressure in the chest decreases significantly and the patient's systolic blood pressure drops 10 mm Hg or more. During expiration, the reverse occurs, and blood pressure increases.

Progression of asthma can lead to emphysema due to hyperinflation. In addition, bacterial infections may result in chronic bronchitis, bronchiectasis, or pneumonia. Cor pulmonale and heart failure manifest in some cases.

LABORATORY ANALYSES AND DIAGNOSIS

Emphysema

Respiratory diseases that must be differentiated from emphysema are bronchial asthma, chronic bronchitis, lung infection, lung tumors, and coronary artery disease. The most useful laboratory analyses in the differential diagnosis of emphysema are pH/blood gas analyses, carbon monoxide (CO)-oximetry, and antitrypsin deficiency tests. Other tests include sputum cytology, monitoring digoxin and theophylline levels, electrolyte measurements and histopathology and hematology (hemoglobin and hematocrit) studies. The arterial blood gas and hematology results reflect the severity of respiratory acidosis and the degree of hypoxemia experienced by the patient.

If AAT deficiency is suspected, then serum electrophoresis may be performed, but it is imperative that quantitative tests (radial immunodiffusion, nephelometry, or electroimmunodiffusion) be used to confirm the diagnosis. In addition, phenotyping may be indicated to determine the allelic variants.

Pulmonary function studies demonstrating hyperinflation and reduced expiratory flows are helpful in evaluating emphysema. Chest radiographs frequently demonstrate little other than hyperinflation.

Asthma

Patients with status asthmaticus who present to an emergency room are often severely compromised and are approaching or are in a state of acute respiratory failure. In these cases there may be little time for more than measure-

ments of arterial pH/blood gases and a complete blood cell count (CBC) to confirm the diagnosis and to determine whether to initiate mechanical ventilation. When patients present in a less severe state, however, more time is available to undertake a more thorough laboratory investigation and differential diagnosis.

The most useful laboratory analyses in the diagnosis of asthma are pH/blood gas analyses, CO-oximetry, and an eosinophil count on peripheral blood.

Other tests typically performed outside of the clinical laboratory include pulmonary function tests, chest radiography, and electrocardiographic studies, which are important in the differential diagnosis and in the prescription for treatment of asthma. Radiographs of the chest are nondiagnostic for asthma but may be helpful in ruling out other conditions, such as lung tumor, emphysema, lung infection, and complications of asthma.

TREATMENT

Emphysema

No cure for emphysema exists because the damage to the lungs is irreversible. Education of patients and their families about preventive measures is among the more important aspects of management. Treatment focuses on the prevention or alleviation of symptoms.

Important preventive measures include the cessation of smoking and avoidance of infections and irritants. Exercise programs do not improve lung function. They can, however, increase endurance but may be contraindicated in patients with concomitant cardiac disorders. Proper nutrition is very important because the energy expended in simply breathing is great. Weight loss for obese patients is important to reduce the body's demand for oxygen. Mobilization of bronchial secretions is essential to improve gas exchange and to prevent recurrent infection.

Drug therapy is primarily symptom-related. Bronchodilators usually produce only slight improvement in emphysema patients unless they have significant airway reactivity. Prophylactic antibiotics may be indicated in patients with frequent bacterial respiratory tract infections. Supplemental oxygen is indicated for patients with severe and persistent hypoxia who meet certain clinical criteria. Oxygen therapy should be carefully administered and titrated for patients with severe dyspnea, because overuse can depress normal respiration.

Asthma

Although there is no cure for asthma, children may recover spontaneously as they mature into adulthood. Treatment is aimed at relieving the symptoms of the existing attack and varies with the individual. Patients and their families must be educated about the causes of the disease to prevent recurrent exposure to either the antigen or the inhaled irritant. In addition, they must be educated about assessment, treatment (including proper use of an inhaler), and control of the disease. Desensitization with small doses of the asthma-inducing antigen has been used, but effectiveness has not been proven in the absence of control studies.

The prevention and treatment of general asthma is primarily reliant on drugs.[8, 9] Adrenergic compounds, methylxanthines, and anticholinergics are bronchodilators that open the airways through a variety of mechanisms. Glucocorticoids are not bronchodilators but reduce airway inflammation, especially with severe obstruction. Mast cell stabilizing agents inhibit mast cell degranulation and the resultant release of chemical mediators. Miscellaneous agents and therapies include immunosuppressants, expectorants, mucolytic agents, oxygen administration (to treat hypoxemia and reduce the work of breathing), and mobilization and removal of bronchial secretions.

Case Study 1

A 35-year-old man presented to the emergency room complaining of shortness of breath. Respirations were 46 breaths per minute (normal = 12 to 20 breaths per minute) and auscultation of the chest indicated bilateral wheezing. Blood pressure was 130/94 mm Hg and heart rate was 120 beats per minute (normal = 60 to 100 beats per minute). The following are the laboratory results on admission, 1 hour later, and 24 hours later:

Laboratory Findings

	Admission	1 Hour Later	24 Hours Later
pH	7.35	7.36	7.44
Pa_{O_2} (mm Hg)	50	106	101
Pa_{CO_2} (mm Hg)	33	35.6	34
HCO_3 (mmol/L) (bicarbonate)	19.5	20.1	22.6
Base excess (mmol/L)	−4.2	−4.0	−0.2
FI_{O_2} (%) (fractional inspired oxygen)	21	85	21
S_{O_2} (calculated %) (oxygen saturation)	83.3	97.9	98.2
O_2Hb (measured %) (oxyhemoglobin)	82	96	98
$COHb$ (%) (carboxyhemoglobin)	1.9	0.9	0.7
tHb (g/dL) (total hemoglobin)	17.3	17.3	14.0

Questions

1. What physical findings particularly suggest asthma as a diagnosis?
2. What accounts for the low Pa_{CO_2}, Pa_{O_2} and HCO_3, the negative base excess, and elevated total hemoglobin found on admission?
3. What precautions must be taken after blood gas levels apparently return to normal?

Discussion

1. Dyspnea and wheezing suggest asthma. This patient was admitted with bronchial asthma and was rehydrated and treated with bronchodilators and oxygen therapy.

2. Upon admission, the patient was hyperventilating secondary to airway restriction and hypoxemia. The elevated total hemoglobin indicated dehydration due to prolonged lack of fluid and food. The low HCO_3 and the negative base excess could indicate the presence of lactate due to prolonged lack of fluid and food. One hour later, with the bronchodilator and oxygen therapy, the arterial blood gas levels begin to return toward normal. Twenty four hours later, the patient's blood gas levels are normal and the normal total hemoglobin concentration indicates the effects of rehydration.

3. Patients with asthma are anxious, hyperventilate, and often have some level of hypoxemia. They are working very hard to move air in and out of the airways and can eventually tire. One indication of significant exhaustion of an asthma patient is when the Pa_{CO_2} level stays in the range of 40 to 45 mm Hg. The level should be watched very carefully and the patient checked for alertness and monitored very closely during such a situation.

Case Study 2

A 62-year-old man was admitted to a hospital emergency room complaining of shortness of breath. The physical examination revealed bilateral wheezing in both lung fields, a barrel chest, and a very long expiratory phase during the breathing cycle. The patient's color was grayish, and he indicated that he had been coughing up copious amounts of very thick, tenacious sputum.

Laboratory Findings

pH	7.36
Pa_{O_2}	58 mm Hg
Pa_{CO_2}	65 mm Hg
HCO_3	36.8 mmol/L
Base excess	8.4 mmol/L
S_{O_2} (calculated)	87%
O_2Hb (measured)	93%
$COHb$	1.9%
Chloride	94 mmol/L
Potassium	3.3 mmol/L
tHb	18.5 g/dL
Sputum Gram stain	gram-negative bacilli

Questions

1. Do the physical findings support a diagnosis of emphysema?
2. What probably triggered this episode?
3. Do the laboratory findings support these conclusions?
4. What precautions must be taken in oxygenating and following this patient?

Discussion

1. Yes. The age range and dyspnea with barrel chest are characteristic, as is a long expiratory phase.

2. This patient has COPD with an exacerbation secondary to infection by gram-negative rods.

3. From a laboratory testing standpoint, one should first be concerned about whether the blood gas values as shown might indicate that the sample is venous rather than arterial because of the elevated $Paco_2$ and the decreased Po_2. The pH is normal (7.35 to 7.45), indicating that the patient has had this problem for a long time and through compensatory (primarily renal reabsorption of bicarbonate) mechanisms has counteracted the hypercapnia. The hemoglobin is elevated in response to low levels of tissue oxygen, which stimulates erythropoietin, a renal hormone.

4. Patients with advanced COPD are usually sensitive to oxygen and breathe on a hypoxic drive. This means that these patients survive on a Pao_2 of 60 mm Hg. If given too much oxygen, respirations can slow down or stop, causing $Paco_2$ to rise and possibly resulting in respiratory and cardiac arrest. Therefore, both the Pao_2 and the acid-base balance should be monitored closely. In this situation, patients usually show a normal pH with a $Paco_2$ between 50 and 60 mm Hg.

References

1. Snider GL, Lucey EC, Stone PJ, et al: The definition of emphysema: Report of the National Heart, Lung, and Blood Institute, Division of Lung Diseases workshop. Am Rev Respir Dis 132:182, 1985.
2. Rubin E, Farber JL: The respiratory system. *In* Rubin E, Farber JL (eds): Pathology, ed 2. Philadelphia, JB Lippincott, 1994.
3. Kobzik L, Schoen FJ: The lung. *In* Cotran RS, Kumar V, Robbins SL (eds): Robbins Pathologic Basis of Disease, ed 5. Philadelphia, WB Saunders, 1994.
4. Lee-Lewandrowski E, Lewandrowski KB: The plasma proteins. *In* McClatchey KD (ed): Clinical Laboratory Medicine. Baltimore, Williams & Wilkins, 1994, p 246.
5. Barnes PJ, Rodger IW, Thomson NC, et al: Asthma: Basic Mechanisms and Clinical Management. London, Academic Press, 1992.
6. Markey J: Immunopharmacology of asthma. Immunol Today 14:3179, 1993.
7. Gailli S: New concepts about the mast cell. N Engl J Med 328:257, 1993.
8. Graziano FM, Lemanske RF: Clinical Immunology. Baltimore, Williams & Wilkins, 1989.
9. McFadden ER: Asthma. *In* Isselbacher KJ, Braunwald E, Wilson JD (eds): Harrison's Principles of Internal Medicine, ed 13. New York, McGraw-Hill, 1994.

Chapter 10

Pulmonary Thromboembolism

Sharon S. Ehrmeyer and Kevin D. Fallon

Occlusion of an artery or vein by material transported by the blood stream is termed *embolism*, and the material that lodges in the blood vessel is the *embolus*. The most common embolus is the thromboembolus, which is caused by circulating fragments or whole blood clots. Pulmonary thromboembolism (PTE) is the occlusion of the main pulmonary artery or its branches. The clinical consequences depend on the size of the embolus, the extent and location of the obstruction, and the general health and circulatory status of the patient.

ETIOLOGY AND PATHOPHYSIOLOGY

PTE is one of the most common preventable causes of death in hospital patients. Each year in the United States, there are more than 500,000 cases of pulmonary emboli. Fewer than 10% of these cases are the sole or major contributing cause of death.[1]

More than 90% of clinically significant PTEs are from thrombi that originate in the deep venous system of the lower extremities. Thrombi can also develop in other veins and in the right ventricle; however, this is uncommon unless some other factor is present to precipitate clot formation. Because most thromboemboli originate in the deep veins, PTE should be viewed as a complication of deep venous thrombosis (DVT). When either part or all of a thrombus dislodges, it becomes a freely moving embolus that flows through the venous system to the right ventricle, and then into pulmonary arterial circulation.

The clinical consequences of PTE can be classified broadly into three categories: (1) massive pulmonary embolism, (2) pulmonary infarction, and (3) pulmonary embolism without infarction.[2] If a large embolus or multiple small emboli lodge in one of the main pulmonary arteries

or span the bifurcation of the main pulmonary artery (saddle embolus), the obstruction results in sudden death. This is common in patients who have undergone major orthopedic surgery, in patients with chronic heart and lung diseases, and in patients subjected to prolonged bedrest.

Small pulmonary emboli usually are not fatal; however, emboli that lodge in peripheral end-arteries can cause pulmonary infarction and subsequent tissue death in the surrounding area as a result of inadequate circulation. Particularly in patients with congestive heart failure or chronic lung disease, pulmonary infarction can lead initially to necrosis and eventually to fibrous scarring.

With the lung's dual blood supply (bronchial and pulmonary arteries), a majority of small pulmonary emboli that obstruct middle-sized arteries do not cause infarction. A rare consequence is mechanical obstruction of the arterial bed by recurrent, numerous small emboli, resulting in pulmonary hypertension. Clinical and radiologic findings in such cases are similar to those seen with pulmonary infarctions.

The three factors—venous stasis, hypercoagulability, and damaged vessel walls—proposed by Virchow in the 19th century are still the primary promoters of DVT (and embolic risk). Venous stasis is caused by a variety of conditions, such as prolonged bedrest, sitting, or standing, and congestive heart failure. *Hypercoagulability*, which is the predisposition to thrombosis due to the alteration of blood coagulation mechanisms, can be caused by primary genetic defects or mutations of the coagulation proteins (antithrombin III, protein C, protein S, and, more rarely, components of the fibrinolytic system). A more difficult association to predict is hypercoagulability due to secondary clinical conditions and factors.[3] These conditions and factors include homocystinuria, nephrotic syndrome, pregnancy, childbirth, estrogen therapy, polycythemia vera, sickle cell disease or trait and other hemoglobinopathies, various malignancies, aging, obesity, and smoking. The third factor that promotes DVT is damaged blood vessel walls. Injury to endothelial cells can originate from alterations in blood flow, infections, hypertension, radiation or chemical agents, autoimmune complex deposits, and other causes. Whatever the origin, damaged blood vessel walls have a potent thrombotic influence.

CLINICAL MANIFESTATIONS

Extreme variability in symptoms occurs depending on the size and location of the PTE and the patient's cardiopulmonary status. It is important to note that symptoms may be clinically silent following the vascular insult; however, many symptoms are apparent and reflect the consequences of the PTE on the pulmonary and cardiovascular systems. Typically, in patients with a normal cardiovascular system, small emboli that do not precipitate pulmonary infarction produce brief chest pain and cough and possibly some hemorrhage. With inadequate pulmonary circulation, small emboli can cause pulmonary infarction, and patients can experience sudden onset of dyspnea and chest pain, bronchospasm, tachypnea, wheezing (rare), cough, hemoptysis, and exercise dyspnea.

For a large PTE, the symptoms—severe chest pain, tachycardia, abnormal heart sounds, signs of shock (pallor, diaphoresis, rapid pulse with low blood pressure), fever, and elevation of enzyme levels—mimic those of a myocardial infarction.

Other associated symptoms may include profound apprehension, fever of unknown origin, confusion, and lightheadedness. Concurrent thrombophlebitis, often manifested by pain, swelling, ankle edema, cyanosis, and tenderness of the affected limb, is clinically suggestive of PTE.

LABORATORY ANALYSES AND DIAGNOSIS

Among the conditions that should be considered in the differential diagnosis of PTE are acute myocardial infarction, angina pectoris, pneumonia, asthma, paradoxical embolism (rare), primary pulmonary hypertension, congestive heart failure, pulmonary edema, undiagnosed sickle cell trait, spontaneous pneumothorax, bronchial carcinoma, and atelectasis.

Clinical Tests

The lung perfusion scan is useful in the diagnosis of PTE. Perfusion studies that display the distribution of blood flow are commonly performed in conjunction with ventilation-perfusion ($\dot{V}/\dot{Q}$) scans. The specificity of the test in resolving abnormalities of ventilation and perfusion abnormalities is greatly enhanced when the two studies are performed simultaneously. When viewed together, the various types of scan patterns allow the determination of a probability estimate for pulmonary embolism. Pulmonary angiography, an invasive procedure that requires experienced personnel, can provide a conclusive diagnosis of PTE. However, an angiogram should be performed as soon as possible after symptoms appear, and it is indicated only when the other diagnostic tests ($\dot{V}/\dot{Q}$ scan, x-ray) are inconclusive and an accurate diagnosis is necessary.[4]

Electrocardiography (ECG) is nonspecific in the diagnosis of PTE because a large percentage of patients with pulmonary embolism present with normal ECG findings. Patients with more severe cases, however, present with ECG evidence of acute strain on the right ventricle. Pulmonary function test findings are nonspecific for pulmonary embolism. Thoracentesis may or may not yield hemorrhagic fluid.

Laboratory Tests

No clinical laboratory test is diagnostic for PTE. The laboratory tests most useful in the diagnosis of massive

PTE are arterial pH and arterial blood gas analyses. These usually indicate a low $PaCO_2$ with an elevated pH (alkalosis) due to hyperventilation. The PaO_2 may be low as well because of arterial hypoxemia, and a normal PaO_2 does not rule out the diagnosis. The leukocyte count and sedimentation rate may be elevated with an infarction. Enzyme levels may be elevated owing to liver or heart damage or the degradation of erythrocytes from hemorrhage as a result of PTE. In addition, coagulation studies can be performed to determine whether a patient is genetically predisposed to thrombus formation.

TREATMENT

Prophylactic Treatment

With PTE, prevention of DVT is extremely important. Approaches include early ambulation in postoperative and postpartum patients and use of elastic stockings and leg exercise therapy for immobilized patients. Anticoagulation therapy is an effective prophylactic treatment and is also used to prevent recurrent venous thromboembolism.

Treatment After Diagnosis of PTE

Goals of therapy for PTE include inhibition of the development of thromboemboli, resolution of the thromboemboli, and prevention of recurrence. Anticoagulant therapy inhibits development of emboli, facilitates resolution, and assists in preventing recurrence. *Fibrinolytic* agents are administered to bring about clot lysis by activating plasminogen to form plasmin. Fibrinolytic agents do help in the resolution of venous thrombi and PTE; however, they do not replace the use of conventional anticoagulants. Fibrinolytic agents are associated with risks, and their effectiveness in altering morbidity, mortality, and recurrence has not been firmly established. The value of continuous monitoring of clotting time and partial thromboplastin time (PTT) and the utility of other clotting studies have not been clearly established; however, many recommend determination of clotting time or PTT just before administering another intermittent dose of anticoagulant.[4]

Case Study

A 56-year-old white female was having a routine recovery from coronary artery bypass surgery. On the third day of postoperative care, the patient's condition was stable and she was discharged from the cardiovascular intensive care unit to the general care floor. At 2:00 AM, a nurse took the vital signs and noticed that the patient was hyperventilating and perspiring and that the nail beds and lips were cyanotic. Blood pressure was slightly elevated (148/92 mm Hg).

Laboratory Findings

	Second Postoperative Day	Third Postoperative Day
PaO_2	87 mm Hg	54 mm Hg
$PaCO_2$	39 mm Hg	28 mm Hg
pH	7.43	7.51

Questions

1. Can the physical and laboratory findings of the third postoperative day be correlated?
2. Do the history, the physical, and the laboratory findings support a diagnosis of PTE?
3. What other procedures should be performed to confirm the diagnosis?
4. What therapy and subsequent monitoring are appropriate?

Discussion

1. Low oxygenation is evidenced by cyanosis, hyperventilation, and PaO_2 value. Hyperventilation leads to low $PaCO_2$ and increased pH.
2. Cardiac surgery is a primary predisposing factor for PTE. Clinical and laboratory findings are consistent with PTE.
3. Pulmonary angiography is performed to confirm the presence of pulmonary embolism.
4. Because results of the angiogram were positive and the patient did have a pulmonary embolism, the patient was immediately given 60% oxygen, and arterial blood gas analyses were repeated and monitored to keep the oxygenation at adequate levels. Heparin was administered intravenously as an anticoagulant to treat the embolism. The patient was already receiving cardiotonic drugs to reduce heart strain. Constant ECG monitoring was undertaken, and the patient was moved back into the intensive care unit. Administration of streptokinase to treat the pulmonary embolism was considered, but the patient's arterial oxygenation was restored to normal levels without such action. The PTT was monitored to minimize the risk of bleeding.

References

1. Kobzik L, Schoen FJ: The lung. *In* Cotran RS, Kumar V, Robbins SL (eds): Robbins Pathologic Basis of Disease, ed 5. Philadelphia, WB Saunders, 1994.
2. Mergner WJ, Trump BF: Hemodynamic disorders. *In* Rubin E, Farber JL (eds): Pathology, ed 2. Philadelphia, JB Lippincott, 1994.
3. Schaffer M: Pathology of thrombosis. *In* Loscaizo J, Creager MA, Dzau VJ (eds): Vascular Medicine, Boston, Little, Brown & Co., 1992.
4. Moser KM: Pulmonary thromboembolism. *In* Isselbacher KJ, Braunwald E, Wilson JD (eds): Harrison's Principles of Internal Medicine, ed 13. New York, McGraw-Hill, 1994.

Chapter 11

Respiratory Tract Infections

Lauren Roberts

The primary purpose of respiration is to take in oxygen and remove unnecessary carbon dioxide (CO_2). When following the course that air must travel the anatomic complexity of the region of the respiratory tract region becomes apparent. As air is taken in through the mouth and nose, it passes the sinuses, flows into the pharynx past the epiglottis, through the larynx, down the trachea and into the bronchioles, and, finally, into the alveoli. In addition to the exchange of air, this region has other functions including the intake and separation of food and liquids from the air flow, the expression of speech, and the senses of taste, smell, and hearing.[1] The entire region is also important in defending the respiratory tract from invading microorganisms.

Infections of the respiratory tract are the most common infections in the United States, ranging from benign conditions, such as the common cold and viral pharyngitis, to life-threatening pneumonia and other significant pulmonary infections. The upper respiratory tract (URT) includes the nasal cavity and sinuses, the nasopharynx, oropharynx, middle ear, epiglottis, and larynx. Most URT infections affect the nasal passages and the pharynx and are usually caused by viruses, although certain bacteria are also pathogens[2] (Table 11–1). The lower respiratory tract (LRT) consists of the trachea, bronchi, bronchioles, and the alveoli. Infection in these areas is caused by a wide variety of etiologic agents including bacteria (e.g., *Chlamydiae, mycoplasmas*), viruses, fungi, and parasites[3] (Table 11–2).

ETIOLOGY AND PATHOPHYSIOLOGY

Host-Parasite Interactions

Numerous mechanisms defend the respiratory tract and protect it from infection.[4,5] Nasal hairs filter air as it passes, and the mucous lining of the nasal passages traps particles. The mechanics of the epiglottis and the reflex closure of the glottis serve as an anatomic barrier to prevent particulate matter from reaching the large airways. Secretory immunoglobulin A (IgA) and other natural antibacterial substances are present in respiratory secretions. Normal bacterial flora reside in the nasopharynx and oropharynx and help to prevent colonization by pathogenic organisms. The mucociliary lining of the trachea, along with coughing, sneezing, and swallowing, provide further defense mechanisms. If organisms breach these barriers and enter the alveoli, they are ingested by macrophages and presented to cells of the immune system. This process produces secretory components that attract polymorphonuclear cells, and inflammation results.

Respiratory tract infections occur when microorganisms

Table 11–1. Etiologic Agents of Upper Respiratory Tract Infections

Clinical Syndrome	Etiologic Agents
Common cold	Rhinoviruses, coronaviruses, adenoviruses, parainfluenza viruses, influenza viruses, respiratory syncytial viruses
Pharyngitis	*Streptococcus pyogenes* (group Aβ-hemolytic streptococcus), *Corynebacterium diphtheriae, Neisseria gonorrhoeae,* adenoviruses, parainfluenza viruses, rhinoviruses, coxsackie viruses, herpes simplex viruses, Epstein-Barr viruses
Epiglottitis	*Haemophilus influenzae* type b (rarely: *Streptococcus pneumoniae, Staphylococcus aureus,* β-hemolytic streptococci)
Sinusitis	*Streptococcus pneumoniae, Haemophilus influenzae, Moraxella catarrhalis, Streptococcus pyogenes, Staphylococcus aureus,* anaerobes, gram-negative bacilli, fungi
Otitis media	*Streptococcus pneumoniae, Haemophilus influenzae, Streptococcus pyogenes, Moraxella catarrhalis, Staphylococcus aureus*
Pertussis	*Bordetella pertussis, Bordetella parapertussis*
Diphtheria	*Corynebacterium diphtheriae*

Table 11–2. Etiologic Agents of Lower Respiratory Tract Infections

Clinical Syndrome	Etiologic Agents
Bronchitis/ bronchiolitis	Respiratory viruses, *Mycoplasma pneumoniae*, *Chlamydia pneumoniae*, *Bordetella pertussis*
Pneumonia	
Community-acquired	*Streptococcus pneumoniae, Staphylococcus aureus, Haemophilus influenzae, Mycoplasma pneumoniae, Legionella* spp., *Chlamydia* spp., respiratory syncytial viruses, parainfluenza viruses, adenoviruses, influenza viruses
Nosocomial	*Pseudomonas aeruginosa*, Enterobacteriaceae, *Staphylococcus aureus*, anaerobes, *Legionella* spp.
Aspiration; lung abscess; empyema	Anaerobes, mixed aerobes and anaerobes
Chronic	*Mycobacterium tuberculosis*, other mycobacteria, *Nocardia* spp., fungi

overcome the natural host defenses and multiply sufficiently to produce symptoms. The virulence factors that enable them to do so include adherence, toxin production, and the evasion of host defenses.[4] For an organism to develop within the respiratory tract, it must first attach itself to the mucosal lining. Successful respiratory pathogens often possess specific adherence properties such as adhesins, fimbriae, hemagglutinins, or certain proteins that mediate attachment. The elaboration of extracellular toxins is another virulence mechanism possessed by certain pathogens of the respiratory tract, *Corynebacterium diphtheriae* and *Bordetella pertussis* are examples of toxin-producing pathogens. The presence of a polysaccharide capsule allows a microorganism to avoid host defenses by preventing phagocytosis and protecting microbial antigens from exposure to immunoglobulins. Other pathogens are protected from the host immune system by multiplying intracellularly. *Chlamydiae*, viruses, and mycobacteria are all examples of intracellular respiratory pathogens.

Mild respiratory tract infections occur in all individuals, whereas life-threatening infections are more often associated with newborns, the elderly, or the immunocompromised host. Other factors that predispose an individual to infection include exposure to aerosol droplets containing infectious microorganisms, long-term hospitalization, antimicrobial or cytotoxic therapy, and smoking. Serious LRT infection (LRTI) can also develop in individuals who experience a loss of consciousness and aspirate oropharyneal contents.

Upper Respiratory Tract Infections

The Common Cold

The common cold is the most prevalent respiratory tract infection of humans. It is an acute syndrome of inflammation in the respiratory mucous membranes and is usually viral in origin. Although usually mild and self-limiting, it is the most frequent cause for work and school absenteeism.[6] Complications are rare, but bacterial infection to the dam-

aged respiratory tissue can lead to sinusitis, otitis media, or LRTIs.

The rhinoviruses are the most important etiologic agents of the common cold, causing approximately 25% of colds in adults. Coronaviruses are involved in approximately 10% of adult infections. Other viruses that have been linked to the common cold include parainfluenza viruses, respiratory syncytial viruses, adenoviruses, and influenza viruses.[6] This heterogeneous group of viruses shares the following common features: worldwide distribution, responsibility for a variety of acute respiratory disease syndromes, a relatively short incubation period of 1 to 4 days, and person-to-person transmission.

The transmission of these respiratory viruses is through direct contact with the respiratory secretions of an infected individual. This can occur directly, by inhalation of aerosols containing infectious particles, or indirectly, by hand transfer of the infectious secretions to the nasal or conjunctival epithelium. The incubation period for most respiratory viruses is from 1 to 4 days, and the symptoms last for approximately 1 week. Viral replication occurs in the ciliated epithelium of the nasal passages and the pharynx. An inflammatory process ensues, resulting in vasodilation, edema, mucous gland secretion, and leukocyte infiltration.

The frequency of colds is increased in the winter months, due to the spread by person-to-person contact. Adults usually average 2 to 3 colds per year, whereas children average 6 to 8 per year, and some preschoolers may experience 10 to 12 cold syndromes per year.[7]

Pharyngitis

Acute pharyngitis is an inflammation in the mucous membranes of the posterior oral cavity involving the throat and, possibly, the uvula, nasopharynx, and soft palate. The majority of cases are of viral etiology and are generally self-limited. Pharyngitis, in these cases, often presents as part of the clinical picture of a common cold or an early sign of influenza. The viruses that cause the common cold are implicated in nonbacterial pharyngitis along with herpes simplex virus (HSV), Epstein-Barr virus (EBV), cytomegalovirus (CMV), coxsackie A virus, and human immunodeficiency virus (HIV).

Streptococcus pyogenes (group A β-hemolytic streptococci) is the most commonly encountered agent of bacterial pharyngitis. Other β-hemolytic streptococci (groups B, C, and G) may also cause pharyngitis, but these groups do not lead to the sequelae that may occur in group A streptococcal infections.[7] Less common bacterial agents of pharyngitis include *Corynebacterium diphtheriae, Co. ulcerans, Co. pyogenes,* and *Neisseria gonorrhoeae. Arcanobacterium haemolyticum* (formerly *Corynebacterium*) is associated with pharyngitis and tonsillitis in patients 10 to 30 years old. *Haemophilus influenzae, Staphylococcus aureus,* and *Streptococcus pneumoniae* can be isolated from throat cultures, but they are not considered a cause of pharyngitis. *Neisseria meningitidis* can also be recovered from the nasopharynx of carriers, but its presence is not significant unless the individual has recently been exposed to a patient with *N. meningitidis* meningitis. Mixed anaerobic bacteria can result in an exudative pharyngitis known as Vincent's angina. Lastly, *Chlamydia pneumoniae, Mycoplasma pneu-*

moniae, and *Treponema pallidum* can also cause pharyngitis.

The transmission of acute pharyngitis occurs in the same fashion as the common cold, direct contact with secretions from an infected individual. Most cases of pharyngitis, including streptococcal pharyngitis occur during the colder months of the year. The pathogenesis is dependent on the etiologic agent involved. Some viruses cause cellular destruction that leads to an inflammatory response, whereas other viruses are not cytopathic but elicit inflammatory mediators. *S. pyogenes* elaborates several extracellular products that lead to an inflammatory process. *C. diphtheriae* multiplies on the epithelial cells in the pharynx and produces damage through the production of an exotoxin.

Acute Laryngitis, Croup, and Epiglottitis

Acute laryngitis is an inflammation of the larynx and usually occurs as part of another upper respiratory illness such as the common cold. The inflammation is localized in the subglottic laryngeal structures, including the vocal cords. Respiratory viruses that are associated with the common cold are responsible, including influenza, parainfluenza, rhinovirus, and adenovirus.[8] The role of bacteria in this condition is not understood. *Moraxella catarrhalis* and *H. influenzae* have been isolated from the nasopharynx of adults with laryngitis, but these organisms may indicate secondary colonization.[7, 8]

A more severe form of laryngitis can develop if the infection extends from the larynx to the trachea and the bronchi, resulting in a condition called *laryngotracheobronchitis* or *croup.* This clinical syndrome is more common in children under the age of 3 years, and the etiology is usually viral.[1] Parainfluenza viruses are the most frequently identified pathogens, but other respiratory viruses and *M. pneumoniae* have also been implicated.

Epiglottitis, also referred to as *supraglottitis,* is a rapidly progressive inflammatory condition of the epiglottis and surrounding tissues in the supraglottic airway.[1] Inflammation and edema, along with the accumulation of mucus inspissated from the bronchi, can lead to an airway obstruction. In the past, this condition has been primarily associated with children, and it can be a life-threatening infection. *H. influenzae* type b is the usual pathogen in this condition, although a viral infection may precede an episode of epiglottitis. Immunization of children against *H. influenzae* type b may be changing the epidemiology of epiglottitis. In recent years, the number of cases in children is decreasing; however, the number of cases in adults is increasing.[9, 10]

Sinusitis

Sinusitis is an acute inflammation of the mucosal lining of one or more of the paranasal sinuses, which are directly contiguous to the nasal cavity. These air-filled cavities are lined with ciliated epithelium and normally remain sterile because of the continuous mucociliary clearance. Acute sinusitis often follows a cold or other acute upper respiratory tract infection (URTI), although respiratory allergies also predispose an individual to sinusitis (Table 11–3). When acute sinusitis recurs and is not completely resolved, the epithelial lining can become irreversibly damaged leading to chronic sinusitis.

Table 11–3. Predisposing Factors for Sinusitis

Predisposing Factor	Examples
Impaired mucociliary function	Viral infections
	Environmental conditions: air, chemicals
	Cystic fibrosis
Sinus obstruction	Viral infections
	Allergies
	Nasal polyps
	Foreign bodies
Immune deficiency	Immunoglobulin A (IgA) deficiency
	Immunoglobulin G (IgG) deficiency
	AIDS
Microbial invasion	Dental infections
	Nasotracheal intubation
	Swimming
	Cocaine sniffing

Obstruction of the osteomeatal area of the nasal cavity is a major risk factor for sinusitis.[7] During viral or allergic rhinitis, mucosal swelling causes obstruction of the sinus ostia and interrupts the normal cleansing process, thus leading to bacterial overgrowth. Other predisposing factors that prevent normal drainage include the presence of mucosal polyps, tumors, or other foreign bodies.[11] Patients with cystic fibrosis, selective immunoglobulin deficiencies, or acquired immunodeficiency syndrome (AIDS) are also predisposed to sinusitis. Lastly, maxillary sinusitis can occur from a dental root abscess.

When cultures are performed on adults with sinusitis, *S. pneumoniae* and unencapsulated strains of *H. influenzae* are the most common pathogens isolated. *M. catarrhalis* is another important pathogen, with a higher incidence of infection in children than in adults.[12] Other pathogens associated with sinusitis include *S. pyogenes, S. aureus,* and gram-negative bacilli. Anaerobes are not usually associated with acute sinusitis, unless the source of the infection is dental, but they are the predominant organisms in chronic sinusitis. Saprophytic fungi can cause acute sinusitis in immunocompromised hosts, whereas chronic fungal sinusitis usually occurs in an immunocompetent host with recurrent sinus problems.

Otitis Media and Otitis Externa

Otitis media, an infection of the middle ear canal, is the most common localized infection of the URT in preschool-age children.[13] Most cases occur during or following a viral URTI. As in sinus infections, when the normal clearance mechanism of the ciliated epithelium and mucus-secreting cells of the middle ear becomes impaired, infection can develop. Young children are predisposed to otitis media because of an anatomic immaturity in the eustachian tube, which allows the middle ear to become contaminated with nasopharyngeal bacteria. Infection can result in damage to the tympanic membrane and hearing loss.

The microbial etiology of otitis media is similar to that of acute sinusitis. *S. pneumoniae* and *H. influenzae* are the most common isolates, although *M. catarrhalis* is increasing in incidence.[13] Other less common pathogens include group A β-hemolytic streptococci and *S. aureus.* Viruses can also be isolated from middle ear fluid; however, the viral agents are probably predisposing the patient to super-infection by bacterial agents.[11]

Otitis externa, also known as "swimmer's ear," is a superficial infection of the external ear canal. It occurs most often in the summer months and is thought to develop from a change in the environmental conditions of the external ear canal with increased alkalinization leading to overgrowth by bacteria. Trauma, boils, and foreign bodies can also result in otitis externa.

Pseudomonas aeruginosa is the most common organism associated with otitis externa. Malignant external otitis, also caused by *P. aeruginosa,* is a more severe form of external ear canal infection that can progress to the inva-sion of cartilage and bone.[11] It is found most often in elderly patients with diabetes mellitus and in immunocom-promised hosts and can result in cranial nerve palsy and death.

Diphtheria, Pertussis, and Other Infections

Diphtheria is a localized and generalized intoxication caused by toxigenic strains of *C. diphtheriae.* The disease is rare today because of widespread immunization. Most cases occur in developing countries, but outbreaks can occur if immunity is not maintained in adults.[14]

The disease has two forms, respiratory and cutaneous. The organism is transmitted by droplet infection, hand-to-mouth contact, or direct skin-to-skin contact. The organism multiplies on the epithelial cells of the respiratory tract or on superficial skin surfaces, resulting in an inflammatory response. Toxigenic strains elaborate a toxin that inhibits intracellular protein synthesis, causing local tissue necrosis and exudate formation. Dissemination of the toxin results in systemic manifestations that affect all tissues. The major organ tissues affected are the kidneys, heart, and nervous system.

Pertussis, meaning intense cough, is a highly contagious infection of the tracheobronchial tree caused by *B. pertus-sis. B. parapertussis* is associated with a similar but milder form of illness. Also referred to as whooping cough, the term pertussis is more appropriate because many patients cough but do not whoop.[15]

The organisms are transmitted through respiratory drop-lets and possess adhesins and pili by which they readily attach to the ciliated respiratory epithelium. A massive production of mucus occurs and results in forceful coughing. Although the pathogenesis of pertussis is not completely understood, several toxins are responsible for the clinical manifestations. The major virulence factor is pertussis toxin, which causes several biologic effects, in-cluding histamine sensitization, promotion of lymphocyto-sis, and secretion of insulin.[16] Complications include LRTI, often caused by a secondary bacterial agent, and central nervous system manifestations.

The key to preventing pertussis is immunization. A dramatic decline in this disease was noted in the United States after the introduction of a vaccine in the 1940s. Additionally, an increase in cases is reported when immuni-zation rates decrease. Vaccine protection is not lifelong, as is the immunity when the natural disease occurs. The highest incidence and the greatest complications of this disease are in young infants. Vaccination has shifted the epidemiology of pertussis. Children with the highest vacci-nation rate, between the ages of 1 and 9 years make up a smaller percentage of cases than in the prevaccine days. The population of young adults is becoming more suscepti-ble as vaccine protection wanes and the number of older persons with lifelong immunity as a result of acquiring the disease from nature is declining. Concern has arisen that this will increase the spread of infection from adults with minimal symptoms to nonimmunized infants.[17, 18]

Stomatitis is an inflammation of the oral cavity with lesions on the oral mucosa, tongue, and lips. Infectious agents that result in stomatitis include HSV and *Candida* species, causing thrush. Thrush is found most commonly in neutropenic patients, diabetic patients, or patients who have received antibiotic therapy. Infants born of mothers who have vaginal candidiasis may develop thrush.

Lower Respiratory Tract Infections

Acute Bronchitis/Tracheobronchitis and Bronchiolitis

Normally, the LRT is sterile, even though it is adjacent to microorganisms residing in the oropharynx and is contin-ually exposed to organisms in the inhaled air. The sterility of the LRT is normally maintained by efficient filtering and clearing mechanisms. Acute bronchitis, or tracheobron-chitis, is a common infectious process involving the air-ways between the larynx and the bronchioles. URTI often precedes the development of acute bronchitis, and most cases are thought to be viral in origin.[19] Acute bronchitis is often considered an extension of the same viral infection that causes URT symptoms. Infection of the trachea and bronchi produces inflammatory changes, increased mucous secretions, and decreased ciliary action.

All of the common viruses that are involved in URTI have been implicated as a cause of acute bronchitis and are frequently found in a seasonal pattern. When influenza viruses are prevalent in the community, these viruses are the most common cause of acute bronchitis. Other viral agents involved in acute bronchitis include rhinovirus, co-ronavirus, and parainfluenza virus. Respiratory syncytial virus (RSV) is an important cause of community-wide outbreaks in infants. Nonviral pathogens associated with acute bronchitis include *M. pneumoniae, C. pneumoniae,* and *B. pertussis.* Acute viral infections can be complicated by secondary bacterial infections. When this occurs, *S. pneumoniae, H. influenzae, S. aureus,* and *M. catarrhalis* are the most common isolates.

Like other acute respiratory tract infections, the inci-dence of acute bronchitis is greatest in the winter months.[19] Children with allergies, poor nutrition, and immunoglobu-lin G (IgG) subclass deficiencies are predisposed to respi-ratory tract infections associated with acute bronchitis. Older patients with emphysema and other chronic respiratory illnesses are also at risk of infection. Air pollution and rapid environmental temperature or humidity changes may also trigger this condition.

Bronchiolitis is an acute respiratory tract infection of young infants in which inflammation of the bronchioles leads to an obstruction. This condition is thought to be an extension of URTI to the trachea, bronchi, and, finally, the terminal branches of the bronchial tree. RSV and parainfluenza virus type 3 are the most common pathogens.[19]

Chronic Bronchitis

Chronic bronchitis is defined as a productive cough present on most days, for at least 3 months of the year, for a minimum of 2 years in succession.[19] Chronic bronchitis is not associated with other pulmonary diseases such as malignancy, cystic fibrosis, bronchiectasis, or primary cardiac disease. This condition is the result of prolonged damage to the bronchial epithelium with a loss of cilated cells. Cigarette smoking is often described as the cause of this disease, but environmental pollution, chronic infections, or other factors that inhibit the normal clearance of bronchial secretions can be responsible as well.

Infectious agents do not cause this disease, except in the patient with a history of frequent respiratory tract infections, but they may perpetuate it. Patients are susceptible to recurrent acute episodes from infection with and colonization by viruses and bacteria. A cycle of repeated infection develops, leading to further damage and an increased potential for pulmonary damage.

Pneumonia

Pneumonia, another LRTI with subtle differences from acute bronchitis, is an inflammation of the pulmonary parenchyma. The distinction between acute bronchitis and acute pneumonia depends on the intensity and extent of the infectious process in the LRT. Typically, patients who have bronchitis do not demonstrate the physical examination and chest radiograph findings indicative of inflammation to the pulmonary parenchyma. Microbial pathogens can reach the lung by three methods: aspiration of organisms that colonize the oropharynx, inhalation of infectious airborne particles, and hematogenous dissemination.[20]

Although not all pneumonia occurs as a result of a defective host defense, most cases of pneumonias are the result of some compromise to the normal pulmonary defense mechanisms. Drugs, anesthesia, stroke, toxic inhalations, cigarette smoking, and alcohol abuse are contributing factors that can compromise the upper airway mechanisms for filtering or clearing inhaled infectious agents. A common precursor to pneumonia in healthy persons is an acute viral infection of the URT that allows oropharyngeal bacteria to reach the LRT.

Pneumonia is caused by a variety of microorganisms including bacteria (e.g., mycoplasmas, chlamydiae, rickettsiae), viruses, fungi, and parasites. Pneumonia can be subdivided into diagnostic categories based on clinical presentation, location of acquisition, and patient age and immune status. Acute pneumonia develops over hours to days, whereas chronic pneumonia has an insidious onset and develops over weeks to months. The location of acquisition (community or hospital) can provide presumptive information as to the etiologic agent involved. Infections that develop in patients in their normal setting are referred to as *community-acquired,* and infections that develop in the hospital are termed *nosocomial.* The incidence of pneumonia is higher in the very young and the very old.

Table 11–4. **Lower Respiratory Tract Pathogens and Age**

Age	Etiologic Agents
Newborn	*Chlamydia trachomatis*
Children	Respiratory syncytial viruses
	Influenza viruses
	Parainfluenza viruses
	Streptococcus pneumoniae
	Haemophilus influenzae
	Chlamydia pneumoniae
Young adults	*Mycoplasma pneumoniae*
	Chlamydia pneumoniae
	Respiratory viruses
Elderly	*Streptococcus pneumoniae*
	Haemophilus influenzae
	Staphylococcus aureus
	Legionella spp.

The etiologic agents of acute pneumonia are strongly related to age (Table 11–4). In the neonate, *Chlamydia trachomatis* is an important pathogen. Most pneumonia cases in infants and young children are caused by viruses, especially RSV and parainfluenza. Bacterial pneumonia is not very common in children, however, viral infections can predispose them to a secondary bacterial infection with *S. pneumoniae* or *H. influenzae* type b. *C. pneumoniae* is a common pathogen of school-age children and young adults. Respiratory viruses and *M. pneumoniae* are responsible for pneumonia in adolescents and young adults.[20]

The majority of the pneumonia in elderly patients is due to bacterial pathogens, with *S. pneumoniae* being the most common cause of acute community-acquired pneumonia.[21] Underlying conditions also affect the bacteria involved. In adults with chronic lung disease, *S. pneumoniae* and *H. influenzae* are the most common isolates. Outbreaks of influenza in the winter months can lead to secondary bacterial pneumonia in the elderly, which is a major cause of death in patients with influenza infection. The bacteria involved include *S. pneumoniae, S. aureus,* and *H. influenzae.* Pneumonia that develops in alcoholics is often due to gram-negative bacilli.

Legionella pneumophila is another pathogen that can be responsible for pneumonia in adults. Legionnaires' disease can occur in sporadic cases as well as in epidemic outbreaks in the community.[22] This organism is acquired through inhalation of aerosolized particles from the environment. Although *Legionella* species can cause disease in healthy hosts, more serious disease occurs in compromised hosts.

Hospitalized patients, especially those with a serious underlying disease, are at increased risk of becoming colonized with gram-negative bacilli. Therefore, enteric gram-negative bacilli and *P. aeruginosa,* are responsible for the majority of nosocomial pneumonia infections.[20] The gram-positive cocci, *S. aureus* and *S. pneumoniae* are also important pathogens in this population. The ability of *L. pneumophila* to contaminate water systems makes it a serious potential pathogen in hospitalized patients. Hospital outbreaks have occurred in which aerosols from sinks and showers have been implicated.[22]

Aspiration pneumonia can occur in the general population or in hopitalized patients through aspiration of oropharyneal or gastric contents into the LRT. Aspiration is more severe in individuals with an impaired level of consciousness, thus this form of pneumonia is more common in alcoholics, drug abusers, seizure or stroke victims, and patients undergoing general anesthesia.[20] The microorganisms involved are those that colonize the URT and include both aerobes and anaerobes. The infections that result range from a simple pneumonia that can be treated easily to necrotizing pneumonitis, lung abscess, and empyema. Lung abscess is a complication of aspiration pneumonia and a majority are caused by anaerobic organisms. The anaerobes most often involved are *Prevotella* species, *Fusobacterium nucleatum,* various anaerobic cocci, and *Bacteroides gracilis.*[23]

Chronic pneumonia differs from acute pneumonia in clinical presentation, radiologic pattern, and etiology. The most common agent of chronic LRTI is *Mycobacterium tuberculosis.*[24] Tuberculosis (TB) represents a classic example of a disease that is transmitted almost exclusively through the inhalation of droplet nuclei that contain *M. tuberculosis.* Most individuals with a competent immune system will mount a cell-mediated response and halt the proliferation of the organism. A defect in cell-mediated immunity will allow the bacteria to progress and disseminate. The incidence of TB in the United States declined steadily from the 1950s through the mid-1980s. A resurgence of this disease was noted in 1985 and cases continue to increase[24] as a result of several factors including the AIDS epidemic, poverty, overcrowded living conditions, and a reduction in public health funds allocated to TB control. The emergence of multi-drug resistant strains of TB has created additional complications in controlling the disease.

Fungal agents constitute another cause of chronic pneumonia. *Coccidioides immitis, Histoplasma capsulatum,* and *Blastomyces dermatitidis* cause pulmonary mycoses that can develop in normal or immunocompromised hosts. *Candida* species, *Aspergillus* species, and *Cryptococcus neoformans* are primarily considered opportunistic fungal infections.

Pneumocystis carinii represents another microorganism that is clinically significant in patients with impaired cellular immunity. A great deal of taxonomic confusion has existed over this organism because it was originally believed to be a yeast, then a protozoan; most recently it has been reclassified as a fungus.[25] *Pneumocystis* was associated with epidemics of interstitial plasma cell pneumonia in malnourished infants in European orphanages after World War II. Following this, infection with this organism was rare until the beginning of the AIDS epidemic, when *P. carinii* pneumonia was recognized as the most common opportunistic infection of these patients. Prophylaxis against *P. carinii* is now being used to decrease the incidence of this infection to patients at risk.

Actinomycotic bacteria can also cause infections of the LRT. *Nocardia* species are aerobic actinomycetes that exist primarily as saprophytes in soil, but inhalation of these organisms can result in an acute necrotizing pneumonia. *Actinomyces* species, are anaerobic bacteria that are found as normal inhabitants of the oropharynx, gastrointestinal tract, and female genital tract of humans. Pulmonary actinomycosis develops through aspiration, extension of a cervicofacial infection, or by hematogenous spread.

Unusual agents responsible for LRTIs include *Yersinia pestis, Francisella tularensis, Brucella* species, and *Coxiella burnetti.* Parasites that cause pulmonary complications are *Entamoeba histolytica, Ascaris lumbricoides, Strongyloides stercoralis,* and *Paragonimus westermani.*

CLINICAL MANIFESTATIONS

Upper Respiratory Tract Infections

The clinical manifestations of the common cold are so typical that most cases are diagnosed by the patient. The initial symptom is a dry, scratchy sore throat, followed by sneezing, nasal stuffiness, and rhinorrea. A low-grade fever, general malaise, and headache may also be present. The individual may also experience hoarseness and a dry, irritating cough.

The most characteristic symptom of pharyngitis is a sore throat accompanied by erythema and swelling of the tonsils and affected tissues. The clinical manifestations of viral and streptococcal pharyngitis are similar and they cannot be differentiated solely by clinical features. Pharyngitis associated with the common cold is usually mild, and other cold symptoms are present. In influenza virus infection a severe sore throat is noted, along with myalgia, headache, cough, and fever.[8] Primary infection with HSV may present as an acute sore throat with vesicular lesions on the buccal mucosa, tongue, palate, and oropharynx. Pharyngitis or exudative tonsillitis, accompanied by cervical and generalized lymphadenopathy, is also noted in patients with infectious mononucleosis (EBV). Primary infection with HIV typically includes pharyngitis, along with fever, myalgia, lethargy, and a rash.

Acute streptococcal pharyngitis is typically manifested by an abrupt onset of sore throat with difficulty swallowing.[26] Fever is more commonly observed in streptococcal pharyngitis than in viral pharyngitis. Other symptoms include chills, headache, tender submandibular lymph nodes, malaise, and, occasionally, nausea. Examination of the pharynx frequently reveals a thick exudate covering the tonsils and posterior pharynx, which is less common in viral pharyngitis. Some patients, however, may experience a mild or a subclinical infection that is indistinguishable from viral pharyngitis. Upper respiratory symptoms of rhinorrhea, cough, and nasal congestion are usually absent in streptococcal pharyngitis.

Vincent's angina represents another bacterial infection presenting with pharyngitis. This infection begins abruptly with pain, foul breath, and gingival or tonsillar bleeding. Tonsillar ulceration, necrosis, and a pseudomembrane are present, along with excessive salivation and fever. Diphtheria also presents as pharyngitis or tonsillitis, and a gray-white membrane develops on the tonsils, uvula, palate, or pharyngeal wall.

The symptoms of laryngitis include hoarseness, difficulty swallowing, and pain. Examination of the larynx reveals inflammation and edema. Croup is characterized by a classic inspiratory stridor and a barking cough. Acute epiglottitis can easily be confused with croup or laryngitis; however, the clinical course of epiglottitis is rapidly progressive. Children with epiglottitis present with sore throat, fever, difficulty swallowing, difficulty speaking, drooling, and airway obstruction.[7] The cough that is typical of croup is generally not present in patients with epiglottitis.

The clinical manifestations of sinusitis vary, depending on whether the infection is acute or chronic, which sinuses are infected, and the age of the patient.[12] Common features include pressure in the sinus area followed by pain and tenderness. The patient may experience fever, headache, a purulent nasal discharge, tonal changes in the voice, and alteration of the sense of smell. The symptoms of acute sinusitis in children may be quite different from those of adults. The major symptoms in young children may be cough, nasal discharge, and a sore throat. Chronic sinusitis patients usually experience less intense symptoms with nasal congestion and a postnasal drainage that may result in a chronic cough. Fever is unusual in chronic sinusitis, but fatigue and general malaise are often noted.

Otitis media is characterized by a severe, throbbing pain in the ear. Fever is usually present, and there may be a slight hearing impairment. Examination of the tympanic membrane will reveal a red, bulging ear drum. A perforation of the tympanic membrane may occur, and purulent secretions may drain into the ear canal. Otitis externa is associated with painful cellulitis that may extend into adjacent soft tissues. A purulent ear drainage is usually present.

Pertussis is divided into three clinical stages with a total duration from 6 to 10 weeks.[15, 18] Following an incubation period of 7 to 10 days, the catarrhal stage begins with symptoms of a common cold, including sneezing, cough, and infected conjunctivae. The disease is not usually recognized during this stage when the condition is most infectious. The paroxysmal stage is characterized by severe coughing episodes that may occur up to 50 times a day for 2 to 4 weeks. An inspiratory whoop may be heard, as air is forcefully inhaled through a narrow glottic opening, however, this whooping sound is not always present during pertussis infection. During the final convalescent stage, the coughing spells gradually diminish in number and severity.

Lower Respiratory Tract Infections

The primary manifestations of acute bronchitis are cough and fever. The cough is initially dry and becomes productive as the illness progresses. The clinical presentation of bronchiolitis in infants is a febrile URTI with signs of LRT airway obstruction. The onset is rather insidious, but as bronchial involvement develops, the infant experiences difficulty breathing, and intercostal retractions during inspiration become increasingly noticeable.[19] These patients also have a severe cough, purulent sputum, chest congestion, and wheezing.

Community-acquired bacterial pneumonia is described as having a typical presentation that consists of a sudden onset of fever and chills. A productive cough is noted, and the sputum is often purulent and may be blood-tinged, rust-colored, or foul smelling. The patient experiences pleuritic pain, difficulty breathing, and hypoxemia that may lead to cyanosis of the lips and nail beds.[21] The clinical presentation in immunocompromised hosts may not be as dramatic as the appearance of symptoms in a patient with a normal immune response.

The presentation of atypical pneumonia syndrome differs from bacterial pneumonia. Atypical pneumonia is characterized by a gradual onset, a dry cough, and more general constitutional symptoms of headache, myalgia, fatigue, nausea, vomiting, and diarrhea. The physical examination may indicate minimal pulmonary involvement, yet the chest radiograph reveals more extensive abnormalities. The atypical pneumonia syndrome is associated with *M. pneumoniae,* viral pneumonia, *C. pneumoniae,* and *L. pneumophila.* Patients with legionnaires' disease often experience gastrointestinal symptoms and mental confusion. Symptoms of lung abscess include cough, chest pain, recurrent fever, and large amounts of sputum production. Hemoptysis may occur in some patients. Radiological evidence of cavitation is present and diagnosis may be confirmed by computed tomography (CT). Empyema may cause radiologic confusion with lung abscess; however, purulent fluid is present in the pleural space in empyema.

Chronic pneumonia has a gradual onset of general constitutional symptoms that develop over weeks to months. Although the patient may experience some symptoms that are observed in patients with acute pneumonia, the symptoms are less dramatic and less intense. Patients with chronic pneumonia will also experience weight loss, insomnia, and night sweats. The development of cough and sputum production may be the first sign that this constitutional illness has a focus in the lung.

LABORATORY ANALYSES AND DIAGNOSIS

Upper Respiratory Tract Infections

Specimen Collection

Throat specimens are collected to aid in the diagnosis of streptococcal pharyngitis, diphtheria, and pharyngeal gonorrhea, and to isolate adenoviruses, herpesviruses, mycoplasmas, and chlamydiae. In the collection of pharyngeal specimens, it is important to vigorously swab the tonsillar areas and the posterior pharynx to recover the pathogen. Nasopharyngeal swabs provide a better recovery for the detection of *B. pertussis,* RSV, parainfluenza virus, and *N. meningitidis.*

Swabs consisting of cotton, Dacron, or calcium alginate are acceptable for most microorganisms. All swabs, however, can be somewhat toxic to *Chlamydia* species, and this should be considered when interpreting a negative culture report. Once collected, the swab must be kept moist to maintain the viability of the organism. Appropriate transport media are recommended for specific agents. The exception to this is group A streptococci, which are resistant to drying and can remain viable on a dry swab for 48 hours.[23]

Direct Microscopic Examination

Direct Gram stain of pharyngeal secretions will not differentiate pathogens from normal microbial flora, and therefore, it is not generally useful for clinical or laboratory diagnosis. However, direct microscopic examinations are helpful in the detection of thrush, Vincent's angina, or a tonsillar abscess. The diagnosis of thrush is based on the detection of yeast cells in a Gram stain, a 10% potassium hydroxide (KOH) preparation, or a calcifluor white stain. In Vincent's angina, a Gram stain will reveal white blood cells, spirochetes, and fusiform bacilli. Direct fluorescent antibody stains are available for the detection of *B. pertussis*, HSV antigen, adenovirus, parainfluenza virus, influenza virus, and RSV.

Culture Methods

Laboratory confirmation by culture is necessary to distinguish streptococcal pharyngitis from pharyngitis due to common cold viruses or influenza.

Throat swabs are routinely cultured for the presence of β-hemolytic streptococci only; therefore, if an unusual cause of pharyngitis is suspected, the laboratory must be notified so that special media can be employed.

Nasopharyngeal specimens for the recovery of *B. pertussis* should be plated onto the appropriate selective media. URT specimens that are submitted for the isolation of *N. gonorrhoeae* or *N. meningitidis* should be plated onto a selective medium such as modified Thayer-Martin or Martin-Lewis agar. The etiologic agent of epiglottitis is not usually confirmed through culture methods because of the danger of airway obstruction while attempting to collect a specimen. If the airway is secure and specimens of the epiglottis are collected, the laboratory should culture for the presence of *H. influenzae*, *S. aureus*, *S. pneumoniae*, and β-hemolytic streptococci. Blood cultures are also collected in cases of epiglottitis. Nasopharyngeal swabs or washes can be cultured for viruses, using various cell culture techniques.

Other Methods

Commercially available antigen detection methods are also utilized in the diagnosis of certain URTIs. The most widely used test is for the detection of group A streptococci in throat samples. Available diagnostic kits employ latex agglutination or some form of solid-phase immunoassay. The advantage of direct antigen tests is the rapidity for detection of positive findings. When performed in the physician's office, patients with positive results can be given antibiotic therapy without having to wait for culture results. Although the specificity of these tests is very high, the sensitivity is not as high as that of culture; therefore, unless the physician has a significant reason to do otherwise negative direct antigen tests ideally should be followed with a culture. Some studies performed on a commercially available optical immunoassay show that its sensitivity and specificity exceed those of other methods,[27] although other studies have not confirmed this difference.

Direct antigen tests are also available to detect certain viruses. In addition to direct fluorescent microscopic methods, enzyme immunoassays (EIA) are available. This has been very useful in the detection of RSV where EIA has become the most frequently used method of RSV antigen detection.

Lower Respiratory Tract Infections

The diagnosis of LRTIs is dependent on physical examination findings, chest radiography results, and laboratory studies. The physical examination provides information on the degree and severity of the illness as evidenced by consolidation. Chest radiographs provide further information on the extent of involvement of the LRT. Characteristic radiographic patterns or pulmonary infiltrates can indicate certain microbial agents, although they cannot reliably establish an etiologic diagnosis.[28] Laboratory studies that are useful in evaluating patients with LRTIs include white blood and differential cell counts and a microbiologic evaluation of the respiratory secretions. The most common specimen that is analyzed is expectorated sputum. In patients who are not able to produce sputum, an induced specimen may be obtained. Other conditions may require specimens that are collected through more invasive procedures, such as bronchoscopy, tracheostomy, endotracheal aspiration, transtracheal aspiration, percutaneous transthoracic lung puncture, and lung biopsy.

Specimen Collection

The expectorated sputum sample is the most easily obtained lower respiratory secretion, but it must be evaluated carefully because it is impossible to collect a specimen of the LRT that is free of contamination from the URT. Patients must be instructed so that they understand that the specimen must represent lung secretions, rather than saliva or drainage from the nasopharynx. Once collected, the specimen must be transported to the laboratory promptly to minimize the deterioration of certain pathogens and to prevent the overgrowth of contaminants.

Direct Microscopic Examination

A direct microscopic examination of lower respiratory secretions is a vital component of the laboratory evaluation. Direct microscopy enables the clinician to substantiate or disprove his or her clinical impression, allowing selection of an appropriate empiric therapy. The microscopic examination is useful to the laboratorian, not only to detect the specific organism involved, but also to assess the quality of the specimen, and, in some situations, to select the most appropriate media to isolate the pathogen.

Gram stain is the most useful procedure for evaluating the quality of an expectorated sputum sample.[29] Culture of a poorly collected sputum specimen provides misleading results to the physician and can have a negative impact on the treatment of the patient. Evaluation of the sputum before culture can eliminate the processing of saliva and improve the quality of the laboratory information. The Gram stained, sputum specimen is examined microscopically for the presence of squamous epithelial cells and polymorphonuclear leukocytes (PMNs). The presence or predominance of PMNs and few or no epithelial cells indicate an acceptable specimen for culture.

Mycobacteria are detected in respiratory specimens with acid-fast staining of a concentrated sputum specimen. The fluorochrome stain, auramine-rhodamine, is recommended for screening specimens because it is more sensitive in detecting acid-fast bacilli (AFB) than the traditional carbolfuchsin stains (Ziehl-Neelsen or Kinyoun's). A modified acid-fast stain will demonstrate the weakly acid-fast property of *Nocardia* and help to differentiate this branching bacteria from the non–acid-fast actinomycete, *Actinomyces*.

The presence of fungi are noted in a direct microscopic examination using the 10% KOH procedure or the calcofluor white stain. Yeast cells are also observed with Gram stain. *P. carinii* is demonstrated by examining lower respiratory specimens such as induced sputum sample, or bronchial alveolar lavage specimens. These organisms are not found in expectorated sputum. The stains available for *P. carinii* include Giemsa, Gomori's methenamine silver, toluidine blue O, and a monoclonal antibody fluorescent technique.

Direct fluorescent antibody staining is used for the detection of *Legionella* species. Direct fluorescent antibody stains are also available to detect viral antigens including HSV, CMV, adenovirus, and RSV. *C. trachomatis* can be detected in the respiratory secretions of infants with pneumonia with a fluorescent monoclonal antibody stain. A fluorescent antibody method is also available for detecting *C. pneumoniae* in respiratory secretions.

Culture Methods

Most of the organisms involved in bacterial pneumonia are recovered on commonly used media including chocolate, sheep blood, and MacConkey's agars. Anaerobic cultures are not performed on most respiratory secretions because of the contamination of oral flora; however specimens obtained by percutaneous lung aspiration or transtracheal aspiration are acceptable for anaerobic work-up. Cultures for *Legionella* species are inoculated to buffered charcoal yeast extract (BCYE) and selective BCYE agars.

Specimens for mycobacteria studies must be digested, decontaminated, and concentrated prior to culture. The conventional method for the isolation of mycobacteria utilizes solid media such as Löwenstein-Jensen and Middlebrook's agars. Broth-based methods demonstrate more rapid growth of these organisms. The radiometric detection system is one broth-based method that has improved the time for the detection of these organisms. Automated mycobacterial detection systems are the most recently introduced broth-based methods. These systems provide continuous monitoring of bottles, therefore improving the time frame for the detection of positive cultures.

Specimens for fungi should be inoculated onto a nonselective fungal media as well as a medium with antibiotics to inhibit bacterial overgrowth. Respiratory secretions that are highly viscous can be treated with a mucolytic agent.

M. pneumoniae can be isolated from respiratory specimens using specialized media. However, recovery of these organisms from culture is difficult and serologic testing is more helpful. Viruses and chlamydiae can be isolated using tissue culture techniques. *C. pneumoniae* is more labile than *C. trachomatis,* and culture methods are not always successful.

Other Methods

The current emphasis in laboratory testing is to use methods that provide a more rapid detection of LRT pathogens than conventional culture methods. One technique that can provide rapid results is direct fluorescent antibody staining, previously described under microscopic methods. Serologic tests are useful in detecting certain pathogens that are difficult to isolate in culture, such as *C. pneumoniae* and *M. pneumoniae.* EIA is available to detect antigens of *C. trachomatis.* Antigens of *L. pneumophila* can be detected in urine specimens with radioimmunoassay.

The most promising techniques being introduced into the clinical laboratory employ nucleic acid methods. *Legionella* species can be tested for directly in respiratory specimens with a commercially available deoxyribonucleic acid (DNA) probe. This method is similar in sensitivity to other more conventional methods, but it detects all species of *Legionella,* not only *L. pneumophila.* DNA probes have been very helpful in the identification of *M. tuberculosis* and *Mycobacterium avium-intracellulare* from cultures. Nucleic acid amplification techniques, such as polymerase chain reaction (PCR), are rapidly evolving into the clinical diagnostic laboratory. Recently, a PCR assay has been developed for rapid detection of *M. tuberculosis* in respiratory secretions that are AFB-smear positive.

TREATMENT

Upper Respiratory Tract Infections

Treatment of an uncomplicated common cold is primarily symptomatic with supportive measures to reduce the discomfort of the patient. Antimicrobial agents do not affect the course of infection and are not indicated.[6] Resting or staying indoors in the beginning of the illness provides comfort for the patient and diminishes the exposure of others during the maximum virus shedding.[7] Handwashing and carefully avoiding contamination of the environment with nasal secretions will also help to prevent the spread. Malaise and headache may be relieved with aspirin, acetaminophen, or naproxen. Saline gargles and nasal decongestants can be used to provide relief from a sore throat, to clear nasal blockage and to provide nasal drainage. Drinking sufficient fluids is also recommended.

The possibility of sequelae to streptococcal infections makes it important to distinguish between viral pharyngitis and streptococcal pharyngitis as treatment of each differs. Viral pharyngitis is treated with supportive measures, whereas streptococcal pharyngitis is treated with antimicrobial agents. Penicillin remains the drug of choice against group A streptococci, and it is also effective in preventing acute rheumatic fever.[26] Erythromycin is an alternative in patients who are penicillin-allergic. Oral cephalosporins are also effective in treating streptococcal pharyngitis.

Acute laryngitis is treated with supportive therapy, including resting the voice and inhaling moist air. Antibiotics are not indicated unless the condition is associated with streptococcal pharyngitis. Croup also requires supportive therapy, and humidification of the air provides some relief. In severe cases of croup, children may require hospitalization. The treatment of epiglottitis involves establishing an airway and administering antibiotics.[8] The antibiotics are primarily directed at *H. influenzae,* but they must also cover *S. pneumoniae* and other streptococci. The conventional therapy is intravenous ampicillin, plus chloramphenicol to cover ampicillin-resistant strains of *H. influenzae.*[8] Alternative therapy is intravenous cefuroxime or a third-generation cephalosporin.

Therapy for sinusitis is directed at eradicating the causative agent, improving sinus function, and providing relief of symptoms.[12] Antimicrobial therapy is selected on an empirical basis, related to the most likely bacterial agents and their usual susceptibility. Ampicillin may no longer be effective because of β-lactamase–producing strains of *H. influenzae* and *M. catarrhalis*. Other antimicrobials that can be administered include trimethoprim-sulfamethoxazole, cefuroxime axetil, or amoxicillin plus clavulanic acid.[7] Vasoconstricting agents in the form of appropriate nasal sprays can be used to decrease nasal swelling. Inhalation of steam and application of warm compresses can help relieve symptoms. Headache and facial pain can be relieved with pain medication.

Acute otitis media is treated with empiric therapy directed against *S. pneumoniae, H. influenzae,* and *M. catarrhalis*. Tympanocentesis is necessary for an accurate bacteriologic diagnosis, but it is not usually performed except in cases in which empiric treatment fails. Amoxicillin plus clavulanic acid, trimethoprim-sulfamethoxazole, and cefuroxime axetil are often administered.[1, 7] Treatment for otitis externa includes topical antibacterial ear drops.

The primary therapy in treating diphtheria is immunotherapy, using antitoxin to neutralize the toxin produced by the organism.[14] Antibiotics are also administered to decrease further sources of toxin production and to eliminate the transmission of infection. Erythromycin is the drug of choice.

Supportive care to prevent hypoxia and pulmonary complications is the main focus of treatment for pertussis.[15] Once the patient has entered the paroxysmal stage of pertussis, antibiotics will not alter the course of the disease, but they will eliminate nasopharyngeal colonization and reduce transmission. Erythromycin is the drug of choice.

Lower Respiratory Tract Infections

Acute bronchitis is usually a self-limiting infection in previously healthy individuals. Supportive treatment, including bedrest and breathing warm, moist air, will alleviate some patient discomfort. Acetaminophen can relieve malaise and fever, and a nonproductive cough can be treated with appropriate formulas. In young children, elderly patients, and individuals with chronic pulmonary disease, antibiotics may be used.

Bacterial pneumonia is treated with empiric antimicrobial agents, until the results of cultures and antimicrobial susceptibility tests are available. The selection is based on the patient's age, history, immune status, physical findings, chest radiographic appearance, and the sputum Gram stain.[5]

S. pneumoniae has shown increasing resistance to penicillin in recent years, and in critically ill patients requiring hospitalization, a second- or third-generation cephalosporin may be indicated. These antimicrobial agents are also effective against *H. influenzae*. Erythromycin provides activity against *M. pneumoniae* and *Legionella* species. Clarithromycin and azithromycin, the newer macrolides, show activity against *Haemophilus* species, *S. pneumoniae, L. pneumophila, M. pneumoniae,* and *C. pneumoniae*. These agents are very useful for outpatient treatment of pneumonia.[5]

The treatment of hospital-acquired pneumonia is more complicated, and a knowledge of the organisms that have caused pneumonia in other hospitalized patients may help select the most appropriate antimicrobial agent. A Gram stain will help to differentiate two major causes of nosocomial pneumonia: *Staphylococcus* or gram-negative bacilli. Initial therapy for these infections includes extended spectrum penicillins, cephalosporins, aztreonam, or imipenem. *S. aureus* is treated with oxacillin or nafcillin, or with a first-generation cephalosporin if the patient is penicillin-allergic. Methicillin-resistant *S. aureus* is treated with vancomycin. Most lung abscesses resolve with antibiotics and postural drainage; however, when these measures fail, surgery is necessary. Empyemas must be drained, either by thoracentesis or surgery if fluid is too viscous.

The emergence of multiple-drug resistant tuberculosis has complicated the treatment of this disease. First-line drugs include isoniazid, rifampin, pyrazinamide, streptomycin, and ethambutol. Patients are placed on a multiple-drug regimen for 6 to 9 months.[23] Treatment for *P. carinii* includes trimethoprim-sulfamethoxazole, trimethoprim-dapsone, clindamycin-primaquine, or pentamidine. The treatment for systemic fungal infections may include amphotericin B or other azole antifungal drugs.

Case Study

A 9-year-old girl was brought to her physician's office complaining of a sore throat and difficulty swallowing. On examination, the nurse practitioner noted that the pharynx was red and an exudate was present and the tonsils were very swollen. She also indicated that the cervical lymph nodes were enlarged and tender. The child had a slight fever of 99.5°F. A throat swab was collected, and a positive result was obtained with a direct streptococcal antigen test. Because of penicillin allergy, the child was given clarithromycin.

The child's symptoms became progressively worse over the next few days. Her lymph nodes became more painful, her tonsils more enlarged, and she had extreme difficulty swallowing water. After 3 days of antibiotics and a worsening of symptoms, she was brought back to the physician's office. The physician examined the patient and indicated that either the *Streptococcus* was resistant to the antibiotic, which was highly unlikely, or that a viral agent was also involved in this infectious process. Further questioning revealed that the child had been lethargic and easily fatigued for the past 10 days. The physician ordered a complete blood cell count (CBC) and a mononucleosis test; both of these laboratory results were consistent with infectious mononucleosis.

Questions

1. What is the diagnosis?
2. Is there any difference in the symptoms of streptococcal pharyngitis and infectious mononucleosis?
3. How common is it for streptococcal pharyngitis and infectious mononucleosis to occur together?
4. What is the recommended treatment?

Discussion

1. The diagnosis is streptococcal pharyngitis and infection with EBV causing infectious mononucleosis.

2. Infectious mononucleosis is usually associated with systemic symptoms and signs of anorexia, malaise, fatigue, pharyngitis, generalized adenopathy, and splenomegaly. Although viral pharyngitis is not usually exudative, up to half of patients with infectious mononucleosis will present with exudative pharyngitis. Exudative pharyngitis can also be found in HSV and adenovirus infection. Infectious mononucleosis can easily be confused with streptococcal pharyngitis, especially in patients who present with a primary complaint of pharyngitis without the typical systemic signs that are usually present in infectious mononucleosis. Therefore, laboratory confirmation is necessary for the accurate diagnosis of these infections.

3. Simultaneous infection with group A *Streptococcus* and EBV can occur. In this case, it was thought that the child was initially infected with LBV, and because of her diminished defenses, the streptococcal infection was secondary.

4. The child continued her course of therapy for streptococcal pharyngitis. The treatment for infectious mononucleosis is mainly supportive. The child was given a short course of prednisone to alleviate the severe tonsillar swelling.

References

1. Lebovics R, Baker AS: Infectious diseases of the upper respiratory tract. *In* Isselbacher KJ, Braunwald E, Wilson JD, et al (eds): Harrison's Principles of Internal Medicine, ed. 13., New York, McGraw-Hill, 1994, pp 515–519.
2. Ray CG: Upper respiratory tract infections and stomatitis. *In* Ryan KJ (ed): Sherris Medical Microbiology, ed 3. Norwalk, Conn. Appleton & Lange, 1994, p 755.
3. Ray CG, Ryan KJ: Middle and lower respiratory tract infections. *In* Ryan KJ (ed): Sherris Medical Microbiology, ed 3. Norwalk, Conn. Appleton & Lange, 1994, p. 763.
4. Falkow S: Host-parasite relationships. *In* Ryan KJ (ed): Sherris Medical Microbiology, ed 3. Norwalk, Conn. Appleton & Lange, 1994, p 143–160.
5. Neu HC: Pneumonia. *In* Stein JH (ed): Internal Medicine, ed 4. St Louis, Mosby–Year Book, 1994, pp 1868–1870, 1874.
6. Liu C: The common cold and nonbacterial pharyngitis. *In* Hoeprich PD, Jordan MC, Ronald AR (eds): Infectious Diseases, ed 5. Philadelphia, JB Lippincott, 1994, pp 336–340.
7. Winther B, Gwaltney JM: Upper respiratory infections (colds, pharyngitis, sinusitis). *In* Stein JH (ed): Internal Medicine, ed 4. St Louis, Mosby–Year Book, 1994. pp 1860–1868.
8. Baker AS, Behlau I, Tierney M: Infections of the pharynx, larynx, epiglottis, trachea, and thyroid. *In* Gorbach SL, Bartlett JG, Blacklow NR (eds): Infectious Diseases, Philadelphia, WB Saunders, 1992, pp 448–451.
9. Carey MJ: Epiglottitis in adults. Am J Emerg Med 14:421–424, 1996.
10. Mayo Smith MF, Spinale JW, Donskey CJ, et al: Acute epiglottitis: An 18-year experience in Rhode Island. Chest 108:1640–1647, 1995.
11. Ray CG: Eye, ear, and sinus infections. *In* Ryan KJ (ed): Sherris Medical Microbiology, ed 3. Norwalk, Conn. Appleton & Lange, 1994, p 743–745.
12. Chow AW, Vortel JJ: Infections of the sinuses and parameningeal structures. *In* Gorbach SL, Bartlett JG, Blacklow NR (eds): Infectious Diseases. Philadelphia, WB Saunders, 1992, pp 434–435.
13. Bluestone CD: The ear and mastoid infections. *In* Gorbach SL, Bartlett JG, Blacklow NR (eds): Infectious Diseases. Philadelphia, WB Saunders, 1992, p 441.
14. Halsey N: Corynebacteria. *In* Gorbach SL, Bartlett JG, Blacklow NR (eds): Infectious Diseases. Philadelphia, WB Saunders, 1992, pp 1429–1432.
15. Bromberg K: Pertussis. *In* Hoeprich PD, Jordan MC, Ronald AR (eds): Infectious Diseases, ed 5. Philadelphia, JB Lippincott, 1994, pp 393, 396.
16. Ryan KJ, Falkow S: *Haemophilus* and *Bordetella*. *In* Ryan KJ (ed): Sherris Medical Microbiology, ed 3. Norwalk, Conn. Appleton & Lange, 1994, p 367.
17. Gershon AA: Present and future challenges of immunizations on the health of our patients. Pediatr Infect Dis J 14:445–449, 1995.
18. Durbin WA: *Bordetella*. *In* Gorbach SL, Bartlett JG, Blacklow NR (eds): Infectious Diseases. Philadelphia, WB Saunders, 1992, p 1539.
19. Liu C: Infections of large and small airways. *In* Hoeprich PD, Jordan MC, Ronald AR (eds): Infectious Diseases, ed 5. Philadelphia, JB Lippincott, 1994, pp 341–348.
20. Levison ME: Pneumonia, including necrotizing pulmonary infections (lung abscess). *In* Isselbacher KJ, Braunwald E, Wilson JD, et al (eds): Harrison's principles of Internal Medicine, ed 13. New York, McGraw-Hill, 1994, pp 1184–1186.
21. Hoeprich PD: Bacterial pneumonias. *In* Hoeprich PD, Jordan MC, Ronald AR (eds): Infectious Diseases, ed 5. Philadelphia, JB Lippincott, 1994, pp 421–426.
22. Plouffe JF: Legionnaires' disease and related infections. *In* Hoeprich PD, Jordan MC, Ronald AR (eds): Infectious Diseases, ed 5. Philadelphia, JB Lippincott, 1994, p 442.
23. Baron EJ, Peterson LR, Finegold SM (eds): Bailey & Scott's Diagnostic Microbiology, ed 9. St Louis, Mosby–Year Book, 1994. p 224–225.
24. Winn RE, Prechter GC: Pulmonary tuberculosis. *In* Hoeprich PD, Jordan MC, Ronald AR (eds): Infectious Diseases, ed 5. Philadelphia, JB Lippincott, 1994, pp 447–460.
25. Stringer JR: *Pneumocystis carinii:* What is it exactly? Clin Microbiol Rev 9:489, 1996.
26. Ayoub EM, Ferrieri P: Group A streptococcal diseases. *In* Hoeprich PD, Jordan MC, Ronald AR (eds): Infectious Diseases; ed 5. Philadelphia, JB Lippincott, 1994, pp 354–356.
27. Smith JM, Bauman MC, Fuchs PC: An optical immunoassay for the direct detection of group A strep antigen. Lab Med 26:408–410, 1995.
28. LaForce FM: Approach to the patient with pleuropulmonary infection. *In* Gorbach SL, Bartlett JG, Blacklow NR (eds): Infectious Diseases. Philadelphia, WB Saunders, 1992, pp 461–462.
29. Morin S, Tetrault J, James L, et al: Specimen acceptablility: Evaluation of specimen quality. *In* Isenberg HD (ed): Clinical Microbiology Procedures Handbook. Washington DC, American Society for Microbiology, 1992, pp 1.3.1–1.3.6.

Lung Cancer

Sharon S. Ehrmeyer

The great majority of primary carcinomas of the lung are bronchogenic in origin, and thus primary lung cancer is synonymous with bronchogenic carcinoma. Lung cancer occurs most frequently between the ages of 45 and 70 years, with peak incidence in the sixth and seventh decades. It is the most common malignancy and cause of death from cancer in men. In 1987 it surpassed breast cancer to become the number one cause of cancer death in women in the United States.[1] The 5-year relative survival rate is only 13% in all lung cancer patients, regardless of the stage at diagnosis.[1] Survival is directly related to early diagnosis and treatment; however, early detection is often difficult. Lung cancer is of particular interest because most cases are a direct result of cigarette smoking.

ETIOLOGY AND PATHOPHYSIOLOGY

Cigarette smoking is considered the primary cause of lung cancer.[2] The risk of lung cancer increases in direct proportion to the number of cigarettes smoked per day, amount of smoke inhaled, and the duration of the habit. The risk of lung cancer diminishes with increasing years of abstention. The rate of lung cancer is very low in nonsmokers, which further implicates smoking as the primary cause of lung cancer. The risk for cigar and pipe smokers is not increased appreciably, perhaps because these products are rarely inhaled. Mounting evidence indicates a link between lung cancer and passive inhalation of cigarette smoke by nonsmokers.

A small proportion of cases of lung cancer are a result of occupational exposure to certain substances. These sub-stances include asbestos, ionizing radiation, nickel, chromates, coal products, mustard gas, arsenic, beryllium, polyvinyl chloride, iron oxides, and bischloromethyl ether.[3–5] It must be recognized, however, that many occupationally exposed workers are also heavy smokers and that certain substances, for example, asbestos and uranium, may act synergistically with the effects of tobacco smoke.

Although air pollution has been implicated as a cause of lung cancer, it is unclear whether this type of pollution alone has an impact on the incidence of lung cancer. Recently, low levels of radon, the ubiquitous and naturally occurring radioactive gas, have been linked to lung tumors.[6] Although the concentration of cancer-causing agents may be increased in an urban environment, the concentration of these carcinogens is much less than that found in cigarette smoke.[7]

Finally, pulmonary scarring, a result of conditions such as scleroderma, granulomatous infection, and wounds, has been associated with pulmonary carcinoma. The tumors are usually adenocarcinomas; however, in most cases, the scar is thought to be a response to the tumor rather than the cause of the tumor.[8]

There are four major histologic types of lung cancer: squamous cell, adenocarcinoma, small cell, and large cell undifferentiated.[9] Table 12–1 shows the incidence, growth rate, metastatic potential, and 5-year survival rate for each type after curative resection.[10, 11] Histologic examination is necessary to confirm the diagnosis, determine the cell type and extent of the disease, and help plan the appropriate therapeutic regimen. Thorough tissue evaluation is necessary because many lung tumors are composed of more than one histologic pattern.

Table 12–1. Bronchogenic Cancer*

Histologic Type	Incidence (%)	Growth Rate	Metastatic Potential	5-yr Survival Rate (%)
Squamous cell	33	Slow	Moderate	37
Adenocarcinoma	50	Fast	High	27
Small cell	15	Fast	High	1
Large cell	<5	Fast	High	27

*Histologic type, incidence, growth rate, metastatic potential, and 5-year survival rate after curative resection.

Squamous Cell Carcinoma

Squamous cell carcinoma originates from altered epithelium of the bronchi. The majority of tumors are located centrally, near the hilum of the lung and at the points of bifurcation of the large bronchi. Histologically the cells can vary from well-differentiated to poorly differentiated. Growth of the tumor into the bronchial lumen may cause obstruction. Local metastases can involve the mediastinum and the superior vena cava. Peripheral lesions may invade the chest wall. Lymphatic spread to the hilar nodes and blood-borne metastasis to the adrenal glands, liver, bone, and brain occurs frequently, especially with poorly differentiated squamous cell carcinoma. The majority of patients do not experience symptoms until the disease has advanced considerably.

Adenocarcinoma

Adenocarcinomas are tumors that form glandular structures. These tumors may arise from surface epithelial cells or from bronchial mucous glands within the respiratory tract. Adenocarcinoma occurs peripherally rather than centrally, and it is frequently associated with pulmonary fibrosis or scars. The cause-and-effect relationship between smoking and this type of tumor is suspected but has not been established. Adenocarcinomas are the most common type of lung cancer in women and nonsmokers. These tumors tend to grow more rapidly than do squamous cell tumors, and blood-borne metastasis may occur early.

Small Cell Carcinoma

Small cell carcinoma is a highly malignant, aggressive tumor characterized by rapid growth and early metastasis via the lymphatics and blood. Patients with this type of tumor are much more likely to have widespread and early disseminated disease with metastasis to the central nervous system, liver, bone, bone marrow, lymph nodes, and adrenal glands. It is the form that is least amenable to surgery. Although most occur centrally, this carcinoma may arise in any part of the bronchial tree. There is a strong correlation between small cell carcinoma and cigarette smoking.

It has been suggested that small cell carcinomas originate in the endocrine cells (Kulchitsky's cells) of the lung. With electron microscopy, some of the lymphocyte-like tumor cells show dense-core, neurosecretory granules similar to those seen in other neuroendocrine tumors of the amine precursor uptake and decarboxylation (APUD) system. Many small cell carcinomas are associated clinically with paraneoplastic syndromes caused by ectopic hormone secretion of substances such as antidiuretic hormone (ADH) and adrenocorticotropic hormone (ACTH). The symptoms of inappropriate hormone secretion may precede pulmonary problems. Some small cell carcinomas have been associated with deletion of the short arm of chromosome 3.[12]

Large Cell Carcinoma

The tumor cells in the large cell form of bronchogenic carcinoma are poorly differentiated. Special stains and ultramicroscopic studies may show that some large cell carcinomas are actually adenocarcinomas or squamous cell carcinomas. They usually arise peripherally and metastasize frequently to the mediastinal lymph nodes, pleurae, adrenals, central nervous system, and bone.

CLINICAL MANIFESTATIONS

Bronchogenic carcinoma manifests in a variety of ways, but it is not uncommon for the diagnosis to be made when an asymptomatic mass is discovered on a chest x-ray ordered as part of a routine physical examination. Patients presenting with asymptomatic tumors that are localized and resectable have a better prognosis. As symptoms become evident, the lung cancer is usually advanced, unresectable, and often incurable.

Pulmonary Symptoms

Early symptoms often mimic those of other pulmonary conditions. Cough is the most common first symptom of bronchogenic cancer. Because most of its victims are smokers, patients may initially consider the cough as a consequence of their habit and ignore it. Weight loss, chest pain, and shortness of breath (dyspnea) are also common complaints. Bleeding may result from invasion of the bronchial wall and vessels by cancer or from chronic bronchitis associated with smoking.

Other pulmonary symptoms correlate with extension of the bronchogenic tumor within the chest. The cough may worsen, and the production of sputum may increase. New onset of wheezing or dyspnea is highly suggestive of bronchial obstruction. Depending on the specific location of the local extension, hoarseness, chest pain, pericardial involvement, and superior vena cava obstruction may occur.

Extrapulmonary Manifestations

Bronchogenic carcinoma commonly metastasizes widely, and no part of the body is exempt. Extrapulmonary manifestations may be seen before the primary cancer produces symptoms. Weight loss and general malaise may be the only evidence that a problem exists. Involvement of the central nervous system can cause the initial manifestation. Metastases to the liver, bone, kidneys, adrenals, and remaining lung tissue are common. A variety of symptoms associated with disease of the organs involved is expected.

Other Manifestations

Paraendocrine syndromes represent various unusual clinical manifestations associated with malignancies, particularly bronchogenic carcinoma.[12] The symptoms are due to the inappropriate production and release of biologically active hormones or hormone-like substances. Identification of these substances can aid in the monitoring of the malignancy. Cushing's syndrome is a rare manifestation resulting from ACTH-like substances secreted primarily by small cell tumors. Symptoms include hypokalemic and hypochloremic alkalosis, weakness, muscle wasting, and hyperglycemia. Ectopic ADH production, also seen with small cell carcinoma, inhibits diuresis, resulting in hyponatremia. A common manifestation of lung cancer is hypercalcemia from the excessive secretion of parathyroid hormone–like substances from squamous cell carcinoma, but hypercalcemia may also result from the osteolytic activity of bone metastases. Symptoms are directly related to the calcium level. Other hormone-like substances (e.g., insulin, calcitonin, thyroid-stimulating hormone, prolactin, renin, glucagon) have also been reported to be secreted by tumor cells.

Systemic manifestations are many and include muscle weakness; peripheral neuropathies (usually sensory); and dermatologic, hematologic, and connective tissue abnormalities.[5, 13] In older patients, bronchogenic carcinoma can manifest as acanthosis nigricans, the thickening and darkening of the basal skin layer, and dermatomyositis, the inflammation and degeneration of the skin, subcutaneous tissue, and muscle. Venous thrombosis and migratory thrombophlebitis are found in 3% to 30% of patients with bronchogenic carcinoma. Nonbacterial thrombotic endocarditis is associated occasionally with mucin-producing adenocarcinoma.

LABORATORY ANALYSES AND DIAGNOSIS

The diagnosis of bronchogenic carcinoma is primarily established by radiologic techniques. The imaging techniques of chest x-ray and computed tomographic (CT) scans are used to detect the pulmonary tumor, and they are useful in staging the tumor for prognostic and treatment purposes. Mediastinoscopy assesses tumor extension to the mediastinal lymph nodes.

Cytologic examination of sputum, bronchial secretions and washings, and pleural fluid is useful for diagnosing lung cancer. Bronchoscopy is the most common method of obtaining tissue for microscopic diagnosis when the tumor is centrally located. Transthoracic needle aspirations, thoracentesis, pleural biopsies, and axillary and supraclavicular node biopsies are used to determine metastatic spread.

Bone marrow aspiration and biopsy are essential, especially with small cell carcinoma, to determine the extent of metastasis. Other conditions have to be considered if a shadow is seen on x-ray and a lung tumor is suspected. These conditions include tuberculous and other granulomatous lesions and infections. Microbiologic studies are needed to differentiate active and chronic bacteriologic processes and malignancies.

Hematologic, chemical, and microbiologic procedures, depending on the specific situation, are sometimes useful in evaluating the lung cancer patient. General laboratory procedures are helpful in screening for abnormalities. A complete blood count (CBC) evaluates the patient's general condition, and mild anemia (hemoglobin level of 10 g/dL or less) is seen in about one-fifth of patients with bronchogenic carcinoma. Leukocytosis may reflect complications such as pneumonia, or it may occur without evidence of infection. A chemistry panel with electrolytes may detect abnormalities resulting from inappropriate hormone secretion and metastatic lesions. Ectopic ADH production results in hyponatremia, hypochloremia, decreased serum osmolality, and elevated urine osmolality. Increased calcium levels also occur in some patients. Microbiologic testing is necessary to monitor infections caused by obstructions by the tumor.

Depending on the specific situation, additional laboratory tests may be warranted. Arterial blood gas and oxygen saturation (CO-oximetry) analyses may be performed when surgery is being considered. A patient with poor oxygen exchange levels and inadequate oxygen saturation levels is not considered a good surgical candidate. Coagulation studies may be necessary to diagnose and monitor coagulopathies that develop. Hypercoagulation and shortened thrombin times associated with disseminated intravascular coagulopathy and thrombocytopenic purpura occur less frequently.

TREATMENT

Many factors influence the treatment of and prognosis for bronchogenic carcinoma. Considerations include the histologic cell type, duration and type of symptoms, age and sex of the patient, presence of other diseases, and growth rate and stage of the tumor. Of these, the histologic cell type and stage of the tumor are the two most important factors.

Stage of the tumor refers to the anatomic extent of the tumor at the time of detection. It describes the location and size of the primary tumor, the presence or absence of spread to the regional lymph nodes, and the presence or absence of metastases to distant lymph nodes and other parts of the body. The patient workup determines whether the cancer is of the type and stage suitable for surgical resection. The treatment of choice for localized, non–small cell carcinomas is surgery. The vast majority of patients with bronchogenic carcinoma, however, have tumor spread and are treated primarily by radiation, with or without adjuvant chemotherapy.

Laboratory tests are primarily used to evaluate the well-being of the patient. Chemistry panels and electrolyte measurements assist in detection of metastatic lesions that cause damage to certain organ systems, detection of recurring inappropriate hormone production, and assessment of the patient's general metabolic state. The CBC is useful in identifying early signs of wasting. Carcinoembryonic antigen (CEA), a tumor-related antigen marker, may be useful in monitoring the effectiveness of therapy. CEA is not useful in screening for small lesions or in differentiating between types of malignancies.

Case Study

A 72-year-old white man, a retired bank clerk, was admitted to the hospital with a chief complaint of muscle weakness and intermittent episodes of confusion and frequent falls within the past 2 to 3 months. His past medical history included chronic obstructive pulmonary disease (since 1988) and a 35 pack-year (1 pack a day for 35 years) smoking history.

Physical examination revealed an elderly man with thin atrophic skin and numerous scattered ecchymoses. Blood pressure was 136/90 mm Hg; pulse, 90/minute; and respirations, 18/minute; the patient was afebrile. Bilateral pitting edema of the extremities was evident. The neurologic examination revealed generalized weakness and muscular atrophy, and proximal weakness greater than distal.

Blood chemistry analyses included the following values: serum potassium, 2.8 mmol/L; plasma cortisol (at 8:00 AM), 45 μg/100 mL; and plasma ACTH (at 8:00 AM), 400 pg/mL.

Chest x-rays showed an enlarging right lower lung infiltrate. Bone marrow examination revealed metastatic malignant cells compatible with small cell carcinoma, and chemotherapy was begun. The patient became more confused and lethargic. Fever and hypotension developed. Several blood cultures grew *Staphylococcus aureus* and enterococci. Despite administration of antibiotics, the patient's condition deteriorated, and pneumonia and hypotension worsened. A chest x-ray showed extensive changes consistent with pneumonia and adult respiratory distress syndrome. The diagnosis was small cell carcinoma, metastatic, with ectopic ACTH production. The patient died 6 weeks after initial diagnosis.

Questions

1. How is muscle weakness related to the bronchogenic carcinoma?
2. What is the relationship of chronic obstructive pulmonary disease (COPD) to bronchogenic carcinoma?
3. Why does this patient have a positive blood culture?

Discussion

1. Muscle weakness is due to two factors. Cancer patients who are not eating properly often develop a negative nitrogen balance. Also, the metabolic derangement due to ectopic hormone production produces hypokalemia.

2. Most lung cancers develop in patients with a history of chronic bronchitis, usually precipitated by smoking. Often the cough and pulmonary symptoms associated with COPD and smoking delay the diagnosis.
3. Bronchogenic carcinomas often partially obstruct the bronchus, which results in an increased susceptibility to infection beyond the obstruction.

References

1. Cancer Facts & Figures—1995. New York, American Cancer Society, 1995.
2. Samet JM: Epidemiology of lung cancer. Chest 1993; 103:20.
3. Fraumeni JF Jr (ed): Persons at High Risk of Cancer: An Approach to Cancer Etiology. New York, American Cancer Society, 1975.
4. Israel L, Chaninian A: Lung Cancer: Natural History, Prognosis, and Therapy. New York, Academic Press, 1976.
5. Rubin E, Farber JL: Neoplasia. *In* Rubin E, Farber JL (eds): Pathology, ed 2. Philadelphia, JB Lippincott, 1994.
6. Harley NH, Harley JH: Potential lung cancer risk from indoor radon exposure. CA Cancer J Clin 1990; 40:265.
7. Abelson PH: Uncertainties about health effects of radon (editorial). Science 1990; 250:353.
8. Barsky SH, Huang SJ, Bhuta S: The extracellular matrix of pulmonary scar carcinomas is suggestive of a desmoplastic origin. Am J Pathol 1986; 124:412.
9. Yesner R, Hirsh FR, Matthews MJ (eds): International Histologic Classification of Tumors, ed 2. vol 1. Geneva, World Health Organization, 1982.
10. Martini N: Operable lung. CA Cancer J Clin 1993; 43:201.
11. Minna JD: Neoplasms of the lung. *In* Isselbacher KJ, Braunwald E, Wilson JD (eds): Harrison's Principles of Internal Medicine, ed 13. New York, McGraw-Hill, 1994.
12. Patel A, Davila DG, Peters SG: Paraneoplastic syndromes associated with lung cancer. Mayo Clin Proc 1993; 68:278.
13. Kobzik L, Schoen FJ: The lung. *In* Cotran RS, Kumar V, Robbins SL (eds): Robbins Pathologic Basis of Disease, ed 5. Philadelphia, WB Saunders, 1994.

Chapter 13

Pleural Effusions

Herb Miller

Etiology and Pathophysiology
Clinical Manifestations
Laboratory Analyses and Diagnosis
Treatment and Management
Case Studies

Pleural fluid, an ultrafiltrate of the blood plasma, is formed continuously in the pleural cavity. This cavity, normally containing from 1 to 10 mL of fluid, is formed by the parietal pleura lining the chest wall, and by the visceral pleura covering the lung.[1] Each lung is enveloped by this double-folded membrane of contiguous mesothelial layers.

The pleural cavity is created between the fourth and the seventh weeks of embryologic development and is lined by the splanchnopleure and somatopleure. These embryonic components of visceral and parietal pleurae, respectively, develop different anatomic characteristics with regard to vascular, lymphatic, and nervous supply. Both the visceral pleura and the parietal pleura have two layers, a superficial mesothelial cell layer facing the pleural space and an underlying connective tissue layer. Fluid is filtered into the pleural space according to the net hydrostatic-oncotic pressure gradients.[2]

Pleural fluid acts as a natural lubricant for the contraction and expansion of the lungs during respiration. It flows downward along a vertical pressure gradient and is reabsorbed by the lymphatics and the venules in the pleura. Regulatory mechanisms involve hydrostatic pressure (blood pressure), colloid osmotic (oncotic) pressure, intrapleural pressure, permeability/constriction of the capillaries, and lymphatic reabsorption. Under normal conditions, the colloid pressure remains constant on both sides of the pleural membrane. The colloid pressure, due mostly to the presence of high-molecular-weight proteins in the blood plasma, holds back water from being filtered. This colloid pressure is an opposing pressure to filtration across the parietal pleura.

Hydrostatic pressure is greater at the parietal pleura and favors filtration. At the visceral pleura, the hydrostatic pressure is decreased, allowing the fluid to pass out of the pleural cavity and to be reabsorbed by the capillaries and lymphatic system.[3, 4] Figure 13-1 illustrates the normal filtration and reabsorption of pleural fluid. Thoracentesis—removal of pleural fluid—is performed for diagnostic reasons, for relief of symptoms associated with the fluid accumulation, or to introduce medication.

ETIOLOGY AND PATHOPHYSIOLOGY

A pleural effusion is an accumulation of fluid in a pleural cavity. Disturbances that interfere with hydrostatic pressure (blood pressure), protein concentration in the blood (oncotic pressure), normal dilation/contraction of the vessels (vasomotion), blockage of the lymphatic drainage system, or other disease states of the lungs result in accumulation of increased amounts of serous fluid in the pleural cavities. Pleural effusions are alternatively referred to as thoracentesis fluid or empyema fluid.

Vasomotion, which affects the normal filtration of blood plasma into the pleural cavities, refers to the dilation/contraction of the capillaries. During dilation, water leaves the capillary, whereas during contraction, water enters the capillary. Inflammation is a cause of increased dilation; decreased cardiac output and thrombosis are causes of constriction.[5] Capillary permeability, the extent to which the capillary blocks the loss of protein, is a third important factor.[5] Damage to the capillary increases the loss of protein, which decreases the oncotic effect, thereby enhancing the transfer of water. Adequate lymphatic drainage of the pleural fluid is also important.[1] Any disruption of lymphatic flow, such as that caused by a neoplasm or other disease process of the lungs, decreases the drainage and enhances the accumulation of fluid.

Effusions are generally classified as either transudates or exudates. A *transudate* is an effusion caused by systemic disturbances (disease) outside the pleural cavity itself. An *exudate* results from a disease state within the pleural cavity or lungs.[3] Classification of a pleural effusion as to type is based on clinical laboratory findings and involves various chemical, microbiologic, immunologic, and cytologic tests.

Physical and radiologic examinations usually precede the removal of pleural fluid and subsequent clinical laboratory testing. It is important for the clinical laboratory scientist to have a basic understanding of the medical terms and abbreviations utilized in reporting both the physical and radiologic results to ensure adequate communication with the physician and other medical personnel. Terms and abbreviations commonly used are listed in Box 13-1.[6]

In the United States, approximately 1 million patients each year develop pleural effusion. Most patients who have

PLEURAL FLUID FORMATION

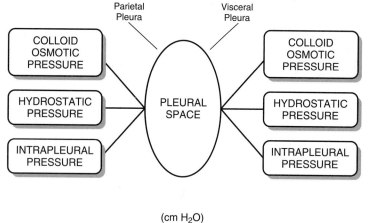

Figure 13–1. Normal filtration and reabsorption of pleural fluid.

(cm H$_2$O)

Hydrostatic Pressure ⟶ 30   11 ⟵ Hydrostatic Pressure
Osmotic Pressure ⟵ 26   26 ⟶ Osmotic Pressure
Intrapleural Pressure ⟶ 5   5 ⟵ Intrapleural Pressure
NET ⟶ 9   10 ⟶ NET

pleural effusion with congestive heart failure have left ventricular failure. The transudation of the pulmonary interstitial fluid across the visceral pleural is believed to overwhelm the capacity of the lymphatics to remove the fluid. Most patients with cirrhosis, who have pleural effusion, also have ascites. In this situation, it is believed, the pleural effusion forms when fluid moves directly from the perito-

neal cavity into the pleural cavity through pores in the diaphragm.[7]

Leading causes of exudative pleural effusions are pneumonia, malignancy, and pulmonary embolization. The principal malignancies that have an associated pleural effusion are breast carcinoma, ovarian cancer, lung carcinoma, lymphomas, and leukemias. The diagnosis of pleural malig-

---

Box 13–1. **Medical Terms and Common Abbreviations**

Medical Terms

Atelectasis	An incomplete expansion of the lungs
Auscultation	Listening to sounds within the body
Dypsnea	Difficult or labored breathing
Hemithorax	One side of the pleural cavity or chest
Hemothorax	The presence of blood in the pleural cavity
Lobectomy	The removal of a lobe of a lung
Opacification	Opaque to radiation
Percussion	The act of striking with sharp, short blows to aid in diagnosis by sound
Pneumonectomy	The removal of a lung
Pneumothorax	A collapsed lung
Rales	An abnormal rattling sound heard on auscultation
Thoracotomy	Cutting into the pleural cavity

Common Abbreviations

A&P	Auscultation and percussion
ARDS	Adult respiratory distress syndrome
COPD	Chronic obstructive pulmonary disease
CXR	Chest x-ray (radiograph)
SOB	Shortness of breath
RUL, RLL	Designate, respectively, right upper and right lower lobes of the lung
LUL, LLL	Designate, respectively, left upper and left lower lobes of the lung

Data from Chabner D: The Language of Medicine. Philadelphia, WB Saunders, 1985.

nancy is made most commonly by means of pleural fluid cytologic analysis. Immunohistochemical tests have also proved invaluable in differentiating benign from malignant pleural effusions.[7]

CLINICAL MANIFESTATIONS

Patients with pleural effusions usually present with pleuritic pain. The pain may be mild to severe and is described as sharp or cutting. Dypsnea is often the presenting symptom. A nonproductive or slightly productive cough is also commonly present. In infectious effusions, a fever is usually present, but fever can also be encountered in pulmonary infarction and in neoplastic or collagen diseases.[8] Typical physical findings include grunting respiration, splinting of the affected chest, shortness of breath, increased abdominal breathing, stifling of deep respiration, coughing, and impaired resonance on percussion. A shifting of the area of impaired resonance with changes in body position is virtually pathognomonic of a pleural effusion.[8] The cutoff in the percussion note during auscultation and percussion (A&P) is strikingly loud and sharp at the fluid level and allows precise delineation of even minimal amounts of pleural effusion. Examination by A&P is highly specific for the detection of free pleural fluid, even in the presence of obesity, pleural thickening, lung masses, pneumonia, and associated lung disease. Pleural effusion undetectable by standard chest radiography can often be detected by the method of A&P.[9]

LABORATORY ANALYSES AND DIAGNOSIS

Pleural fluid specimens are usually of large volume and are collected by needle aspiration. It is important to collect anticoagulated, sterile, and nonanticoagulated specimens.[4] The anticoagulated specimen is used for cell counts, the sterile specimen is used for microbiologic examination, and the nonanticoagulated specimen is observed for spontaneous clotting and chemical testing. Before cytologic and microbiologic tests are performed on large samples, it is important to concentrate the specimen by centrifugation.[4]

Diagnostic thoracentesis is most valuable in separating exudative fluids from transudates. Analysis of the exudative fluid has the highest yield when infection or malignancy is likely. Pneumothorax, the most common major complication, can be minimized by the use of small-diameter needles when a small amount of fluid is removed (35 to 50 mL). Ultrasonography may be of value to decrease morbidity when small or loculated volumes of fluid are present. Therapeutic thoracentesis offers relief of symptoms of dyspnea, but should be performed with particular caution because large needles and removal of large volumes of fluid may increase morbidity.[10]

Gross evaluation of a pleural fluid can reveal information useful in classifying it as either a transudate or exudate, and its color and turbidity as well as the presence of clotting are valuable in this regard. Transudates are usually pale yellow and clear with no clot formation, whereas exudates are usually cloudy and dark and tend to clot owing to the presence of fibrinogen. Hemorrhagic specimens may be due to a traumatic tap, malignancy, pulmonary in-

farction, trauma, pancreatitis, or tuberculosis.[1] Specimens from traumatic taps must be distinguished from true hemorrhagic specimens. In true hemothorax, the hematocrit of the specimen is similar to that of peripheral blood, whereas with a traumatic tap, the amount of blood diminishes as the aspiration continues and the hematocrit is lower with uneven distribution of blood throughout the specimen.[1] Icteric or hemolyzed fluid in a centrifuged hematocrit tube containing the specimen usually indicates a true hemothorax.

Transudative pleural effusions can be differentiated from exudative pleural effusions by measurement of the pleural fluid protein and lactic dehydrogenase (LD) levels. In transudative pleural effusions, the ratio of pleural fluid protein to serum protein is less than 0.5, the ratio of pleural fluid LD to serum LD is less than 0.6, and the absolute value of the pleural fluid LD level is less than two thirds of the upper normal limit.[7] Malignancies have been observed to exhibit both increased and normal LD_4 and LD_5 levels.[1, 11]

Transudates have a low cholesterol content because of low levels of low-density lipoprotein (LDL) cholesterol, whereas inflammatory exudates and malignant exudates exhibit high levels of LDL. LDL levels in effusions correlate with serum levels in exudates but not in transudates. Transudates have been found to have cholesterol-rich high-density lipoprotein (HDL) compared with serum. HDL particles of malignant exudates are poor in cholesterol. A strongly abnormal HDL cholesterol level has been found in a long-standing tuberculous effusion.[12]

Cholesterol in acute effusions is bound to lipoproteins and derived from the blood. Transudates show the lipoprotein characteristics of interstitial fluid. Alterations of lipoproteins occur in chronic inflammation and in malignancy. Lipoprotein Lp(a) accumulates independently from LDL in the pleural space, a finding that supports the view that the physiologic function of lipoprotein Lp(a) is located in the interstitial space.[12]

Chylous is a third classification used to denote milky-white to greenish appearing effusions. A true chylous effusion is rare and is usually caused by leakage from the thoracic ducts or by lymphatic obstruction. Complications of thoracic surgery, cancer, thrombosis of the great veins, or filariasis can also cause chylous effusions.[8] Chylous effusions are characterized by a high number of chylomicrons.

Pseudochylous effusions, appearing whitish to greenish, are seen in cases of tuberculosis and rheumatoid arthritis. These do not contain large amounts of chylomicrons but exhibit high levels of cholesterol with cholesterol crystals often found.[1]

Specific gravity tests are useful for classifying effusions. Exudates exhibit an increased specific gravity, usually greater than 1.015. Glucose levels are expected to be low in cases of higher utilization, as seen in malignancies and bacterial infections, and pH values are decreased in exudates. Pleural fluid C-reactive protein (CRP) values greater than 10 mg/L have a good predictive value in identifying exudate effusions. Transudates tend to have lower ratios of pleural to serum CRP levels than exudates. Malignant effusions have lower ratios than pneumonic and tuberculous effusions.[13]

Carcinoembryonic antigen (CEA) levels in malignant

effusions have been found to be significantly higher than in benign effusions, and their measurement has been proven to be a valuable tool in the detection of pleural malignancy.[14] Monoclonal antibody MOC-31, which recognizes a membrane glycoprotein of 40-kD molecular weight present on epithelial cells and not on mesothelial cells, is a highly sensitive and reliable reagent in the differential diagnosis of reactive pleural or ascitic fluids and adenocarcinoma. Adenocarcinomas stain positive, whereas reactive mesothelial hyperplasias stain negative.[15]

The laboratory findings just described are helpful but must be considered together before a definite classification of pleural effusion can be made. Table 13–1 summarizes the laboratory tests most often performed to differentiate pleural transudates from pleural exudates.[1, 4, 11]

All effusion specimens should be examined as soon as possible. Prolonged standing can interfere with test results, especially glucose, pH, and cytologic parameters.

Red and white blood cell counts are generally performed on the pleural fluid with a hemocytometer. A high red blood cell (RBC) count can indicate a hemothorax, traumatic tap, or malignancy. A high white blood cell (WBC) count is indicative of inflammation. As to the etiology of inflammation, it is beneficial to utilize a cytocentrifuge in preparing the specimen for a cell differential count. Traditional Wright's stain, Papanicolaou's stain, and hematoxylin-eosin stain are used in the cytocentrifuge preparations. Enumeration and cytologic evaluation of the cells after cytocentrifuge concentration have allowed the laboratory to detect early malignancies and to classify the various white blood cell types seen in different transudates and exudates. For example, a moderately increased count with a predominance of lymphocytes is seen in tuberculosis, whereas higher counts with a predominance of neutrophils is seen in bacterial infections. It has been suggested that the presence of eosinophils is a good prognostic sign, because fluids containing eosinophils seldom become infected.[16]

Systemic lupus erythematosus (SLE) commonly involves the pleura, with resultant pleural effusion. Studies indicate that detection of antinuclear antibodies (ANAs) in

Table 13–2. Cytologic Laboratory Tests for Differentiating Transudates From Exudates in Pleural Effusion

Cell Count	Transudates	Exudates
White blood cells	<1000/μL	>1000/μL
Red blood cells	Few	>10,000/μL
Differential		
Mesothelial	Variable	Increases seen in pneumonias, infarctions, and malignancies; scarce in pyogenic diseases
Polymorphonuclear neutrophils	Variable	Predominant in bacterial pneumonia and infarctions
Lymphocytes	Variable	Predominant in tuberculosis and malignancies
Mononuclear	Variable	Variable

pleural fluid is a sensitive indicator for distinguishing SLE from other etiologies. Negative or low titers of ANAs and a speckled staining pattern in a specimen from a patient with suspected lupus pleuritis suggest an alternative diagnosis. High pleural titers (up to 1:640) have been seen in patients with inflammatory pleural effusions in the absence of SLE.[17] Table 13–2 summarizes the most common cytologic parameters helpful in differentiating pleural transudates and exudates.[11, 16, 17]

Microbiologic studies of pleural fluid to search for aerobic and anaerobic bacteria are an important part of a pleural fluid workup. Mycobacterial (acid-fast bacilli), fungal, and parasitologic studies may also be performed. Systemic fungi such as *Histoplasma, Blastomyces,* and *Coccidioides* are very dangerous and usually enter through the lungs before spreading throughout the body. Pulmonary candidiasis, cryptococcosis, aspergillosis, and *Pneumocystis carinii* infections are opportunistic infections encountered.[18] Cryptococcal pneumonia should be considered in the differential diagnosis of *P. carinii* pneumonia, bacterial pneumonia, and tuberculosis in patients positive for human immunodeficiency virus (HIV).[19] Parasitologic studies may also be ordered. Rarely, *Echinococcus granulosus, Entamoeba histolytica,* and *Paragonimus westermani* are found.[1, 8]

TREATMENT AND MANAGEMENT

Resolution of or improvement in the underlying cause of a pleural effusion generally results in its disappearance. If the etiology of the effusion is unknown or if there is dyspnea, however, aspiration is performed. Hemothorax usually improves upon draining of the pleural space; however, thoracotomy is sometimes necessary if bleeding continues. Neoplastic effusions often reaccumulate rapidly after aspiration. To avoid the necessity of multiple aspirations, sclerosing compounds are sometimes instilled to reduce the rate of liquid accumulation.[20]

Video-assisted thoracic surgery (VATS) has assumed greater importance in the management of pleural disease. It has been found to be highly successful in the early management of empyemas and hemothoraces.[21] In the management of three groups of patients: (1) patients with cryptogenic pleural effusions, for the purpose of diagnosis; (2) patients with established malignant effusions, for talc

Table 13–1. Pleural Transudates versus Pleural Exudates

Laboratory Finding	Transudates	Exudates
Color/transparency	Clear/pale yellow	Cloudy/dark
Spontaneous clotting	No	Yes
Total protein	<3 g/dL	>3 g/dL
Lactate dehydrogenase (LD)	<200 IU/L	>200 IU/L
Fluid-serum protein ratio	<0.5	>0.5
Fluid-serum LD ratio	<0.6	>0.6
Specific gravity	<1.015	>1.015
pH	7.3–7.4	<7.2; <6 seen in esophageal rupture
Glucose amylase	Similar to that of serum	Normal to decreased; elevated in pancreatitis, malignancies, and esophageal rupture
Carcinoembryonic antigen	No	Can be found in malignant conditions

insufflation and limited decortication; and (3) patients with early empyema, for debridement and drainage, VATS was found to be a safe and effective way to manage patients.[22]

Case Study 1

A 41-year-old white male was admitted, confused but responsive. He complained of shortness of breath (SOB), urinary incontinence, and bleeding per rectum for 4 days. His temperature was 102.6 °F, respiration rate 20/minute, and blood pressure (BP) of 124/82 mm Hg. Liver function tests showed an elevated alkaline phosphatase of 157 IU/L, LD of 124 IU/L, and serum aspartate transaminase (AST) of 47 IU/L. An oral examination revealed candidiasis. Chest x-ray (CXR) results were as follows: Complete opacification of left hemithorax with pleural effusion. 150 mL of pleural fluid was removed by needle aspiration. On examination, the fluid was dark and cloudy, with a specific gravity of 1.022. Chronic inflammatory cells, including lymphocytes, plasma cells, macrophages, and eosinophils, were found. *P. carinii* and *Candida* species were noted. *Enterobacter aerogenes* grew in thioglycollate broth. The specimen was negative for malignant cells, viral inclusions, and acid-fast bacilli.

Questions

1. Given the physical and laboratory findings, is this an exudative or transudative effusion?
2. What is the significance of the chronic inflammatory cells?
3. What is the significance of the opportunistic fungus found?
4. Is the presence of eosinophils important?
5. What is the probable diagnosis?

Discussion

1. This is an exudate.
2. This is not a specific finding because chronic inflammatory cells are seen in a number of disorders.
3. Opportunistic fungi are often found in immunocompromised patients.
4. This is not a specific finding because eosinophils are seen in a number of disorders.
5. This is an acute bronchopneumonia caused by *P. carinii*, secondary to AIDS.

Case Study 2

A 30-year-old black woman presented with painful micturition, polyuria, and periorbital, peritibial, and generalized edema. BP was 220/90 mm Hg; respirations, 28 per minute with shortness of breath (SOB). Urinalysis revealed massive proteinuria with a variety of renal casts, oval fat bodies, and renal epithelial cells. Clinical chemistry results were as follows: creatinine, 8.1 mg/dL;

blood urea nitrogen (BUN) 80 mg/dL; decreased total protein and albumin. Chest x-ray (CXR) showed diffuse opacification of right and left lower lungs. Thoracentesis analysis revealed a pale, clear, acellular effusion, in which no microorganisms were found.

Questions

1. Is this an exudative or transudative effusion?
2. What is the significance of the elevated creatinine and BUN?
3. What is the significance of the proteinuria, renal casts, and oval fat bodies?
4. What is the significance of the effusion's being acellular?

Discussion

1. This is a transudate.
2. This patient has kidney disease, probably nephrosis.
3. Loss of protein due to kidney damage in nephrosis reduces oncotic pressure, enhancing movement of water into tissues and serous cavities. Renal casts and oval fat bodies are common findings in the urine of such patients.
4. Very few cellular components are found in effusions caused by nephrosis.

References

1. Kjeldsberg CR, Knight JA: Body Fluids: Laboratory Examination of Cerebrospinal, Synovial and Serous Fluids: A Textbook Atlas. Chicago, American Society of Clinical Pathologists Press, 1982.
2. Lee KF: Anatomy and physiology of the pleural space. Chest Surg North Am 4:391–403, 1994.
3. Glasser L: Evaluation: Serous fluids. Diagn Med 3:80, 1980.
4. Strasinger SK: Urinalysis and Body Fluids: A Self-Instructional Text. Philadelphia, FA Davis, 1985.
5. Valtin H: Renal Function: Mechanisms Preserving Fluid and Solute Balance in Health, ed 2. Boston, Little, Brown & Co, 1983.
6. Chabner D: The Language of Medicine. Philadelphia, WB Saunders, 1985.
7. Light RW: Pleural diseases. Disease-A-Month 38:261–331, 1992.
8. Lowell JR: Pleural Effusions: A Comprehensive Review. Baltimore, University Park Press, 1977.
9. Guarino JR, Guarino JC: Auscultatory percussion: A simple method to detect pleural effusion. J Intern Med 9:71–74, 1994.
10. Qureshi N, Momin ZA, Brandstetter RD: Thoracentesis in clinical practice. Heart Lung 23:376–383, 1993.
11. Ross DL, Neely AE: Textbook of Urinalysis and Body Fluids. Norwalk, Conn. Appleton-Century-Crofts, 1983.
12. Pfalzer B, Hamm H, Beisiegel U, et al: Lipoproteins and apolipoproteins in human pleural effusions. J Lab Clin Med 120:483–493, 1992.
13. Castano Vidriales JL, Amores Antequera C: Use of pleural fluid C-reactive protein in laboratory diagnosis of pleural effusions. Eur J Med 1:2201–2207, 1992.
14. Toumbis M, Chondros K, Ferderigos AS, et al: Clinical evaluation of four markers in malignant and benign pleural effusions. Anticancer Res 12:1267–1270, 1992.
15. Ruitenbeek T, Gouw AS, Poppema S: Immunocytology of body cavity fluids: MOC-31, a monoclonal antibody discriminating between mesothelial and epithelial cells. Arch Pathol Lab Med 118:265–269, 1994.

16. Light R: Management of pleural effusions. *In* Chretien J, Bignon J, Hirsch A (eds): The Pleura in Health and Disease. New York, Marcel Dekker, 1985.

17. Khare V, Baethge B, Lang S, et al: Antinuclear antibodies in pleural fluid. Chest 106:866–871, 1994.

18. Rippon JW: Medical mycology: The pathogenic fungi and the pathogenic actinomycetes. *In* Freeman BA: Burrows Textbook of Microbiology, ed 22. Philadelphia, WB Saunders, 1985.

19. Friedman EP, Miller RF, Severn A, et al: Cryptococcal pneumonia in patients with acquired immunodeficiency syndrome. Clin Radiol 50:756–760, 1995.

20. Light RW: Disorders of the pleura, mediastinum, and diaphragm. *In* Isselbacher KJ, Braunwald E, Wilson JD, et al (eds): Harrison's Principles of Internal Medicine. New York, McGraw-Hill, 1994.

21. Landreneau RJ, Keenam RJ, Hazelrigg SR, et al: Thoracoscopy for empyema and hemothorax. Chest 109:18–24, 1996.

22. Yim AP, Ho JK, Lee TW, et al: Thoracosopic management of pleural effusions revisited. Austr N Z J Surg 65:308–311, 1995.

Renal Disorders

Chapter **14**

Renal Failure

Martha Savage Payne

ETIOLOGY AND PATHOPHYSIOLOGY

Renal disease is a significant problem in the U.S. population, and a common result is end-stage renal disease (ESRD) and renal failure. The incidence of ESRD has increased over the past 20 years, probably owing to an aging population, because renal function tends to decrease with age, and to better survival of those with chronic diseases that affect renal function, such as diabetes mellitus. Renal disease is more common in certain ethnic groups, including blacks, native Americans, and possibly Hispanic Americans.[1]

Acute Renal Failure

Acute renal failure (ARF) can be defined as a rapid deterioration of the renal function of glomerular filtration. It is associated with *azotemia*, the accumulation of nitrogenous wastes that are normally excreted by the kidney, such as blood urea nitrogen (BUN) and creatinine.[2] High morbidity and mortality rates are associated with this condition, and because some of the causes may be reversed, a diagnosis must be obtained and appropriate treatment instituted immediately. The azotemia of acute renal failure is usually, but not always, accompanied by *oliguria,* defined as a urine volume of less than 400 mL/24 hours. There are many specific causes of ARF, including various parenchymal renal diseases as well as several extrarenal disorders. These disorders may be divided into three groups:

1. Prerenal azotemia is caused by renal hypoperfusion, which can be reversed immediately upon restoration of renal blood flow with no structural damage in the kidney.
2. Acute intrinsic renal failure results from diseases involving renal parenchymal tissue; this is usually a result of renal hypofusion or a nephrotoxin and is associated with tubular cell damage (acute tubular necrosis, ATN).
3. Postrenal azotemia (obstructive uropathy), resulting from obstruction in the urinary collecting system.

Other syndromes, such as acute interstitial nephritis, acute glomeruonephritis or vasculitis, and acute renovascular disease resulting from obstruction of the renal artery or vein of both kidneys (or of one kidney functioning alone) can cause ARF. It is important to determine which of these broad categories is the cause of ARF, because both prerenal and postrenal ARF require rapid intervention to prevent permanent renal damage.[3]

Both prerenal and postrenal factors can lead to the deterioration of renal function, resulting in azotemia and oliguria, but they are immediately reversible when the initiating disturbance is eliminated, in contrast to acute intrinsic renal failure. Reversal is accomplished by modifying the causative factors external to the kidney, such as instituting volume repletion therapy or removing obstructions in the urinary tract. If the situation is managed properly and expeditiously, no renal damage results. Intrinsic renal failure, in which there is actual tubular cell damage, however, continues for one to several weeks before renal function is restored, while tubular cells regenerate.[4] The history, physical examination, and urine analysis, discussed later in this chapter, should establish the diagnosis in about 90% of all patients with acute renal failure.

Prerenal azotemia, the most common cause of ARF, results from events leading to a decrease in renal perfusion pressure and/or an increase in renal vascular resistance (Box 14–1). Either circumstance can decrease the glomerular filtration rate (GFR) to such an extent that the daily endogenous load of nitrogenous wastes cannot be excreted.[2] This azotemic state is not associated with structural damage in the kidney and can be corrected if the extrarenal circumstances causing the renal ischemia are reversed. Improvement in renal function may involve increasing the intravascular fluid volume, enhancing cardiac output, or correcting the cause of systemic vasodilation, such as bacteremia or excessive use of antihypertensive drugs.[2] Improvement after anesthesia or surgical trauma may reverse a state of prerenal azotemia. Because some of the same factors that cause prerenal azotemia can lead to intrinsic acute renal failure, distinguishing between these two disease states may become possible only after the outcome of therapy is observed. If a patient immediately improves, then prerenal azotemia was present.

Postrenal azotemia occurs subsequent to urine formation and as a result of obstruction to the elimination of urine from the urinary tract.[3] Common causes are listed in Box 14–2. They are diagnosed with various radiologic procedures. Postrenal azotemia is immediately reversible when the obstruction is removed or corrected, unlike acute intrinsic renal failure (see also Chapter 18).

The diagnosis of acute intrinsic renal failure is a diagnosis of exclusion (Fig. 14–1). Primary renal disturbances that result in actual renal damage, causing acute azotemia, cannot be changed immediately by volume repletion, removal of urinary tract obstructions, or changing of other factors outside the kidney. Numerous clinical situations can be associated with acute intrinsic renal failure.[5] Those that are unassociated with primary glomerular or vascular disorders have been referred to as acute tubular necrosis (ATN). Although proximal tubular necrosis is often present, it is not consistently present in patients with acute intrinsic renal failure, and the terms should not be used interchangeably. The term "vasomotor nephropathy" has also been applied to acute renal failure in which the central cause is a microvascular regulation abnormality. The categories and specific disorders that cause acute intrinsic renal failure are shown in Box 14–3.

Ischemic disorders predispose to the development of

Box 14–1. Prerenal Azotemia (Decrease in GFR, Resulting in Renal Hypoperfusion)

Intravascular Volume Depletion

Excessive diuresis (diuretic use)
Hemorrhage (postpartum, gastrointestinal, surgical)
Gastrointestinal losses (vomiting, diarrhea, dehydration)
Major trauma, burns, crush syndrome
Pancreatitis, peritonitis
Hypoalbuminemia
Decreased intake

Cardiac and Vascular Disorders

Congestive heart failure
Acute myocardial infarction
Pericardial diffusion with tamponade
Pulmonary hypertension, massive pulmonary embolism
Renal artery: emboli, thrombosis, stenosis, dissecting aneurysm, vasculitis
Renal vein: thrombosis, compression
Cardiac arrhythmia

Peripheral Vasodilation

Sepsis
Antihypertensive medications (norepinephrine, ergotamine)
Shock
Liver failure
Drug overdose

Increased Renal Vascular Resistance

Surgery
Anesthesia
Hepatorenal syndrome
Prostaglandin inhibitors (nonsteroidal anti-inflammatory drugs), aspirin, indomethacin, ibuprofen during renal hypoperfusion
Inhibitors of angiotensin-converting enzyme (ACT inhibitors) in renal artery stenosis

---

ARF because of reduced blood flow to the kidneys. The loss of blood supply has its greatest impact on the proximal tubule, resulting in the death of the tubular epithelium. Damage to the epithelium, both during the initial ischemic period and afterwards, may compromise nephronal function through obstruction and back-leakage of glomerular filtrate. Obstruction results from accumulation of the cellular debris from the sloughed proximal tubular epithelium. The increased tubular pressure reduces the net driving force for glomerular filtration. In areas void of the epithelium, back-leakage of glomerular filtrate occurs. As a result, net glomerular filtration is considerably reduced or eliminated in the severely affected nephrons. Recovery of renal function and maintenance of normal GFR depend on (1) restored patency of obstructed nephrons and successful proliferation

Box 14–2. Postrenal Azotemia

Urethral Obstruction

Congenital valve
Stricture
Phimosis
Tumor

Bladder Neck Obstruction

Stones
Clots
Prostatic hypertrophy or malignancy
Bladder carcinoma
Bladder infection
Autonomic neuropathy or ganglionic blocking agents

Ureteral Obstruction (Bilateral, or Unilateral Functional Kidney)

Intraureteral
   Stones
   Blood clots
   Pyogenic debris or sloughed necrotic papillae
   Edema (following retrograde pyelography)
   Fungus balls
   Sulfonamide and uric acid crystals
Extraureteral
   Prostatic, bladder cervical cancer
   Endometriosis
   Periureteral fibrosis
   Accidental ureteral ligation or trauma during pelvic
     surgery
   Retroperitoneal hemorrhage

of tubule cells to replace those lost and (2) reestablished continuity of a fully differentiated and functional epithelium. ARF due to ischemic disorders is seen most commonly in postoperative patients, following trauma, during severe hypovolemia, and in overwhelming sepsis and burns.[5]

Rhabdomyolysis-induced ARF is being recognized with greater frequency, and may account for many cases of acute renal failure previously classified as "etiology unknown." Rhabdomyolysis results from muscle injury and the release of muscle contents (myoglobin) into the circulation.[6] Myoglobin is not bound by serum proteins and is filtered freely by the glomerulus because of its small size. Various causes of myoglobinuria or rhabdomyolysis are crush injuries, coma (lying in one position without moving for prolonged periods, especially after drug overdose or alcohol ingestion), burns, ischemia to large muscles, toxins, drugs, metabolic disorders, infectious diseases, and, in some normal individuals, very vigorous exercise. Myoglobinuria should be considered in patients who present with acute azotemia accompanied by brown urine with a positive hemoglobin test and no intact red cells observed on the urine microscopic examination. More specific tests can be performed to identify the pigment. Brown debris and pigment casts are commonly seen. Serum enzymes are elevated, including creatine kinase (CK), transaminases, and lactate dehydrogenase (LD).[5]

Nephrotoxic disorders are caused by the ingestion or the administration of certain drugs (see Box 14–3).[7] Because the kidneys are exposed to a large blood volume (25% of cardiac output), they are exposed to higher concentrations of blood-borne substances than most body tissues. The renal tubular cells are prime targets of these substances. In hospitalized patients, nephrotoxins have become a major cause of acute renal failure.[8] Antibiotics, especially the aminoglycosides, are commonly implicated in acute renal failure, and it has been estimated that 10% to 30% of all patients treated with aminoglycosides have some degree of nephrotoxicity.[9] Radiocontrast agents and cyclosporin have been implicated in ARF as well as chemotherapeutic agents such as cisplatin and ifosfamide.[10-12] Angiotensin-converting enzyme (ACE) inhibitors can lead to ischemic ARF, especially in the presence of renal artery stenosis and diuretics with sodium depletion. Nonsteroidal anti-inflammatory agents may cause ARF in the patient with decreased effective intravascular volume, because they inhibit prostaglandins, which help maintain renal blood flow in volume-depleted states.[8]

Acute urate nephropathy occurs from the intrarenal deposition of urate crystals. It occurs most often in leukemic or lymphoproliferative states during tumor lysis syndrome. The destruction of these abnormal cells, especially after treatment with radiation or chemotherapy, may cause severe ARF with oliguria, hyperphosphatemia, hypocalcemia, and hyperkalemia as well as hyperuricemia.

Ingestion of ethylene glycol, usually in the form of antifreeze, produces ARF after 48 to 72 hours. In addition, a severe metabolic acidosis with a profound increase in the serum anion gap is also present. Neurologic manifestations may occur. Urinalysis reveals many envelope-shaped calcium oxalate crystals.

In some disease states, especially multiple myeloma and diabetes mellitus, intravenous x-ray contrast administration is a major cause of acute renal failure.[11] Many of these patients probably have preexisting renal insufficiency, proteinuria, and vascular disease.

Various therapeutic agents also may cause interstitial nephritis.[13] The area of the kidney primarily affected is the interstitial space, which in acute interstitial nephritis is markedly edematous and is infiltrated with white blood cells. The mechanism is mediated immunologically. Loss of renal function from drug sensitivity tends to be less severe than in classic renal failure. Recovery of renal function following withdrawal of the drug is sometimes slow and may be incomplete.

Other causes of acute renal failure are primary renal diseases (e.g., glomerulonephritis), systemic diseases (e.g., Goodpasture's syndrome, systemic lupus erythematosus), and vascular diseases (e.g., renal arterial thrombosis, malignant hypertension) (see Box 14–3). The acute azotemia associated with these disorders is often only one of many serious complications of underlying disease. In these cases, the glomerulus is the primary site of injury, and the tubules and interstitial areas are relatively uninvolved. Fever, extrarenal systemic manifestations, and nephritic urinary sediment and composition help in the differentiation from other types of ARF.[2]

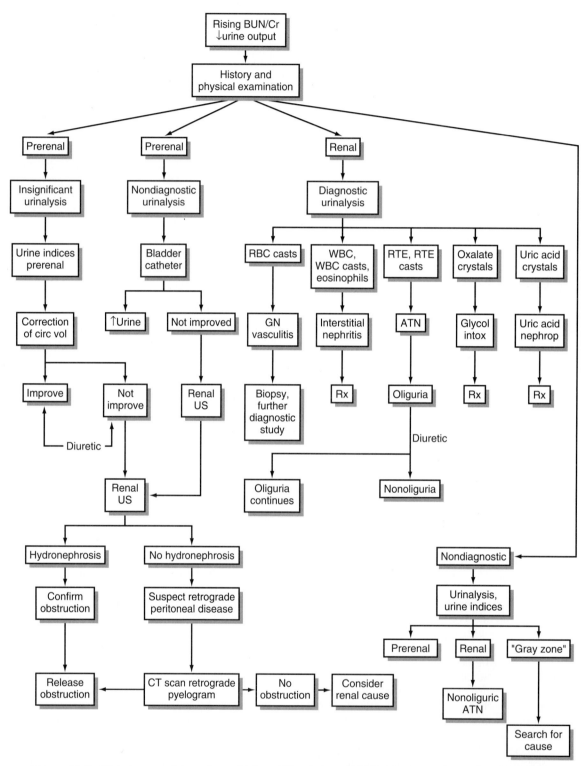

Figure 14–1. Clinical approach to acute renal failure. Abbreviations: BUN/Cr, blood urea nitrogen/creatinine; RBC, red blood cell; WBC, white blood cell; RTE, renal tubular epithelial cells; circ vol, circulating volume; GN, glomerulonephritis; ATN, acute tubular necrosis; intox, intoxication; nephrop, nephropathy; US, ultrasonography; Rx, therapy; CT, computed tomography. (Redrawn with permission from Jacobson HR, Striker GE, Klahr S (eds): Principles and Practice of Nephrology, ed 2. St Louis, Mosby–Year Book, 1995.)

Box 14–3. **Acute Intrinsic Renal Failure (Decrease in GFR, Resulting from Renal Parenchymal Damage)**

Ischemic Disorders

Complication of surgery
Hemorrhage
Trauma
Sepsis
Postpartum hemorrhage
Prolonged prerenal azotemia

Pigment Injury

Myoglobinuria
Hemoglobinuria

Crystal-Induced Injury

Uric acid nephropathy
Oxalate

Nephrotoxic Disorders

Antibiotics
  Aminoglycosides (neomycin, kanamycin, gentamicin, tobramycin, amikacin, netilmicin, and streptomycin)
  Cephalosporins
  Tetracyclines
  Sulfonamides
  Amphotericin B
  Polymyxins
  Bacitracin
  Pentamidine
Iodine-containing radiographic contrast media
Heavy metals (arsenic, lead, cadmium, mercury, bismuth, uranium)
Organic solvents
Glycols (ethylene glycol [antifreeze] and diethylene glycol)
Carbon tetrachloride and other halogenated hydrocarbons

Toluene
Hydrocarbons (gasoline, kerosene, turpentine, paraphenylene diamine [hair dye])
Anesthetics (methoxyflurane, enflurane)
Analgesics (aspirin, ibuprofen, indomethacin)
Antiulcer regimens (cimetidine)
Diuretics
Chemotherapeutic agents
Cyclosporine
Poisons
Recreational drugs (heroin, amphetamines)

Primary Renal Systemic and Vascular Diseases That May be Associated With Acute Azotemia

Glomerular and small-vessel obstruction
  Acute post-streptococcal glomerulonephritis
  Rapidly progressive glomerulonephritis
  Vasculitis
  Pregnancy-induced hypertension (toxemia of pregnancy)
  Hemolytic-uremic syndrome
  Disseminated intravascular coagulation
  Malignant hypertension
  Radiation injury
Renovascular obstruction
  Renal artery: atherosclerosis, embolism, thrombosis, dissecting aneurysm, vasculitis
  Renal vein: thrombosis, compression
Other
  Goodpasture's syndrome
  Systemic lupus erythematosus
  Subacute bacterial endocarditis
  Postpartum renal failure
  Multiple myeloma
  Macroglobulinemia
  Polycythemia

Chronic Renal Failure

Chronic renal failure (CRF) may result from many processes that have a prolonged downhill course with progressive loss of nephron mass. Not a specific disease, CRF refers to any situation in which there is a permanent reduction of renal function, causing significant abnormal chemical findings in the blood of a patient. Although the condition usually begins with minor alterations in blood analytes, it is almost always a progressive process that eventually becomes life threatening.[14] Even as nephrons are being destroyed, however, the surviving nephrons and the rest of the body adapt; an individual can survive even if 90% of the original nephron population is destroyed.

Renal disease progresses through four overlapping stages. The first is a diminution of renal reserve in which renal function is reduced by 25%, the GFR is reduced but azotemia is not present, and electrolyte and acid-base balance are maintained. Next is renal insufficiency, which is associated with a reduction in renal function of up to 75%. Azotemia is present, and anemia develops owing to decreased production of erythropoietin. Overt renal failure, the third stage, is characterized by worsening azotemia and anemia along with acidemia, hypocalcemia, hyperphosphatemia, and isosthenuria. This stage rapidly progresses to uremia or end-stage renal failure with hyperkalemia.

In adults, the common causes of CRF are glomerulonephritis, polycystic kidney disease, interstitial nephritis, diabetic glomerulosclerosis, and hypertension (nephrosclerosis). In pediatric patients, common causes also are glomerulonephritis, polycystic kidney disease, and interstitial nephritis, as well as renal hypoplasia, obstruction in the urinary tract, and a variety of individually rare hereditary disorders. Some less common causes of CRF are amyloidosis, sickle cell anemia, tuberculosis, hemolytic-uremic syndrome, and renal artery or vein occlusion.

End-Stage Renal Disease (Uremic Syndrome)

The decline in renal function in a patient with CRF occurs over a long period and culminates in end-stage renal disease with physiologic symptoms of the uremic syndrome. Many pathophysiologic adjustments are made by the kidney because of the progressive loss of nephrons. Other organ system problems also occur in response to renal failure. The patient becomes unable to maintain electrolyte balance with deficiencies or excesses of salt, and hypertension usually develops. Calcium metabolism becomes impaired, leading to adverse adjustments by the parathyroid and skeletal systems. Anemia occurs, as do metabolic acidosis and the associated buffer-base depletion. The kidneys fail to maintain adequate excretory, regulatory, and endocrine function, and the need arises for renal replacement therapy in the form of dialysis or transplantation.[15]

CLINICAL MANIFESTATIONS
Acute Renal Failure

ARF may manifest in one of the following four ways:

- An unexpected elevation in the BUN and serum creatinine
- An alteration in urine flow rate (oliguria)
- Clinical features of the underlying precipitating cause
- Clinical or biochemical complication of uremia

Because hospital patients are monitored daily with many biochemical tests, nonoliguric acute renal failure is now being recognized much more commonly, even before other symptoms appear. The early identification of patients at risk, with prompt elimination of potential insults, can save many lives. Nonoliguric renal failure may account for up to 50% of all cases and is common after aminoglycoside nephrotoxicity, burns, and the administration of intravenous contrast dye.

The clinical course of ARF can be divided into three phases: an oliguric phase, a diuretic phase, and a recovery phase. The oliguria may last from a few hours to several weeks or months; the longer the oliguric phase, the poorer the prognosis. The diuretic phase begins with an increase in urine flow to more than 4000 mL/day, and sometimes there is profuse diuresis of several liters a day. Usually, the blood urea nitrogen (BUN) and creatinine levels continue to rise, but they fall after several days of urine output greater than 1000 mL/day. In the diuretic phase, the patient is still in danger of complications, because electrolyte and other biochemical abnormalities persist. Both glomerular filtration and tubule function improve as diuresis progresses.

The prognosis of a patient with acute renal failure depends on the condition that precipitated the problem. About 50% of patients with postoperative acute renal failure, about 33% of patients with medical ARF, and about 15% of patients with obstetric ARF die in the course of the syndrome. Patients who are nonoliguric have the best prognosis. The primary causes of death are infectious, cardiovascular, and respiratory complications. The majority of the patients who recover have nearly normal renal function.[3]

Chronic Renal Failure

In chronic renal failure, a patient with 25% or more of normal kidney function is likely to have few physical symptoms. As the nephron population decreases, the glomerular filtration rate falls, and the first chemical abnormalities noted are an increase in urea and creatinine in the blood (azotemia). Early chronic renal disease is, therefore, often found incidentally through routine laboratory analyses of blood and urine. As the GFR decreases below 25% of normal, physical symptoms appear. At this point, other solutes that are normally either filtered, reabsorbed, or secreted, such as phosphate, sulfate, and urate may also be retained in body fluids. This may lead to bone disease, a well-recognized complication of chronic renal failure. The abnormal divalent ion metabolism plus increased parathyroid activity and disordered vitamin D metabolism can lead to many forms of skeletal abnormalities; however, patients usually manage quite well until renal function is reduced to about 10% of normal. At this level, the patient usually begins to experience symptoms of *uremia,* a toxic state caused by retention of waste products, such as organic acids, phenolic compounds, indoles, guanidines, various metabolic intermediates, and certain peptides. Many of these substances have toxic potential and could possibly contribute to the symptoms of chronic renal disease.

Classic clinical signs of uremia are progressive weakness and easy fatigability, loss of appetite followed by nausea and vomiting, muscle wasting, tremors, abnormal mental function, frequent but shallow respirations, and metabolic acidosis. The patient progresses to a state of stupor, coma, and, ultimately, death unless dialysis or successful renal transplantation is provided.[14]

LABORATORY ANALYSES AND DIAGNOSIS

The clinical laboratory is vital in the diagnosis of renal disease in general and in following the course of patients with both acute and chronic renal failure. Laboratory measurements needed to detect the various renal syndromes are urinalysis, measurement of serum creatinine and blood urea nitrogen (BUN), a chemistry profile including electrolytes and other analytes described later, and a complete blood cell count.

Urinalysis

The examination of urine is one of the simplest yet most important procedures in detecting and monitoring renal parenchymal or urinary tract disease. Especially important for the diagnosis of these disorders are tests for protein and hemoglobin and the examination of the urinary sediment.

The screening test for protein usually is a reagent strip, which changes color in the presence of albumin but does not react as well, or at all, with globulin or Bence Jones protein. The sulfosalicylic acid test should also be done to detect these other proteins, especially when renal disease is suspected. Subsequent protein immunoelectrophoresis confirms the presence of light chains (Bence Jones proteinuria). Although Bence Jones proteinuria is most commonly associated with multiple myeloma, it may also be found in other malignancies.

The urine protein test is the most important screening test for renal function, because proteinuria signals chronic renal disease before symptoms appear or serum creatinine or BUN levels become abnormal. A positive protein test result may be the first indication that a patient will ultimately go into chronic renal failure. It should be remembered, however, that the presence of proteins in the urine may sometimes occur in healthy individuals. This functional proteinuria may result from such physiologic processes as fever, strenuous exercise, emotional stress, salicylate therapy, and exposure to cold.

In teenagers and in patients recovering from glomerular disease, orthostatic (postural) proteinuria should be considered. This condition is characterized by increased excretion of protein while a person is standing but not while he or she is in the prone position. A first-morning urine specimen is normal in protein content, but those collected during the day contain elevated protein. Orthostatic proteinuria is not usually associated with chronic renal failure.[15]

Researchers have found that small amounts of albumin—*microalbuminema*—in the patient with insulin-dependent diabetes mellitus predict the future development of renal disease with considerable accuracy.[16] Assays such as radioimmunoassay, radial immunodiffusion, enzyme-linked immunoabsorbent assay (ELISA), immunofixation electrophoresis, and immunoturbidimetry (nephelometry) are used to detect the albumin. Normal 24-hour albumin excretion is below 30 mg/day. Several screening methods using reagent strips have been developed to screen qualitatively for urinary albumin excretion. Although albumin reagent strips were found to be more sensitive than standard dipsticks, they appeared to have a relatively high rate of false-positive results.

If all nonrenal causes for proteinuria and orthostatic proteinuria have been excluded, renal disease must be considered. A quantitative protein determination should be performed on a 24-hour sample and should be repeated three or four times to determine whether the proteinuria is persistent or intermittent. Intermittent proteinuria is usually associated with a benign course, whereas persistent proteinuria is associated with renal disease.

Repeated measurements of protein excretion are a valuable tool for following the course of patients with renal disease. A return to normal protein excretion indicates healing of the glomerular lesion, and conversion from persistent to postural proteinuria indicates a good prognosis. By contrast, persistence of proteinuria increases the likelihood that progressive renal insufficiency and renal failure will develop.[15] In lupus nephritis, a rise in protein excretion suggests heightened immunologic activity.

Once proteinuria is detected by screening methods, it should be quantified by timed urine collection, and the composition of the urinary protein evaluated by electrophoresis. An increased amount of albumin and high-molecular-weight proteins suggests glomerular proteinuria, whereas increases in low-molecular-weight protein fractions (such as β_2-microglobulin) are more suggestive of tubular proteinuria. Aminoglycoside-induced kidney damage, heavy metal nephropathies, intravenous contrast nephropathy, and kidney transplant rejection are among the many acute and chronic tubulointerstitial nephropathies associated with high urinary β_2-microglobulin levels. When proteinuria is greater than 2 g/day, selectivity, which determines whether the protein is mainly albumin or is albumin and globulin, may be assessed by electrophoresis of the urine and a comparison of clearance of proteins of differing molecular weights, such as the ratio of immunoglobulin G (IgG) and albumin (IgG/albumin ratio). When selectivity is high (IgG/albumin ratio <0.10), as it often is in children with minimal lesion disease, treatment with corticosteroids is likely to be successful (see Chapters 15 and 16). Patients with immunoglobulin G/albumin clearance ratios greater than 0.50 have a nonselective pattern.[16]

The methods for quantitation of urinary total protein all have some disadvantages. Dye-binding methods, the most popular methods of measuring protein, use such dyes as Ponceau S dye, pyrogallol red, and Coomassie brilliant blue. The range for protein concentration is 1 to 14 mg/dL. The reference range for 24-hour (day) excretion is less than 100 mg/d (<150 mg/day in pregnancy). The concentration may reach 300 mg/day in urine of healthy subjects after exercise.[17]

Studies have shown that the protein (albumin)–creatinine ratios from random or timed specimens may be used to estimate the 24-hour urinary protein excretion. The normal ratio is near 0.1, with 110 to 150 mg of protein and 1000 to 1500 mg of creatinine per 24 hours. A urine protein-creatinine ratio of 1.0 would correlate with a quantitative proteinuria of approximately 1 gm/24 hours, and a ratio of 2.0 would correlate with 2 gm/24 hours, and so on. In individuals in whom timed collections are difficult, this correlation may be especially useful.[16]

Hematuria is the second most important clue to the presence of kidney disease or diseases of the urinary tract. A positive reaction on a dipstick test can indicate the presence of free hemoglobin (hemoglobinuria), intact red blood cells (hematuria), or myoglobin (myoglobinuria) in the urine.[15] Sediment from a fresh, concentrated urine sample with low pH should also be examined for the presence of red blood cells to confirm hematuria. If few or no intact red cells are found, hemoglobinuria or myoglobinuria should be suspected and may be the cause of acute renal failure. Other more specific tests may be ordered to identify hemolysis. These include examination of the peripheral blood smear and measurement of blood lactate dehydrogenase, haptoglobin, or serum free hemoglobin. Rhabdomyolysis can be detected with serum creatine kinase. Hematuria along with red blood cell casts may indicate acute glomerulonephritis, which may also manifest as acute renal failure.

A microscopic examination of the urine provides invaluable information concerning renal disease. The finding of specific type casts, cells, or crystals in urine sediment is associated with various renal diseases and causes of renal failure, as indicated in Box 14–4. These characteristic urine sediments are discussed in detail in the chapters on the specific disorders; however, a general discussion appears here.

White blood cells, red blood cells, and tubular epithelial cells may appear in urine sediment and are associated with various pathologic processes.[15] Increased red blood cells (more than 5 per high-power field [hpf]) are associated with bleeding into the urine from various causes, such as cystitis, renal tumors, calculi, hemoglobinopathies, and

┌───┐
Box 14–4. Characteristic Urine Sediments

Glomerular inflammatory diseases (in association with
    2+ to 4+ proteinuria)
  Nephritic (active sediment)
  Hematuria
  Red blood cell casts
Nephrotic syndrome (in association with 3+ to 4+
    proteinuria)
  Nephrotic syndrome
  Free fat
  Fatty casts
  Oval fat bodies
End-stage chronic renal disease (degree of proteinuria
    varies)
  Broad casts (with many inclusions)
  Waxy casts
  Increased numbers of white and red cells
Combination of nephritic, nephrotic, and chronic renal
    failure sediments (telescoped sediment) (seen in
    vasculitis, collagen vascular disease [SLE])
  Hematuria
  Red blood cell casts
  Free fat
  Oval fat bodies
  Waxy casts
  Broad casts
Acute renal failure (acute tubular necrosis) (in associa-
    tion with 1+ to 2+ proteinuria)
  Many narrow, pigmented, granular (dirty brown)
    casts
  Renal tubular epithelial cells
  Epithelial cell casts
  Hyaline casts
└───┘

bleeding across the glomerular membrane in inflammatory glomerular disease, all of which may be involved in causing renal failure. In a specimen with increased white blood cells (>3/hpf), the extra cells are usually segmented neutrophils and are most commonly associated with bacterial infection of the urinary tract. Eosinophils may also be present and are associated with allergic interstitial nephritis. Hansel's stain (methylene blue and eosin Y in methanol) of dried sediment is recommended when eosinophiluria is suspected.[18] Increased numbers of tubular epithelial cells (>1/hpf) may appear in the urinary sediment of acute renal failure from numerous causes, including drug nephrotoxicity and tubular interstitial inflammation.

Casts are cylindrical elements formed in the tubules and found in urine sediment. The major component of their matrix is Tamm-Horsfall protein, which is excreted in the urinary tract.[15] Because casts are formed in the renal parenchyma, they are of particular significance, indicating intrinsic renal disorders. The cellular composition inside casts may help indicate various processes occurring in the renal parenchyma.

Hyaline casts are transparent cylinders without cellular components. Greater numbers of hyaline casts are excreted after exercise, fever, or dehydration and in many circum-

stances in which protein excretion is increased. Granular casts are semitransparent cylinders containing fine refractile granules that are probably aggregates of serum proteins. This finding is contrary to the assumption made for many years that granular casts consist of degenerating cellular material.[19] They are seen in the same physiologic settings as hyaline casts. Presence of both of these casts is nonspecific and occurs with proteinuria, so is a common finding in many types of renal disease and in renal failure.

Waxy casts have a highly refractile, yellow surface with a waxy appearance. Their presence signifies chronic renal disease. Broad casts have a diameter 2 to 6 times that of other casts because of decline in urine flow and indicate advanced chronic renal disease. Fatty casts, containing lipid droplets along with free fat in the urine, may be seen in nephrotic syndrome. This fat, called oval fat bodies, may also be contained in renal tubular epithelial cells. With polarization, the cholesterol takes on a brilliant four-lobed "maltese cross" appearance. Neutral fat can be identified with special lipid stains.[15]

Cellular casts have cells (red, white, or renal tubular cells) that are deposited within their matrix in the parenchyma of the kidney. Red cell (erythrocyte) casts (along with degenerated red cells in casts or hemoglobin casts) are diagnostic of glomerulonephritis or vasculitis of the kidney. White cell (leukocyte) casts are seen in acute and chronic interstitial nephritis and may be found in large numbers in glomerulonephritis.

Patients with acute renal failure often have many narrow, pigmented ("dirty" or "muddy brown"), granular casts, and have renal tubular epithelial cells, both free and in casts, in their urine.[15] Hyaline casts may also appear, along with increases in red and white cells. The urine of chronic renal failure may exhibit granular and hyaline casts but usually also contains broad and waxy casts. In the nephrotic syndrome, oval fat bodies and fatty casts may be present. When nephritic, nephrotic, acute, and chronic elements are found together in a single sediment, the sediment is referred to as "telescoped." This finding usually indicates a rapidly progressive nephritis or a collagen vascular disease such as lupus erythematosus.

Renal Function Tests

The *glomerular filtration rate* is the rate at which plasma water crosses all the glomeruli into the tubular system of the nephron. It can best be measured by calculating the amount of a substance that is totally filtered across the glomeruli without being reabsorbed from the tubules or secreted into them. Inulin and iothalamate are the substances used in clearance tests. Clearance (C_x) is calculated using the following formula:

$$C \times \text{(mL/min)} = \frac{U_x \times V \text{ (mL/min)}}{P_x}$$

where U_x is the concentration of substance x in the urine, P_x is the concentration of x in the plasma, and V is the rate of urine flow.

Although the clearance of any substance excreted by the kidney can be measured with the same formula, such clearances are equal to the GFR only when the substance is totally filtered across the glomeruli and is not reabsorbed from the tubules. Inulin and iothalamate are good indicators of renal function, but they are not products of human metabolism. Their use in clearance tests involves intravenous administration over a long period to achieve a stable blood concentration; this is very time consuming and expensive.

As a compromise among convenience, expense, and accuracy in clinical situations, the creatinine clearance test has been used. Creatinine is a natural product of muscle metabolism that is produced in the body at a constant rate and filtered easily through the glomeruli. It is eliminated from the body only through the kidney. For these reasons, the creatinine clearance is often used to provide an approximate measure of GFR. Some creatinine is also secreted by the renal tubules, resulting in creatinine clearances that are slightly higher than inulin clearances. This is not clinically significant until severe renal failure is present. The creatinine clearance is calculated by the following formula:

$$C_{cr} \text{ (mL/min)} =$$
$$\frac{U_{cr} \text{ (mg/dL)} \times V \text{ urine (mL/24 hr)}}{P_{cr} \text{ (mg/dL)} \times 1440 \text{ min/24 hr}} \times \frac{1.73}{m^2} = GFR$$

where:

C_{cr} = creatinine clearance
V urine = volume of urine excreted in 24 hours
U_{cr} = concentration of creatinine in urine
P_{cr} = concentration of creatinine in serum
$1.73/m^2$ = normalization factor for body surface area
GFR = glomerular filtration rate

The reference ranges for creatinine clearance in persons of average body surface area are, for males, 97 to 137 mL/min/1.73m² and, for females, 88 to 128 mL/min./1.73m². This decreases 6.5 mL/min/1.73m² per decade.[20]

Other Chemical Analyses for Renal Function

Other analyses used to evaluate renal function include measurements of urea and of creatinine. Urea, a catabolic byproduct of protein, increases in the plasma in renal disease because more than 90% of urea is normally excreted through the kidney. Urea is neither actively reabsorbed nor secreted by the tubules and is filtered freely by the glomerulus. In the normal kidney, 40% to 70% of the highly diffusible urea moves passively out of the renal tubule and reenters the plasma. More urea flows back when blood flow is slow; therefore, the urea clearance rate underestimates GFR. Urea production is also very dependent on diet and synthesis by the liver; therefore, the blood level of urea is not a very good independent indicator of renal function. Other nonrenal factors, such as mild dehydration, high-protein diet, increased protein catabolism, muscle wasting, reabsorption of blood protein after a gastrointestinal (GI) bleed, certain drugs (such as cortisol), and decreased renal perfusion can also cause increases in blood urea (azotemia). Postrenal azotemia is caused by obstruction of the flow in the urinary tract by renal stones, tumors of the bladder or prostate, or severe infection.

Although current methods for measurement of urea use serum or plasma, the measurement of urea was originally performed on a filtrate of whole blood and was based on the amount of nitrogen present. Thus, the assay was called a blood urea nitrogen (BUN), and the term is still commonly used to denote this assay. In the United States, urea assays are still reported as urea nitrogen. The reference range is 7 to 18 mg/dL.[19]

The BUN can be used in conjunction with the measurement of plasma creatinine to help distinguish between prerenal and postrenal azotemia, by calculating the urea nitrogen-creatinine ratio.[20] For a normal individual on a normal diet, the ratio ranges between 12 and 20. Very low ratios usually denote acute renal failure, low protein intake, starvation, or severe liver disease with decreased urea synthesis. High ratios with normal creatinine levels may be seen with catabolic states of tissue breakdown, prerenal azotemia, and high protein intake, and following gastrointestinal bleeds. High ratios associated with elevated creatinine concentrations may denote either postrenal obstruction or prerenal azotemia superimposed on renal disease. The ratio may be affected by the specificity of the laboratory method used to measure both urea and creatinine and can show great variability.

Two analytical approaches have been used to assay for urea. The method involving hydrolysis of urea to ammonia and the subsequent measurement of NH_4^+ has the disadvantage of being very sensitive to ammonia contamination, and endogenous ammonia (NH_3) must be removed from urine samples before they are assayed; however, this method demonstrates good specificity and sensitivity when done as a kinetic assay. The other approach measures the rate of increase in conductivity in the sample as the nonionic urea is hydrolyzed by urease to the ionic species NH_4^+ and HCO_3^-. Ammonia contamination is not a problem in this method. Direct condensation methods have the disadvantages of caustic chemical use and limited linearity.

Creatinine, a byproduct of muscle metabolism, is excreted into the plasma at a relatively constant rate. The generation of creatinine in an individual can be derived from estimates of total muscle mass based on age, sex, and weight. This substance is continuously excreted, almost entirely by glomerular filtration. The creatinine excretion rate in any one individual is relatively constant in the absence of renal disease, and parallels endogenous production, because creatinine has a low molecular weight, does not bind to plasma proteins, and is freely filtered by the renal glomerulus. Although tubular secretion of creatinine is variable, the linear decrease of creatinine clearance over time, as renal function fails, has been thoroughly documented for several forms of chronic glomerulonephritis, diabetic nephropathy, chronic interstitial nephritis, and chronic pyelonephritis. Creatinine clearance is initially used by physicians to estimate the severity of renal failure and to make decisions about dialysis. Other than this important use, creatinine clearance is a time-consuming and expensive index of glomerular function.

It has been shown that the creatinine clearance of a patient increases (or decreases) as the reciprocal of plasma creatinine increases (or decreases) linearly. Therefore, the serum creatinine level is probably the most widely used indirect measure of glomerular filtration rate. The correct interpretation of serum creatinine levels is a problem, how-

Table 14–1. Biochemical Abnormalities in Renal Disease and Renal Failure

	Acute Renal Failure	Chronic Renal Failure	Acute Glomerulonephritis	Nephrotic Syndrome
Blood urea nitrogen	↑	↑	↑	NL
Serum creatinine	↑	↑	↑	NL
Serum potassium	↑	↑	↑ or NL	↑ or NL
Serum phosphorus	↑	↑	↑ or NL	NL
Serum calcium	↑	↑	NL	↑
Serum uric acid	↑	↑	NL	NL
Acidosis	P	P	Abs	Abs
Proteinuria	↑ or NL	↑	↑	↑↑↑↑
Hematuria	P	↑	↑↑	↑

Abbreviations and symbols: ↑, increased; P, present; Abs, absent; NL, normal.

ever, because they vary with differences in muscle mass and because of the variations of interferences in creatinine testing methodology explained later. This relationship also does not hold as true for patients with near end-stage renal disease, because the percentage of creatinine secreted by the tubules may rise greatly, making the clearance rate look better than it is. It has, however, been suggested that plasma creatinine alone may be used as an index of glomerular function, especially after an initial clearance rate has been determined.

The American College of Physicians recommends that serum creatinine evaluation be used as a screening test in asymptomatic adults, even though the sensitivity of serum creatinine is low, especially in patients who have mild renal insufficiency. This is because more sophisticated measures are so expensive and difficult to perform. Serum creatinine should be measured in all acutely ill, hospitalized patients and in any patient with known or suspected renal disease. All patients who are to receive potentially nephrotoxic agents, such as aminoglycosides, contrast media, and nonsteroidal anti-inflammatory agents, and who have the potential of renal disease should be screened with a serum creatinine measurement before treatment.

The methods used most commonly to measure creatinine are somewhat nonspecific and subject to interference by many compounds present in blood. These methods are based on the Jaffe picrate reaction, which also reacts with glucose, ascorbic acid, guanidine, acetone, cephalosporins and α-keto acids. Various methods and procedures, such as kinetically based methods, have been used to eliminate these interferences in the Jaffe reaction. Automated enzyme kinetic slide based methods have been developed that eliminate such positive interferences as α-keto acids, which are often found in diabetic serum. Bilirubin in icteric serum samples, however, has been shown to give low creatinine results when measured by the slide kinetic method.

Clinical laboratory scientists who serve an active renal disease center must recognize how the specificity of the method used in their facility affects the clinical application of results. Reference ranges for creatinine clearance, the reciprocal of plasma creatinine concentration, and the urea nitrogen-creatinine ratio vary according to the specificity of the method for creatinine that is used in the calculation. The more a method overestimates true creatinine, the greater the underestimation of creatinine clearance. Reference ranges for serum or plasma creatinine measured by

Jaffe methods similar to those discussed are 0.6 to 1.2 mg/dL in men and 0.5 to 1.1 mg/dL in women. The upper end of the range for the slide method is slightly lower.[19] Other biochemical abnormalities present in renal failure are listed in Table 14–1.

Laboratory Results in Acute Renal Failure

Acute renal failure is associated with a daily elevation of the BUN level of 10 to 20 mg/dL (azotemia) and a daily elevation of the serum creatinine level of 0.5 to 1.0 mg/dL.[2] As discussed previously, the creatinine value reflects kidney function better than the urea level, because urea production is altered by so many factors. Oliguria is commonly present, but not always. Nonoliguric acute renal failure has increasingly been recognized in nephrotoxin-induced as well as hypoperfusion-induced disease. It is usually associated with a less severe insult to the kidney, as well as with lower morbidity and mortality, than oliguric acute renal failure.[2]

Differentiating between prerenal azotemia and acute renal failure is facilitated by several laboratory tests. The urinary indices show concentrated urine (specific gravity often higher than 1.020 and high osmolality) in prerenal failure, but lower specific gravity (less than 1.012, similar to that of blood plasma, in acute renal failure (Table 14–2). The urine sodium level is lower in prerenal than in acute renal failure, and the urine-to-plasma creatinine ratio is higher in prerenal azotemia. It should be emphasized that diuretics may invalidate the use of these indices for up to 24 hours, so these agents should not be used prior to collection of urine for these analyses.[2, 3]

Patients with acute renal failure exhibit the biochemical abnormalities associated with uremic syndrome, but with a more rapid onset. The patient may be hyperkalemic even without an exogenous source of potassium because of the catabolic release of potassium from tissues. Hyponatremia is present because of water retention. Acidosis may occur as the kidneys lose their capacity to regulate the acid-base balance of the body. Metabolic alkalosis may also be found if the patient is losing large amounts of acidic gastric juice from vomiting.

Divalent ion disturbances are commonly seen in acute renal failure. Owing to retention of the ions, hyperphosphatemia and hypermagnesemia are almost always present in

Table 14–2. Urinary Diagnostic Indices

Index	Prerenal	ARF (Acute Tubular Necrosis)
U_{Na} (mEq/L)	<20	>40
U_{Cr} (mg/dL)P_{Cr} (mg/dL)	>40	<20
U_{OSM} (mOsm/kg H_2O)	>500	<350
Renal failure index (RFI): $$RFI = \frac{U_{Na}}{U_{Cr}/P_{Cr}}$$	<1	>1
Fractional excretion of filtered sodium (Fe_{Na}): $$Fe_{Na} = \frac{U_{Na} \times P_{Cr}}{P_{Na} \times U_{Cr}} \times 100$$	<1	>1
Urine specific gravity	1.020	1.012

Abbreviations: Fe_{Na}, fractional excretion of filtered sodium; P_{Cr}, plasma creatinine; P_{Na}, plasma sodium; RFI, renal failure index; U_{Cr}, urine creatine; U_{Na}, urine sodium; U_{OSM}, urine osmolality.

oliguric acute renal failure.[2] Hyperphosphatemia (up to 20 mg/dL) may be very severe in patients with renal failure, because of tissue breakdown or rhabdomyolysis. Patients with acute renal failure who are given magnesium-containing medications such as antacids or laxatives may have very high magnesium levels. Hypocalcemia, in the range of 5 to 8 mg/dL, is also common.[4]

Anemia is common in acute renal failure and may occur rapidly owing to suppressed erythropoiesis, hemolysis, bleeding, and hemodilution. A low white count is usually the result of the precipitating illness. A bleeding problem may also exist, as in chronic uremia, because of platelet dysfunction and factor VII dysfunction.

The microscopic evaluation of urine sediment is helpful in the diagnosis of acute renal failure. A sediment that contains renal tubular epithelial cell debris and casts supports the diagnosis of acute renal failure. Sometimes there are only "muddy" brown granular casts, and there may or may not be accompanying free renal tubular epithelial cells. A few red blood cells and white blood cells per high power field may be present. A 1+ or 2+ proteinuria level on a urinary reagent test strip is also compatible with ARF. These results contrast with the large amounts of urine protein and numerous red blood cell casts found in acute renal failure secondary to renal disorders such as glomerulonephritis (see Box 14–3). Hyaline casts in large numbers may be seen in prerenal azotemia. The absence of cellular elements and protein in the urine is most compatible with prerenal and postrenal azotemia. Numerous crystals, such as uric acid, oxalate, or hippuric acid crystals, may occur with ethylene glycol, methoxyflurane, or other chemical toxicity when the cause of acute renal failure is a nephrotoxic agent.[2, 3, 20]

Myoglobinuria as the cause of the ARF should be suspected in a patient with a history of muscle injury, prolonged periods of unconsciousness, alcohol or drug abuse, or seizures.[6] The urinary reagent test strip does not distinguish between myoglobin and hemoglobin. Myoglobin should be suspected, however, with a heme-positive urine in the absence of intact red cells and with normal serum color (which would be pink if intravascular hemolysis had occurred). Myoglobin, a low-molecular-weight protein, is cleared from the circulation much faster than hemoglobin. The patient with myoglobinuria also has elevations of serum creatinine phosphokinase (CK) and aldolase. Precise identification of myoglobin depends on sophisticated absorption spectrophotometry, electrophoresis, or immunochemical methods.

In acute drug-induced interstitial nephritis, the laboratory finding of a 10% to 60% eosinophilia usually accompanies the clinical symptoms of fever and maculopapular skin rash. Also present are proteinuria, and the presence of casts, hematuria, and white blood cells, many of which may be eosinophils, in the urinary sediment. A Hansel's stain preparation of a sediment of freshly voided urine is useful in demonstrating the eosinophils.[18]

Finally, a blood screen for toxic chemicals and drugs may give valuable information in acute renal failure if no other causes can be detected from the patient's history and laboratory results.

Laboratory Results in Chronic Renal Failure

Chronic progressive renal disease that ultimately results in CRF can be divided into four stages associated with various laboratory abnormalities. In the first stage, the only abnormalities present may be proteinuria and an abnormal urine sediment. Renal function (GFR) is usually nearly normal or is reduced by less than 25%, and there is only a slight decrease in renal reserve. The second stage evolves with mild renal insufficiency. At least 50% of normal function must be lost before the concentration of urea nitrogen or creatinine rises above the normal range. In the third stage, frank renal failure develops. Anemia, acidosis, worsening azotemia, isosthenuria, hypocalcemia, hyperphosphatemia, and osteodystrophy are present. Development of end-stage renal disease accompanied by the uremic syndrome is the fourth stage.

The characteristic physiologic and laboratory findings are the same in end-stage renal disease (the uremic syndrome), regardless of the initiating disease process. The most characteristic findings are higher concentrations of nitrogen compounds, such as urea nitrogen and creatinine, as a result of reduced GFR and decreased tubular function. Retention of these compounds and of metabolic acids is followed by progressive hyperphosphatemia, hypercalcemia, and hyperkalemia. Hyperkalemia is potentially very dangerous because it raises the risk of cardiac arrest. Reduced endocrine function manifests as inadequate synthesis of erythropoietin, resulting in anemia, and inadequate synthesis of vitamin D, resulting in osteomalacia. Hypertension is usually a problem, because regulation of blood sodium is disordered (Fig. 14–2).

TREATMENT

Acute Renal Failure

Treatment of ARF involves diagnosing and treating the underlying cause of renal failure, restoring fluid and electrolyte balance, preventing or delaying metabolic complications, and treating any infections promptly.[21] The clinical

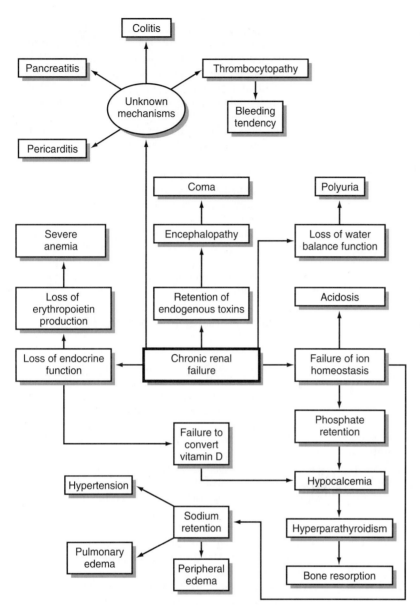

Figure 14–2. Pathophysiology of chronic renal failure. (From Creech, CL: Renal function. *In* Bishop ML, Duben-von Laufen JL, Fody EP (eds): Clinical Chemistry. Philadelphia, JB Lippincott, 1992.)

laboratory plays an important role in the management of affected patients by performing daily serum electrolyte measurements. The management of electrolytes is concerned principally with sodium and potassium. Serum sodium concentrations should remain between 135 and 145 mEq/L. Changes in sodium concentration indicate changes in water balance. A rising serum sodium value is generally an indication of a water deficit, and a falling serum sodium is an indicator of excessive water administration. Hyperkalemia is one of the more common complications of renal failure, and can cause death through induction of cardiac arrhythmias. Usually, potassium can be controlled with dialysis, which can also control fluid balance and correct other electrolyte abnormalities. Patients can undergo either peritoneal dialysis or hemodialysis. Even when patients enter the diuretic phase of ARF, careful management is necessary, because glomerular filtration rates remain low. Daily serum sodium and potassium concentration measurements remain essential to proper management of the patient with acute renal failure.

Chronic Renal Failure

The abnormal laboratory results of proteinuria and, at a later stage, elevated BUN and creatinine levels may be the only indication in CRF of silent but progressive progress toward end-stage renal disease. In the management of any patient with renal insufficiency, the first goal is to identify and treat the underlying cause if possible. The laboratory plays an important role in this phase, because abnormal laboratory parameters, rather than clinical symptoms, may be the first clue to renal disease. The second goal is to identify and treat any conditions that aggravate the underlying renal disease or have adverse effects on renal function. Some commonly found conditions that the laboratory can play a role in detecting are urinary tract infections, sodium and water depletion, and metabolic derangements, such as electrolyte imbalance produced by anorexia and vomiting. Metabolic acidosis can also adversely affect renal function and should be controlled. Phosphorus excretion should be monitored in patients with chronic renal disease, because abnormalities of phosphorus excretion are central to the problems of uremic osteodystrophy. Both calcium and phosphorus levels are also important in the prevention and management of renal disease–induced bone problems.

When renal failure can no longer be managed through diet and medication, the treatment must involve dialysis to prolong life. Laboratory data is still vital in following and managing patients undergoing dialysis. Renal transplantation may be considered finally in the management of some patients with chronic renal failure.

Case Study

A 39-year-old white man with no significant past history presented to a small community hospital with a 2-day history of nausea and vomiting. He was found on initial examination to be moderately icteric. The patient had a history of chronic headaches and had been taking 4 to 10 extra-strength acetaminophen tablets every day throughout the past year. His alcohol consumption consisted of three to four drinks of rum and cola routinely on weekday evenings, with a higher intake on weekends. The patient was transferred to a tertiary care hospital and admitted to the intensive care unit. He received 2 units of fresh-frozen plasma and 20 mg of vitamin K intravenously. His hepatitis profile was negative. Laboratory findings (including reference ranges) were as follows:

AST (aspartate aminotransferase):	>19,000 IU/L (8–20)
ALT (alanine aminotransferase):	>6,000 IU/L (8–20)
Creatinine:	7.2 mg/dL (0.7–1.5)
BUN:	48 mg/dL (10–20)
Prothrombin time:	20 sec. (10–14)

Urinalysis revealed the abnormal presence of protein (4+), bilirubin, blood (a large amount of hemoglobin), and 8 to 11 coarsely granular casts per high-power field.

Urine output was initially only 300 mL per 24 hours. Repeated testing of renal parameters revealed that the creatinine value was increasing rapidly, with a reading of 14.3 mg/dL by the third day of hospitalization. Consultation with the Nephrology Service was obtained. Because of the severe nature of the liver insult, consultation was also obtained with liver transplant team. However, liver function values began a slow descent toward normal. On the third day, acute dialysis was initiated, and urine output began to increase. The creatinine value returned toward the normal range.

The patient was discharged on the fourteenth hospital day with the following laboratory results:

AST:	19 IU/L
ALT:	16 IU/L
Creatinine:	2.3 mg/dL
BUN:	32 mg/dL

Questions

1. What is the diagnosis?
2. What is the cause of the renal failure?

Discussion

1. The patient was diagnosed as having severe hepatocellular necrosis secondary to acetaminophen abuse and acute renal failure.
2. The renal failure possibly could be secondary to the acetaminophen abuse and be a drug-induced interstitial acute renal failure. More likely, it is a volume depletion prerenal azotemia caused by the severe vomiting secondary to the liver problem. The patient responded promptly to fluids and acute hemodialysis. No renal biopsy was performed, so interstitial nephritis was not definitely ruled out. The patient refused to return to the hospital at a later time for reevaluation of either renal function or liver status.

References

1. Agodoa LYC, Jones CA, Striker GE: Scope, prevalence and incidence of renal disease. *In* Jacobson HR, Striker GE, Klahr S (eds): Principles and Practice of Nephrology, ed 2. St Louis, Mosby–Year Book, 1995.
2. Brady HR, Brenner BM, Lieberthal W: Acute renal failure. *In* Brenner BM (ed): The Kidney, ed 5, vol II. Philadelphia, WB Saunders, 1996.
3. Lazarus JM, Brenner BM (eds): Acute Renal Failure, ed 3. New York, Churchill Livingstone, 1993.
4. Schrier RW: Acute renal failure: Pathogenesis, diagnosis, and management. Hosp Pract 16:93–112, 1981.
5. Pavit C, Ram KA, McDonald FD: Differential diagnosis of acute renal failure. *In* Jacobson HR, Striker GE, Klahr S (eds): In The Principle and Practice of Nephrology, ed 2. St Louis, Mosby-Year Book, 1995.
6. Honda N, Kurokawa K: Acute renal failure and rhabdomyolysis. Kidney Int 23:888, 1983.
7. Bennett WM, Porter GA: Nephrotoxic acute renal failure due to common drugs. Am J Physiol 241:F1–F8, 1981.
8. Swan SK, Bennett WM: Nephrotoxic acute renal failure. *In* Lazarus JM, Brenner BM (eds): Acute Renal Failure, ed 3. New York, Churchill Livingstone, 1993.
9. Smith CR, Lipsky JJ, Laskin OL, et al: Double blind comparison of the nephrotoxicity and auditory toxicity of gentamycin and tobramycin. N Engl J Med 302:1106, 1983.
10. D'Elia JA, Gleason RE, Alday M, et al: Nephrotoxicity from angiographic contrast material. Am J Med 72:719, 1982.
11. Margulies KB, Schirger J, Burnell JC Jr: Radiocontrast-induced nephropathy: Current status and future prospect: Int Angiol 2:20, 1991.
12. Hannerman J, Baumann K: Nephrotoxicity of cisplatin, carboplatin and transplatin. Arch Toxicol 64:393, 1990.
13. Linton AL, Clark WF, Driedger AA, et al: Acute interstitial nephritis due to drugs: Review of the literature with a report of nine cases. Ann Intern Med 93:735, 1980.
14. Suki WN, Eknoyan G: Pathophysiology and clinical manifestations of chronic renal failure and the uremic syndrome. *In* Jacobson HR, Striker GE, Klahr S (eds): The Principles and Practice of Nephrology, ed 2. St Louis, Mosby-Year Book, 1995.
15. Brunzel NA: Fundamentals of Urine and Body Fluid Analysis. Philadelphia, WB Saunders, 1994.
16. Kasisho BL, Keane WF: Laboratory assessment of renal disease: Clearance, urinalysis and renal biopsy. *In* Jacobson HR, Striker GE, Klahr S (eds): The Principles and Practice of Nephrology, ed 2. St Louis, Mosby-Year Book, 1995.
17. Silverman LM, Christensen RH, Grant GH: Amino acids and proteins. *In* Tietz NW (ed): Textbook of Clinical Chemistry. Philadelphia, WB Saunders, 1994.

18. Corwin HL, Bray RA, Haber MH: The detection and interpretation of urinary eosinophils. Arch Pathol Lab Med 113:1256, 1989.

19. Whelton A, Watson AJ, Rock RC: Nitrogen metabolites and renal function. *In* Tietz NW (ed.): Textbook of Clinical Chemistry. Philadelphia, WB Saunders, 1994.

20. Frommer JP, Ayus JC: Acute ethylene glycol intoxication. Am J Nephrol 2:1, 1982.

21. Dougherty JC: Acute renal failure. *In* Forland M (ed): Nephrology. New Hyde Park, NY, Medical Examination Publishing, 1983.

Glomerulonephritis

Martha Savage Payne

Glomerulonephritis refers to an inflammatory process affecting the renal glomerulus. The structural and functional disorders of the glomeruli constitute the majority of cases of chronic renal failure.[1] These include both the primary glomerular diseases, in which the glomeruli are the sole or predominant tissue involved, and secondary glomerular disorders associated with many systemic diseases.

Glomerular diseases may be grouped into patterns primarily on the basis of clinical onset, progression, and pathologic condition found on renal biopsy. These are acute glomerulonephritis, rapidly progressive glomerulonephritis, chronic glomerulonephritis, recurrent or primary hematuria with few or no symptoms, and nephrotic syndrome.[1] These syndromes may appear with primary glomerular disease or in association with various multisystem, infectious, drug-induced or hereditary diseases.

The nomenclature of glomerular disease is constantly undergoing revision as new clinicopathologic entities emerge, arising from studies using various sophisticated techniques. Renal biopsy has become a very important tool in the diagnosis of glomerular disease, and there are terms commonly used to describe the pathologic lesions seen in renal biopsy. *Focal* has been used to indicate changes present only in some glomeruli, whereas *generalized* means that all the glomeruli are involved. *Segmental* refers to changes that are present only in part of the glomerulus, other parts being spared. For example, most focal lesions are also segmental. *Diffuse,* on the other hand, describes changes involving most or all of the glomeruli in their entirety. *Membranous* refers to the thickening of the glomerular capillary wall that may result from the development of immune deposits in the glomerular structures. In electron microscopy, deposits are described according to their location. *Subendothelial deposits* are within the basement membrane underneath the epithelial cell (see Fig. 15–1).

A *crescent* is a sickle-shaped collection of epithelial cells and macrophages along the inside wall of Bowman's capsule but external to the glomerular capillaries. Leakage of fibrin into the capsule is believed to cause this inflammatory response. The finding of crescents on renal biopsy indicates severe glomerular injury.

Proliferative changes in the glomerulus refers to an increased number of endocapillary or extracapillary cells. The endocapillary cells may be either endothelial or mesangial cells. The extracapillary cells may be either epithelial cells or blood-derived cells, such as neutrophils or macrophages.

ETIOLOGY AND PATHOPHYSIOLOGY
Immunologic Mechanisms

Current theory, based on experimental animal models, clinical observation, immunohistochemical detection of immunoglobulin (Ig) G and mediators such as complement, and other serologic evidence, suggests that most, if not all, forms of human glomerulonephritis are mediated by an immunologic mechanism.[2] Both humoral and cellular immune mechanisms as well as activation of mediator systems have been implicated.[3] Most cases of glomerulonephritis are associated with some form of immune deposits. These deposits may be antibodies to circulating antigens that form soluble immune complexes in the circulation and

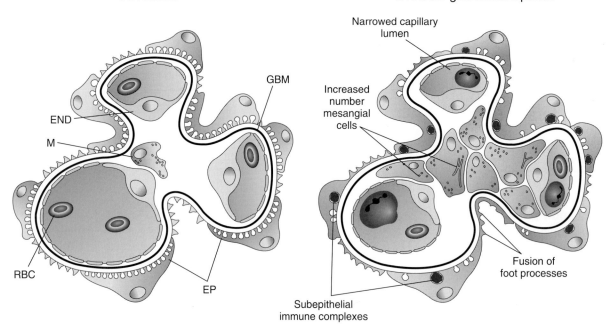

Figure 15–1. Diagrammatic representation of three glomerular capillary loops of normal glomerulus *(A)* and a mesangial area *(dark shading)* illustrating the types of immune deposits seen in glomerulonephritis *(B)*. Deposits in the mesangium and along the subendothelial surface of the basement membrane may result from trapping of circulating immune complexes. These deposits are either characteristic of focal nephritis (mesangial deposits) or of diffuse proliferative lupus nephritis and type I mesangiocapillary glomerulonephritis (subendothelial deposits). The linear deposits shown by immunofluorescence in anti-GBM antibody disease, the finely granular deposits on the subepithelial surface of the capillary wall characteristic of membranous nephropathy, and the subepithelial humps of poststreptococcal glomerulonephritis probably form locally. Abbreviations: END, endothelial cell; EP, epithelial cell; GBM, glomerular basement membrane; M, mesangium; RBC, red blood cell.

are subsequently trapped in the glomerulus, or they may be antibodies to antigens that have been trapped nonimmunologically in the glomerulus. In other cases, the deposits may be antibodies to portions of the glomerular basement membrane itself. Glomerular injury sometimes occurs in the absence of detected antibody deposition (IgG), but complement deposition may be impressive and the patient hypocomplementemic.

These immune deposits may damage the glomeruli and may also activate other portions of the immune system, such as the complement system, leukocytes (neutrophils, monocytes, and T lymphocytes), coagulation factors, and, possibly, kinins and prostaglandins.[4] Neutrophils are drawn to and accumulate at the site of the antigen-antibody-complement localization in the glomeruli by chemoattractants. The neutrophils can then displace the endothelial lining of the glomerular capillary and even cause gaps in the glomerular basement membrane. Neutrophils then destroy glomerular tissue by releasing lysosomal materials. Macrophage/monocytes are attracted to the site, also involving the T lymphocytes. All of these cells can react in an inflammatory response that damages the glomeruli. This damage results in hematuria, proteinuria, reduced glomerular filtration rate (GFR), and alteration in sodium excretion leading to edema, circulatory congestion, and/or hypertension associated with glomerular diseases.

Proteinuria

The glomerular capillary wall normally permits a high rate of fluid filtration but markedly restricts the passage of macromolecules such as protein; therefore, the urine of a normal individual contains very little protein. Experimental evidence suggests that this restriction results from a discrete structural barrier of the glomerulus as well as a charge-selective characteristic of the capillary wall.[5] Negatively charged component(s) of the capillary wall may constitute an electrostatic hindrance to circulating, negatively charged proteins. The large size and shape of the proteins are also factors in their restricted passage through the small pores of the glomerular membrane. In glomerular disease such as minimal change lesion, little structural damage is noted in the glomerulus, but massive amounts of negatively charged albumin are excreted. Experimental evidence suggests that this excretion is due to loss of glomerular fixed-negative charges.[3] No evidence exists for change in the structural barrier or pore size of the glomerulus in this instance.

In more severe inflammatory diseases of the glomerulus, greater structural damage occurs within the glomerulus, and large, protein-permeable pores develop. A size and charge-dependent flux of protein ensues, evidenced by large amounts of both albumin and large proteins such as IgG.[5]

Hematuria

The hematuria of glomerulonephritis is also associated with the immunologically damaged glomerular membrane barrier. Marked disruption in its integrity allows red cells to be pushed through these gaps in the glomerular basement membrane because of the pulsatile capillary hydraulic pressure and the deformability of the red cell.[6]

The reduction in total kidney glomerular filtration rate is a result of the alteration in the filtering surface area or intrinsic hydraulic conductivity of the capillary wall of the glomerulus or of the loss of entire nephron units in a focal manner. The edema, circulatory congestion, and hypertension are manifestations of the salt and water retention leading to the expansion of extracellular fluid volume in the peripheral capillary circulation.[1]

Acute Glomerulonephris

Acute glomerulonephritis or the nephritic syndrome is a clinical pattern characterized by a relatively abrupt onset of variable degrees of hematuria, proteinuria, diminished GFR, sodium and fluid retention, circulatory congestion, hypertension, and, occasionally, oliguria. This syndrome is also typified by a tendency for spontaneous recovery and a common association with preceding microbial infection (Box 15–1).

Poststreptococcal glomerulonephritis (PSGN) is a common acute glomerulonephritis related to a recent group A β-hemolytic streptococcal infection of the skin or the pharynx.[7] Only certain strains of group A β-hemolytic streptococci are capable of inducing nephritis. M type 12 is the nephritogenic strain most commonly encountered, but more than 12 others have been identified.[1] The latent period between the pharyngitis and the ensuing nephritis is usually 6 to 21 days, with the attack rate being less than 5%. In skin infection caused by group A β-hemolytic streptococcal infection, the latent period is usually longer (3 weeks), and the attack rate usually higher.[7] Children are most commonly affected, with a peak age of 2 to 6 years, but PSGN can occur at any age.

The exact mechanism of the pathogenesis of poststreptococcal glomerulonephritis is unknown. The latent period between infection and onset of nephritis, the granular immune deposits in glomeruli seen on renal biopsy, and the hypocomplementemia implicate it as an immune complex disease. The sequence of events leading to the immune deposit formation and inflammation is not fully understood, although three mechanisms have been proposed. One suggests that nephritogenic streptococci release an enzyme capable of altering IgG to the extent that affected patients develop antibody to their own altered IgG. The second possibility proposed is that circulating streptococcal antigens bind to the glomeruli and serve as planted antigen for circulating antistreptococcal antibodies. The third mechanism proposes that antibodies to the streptococcal antigen cross-react with glomerular antigen. These immune complexes, however formed, are involved in the pathogenesis of the disease.[8]

Although renal biopsies are not usually performed when poststreptococcal glomerulonephritis is the presumptive diagnosis, much has been learned of the pathology of PSGN from percutaneous renal biopsies that have been performed on a widespread basis in the last several decades. Early in the course of the disease, a typical picture emerges. On tissue sections using light microscopy, all the glomeruli are shown to be uniformly involved, and they appear bloodless and hypercellular as a result of proliferation of mesangial

Box 15–1. Infectious Agents/ Syndromes Associated with Acute Glomerulonephritis

Bacterial

Group A streptococci
Viridans streptococcus
Pneumococcal infections
Klebsiella pneumoniae
Staphylococcal or gram-negative sepsis (meningococcemia, gonococcemia)
Haemophilus influenzae
H. aphrophilus
Shunt infections with staphylococci, diphtheroids, *Corynebacterium bovis, Propionibacterium acnes*
Brucellosis
Typhoid fever
Legionnaires' disease
Rocky Mountain spotted fever
Typhus
Chlamydia psittaci

Viral and Mycoplasmal

Hepatitis B
Mumps
Measles
Varicella-zoster
Coxsackievirus
Infectious mononucleosis
Hantavirus
Mycoplasma pneumoniae

Fungal

Candida albicans
Histoplasmosis

Protozoal

Plasmodium malariae
Plasmodium falciparum
Toxoplasma gondii

Helminthic

Schistosoma mansoni
Trichinosis

Spirochetal

Treponema pallidum
Leptospirosis

and endothelial cells and the infiltration of neutrophils, monocytes, and sometimes eosinophils in the glomerular capillaries.[9] In some cases, cellular crescents may form from extensive accumulation of cells in Bowman's capsule; this is the exception rather than the rule and may be associated with a more grave prognosis.

Electron microscopy shows discrete electron-dense, dome-shaped deposits projecting outward from the epithelial side of the basement membrane (see Fig. 15–1). With immunofluorescence, bright diffuse granular staining for IgG or complement component C3 is found along the glomerular basement membrane and, in early glomerulonephritis, in mesangial deposits.[1]

Although PSGN is the most common postinfectious glomerulonephritis, its incidence has significantly decreased in developed countries, making other forms of postinfectious glomerulonephritis relatively more common in those countries. In the majority of infections associated with glomerulonephritis, kidney involvement is mild and reversible. Occasionally, however, progression to renal failure occurs, even when the infection is controlled.[1]

Rapidly Progressive Glomerulonephritis

Rapidly progressive glomerulonephritis (RPGN), also referred to subacute glomerulonephritis or extracapillary proliferative glomerulonephritis, is a clinical syndrome that manifests as an abrupt or insidious onset of acute nephritis accompanied by a rapid and progressive decline in renal function.[10] Without treatment, this syndrome progresses to end-stage renal disease in a short time (weeks or months). This syndrome may accompany a number of infectious diseases or multisystem diseases, such as Goodpasture's syndrome, or it may be a primary (idiopathic) renal disease. The diseases that have been associated with RPGN are listed in Box 15–2. Idiopathic RPGN, which is a primary glomerular disease, affects older persons and has a male preponderance, of 2:1.[1] It is a relatively uncommon disorder. Autoantibodies such as anti–glomerular basement membrane (anti-GBM) antibody and anti–neutrophil cytoplasmic autoantibodies (ANCAS) have been discovered in various forms of crescentic glomerulonephritis and have helped classify the disorder according to its pathogenic mechanism or associated serologic findings.

One type of RPGN is associated with Goodpasture's syndrome, which is clearly mediated by antibodies directed against the glomerular basement membrane. In addition to the glomerulonephritis, there is lung hemorrhage. The diagnosis of Goodpasture's syndrome requires the presence of all three of the following elements: (1) glomerulonephritis, commonly of the rapidly progressive and crescentic variety, (2) anti-GBM antibody, and (3) pulmonary hemorrhage.[11]

Renal biopsy reveals extensive extracapillary proliferation or crescent formation in Bowman's capsule.[12] The infiltrated cells that form the crescents along with fibrin are probably macrophages derived from blood monocytes. These cells undergo proliferation and epithelioid transformation upon exposure to the fibrinogen and fibrin polymers that have escaped into Bowman's capsule.

The variability of the immunofluorescence findings reflects the variation in the underlying mechanisms of this disease syndrome.[13] Linear deposits of IgG and C3 indicate involvement of anti-GBM antibodies (see Fig. 15–1). Circulating anti-GBM antibodies are also found in these cases. Another type has granular deposits of immunoglobulin (IgG and/or IgM, sometimes with C3), suggesting an immune complex–mediated disease. Another type contains only scant deposits of IgG (pauci immune) but has ANCAs.

Box 15–2. Disorders Associated With Rapidly Progressive Glomerulonephritis

In Primary Glomerular Diseases

Primary diffuse crescentic glomerulonephritis:
   Type I—with anti-GBM (no pulmonary hemorrhage)
   Type II—immune complex associated disease without anti-GBM or ANCAs
   Type III—pauci immune with ANCAs
   Type IV—with anti-AMB and ANCAs
   Type V—pauci immune without ANCAs or anti-GBM
Anti–glomerular basement membrane disease
Immune complex disease
Mesangiocapillary glomerulonephritis (MCGN)
IgA nephropathy (Berger's disease)
Focal and segmental glomerulosclerosis

After Infectious Diseases

Poststreptococcal glomerulonephritis
Bacterial endocarditis
Visceral abscesses
Shunt nephritis
Other infection (e.g., hepatitis B)

In Association With Multisystem Diseases

Systemic lupus erythematosus
Henoch-Schönlein syndrome
Cryoglobulinemia
Polyarteritis and other vasculitides
Wegener's granulomatosis
Lung cancer, lymphoma

A fourth type has linear deposits of IgG and both the anti-GBM and the ANCAs. A fifth type has scant deposits of IgG and no anti-GBM or ANCA[1] (see Box 15–2).

Chronic Glomerulonephritis

Chronic glomerulonephritis is a vague, all-inclusive term referring to progressive diminished renal function that often has an insidious onset and, over 5 to 10 years or longer, leads to end-stage renal disease. Thus, chronic glomerulonephritis is not a disease entity but can be caused by many glomerular diseases and results in persistent and usually deteriorating renal functional abnormalities.[1] When it is detected early by routine screening, the only manifestations may be abnormal urine sediment, proteinuria, and mildly reduced renal function. The final stage of this syndrome is total renal failure with uremia.

The basic initiating process may subside, but the progressive loss of renal function through destruction of the glomerular capillary bed may persist.[14] Although the exact mechanism is unknown, it may be related to the adaptive hemodynamic events arising from the initial loss of filtering surface area, which include increases in glomerular capillary pressure and flow. This process may then damage the remaining capillaries and set up a vicious circle of destruction of the glomerular capillary beds.

Recurrent or Primary Hematuria

Recurrent or primary hematuria is a clinical syndrome characterized by persistent or repeated episodes of hematuria (gross or microscopic), caused by glomerular capillary hemorrhage,[1, 15] in the absence of systemic diseases involving renal tissue, lesions within the lower urinary tract, and other major signs of renal disease. Proteinuria may be present but is mild. Renal biopsy is probably unnecessary in the evaluation of every patient with primary hematuria, but when it is performed, many patients (30% to 50%) with recurrent hematuria of a glomerular origin are found to have focal glomerulonephritis.[16]

These changes are also seen in association with such systemic diseases as systemic lupus erythematosus, polyarteritis nodosa, Wegener's granulomatosis, subacute bacterial endocarditis, Henoch-Schönlein syndrome, and early Goodpasture's syndrome.[1] The diseases must be ruled out in a patient with recurrent hematuria by clinical and laboratory data. From 20% to 50% of patients with hematuria have a diffuse mesangial proliferation sometimes resembling that seen in poststreptococcal glomerulonephritis.[1] The remaining patients have more advanced lesions, such as diffuse proliferative glomerulonephritis with variable crescentic involvement.

The immunofluorescence patterns in primary hematuria have also been variable. Some patients may have IgM or IgG with C3 deposits.[1] Some studies have shown that as many as 50% of patients have extensive granular deposits of IgA in the mesangium, usually in association with IgG and C3; this syndrome is referred to as IgA nephropathy or Berger's disease (discussed later). Other patterns of IgG and/or C3 deposits may be seen, but in some cases, no IgG or C3 deposits at all are seen.

IgA Nephropathy

IgA nephropathy (Berger's disease) is a primary renal disease in which IgA is the principal glomerular immunoglobulin. IgA nephropathy is believed to be the most common cause of hematuria of glomerular origin in the world. Renal biopsy usually reveals a focal and segmental proliferative glomerulonephritis. Electron microscopy usually demonstrates homogeneous electron-dense deposits in the mesangium of the glomeruli. The diagnostic immunofluorescence pattern appears as granular deposits of IgA in the mesangium.[17] In a high percentage of the biopsy specimens, IgG is found in the same pattern as IgA, leading some to call the entity IgA/IgG nephropathy. IgM, C3, properdin, and fibrin deposits have also been found in the mesangial areas. The pathogenesis of this disease is unknown; however, the presence of IgA and C3, but not early-acting C components, suggests that it is a circulatory immune complex–mediated disease involving prominent activation of the alternative C pathway.

Henoch-Schönlein Syndrome

Henoch-Schönlein syndrome is characterized by multiorgan involvement: dermal (purpura), gastrointestinal (colic and bleeding), musculoskeletal (arthritis of the ankles and knees), and renal (IgA nephropathy). The renal biopsy reveals findings similar to those seen in IgA nephropathy.[18]

Hereditary Nephritis

Hereditary nephritis (Alport's syndrome) occurs in families and is X-linked in the large majority of affected families. Initially there is hematuria, but the nephrotic syndrome develops in 30% to 40% of patients. Hearing loss is associated with this syndrome as well as ocular defects in some patients. Renal failure results from deteriorating renal function in the second decade of life in severely affected men.[18] Renal failure is uncommon in women. The glomerular alterations are nondescript on light microscopy, and immunofluorescence studies are generally negative. The electron microscopy picture is the most diagnostic, showing thinning, splitting, and a moth-eaten appearance of the glomerular capillary basement membrane.[18]

CLINICAL MANIFESTATIONS

Acute glomerulonephritis, or the nephritic syndrome, is typified by the sudden onset (a matter of hours to days) of hematuria, oliguria, hypertension, proteinuria, and symptoms of uremia. It is not necessary for all five abnormalities to be present to establish the diagnosis, but hematuria must be present in combination with at least one of the other four components. The syndrome of acute renal failure may supervene, and systemic complications of azotemia and hypertension may occur. These include congestive heart failure, salt and water retention, edema, central nervous system manifestations, and electrolyte and acid-base disturbances. These complications are not unique to glomerular diseases and can result from any form of renal injury sufficient to produce acute renal failure. When the signs and symptoms develop over a 4 to 8 weeks, the resulting syndrome is often referred to as subacute or rapidly progressive renal failure.

A number of patients may present with persistent hematuria (with or without proteinuria). These individuals may have mild renal insufficiency that may ultimately progress to result in a nephrotic or a nephritic syndrome, or there may be a relentless progressive deterioration in renal function ultimately leading to end-stage renal failure.

Poststreptococcal glomerulonephritis classically manifests as an abrupt onset of hematuria (microscopic or gross), proteinuria (less than 3.0 grams per day in 80% of cases), edema, hypertension, and varying degrees of renal dysfunction.[1] A broad range of severity of disease exists, however, from entirely asymptomatic cases detected by the incidental finding of microscopic hematuria, to oliguric acute renal failure. The patient usually reports a low amount of urine (oliguria) and a smoky or rusty appearance to the urine (hematuria). Dysuria may be present in a few cases with gross hematuria, but severe loin or abdominal pain is generally not a presenting symptom. Since there is considerable variability in the presenting features of acute PSGN, anyone presenting with edema, oliguria, hypertension, and circulatory congestion should have a urine sediment examination and urine protein quantitation.

Clinically, *rapidly progressive glomerulonephritis*

(RPGN) presents with a 4- to 8-week or more abrupt onset of severe oliguria or even anuria. The presenting complaints usually relate primarily to the uremia or fluid retention. Fever, myalgia, and abdominal pain are also sometimes present. Hypertension is typically mild. In the RPGN associated with Goodpasture's syndrome, lung hemorrhage is a clinical finding in addition to the symptoms associated with the glomerulonephritis.

In *recurrent hematuria,* the patient presents with either persistent or repeated hematuria with or without mild proteinuria and may otherwise be asymptomatic. Other primary renal diseases and systemic diseases that involve the kidney and lower urinary tract bleeding must be excluded by laboratory evaluation and radiologic and endoscopic examinations.

IgA nephropathy occurs most commonly in patients between the ages of 16 and 35 years. The male-to-female ratio of occurrence is 2:1.[19] The most common clinical presentation of IgA nephropathy is recurring episodes of gross hematuria immediately following or concurrent with upper respiratory infections, which may confuse the initial diagnosis with PSGN. Low-grade fever along with a loin pain or dysuria may accompany the hematuria; therefore, bacterial hemorrhagic cystitis must be ruled out. Blood pressure is usually normal but may be elevated, especially in advanced disease. Reversible acute renal failure may occur with episodes of macroscopic hematuria.

Most patients with IgA nephropathy have a chronic course, with recurrent episodes of gross or microscopic hematuria that may last for years. Up to 25% of patients show a progressive loss of renal failure over several years. It has been estimated that 1% to 2% of patients diagnosed with IgA nephropathy progress to end-stage renal failure each year from the time of diagnosis.[1] Clinical features that indicate a poorer prognosis are older age, decreased GFR at time of onset, hypertension, and proteinuria in the nephrotic range.

LABORATORY ANALYSES AND DIAGNOSIS

Urinalysis, Hematology, and Clinical Chemistry Analyses

The laboratory findings in acute glomerulonephritis include hematuria, red blood cell (RBC) casts in the urine sediment, proteinuria, decreased clearances due to a diminished GFR, and imbalance in serum electrolytes due to sodium and fluid retention. The renal dysfunction involving sodium and water retention probably reflects a reduction in glomerular function with intact tubular function. Clinically, this dysfunction results in edema and, in severe cases, massive fluid retention with circulatory overload and congestive heart failure. Urinary sodium and calcium levels are reduced. The patient may exhibit a mild dilutional hyponatremia and hyperchloremia and acidosis with mild hyperkalemia. The blood urea nitrogen (BUN) value may be increased disproportionately to the serum creatinine level[1] (see Chapter 14).

The presence of hematuria is essential to the diagnosis of the nephritic syndrome. Hematuria may be associated with many other urinary tract abnormalities (Fig. 15–2),

but if red cell casts are found, the RBCs are known to have a renal origin (see Chapter 14 for discussion of cast formation). An inflammatory glomerulonephritic urine that contains RBCs, especially with RBC casts, is said to have an "active" sediment, because these findings suggest an active inflammatory process in the kidney. The combination of RBCs, RBC casts, and proteinuria is also commonly called a *nephritic sediment.*

It should be noted that for best identification of RBC casts on urine microscopic examination, a large aliquot of fresh, acidic urine should be spun lightly and the sediment gently resuspended. Scanning along the edge of the coverslip also facilitates the important finding of RBC casts.

Several authorities have noted that the RBCs in acute glomerulonephritis are dysmorphic (fragmented, distorted, and poorly hemoglobinized)[20–23] because of the shearing stresses on their surfaces when they are forced through the gaps in the glomerular basement membrane of the immunologically damaged glomerulus. This finding can be important, especially in primary or recurrent hematuria, because it helps to establish that the RBCs are of glomerular origin rather than from the lower urinary tract.

Most patients with glomerulonephritis present with proteinuria due to increased permeability of the glomerulus. For selective proteinuria with mostly albumin in the urine, the cause is probably the loss of glomerular fixed charge. In unselective proteinuria, both the albumin and the high-molecular weight proteins are in the urine because of the loss of the glomerular fixed charge as well as the large pores in the damaged glomerular membrane. Either moderate amounts of protein loss (<3.0 g/day) or heavy proteinuria (>3.5 g/day) may be seen in the nephrotic syndrome[1] (Fig. 15–3).

The patient with acute glomerulonephritis usually has a slight normocytic, normochromic anemia and hypoalbuminemia, probably as a result of the retention of fluid and circulatory congestion. About 20% of patients hospitalized with acute PSGN have a frank nephrotic syndrome.[1] They may also exhibit hyperlipemia, which occurs in nephrotic syndrome for a short time.

In RPGN, the urinalysis reveals a nephritic (active) sediment with hematuria, dysmorphic red blood cells, and RBC casts. Proteinuria, which is nonselective, is a consistent finding but usually is not in the nephrotic range. Azotemia develops early in the course of the disease and increases at a rapid rate. Goodpasture's syndrome engenders similar laboratory findings. The laboratory findings related to the renal involvement in Henoch-Schönlein syndrome are hematuria and proteinuria.[18]

Early in the course of chronic glomerulonephritis, when there are no clinical symptoms, routine laboratory test abnormalities (urinalysis and chemistry profile) are the only detectable manifestations of the disease. Any combination of abnormal urine sediment with RBCs and RBC casts, proteinuria, or mildly reduced renal function with elevated creatinine or BUN values may be present. The final stage of this syndrome is total renal failure with uremia.

Laboratory findings in IgA nephropathy (Berger's disease) reveal recurrent macroscopic hematuria, usually with persistent microscopic hematuria. Dysmorphic erythrocytes may be seen in the urine. Proteinuria is absent or mild, with excretion of less than 1 gram per day in 60% of cases.

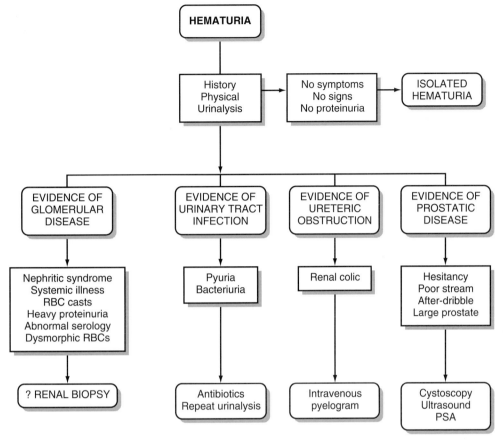

Figure 15–2. Clinical approach to a patient with symptomatic hematuria. Abbreviations: PSA, prostate-specific antigen. (Redrawn with permission from Jacobson HR, Striker GE, Klahr S (eds): Principles and Practice of Nephrology, ed 2. St Louis, Mosby–Year Book, 1995.)

The GFR is usually normal on presentation but, in the majority of cases, shows a slowly progressive decline over many years.[24, 25]

Microbiologic and Serologic Evaluations

In PSGN, throat cultures for group A streptococci are positive commonly, but not always in patients appearing with nephritis. Many (90%) have antistreptolysin O (ASO) titers above 200 Todd units.[1, 26] Patients with streptococcal skin infections may have elevations of ASO titers as well as of titers of other streptococcal antibodies, such as antistreptokinase, antihyaluronidase, and antiDNase B and antiNADase.[27] The Streptozyme test (Wampole Laboratories) may also be used. It detects five antibodies to extracellular breakdown products of the organism. Although less specific, this test is more sensitive to streptococcal infection than any of the tests used to detect the streptococcal antibodies listed here when it is used alone.

Serologic tests aid in the differential diagnosis and management of glomerular disorders.[28] This is especially true in the glomerular diseases with a presumed immunologically mediated cause. The most common clinically relevant complement studies are C3 and C4 assays and the total hemolytic assay CH_{50}. C3 is the most plentiful complement component and its assay is most widely available. Hypocomplementemia occurs when consumption of complement

exceeds its production.[29] Low serum complement levels are seen in acute glomerulonephritis associated with membranoproliferative disease and acute poststreptococcal infections as well as in systemic diseases such as systemic lupus erythematosus, subacute bacterial endocarditis, "shunt" nephritis, and cryoglobulinemia.

In PSGN, serum C3 levels are very depressed; however, Clq, C4, and C2 levels are only slightly decreased or normal. Properdin levels are decreased in about 60% of cases. This pattern suggests complement activation by the alternative pathway.[29] The serum C3 levels are depressed for 2 to 12 weeks, and then usually return to normal.[30] Failure of C3 levels to return to normal suggests a poor prognosis or possibly a different glomerular disease, such as mesangiocapillary glomerulonephritis (MCGN), also known as membranoproliferative glomerulonephritis (MPGN). The extent of depression of C3 level is not related to disease severity or prognosis. Elevations of cryoglobulins and immune complexes are commonly detectable.[31]

Normocomplementemia indicates that complement production is keeping pace with consumption but does not exclude a role for complement in the pathogenesis of the underlying renal disease. Normal serum complement levels are seen in glomerulonephritis caused by IgA nephropathy and RPGN and in the systemic disorders—polyarteritis nodosa group, hypersensitivity vasculitis, Wegener's granulomatosis, Henoch-Schönlein purpura, Goodpasture's syn-

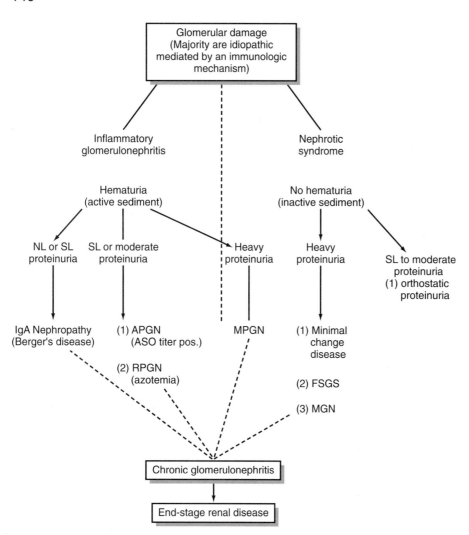

Figure 15–3. Glomerular disorder. Abbreviations: NL, normal; SL, slight; IgA, immunoglobulin A; APGN, acute poststreptococcal glomerulonephritis; ASO, antistreptolysin O; MPGN, mesangioproliferative glomerulonephritis; RPGN, rapidly progressive glomerulonephritis; FSGS, focal segmental glomerulosclerosis; MGN, membranous glomerulonephritis, *broken line,* leading to chronic glomerulonephritis.

drome and visceral abscesses. Serial complement levels are useful in assessing disease activity and response to therapy for some entities.

C3 nephritic factor (C3NeF) is an IgG autoantibody to a neoantigen of the C3 convertase C3bBb of the alternative pathway of complement activation.[32] Its presence is associated with stabilization of C3bBb and leads to continuous C3 breakdown and a decrease in serum C3 but no decrease in other complement components. Pronounced or persistently elevated levels of C3NeF indicate MCGN. C3NeF is occasionally found in low amounts in patients with PSGN. C4 nephritic factor, an autoantibody that stabilizes the C4b2a convertase of the classical pathway, has been reported in SLE, chronic glomerulonephritis, MCGN, and PSGN.[32]

Antineutrophil cytoplasmic antibodies (ANCAs) are serum specific for constituents of neutrophil primary granules and monocyte lysosomes. The detection and characterization of these antibodies over the last few years constitutes an advance in the diagnosis and management of systemic and renal vasculitis.[32] Two definite staining patterns are observable with indirect immunofluorescence microscopy when ANCAs are incubated with ethanol-fixed human neutrophils. One is a diffuse cytoplasmic staining pattern (c-ANCA) and the other is a perinuclear staining pattern

(p-ANCA). The cytoplasmic staining pattern is strongly associated with Wegener's granulomatosis and microscopic polyarteritis. Both c-ANCA and p-ANCA have been associated with RPGN, in approximate proportions of 60% and 40%, respectively.[33]

Anti-GMB antibody can be detected by radioimmunoassay (RIA), enzyme-linked immunosorbent assay (ELISA), and immunoblotting. Testing for anti-GBM should be performed to aid in diagnosing RPGN, Goodpasture's syndrome, and unexplained hemoptysis.[34]

Other serologic testing, including antinuclear antibodies (ANAs), is important in autoimmune diseases, such as lupus, that have renal manifestations. Cryoglobulins can be found in the serum of patients with diverse disorders, including primary glomerulopathies.[32] These are immunoglobulins with abnormal solubility that form a precipitate in the cold (4 °C) and redissolve on warming to 37 °C.

Results of serologic studies in IgA nephropathy (cryoglobulins, rheumatoid factor, and antinuclear factors) are usually normal. In 50% of patients, there is an increased IgA concentration in the serum.[35] Complement component levels are usually either normal or elevated, but C3 fragments may be increased in 50% to 75% of patients. This finding suggests C3 activation in vivo, perhaps by the alternative pathway.[36] Skin biopsy usually reveals dermal capillary deposits of IgA, C3, properdin, and fibrin, similar to the pattern seen in the renal biopsy.[37]

Laboratory Monitoring and Follow-Up

The laboratory plays a key role in both diagnosis of glomerulonephritis and follow-up of glomerular disease syndromes. Laboratory studies are needed to monitor the severity of renal impairment and to manage fluid and electrolyte disorders. To help in identifying the clinical syndromes, the laboratory database should consist of a complete urinalysis, complete blood count, and the following analyses of blood or serum: urea nitrogen, creatinine, sodium, potassium, chloride, CO_2, phosphorus, calcium, and uric acid.[38] Supplemental data are 24-hour protein excretion measurement, urine protein electrophoresis, urine cultures, and serial measurements of serum creatinine or GFR and a 24-hour urine volume determination.[38] The serial estimation of complement components along with other appropriate serologic testing as discussed previously is a very important laboratory parameter utilized in the investigation of patients with glomerulonephritis.

Diagnosis of glomerular disease is made from the history and physical findings along with the data provided by the laboratory. Selected laboratory tests, including urea nitrogen, creatinine, and electrolyte analyses, are used to follow the progress of the disease and to determine and evaluate whether supportive therapy, such as hemodialysis, is needed.

SECONDARY GLOMERULAR DISEASES THAT MANIFEST AS A NEPHRITIC PICTURE

Many diseases have a renal component with manifestations of glomerular disease, but the renal involvement is only one part of the total clinical picture. Sometimes the renal involvement may be subtle or may be responsible for the presenting symptoms. Thus, it is very important to consider the possibility of these disorders when a patient presents with renal abnormalities, and appropriate laboratory tests such as ANA measurement for systemic lupus erythematosus, blood cultures for bacterial endocarditis, ANCA determination for necrotizing vasculitis, and cryoglobulin measurements should be performed to facilitate the differential diagnosis.

Systemic Lupus Erythematosus (SLE)

Renal involvement in SLE can manifest in several different clinicopathologic ways. The disease is clearly immunologically predicated, with the antibodies to nuclear antigens, particularly DNA. Antinuclear antibody detected by fluorescence (FANA) is found in most patients with active disease. One mechanism of renal damage involves immune complexes composed of DNA and antibodies to DNA. These are localized in glomerular capillaries, where they bind and activate complement, initially via the classic pathway. When glomerular injury is intense, a typical "nephritic urine sediment" of RBC and RBC casts is found,

commonly accompanied by proteinuria, hypertension, and varying degrees of renal failure.[39]

Several histologic types of lesions are seen on renal biopsy and have been classified into six categories by the World Health Organization (WHO). Type I involves normal glomeruli, and type II involves pure mesangial alterations. Type III, focal segmental glomerulonephritis, is characterized by areas of focal and segmental cellular proliferation, with or without polymorphonuclear leukocyte infiltration. Type IV, diffuse proliferative glomerulonephritis, is a much more serious disorder, with a high mortality rate unless reversed either spontaneously or by intervention with immunosuppressive agents. Type V, the membranous form of SLE glomerulonephritis, is discussed in Chapter 16. Type VI is an extremely advanced sclerosing phase of glomerulonephritis with widespread glomerular scarring. Immunofluorescence demonstrates variable results, usually with any combination of the immunoglobulins being present. Electron microscopy may show large, dense deposits that are usually subendothelial in location[26] (see Fig. 15–1).

Renal failure is the leading cause of death from lupus nephritis, even though the course is highly variable and is sometimes punctuated by spontaneous remissions and exacerbations. Many cases respond dramatically to the use of high doses of corticosteroids.

Necrotizing Vasculitis

Vasculitic disorders occur in several distinct clinical forms, including polyarteritis nodosa, microscopic polyarteritis (hypersensitivity angiitis), Wegener's granulomatosis, and mixed cryoglobulins.[40] Patients with Wegener's granulomatosis have necrotizing granulomatous arteritis of the upper and lower respiratory tracts, which often is associated with evidence of glomerular injury. All of these vasculitic disorders may have an associated glomerulonephritis, with the typical clinical findings of a nephritic urine sediment and elevations in BUN and creatinine. The histologic appearance is often characterized by the presence of numerous crescents, and the patient's condition often progresses rapidly to uremia. About 50% of cases demonstrate immune deposits on immunofluorescence.[18]

Tests for ANCAs and cryoglobulins are important diagnostic parameters. The majority of patients with a c-ANCA pattern have Wegener's granulomatosis, and the majority of patients with a p-ANCA pattern have non-Wegener's vasculitis. Titers of c-ANCA can be helpful in guiding long-term management of patients with Wegener's granulomatosis.

Aggressive treatment with corticosteroids and cyclophosphamide may produce dramatic improvement, especially in small-vessel diseases.[18]

Bacterial Endocarditis

Bacterial endocarditis produces several types of vessel injury, ranging from gross infarctions secondary to emboli, to renal abscesses, focal and segmental glomerular injury, and diffuse proliferative glomerulonephritis.[41] The last two forms of glomerulonephritis result from immune complex injury and are associated with reduced levels of serum complement. Each of the forms of glomerulonephritis is accompanied by variable degrees of renal impairment, which is usually less severe in the focal segmental form. All of these types of bacterial endocarditis respond to eradication of the bacterial antigen by appropriate antibiotic therapy.

TREATMENT

The therapy for most of the glomerulonephritis syndromes is predominantly supportive and directed toward prevention and management of the potentially lethal complications—uremia, hyperkalemia, hypertensive encephalopathy, and pulmonary edema. The laboratory provides the data (serum potassium and urea nitrogen levels) to monitor the first two complications.

The treatment for PSGN and other infective types of glomerulonephritis is primarily symptomatic and supportive. Appropriate antibiotic therapy is given if infection persists. Sodium restriction is critical in managing hypertension, congestive heart failure, and edema. Temporary dialysis may be required if the renal failure is severe enough. The prognosis, especially in children, is quite favorable, with 95% of patients recovering normal renal function within 2 months. Some, however, may exhibit minimal hematuria and proteinuria for more than 2 years, and rarely, a patient develops end-stage renal failure. The more severe cases usually occur in older patients. The vast majority of patients experience a spontaneous diuresis accompanied by resolution of circulatory congestion, edema, and hypertension within a week of onset. Prolonged oliguria (exceeding 1 week in duration) is observed in only 5% to 10% of patients.[33] No therapeutic maneuver influences the severity of renal dysfunction or promotes histologic healing.[42]

The prognosis in rapidly progressive glomerulonephritis is poor, and 50% to 70% of patients require maintenance hemodialysis within 6 months of the onset of symptoms. Various treatments, including intermittent "pulse" high-dose steroids, plasma exchange, cytotoxic agents, and anticoagulant therapy, have been tried, with varying success.[42] Current evidence seems to indicate a favorable role for the use of plasmapheresis and immunosuppression in the RPGN of Goodpasture's syndrome.[34]

No specific therapy is indicated for patients who have recurrent hematuria or IgA nephropathy, because most patients do not have the progressive form of the disease. Treatment for this syndrome is supportive only.

Case Study

A 54-year-old man was admitted to the hospital with marked cellulitis of the left knee. Five to 6 weeks prior to admission, he had injured ("scraped") that knee. The injury was followed by minimal erythema and tenderness, progressing to a more widespread area over the next 4 weeks. One week prior to admission, the patient developed fever, chills, and progressive edema. He was found to be oliguric and in acute renal failure. His blood pressure was 70/50 mm Hg.

The patient was started on acute dialysis. His urine volume increased on day 26 of treatment, and hemodial-

ysis was stopped. He was discharged 32 days after admission, when the acute renal failure had resolved. Pertinent laboratory data areas follow:

Parameter	Reference Range	Day 1	Day 2	Day 19	Day 26	Day 32
BUN (mg/dL)	10–20	135	153	88	72	41
Creatinine (mg/dL)	0.7–1.5	8.6	9.0	9.2	7.4	3.0
Sodium (mEq/L)	135–145	131	133	131	135	141
Potassium (mEq/L)	3.5–5.0	4.9	5.0	5.1	4.0	3.6
Chloride (mEq/L)	95–105	86	91	99	66	112
Culture of fluid from wound:	—	Negative —		—	—	—
WBC (× 10⁹/L)	5–10.0	37.3	51.5	13.6	10.5	8.6
Urine blood	Negative	Large	Large	Moderate	Small	Negative
Urine RBC (/hpf)	2–3	40–50	100–150	15–20	2–4	Negative
RBC casts (/1pf)	0	1–2	2–4	0	0	0
Urine albumin	Negative	4+	4+	2+	1+	Negative
ASO (Todd units)	0–166	333	—	—	—	—
Streptozyme (STZ units)	0–100	300	—	—	—	—
Complement C3 (mg/dL)	83–177	87.2	—	99.0	—	—

Questions

1. What is the most probable cause of acute renal failure?

2. Are the negative results of culture on the fluid from the wound unexpected?

3. Is the patient's presenting blood pressure unexpectedly low?

4. What is the patient's prognosis?

5. Is it likely that the patient will experience acute renal failure from this cause again?

Discussion

1. The most probable cause of acute renal failure is acute poststreptococcal glomerulonephritis.

2. The negative wound culture results are not unexpected. In group A β-hemolytic streptococcal skin infections, the latent period is usually 3 weeks. The positive Streptozyme and ASO titer results give evidence of a streptococcal infection.

3. Hypertension is usually present; however, when this patient first was admitted to the hospital, he was very ill and in acute distress. His blood pressure was somewhat elevated at a later time.

4. The patient's prognosis is favorable. Because he is older, however, and because his renal function did not improve until 4 weeks after admission, his renal

function status should be followed with periodic urine protein measurements and microscopic examinations of the urine sediment.

5. Patients do not usually experience poststreptococcal glomerulonephritis a second time; however, the first episode may damage the kidney and possibly begin a chronic process in a small percentage of patients.

References

1. Glassock RJ, Cohen AH, Adler SG: Primary glomerular diseases. *In* Brenner BM (ed): The Kidney, ed 5. Philadelphia, WB Saunders, 1996.
2. Dixon FJ, Wilson CB: The development immunopathologic investigation of kidney disease. Am J Kidney Dis 16:574–578, 1990.
3. Wilson CB: Immunologic aspects of renal diseases. JAMA 268:2904–2909, 1992.
4. Couser WG: New insights into mechanisms of immune glomerular injury. West J Med 160:440–446, 1994.
5. Myers B, Okarma T, Friedman S, et al: Mechanisms of proteinuria in human glomerulonephritis. J Clin Invest 70:732, 1982.
6. Lin JT, Wada H, Maed H, et al: Mechanisms of hematuria in glomerular disease: An electron microscopic study in the case of diffuse membranous glomerulonephritis, Nephron 35:68, 1983.
7. Tejani A, Inguilli A: Post streptococcal glomerulonephritis: Current clinical and pathologic concepts. Nephron 55:1–5, 1990.
8. Madaio MP: Postinfectious glomerulonephritis. *In* Jacobson HR, Striker GE, Klahr S (eds): The Principles and Practice of Nephrology. St Louis, CV Mosby, 1995.
9. Sagel I, Treser G, Ty A, et al: Occurrences and nature of glomerular lesions after group A streptococcal infections in children. Ann Intern Med 70:492, 1973.
10. Andrassy K, Kuster S, Waldherr R, Ritz E: Rapidly progressive glomerulonephritis: Analysis of prevalence and clinical course. Nephron 59:206–212, 1991.
11. Biggs WA, Johnson JO, Tiechman S, et al: Antiglomerular basement membrane antibody in the pathogenesis of human glomerulonephritis and Goodpastures's syndrome. Medicine 58:348, 1979.
12. Couser WG: Rapidly progressive glomerulonephritis: Classification, pathogenetic mechanisms and therapy. Am J Kidney Dis 11:449, 1988.
13. Glassock R: A clinical and immunopathologic dissection of rapidly progressive glomerulonephritis. Nephron 22:253, 1978.
14. Brenner BM: Hemodynamically-mediated glomerular injury and the progressive nature of kidney disease. Kidney Int 23:647, 1983.
15. Glassock RJ: Hematuria and pigmenturia. *In* Massry S, Glassock R (eds): Textbook of Nephrology, ed 3. Baltimore, Williams & Wilkins, 1995.
16. Hendler E, Kashgarian M, Haslett J: Clinicopathological correlation of primary hematuria. Lancet 1:458, 1972.
17. Berger J: IgA glomerular deposits in renal disease. Transplant Proc 1:939, 1969.
18. Adler, SG, Arthur HC, Glassock RJ: Secondary glomerular diseases. *In* Brenner BM (ed): The Kidney, ed 5. Philadelphia, WB Saunders, 1996.
19. Clarkson AR, Woodroffe AJ, Bannister KM, et al: The syndrome of IgA nephropathy. Clin Nephrol 21:7, 1984.
20. Fairley KF, Birch DF: Microscopic urinalysis in glomerulonephritis. Kidney Int 44(suppl):S9–S12, 1993.
21. Tomita M, Kitamoto Y, Nakayama M, Sato T: A new morphological classification of urinary erythrocytes for differential diagnosis of glomerular hematuria. Clin Nephrol 37:84–89, 1992.
22. Kohler H, Wandel E, Brunck B: Acanthocyturia: A characteristic marker for glomerular bleeding. Kidney Int 40:115–120, 1991.
23. Kohler H, Wandel E: Acanthocyturia detects glomerular bleeding. Nephrol Dial Transplant 8:879, 1993.
24. Glassock RJ: IgA nephropathy: 25 years of progress. Contrib Nephrol 104:212–219, 1993.
25. Glassock RJ: Highlights and trends: IgA symposium. Contrib Nephrol 111:201–208, 1995.
26. Rodriguez-Iturbe B: Epidemic post-streptococcal glomerulonephritis. Kidney Int 25:129, 1984.
27. Dillion HC: Pyoderma and nephritis. Ann Rev Med 18:207, 1967.
28. Madaio MP, Harrington JT: The diagnosis of acute glomerulonephritis. N Engl J Med 309:1200, 1983.
29. Hebert LA, Cosio FG, Neff JC: Diagnostic significance of hypocomplementemia. Kidney Int 39:811–821, 1991.
30. Sjoholm AG: Complement components and complement activation in acute poststreptococcal glomerulonephritis. Am J Nephrol 3:23, 1983.
31. Yoshizawa N, Treser G, McClung JA, et al: Circulating immune complexes in patients with uncomplicated Group A streptococci pharyngitis and patients with acute poststreptococcal glomerulonephritis. Am J Nephrol 3:23, 1983.
32. Foster MH: Serologic evaluation of the renal patient. *In* Jacobson HJ, Stricker GE, Saulo K (eds): The Principles and Practice of Nephrology, ed 2. St Louis, CV Mosby, 1995.
33. Folk RJ: ANCA-associated renal disease. Kidney Int 38:998–1010, 1990.
34. Turner N, Rees AJ: Antiglomerular basement membrane disease. *In* Cameron J, Davison A, Grunfeld JP, Rits E (eds): Oxford Textbook of Clinical Nephrology. London, Oxford Medical Publishers, 1992.
35. Jones CL, Powell HR, Kincaid-Smith P, Roberton DM: Polymeric IgA and immune complex concentrations in IgA-related renal disease. Kidney Int 38:323–331, 1990.
36. Hasbargen J, Copley J: Utility of skin biopsy in the diagnosis of IgA nephropathy. Am J Kidney Dis 6:100, 1985.
37. Whelton A, Watson AJ, Rock RC: Nitrogen metabolites and renal function. *In* Burtis CA, Ashwood ER (eds): Tietz Fundamentals of Clinical Chemistry, ed 4. Philadelphia, WB Saunders, 1996.
38. Appel GB, D'Agati V: Lupus nephritis. *In* Jacobson, HJ, Stricker GE, Saulo K (eds): The Principles and Practice of Nephrology, ed 2. St Louis, CV Mosby, 1995.
39. Furlong TJ, Ibels LS, Eckstein RP: The clinical spectrum of necrotizing glomerulonephritis. Medicine 66:192, 1987.
40. Neugarten J, Baldwin DS: Glomerulonephritis in bacterial endocarditis. Am J Med 77:297, 1984.
41. Vogl W, Renke M, Mayer-Eichberger D, et al: Long-term prognosis in endocapillary glomerulonephritis of poststreptococcal type in children and adults. Nephron 74:58, 1986.
42. O'Meara Y, Salant D: Management of glomerular disease of primary and secondary origin. Curr Opin Nephrol Hypertens 1:124–132, 1992.

Chapter 16

Nephrotic Syndrome

Martha Savage Payne

ETIOLOGY AND PATHOPHYSIOLOGY

Nephrotic syndrome, one of the major clinical syndromes of glomerular disease, can be associated with many different pathogenic mechanisms of both primary renal disorders and of systemic disease (Box 16–1).

Nephrotic syndrome is primarily a defect of glomerular permeability that causes abnormal leaking of massive amounts of protein, lipids, and other macromolecules. There is a variable tendency toward edema, hypoalbuminemia, hyperlipidemia, and hypercoagulability.[1] The daily urinary protein excretion is greater than 3.5 g per 1.73 m^2 of body surface area in the absence of a depressed glomerular filtration rate (GFR).[2]

The proteinuria of nephrotic syndrome can result from abnormalities in the charge-selective or size-selective barrier (see Chapter 15). Charge-selective barrier abnormalities are often unrecognizable with light microscopy of a kidney biopsy specimen; however, special staining techniques may show slight abnormalities. The nephrotic syndrome of minimal change disease results from charge-selective barrier abnormalities. However, size-selective barrier abnormalities are usually associated with abnormalities of the glomerular structure, easily seen by a light microscope, which include deposition of proteins, alterations in the basement membrane structure, and mesangial abnormalities. The major component of the urine protein is albumin (60% to 90%). Larger-weight molecules are excreted to a variable degree.

Hypoalbuminemia is almost always present at some phase during the course of nephrotic syndrome.[3] This is caused by the increased excretion of albumin. Although normal or increased hepatic synthesis occurs, it cannot replace the volume of albumin excreted. An increased rate of renal albumin catabolism is also present. Hypoalbuminemia can put the patient with nephrotic syndrome at risk for drug overdose problems after usual therapeutic doses, because with lower plasma albumin levels, less drug is bound, leaving a greater amount of active free drug in the plasma.[4] In addition, low albumin levels put the patient at risk of prerenal azotemia and acute renal failure caused by renal hypoperfusion or drug toxicity. Increased platelet aggregability, causing a hypercoagulable state, hyperlipoproteinemia, and edema, also results from hypoalbuminemia.[1, 2, 5] The edema is caused by reduced plasma oncotic pressure due to the loss of serum albumin to the urine.[6] A translocation of fluid to the interstitium of body tissue occurs, probably as a result of sodium retention by the kidney. The exact mechanism has not been identified. The hyperlipidemia in nephrotic syndrome is inversely proportional to the serum albumin concentration. Nearly all blood lipid and lipoprotein fractions are elevated in nephrotic syndrome, including serum total cholesterol, phospholipid, very-low-density lipoprotein (VLDL), intermediate-density lipoprotein (IDL), and low-density lipoprotein (LDL).[7] The main mechanism of hyperlipoproteinemia is enhanced hepatic synthesis of the lipid and protein moieties of the lipoprotein molecule, stimulated by the hypoalbuminemia.

Immune responses are deficient in nephrotic syndrome. Reduced levels of immunoglobulin G (IgG) and various components of complement are seen along with defective cell-mediated immunity.[1, 2] The decreased immunoglobulins are partially due to loss of protein in the urine. The cause of the cell-mediated immunity problem is unknown but is probably a result of trace metal deficiencies in the urine. Infections are an important cause of morbidity and mortality in nephrotic syndrome.

A tendency for spontaneous thrombosis is present in nephrotic syndrome because of changes in the coagulation system proteins in combination with increased aggregabil-

<hr>

Box 16–1. **Classification of the Disease States Most Commonly Associated With Nephrotic Syndrome**

Primary Glomerular Diseases

Membranous
Proliferative and focal
    Acute (poststreptococcal) glomerulonephritis (rare)
    Rapidly progressive glomerulonephritis
    FSG
Membranoproliferative
Minimal lesion

Other Disorders

Medications and drugs
    Mercury
    Gold
    Penicillamine
    "Street" heroin
    Probenicid
    Trimethadione
    Anticonvulsant agents
    Nonsteroidal antiinflammatory drugs (rare)
Allergens
    Bee sting
    Pollens
Infections
    Bacterial endocarditis and shunt infections
    Malaria
    Syphilis
    Hepatitis B and C
    Schistosomiasis
    HIV
Neoplasms
    Solid tumors
        Lung, colon, stomach, breast, esophagus, melanoma, renal cell, neuroblastoma
    Leukemia and lymphoma
    Non-Hodgkin's
    Hodgkin's
    Chronic lymphocytic leukemia
Multisystem disease
    Diabetes mellitus
    Systemic lupus erythematosus
    Amyloidosis
    Polyarteritis
    Henoch-Shönlein purpura
    Cryoglobulinemia
    Sickle cell anemia
    Sarcoidosis
Pregnancy-associated
Chronic renal allograft rejection

<hr>

ity of the platelets and hyperlipidemia.[8] Fibrinogen levels along with factors V, VII, VIII–von Willebrand's, and X may be increased.[9] Antithrombin III levels may greatly decrease, and protein C and S levels are usually normal, but the functional activity of these proteins may be reduced.

Factors XI and XII, prekallikrein, and kallikrein levels may be depressed. Antiplasmin, α_1-antitrypsin, plasminogen activator, and endothelial prostacyclin-stimulating factor levels may be decreased. Overall, proaggregatory and procoagulant factors are enhanced, and antiaggregatory, anticoagulant, and fibrinolytic mechanisms are impaired.[10]

Urinary loss of proteins having important metal-binding or hormone-binding function may cause various clinical manifestations.[1] Loss of erythropoietin may contribute to anemia and the extreme depression of serum transferrin concentration, leading to a microcytic, hypochromic anemia resistant to iron therapy. Loss of cholecalciferol-binding globulin may result in an acquired vitamin D deficiency. Urinary losses of lecithin–cholesterol acyltransferase may contribute to the disordered lipoprotein metabolism in nephrotic syndrome. Thyroxine-binding globulin deficiency may affect thyroid function tests (Fig. 16-1).

Minimal Change Disease

The patient presenting with nephrotic syndrome due to *minimal change disease,* also called *minimal lesion nephrotic syndrome* or *minimal change nephropathy,* will show swelling of the epithelial cell foot processes on renal biopsy.[1, 11] Under light microscopy, little alteration of the glomerular basement membrane or the glomerulus itself is present. The proximal tubules may contain fine lipid droplets that are doubly refractile and similar to the oval fat bodies found in urine. With electron microscopy, the characteristic glomerular lesion is identified and is shown to consist of swollen foot processes of the glomerular epithelial cells (podocytes), with fusion over the surface of the basement membrane. There is juxtaposition of the club-shaped foot processes and obliteration of the slit-pore membrane complex. Immunofluorescent microscopy findings are noteworthy for showing the absence of IgG and complement deposition in the glomeruli.[11] The cause of minimal change lesion is entirely unknown. The basic abnormality may reside in the glomerular basement membrane or the epithelial cell. A charge-selection barrier defect has been suggested, but the reason for this is unknown.[12] Because patients with Hodgkin's disease, in whom nephrotic syndrome is present, have an identical lesion, a role of lymphocytes, especially a T cell dysfunction, has been suggested in its pathogenesis.[13, 14]

Mesangioproliferative Glomerulonephritis

Mesangioproliferative glomerulonephritis (MPGN) is a rather rare glomerular lesion that is associated with nephrotic syndrome. Light microscopy shows glomeruli characterized by variable degrees of increased cellularity of the mesangium.[15] This cellularity separates the diagnosis of MPGN from that of minimal change disease, even though an overlap in the diagnosis may have been obtained from biopsy results alone.[1] Electron microscopy shows epithelial foot processes diffusely swollen and effaced. Finely granular or homogenous electron-dense deposits are identified in the mesangium in up to 50% of patients. Immunofluorescence frequently shows immunoglobulin M (IgM) deposits, primarily in the mesangium.[15] This type of lesion with

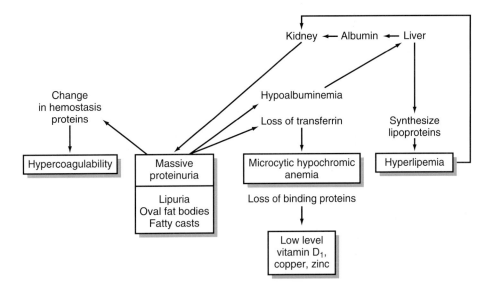

Figure 16–1. Pathophysiologic changes in nephrotic syndrome.

immunoglobulin A (IgA) deposits is classified as IgA nephropathy or Berger's disease (see Chapter 15).

Focal and Segmental Glomerulosclerosis

Focal and segmental glomerulosclerosis (FSG) is characterized by a lesion seen on renal biopsy that consists of sclerosis and hyalinization of some, but not all, glomeruli (focal) and not involving the whole glomerulus (segmental).[16] Patients may initially present with minimal lesion nephrotic syndrome but later develop hypertension and increasing impairment of renal functions. In many patients, characteristic lesions first develop in the deep juxtamedullary cortex region and progressively involve glomeruli farther outward in the cortex. The remaining glomeruli may appear normal, as in minimal change disease, or may reveal diffuse mesangioproliferation. By electron microscopy, most of the glomeruli show diffuse or segmental foot process alterations. IgM, C1q, and C3 deposits may be seen by immunofluorescence but only in association with focal sclerotic lesions. The cause of this disorder is unknown, but the mesangial deposits of immunoglobulin suggest an immune complex disease. A high incidence of similar lesions occurs in the allograph following transplantation.[1]

Membranous Glomerulonephritis

The most common cause of idiopathic nephrotic syndrome in adults, *membranous glomerulonephritis* (MGN) accounts for 25% to 30% of all cases. It occurs less frequently in childhood but has a high association with hepatitis B infection when it does occur in older children.[2] The term *membranous* refers to the characteristic pathologic lesion of diffuse thickening of the glomerular basement membrane. MGN may be primary glomerulonephritis (idiopathic), or it may be secondary to various underlying diseases. A very strong association exists with solid tumors (6% to 11% of patients with MGN).[1, 2] The malignancy may be overt at presentation of MGN or occult, which occurs in many cases, at the time of nephrotic syndrome

discovery. Thus a differential diagnosis must be made between idiopathic and secondary MGN. MGN may also be the initial manifestation of an infection, such as chronic, hepatitis B or a multisystem disease such as systemic lupus erythematosus (SLE).

The characteristic light microscopic finding in MGN is diffuse and uniform thickening of the basement membrane (capillary wall), usually without significant proliferation of endothelial, mesangial, or epithelial cells. Although this finding may be absent early in the course of the disease, it enables easy diagnosis of advanced MGN.[17] On silver stain examination, basement membrane spikes may be seen projecting toward the urinary space. Electron microscopic findings are consistent with light microscopic findings. Early in the disease the glomerular basement membrane may be normal in thickness, but small, dense, and discrete subepithelial deposits appear at the level of the slit-pore membrane. In more advanced cases the membrane thickens, the deposits increase in number, and projections of basement membrane extend between deposits, corresponding to the silver-positive spikes seen with light microscopy. Immunofluorescence findings are typical of MGN, with IgG nearly always present in a uniform granular distribution outlining all of the capillary loops. C3 is usually present in a pattern and an intensity that are similar to IgG.[1, 17]

The cause of MGN is unknown, but human leukocyte antigen (HLA) studies suggest that a genetic basis of susceptibility exists.[17] It has been suggested that (1) immune deposits on the capillary wall form from a reaction of circulating antibodies with either exogenous or endogenous antigens previously localized on the epithelial surface of the capillary, or (2) the lesions may arise consequent to a reaction of circulating antibody with intrinsic glomerular antigen. Some antigens have been identified in association with secondary MGN caused by hepatitis and tumors. The mechanism of proteinuria in MGN involves the appearance of large-radius pores leading to increased permeability of the capillary wall. Experimental evidence suggests that complement deposits may play a role in the increased glomerular permeability.

Mesangiocapillary Glomerulonephritis

Also known as membranoproliferative glomerulonephritis, mesangiocapillary glomerulonephritis (MCGN) is characterized by a lesion with a prominent increase in mesangial cellularity and a change in segmental capillary wall that lead to a thickened and reduplicated ("tram-track") capillary wall as seen by light microscopy. MCGN may be a primary renal disease or a manifestation of a multisystem disease such as SLE. The primary forms are heterogeneous and have been subgrouped on the basis of light microscopic, electron microscopic, and immunofluorescent appearance.[18] Type I MCGN is typified by abundant subendothelial electron-dense deposits that frequently contain C3 component of complement and immunoglobulin. Type II characteristically shows dense deposits within the glomerular basement membrane that contain C3 in a linear pattern in peripheral glomerular capillary walls. Other variants have been described, and some authors include a type III that has electron-dense subepithelial deposits and immunoglobulin granular deposits in the glomerular capillary walls and mesangium and has the features of membranous glomerulopathy.[19]

The pathologic hallmarks of this group of glomerular lesions are pronounced abnormalities of mesangial areas and the peripheral capillary walls. Diffuse glomerular cell proliferation is present, and the glomeruli frequently contain numerous polymorphonuclear leukocytes. Silver methenamine–stained sections demonstrate thickened capillary walls, resulting in a "double-contoured" or "tram-track" appearance caused by extension and interposition of the mesangial matrix. A few cases of MCGN are complicated by the formation of cellular crescents in Bowman's space. In electron microscopy, both types of MCGN show an extension of the mesangial cell cytoplasm and mesangial matrix between the basement membrane and the endothelial cell, which accounts for the splitting of the basement membrane seen on light microscopy. In type I MCGN, discrete subendothelial electron-dense deposits are seen along some of the capillary loops. Many cells, either mesangial or monocytic, infiltrate the space between the mesangial matrix and the basement membrane.[18] In type II MCGN, the basement membranes are widened by ribbon-like, continuous, dense intramembrane deposits, which is the reason this disease received its common name, "dense deposit disease." The immunofluorescent findings vary widely. C3 is usually present and may be accompanied by variable amounts of IgG or IgM in type I disease. In type II disease, C3 is nearly always heavily deposited in the glomeruli (basement membrane and mesangium).[18]

The pathogenesis of MCGN is unknown. The depression of serum complement and subendothelial deposits in type I suggest an immune complex disorder.[20] However, no direct link of hypocomplementemia to renal disease is shown, and part of this phenomenon may be related to decreased synthesis and increased activation. Type II disease appears to be a structural alteration of renal basement membranes that activates the alternative pathway of complement. A high incidence of recurrent disease occurs in kidney transplant patients with MCGN, which suggests a circulating factor as the genesis of the glomerular lesion.

CLINICAL MANIFESTATIONS

The patient with nephrotic syndrome usually presents with generalized edema. The edema is usually manifested by puffiness around the eyes in the mornings and ankle swelling when the patient is up and walking about. As the condition progresses, massive fluid retention, or anasarca, may result, and genital swelling, ascites, and pleural effusions may develop. Symptoms such as dyspnea and othopnea do not occur until anasarca is marked or pleural effusion is present. Venous pressure is usually normal. Common physical complaints are anorexia and fatigue.

Minimal change disease occurs predominantly in young children, with peak occurrences between ages 2 and 6 years. In fact, 80% of the nephrotic syndrome in children is of the minimal change variety. Conversely, in adults, only 15% to 20% of cases of nephrotic syndrome are a result of minimal change disease. Boys predominate by about 2:1 in cases of children, whereas in adults the male-to-female ratio is closer to 1:1.[11] The onset of symptoms sometimes immediately follows an upper respiratory tract viral infection. The illness often presents suddenly, and a full-blown nephrotic syndrome with heavy proteinuria, hypoalbuminuria, and hyperlipidemia is the rule. The edema is frequently massive and rarely may be accompanied by ascites and pleural effusion. Gross hematuria and hypertension are uncommon.[11]

MPGN can affect any age, but older children and young adults are most frequently represented. There is a slight male-to-female predominance. Hematuria is present in the majority of cases. Mild hypertension is present in 30% of cases. Clinically, this entity is very difficult to separate from minimal change disease.[21]

Patients with FSG are usually older than the typical patient with minimal change disease. Overall, FSG is found in 7% to 15% of children and 15% to 20% of adults with nephrotic syndrome. Hypertension and microscopic hematuria occur more frequently and severely. Fifty percent to 70% of these patients have a progressive course to renal failure without responding to steroid therapy.[1]

Idiopathic MGN presents as nephrotic syndrome in 80% of cases and as asymptomatic proteinuria in the remaining 20%. Occurrence of MGN is unusual in children, with about 80% to 90% of patients being older than 30 years at time of diagnosis. A male predominance is usually reported. Renal function is usually normal at presentation, with azotemia occurring late in the course of the disease. Overt diabetes mellitus appears to be more common than might be expected by chance alone, and some authors have suggested a common underlying phenotype related to susceptibility to both disorders.[1]

The course of idiopathic MGN is variable, but it is usually indolent and slowly progressive. Patients may have both clinical remissions and relapses of the nephrotic syndrome. The overall prognosis in children is good. In adults, 50% of patients have spontaneous complete or partial remissions, although the other half have chronic renal failure or end-stage renal disease.[1, 17] Hypertension is usually a late finding, and microscopic hematuria without red cell casts is common.

The majority of patients with MCGN have the onset of the disease after age 5 years and before age 30 years.[1] A slight predominance of females occurs in type I and nearly an equal sex ratio in type II. The initial clinical presentation is varied. Forty percent to 50% of patients present with well-developed nephrotic syndrome; 30% to 40% present with asymptomatic proteinuria or hematuria; and another 20% to 30% present with features of acute nephritic syndrome.[1] Acute nephritic syndrome is more common in type II disease. An upper respiratory illness precedes the onset of renal disease in approximately one-half of cases. Hypertension, usually mild, is present in about 30% of patients. Type I MCGN is a slowly progressive disease. Some patients remain stable for years with nephrotic range proteinuria. Type II MCGN is usually a more aggressive disease. The median time from diagnosis to renal failure ranges from 5 to 10 years.[19]

LABORATORY ANALYSES AND DIAGNOSIS

When a patient presents with massive proteinuria on the screening reagent strip, and medical history and physical examination by the physician indicate probable renal abnormalities, the following laboratory data should be obtained: 24-hour urine quantitative protein excretion, blood urea nitrogen (BUN), serum creatinine, glucose, electrolytes, creatinine clearance, protein electrophoresis, and complete blood cell count. In addition, the physician may perform a renal biopsy and order additional serologic tests such as Streptozyme, fluorescent antinuclear antibody (FANA), total complement, VDRL, hepatitis B surface antigen, and cryoglobulins, to facilitate the differential diagnosis of multiple causes of nephrotic syndrome (Table 16–1).

The most prominent laboratory changes in nephrotic syndrome are massive proteinuria, hypoalbuminemia, and hyperlipidemia. Protein excretion in the urine usually exceeds 3.5 g/day per 1.73 m^2 of body surface area in the absence of depressed GRF. It must be remembered that profound hypoalbuminemia often leads to a reduction in urine protein excretion, in which the urine protein level is not in the nephrotic range, even though no change in the fundamental glomerular defect occurs. Also, an infusion of albumin to raise the serum albumin level causes a dramatic rise in the albumin excreted. For these reasons it has been suggested that protein excretion rates should be expressed as clearance ratios for specific proteins, such as albumin or as clearance ratios, such as clearance of albumin/clearance of creatinine.[1, 21]

Other changes in protein levels in the serum include increased α_2- and β-globulins. IgG levels may be significantly decreased, although levels of other immunoglobulins are usually normal. Factor B of the alternative pathway of complement may be significantly decreased. These factors, especially in children, may lead to an increased susceptibil-

Table 16–1. Nephrotic Syndrome

	Age	Renal Function at Presentation	Serum C3	Serum C4	Prognosis	Other
Presenting findings						
Massive proteinuria						
Hypoalbuminemia						
Increased blood lipids						
Active sediment with RBC and/or RBC casts						
PRIMARY						
Mesangiocapillary glomerulonephritis	Young usually	N1 or ↓	Often ↓	Often ↓	Renal failure in 70%–90%	C3 nephritic factor in serum of some
MULTISYSTEM						
Systemic lupus erythematosus	Young adults, usually female	N1 usually	↓	↓	Often responds to therapy if early SLE remission	
Presenting findings						
Massive proteinuria (>3.5 g/day in adult)						
Hypoalbuminemia						
Increased blood lipids						
Minimal or no hematuria (inactive urine sediment)						
PRIMARY						
Minimal change disease	Children more common but any age	N1	N1	N1	Good	—
Focal sclerosing glomerulonephritis	Children more common but any age	Usually N1	N1	N1	Renal failure in 70%–80%	—
Membranous glomerulonephritis	Adults usually	Usually N1	N1	N1	20% remission, renal failure in 80%; slowly progressive	—
MULTISYSTEM						
Diabetic glomerulonephropathy	Adults	Decreased	N1	N1	Very poor	—
Amyloidosis	Adults usually	Decreased	N1	N1	Very poor	—

ity to infection with such organisms as *Streptococcus pneumoniae.* Other complement components are not significantly decreased. Hypercholesterolemia and elevated phospholipid and triglyceride levels are the usual laboratory abnormalities, in addition to increased levels of LDL and VLDL.

Serum levels of several binding proteins including transferrin, transcortin, and thyroxine-binding globulin are decreased.[1, 22] These serum abnormalities in turn affect other laboratory tests such as total iron-binding capacity, total serum iron, and total triiodothyronine (T_3) and thyroxine (T_4). A microcytic hypochromic anemia that is resistant to iron therapy may develop because of decreased levels of transferrin. In addition, nephrotic syndrome patients may have reduced concentrations of various vitamins and minerals, including vitamin D, copper, and zinc, due to loss of their respective binding proteins.[22]

The urine from a patient with nephrotic syndrome shows heavy proteinuria and abnormal urinary sediment. Lipuria occurs and manifests in the urine sediment as free fat, oval fat bodies (renal tubular epithelial cells containing cholesterol esters), and fatty casts. All of these exhibit a Maltese cross pattern under polarizing light. A positive stain with Sudan IV on the sediment will also occur with the fat. Lipuria parallels the level of urine protein excretion rather than levels of serum lipids.[1]

In children with minimal change disease, the usual findings are a highly selective type of heavy proteinuria containing mostly albumin, a normal or near normal GFR, a normal or increased serum C3 concentration, and an unremarkable urine sediment. Microscopic hematuria is seen in only 15% to 20% of cases.[1, 8] Serum albumin levels are low. Serum creatinine levels may be mildly increased in as many as one-third of the cases at the time of initial presentation. Serum sodium levels may be decreased.[1] Hematocrit and hemoglobin may be increased if plasma volume is greatly reduced. Platelet counts are modestly increased. The erythrocyte sedimentation rate is increased. Total cholesterol, triglycerides, VLDL, and LDL levels are increased. High-density lipoprotein (HDL) levels may be increased as well.[1, 8]

IgG levels may be profoundly depressed during relapse, and this may account for the susceptibility of such children to infection with pneumococci. The complement fractions C3 and C4 and properdin levels are usually within normal limits. IgM levels are modestly increased during both remission and relapse.[1]

Certain HLA types are associated with minimal change disease. HLA-B12 antigen is associated with patients with atopy and a frequently relapsing, steroid-dependent course. Increase in other HLA types, including HLA-DR7, have been associated with nephrotic syndrome due to the minimal change lesion.[1]

In MPGN, typical nephrotic syndrome features are present. Proteinuria is nonselective, and hematuria is frequently present. Renal function tests are decreased in about 25% of patients. IgG levels may be modestly reduced, and complement levels are most often normal. No association with HLA antigens is known.[1]

In FSG, heavy proteinuria that is nonselective is nearly always present, and hematuria is common.[1, 16] C3 levels are nearly always normal, whereas IgG levels may be significantly depressed. Tubular malfunctions are more common in this syndrome than in other causes of nephrotic syndrome, which may be evidenced by pyuria, glycosuria, aminoaciduria, and phosphaturia. Circulating immune complexes may be found in 10% to 30% of cases. A circulating vascular permeability factor may be present in some patients. Some of these patients have an increased frequency of HLA-DR4 and HLA-DR8 types.[1]

Proteinuria in MGN is usually, but not always, nonselective, and is in the nephrotic range of greater than 3.5 g/day in more than 80% of cases. Proteinuria of more than 20 g/day has been reported.[1, 17] Microscopic hematuria is common.[1] The C3 and other complement component levels are usually normal in idiopathic MGN.[17] The urinary sediment and GFR are usually normal in the early course of the disease. Certain HLA types, especially HLA-DR3 and HLA-B8, are increased in this disorder.[1]

Proteinuria and microscopic hematuria are almost universal features of MCGN. In about 50% of the cases, the proteinuria is in the nephrotic range.[1, 19] Urine protein selectivity is usually moderate or poor.[1] In about 90% of cases, an important diagnostic marker for MCGN is the depression of hemolytic complement activity of serum, accompanied by the lowering of the C3 component.[19] This is an important differential diagnostic feature, because both the serum hemolytic complement activity and the C3 component are lowered in acute postinfectious glomerulonephritis but characteristically return to normal within 3 to 8 weeks. The failure of complement levels to return to normal within 2 months of onset of acute nephritic syndrome is highly suggestive of underlying MCGN. In general, type I MCGN, is associated with a depressed serum C3 concentration, accompanied by low levels of C1q, C4, and C2, which are early complement components. This is suggestive of activation of the alternative complement pathway. In type II, an isolated C3 and factor B depression occurs in 80% of patients. Some type II patients have a heat-stable factor called C3 nephritic factor (C3NF) that is capable of cleaving C3 in fresh normal plasma.[1] C3NF is an IgG autoantibody to the C3 convertase of the alternate C pathway. It apparently stabilizes this converting enzyme, resulting in the continuous degradation of native C3.

The GFR in MCGN is frequently decreased but may be normal. Normocytic, normochromic anemia is found in more than 50% of cases and may be severe and out of proportion to the degree of azotemia.[1]

SECONDARY GLOMERULAR DISEASES THAT PRESENT WITH A "NEPHROTIC" PICTURE

Diabetic Nephropathy

Nephropathy is a major cause of illness and death in diabetes and is the single most common cause of end-stage renal disease (ESRD) in the United States.[23] As the disease progresses, a nephrotic syndrome develops. Since 1988, a predictor of nephropathy in diabetic patients has been established. *Microalbuminemia,* or urinary albumin excretion greater than 30 mg/24 hours and less than or equal to 30 mg/24 hours, predicts the development of diabetic nephropathy.[23] A single measurement below the level of clinical albuminuria is also strongly predictive of nephropathy. In insulin-dependent diabetes mellitus, 30% to 50% of patients ultimately have nephropathy, whereas 10% to 15% of non–insulin-dependent diabetics do.[24] Without aggressive treatment, approximately 1 to 5 years after the onset of microalbuminemia, proteinuria increases and can be detected by protein dipstick measurement in routine urinalysis. Small serum creatinine concentration increases may represent a decline in GFR and also a progression of nephropathy. Several interventions slow the progression of kidney disease in diabetes, so close laboratory monitoring is extremely important. Hyperkalemia is common in diabetes when significant nephropathology has occurred and potassium levels should be monitored closely.[23] Once ESRD has developed, patients become candidates for hemodialysis, peritoneal dialysis, or transplantation.

The glomerular lesion in diabetic nephropathy is a nodular glomerulosclerosis, with an increase in mesangial matrix and a decrease in mesangial endothelial and epithelial cells.[23]

Amyloidosis

Amyloidosis includes a number of multisystem diseases that are characterized by extracellular deposition of insoluble fibrillar proteins and are termed primary, secondary, and hereditary.[25, 26] Up to 80% of patients with amyloidosis can have kidney involvement. Nephrotic syndrome is the initial feature in almost 75% of patients with secondary amyloidosis and in approximately 25% of patients with primary amyloidosis, but it is a rare, late complication of most types of hereditary amyloidosis.[25] The primary form of amyloidosis is much more common in elderly patients and is frequently associated with disorders involving other organs, such as hepatomegaly and restrictive cardiomyopathy with congestive heart failure.[26] The secondary form of amyloid renal involvement can be seen with any longstanding chronic inflammatory process such as tuberculosis, bronchiectasis, rheumatoid arthritis, chronic urinary tract infections, osteomyelitis or in patients with multiple myeloma.[25] There is no satisfactory evidence that any form of treatment ameliorates either the proteinuria or the renal failure that develops, which usually occurs in a period of a month to 2 years. Renal disease appears to be secondary to deposition of amyloid protein within the kidney.

Light microscopy shows infiltration, with the amyloid glycoprotein replacing the mesangial matrix of the glomeruli and, in advanced cases, obliterating the capillary loops. Amyloid substances may also be noted in vessel walls and interstitium. Congo red stain is used to demonstrate reddish pink deposits in the mesangium, peripheral capillary walls, and blood vessels. Such deposits show apple-green birefringence under polarization.[26] Electron microscopy shows that the deposits contain fibrils with characteristics specific for amyloid.

Multiple Myeloma

Nephrotic syndrome in multiple myeloma most commonly represents an "overflow" proteinuria, that is, the presence in the urine of light chains that are easily filtered by the glomerulus. These are usually picked up in quantitative determinations of proteinuria by the sulfosalicylic acid test but may be missed with the reagent strip test that reacts with albumin. There are no characteristic glomerular abnormalities in multiple myeloma, as the glomerulus tends not to be primarily involved, and the myeloma is more a tubulointerstitial disease in the form of acute renal failure. The kidney biopsy shows "cast nephropathy," which results from the light chains (Bence Jones protein) binding to the Tamm-Horsfall glycoprotein in the tubules. These casts are large tubular casts surrounded by macrophages.[27]

Pregnancy-Induced Hypertension (Preeclampsia of Pregnancy)

Severe preeclampsia of pregnancy may be associated with massive proteinuria and biochemical features of nephrotic syndrome. It is usually accompanied by significant edema and hypertension in the third trimester of pregnancy. As seen by light microscopy, the glomerular lesion is predominantly characterized by endothelial cell swelling, which is thought to be a response to fibrin deposition in the glomerular capillaries and mesangial cell prominence.[26] The lesion usually undergoes complete remission following termination of pregnancy.

Systemic Lupus Erythematosus

Renal involvement in SLE can present in several different clinicopathologic ways and has been classified into six types by the World Health Organization (WHO). The renal disease of lupus is immunologically mediated. The nephrotic syndrome occurs in 66% of lupus patients with renal involvement. One form of lupus nephritis associated with nephrotic syndrome is diffuse MGN (WHO class V), a form that is clinically and pathologically very difficult to differentiate from the idiopathic form of MGN. Its clinical manifestations are predominantly those of proteinuria and nephrotic syndrome, with variable degrees of hypertension, hematuria, and renal insufficiency.[26] The serologic parameters of SLE are frequently helpful in making the differential diagnosis, as are the systemic features of this disorder. This lesion may evolve in the absence of striking extrarenal manifestation of SLE. Evidence of active complement consumption is less common in the membranous form of lupus than it is in other forms of lupus nephritis. By light microscopy, the lesion in SLE is indistinguishable from idiopathic membranous glomerulonephritis. Immunofluorescence may demonstrate the presence of multiple immunoglobulins (IgA, IgG, and IgM) and complement (C3). Electron microscopy usually shows a similar pattern.[26] Patients with pure MGN usually do well even without specific therapy. Treatment with glucocorticoid or immunosuppressive regimens induces complete or partial remission in 35% to 50% of patients. Progression to renal insufficiency may occur in patients with persisting heavy proteinuria. The course of this disease is similar to that in idiopathic membranous changes. The diffuse proliferative glomerular lesions (WHO class IV) are also associated with nephrotic syndrome. Renal failure often occurs and severe hypertension or vasculitis may be present, but clinically "silent" diffuse proliferative glomerulonephritis also occurs.

Viral Infections

Nephrotic syndrome has been associated with various liver diseases, including viral hepatitis B and C and cirrhosis of the liver.[26] Membranous nephropathy is associated with all three hepatitis B antigens—hepatitis B surface (HB_s), core (HB_c), and early (HB_e) antigens. These antigens have been identified in the subepithelial complexes at renal biopsy. In children, most of whom are from Asia, proteinuria and hematuria occur, but hypertension is uncommon. In children, spontaneous remission is the rule as the hepatitis resolves. Adults with nephrotic syndrome membranous nephropathy associated with hepatitis B are less likely to have a spontaneous remission. Type I MCGN is the most common type of nephrotic syndrome associated with hepatitis C.[26] Nearly all patients have microscopic hematuria and proteinuria, and more than half are in the nephrotic range. Other clinical characteristics are hypertension, edema, hepatomegaly, and palpable purpura. Cirrhosis of the liver may occasionally be associated with a diffuse glomerular sclerotic process, but the proteinuria and hematuria are usually mild.

An HIV-associated nephropathy may occur in asymptomatic carriers of HIV or patients with AIDS.[26] It presents with nonselective proteinuria often in the nephrotic range and usually without edema, hypercholesterolemia, or hypertension. This is a relatively uncommon occurrence. The majority of patients have a variant of segmental glomerulosclerosis with degeneration or necrosis of the tubular cells. The prognosis is poor for both renal function and survival of the patients with HIV-associated nephropathy. Often, rapid progression to renal failure occurs, and patients succumb to complications of AIDS regardless of whether they are maintained by dialysis.

Nephrotic syndrome rarely appears in association with other viral infections, including herpes zoster, infectious mononucleosis, and cytomegalovirus, among others.

Drugs and Medications

Nephrotic syndrome occurs in association with various drugs and medications.[26] The nephrotic syndrome of intravenous heroin abuse is associated with several types of glomerular lesions, and focal glomerular sclerosis with mesangiocapillary is most common. Patients have a poor prognosis, with more than three-fourths progressing to ESRD within 4 years. Use of various medications, such as probenicid, trimethadione, gold, anticonvulsant agents, and, rarely, various nonsteroidal antiinflammatory drugs, has occasionally been associated with nephrotic syndrome.

TREATMENT

The course and treatment of nephrotic syndrome vary with the particular lesion associated with it. The urine protein can be used as a measure of response to treatment. Laboratory data can also be used to monitor both kidney function and biochemical abnormalities associated with deteriorating function.

Minimal change disease is characterized by a remitting and relapsing course. A large body of evidence indicates that corticosteroids enhance the natural tendency to undergo remission.[1, 11] Most children who respond to steroid therapy do so within 4 weeks. Adults respond more slowly, and 8 weeks of therapy may be needed to ascertain steroid sensitivity. The long-term prognosis for idiopathic nephrotic syndrome with minimal change lesions is excellent. Most patients, given time, will undergo spontaneous remission. Chronic renal failure is a rare outcome and is usually associated with the development of a glomerular lesion of FSG.

Among MPGN patients, the progression to renal failure does occur, especially in patients with well-developed nephrotic syndrome who have failed to respond to glucocorticoids, and in whom superimposed focal and segmental sclerosis have developed. However, 50% or more of patients respond to glucocorticoid therapy and have a complete remission of proteinuria.[15] Hematuria findings may predict a poorer response to steroids. Most of the patients who present with FSG demonstrate a progressive decline in GFR, hypertension, and persistent proteinuria.[1] The course of idiopathic MGN is variable, but usually it is an indolent and slowly progressive one.[17] Patients may have both clinical remissions and relapses of nephrotic syndrome. The overall prognosis in children is good. In adults, however, 40% to 60% of patients who present with nephrotic syndrome have progressive deterioration of renal function over several years. Steroid therapy studies have been difficult to interpret, but steroids and cytotoxic agents may be helpful in some cases. Focal sclerosis is a partially steroid-responsive lesion but requires prolonged and high-dosage treatment. Cyclosporine has shown positive results in some patients. The course of MCGN is slowly progressive, with the majority of cases culminating in ESRF within several years.[19] Once azotemia develops, deterioration toward end-stage disease generally occurs within 1 to 2 years. No form of treatment has proven to be beneficial, although steroids, immunosuppressants, aspirin, and dipyridamole, and plasma exchange have been used. Recurrent disease in renal allographs is common in type I MCGN and perhaps universal in type II MCGN.

Case Study

A 22-year-old man with a history of acute glomerulonephritis, type unknown, was admitted to the hospital to have a renal biopsy because of continued proteinuria. Blood pressure was 130/84 mm Hg. Extremities revealed no edema. The biopsy revealed some MPGN, which was thought to be related to his previous glomerulonephritis.

Laboratory Findings (Reference Ranges)

Urine blood (Negative)	Negative
Urine albumin (Negative)	4+
24-hour urine protein (0–150 mg/24 hr)	15
Creatine clearance (97–137 mL/min)	115

One year later the patient returned for a follow-up visit. He had no complaints. Blood pressure was normal and his extremities revealed no edema.

Laboratory Findings
(Reference Ranges)

Urine blood (Negative)	Negative
Urine albumin (Negative)	4+
24-hour urine protein (0–150 mg/24 hr)	1577
Creatine clearance (97–137 mL/min)	95

The patient did not come for follow-up for 5 years. At this time, the patient presented with edema, which had been present less than 1 year. His blood pressure was 137/80 mm Hg. Pertinent laboratory data are shown. Another renal biopsy was performed and revealed FSG.

Laboratory Findings
(Reference Ranges)

Urine blood (Negative)	Small
Urine albumin (Negative)	4+
Urine electrophoresis	
Albumin (6.28–8.48 mg/dL)	4.60
α-$_1$ (0.11–0.25 mg/dL)	0.17
α-$_2$ (0.32–0.76 mg/dL)	0.93
β (0.53–0.92 mg/dL)	0.90
γ (0.43–1.30 mg/dL)	0.29
Total protein (6.28–8.48 mg/dL)	4.60
Albumin-globulin (A/G) ratio	1.0
24-hr urine protein (0–150 mg/24 hr)	10,462
Creatine clearance (97–137 cc/min)	90
Cholesterol (125–200 mg dL)	483

The physician discussed in detail with the patient the diagnosis and therapeutic options. Although this glomerular process is not known for its response to steroids, both physician and patient agreed that a trial of steroids should be undertaken, considering the severity of the nephrotic state. After a 2-month trial of steroids, the patient's urine protein was 6090 mg/24 hr and the creatinine clearance was normal. He was still experiencing edema and was also experiencing recurrent upper respiratory infections, which were treated with antibiotics.

Questions

1. What abnormal laboratory values obtained from this patient are consistent with a nephrotic syndrome?
2. What type of urine sediment would be expected from this patient?
3. Could the recurrent respiratory infections be related to the nephrotic syndrome?
4. What is the patient's prognosis?

Discussion

1. The very high 24-hour urine protein value, the hyperlipidemia, and the low serum albumin values are consistent with a nephrotic syndrome.
2. The patient would probably have free fat, oval fat bodies, and fatty casts, which would exhibit a Maltese cross pattern under polarizing light.
3. Yes; IgG levels are decreased, which may lead to increased susceptibility to infections.
4. Patients with FSG usually run a progressive course to renal failure without responding to steroid therapy.

References

1. Glassock RJ, Cohen AH, Adler SG: Primary glomerular diseases. *In* Brenner MB (ed): The Kidney, ed 5. Philadelphia, WB Saunders, 1996, p 1392.
2. Bernard DB, Salant DJ: Clinical approach to the patient with proteinuria and the nephrotic syndrome. *In* Jacobson HR, Striker GE, Saulo K (eds): Principles and Practices of Nephrology, ed 2. St Louis, Mosby–Year Book, 1995, p 110.
3. Glassock R: Proteinuria. *In* Massry S, Glassock R (eds): Textbook of Nephrology, ed 3. Baltimore, Williams & Wilkins, 1995, p 600.
4. Bernard DB: The nephrotic syndrome: A clinical approach, Hosp Prac 15:114–130, 1990.
5. Kuhlmann U, Steuser J, Rhyner K, et al: Platelet aggregation and β-thromboglobulin levels in nephrotic patients with and without thrombosis. Clin Nephrol 15:229, 1981.
6. Humphreys MH: Mechanisms and management of nephrotic edema. Kidney Int 45:266–281, 1994.
7. Wheeler DC, Bernard DB: Lipid abnormalities in the nephrotic syndrome: Causes, consequences and treatment. Am J Kidney Dis 23:331–346, 1994.
8. Llach F: Hypercoagulability, renal vein thrombosis and other thrombotic complications of nephrotic syndrome. Kidney Int 28:429–439, 1985.
9. Harris RC, Ismail N: Extrarenal complications of the nephrotic syndrome. Am J Kidney Dis 23:447–497, 1994.
10. Cameron JS: Coagulation and thromboembolic complications in the nephrotic syndrome. Adv Nephrol 13:75, 1984.
11. Grupe WE: Minimal change disease. Semin Nephrol 2:241, 1982.
12. Bridges CR, Myers BD, Brenner BM, et al: Glomerular charge alterations in human minimal change nephropathy. Kidney Int 22:677, 1982.
13. Walker F, O'Neill S, Carmody M, et al: Nephrotic syndrome in Hodgkin's disease. Int J Pediatr Nephrol 4:35, 1983.
14. Mallick NP: The pathogenesis of minimal change nephropathy. Clin Nephrol 7:87, 1977.
15. Cohen AH, Border WA: Mesangial proliferative glomerulonephritis. Semin Nephrol 2:228, 1982.

16. Schwartz MM, Korbet SM: Primary focal segmental glomerulosclerosis: Pathology, histological variants and pathogenesis. Am J Kidney Dis 22:847–883, 1993.
17. Remuzzi G, Bertani T, Schieppati A: Idiopathic membranous nephropathy. Lancet 342:1277–1289, 1993.
18. D'Amico G, Ferrario F: Mesangiocapillary glomerulonephritis. J Am Soc Nephrol 2:S159–S166, 1993.
19. Donadio J Jr: Membranoproliferative glomerulonephritis. *In* Jacobson HR, Striker GE, Saulo K (eds): Principles and Practices of Nephrology, ed 2. St Louis, Mosby–Year Book, 1995, p 155.
20. Varade WS, Forristal J, West CD: Patterns of complement activation in idiopathic membranoproliferative glomerulonephritis, types I, II and III. Am J Kidney Dis 16:196–206, 1990.
21. Shaw AB, Pisdon P, Lewis-Jackson J: Protein-creatinine index and Albusitx in assessment of proteinuria. Br Med J 287:929, 1983.
22. Bernard DB: Metabolic abnormalities in nephrotic syndrome. *In* Brenner BM, Stein JH (eds): Pathophysiology and Complication in Nephrotic Syndrome: Contemporary Issues in Nephrology. New York, Churchill Livingstone, 1982, p 89.
23. Hans-Henrik P, Osterby R, Anderson PW, et al: Diabetic nephropathy. *In* Brenner MB (ed): The Kidney, ed 5. Philadelphia, WB Saunders, 1996, p 1864.
24. Rosenberg ME, Correa-Rotter R, Pathogenesis and risk factors for diabetic nephropathy. *In* Jacobson HR, Striker GE, Saulo K (eds): Principles and Practices of Nephrology, ed. 2. St Louis, Mosby–Year Book, 1995, p 330.
25. Skinner M: Amyloidosis of the kidney. *In* Jacobson HR, Striker GE, Saulo K (eds): Principles and Practices of Nephrology, ed 2. St Louis, Mosby–Year Book, 1995, p 192.
26. Adler SG, Cohen AH, Glassock RJ: Secondary glomerular diseases. *In* Brenner MB (ed): The Kidney, ed 5. Philadelphia, WB Saunders, 1996, p 1498.

Chapter 17

Renal Hypertension

Martha Savage Payne

ETIOLOGY AND PATHOPHYSIOLOGY

Essential or Primary Hypertension

Hypertension as defined in Chapter 6 is characterized by systolic and diastolic blood pressures exceeding 140/90 mm Hg. In the vast majority of cases, hypertension has no identified specific etiology, and this form is classified as primary, or essential, hypertension. Hypertension appears to be a disease of regulation in which several of the mechanisms that control blood pressure are disordered or reset.[1] Many variables control and regulate blood pressure, and near the center of the schema is the kidney.[2] The kidney produces both vasopressor and vasodepressor substances and is the excretory organ for sodium. The kidney may be damaged by elevated blood pressure, even to the point of renal failure.[3]

There are three major mechanisms through which the kidney can affect blood pressure: (1) production of the hormone renin, which helps maintain blood pressure; (2) the effector mechanism for the control of sodium and fluid volume; and (3) production of prostaglandins, which may have vasodepressor or blood pressure–lowering properties. Any disease, either primary in the kidney or one to which the kidney may be responding, can cause hypertension.[4]

Renin is a proteolytic enzyme that is synthesized, stored, and secreted by the kidney. It is a highly specific enzyme that cleaves a decapeptide from an α_2-globulin synthesized by the liver to produce angiotensin I. This is converted to angiotensin II, an octapeptide, by a converting enzyme located primarily in the lung. Angiotensin II is both a potent vasoconstrictor and an aldosterone production stimulator (see Fig. 6–1, Chapter 6). Renin release is the rate-limiting step in angiotensin production. This release is subject to feedback control by angiotensin II, directly and indirectly, through the effect of angiotensin on blood volume, blood pressure, and sodium balance. The renin-angio-tensin system is complex, and it interrelates with various other systems for the control of vascular volume and resistance. The measurements of renin activity are made by using specific, precise, and reproducible radioimmunoassays for angiotensin I and II, which can be used to identify significant renal artery stenosis and to categorize patients with other forms of hypertension.

The second group of mechanisms through which the kidney can influence blood pressure are the factors that control sodium excretion.[5] Epidemiologic studies have demonstrated a direct correlation between the level of sodium intake and the incidence of hypertension in population groups. The factors that control sodium excretion in the kidney are glomerular filtration rate (GFR), aldosterone, and the peritubular capillary Starling forces. Under normal circumstances, the sodium balance in humans is not regulated by variation in the GFR. In renal failure, however, the GFR may be so depressed that it is the rate-limiting step for sodium excretion. Sodium and water retention will, therefore, produce volume-dependent hypertension. Aldosterone, a corticoid steroid produced in the adrenals, facilitates sodium reabsorption and potassium excretion by the distal tubules. Sodium depletion, potassium excess, and elevated angiotensin II stimulate aldosterone secretion. Aldosterone can participate in hypertensive disease either by primary adrenal overproduction or, secondarily, in response to renal renin secretion. The third factor controlling sodium excretion is the Starling forces in the peritubular capillaries. An increase in pressure inhibits sodium reabsorption and enhances sodium excretion. This may not be a cause of hypertension, but rather a mechanism to achieve sodium homeostasis. When patients with renal failure are unable to excrete sodium equivalent to their intake due to a low GFR, volume-expansive hypertension will increase peritubular capillary pressure and facilitate sodium excretion.

Prostaglandins produced by the renal medulla (prostaglandin E_2 [PGE_2] and possibly prostaglandin I_2 [PGI_2]) may have the capacity to lower blood pressure by dilating peripheral arteries.[6] It has also been postulated that these compounds may influence sodium and water reabsorption by redistribution of blood flow within the kidney. The relevance and importance of these compounds to hypertension in humans is not clearly understood. The administration of nonsteroidal anti-inflammatory drugs to patients with renal parenchymal hypertension has been shown to increase blood pressure, reduce GFR, and decrease urinary prostaglandin excretion. It is unlikely that a deficiency of renal prostaglandin synthesis contributes to hypertension in renal disease.

Essential hypertension seems to involve the kidney or some aspect of renal function, but the exact mechanism in most cases is elusive.[3] Changes in arterial pressure involve changes in vascular resistance. The development of hypertension is associated with vasoconstriction, although cardiac output remains relatively unchanged. Vascular smooth muscle responds both to local conditions and to systemic neural and humoral signals. The local response is called autoregulation of blood flow; normal blood flow and elevated vascular resistance might be expected in hypertension.[2] Autoregulation is difficult to connect with the general contention that the kidney dominates blood pressure control. One explanation that connects the renal involvement with autoregulation is that salt and water are retained when the excretory load exceeds the kidney's excretory capability. Some of this retained fluid in the circulation tends to increase venous return and cardiac output. Elevated cardiac output increases arterial pressure while triggering autoregulatory vasoconstriction. Rising pressure facilitates salt and water excretion and helps reestablish salt and water balance. The eventual hemodynamic picture is one of sodium balance, elevated arterial pressure, vasoconstriction, and normal cardiac output. It is not clearly understood which is the cause and which is the result in the relationship between arteriolar nephrosclerosis and hypertension. Evidence exists that can be used to support the view that hypertension is responsible for nephrosclerosis. However, some of the same evidence can be interpreted differently to be consistent with the view that hypertension is secondary to arteriolar nephrosclerosis. At this time the evidence is not conclusive.

Renal Artery Stenosis

Renal artery stenosis (RAS) can cause hypertension.[7] Some authors have estimated that approximately 5% of the hypertensive population have RAS. Many lesions can produce RAS, with atherosclerosis being more common in older men and fibromuscular dysplasia more common in women whose average age is 40 years. RAS can be unilateral or bilateral. The altered pressure-flow relationships within the kidney due to RAS activate compensatory mechanisms that produce the hypertension and metabolic and physiologic abnormalities. Total renal blood flow is decreased by the stenosis when the diameter of the renal artery is reduced by 60% or more. This leads to an increase in angiotensin II via renin production, with a subsequent increase in peripheral vascular resistance. Aldosterone secretion is increased by the angiotensin, which favors potassium excretion and sodium and water retention. The other normal kidney excretes the sodium and water, decreasing plasma volume. The flow and pressure are not restored to the affected kidney, and renin secretion continues.

Hypertension Associated With Other Forms of Renal Disease

All forms of chronic renal disease and acute renal failure may be associated with an increased incidence of hypertension. Chronic glomerulonephritis, chronic pyelonephritis, vascular lesions such as in polyarteritis nodosa, lupus erythematosus, polycystic disease, and renal carcinoma can cause hypertension.[8] Obstructive uropathies, analgesic abuse, and renal calculi can also cause hypertension. Acute renal failure can cause rapid elevation of blood pressure, especially in fluid overloaded patients.

Patients without kidneys or those in terminal renal failure with very low GFR values are extremely sensitive to changes in salt and water balance. Plasma renin and angiotensin levels are usually low. This form of hypertension must be managed by salt and water restriction and elimination of excess by dialysis.

CLINICAL MANIFESTATIONS

Clinically, it is very difficult to distinguish essential hypertension from RAS hypertension.[9] Patients with RAS usually have hypertension of short duration that is severe and accelerated in nature. RAS frequently occurs in patients younger than 25 years or older than 45 years. In general, those with RAS caused by fibromuscular hyperplasia are younger and female, and those with RAS caused by atherosclerosis are older than patients with essential hypertension and are predominantly male. The onset of hypertension outside of the usual age range for essential hypertension or the absence of a family history of hypertension are important clues in the differential diagnosis. Associated with hypertension caused by RAS due to either atherosclerosis or fibromuscular dysplasia is an accelerated increase in the level of blood pressure, difficult-to-control blood pressure, and/or headaches associated with elevated blood pressure.

LABORATORY ANALYSES AND DIAGNOSIS

Diagnostic evaluation of patients with hypertension should help to stage organ damage, to identify factors that will affect treatment and prognosis, and to identify any correctable etiology. RAS comprises more than half of the correctable causes. The majority of the other correctable causes (e.g. pheochromocytoma) may be strongly suspected based on initial history and physical examination. The crucial decision in these patients is usually whether to carry out diagnostic studies for renovascular hypertension. Each of these studies should be done only after the risks are assessed in relation to the specificity and sensitivity of the study. If renovascular hypertension is the diagnosis, then surgical or medical therapy must be chosen. If the patient is known to be an unsuitable candidate for surgery, then the expensive diagnostic evaluation is of little use and is not cost-effective. The first step in diagnosis is the history, followed by routine laboratory tests (urinalysis, blood chemistry analyses) and then by special tests, such as baseline venous plasma renin activity, scintigraphy with angiotensin-converting enzyme (ACE) inhibitors, flow study with duplex ultrasound, and stimulated plasmin renin activity.[8, 9]

In hypertension secondary to specific renal disease, the laboratory values will correspond to the particular disease entity. Chapter 6 provides a detailed discussion of hypertension, with suggested treatment and representative case studies.

References

1. Dougherty JC: Hypertension and the kidney. *In* Farland M (ed): Nephrology. New Hyde Park, NY, Medical Examination Publishing, 1983.
2. Guyton AC: Dominant role of the kidney and accessory role of the whole body autoregulation in the pathogenesis of hypertension. Am J Hypertens 2:575–585, 1989.
3. Laragh JH, Blumenfeld JD: Essential hypertension. *In* Brenner BM (ed): The Kidney. Philadelphia, WB Saunders, 1996, p 2071.
4. Smith MC, Dunn MJ: Role of the kidney in blood pressure regulation. *In* Jacobson HR, Striker GE, Klahr S (eds): The Principles and Practice of Nephrology. St Louis, Mosby–Year Book, 1995, p 362.
5. Luft FC: Salt and hypertension: Recent advances and perspectives. J Lab Clin Med 114:215–221, 1989.
6. Mene P, Dunn MJ: Vascular, glomerular, and tubular effecs of angiotensin II, kinins, and prostaglandins. *In* Seldin DW, Giebisch G (eds): The Kidney: Physiology and Pathophysiology. New York, Raven Press, 1992, p 1205.
7. Laragh JH: Renovascular hypertension: A paradigm for all hypertension. J Hypertens Suppl 4:S79, 1986.
8. Acosta JH: Hypertension in chronic renal failure. Kidney Int 22:702–712, 1982.
9. Ploth DW: Renovascular hypertension. *In* Jacobson HR, Striker GE, Klahr S (eds): The Principles and Practice of Nephrology. St Louis, Mosby–Year Book, 1995, p 379.

Chapter 18

Urinary Obstructive Disorders

Catherine Downs

Obstruction can occur anywhere in the urinary tract from the renal tubules to the distal urethra. Obstruction of the urinary tract is an important clinical problem because when the normal flow of urine is impeded by an obstructive lesion, the potential exists for impairment of renal function and urinary tract infection.[1] The patient's clinical presentation and the degree of renal function impairment vary according to the location of the obstruction, whether it is acute or chronic, partial or complete, unilateral or bilateral, and whether an infection is present.[2] Urinary tract obstruction requires early diagnosis and prompt, appropriate treatment in order to minimize the structural and functional changes that the obstruction may produce in the kidneys. If uncorrected, the obstruction may lead to complete, irreversible loss of renal function.[3]

ETIOLOGY AND PATHOPHYSIOLOGY
Terminology and Classification

Obstructive uropathy is a general term used to describe the obstruction of urinary flow. Initially, obstructive uropathy results in dilation of the ureter, renal pelvis, and calyces with urine. This dilation is referred to as *hydronephrosis*. If uncorrected, obstructive uropathy may lead to *obstructive nephropathy*—the functional and histopathologic changes in the kidney resulting from obstruction of urinary flow. It should be noted that the definitions of these terms may vary from writer to writer.[1]

Urinary tract obstructions are described using three classifications. These are (1) *duration*, as acute (having short duration and abrupt onset), subacute (lasting from days to weeks), or chronic (months to years); (2) *degree*, as high grade (total or complete obstruction) or low grade (partial or incomplete obstruction); and (3) *location*, in the renal tubule, upper urinary tract, or lower urinary tract. Upper urinary tract obstruction is most commonly unilateral and may involve the renal pelvis, the ureter, or the ureter's junction with the pelvis (ureteropelvic) or bladder (ureterovesical). Obstruction involving the bladder or urethra is described as lower urinary tract obstruction and thus is bilateral, affecting the upper urinary tract of both kidneys.[4]

Various causes of urinary tract obstruction appear in Table 18–1. Urinary tract obstruction can have intrinsic (intraluminal or intramural) or extrinsic causes. The obstructive lesion may occur in the renal tubule or the upper or lower urinary tract. Patient age and gender affect the predominant likely causes of urinary tract obstruction.

Intraluminal Causes

Intraluminal obstruction is caused by a mechanical obstruction of the lumen at any level of the urinary tract.[2] The deposition of uric acid crystals in the tubules, seen most commonly in hematologic malignancies, is a common cause of intraluminal obstruction arising within the renal

Table 18–1. Various Causes of Urinary Tract Obstruction

	Intrinsic Causes	Extrinsic Causes
Upper urinary tract obstruction	Calculi Sloughed papillae Ureteropelvic dysfunction Ureteral tumor Ureteral stricture	Pregnancy Pelvic malignancies Ureteral ligation Retroperitoneal fibrosis
Lower urinary tract obstruction	Posterior urethral valve Neurogenic bladder Urethral stricture	Prostatic obstruction

parenchyma. Patients with multiple myeloma may also develop intraluminal obstruction, caused by the deposition of Bence Jones protein in the renal tubule. Renal failure is a common cause of death in such patients; however, controversy exists as to whether the renal insufficiency results from toxic effects or from obstructive effects of Bence Jones protein.[4] Other causes include sulfonamide or acyclovir crystal deposition.[5]

Urinary tract calculi are a predominant cause of intraluminal obstruction, especially in the young adult male. Most stones are composed of one or more of the following substances: calcium oxalate, calcium phosphate, uric acid, cystine, and magnesium ammonium phosphate (struvite). The most common stones are composed of calcium oxalate. A multitude of factors are probably responsible for stone formation, including reduction in urine volume, increased urinary excretion of the relatively insoluble substances just listed, urine pH, and the absence of inhibitors to precipitation of these insoluble agents.[6]

Sloughed papillae resulting from necrosis of renal papillae may also cause intraluminal obstruction. Papillary necrosis is associated with a number of conditions, including analgesic abuse, sickle cell disease or trait, diabetes mellitus, and severe pyelonephritis. In addition, blood clots and fungus balls have been known to obstruct the ureter.[4]

Intramural Causes

Intramural obstruction can be caused by either functional or anatomic abnormalities of the ureter, bladder, or urethra. These can be the result of congenital conditions, seen most commonly in children, or acquired conditions, which occur most commonly in adults. In childhood, posterior urethral valves and anomalies of the ureteropelvic junction are two conditions that produce obstruction.

Neurogenic bladder dysfunction is a common cause of an acquired functional obstruction. It results from metabolic and neurologic disorders of or injuries to the spinal cord. A significant number of individuals with diabetes mellitus or multiple sclerosis develop neurogenic bladder dysfunction.[4]

Examples of anatomic alterations that lead to obstruction are ureteral strictures (as a consequence of surgical procedures in the retroperitoneum, complication of radiation therapy in cervical carcinoma, or treatment of tuberculosis that has directly involved the ureter) and urethral strictures (secondary to long-term instrumentation, surgery, or gonococcal infections). In addition, urinary tract obstruction

may result from tumors of the renal pelvis, ureter, or bladder.[4]

Extrinsic (Extramural) Causes

Extrinsic causes of urinary tract obstruction are the result of pressure from masses or of processes extrinsic to the urinary tract. In elderly men, benign prostatic hypertrophy and carcinoma of the prostate are the most common causes of extrinsic obstruction of the urinary tract. In women, pregnancy and pelvic malignancies are the most common causes of obstruction. A variety of gastrointestinal processes (e.g., Crohn's disease) and vascular abnormalities or diseases (e.g., abdominal aortic aneurysms) may also cause obstruction. Accidental ureteral ligation during surgery can result in obstruction. Retroperitoneal fibrosis, which may be idiopathic, drug induced, or associated with a wide variety of conditions, can also cause ureteral compression.[4, 7]

Increased Pressure and Decreased Renal Blood Flow

When the urinary tract is obstructed, there is an increase in pressure throughout the urinary tract proximal to the obstruction as the formation of urine continues. The pressure increase is transmitted to the kidney, where it initially affects distal tubule function, and thus, an early manifestation may be inability to concentrate the urine. Inability to acidify the urine then follows.[8]

Elevated pressure also results in reductions in glomerular filtration rate and renal blood flow, although in the initial period following obstruction, renal blood flow may increase.[8]

Renal Damage

The longer the obstruction persists, the more likely it is that renal damage will occur.[9] If obstruction is not relieved, ischemic atrophy of the kidney results, with subsequent renal failure. Unilateral obstruction results in destruction of only one kidney, with the remaining kidney able to maintain normal excretory function. Bilateral obstructive disease, if uncorrected, leads to progressive renal failure, uremia, and, possibly, death. If the obstruction is prolonged, permanent damage to the kidneys may result, although renal function may significantly improve or at least stabilize if the obstruction is relieved prior to the stage of irreversible damage.[2, 10] Studies have shown that glomerular filtration rate improves over a period of 1 to 4 weeks after relief of the obstruction, if the obstruction is of recent onset.[1]

Diabetes Insipidus

A syndrome of vasopressin-resistant diabetes insipidus may arise secondary to the obstructive disorder.[11] Acquired nephrogenic diabetes insipidus may be the presenting manifestation of the obstructive disorder in affected patients. The mechanism whereby the nephron does not respond to vasopressin is unknown.[1]

Infection

Although obstruction alone may injure the kidney, an additional risk is the predisposition of the urinary tract to infection. Urinary tract infection superimposed on the obstruction inevitably contributes to the increased rate of nephron destruction.[1] Infection, once established in the obstructed urinary tract, is difficult to eliminate and may contribute significantly to morbidity.[2]

CLINICAL MANIFESTATIONS

The clinical manifestations observed in urinary tract obstruction depend on the duration, location, and degree of obstruction. They can be nonspecific, although some signs and symptoms, when they exist, are sufficiently definitive to suggest to the physician that an obstructive disorder is the most likely diagnosis.[4] Urinary tract obstruction usually causes changes in patterns of urination (i.e., oliguria, anuria, polyuria, nocturia) and may also result in localized pain.[12] If the obstruction develops gradually, however, patients may be asymptomatic even with severe obstruction.[7]

Presenting Signs and Symptoms

The diagnostic approach to a patient presenting with possible urinary tract obstruction varies with the initial symptoms,[4] which may range from acute onset of pain to acute renal failure.[5] Common complaints include difficulty in voiding, pain, infection, and changes in urinary volume.[13] Obstruction at or below the bladder is commonly associated with low abdominal pain due to bladder distention. Mild obstruction results in hesitancy, urinary frequency, overflow incontinence, and postvoid dribbling.[3] Pain in the flank, groin, or lower abdomen is often the presenting symptom that causes the patient to seek medical advice. It is important to remember, however, that with chronic, low-grade obstruction, pain may be nonexistent. Symptoms may be totally absent until kidney damage is so severe that renal failure becomes the initial manifestation of the obstructive disorder. Evidence of recurrent urinary tract infections should lead to the suspicion of urinary tract obstruction. Affected patients present with the typical symptoms of fever, flank tenderness, and dysuria. In addition, gastrointestinal symptoms such as nausea, vomiting, and abdominal fullness are common.[1]

Obstructive disorders generally represent treatable causes of renal failure. Because the extent of renal impairment is related to the severity and duration of the obstruction, timely diagnosis is a major goal.[14] Urinary tract obstructions may be caused by such a wide variety of lesions that, in order for a diagnosis to be made, consideration must be given to the entire urinary tract. Certain preliminary information is important in the diagnostic process and in the choice of laboratory and radiologic tests.

Pain

Patients with urinary tract obstruction most commonly seek medical attention because of pain caused by distention of the renal capsule or urinary collecting system. The intensity of the pain, however, is influenced more by how rapidly the distention develops than by the degree of disten-

tion. Thus, pain is more commonly associated with obstruction of sudden onset, whereas chronic obstruction may not produce pain or may be associated with only mild discomfort.[7] The severe pain experienced with acute urinary tract obstruction due to renal calculi is referred to as *renal colic*. This pain often radiates from the flank into the groin, depending on the location of the obstruction.[3, 4]

Changes in Urinary Output

A common presenting sign of urinary tract obstruction is a change in urinary habits.[12] Total anuria or fluctuation in urine volume from oliguria to polyuria is highly suggestive of an obstructive disorder. Total anuria may result if obstruction is complete and bilateral. Urine output may be normal if the obstruction is partial, although polyuria may occur as a result of the kidney's impaired concentrating ability. This concentrating defect may also result in nocturia as an early symptom when there is significant obstruction. If the patient is hospitalized, it is wise to determine the pattern of urinary output. Recognition of abrupt changes, gradual decline, or fluctuation may aid in the diagnostic process. Sudden cessation of voiding may point to a bladder outlet obstruction.[1, 4]

Recurrent Urinary Tract Infections

The presence of a urinary tract obstruction must be investigated in any patient who presents with a history of repeated urinary tract infections or resistance of the infection to normal antibiotic therapy. In such a patient, it may be extremely difficult to clear the infection as long as the obstruction continues.[4]

Renal Failure

Acute or chronic renal failure can result from bilateral obstruction or from unilateral obstruction in patients with only one functioning kidney.[2] It is therefore important to suspect urinary tract obstruction in patients presenting with signs and symptoms of renal failure. This is especially true when there is no previous history of renal disease and routine urinalysis results are negative, or when there is sudden deterioration of renal function for no reason in a patient with known renal disease.[4]

Urolithiasis

The stasis resulting from obstruction of the urinary tract may encourage stone formation.[3]

Hypertension

Elevated blood pressure may be present in patients with acute unilateral obstruction and is usually due to increased renin secretion.[13] Abnormal salt and water retention appears to be responsible for the hypertensive state in cases of chronic, bilateral hydronephrosis. Thus, these patients have a volume-dependent form of hypertension, and their circulating levels of renin are often suppressed.[5, 15]

Renal Enlargement and Palpable Masses

Patients with long-standing obstruction may note increased abdominal girth or may present with a palpable flank mass due to increased kidney size.[5]

Lower Urinary Tract Symptoms

Obstruction of the lower urinary tract often results in changes in micturition. Common symptoms are hesitancy, postvoid dribbling, incontinence, and decreased force and size of urine stream.[5]

Hyperkalemic, Hyperchloremic Metabolic Acidosis

A hyperkalemic, hyperchloremic metabolic acidosis may develop in patients with obstruction. It is due to a decrease in hydrogen ion and potassium secretion by the distal segments of the nephron. This disorder occurs more commonly in the elderly.[11]

Gross Hematuria

Gross hematuria may be associated with specific etiologies of urinary tract obstruction, such as urinary tract stones, neoplasms, and infection.

Polycythemia

The polycythemia manifested in a few instances of obstructive disorders is believed to be caused by abnormal erythropoietin production by the obstructed kidney. This belief has been supported by the resolution of the erythrocytosis once the obstruction is relieved.[2]

LABORATORY ANALYSES AND DIAGNOSIS

Assessment of the patient's condition generally proceeds along two lines. The first involves assessment by clinical laboratory evaluation of urine and blood samples. The results of these tests may suggest an obstructive disorder, although it is the second line of assessment, involving radiologic evaluation of the urinary tract, upon which a diagnosis is generally based.[9] Several laboratory tests are considered particularly useful in evaluating urinary tract obstruction; they are routine urinalysis, urine culture, complete blood count, and serum urea nitrogen and creatinine determinations. Laboratory evaluation for possible systemic conditions or diseases (e.g., hypercalcemia, gout, or multiple myeloma) that predispose the patient to obstructive disorders is also important to consider.[16]

Urine Studies

A complete urinalysis that includes microscopic evaluation of the urinary sediment can be a helpful tool for assessing urinary tract obstruction. The results are generally nonspecific but may occasionally be diagnostic, as in the observation of fragments of necrosed renal papillae or bladder tumor in the urinary sediment. The urinalysis results may even be completely normal, especially in complete unilateral obstruction, in which abnormal urine cannot reach the bladder.[1] An unremarkable urinalysis result in a patient with unexplained renal failure correlates highly with the presence of urinary tract obstruction.[7, 12]

The finding of hematuria without other positive findings may suggest renal or ureteral calculi, papillary necrosis, or a tumor as the cause of obstruction.[4] Hematuria has been found to occur consistently when stones are present, even asymptomatically.[17] With the presence of bacteria and leukocytes, urinary tract infection should be suspected, and urine culture and sensitivity testing should be performed. Bacteriuria alone may indicate stasis. The urine sediment should also be carefully examined for the presence of crystals that may suggest the possible source for urinary tract obstruction or may provide information regarding the etiology of urinary tract stones. Proteinuria, if present, is generally mild (less than 1.5 to 2 g/day), which is in contrast with proteinuria in glomerular diseases.[7, 14]

Urinary pH measurement, on a fresh sample from a patient in a fasting state, may be valuable in determining the kinds of crystals precipitating urinary tract calculi. The ionization and, thus, solubility of some urinary constituents may be affected by changes in urinary pH. Calcium oxalate forms stones at a pH less than 7.5, calcium phosphate at pH 6.0 to 6.5, and uric acid at pH 5.3. Magnesium ammonium phosphate forms stones (struvite or infection stones) at an alkaline pH. These stones are produced when there is an infection from urea-splitting organisms, such as *Proteus* species, which cause alkalinization of the urine.[17, 18]

Urinary cytology studies, although not part of the routine urinalysis, may offer useful diagnostic information in patients with bladder tumors.[19]

Evaluation of renal concentrating ability, the earliest functional abnormality in obstruction, can be estimated with the measurement of urinary specific gravity and/or osmolality, osmolality being the preferred measurement. Urine concentration varies widely according to several factors, especially water intake; therefore, a random urine concentration measurement provides little information about renal concentrating ability unless a period of water deprivation ranging from 18 to 24 hours precedes the sample collection. A urine osmolality greater than 900 mOsm/kg and/or a urine specific gravity greater than 1.023 (in the absence of glucose, protein, or contrast dyes) would indicate a normal renal concentrating mechanism.[20]

Information about the kidney's ability to acidify the urine, which may be impaired in urinary tract obstruction, can be obtained by measuring the lowest urinary pH measured when the patient is in a state of metabolic acidosis. The acidosis either may be spontaneous or may be induced with administration of ammonium chloride. An abnormal response is indicated when the urinary pH does not drop below 5.4.[21]

Observations of urine volume output can be an important diagnostic tool, and measurement of 24-hour urine volume may be indicated. In the hospitalized patient, evaluation of the input and output records for even hourly changes can be helpful. This information can establish whether urine output has changed abruptly, has gradually declined, or has fluctuated.[5] Additionally, bladder catheterization to measure residual urine volume after voiding may be helpful in diagnosing lower urinary tract obstruction, which is suggested by the presence of increased residual urine in the bladder.[2] This form of obstruction may also be observed with postvoiding radiographs of the bladder.[22]

Urine culture may be indicated to determine the status of infection. It should be performed for all patients with obstruction, even in the absence of pyuria.[14]

Assessment of Renal Function

To assess renal function, blood urea nitrogen (BUN) and serum creatinine levels should be measured (see also Chapter 15). These values vary with the extent of the obstruction but may be elevated when obstruction is severe enough to have compromised renal function. The BUN-creatinine ratio can be an important clue to diagnosis, in that it is often elevated in disease caused by urinary tract obstruction. The normal ratio is between 10:1 and 20:1, but in postrenal azotemia (resulting from obstructive disorders), the BUN rises out of proportion to the serum creatinine, owing to the greater reabsorption of urea that occurs with a low rate of urine flow.[1]

An additional evaluative tool is measurement of the glomerular filtration rate to estimate the number of functioning nephrons. There is no ideal material of endogenous origin for use in measuring glomerular filtration rate, but the determination of creatinine clearance is, overall, the most useful and convenient indicator of glomerular filtration rate. A clearance test using an exogenous substance such as inulin is the method of choice when a more accurate assessment of glomerular filtration rate is required.[21] The results depend on the etiology of the urinary tract obstruction and thus reflect the extent of renal function impairment induced by the obstruction.

Other Blood Studies

Information regarding underlying metabolic disorders may be obtained by performing selected chemistry tests. The results should be evaluated for indications of abnormalities that may give rise to obstructive disorders, such as hypercalcemia, gout, and diabetes. Specific analytes that should be measured include serum electrolytes, calcium, phosphorus, magnesium, uric acid, and albumin.[7] Protein abnormalities present in multiple myeloma should be considered as a cause of urinary tract obstruction.

A white blood cell count should be performed to investigate the possibility of a hematologic malignancy. In addition, the hematocrit should be measured to identify anemia due to chronic renal disease.[7]

Evaluation of Urinary Tract Calculi (Stones)

Analysis of urinary calculi is essential to establish etiology and to prevent their recurrence. A number of physical and chemical techniques have been used to analyze the composition of urinary tract stones. Among these are x-ray diffraction and infrared spectroscopy, which provide quantitative data regarding stone composition and offer the

---

Box 18–1. Laboratory Studies Recommended for Patient Evaluation in Stone Formation

On each urine and serum sample:

> Calcium
> Phosphate
> Uric acid
> Creatinine

On one serum sample:

> Sodium
> Potassium

On three urine samples:

> Oxalate
> Citrate
> pH
> Volume

---

most complete and accurate analysis.[23] They are gradually replacing the less specific qualitative chemical methods that assess only the elemental composition of the calculi.[16] Separate analyses can also be performed on the center of the stone and on the rim, to aid in identifying the factors contributing to stone formation.[24]

Prevention of stone recurrence requires a diagnosis of the cause of stone formation. In addition to identifying the composition of urinary tract stones, chemical analyses of serum and urine can reveal metabolic disorders that may be responsible for stone formation. Specimen requirements for this diagnosis are a 24-hour urine specimen and a corresponding fasting blood sample. Some authorities recommend collecting these specimens on three separate occasions to estimate variability. The analytes most commonly measured are listed in Box 18–1. It is also recommended that cystine screening be performed on all patients.[25, 26] Patients should eat their usual diet during this evaluation process because controlling the diet could obscure abnormalities.[27]

Radiologic Evaluation

A wide range of radiologic techniques are available to evaluate a suspected urinary tract obstruction. The results of the history, physical examination findings, and laboratory data should guide the selection of radiologic procedures for diagnosis.[7] Two important considerations are the presence of pain and evidence of diminished renal function. For example, in patients who present with abdominal or flank pain without evidence of renal dysfunction, plain films of the abdomen (kidney, ureter, and bladder) and intravenous urography (also known as intravenous pyelography) are required as the initial, and possibly only, tests; the initial procedures in patients who present with acute or chronic renal failure, however, are abdominal plain films and ultrasonography. If dilation of the urinary tract is detected, other procedures are required to determine the cause and severity of the obstruction.[5, 14]

Plain films of the abdomen provide useful information on renal and bladder morphology and may reveal the presence of calculi. Most renal calculi are radiopaque and thus are visible on a plain film of the abdomen. If a calculus is found, or other evidence suggests passage of a stone, intravenous pyelography (IVP) is performed as the next step.[5] Intravenous urography or pyelography is the procedure of choice in most cases of urinary tract obstruction, especially for investigation of acute renal colic or suspicion of upper urinary tract obstruction.[14, 15]

Because IVP is not useful in patients with compromised renal function and because of the complications associated with this procedure (e.g., allergic reactions to the iodinated contrast material, renal failure), other techniques may be required as alternative diagnostic tools. Ultrasonography is a useful screening procedure to detect hydronephrosis and thus to suggest urinary tract obstruction. Because it is noninvasive and does not depend on renal function, ultrasonography is especially useful in patients presenting with renal failure. Further studies are then indicated to determine whether dilation is a consequence of obstruction or of another condition. It is important to note, however, that in some instances, the ultrasound evaluation may give false-negative results and thus cannot be used to completely rule out the presence of obstruction. Computed tomography may be useful in determining the cause of obstruction, especially when the etiology remains uncertain after ultrasonography or IVP. Other techniques that can be used to further assess the presence of obstruction are retrograde and antegrade pyelography, isotopic renography, and magnetic resonance imaging. Also, a number of tests are useful in diagnosing lower urinary tract obstruction, such as a voiding cystourethrogram and various urodynamic tests.[10, 14, 15]

TREATMENT

Once a urinary tract obstruction has been diagnosed, it is necessary to decide when and how to decompress the obstruction.[5] The primary goals of therapy are to relieve the symptoms of obstruction, to control or prevent infection, and to preserve renal function. The specific medical (nonsurgical) or surgical intervention expected to relieve the obstruction must be chosen on an individual basis. Among other things, the general status of the patient, the specific etiology and location of the obstruction, whether the procedure is a emergent or elective, and the state of renal function in the obstructed kidney must all be taken into consideration by the physician in choosing the appropriate intervention.[8] The severely ill patient may, on occasion, need to be treated with dialysis or temporary drainage of urine through nephrostomy or other bypass procedures.[22] Furthermore, management of pain and urolithiasis is necessary.

Medical treatments include management of fluid and electrolytes (e.g., for nephrogenic diabetes insipidus), treatment of complications such as hypertension, and antibiotic therapy for urinary tract infections.[14] A patient with urinary tract obstruction complicated by infection is at great risk for developing generalized sepsis. This situation constitutes a urologic emergency, and the obstruction must be relieved as soon as possible.[13]

The most common cause of ureteral obstruction is urinary tract calculi (stones). Most ureteral stones less than 5 mm in diameter pass spontaneously and do not require surgical intervention or instrumentation. Thus, in the absence of infection, such calculi can initially be treated conservatively with administration of analgesics for pain and increased hydration. High fluid intake, to ensure a minimum urine volume of 2 L per day, can help the stone pass. It is important that the patient collect and strain all urine to attempt to recover even the smallest stone for analysis. The likelihood of spontaneous passage decreases as the stone size increases, especially beyond 7 mm. Such stones usually require surgery or instrumentation of the urinary tract, depending on their location and size, the extent of obstruction, and the presence or absence of infection.

The approach to treatment of ureteral calculi has undergone significant change in the last decade, and the number of options has increased. The introduction of newer, less invasive techniques such as lithotripsy (stone fragmentation), has greatly reduced the necessity for open surgical procedures.[5, 7] Lithotripsy utilizes either shock waves or ultrasonic energy to fragment the stone, with subsequent passage of stone fragments into the urine. In one of these techniques useful for renal stones, extracorporeal shock-wave lithotripsy (ESWL), the patient is submerged in a water tank, and shock waves are directed at the stone to fragment it.[26, 28] Distal ureteral stones can be removed ureteroscopically by use of a variety of loops or baskets or can be fragmented by special lithotripsy techniques.[7]

Prevention of further stone formation is the primary aim in treatment. Dietary modifications, forcing of fluids, and acidification or alkalinization of the urine may constitute an appropriate treatment regimen, along with management of underlying conditions that contribute to stone formation (e.g., primary hyperparathyroidism, cystinuria, gout). Regardless of what disorders are found in patients with renal calculi, every patient should be instructed to drink 12 to 16 glasses of water daily and to avoid dehydration.[26]

A syndrome of postobstructive diuresis may be observed after relief of bilateral urinary tract obstruction. It is caused by the unloading of retained water and solute, and the osmotic effect of excretion of retained urea. The diuresis is usually transient, but careful monitoring of the patient's fluid and electrolyte balance is necessary to determine whether fluid and salt replacement are required.[4]

Tests used for long-term follow-up of patients who underwent surgical treatment for obstruction or who have chronic obstruction are urinalysis and urine culture, periodic radiologic evaluation, and assessment of renal function, usually by creatinine clearance.[14]

The prognosis for the patient with urinary tract obstruction depends largely on whether irreversible renal damage has occurred before treatment is begun. The duration and completeness of the obstruction and the presence or absence of infection greatly influence the extent of renal damage and, thus, the prognosis. The ultimate result for the patient may also depend on the underlying condition that has led to the obstruction.[9, 10]

Case Study

A 31-year-old white male presented to the emergency room with the chief complaint of intermittent pain that began in the flank but moved to the groin. The patient reported feeling fine until an hour before, when the pain began and increased in severity, forcing him to seek medical attention. A urinalysis was ordered, and the results indicated a urine pH of 6.5 and the presence of a microscopic hematuria (20 to 30 red blood cells per high-power field [rbc/hpf]); all other results appeared normal.

Questions

1. What additional test should be performed to determine the patient's diagnosis?
2. If the test reveals an obstruction in the urinary tract, what would be the most common cause, given the age, gender, and presenting symptoms and signs of this patient?
3. If an obstruction due to urinary tract calculi were found in this patient, what additional laboratory tests should be performed?
4. What would be the appropriate treatment for the prevention of further stone formation?

Discussion

1. Diagnosis of a urinary tract obstruction is generally based on the results of radiologic examination of the urinary tract, including intravenous pyelography.
2. Urinary tract calculi are a predominant cause of intraluminal obstruction, especially in the young adult male.
3. Serum and urine (24-hour) calcium, phosphorus, uric acid, and creatinine measurements should be performed. Tests for urinary oxalate and citrate may also be indicated. Some patients with urinary tract calculi have underlying metabolic disorders that cause stone formation. These can be detected by chemical analyses performed on serum and urine. In addition, the composition of any stones that might pass spontaneously should be analyzed to help establish etiology and define appropriate treatment. In many instances, physicians delay an investigation as complete and costly as the foregoing until a second episode of stone formation. This is because only 40% of patients ever have a subsequent episode.
4. No matter what disorder(s) is found, the patient should be instructed to avoid dehydration and to increase water intake. Use of dietary modification, acidification/alkalinization of the urine, or medications depends on stone type. This patient had a calcium phosphate stone, and the cause was identified as idiopathic hypercalciuria (normal serum calcium, unexplained hypercalciuria [urine calcium greater than 300 mg/24 hours]). A thiazide diuretic agent was prescribed as the appropriate treatment to prevent further stone formation.

References

1. Beck LH, Stein JH, Earley LE: Obstructive uropathy. *In* Early LE, Gottschalk CW (eds): Strauss and Welt's Diseases of the Kidney, ed 3. Boston, Little, Brown & Co, 1979.
2. Rector FC: Obstructive nephropathy. *In* Wyngaarden JB, Smith LH (eds): Cecil Textbook of Medicine, ed 17. Philadelphia, WB Saunders, 1985.
3. Brenner BM, Humes HD: Urinary tract obstruction. *In* Isselbacher KJ, Adams RD, Braunwald E, et al (eds): Harrison's Principles of Internal Medicine, ed 9. New York, McGraw-Hill, 1980.
4. Klahr S, Buerkert J, Morrison A: Urinary tract obstruction. *In* Brenner BM, Rector FC Jr (eds): The Kidney, ed 3. Philadelphia, WB Saunders, 1986.
5. Klahr S: Obstructive nephropathy. *In* Massry SG, Glassock RJ (eds): Massry and Glassock's Textbook of Nephrology, ed 3, vol 2. Baltimore, Williams & Wilkins, 1995.
6. Pak CYC: Renal calculi. *In* Wyngaarden JB, Smith LH (eds): Cecil Textbook of Medicine, ed 17. Philadelphia, WB Saunders, 1985.
7. Curhan GC, Zeidel ML: Urinary tract obstruction. *In* Brenner BM (ed): Brenner and Rector's The Kidney, ed 5, vol 2. Philadelphia, WB Saunders, 1996.
8. Wright FS, Howards SS: Obstructive injury. *In* Brenner BM, Rector FC Jr (eds): The Kidney, ed 2. Philadelphia, WB Saunders, 1981.
9. Muldowney FP: Obstructive nephropathy. *In* Beeson PB, McDermott W, Wyngaarden JB (eds): Cecil Textbook of Medicine, ed 15. Philadelphia, WB Saunders, 1979.
10. Boyd JC, Boyce WH: Obstructive nephropathy. *In* Conn RB (ed): Current Diagnosis, ed 7. Philadelphia, WB Saunders, 1985.
11. Yarger WE, Harris RH: Urinary tract obstruction. *In* Seldin DW, Giebisch G (eds): The Kidney: Physiology and Pathophysiology. New York, Raven Press, 1985.
12. Andreoli TE, Carpenter CCJ, Plum F, et al: Cecil Essentials of Medicine, ed 2. Philadelphia, WB Saunders, 1990.
13. Seifter JL, Brenner BM: Urinary tract obstruction. *In* Isselbacher KJ, Braunwald E, Wilson JD, et al (eds): Harrison's Principles of Internal Medicine, ed 13, vol 2. New York, McGraw-Hill, 1994.
14. Wilson DR, Klahr S: Urinary tract obstruction. *In* Schrier RW, Gottschalk CW (eds): Diseases of the Kidney, ed 5. Boston, Little, Brown & Co., 1993.
15. Klahr S: Obstructive uropathy. *In* Bennett JC, Plum F (eds): Cecil Textbook of Medicine, ed 20. Philadelphia, WB Saunders, 1996.
16. Whelton A, Watson AJ, Rock RC: Nitrogen metabolites and renal function. *In* Burtis CA, Ashwood ER (eds): Tietz Textbook of Clinical Chemistry, ed 2. Philadelphia, WB Saunders, 1994.
17. Schumann GB, Schweitzer SC: Examination of urine. *In* Henry BH: Clinical Diagnosis and Management by Laboratory Methods, ed 18. Philadelphia, WB Saunders, 1991.
18. Worcester EM, Lemann J: Nephrolithiasis. *In* Massry SG, Glassock RJ (eds): Massry and Glassock's Textbook of Nephrology, ed 3, vol 2. Baltimore, Williams & Wilkins, 1995.
19. Rowland RG, Garrett RA: Tumors of the ureter and urinary bladder. *In* Conn RB (ed): Current Diagnosis, ed 7. Philadelphia, WB Saunders, 1985.
20. Kassirer JP, Gennari FJ: Laboratory evaluation of renal function. *In* Earley LE, Gottschalk CW (eds): Strauss and Welt's Diseases of the Kidney, ed 3. Boston, Little, Brown & Co., 1979.
21. Dennis VW: Investigations of renal function. *In* Wyngaarden JB, Smith LH (eds): Cecil Textbook of Medicine, ed 17. Philadelphia, WB Saunders, 1985.
22. Stein MF: The kidney. *In* Taylor RB (ed): Family Medicine: Principles and Practice. New York City, Springer-Verlag, 1983.
23. Mandel, N: Urinary tract calculi. Lab Med 17:450–451, 1986.
24. Resnick MI, Freidland GW: Urinary stone disease. *In* Resnick MI, Older RA (eds): Diagnosis of Genitourinary Disease. New York, Thieme-Stratton, 1982.
25. Coe FL, Parks JH, Asplin JR: The pathogenesis and treatment of kidney stones. N Engl J Med 327:1141–1144, 1992.
26. Coe FL, Favus MJ: Nephrolithiasis. *In* Isselbacher KJ, Braunwald E, Wilson JD, et al (eds): Harrison's Principles of Internal Medicine, ed 13, vol 2. New York, McGraw-Hill, 1994.
27. Coe FL: Clinical and laboratory assessment of the patient with renal disease. *In* Brenner BM, Rector FC Jr (eds): The Kidney, ed 2. Philadelphia, WB Saunders, 1981.
28. Health and Public Policy Committee, American College of Physicians: Lithotripsy. Ann Intern Med 103:626, 1985.

Urinary Tract Infections

Lauren Roberts

The urinary tract is lined with a sheet of epithelium that is continuous with the skin, extending from the distal urethra to the calyces of the kidney. This epithelial surface serves as a potential pathway for the entry of microorganisms. Although the flushing of urine and sloughing of epithelial cells provide a protective measure for the urinary tract, microorganisms occasionally overcome these features, and infection results.[1] Infections of the urinary tract are the second most common infections in the United States, exceeded only by respiratory infections.

Urinary tract infection (UTI) refers to the presence of microorganisms in the urinary tract, whether in the bladder, prostate, ureters, or kidneys.[2] Acute infections are subdivided into two general anatomic categories, lower UTI and upper UTI. Lower UTIs involve the bladder (cystitis), urethra (urethritis), or prostate (prostatitis), whereas upper UTIs involve the renal parenchyma (pyelonephritis) or the ureters (ureteritis). All anatomic areas of the urinary tract are joined by a liquid medium; therefore, infection at any site may spread to involve other areas of the system. Uncomplicated UTIs occur in patients with a normal urinary tract structure; infections in patients with anatomic abnormalities, stones, or indwelling catheters are considered complicated infections.

The urinary tract is normally free of microorganisms, and under normal conditions, urine should be a sterile body fluid. The microorganisms involved in UTI are most commonly bacteria, although fungi, parasites, and viruses can be involved. The presence of bacteria in urine is referred to as *bacteriuria*, and the presence of white blood cells as *pyuria*. Urinary tract infections include a wide range of clinical entities, from asymptomatic bacteriuria to serious symptomatic infections that may result in septicemia, renal damage, and renal failure. These infections may be acute or chronic, and they may recur through relapse or reinfection.

ETIOLOGY AND PATHOPHYSIOLOGY
Mechanisms of Invasion

Infectious agents can gain access to and spread throughout the urinary tract by three routes: ascending route, hematogenous route, and lymphatic pathways.

The majority of infections, especially in women, occur by the ascending route.[3] The anatomy of the female urethra is of particular importance in the pathogenesis of urinary tract infection. Bacteria can reach the bladder more easily in females than in males, because the urethra is shorter, is in close proximity to the perirectal area, and is subjected to the massaging effect of sexual intercourse. Fecal flora colonize the vaginal area, the external periurethral area, and the distal urethra. These organisms can be easily inoculated into the short urethra and bladder following minor trauma during instrumentation or through sexual intercourse. Once the organism enters the bladder, it may extend via the ureter to the kidneys. This extension occurs in 30% to 50% of women with normal urinary anatomy, and it may be due to vesicoureteral reflex.[3] Infection in the kidney begins in the medulla and extends to the cortex and capsule of the kidney. Men are protected from ascending infection by the length of the urethra and by the antibacterial properties of prostatic secretions. Ascending infection associated with catheterization or other instrumentation is common in both sexes.

Infection by the hematogenous route is less common than by the ascending route but it is a significant pathway. These blood-borne infections result in renal abscesses rather than in ordinary UTI. Large volumes of blood flow through the kidney, and any systemic infection can seed this organ. Hematogenous pyelonephritis is more commonly found in patients with staphylococcal bacteremia or endocarditis, mycobacterial infection, or systemic infection with *Candida* species. Lymphatic flow can be directed toward the kidney because of increased pressure on the bladder. There is little evidence, however, that the lymphatic route plays a significant role in the pathogenesis of urinary tract infection, although it may contribute to prostatitis.[4]

Host Defense Mechanisms

The main defense mechanisms against infection of the urinary tract are attributed to the urinary bladder. The normal flow of urine and other anatomic factors are more important in the defense against UTI than cellular and humoral immunity. The primary defense mechanism of the bladder is the act of voiding. The constant flushing of urine from the body, and its dilution with newly formed urine, efficiently eliminates bacteria or keeps their numbers low. The bladder mucosa also provides defense against infection by a poorly understood intrinsic mechanism that prevents bacterial multiplication in the thin film of urine residing on the bladder mucosa after voiding.[5]

In addition, the antimicrobial properties of urine are important in preventing the multiplication of organisms. Urine is inhibitory to anaerobes and other fastidious organisms that constitute the normal flora of the urethral mucosa. Even bacteria that are known to multiply in urine are inhibited when exposed to the low pH and high osmolarity. Other nonbladder defense mechanisms are cervicovaginal antibodies that prevent colonization of typical uropathogens, antibacterial properties found in prostatic fluid, and normal flora of the periurethral area that may inhibit growth of coliform bacteria.[3]

Microbial Virulence Factors

In spite of the defense mechanisms of the host, some microorganisms possess specific virulence mechanisms that enable them to overcome the host factors, and infection can result. Urinary tract infections are usually endogenous infections, because they develop from bacteria in the patient's fecal flora. One of the most important bacterial factors contributing to UTI is adherence, or the ability of the organism to stick to the mucosa of the urinary tract.[6] Adhesion to epithelial cells ensures that the organism will not be removed by the flow of urine. Adherence of bacteria is a specific binding process that involves adhesins (bacterial surface structures) and receptor molecules on vaginal or uroepithelial cells. The most common adhesins involved in attachment are fimbriae or pili.

Once the bacterial attachment takes place, other virulence factors are involved. Most uropathogens that cause pyelonephritis produce hemolysin, have siderophores for scavenging iron, and are resistant to the bactericidal action of human serum. Other contributing factors are capsular polysaccharide, endotoxin, and calculi formation.

Epidemiology and Predisposing Factors

Because the microorganisms that are usually responsible for causing UTIs are a part of the patient's normal flora,

the epidemiology of UTIs are related to factors in the host that make infection possible. All individuals are susceptible to UTIs, but the prevalence varies with age, sex, and certain predisposing factors. Infections can begin as early as the first few days of life and may continue throughout life. The incidence of infection peaks at certain times during life and is affected by both age and sex (Table 19–1).

The prevalence of bacteriuria in the newborn is 1% to 2%, and infections in this age group are often associated with life-threatening gram-negative sepsis. A septic or febrile infant who fails to thrive should be evaluated for a possible UTI. In the first year of life, bacteriuria is more common in males than in females, and such infections are often associated with abnormalities in the urinary tract.[7]

Symptomatic infections in preschool children are more common in girls and are often associated with congenital anomalies of the urinary tract. Most of the renal damage that occurs from a UTI is thought to occur during this period. Vesicoureteral reflux is a functional impairment and is associated with UTIs in girls during the first 5 years of life.[8] In this condition, reflux of urine occurs from the bladder into the ureters and possibly into the renal pelvis. Contaminated urine is introduced into these sterile tissues, and thus, the potential for infection is great. The prevalence of bacteriuria in school-age girls is approximately 1%. Approximately 5% of all girls have at least one episode of UTI prior to completion of high school.[8]

Urinary tract infection is the most common infection among adult women, accounting for 5 million outpatient visits each year in the United States. The onset of UTI often coincides with the beginning of sexual activity in women. Approximately 20% of women have at least one episode of dysuria each year. Some of these infections resolve spontaneously, although many patients may become reinfected. The uses of a diaphragm and spermicidal agents raise the risk of infection, because they alter the normal vaginal flora and are associated with an increase in vaginal colonization with *Escherichia coli*.

The prevalence of bacteriuria during pregnancy varies from 2% to 8%, depending on the age, parity, and socioeconomic status of the patient. Pregnant women with a history of UTI during childhood are more likely to have bacteriuria during pregnancy. Changes in the urinary tract during the later stages of pregnancy can allow any bacteria in the urine easy access to invasion of the kidney, leading to symptomatic pyelonephritis. Thus, undetected asymptomatic bacteriuria in pregnant women is of great concern, because 20% to 30% develop pyelonephritis. Pyelonephri-

Table 19–1. Incidence of Urinary Tract Infection

Age Group	Incidence (%)	
	Females	*Males*
Newborn	1	1–2
Preschool	4–5	0.5
School-age	10–20	<1
Young adult	20–35	1–3
Elderly	15–30	15–30

tis during pregnancy is associated with increases in newborn mortality and prematurity.

From the age of 1 year to 50 years, the incidence of UTI is far greater in females than in males. Bacteriuria in men is uncommon until they reach the age at which prostatic obstruction is common. Impaired bladder emptying and seeding of the urine with organisms from the prostate can result in persistent or recurrent infection. After age 70 years, the incidence of infection in men approaches or exceeds that in women. In elderly patients, the incidence of UTI rises in both sexes. Predisposing factors in this population include catheterization or instrumentation, obstruction, poor bladder emptying, stroke, dementia, and cardiovascular disorders.

The most common cause of hospital-acquired UTI is catheterization. The risk of infection from a single catheterization is 1% in ambulatory patients and up to 10% for bedridden patients. Drainage of indwelling catheters into an open system leads to bacteriuria in more than 90% of patients after 4 days. The use of a closed system reduces the risk of infection significantly.[9]

Despite treatment with antimicrobial agents, urinary tract infections can be recurrent. *Reinfection* or *recurrence*, which refers to the reappearance of infection due to a different organism, can occur any time after treatment has concluded for the previous infection. *Relapse* refers to a recurrence of infection with the same organism as originally isolated and usually occurs shortly after cessation of therapy. Relapse indicates persistence of the organism in the urinary tract and may be associated with an anatomic abnormality such as an obstruction. Reinfection indicates infection with a new pathogen and can occur any time after treatment is stopped. Occasionally, a patient may become reinfected with the same organism; thus, it is not always possible to distinguish between a relapse and a reinfection. *Chronic urinary tract infection* describes multiple relapses of infection in a patient over months or years.

Causative Agents

The majority of urinary tract infections are caused by bacteria, especially facultative gram-negative bacilli of the family Enterobacteriaceae. *E. coli* is responsible for more than 80% of acute uncomplicated infections in the outpatient population.[10] It is isolated less often, however, in specimens from outpatients with recurrent infections, or from hospitalized patients. Other gram-negative bacilli, including *Proteus mirabilis,* and members of the *Klebsiella-Enterobacter* group, along with gram-positive cocci, are responsible for the remainder of infections in outpatients. The same organisms are responsible for infection in hospitalized patients, but the frequency changes, with more resistant isolates being found. This difference is due to catheterization, the use of broad-spectrum antimicrobial agents, and the overall immune status of the patient. Although *E. coli* remains the most common cause of infection in hospitalized patients, the frequency is less than 50%, and *P. mirabilis, Klebsiella-Enterobacter* group, and other Enterobacteriaceae are more significant. In addition, *Pseudomonas aeruginosa* and *Enterococcus* species are rarely found in outpatients, except for nursing home patients,

but they are common isolates in the hospital environment (Table 19–2).

The majority of infections are due to gram-negative bacilli, but gram-positive cocci can play a significant role as nosocomial agents and in certain nonhospitalized patients. *Enterococcus* species are a growing cause of nosocomial infections, especially in catheterized males. *Enterococcus faecalis* is an important pathogen of prostatitis, causing relapsing urinary tract infections. *Staphylococcus aureus,* less commonly found, is associated with urinary tract obstruction, neoplasm, or manipulation. The presence of *S. aureus* in urine is often an indication of a hematogenous renal infection, and its isolation should prompt an evaluation for a potential bacteremia. *Staphylococcus saprophyticus* accounts for 10% to 15% of acute cystitis in young, sexually active females in the United States. Other coagulase-negative staphylococci that are found as normal flora in the vaginal, perineal area, and urethra cause infection in patients with predisposing factors that allow these bacteria to colonize the bladder. *Streptococcus agalactiae* (group B streptococci) is an uncommon cause of UTIs, although it can result in such an infection during pregnancy in a colonized woman.

Other, less common isolates from the urinary tract are anaerobes, sexually transmitted pathogens, *Mycobacterium* species, and yeast. Anaerobic bacteria are found as normal flora in the distal urethra, vagina, and the intestines. These bacteria are rarely involved in urinary tract infections. Anaerobes may play a role in complicated infections, and if aerobic cultures are negative, a suprapubic bladder aspirate may be analyzed. Acute urethral syndrome is another type of urinary tract infection found primarily in young, sexually active women. *Chlamydia trachomatis, Neisseria gonorrhoeae, Ureaplasma urealyticum,* herpes simplex virus, and other sexually transmitted agents can be associated with this infection. *Mycobacterium tuberculosis* is rarely found in the urinary tract, but its presence indicates a hematogenous spread. Funguria is also a rare type of urinary tract infection; the most common organisms are yeasts, primarily *Candida albicans* and *Torulopsis glabrata.* Yeasts can gain entrance to the bladder in catheterization, but their presence can also indicate a hematogenous infection. The parasites *Trichomonas vaginalis* and *Schistosoma haematobium* can also be detected in urine. *Trichomonas vaginalis* is a sexually transmitted pathogen that can be associated with urinary frequency and dysuria. *Schisto-*

Table 19–2. Causative Agents in Urinary Tract Infections

Organism	Rate of Infection (%)	
	Outpatients	**Hospitalized Patients**
Escherichia coli	80–85	30–40
Proteus species	3–5	15–20
Klebsiella and *Enterobacter* species	2–3	10–15
Staphylococcus saprophyticus	10–12	0
Enterococcus species	1–2	10–15
Pseudomonas aeruginosa	0	10–15
Other	1–2	10

soma haemotobium is a bladder fluke that releases its eggs into urine.

CLINICAL MANIFESTATIONS

Asymptomatic Bacteriuria; Bacteriuria with Nonspecific Symptoms

Because the clinical manifestations of urinary tract infections are quite variable, they cannot be relied upon to accurately diagnose infection or to localize the site, and many patients may be asymptomatic. Asymptomatic bacteriuria is most problematic in young children, pregnant women, and the elderly. In children younger than 2 years, UTIs manifest as nonspecific symptoms, including fever, poor feeding, and vomiting. Pregnant women with asymptomatic bacteriuria are at risk for developing serious infection and obstetric complications. As in young children, UTIs in the elderly are often asymptomatic, and when symptoms are present, they are often nonspecific. Because of the potential for ascending infection in these populations, the presence of such nonspecific symptoms warrant an evaluation.

Lower Urinary Tract Infection

Lower UTIs are urethritis, cystitis, and prostatitis. Urethritis without cystitis is most commonly associated with sexually transmitted agents and is characterized by painful urination and the presence of a purulent discharge from the urethral opening. Acute urethral syndrome is a UTI found in young, sexually active women who experience dysuria (burning upon urination), frequency, and urgency. Urine culture for these patients does not usually yield a significant number of bacteria—$<10^5$ CFU/mL (colony-forming units per mL)—but pyuria is present. Patients with cystitis experience pain, dysuria, and increased frequency of urination. Cystitis has a more acute onset and more severe symptoms than are experienced with urethritis. These symptoms are caused by the inflammation of the mucosa in the lower urinary tract due to infection. Some patients may notice hematuria or turbid urine that is malodorous. Pain and tenderness in the suprapubic area may also be noted; however, fever and other systemic symptoms are not present if the infection is limited to the lower urinary tract.

Upper Urinary Tract Infection

In contrast to cystitis, upper UTI or pyelonephritis is an invasive infection that leads to flank pain and fever that exceeds 38.5 °C (101 °F). These manifestations are due to inflammation of the renal pelvis and parenchyma. The signs and symptoms have an acute onset, and in addition to fever and pain, chills, headache, nausea, and vomiting may be present. Symptoms of cystitis are not always reported; if they do occur, they may be present a few days before the systemic symptoms, or they may develop at the same time. Rigors and tachycardia are present in the severely ill patients and often indicate bacteremia.

Prostatitis

Acute bacterial prostatitis is a common cause of urinary tract infections in males. It is a febrile illness associated with pain in the lower back and perirectal area. Cystitis symptoms, that is, dysuria and frequency, may occur and inflammatory swelling of the prostate gland can lead to urinary obstruction.[4] Acute prostatitis is typically found in young adults, but it can follow catheterization in older men. Chronic prostatitis is a common cause of relapsing urinary tract infections. Patients with chronic bacterial prostatitis may be asymptomatic, with normal prostate glands, or they may experience urgency and frequency with back pain and a low-grade fever[4] (Table 19–3).

LABORATORY ANALYSES AND DIAGNOSIS

Urine laboratory studies are essential tools in the diagnosis of UTI and are important in screening asymptomatic individuals who are at high risk of developing significant complications from a UTI. Laboratory testing usually consists of routine urinalysis, assessment of pyuria and bacteriuria, and quantitative urine cultures. Methods to distinguish between upper and lower UTI, or localization techniques, may also be performed to assist the physician in the management of patients with UTIs. A microbiologic evaluation of urine is warranted for patients with acute symptoms of infection, bacteremia of unknown source, or prostatitis, for follow-up after catheter removal, and after treatment of UTI. In an outpatient setting, when symptoms of dysuria and frequency are present, or if blood and protein are found in the urine of otherwise healthy individuals, microbiology

Table 19–3. Clinical Manifestations and Etiology of Urinary Tract Infections

	Cystitis	Urethritis	Prostatitis	Pyelonephritis
Symptoms	Asymptomatic, internal dysuria, frequency, hematuria	Internal dysuria, frequency, discharge	Asymptomatic, fever, chills, back pain	Asymptomatic, fever, chills, flank pain, nausea
Organisms	*Escherichia coli* Other Enterobacteriaceae *Staphylococcus saprophyticus*	*E. coli* *Chlamydia trachomatis* *Neisseria gonorrhoeae* *Trichomonas vaginalis* Herpes simplex virus *S. saprophyticus*	Enterobacteriaceae *C. trachomatis* *Ureaplasma urealyticum*	Enterobacteriaceae *Staphylococcus aureus* Coagulase-negative staphylococci *Myobacterium* species *Mycoplasma hominis* *Candida* species

studies may not be performed before treatment is initiated. Proper evaluation of the specimen by the microbiology laboratory requires information about the method of collection, clinical diagnosis, and antimicrobial therapy.

Specimen Collection and Transport

Appropriate specimen collection and transport are critical to the accurate examination of a urine sample. A voided urine specimen is the easiest sample to obtain, but it is invariably contaminated by bacteria from the urethra, vagina, and perianal areas. The clean-voided midstream urine collection procedure is the least invasive method of specimen collection. In this method, the number of contaminants is reduced through cleansing the periurethral area before voiding. Further contaminants are flushed from the urethra by discarding the first portion of urine and then collecting a specimen. Because the laboratory results are greatly affected by the collection technique, patient education is extremely important, and detailed instructions must be provided.

Urinary catheterization is a more invasive procedure but obtains bladder urine with less urethral colonization. The process of catheterization, however, may introduce urethral organisms into the bladder, thereby causing further problems. Suprapubic bladder aspiration yields the least contaminated specimen, but it is the most invasive technique. This procedure is recommended in patients for whom the interpretation of results from voided urine is difficult, such as infants and small children.

First-morning specimens are recommended, because the urine has been incubating in the bladder overnight, and the bacterial count will be most accurate. The urine should be cultured within 2 hours of collection, or should be refrigerated immediately and cultured within 24 hours.[11] If urine specimens are collected in transport tubes with preservatives, refrigeration is not necessary. Specimens in preservative tubes should be processed within 24 hours.

Specimen Screening

Urine specimens are one of the most common samples processed in the clinical microbiology laboratory, and culture of as many as 60% to 80% of these specimens may be negative for significant bacteria.[12] In order to provide quality, cost-effective patient care, laboratories attempt to process these specimens in a timely and cost-effective fashion. Culture methods are time-consuming; therefore, a rapid screen test to identify urine specimens for which culture will be negative may be indicated. Rapid elimination of negative specimens is cost effective, because it prevents excessive use of media and technologist time, and provides same-day results from negative specimens. Screening tests should not be used indiscriminantly, however. Specimens from hospitalized patients with UTI symptoms, patients at risk of asymptomatic bacteriuria, and specimens collected by straight catheterization, cystoscopy, or suprapubic aspiration should be cultured.

Urine specimens can also be screened for indications of infection by detection of bacteriuria and pyuria. Screening methods for detection of bacteriuria and pyuria include microscopic, chemical, and automated techniques. If chem-

ical testing (described later) does not suggest the possibility of infection, the more labor-intensive microscopic examinations are often not performed unless warranted by special circumstances. Gram staining is a rapid and reliable procedure for the detection of significant bacteriuria. The presence of at least one organism per oil immersion field in a drop of uncentrifuged, well-mixed urine correlates with 10^5 CFU/mL. The presence of squamous epithelial cells and different microbial morphologies usually indicates contamination. Gram staining, however, does not reliably detect bacteriuria below the rate of 10^5 CFU/mL. Gram stains are not performed routinely on all urine specimens because of the low number of positive results, but they should be available upon request. A positive result provides the Gram reaction and morphology of the organism, thus guiding the clinician in the selection of appropriate empiric antimicrobial therapy.

Another microscopic examination that can be an indicator of UTI is screening for white blood cells (WBCs) (pyuria). Patients with a UTI usually excrete more than 400,000 WBCs per hour into their urine; the presence of 8 to 10 or more WBCs per μL of uncentrifuged urine correlates with this WBC excretion rate. The most precise method for measuring this parameter is the examination of a fresh, uncentrifuged urine specimen in a hemocytometer chamber. This method, however is time consuming and is not practical for incorporation into most microbiology laboratories. The quantity of WBCs is often estimated from the routine urinalysis examination of the centrifuged sediment of urine. Unfortunately, these results are far less accurate and reproducible than the hemocytometer method. Accurate measurement of urine volume, standard centrifuge speed and time, and consistent counting techniques can help to improve the use of the routine microscopic examination of urinary sediment.[13]

Several chemical tests are available as dipsticks to measure parameters that may indicate UTI. Common enzyme tests for the detection of bacteriuria and pyuria are nitrate reductase (Griess' test), and leukocyte esterase. Chemstrip, a combination test containing leukocyte esterase and nitrite, has a sensitivity beyond that of either test alone. The tube enzyme catalase test and colorimetric filtration with safranin O dye are methods that detect both bacteria and the extracellular products of WBCs.[14, 15] Chemical tests should not be used alone because of false-positive and false-negative results. False-negative results can occur because the concentration of enzyme present is lower than the detection threshold of the method employed. For this reason, urine to be tested should be allowed to incubate in the bladder overnight, or for at least 4 hours, to increase the concentration of enzyme being tested for.

Automated methodologies have also been developed for screening urine specimens. Bioluminescence systems detect bacterial adenosine triphosphate (ATP) by measuring light emitted by the reaction of luciferin and luciferase. These luminescent tests are expensive, usually require batching of specimens, and therefore may not be performed soon enough to contribute to diagnosis and treatment; they are not widely used. Other systems measure growth through photometric methods. If a significant number of organisms are present in the urine, rapid growth is detected in the substrate wells within 6 to 8 hours. These systems may not detect low counts of bacteria or yeast, however, and their sensitivity is less than optimum.

Quantitative Culture

The confirmation of a UTI is based on the documentation of bacteriuria through culture. Quantitative urine cultures were developed to distinguish simple contaminants introduced during collection from actual infection of the urinary tract. The premise of this method was that contaminants are usually found in small numbers and are nonpathogenic organisms that constitute the normal flora, whereas the true uropathogen is usually present in large numbers. The calibrated loop method is the technique most widely used for quantitating bacteria in urine. This technique is a semiquantitative method, and several variables affect its accuracy. It is still the most practical and widely used culture method for bacteriuria, however.

Early studies indicated that detecting more than 10^5 bacteria per mL of voided urine was indicative of infection. Thus, a urine colony count of 10^5 CFU/mL or higher was adopted as the diagnostic standard for significant bacteriuria. Although this threshold can be applied to the majority of specimens for urine culture, it soon became apparent that it was not applicable in all cases, and that lower colony counts were "significant" in certain populations. Patients with true UTIs whose urine may yield lower colony counts include infants and children, males, and catheterized patients. Other factors that may contribute to low bacterial counts, are early infection, dilute urine due to forced fluids, rapid urine flow, acute urethral syndrome, and use of antimicrobial agents. There has been a great deal of controversy over the interpretation of urine colony counts, and later guidelines address the variations in significant bacteriuria associated with certain clinical conditions and methods of specimen collection (Table 19–4).

The following list is an overview of the interpretive criteria for voided urine specimens:

- Growth of more than 10^5 CFU/mL of one or two uropathogens should be considered clinically significant, and the laboratory should identify the organism(s) and perform antimicrobial susceptibility testing.
- One or two uropathogens in small numbers ($\geq 10^2$ CFU/mL) should be identified, and the culture plates should

be held for 2 to 3 days in case the physician requests further evaluation.
- Growth of more than two species in a specimen usually indicates contamination, and the laboratory should report multiple species present, with no identification.

A variety of commercial culture methods, such as dipsticks and dipslides, are available and are used primarily in the physician's office. These methods are not recommended for use in diagnostic laboratories, where transport of specimens is readily available. These devices make it possible for physicians to rule out negative specimens and submit positive results to a diagnostic laboratory for identification and antimicrobial susceptibility testing. They are not accurate colony counts below 10^3 CFU/mL, however, so they should not be used when there is a possibility of low-count bacteriuria (10^2 CFU/mL). Use of these techniques may be necessary when transport to a laboratory is delayed and refrigeration is not available.

Certain culture methods should not be employed for processing urine specimens in the microbiology laboratory, because they lead to inaccurate or unreliable results. They include inoculation of the urine directly into a broth culture medium, culture of urine sediment, culture of voided or catheterized urine specimens for anaerobes, performing antimicrobial susceptibility testing directly from the urine, and culturing of Foley catheter tips.[11]

Localization of Infection

Characteristic symptoms may be helpful in distinguishing between upper and lower urinary tract infection, but unfortunately, the distinction is not always clear. Definitive methods of determining the location of infection are ureteral catheterization and the bladder washout technique. The complexity and invasiveness of these procedures, however, prevent their use in routine clinical practice. The antibody-coated bacteria technique is less invasive than these other methods, but a lack of standardization and available reagents has lead to confusion in the interpretation of results.[16] A more practical approach for identifying the location of infection is the response to single-dose therapy. After single-dose therapy, the concentration of antimicrobials present in the urine is usually sufficient to

Table 19–4. Interpretive Guidelines and Suggested Laboratory Work-Up For Urine Cultures

Colony Count (CFU/mL)	Clinical Situation or Urine Source	No. of Organisms	Suggested Work-Up
0		None	None
$\geq 10^2$	Symptomatic female, urethritis	Pure culture	Identification and antimicrobial susceptibility testing
$\geq 10^2$	Suprapubic bladder aspirate	All species	Identification and antimicrobial susceptibility testing
$\geq 10^3$	Symptomatic male, catheter urine	Pure culture or 2 species of probable pathogen	Identification and antimicrobial susceptibility testing
$\geq 10^4$	Catheter urine	Pure culture or 2 species of probable pathogens	Identification and antimicrobial susceptibility testing
		≥ 3 species	No work-up; report multiple species present
$\geq 10^5$	Voided urine	Pure culture or two species of probable pathogens in symptomatic patient	Identification and antimicrobial susceptibility testing
		≥ 3 species	No work-up; report multiple species present

cure cystitis but is not usually adequate to treat renal infection, and a relapse will occur.[17]

The presence of WBC casts may indicate pyelonephritis. Nonspecific indicators of inflammation that may accompany acute pyelonephritis include C-reactive protein, an elevated sedimentation rate, urinary β_2-microglobulin, and antibodies to Tamm-Horsfall protein.

TREATMENT

Many antimicrobial agents are effective in the treatment of UTI. The goal of therapy is to eradicate the organism from the urinary tract, to relieve symptoms, and to prevent further spread of infection and renal damage. The ideal antimicrobial agent should be the least toxic, least expensive agent that is effective, and it should be administered for a long enough period to eradicate the infection. Following culture, antimicrobial susceptibility testing should be used to select therapy. Generally, uncomplicated infections of the lower urinary tract respond to low doses and short courses of therapy, whereas upper urinary tract infections require longer treatment.

Treatment of uncomplicated lower UTI requires achieving an inhibitory concentration of antimicrobial agent in the urine, not in the plasma or tissue. Some agents that are used to treat cystitis do not achieve inhibitory concentrations in blood or tissue, but they are excreted in high concentrations in urine. Most cases of community-acquired cystitis are due to bacteria that are relatively sensitive to antibacterial agents. Single-dose therapy has been shown to be effective in patients with acute cystitis and no known complicating factors. It is appropriate in patients with an acute onset of lower urinary tract symptoms, but no signs of upper tract involvement and who can be monitored with follow-up.[18] Single-dose therapy is advantageous because of fewer side effects, better patient compliance, relatively low cost, and less chance of developing bacterial resistance. The agents utilized in single-dose therapy are cefadroxil, trimethoprim-sulfamethoxazole, norfloxacin, and ciprofloxacin. In some areas, approximately 30% of *E. coli* strains are resistant to amoxicillin; therefore, lower cure rates are observed when ampicillin or amoxicillin is prescribed.

The potential disadvantage of single-dose therapy is a higher rate of relapse and a higher incidence of pyelonephritis if an upper urinary tract infection is present. Relapses occur with single-dose therapy, because the therapy is not effective in eliminating the pathogen from the vaginal area. The use of 3-day treatment has been more effective in eliminating relapses. Sulfonamides and trimethoprim either alone or in combination, fluoroquinolones, and nitrofurantoin are the agents most commonly used for a 3-day regimen. Short-course (3-day) therapy should be utilized for treatment of patients with no known complicating factors. Therapy must be prolonged to treat cystitis in children, pregnant women, men, diabetic patients, and immunocompromised hosts.

Patients experiencing acute pyelonephritis often require hospitalization and are preferably treated with bactericidal agents. In acute, uncomplicated pyelonephritis, a 2-week course of therapy is usually effective. The choice of oral or intravenous therapy depends on the severity of the infection. Patients with structural abnormalities or obstruction may require surgery and prolonged therapy.

Patients with acute bacterial prostatitis respond promptly to antimicrobial therapy, which usually lasts 2 to 4 weeks. Chronic prostatitis is more difficult to treat, because the chronically inflamed prostate does not allow rapid diffusion of antimicrobial into the prostatic fluid. Patients with chronic prostatitis often require 6 to 12 weeks of therapy.

In asymptomatic patients with bacteriuria, the decision to treat is based on the potential for further complication. Treatment for asymptomatic bacteriuria is important in three groups of patients: children, pregnant women, and patients who are about to undergo instrumentation of the urinary tract. All symptomatic patients should be treated, regardless of age. Bacteriuria should disappear or should be greatly reduced within 48 hours of therapy. If bacteria persist, they are most likely resistant to the antimicrobial agent. It is sometimes possible to demonstrate moderate resistance with antimicrobial susceptibility testing, even though the clinical disease seems to have responded to therapy. The reason is that most antimicrobials are excreted in the urine, and the concentrations are much higher than those used in antimicrobial susceptibility testing. If the patient's symptoms have not responded, however, the antimicrobial should be changed.

Except in patients with simple cystitis, repeat urine cultures should be performed 48 hours after initiation of therapy and 1 to 2 weeks after treatment is completed. The 48-hour follow-up culture determines the efficacy of the therapy, and a follow-up culture performed after therapy has ended can detect a relapse.

Case Study

A 23-year-old woman presented to her physician with complaints of dysuria, urgency, and increased frequency. These symptoms had appeared early that morning. She immediately recognized them as signs of cystitis, because this was her fourth experience in the past year. It had been 3 months since she had completed therapy from her last urinary tract infection.

Physical examination revealed an otherwise healthy female with suprapubic pain but no flank pain or fever. The patient had no history of childhood UTIs, kidney stones, diabetes, or urologic abnormalities. Laboratory results from her first two episodes demonstrated *E. coli* with colony counts between 10^2 and 10^5 CFU/mL. Her previous infection was due to *S. saprophyticus*.

A routine urinalysis demonstrated positive nitrite and leukocyte esterase tests and a microscopic examination of centrifuged urine sediment contained 20 to 25 WBC/HPF (per high power field). A urine culture was performed, and *P. mirabilis* was isolated, with a colony count of 70,000 CFU/mL.

Questions

1. What is the probable diagnosis?
2. When there is a recurrence of UTI, what is the difference between relapse and reinfection?

3. Are further urologic studies indicated in this patient?
4. What forms of therapy are recommended in this patient?

Discussion

1. This case illustrates an example of recurrent urinary tract infection in a young female. Many women experience an occasional episode of cystitis, but in some, recurrent episodes occur with a frequency of three or more per year. This patient's symptoms were indicative of infection confined to the lower urinary tract. Other clinical conditions that must be included in the differential diagnosis are subclinical pyelonephritis, chlamydial urethritis, vaginitis, and dysuria without urinary tract or vaginal infection.

2. Recurrent UTIs may be either a relapse or a reinfection. A relapse usually occurs shortly after completion of antimicrobial therapy, and it is usually due to the same strain of bacteria that originally caused the infection. Reinfection, on the other hand, may be caused by the same organism or by a different organism, and it can occur any time after therapy is stopped.

3. This patient was experiencing reinfection of the urinary tract, because different bacteria were involved. In some women who are prone to recurrent UTIs the density of bacterial receptors on epithelial cells is greater than normal. In these patients, an increasing number of fecal bacteria colonize the introitus and work their way into the urinary bladder, often during sexual intercourse. Reinfection does not indicate an anatomic abnormality, and urologic studies are not indicated.

4. When patients experience reinfection, the major goal should be to interrupt the cycle of colonization of the introitus that leads to infection of the bladder. Females with a propensity for frequent reinfection may be treated with antimicrobial prophylaxis. The following three strategies can be employed: (a) continuous low-dose prophylaxis is recommended for women who experience 3 or more infections per year; (b) self-administered single-dose therapy is utilized in patients who experience 2 to 3 infections per year; (c) postcoital antimicrobial prophylaxis is administered to patients who relate their infections to sexual activity. The patient in this case was treated with long-term antimicrobial prophylaxis, and she did well, with no further recurrences.

References

1. Barza M: Urinary tract. *In* Schaechter M, Medoff G, Schlessinger D (eds): Mechanisms of Microbial Disease. Baltimore, Williams & Wilkins, 1989.
2. Johnson CC: Definitions, classification, and clinical presentation of urinary tract infection. Med Clin North Am 75:241–252, 1991.
3. Brucker PC: Urinary tract infections. Primary Care 17:825–832, 1990.
4. Meares EM: Bacterial prostatitis. *In* Hoeprich PD, Jordan MC, Ronald AR (eds): Infectious Diseases, ed 5. Philadelphia, JB Lippincott, 1994.
5. Ronald AR: Urethritis and cystitis. *In* Hoeprich PD, Jordan MC, Ronald AR (eds): Infectious Diseases, ed 5. Philadelphia, JB Lippincott, 1994.
6. Plorde JJ: Urinary tract infections. *In* Ryan KJ (ed): Sherris Medical Microbiology, ed 3. Norwalk, CT, Appleton & Lange, 1994.
7. Thomas JG: Urinary tract infections. *In* Mahon CR, Manuselis G (eds): Textbook of Diagnostic Microbiology. Philadelphia, WB Saunders, 1995.
8. Stamm WE: Urinary Tract Infections. *In* Gorbach SL, Bartlett JG, Blacklow NR (eds): Infectious Disease. Philadelphia, WB Saunders, 1992.
9. Andriole VT: Pyelonephritis. *In* Hoeprich PD, Jordan MC, Ronald AR (eds): Infectious Diseases, ed 5. Philadelphia, JB Lippincott, 1994.
10. Stamm WE: Urinary tract infections and pyelonephritis. *In* Isselbacher KJ, Braunwald E, Wilson, JD et al (eds): Harrison's Principles of Internal Medicine, ed 13. New York, McGraw-Hill, 1994.
11. Pezzlo M: Urine culture procedure. *In* Isenberg HD (ed): Clinical Microbiology Procedures Handbook. Washington, DC, American Society for Microbiology, 1992.
12. Baron EJ, Peterson LR, Finegold SM: Bailey & Scott's Diagnostic Microbiology, ed 9. St Louis, CV Mosby, 1994.
13. Pappas PG: Laboratory in the diagnosis and management of urinary tract infections. Med Clin North Am 75:314, 1991.
14. Pezzlo M: Detection of urinary tract infections by rapid methods. Clin Microbiol Rev 1:268, 1988.
15. Pezzlo MT, Amsterdam D, Anhalt JP, et al. Detection of bacteriuria and pyuria by URISCREEN, a rapid enzymatic screening test. J Clin Microbiol 30:680–684, 1992.
16. Thomas VL: The antibody-coated bacteria test: Uses and findings. Lab Management 21:132, 1983.
17. Stamm WE: Urinary tract infections and pyelonephritis. *In* Isselbacher KJ, Braunwald E, Wilson JD, Martin JB, et al (eds): Harrison's Principles of Internal Medicine, ed 15. New York, McGraw-Hill, 1994.
18. Sheehan G, Harding GKM, Ronald AR: Advances in the treatment of urinary tract infection. Am J Med 76:141, 1984.

Gastrointestinal Disorders

Chapter **20**

Ulcers

Douglas W. Estry and David P. Thorne

Until recently, the role of the clinical laboratory in the diagnosis of ulcer diseases has been relatively obscure and, at best, difficult to define. This lack of focus is because historically, a large variety of factors (environmental and pathophysiologic) appeared to contribute to the development of gastritis and ulcers. However, in 1983, following the description by Warren and Marshall[1] of gram-negative curved bacilli on the gastric mucosa, physicians and clinical laboratory scientists began to focus on an infectious disease process as a major causative factor. As a result of this significant change in the understanding of the etiology

of gastric inflammation and peptic ulcers, it is now possible to reclassify these disorders, with only a few exceptions, as related to the following conditions: (1) the use of nonsteroidal anti-inflammatory drugs (NSAIDs), (2) infection with *Helicobacter pylori*, or (3) Zollinger-Ellison syndrome (Z-E).

The development of gastritis or peptic ulcer disease is predicated on a breakdown of the normal gastric defense mechanisms. At the surface of the gastric mucosa, these defense mechanisms include the mucous layer secreted by gastric epithelial cells and the secreted bicarbonate, which is normally responsive to changes in gastric acidity.[2] In addition, the normal ability of the gastric epithelium to undergo rapid repair following injury and to maintain intracellular pH and transmembrane ion exchange constitute critical defense mechanisms.[3, 4] Finally, the maintenance of normal gastric blood flow and vascular pH is important. The latter factor plays a central role in the potential development of ischemic injury and the delivery of cellular mediators of the inflammatory response, and it affects the ability of the cell to regulate ion exchange and the normal intracellular environment.

GASTRITIS

Gastritis is a multipurpose term that has been applied to both trivial and more severe gastric inflammatory disorders. As used in this chapter, the term gastritis is confined to a more limited scope of problems having specific histologic and pathophysiologic consequences.

Gastritis can be classified as either acute or chronic. Although overlap occurs within the parameters that differentiate acute from chronic gastritis, general characteristics define the various stages in the gastric inflammatory process. The acute inflammatory response is characterized by a transient mucosal inflammation.[5] The process has been related to a variety of etiologic agents commonly implicated in gastric inflammation and ulcer formation. Acute gastritis is characterized by neutrophilic infiltration and clinical manifestations that range from virtually no symptoms to epigastric pain, nausea, acute abdominal pain, and hematemesis or melena.

Strickland and Mackay[6] defined two types of chronic gastritis. Type A, an autoimmune type, involves the fundus-body of the stomach and is characterized by antiparietal antibodies, increased gastrin, and hypochlorhydria or achlorhydria. A second type, type B, involves the antral portion of the stomach, is not characterized by the presence of antiparietal antibodies, is much more common than type A, and has a less clearly defined etiology. This type of gastritis has often been associated with gastric mucosal changes that accompany infections with *H. pylori*. A third type of chronic gastritis, proposed by Glass and Pitchumoni[7], is characterized by patchy areas of gastric inflammation, atrophy in both the antrum and body of the stomach, intestinal metaplasia, and an increased risk of gastric ulceration and carcinoma. This type is referred to as type AB.[7]

In 1991, further clarifying the classification of gastritis, Misiewicz[8] proposed the "Sydney system." This system is based on the use of five variables (inflammation, neutrophil activity, glandular atrophy, intestinal metaplasia, and *H. pylori* density), each of which is graded on a four-point scale (absent/normal, mild, moderate, or severe).

PEPTIC ULCERATION

Peptic ulceration is a localized lesion in the mucous membrane of the stomach, duodenum, or esophagus. Many instances of ulceration are associated with increased acid output; however, changes in blood flow and ion transport are also important contributing factors. The onset and progression of peptic ulcer development is dependent on a variety of factors overcoming normal host defenses.[9] These factors include the following:

1. Breakdown of the gastric mucosal barrier, with resulting back-diffusion of hydrochloric acid into the mucosa
2. Failure of intracellular metabolism to maintain normal ionic equilibrium
3. Local ischemia of the mucosa with necrosis
4. Failure of bicarbonate and mucus secretions to buffer the affected area

Peptic ulcers are associated with deep invasion of the mucosal lining and are therefore of primary clinical importance. The peptic ulcer has a defined border, from 1 to 3 cm in diameter and is located in the stomach or, more frequently, in the duodenum. In addition, peptic ulcers are often chronic or recurring. Duodenal peptic ulcers occur 5 to 10 times more frequently than do gastric ulcers.[10] Major factors in the development of peptic ulcers are the concentration of secreted hydrogen ions and the integrity of the defense mechanisms of the mucosal lining. Normal epithelial cells of the mucosa have tight junctions that prevent a significant flow of hydrogen ions into the gastrointestinal (GI) walls. Damage to these junctions is minimized by a constant replacement of the epithelial cells as a function of

the normal defense mechanisms.[10] In peptic ulcers, the defense system breaks down, acid damages the junctions, and erosion of the mucosal wall occurs.

In considering the etiology of gastritis and peptic ulcer disease, it is important to remember that the initial concept of "no acid equals no ulcer"[11] still holds true. With the exception of Z-E, however, the direct relationship between increased gastric acidity and ulceration no longer stands. In a recent review on the management of duodenal and gastric ulcers, Rex describes gastric acid as an "essential permissive factor" because ulceration due to either *H. pylori* or NSAIDs will not develop without it.[12]

ETIOLOGY

A variety of risk factors have been implicated in the development of inflammation and ulcerative lesions of the stomach and duodenum. These included gender,[13] alcohol consumption and smoking,[14, 15] NSAIDs,[16–18] stress,[19, 20] blood group,[21] and age.[17] The primary focus of this chapter is on the central role that *H. pylori* plays in the development of gastritis and peptic ulcer disease; however, both NSAIDs and Z-E are discussed as well as the role that risk factors play in the pathophysiologic processes of ulcer disease.

Helicobacter pylori

Although *H. pylori* is considered to be the primary etiologic agent of gastritis and, potentially, peptic ulcer disease, other species of the genus *Helicobacter* have been identified in humans and in some cases demonstrated to be related to disease (Table 20–1). Only three species (*H. pylori*, *H. cinaedi*, and *H. fennelliae*) have been commonly demonstrated to be involved in human disease. Recently, many of the symptoms associated with acute gastritis were demonstrated in an individual who worked with cats and was shown to be infected with *Gastrospirillum hominis* (*H. heilmanni*).[24]

The primary habitat of *H. pylori* is the gastric mucosa, and because of the normal gastric acidity, *H. pylori* encounters very little competition in this environment. Gastric acidity appears to be an important environmental prerequisite. Most likely this is due to the marked urease activity

Table 20–1. Species of *Helicobacter* and Their Associated Disease Relationships

Species	Disease Relationship
H. pylori	Type B gastritis, peptic ulcers, gastric carcinoma
H. cinaedi	Bacteremia
H. fennelliae	Bacteremia, proctitis, proctocolitis, enteritis
H. heilmanni (*Gastrospirillum hominis*)	Gastritis and gastric ulcer
H. canis	Rarely involved in human infection
H. pullorum	Gastroenteritis in humans

Data from Carnahan AM, Kaplan RL: *Vibrio, Aeromonas, Plesiomonas,* and *Campylobacter. In* Mahon CR, Manuselis G (eds): Diagnostic Microbiology. Philadelphia, WB Saunders, 1995; Owen RJ: Bacteriology of *Helicobacter pylori.* Baillieres Clin Gastroenterol 9:415, 1995.

of *H. pylori*, which results in the production of significant amounts of ammonia. The pH balance, which is achieved as a result of gastric acid and *H. pylori*–produced ammonia, is most likely an adaptive response facilitating the survival of *H. pylori*. Normally, *H. pylori* is found lying between the mucous layer and the epithelial cells of the gastric mucosa with extension into the gastric pits.[5] The importance of this specific environment is underscored by the fact that *H. pylori* is found neither in the duodenum, except at sites of gastric metaplasia, nor in the stomach at sites of intestinal metaplasia. Although originally thought to inhabit primarily the antral portion of the stomach, *H. pylori* has also been found in the body and fundus-body of the stomach and has a tendency to locate in areas of high gastric acidity.[25] In addition, *H. pylori* has been isolated from various sites within the GI tract, including the metaplastic gastric epithelium of the duodenum and of the esophagus, as well as in gastric fluid,[26] saliva and dental plaque in the oral cavity,[27, 28] and feces.[29] However, isolation from this latter group of GI sites is rare.

Although spiral organisms have been observed in the GI tract for many years, Marshall and Warren were the first to describe the association between these organisms (originally referred to as *Campylobacter pylori*) and the histologic findings of gastritis.[30, 31]

H. pylori has been isolated from approximately 80% to 100% of the cases of duodenal peptic ulcer and between 60% and 100% of the cases of gastric peptic ulcer.[32] In the latter case, the decreased percentage may be due in part to the lack of a direct correlation between organism density and the extent of disease (i.e., the decreased number of organisms found in atrophic gastritis), and the variable distribution of *H. pylori* within the various anatomic locations of the gastric mucosa. In addition to peptic ulcer formation, the presence of *H. pylori* in the gastric mucosa results in gastritis.

Although the mode of transmission of *H. pylori* has not been clearly delineated, it appears to result either from person-to-person transmission or via contamination from specific environmental sources. Many cases would suggest a fecal-oral route. As evidence of this, reports have documented clustering of the infection among siblings of *H. pylori*–infected individuals.[33, 34] In addition, increased infection rates have been noted among institutionalized individuals, patients in chronic care facilities,[35] and patients who have undergone endoscopic examinations with improperly cleaned instruments.[36] Environmental factors such as the absence of a hot water supply, improper waste disposal, and overcrowded living conditions have all been associated with a higher incidence of *H. pylori* infection.[37,38] *H. pylori* has been demonstrated to survive in chilled foods and in water,[39] although an animal reservoir or spread by food does not seem likely.

Age is also an important risk factor in gastritis and peptic ulcer disease. The most significant period for infection is in childhood,[40] although increasing age is a primary risk factor for increased seroconversion from negative to positive.[41] Alcohol consumption, ABO blood group, gender, and smoking do not appear to be related to any change in the incidence of *H. pylori* infection.[42, 43] However, certain of these factors may facilitate the development of gastritis and ulcer disease following infection with *H. pylori*.

In a recent National Institutes of Health (NIH) Consensus Development Conference, questions regarding the relationship of *H. pylori* to gastritis and peptic ulcer disease were addressed. In regard to the causal relationship between *H. pylori* and upper GI disease, it was found that: "(1) Virtually all *H. pylori*–positive patients demonstrate antral gastritis. (2) Eradication of *H. pylori* infection results in resolution of gastritis. (3) The lesion of chronic superficial gastritis has been reproduced following intragastric administration of the isolated organism in some animal models and oral administration in two humans."[44] The report goes on to indicate that although it is more difficult to infer a direct relationship between *H. pylori* infection and peptic ulcer disease, at a minimum, *H. pylori* is most likely a predisposing factor.

Nonsteroidal Anti-inflammatory Drugs

GI complications associated with the use of NSAIDs are well documented. In addition to the widespread use of over-the-counter NSAIDs (e.g., aspirin), millions of prescriptions are written annually for a variety of NSAIDs to treat a great variety of inflammatory disorders (Box 20–1). In addition, aspirin is used in low doses as prophylactic treatment for conditions such as stroke, myocardial infarction, and thrombosis.

Zollinger-Ellison Syndrome

Z-E spans the pathologic distance between ulcers and cancers.[1, 7] It is a hormonally induced peptic ulcer disease

---

Box 20–1. Partial Listing of NSAIDs*

Analgesic	Anti-inflammatory	Anti-arthritic
Aspirin	Nonsteroidal	NSAIDs
Bufferin	Advil	Aleve
Easprin	Aleve	Anaprox
Ecotrin	Anaprox	Ansaid
Excedrin	Ansaid	Cataflam
Norgesic	Clinoril	Clinoril
Alka-Seltzer	Dolobid	Daypro
NSAIDs	Feldene	Dolobid
Advil	Indocin	Ecotrin
Aleve	Lodine	Feldene
Anaprox	Motrin	Indocin
Cataflam	Nalfon	Lodine
Lodine	Naprosyn	Motrin
Motrin	Nuprin	Nalfon
Nalfon	Orudis	Naprosyn
Naprosyn	Oruvail	Orudis
Nuprin	Ponstel	Oruvail
Ponstel	Relafen	Relafen
Relafen	Tolectin	Tolectin
Toradol	Toradol	Voltaren
	Voltaren	

*Organized by product category and manufacturers' brand names.
Data from Physicians Desk Reference, ed 49. Des Moines, Iowa, Medical Economics, 1995.

originally characterized by benign ulceration of the upper jejunum, extremely elevated gastric acid secretion, and a gastrin-secreting non–β-cell pancreatic islet tumor.[46] It is extremely rare, with an incidence ranging from 0.1% to 1% of patients with peptic ulcers.[47] Many progressive ulcer disease patients with hypertension, an increased basal acid output–peak acid output (BAO/PAO) ratio, and elevated serum gastrin levels are classified as having duodenal ulcer, but they may actually have Z-E.

Miscellaneous Etiologic Agents

In addition to *H. pylori*, several other infectious agents have been demonstrated to be associated with gastric ulcerations. These include cytomegalovirus,[48] *Candida albicans*,[21] herpes simplex virus types 1 and 2,[49, 50] and the variety of species of *Helicobacter* previously noted.

PATHOPHYSIOLOGY
Helicobacter pylori

All infections with *H. pylori* result in the development of gastritis; however, not all progress to peptic ulcer disease. Most investigators agree that the initial infection with *H. pylori* is characterized by bacterial proliferation and transient acute gastritis lasting from 7 to 10 days.[51] Symptoms of upper GI tract problems may be transiently present or completely absent. The initial infection is characterized by hypochlorhydria (which may last for months), mucin depletion, and exfoliation of surface cells.[52] In addition, maximum fecal shedding of the organism appears to occur during this period, thus enhancing transmission and spread.[53] The motility of *H. pylori*, along with its microaerophilic characteristics, likely aid in resisting the peristaltic movement of the GI tract, thus facilitating its survival in the epithelial layer underlying the mucous lining of the stomach.[54]

A variety of *H. pylori*–related toxic factors have been implicated in the pathogenesis of gastric damage occurring during this stage. Approximately 50% of the isolates of *H. pylori* have been shown to produce a vacuolating toxin that is encoded by the *vacA* gene.[55] This vacuolating cytotoxin is an 87 to 94 kD protein that is synthesized as a 140 kD precursor.[56, 57] This toxin produces acid vacuoles in a variety of cell types, accounting, in part, for some of the toxic affects of *H. pylori*. The vacuolating cytotoxin is produced by a subset (VacA+) of *H. pylori*. Most strains that do not produce the vacuolating cytotoxin (VacA−) still carry the gene.[58, 59] Various combinations of these *vacA* regions were identified in different strains, and the level of vacuolating cytotoxin activity was associated with specific combinations.

Besides VacA, approximately 60% of the strains of *H. pylori* produce a cytotoxin-associated protein (CagA). The CagA protein has been demonstrated to up-regulate interleukin-8 (IL-8). Crabtree and colleagues demonstrated that CagA+ strains of *H. pylori*, whether VacA+ or VacA−, up-regulated IL-8 secretion and gene expression.[60] Alternatively, CagA− strains, even those expressing the vacuolating cytotoxin, had no effect on IL-8 up-regulation

above baseline levels. IL-8 is an important chemotactic mediator as well as activating factor for neutrophils. This can be considered an essential host defense mechanism, calling into play macrophages and other mononuclear cells. Toxin production associated with the *vacA* and *cagA* gene may help to explain why some patients develop peptic ulcer whereas others do not progress beyond symptoms associated with gastritis.

Infection with *H. pylori* results in an immune response consisting primarily of immunoglobulin G (IgG) and immunoglobulin A (IgA) antibodies. Sugiyama and colleagues demonstrated the appearance of immunocompetent antibody-producing cells in the gastric mucosa in response to *H. pylori*.[61] The antibody class produced was IgG with the potential, through antigen-antibody complex formation, of damaging epithelial cells. In addition, CD4+ T cells have been localized at the site of disease, suggesting their involvement in the immune response.[62] An evaluation of various body fluids demonstrated higher IgG than IgA titers in serum in contrast to higher salivary IgA titers.[63] Antibodies to a variety of different molecular weight proteins have been identified, including those ranging in size from approximately 19 to 180 kD.[64, 65] Interestingly, among these is a 54 to 58 kD protein demonstrated to belong to the Hsp60 family of heat-shock proteins.[66, 67] The homology between this 54 to 58 kD protein and the human Hsp60 family may represent a cross-reactive autoimmunizing protein with pathogenic potential. Antibodies to this homologous heat-shock protein and the vacuolating cytotoxin have been shown to be directly correlated with the severity of acute mucosal inflammation.[67]

Several other factors have been identified as being associated with acute tissue damage following infection with *H. pylori*. One unique and identifying characteristic of *H. pylori* is its extremely strong urease activity, which produces a significant amount of ammonia. Ammonium ions have been shown to cause gastritis[68] and to augment and/or potentiate the effect of vacuolating cytotoxin.[69] In addition, bacteria-derived phospholipases and alcohol dehydrogenase directly damage the epithelial layer.[70, 71] Cytokines released from activated macrophages and substances such as tumor necrosis factor α, interleukin-6 (IL-6), and interleukin-10 (IL-10), plays an important role in the inflammation-mediated host tissue damage associated with *H. pylori* infection. Finally, the release of platelet-activating factor (PAF) from mast cells and mononuclear cells could result in thrombosis within the microvasculature, accounting for ischemic tissue damage and activation of the alternate complement pathway. Although this characteristic inflammatory process constitutes a normal host defense mechanism, it can also result in significant tissue damage.

Although some individuals may be able to clear the organism during the initial infectious stage, most progress to chronic superficial gastritis consistent with type B gastritis.[54] There appear to be variable degrees of epithelial degeneration, possibly related to variations in the virulence of the strain of *H. pylori* (i.e., CagA+/VacA+ type I strains vs. CagA−/VacA− type II strains).[72] This phase may last from years to decades; it does not necessarily progress to ulcer formation and it is characterized by both a neutrophilic and a mononuclear (chronic) cell infiltrate. This latter histologic picture is often referred to as *active chronic gastritis.* Depending on the duration and severity of the inflammation, the process may result in glandular atrophy. This is noted primarily in the antral portion of the stomach, potentially the area of heaviest bacterial load. Continued epithelial damage is due in part to the production of toxic oxygen radicals and cytokine production that further up-regulates IL-8. Although a gradual rise in acid production has been noted, a consistent finding of gastric hyperacidity is not characteristic of *H. pylori* infections. The origin of the increased acid secretion is related to the *H. pylori*–induced hypergastrinemia, which has been suggested as being secondary to a decreased release of inhibitory somatostatin.[73] It has been suggested that other bacteria-related factors are capable of down-regulating acid production, but these may, in fact, be related to the initial hypochlorhydria previously noted following initial infection with *H. pylori.*

Beyond the chronic superficial gastritis, which may persist well into the seventh decade of life, various, yet less common, pathways for disease progression have been proposed by Blaser and Parsonnet.[54] One possible scenario is the formation of peptic ulcers. Atherton and colleagues noted that among individuals with past or present peptic ulceration, 91% harbored CagA + /VacA + strains.[59] In contrast, only 2% of individuals with CagA − /VacA − strains had a history of peptic ulcer.

Another route leads to the formation of chronic atrophic gastritis. In this case, it has been hypothesized that, as a result of the increased acidity related to the hypergastrinemia, intestinal metaplasia occurs as a protective response of the gastric epithelium. The increasing glandular atrophy and intestinal metaplasia is accompanied by a decrease in the presence of viable *H. pylori* organisms. This is due to the fact that (1) *H. pylori* requires gastric mucosa, (2) *H. pylori* requires an acidic environment, and (3) acidic glycoproteins produced by the metaplastic intestinal epithelium may significantly alter the ability of *H. pylori* to adhere. The metaplastic changes associated with chronic atrophic gastritis may represent a precancerous condition, eventually leading to gastric adenocarcinoma.

Gastric cancers are one of the most common malignancies worldwide. In the United States, gastric carcinoma is the seventh most common cause of cancer death.[74] A variety of studies have implicated infection with *H. pylori* as a risk factor for the development of adenocarcinoma.[75-78] Although the pathophysiologic mechanisms are not clearly delineated, possibilities include increased cell turnover, thereby increasing the opportunity for cell mutagenesis. In addition, there appears to be an association between CagA + strains of *H. pylori* and increased risk of gastric cancer.[79] Lin and associates have devised a new scoring system for evaluating gastric adenocarcinoma.[80] The system includes serum pepsinogen I levels, *H. pylori* seropositivity, and gastric ulcer as indicators. Recently, the World Health Organization and the International Agency for Research on Cancer classified *H. pylori* as a "definite" carcinogen.[81] Even though the data relating *H. pylori* infection with gastric malignancy are compelling, the NIH Consensus Development Conference on *H. pylori* concluded that as of yet, the eradication of *H. pylori* for the purpose of preventing gastric cancer cannot be recommended.[44]

Nonsteroidal Anti-inflammatory Drugs

NSAIDS appear to have both an immediate, localized impact on the gastric mucosa and a more long-term systemic impact. The latter is primarily related to the inhibition of cyclooxygenase and prostaglandin synthesis. The most severe localized effect is the development of superficial lesions, primarily in the antrum of the stomach.[82] Generally asymptomatic in nature, these localized effects consist of the immediate development of petechiae, followed by the development of gastric erosions. However, over a period of days, these erosions usually disappear.[83] Aspirin is a weak acid capable of crossing the lipid membranes of gastric mucosa as an un-ionized compound. Once inside the cell, dissociation of these compounds increases hydrogen ion concentration, thus damaging gastric mucosa. Kuo and Shanboar[84] found that aspirin inhibited mucosal transport of sodium and chloride ions by initially reducing the adenosine triphosphate (ATP) content of the mucosa. In addition, prostaglandins, important to mucosal defense mechanisms, are also inhibited by aspirin, and mucus secretion is reduced.[85] It has been demonstrated that the use of enteric-coated NSAIDs can reduce or eliminate most of these initial localized effects[85]; however, these compounds do not prevent the potential for more severe gastric problems associated with eventual ulcer formation.

The long-term ulcer-related impact of NSAIDs appears to be related to the ability of these compounds to inhibit cyclooxygenase. Figure 20–1 illustrates the normal pathway for prostaglandin production and the point at which cyclooxygenase, and therefore aspirin, has its impact. The final compounds (i.e., prostaglandins I_2 [PGI_2], E_2 [PGE_2], or $F_{2\alpha}$ [$PGF_{2\alpha}$]) are tissue specific, and their production is based on the presence of the appropriate enzyme. The inhibition of prostaglandin production has the effect of

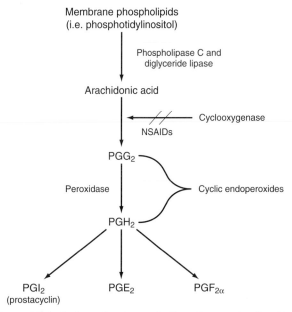

Figure 20–1. Pathway for the production of prostaglandins illustrating the point at which NSAIDs block the production of cyclic endoperoxides. The end products are related to the availability of specific enzymes within each cell type.

decreasing bicarbonate production in the stomach and duodenum and decreasing mucus secretion. In addition, decreases in mucosal blood flow occur, which result in increases in leukocyte adherence, alterations in the normal inhibition of acid secretion, and potential increases in cell turnover.[85] The combined impact of all of these factors is to compromise many of the normal gastric defense mechanisms, thus predisposing the gastric mucosa to ulcer formation.

The severity of the antral gastritis appears to be related to the presence or absence of *H. pylori*. In general, patients taking NSAIDs with an associated *H. pylori* infection had much more severe gastritis than noninfected patients taking NSAIDs.[86] Controversy exists over whether a concomitant infection with *H. pylori* increases the risk of ulcer formation in patients taking NSAIDs.[87, 88]

Zollinger-Ellison Syndrome

Z-E has classically been defined as a triad of symptoms that include recurring peptic ulcer disease, hypersecretion of gastric acid, and a gastrin-secreting non–β-cell pancreatic islet tumor. The term *gastrinoma* is used to refer to the tumor because a primary characteristic is the excess production of gastrin. Although originally described as a tumor of the pancreas, a significant number of gastrin-secreting tumors have been associated with extrapancreatic sites.[89] These include the duodenum, stomach, liver, bile duct, lymph nodes, and bone.[90–92]

The major impact of increased gastrin secretion is twofold. First, gastrin stimulates parietal cells to secrete acid. It has been suggested that this occurs via both a direct, receptor-mediated effect on the parietal cells and indirect methods that involve histamine release, evidenced by the fact that antagonists to histamine H_2 receptors block acid secretion.[93, 94] Second, gastrin has a hyperplastic effect, increasing the total mass of parietal cells.

Approximately 25% of gastrinomas result from an autosomal dominant genetic disorder known as *multiple endocrine neoplasia, type 1* (MEN-I). This disorder is characterized by tumor development in a variety of organ site, including the pancreas, the parathyroid, the pituitary, the adrenal cortex, and the thyroid.[95]

Miscellaneous Etiologic Agents

A variety of risk factors have been historically associated with the development of peptic ulcer disease. Alcohol has long been associated with the development of gastric mucosal damage. Although alcohol is lipid soluble and has the ability to directly damage the gastric mucosa, most evidence would indicate that alcohol plays very little role in the development of ulcers, except in alcoholic cirrhosis and the resulting increased portal hypertension.[96] Smoking, however, has been demonstrated to have a variety of effects ranging from inhibition of bicarbonate secretion, increased production of tissue-damaging free radicals, changes in mucosal blood flow, and increased levels of serum pepsinogen I. Some of these symptoms are similar to those associated with the inhibition of prostaglandin synthesis.[97, 98]

Stress ulcers are associated with diseases such as respiratory failure, hypotension, sepsis, and jaundice.[99, 100] The acute erosions of stress ulcers often occur in the fundus and corpus of the stomach.[9] They are often difficult to detect because of the increased gastric secretions that cross the mucosal barrier and are not reflected in increased BAO and maximum acid output (MAO) levels by pentagastrin stimulation. Stress ulcers may occur in both very young and elderly persons. In children younger than 12 years, acute ulcers may progress to perforation and subsequent life-threatening hemorrhage. After 12 years of age, the clinical presentation is similar to that of adults. Elderly persons may also present with an acute stress ulcer complicated by hemorrhage. After the acute episode, however, the ulcer often persists as a chronic ulcerative condition. It is possible, because of the cephalic stimulation of acid secretion, that stress does play a role in ulcer formation. There does not seem to be a direct relationship between personality type and the development of ulcers.

Blood group O nonsecretors have been thought to be predisposed to ulcer formation. It has been suggested that one of the adhesive factors associated with *H. pylori* binds to Lewis' blood group (Le^b) antigen particularly when associated with the O blood group.[101] Secretion of the Le^b antigen would coat *H. pylori*, thus reducing its adhesion. Nonsecretors would be without this advantage, thus enhancing the potential for cellular damage. Finally, although dietary substances are known to increase gastric acid output in general, dietary restrictions, beyond avoiding substances that may cause increased discomfort, are not specifically warranted.

CLINICAL MANIFESTATIONS

A great deal of variation occurs in the presenting symptoms associated with the development of gastritis and peptic ulcer disease. Most patients have experienced some form of abdominal pain. This may have included a burning sensation that is localized in the epigastric area and is relieved by antacids and/or food. In addition, some patients experience abdominal pain while sleeping. A significant number of these patients may have duodenal or gastric ulcer.[102]

Although abdominal and epigastric pain are one of the primary presenting symptoms of patients with gastritis and peptic ulcer, this finding has relatively low specificity and sensitivity. In fact, a significant number of patients may have no presenting symptoms or only minor discomfort and increased gas following a meal.

A more overt symptom related to complications associated with ulcer formation includes hemorrhage, either hematemesis or melena, or both. In addition, particularly in patients with Z-E, diarrhea may occur, likely related to excessive amounts of acid, inadequate digestion, and possible malabsorption problems. Diarrhea may present long before any other symptoms manifest. In the case of Z-E, additional characteristics might include resistance to standard ulcer treatment with H_2 blockers, ulcers at sites other than the more common gastric and duodenal sites, multiple ulcers, ulcer recurrence, or family history of ulcers and/or endocrine tumors.

LABORATORY ANALYSES AND DIAGNOSIS

As a result of an increased understanding of the pathophysiology of ulcer disease, a variety of new testing protocols have been developed. Although the clinical utility of some of these tests is clear, consensus on the use of others is lacking. In a 1994 review, Plebani and colleagues[103] evaluated the laboratory tests available for the diagnosis of ulcer disease. This section will focus on a limited subset of these tests. Testing will be divided according to the suspected diagnosis and, where appropriate, invasive or noninvasive tests.

Helicobacter pylori

Invasive Tests

ENDOSCOPY AND BIOPSY

The "gold standard" for the determination of ulcer disease is considered to be endoscopy with biopsy. The recommended site for biopsy is the antral region of the stomach; however, sensitivity and specificity can be increased by obtaining samples from two or more sites including the greater curvature of the body of the stomach. The biopsy sample is used for histologic examination, culture, and urease testing.[104]

For purposes of grading or classifying the gastritis, histologic examination can be performed using samples stained with hematoxylin and eosin. However, the Warthin-Starry silver stain is better for visualizing *H. pylori*. Generally Gram's stain is considered to have lower sensitivity than stains for histologic observations. A careful search for the organism must be made using high magnification where it can be found in or underlying the gastric mucus, along the epithelium, and in the gastric pits. The organism is approximately 4 μm in length and spiral shaped. Occasionally, coccoidal forms of the organism can be observed.

CULTURE

Biopsy samples can be cultured following the procedures recommended for this organism.[105] It is best to culture these samples immediately. If this is not possible, samples can be kept in transport media at 4 °C; however, long-term storage can only be achieved by freezing in liquid nitrogen at −70 °C. It is important to use fresh media and to keep the cultures in a moist environment.

CLO TEST AND GASTRIC AMMONIA

A rapid method for the detection of *H. pylori* is the urease or campylobacter-like organism (CLO) test (Delta West Ltd, Bently, Australia), which takes advantage of the very high urease activity of *H. pylori*. The sensitivity of this test has been reported to vary between approximately 68% at 1 hour to almost 90% at 3 hours[106]; however, the specificity significantly drops over time because other species of weakly positive urease organisms begin to grow after prolonged incubation.

Yang and colleagues have proposed the analysis of gastric juice ammonia for the detection of *H. pylori*.[106] When compared to the CLO test, gastric juice ammonia analysis demonstrates more true-positive and fewer false-positive results. At a cutoff value of 6.0 mg/dL of NH_4^+, the test had a sensitivity of 100% and a specificity of 61.8%. At a cutoff value of 8.0 mg/dL, the sensitivity dropped to 90.2% and the specificity increased to 94.1%.[106]

POLYMERASE CHAIN REACTION

Recently, the polymerase chain reaction (PCR) has been applied to the diagnosis of *H. pylori*. Fabre and colleagues found PCR to be the most sensitive and specific test when compared with culture, the CLO test, and histologic examination.[107] This analysis has been performed on biopsy samples[107] and feces,[108] although van Zwet and colleagues reported no success in detecting DNA in feces.[108]

Noninvasive Tests

UREA BREATH TEST

The urea breath test (UBT) appears to be gaining popularity as a simplified and standardized method for the determination of *H. pylori*. Like the CLO test, UBT is based on the very high urease activity of *H. pylori*. In this procedure, a fasting patient ingests a solution of urea labeled with either carbon-13 (^{13}C) or carbon 14 (^{14}C). The ingested, labeled urea is broken down into ammonia and labeled carbon dioxide (CO_2). The labeled CO_2 is absorbed into the blood and then exhaled through the lungs. The labeled CO_2 has been detected using either a nondispersive infrared spectrometer or an isotope-ratio mass spectrometer.[109]

In a double-blind study, Fallone and colleagues determined the relative sensitivity and specificity for ^{14}C UBT and hematoxylin-phloxin-saffron and Giemsa stains for the detection of *H. pylori*. The sensitivities were 95.8%, 75%, and 95.8%, respectively, with a specificity of 100%.[110] Similarly, Cutler and colleagues evaluated ^{13}C UBT, serum IgG and IgA antibodies, biopsy with CLO test, and Warthin-Starry staining. They found that although the Warthin-Starry staining had the best sensitivity and specificity, the CLO test, UBT, and IgG results were not statistically different.[111] The noninvasive nature of the $^{13-14}$C UBT is particularly important in diagnosing disease in pediatric patients, and its effectiveness in the population has been demonstrated.[112] Recently, the Food and Drug Administration has considered approval of the PYTEST (^{14}C-labeled UBT) (Tri-Med Specialties, Lenexa, Kansas).[113] The cost of this test is predicted to be far less than the use of the current "gold standard" of endoscopy.

SEROLOGY

An infection with *H. pylori* is accompanied by an increased level of specific serum IgG and IgA antibodies. These antibodies can often be detected using specific enzyme immunoassays or agglutination assays. Best and colleagues compared a flow microsphere immunofluorescent assay (FIMA) with the Pyloriset enzyme-linked immunosorbent assay (ELISA) for IgG.[114] The FIMA had a sensitivity, specificity, and positive and negative predictive value of 100%, 97%, 96%, and 100%, respectively, with the Pyloriset ELISA having comparative values of 96%, 94%, 92%, and 97%. As previously noted,[111] these antibody tests have sensitivities and specificities similar to the UBT, CLO test, and Warthin-Starry silver stain technique. In addition,

FIMA and ELISA are significantly less expensive to perform than a biopsy.[115] Although these tests are often based on the use of a heterogenous mixture of *H. pylori* antigens, specific antigen fragments for either CagA or VacA could be used to detect strains that have a greater likelihood of causing more severe inflammation and, potentially, peptic ulcer disease.[116] For cases in which serum samples may be difficult to obtain, Luzza and colleagues used an ELISA to demonstrate concordance between the serum IgG markers for *H. pylori* and salivary IgG concentrations.[117]

In contrast to the UBT that quickly becomes negative following eradication therapy, antibody titers detected by serologic testing remain elevated for months. This is a drawback when trying to determine the efficacy of *H. pylori* eradication therapy; however, in cases of atrophic gastritis, because of the decrease in the gastric acidity and the intestinal metaplasia, *H. pylori* may be undetectable by culture while antibody titers still remain elevated.[100]

Zollinger-Ellison Syndrome

The problems with diagnosing Z-E lie in differentiating it from other causes of ulcer disease and in locating the site of the tumor. The key to the determination of Z-E includes identifying gastric hyperacidity secondary to elevated gastrin levels. Plebani and colleagues noted that although gastric acidity is not useful in diagnosing ulcer disease "it is a basic diagnostic test for suspected cases of ZE and hypergastrinemia. It is (also) useful in evaluating parietal cell H_2 histaminergic receptor regulation."[103]

Invasive Tests

Gastric Acid

Because acid output is related to ulceration, performing gastric acid content analyses is helpful for diagnostic purposes but uncomfortable for the patient. It is important to note that because of increased understanding of the pathophysiologic mechanisms of ulcer disease, the data on gastric acidity are not obsolete. According to Tietz,[118] with no stimulation, normal gastric acidity varies up to approximately 40 mmol/L, with a pH between 1.5 and 3.5. This is based on total content and measurement after a 12-hour fast, with attention being paid to intake of any substance known to alter acid output. These values may be elevated in duodenal and gastric ulcers as well as in Z-E. Gastric stimulation tests can be performed following a dose of pentagastrin. In this situation the initial BAO is measured prior to pentagastrin administration. The normal BAO is less than approximately 6 mmol/hour in females and approximately 10 mmol/hour in males.[118] Following pentagastrin stimulation, PAO is less than 40 mmol/hour in females and less than approximately 60 mmol/hour in males. These values appear to be related to the route (subcutaneous or intramuscular) of pentagastrin administration. The BAO/PAO ratio should be less than 0.2.[118]

Duodenal ulcer patients have increased acid secretion and will have BAOs that are elevated but less than 15 mmol/hour, with 25% to 50% of patients having MAOs greater than 40 mmol/hour.[7] Seventy percent of patients with Z-E have BAOs of 15 mmol/hour or higher without stimulation. A BAO/PAO ratio greater than 0.6 suggests Z-E, indicating a need for serum gastrin analysis.[118]

Noninvasive Tests

Gastrin

Although hypergastrinemia is characteristic of Z-E, interpretation of the results of a serum gastrin analysis must be made carefully and in light of other diagnostic information. Taken alone, increased gastrin levels can be seen secondary to disorders that affect end-organ responsiveness. This would include such things as atrophic gastritis and the accompanying inability to secrete adequate amounts of gastric acid; long-term maintenance therapy with H_2 blockers; pernicious anemia, because of the atrophy of the acid-secreting mucosa and the accompanying hyperplasia of G-cells (gastrin-secreting cells) secondary to decreased acid secretion; G-cell hyperplasia due to a relatively uncommon inherited trait[119]; G-cell hyperplasia secondary to retained antrum following a Billroth II gastrectomy[120]; chronic renal failure; gastric carcinomas; or gastrectomy.

Gastrin is secreted by the G-cells and exists in three forms—a 34 amino acid polypeptide (G-34, big gastrin), a 17 amino acid peptide (G-17, little gastrin), and a 14 amino acid peptide (G-14, minigastrin).[121] Although there were indications that the determination of the various forms of these peptides might help to distinguish the site of gastrin production (i.e., antrum, duodenum, or pancreas), this has not proven to be the case. According to Tietz,[118] serum gastrin values vary depending on age, with normal adult values for a fasting specimen ranging from 25 to 90 pg/mL. DelValle and Yamada[122] report that most fasting levels in patients with Z-E are greater than 150 pg/mL. Gastrin levels can also be measured following stimulation with either a meal, calcium infusion, or the administration of secretin. The secretin stimulation test is considered to be the more provocative test when considering Z-E or gastrinomas. Gastrin levels, unassociated with a gastrinoma, either decrease or do not change; however, in Z-E or gastrinomas, gastrin levels increase in response to secretin injection.[122] When Z-E is expected, a combination of key clinical data, including patient symptoms, increased gastric acidity, and hypergastrinemia, must be considered.

TREATMENT

The primary mainstay for the treatment of ulcer disease has been the use of H_2 receptor antagonists. These compounds include ranitidine, famotidine, cimetidine, and nizatidine. These are reversible inhibitors of histamine action at the H_2 receptor on gastric cells. Each of these compounds inhibits basal gastric acid secretion but has little, if any, impact on fasting serum gastrin levels, pepsin secretion, or the secretions of intrinsic factor.

A new compound, omeprazole, has been demonstrated to be very effective at inhibiting gastric acid secretion by blocking the H^+/K^+ adenosine triphosphatase (ATPase) enzyme essential in the final stage of acid secretion from the gastric parietal cell. The effects of omeprazole increase following daily dosage over a period of 3 to 4 days, and the antisecretory effects of omeprazole last for several days after discontinuation of the drug.

Although H₂ antagonists and omeprazole have, for many years, been considered the treatment of choice for peptic ulcer disease, their use is being called into question in some situations. Clearly, ulcer healing occurs following the use of these drugs, but discontinuation often results in a recurrence of the ulcer. In the case of gastritis or ulcer disease precipitated by infection with *H. pylori*, these drugs treat the symptoms rather than the cause of the disease. The NIH Consensus Development Conference concluded the following: (1) "Ulcer patients with *H. pylori* infection require treatment with antimicrobial agents in addition to antisecretory drugs whether on first presentation with the illness or on recurrence," and (2) "the value of treatment of patients with nonulcerative dyspepsia and *H. pylori* infection remains to be determined."[44]

Eradication protocols for *H. pylori* include a combination of either H₂ receptor antagonists or proton pump inhibitors (omeprazole) coupled with antibiotic therapy. Hentschel and colleagues demonstrated a dramatic difference in ulcer recurrence in a group of patients taking ranitidine and amoxicillin plus metronidazole versus a control group taking only the H₂ antagonist.[123] In 1994, Karita and colleagues reported the eradication of *H. pylori* with a treatment regimen consisting of omeprazole followed by plaunotol for 4 weeks with amoxicillin and metronidazole for 7 days.[124] An important aspect of these treatments is the very low ulcer recurrence rate. In addition, a 3 to 4 week regimen of gastric acid blockers coupled with antimicrobial agents (triple therapy) is likely to be less costly than prolonged and recurring periods requiring the use of either H₂ antagonists or proton pump inhibitors.

The case for the use of gastric acid inhibitors is, however, different when it comes to the treatment of gastrinomas, such as in Z-E. Although there have been improvements in the clinician's ability to identify the source of the tumor,[125–129] the recurrence rate following surgical removal is still fairly high. Therefore, even though control of the hyperacidity does not treat the cause of the disease, in this case, treating the symptoms of the disease is an important factor, and the use of H₂ antagonists and proton pump inhibitors is indicated.

Case Study

This patient is a 42-year-old man with a history of alcohol abuse. Twelve years earlier, a diagnosis of peptic ulcer disease was made by endoscopy. Prior to admission the patient had a 3 week history of nausea and "coffee ground" emesis (×3) with increased abdominal blotting. The patient indicated taking no ethanol for the last 3 weeks and denied the use of any NSAIDs. The patient was currently taking Zantac (ranitidine). The following results were obtained on physical and clinical laboratory examination:

Blood Pressure	157/76 mm Hg
Pulse	96/minute
Respirations	18/minute
Not ecteric	
No ascites	
Liver	9 cm
No splenomegaly	
Hemoglobin	10 mg/dL
Platelet count	548 × 10⁹/L
Mean corpuscular volume (MCV)	82 fL
White blood cell count (WBC)	8.4 × 10⁹/L

Endoscopy was performed, and a gastric antral biopsy was taken from the crater of the ulcer. A CLO test was performed to determine urease activity and the sample was positive at 24 hours.

Questions

1. What is the most likely diagnosis in this case?
2. What other possibilities should be considered and why?
3. What other laboratory analysis might be helpful in this case?

Discussion

Although it was determined that this patient represented a case of peptic ulcer disease due to *H. pylori* infection, this particular case presents a rather interesting dilemma. The patient had been diagnosed several years earlier with peptic ulcer disease, and the question being addressed currently was whether this was due to infection with *H. pylori*. In order for the results of the CLO test on the biopsy sample to be diagnostic, you would prefer to see the rapid (3 hour) development of a pink color, indicating a very strong urease reaction. The problem with this patient is that the CLO test was positive at 24 hours, leaving open the possibility of a false-positive result due to interference from other, much more weakly urease-positive, gastric organisms. Although other complicating factors (i.e., alcohol and possible NSAID use) need to be considered, physical examination shows no evidence of either an enlarged or cirrhotic liver, which might suggest changes in portal circulation that would subsequently compromise gastric function and potentially result in ulcer formation. In addition, many instances of peptic ulcer due to NSAID use have, as a precipitating factor, an associated infection with *H. pylori*.

This particular case points out the need for an alternate mechanism for the diagnosis of *H. pylori* infection. Serologic examination of patients suspected of *H. pylori* infection has been demonstrated to have sensitivity and specificity as high as 95% to 99%. In addition, serologic examination is not affected by changes in the gastric environment due to such lesions as intestinal metaplasia and chronic gastritis. Both of these would alter the gastric environment and tend to decrease the bacterial load, reducing the possibility of detecting *H. pylori* by either the CLO test or a UBT. Although endoscopy with biopsy has been considered the "gold standard" for the diagnosis of peptic ulcer disease, particularly in those patients with a history of recurring ulcer disease, it may be appropriate to determine the *H. pylori* status with some noninvasive serologic test prior to the evaluation of ulcer status by endoscopy.

References

1. Warren JR, Marshall BJ: Unidentified curved bacilli on gastric epithelium in active chronic gastritis. Lancet i:1273–1275, 1983.
2. Isenberg JI, Hogan DL, Koss MA, et al: Human duodenal mucosal bicarbonate secretion: Evidence for basal secretion and stimulation by hydrochloric acid and a synthetic prostaglandin E_1 analogue. Gastroenterology 91:370–378, 1986.
3. Lacy ER: Epithelial restitution in the gastrointestinal tract. J Clin Gastroenterol 10(suppl 1):S72–S77, 1988.
4. Feil W, Lacy ER, Wong YM, et al: Rapid epithelial restitution of human and rabbit colonic mucosa. Gastroenterology 97:685–701, 1989.
5. Yogeshwar D, DeLellis RA: The gastrointestinal tract. *In* Cotran RS, Kumar V, Robbins SL (eds): Pathologic Basis of Disease, Philadelphia, WB Saunders, 1989, p 827.
6. Strickland RG, Mackay JR: A reappraisal of the nature and significance of chronic atrophic gastritis. Am J Dig Dis 18:426–440, 1973.
7. Glass GBJ, Pitchumoni CS: Atrophic gastritis. Human Pathology 6:219–250, 1975.
8. Misiewicz JJ: The Sydney System: A new classification of gastritis. J Gastroenterol Hepatol 6:207–208, 1991.
9. Brooks FP, Cohen S, Soloway RD (eds): Peptic Ulcer Disease. New York, Churchill Livingstone, 1985.
10. Emes JH, Novak TF: Introduction to Pathophysiology. Baltimore, University Park Press, 1984.
11. Schwarz K: Über penetrierende Magen-und sejunal-geschwüre. Beiträge zur Klinischen Chirurgie 67:96–128, 1910.
12. Rex DK: An etiologic approach to management of duodenal and gastric ulcers. J Fam Pract 38:60–67, 1994.
13. Kurata JH, Haile BM, Elashoff JD: Sex differences in peptic ulcer disease. Gastroenterology 88:96–100, 1985.
14. Piper DW, Nasiry R, McIntosh J, et al: Smoking, alcohol, analgesics and chronic duodenal ulcer. Scand J Gastroenterol 19:1015–1021, 1984.
15. Friedman GD, Siegelaub AB, Seltzer CC: Cigarettes, alcohol, coffee and peptic ulcer. N Engl J Med 290:469–473, 1974.
16. Keenan GF, Giannini EH, Athreya BH: Clinically significant gastropathy associated with nonsteroidal antiinflammatory drug use in children with juvenile rheumatoid arthritis. J Rheumatol 22:1149–1151, 1995.
17. Roth SH: From peptic ulcer disease to NSAID gastropathy: An evolving nosology. Drugs Aging 6:358–367, 1995.
18. McCarthy DM: Mechanisms of mucosal injury and healing: The role of non-steroidal anti-inflammatory drugs. Scand J Gastroenterol Suppl 208:24–29, 1995.
19. Levi L: Society, brain and gut—a psychosocial approach to dyspepsia. Scand J Gastroenterol 22(suppl 128):120–127, 1987.
20. Susser M: Causes of peptic ulcer: A selective epidemiological approach. J Chronic Dis 20:435–456, 1967.
21. Burford-Mason AP, Willoughby JMT, Weber JCP: Association between gastrointestinal tract carriage of *Candida*, blood group O, and nonsecretion of blood group antigens in patients with peptic ulcer. Dig Dis Sci 38:1453–1458, 1993.
22. Carnahan AM, Kaplan RL: *Vibrio, Aeromonas, Plesiomonas,* and *Campylobacter. In* Mahon CR, Manuselis G (eds): Diagnostic Microbiology. Philadelphia, WB Saunders, 1995, p 491.
23. Owen RJ: Bacteriology of *Helicobacter pylori.* Baillieres Clin Gastroenterol 9:415, 1995.
24. Lavelle JP, Landas S, Mitros FA, et al: Acute gastritis associated with spril organisms from cats. Dig Dis Sci 39:744–750, 1994.
25. Louw JA, Falck V, van Rensburg C, et al: Distribution of *Helicobacter pylori* colonization and associated gastric inflammatory changes: Difference between patients with duodenal and gastric ulcers. J Clin Pathol 46:754–756, 1993.
26. Cover TL, Blaser MJ: The pathobiology of *Campylobacter* infections in humans. Annu Rev Med 40:269–285, 1989.
27. Krajden S, Fuksa M, Anderson J, et al: Examination of human stomach biopsies, saliva, and dental plaque for *Campylobacter pylori.* J Clin Microbiol 27:1397–1398, 1989.
28. Majumdar P, Shah SM, Dhunjibhoy KR, et al: Isolation of *Helicobacter pylori* from dental plaques in healthy volunteers. Indian J Gastroenterol 9:271–272, 1990.
29. Thomas JE, Gibson GR, Darboe MK, et al: Isolation of *Helicobacter pylori* human feces. Lancet 340:1994–1995, 1992.
30. Marshall BJ, Warren JR: Unidentified curved bacilli in the stomach of patients with gastritis and peptic ulceration. Lancet 1:1311–1315, 1984.
31. Marshall BJ, Armstrong JA, McGechie GB, et al: Attempt to fulfill Koch's postulates for pyloric campylobacter. Med J Aust 142:436–439, 1985.
32. Taylor DN, Blaser MJ: The epidemiology of *Helicobacter pylori* infection. Epidemiol Rev 13:42–59, 1991.
33. Mitchell HM, Lee A, Bohane TD: Evidence of person-to-person spread of *Campylobacter pylori. In* Rathbone BJ, Heatley RV (eds): *Campylobacter pylori* and Gastroduodenal Disease. London, Blackwell, 1989, p 197.
34. Drumm B, Perez-Perez GI, Blaser MJ, et al: Intrafamilial clustering of *Helicobacter pylori* infection. N Engl J Med 322:359–363, 1990.
35. Berkowicz J, Lee A: Person-to-person transmission of *Campylobacter pylori.* Lancet 2:680–681, 1987.
36. Graham DY, Alpert CC, Smith JL, et al: Iatrogenic *Campylobacter pylori* infection is a cause of epidemic achlorhydria. Am J Gastroenterol 83:974–980, 1988.
37. Mendall MA, Goggin PM, Molineaux N, et al: Childhood living conditions and *Helicobacter pylori* seropositivity in adult life. Lancet 339:896–897, 1992.
38. Klein PD, Graham DY, Opekun AR, et al: High prevalence of *Campylobacter pylori* infection in poor and rich Peruvian children determined by ^{13}C urea breath test. Gastroenterol 96:260, 1989.
39. Park CE, Stankicwicz ZK, Lior H: Survival of *Campylobacter pylori (pyloridis)* in food and water. *In* Abstracts of the 87th Annual Meeting of the American Society for Microbiology. Washington, DC, American Society for Microbiology, 1987, p 275.
40. Banatvala N, Mayo K, Megraud F, et al: The cohort effect and *Helicobacter pylori.* J Infect Dis 168:219–221, 1993.
41. Veldhuyzen van Zanten SJ, Pollak PT, Best LM: Increasing prevalence of *Helicobacter pylori* infection with age: Continuous risk of infection in adults rather than cohort effect. J Infect Dis 169:434–437, 1994.
42. Hook-Nikanne J: Effect of alcohol consumption on the risk of *Helicobacter pylori* infection. Digestion 50:92–98, 1991.
43. Hook-Nikanne J, Sistonen P, Kosunen TU: Effect of ABO blood group and secretor status on the frequency of *Helicobacter pylori* antibodies. Scand J Gastroenterol 25:815–818, 1990.
44. NIH consensus conference: *Helicobacter pylori* in peptic ulcer disease. JAMA 272:65–69, 1994.
45. Physicians Desk Reference, ed 49. Des Moines, Iowa, Medical Economics, 1995.
46. Zollinger RM, Ellison EH: Primary peptic ulceration of the jejunum associated with islet cell tumors of the pancreas. Ann Surg 142:709, 1955.
47. Isenberg JI, Walsh JH, Grossman MI: Zollinger-Ellison syndrome. Gastroenterology 65:140–165, 1973.
48. Yoshinaga M, Nakate S, Motomura S, et al: Cytomegalovirus-associated gastric ulcerations in a normal host. Am J Gastroenterol 89:448–449, 1994.
49. Archimandritis A, Markoulatos P, Tjivras M, et al: Herpes simplex virus types 1 and 2 and cytomegalovirus in peptic ulcer disease and non-ulcer dyspepsia. Hepatogastroenterology 39:540–541, 1992.
50. al-Samman M, Zuckerman MJ, Verghese A, et al: Gastric ulcers associated with herpes simplex esophagitis in a nonimmunocompromised patient. J Clin Gastroenterol 18:160, 1994.
51. Morris A, Nicholson G: Ingestion of *Campylobacter pyloridis* causes gastritis and raised fasting gastric pH. Am J Gastroenterol 82:192–199, 1987.
52. Cater RE: *Helicobacter* (aka *Campylobacter*) *pylori* as the major causal factor in chronic hypochlorhydria. Med Hypotheses 39:367–374, 1002.
53. Thomas JE, Gibson GR, Darboe A, et al: Isolation of *Helicobacter pylori* from human feces. Lancet 340:1194–1195, 1992.
54. Blaser MJ, Parsonnet J: Parasitism by the "slow" bacterium *Helico-*

bacter pylori leads to altered gastric homeostasis and neoplasia. J Clin Invest 94:4–8, 1994.

55. Cover TL, Tammuru MK, Cao P, et al: Divergence of genetic sequences for the vacuolating cytotoxin among *Helicobacter pylori* strains. J Biol Chem 269:10566–10573, 1994.

56. Cover TL, Blaser MJ: Purification and characterization of the vacuolating toxin from *Helicobacter pylori*. J Biol Chem 267:10570–10575, 1992.

57. Telfor JL, Ghiara P, Dell'Orco M, et al: Gene structure of the *Helicobacter pylori* cytotoxin and evidence of its key role in gastric disease. J Exp Med 179:1653–1658, 1994.

58. Schmitt W, Haas R: Genetic analysis of the *Helicobacter pylori* vacuolating cytotoxin: Structural similarities with the IgA protease of exported protein. Mol Microbiol 12:307–319, 1994.

59. Atherton JC, Cao P, Peek RM Jr, et al: Mosaicism in vacuolating cytotoxin alleles of *Helicobacter pylori*. Association of specific vacA types with cytotoxin production and peptic ulceration. J Biol Chem 270:17771–17777, 1995.

60. Crabtree JE, Covacci A, Farmery SM, et al: *Helicobacter pylori* induced interleukin-8 expression in gastric epithelial cells is associated with CagA positive phenotype. J Clin Pathol 48:41–45, 1995.

61. Sugiyama T, Awakawa T, Hayashi S, et al: The effect of the immune response to *Helicobacter pylori* in the development of intestinal metaplasia. Eur J Gastroenterol Hepatol 6(suppl 1):S89–S92, 1994.

62. Di-Tommaso A, Xiang Z, Bugnoli M, et al: *Helicobacter pylori*-specific CD4+ T-cell clones from peripheral blood and gastric biopsies. Infect Immun 63:1102–1106, 1995.

63. Luzza F, Imeneo M, Maletta M, et al: Isotypic analysis of specific antibody response in serum, saliva, gastric and rectal homogenates of *Helicobacter pylori*-infected patients. FEMS Immunol Med Microbiol 10:285–288, 1995.

64. Faulde M, Cremer J, Zoller L: Humoral immune response against *Helicobacter pylori* as determined by immunoblot. Electrophoresis 14:945–951, 1993.

65. Haque M, Rahman KM, Khan AK, et al: Antigen profile of *Helicobacter pylori* strains isolated from peptic ulcer patients in Dhaka, Bangladesh. Bangladesh Med Res Counc Bull 19:71–78, 1993.

66. Macchia G, Massone A, Burroni D, et al: The Hsp60 protein of *Helicobacter pylori*: Structure and immune response in patients with gastroduodenal diseases. Mol Microbiol 9:645–652, 1993.

67. Perez-Perez GI, Brown WR, Cover TL, et al: Correlation between serological and mucosal inflammatory responses to *Helicobacter pylori*. Clin Diagn Lab Immunol 1:325–329, 1994.

68. Mégraud F, Neman SV, Brugmann D: Further evidence of the toxic effect of ammonia produced by *Helicobacter pylori* urease on human epithelial cells. Infect Immun 60:1858–1863, 1992.

69. Cover TL, Vaughn SG, Cao P, et al.: Potentiation of *Helicobacter pylori* vacuolating toxin activity by nicotine and other weak bases. J Infect Dis 166:1073–1078, 1992.

70. Dixon MF: Pathophysiology of *Helicobacter pylori* infection. Scand J Gastroenterol Suppl 201:7–10, 1994.

71. Mégraud F: Toxic factors of *Helicobacter pylori*. Eur J Gastroenterol Hepatol 6(suppl 1):S5–S10, 1994.

72. Figura N: Progress in defining the inflammatory cascade. Eur J Gastroenterol Hepatol 7:296–302, 1995.

73. Kaneko H, Nakada K, Mitsuma T, et al: *Helicobacter pylori* infection induces a decrease in immunoreactive-somatostatin concentrations of human stomach. Dig Dis Sci 37:409–416, 1992.

74. Woodward TA, Levin B: Cancers of the stomach and the duodenum. Gastroenterologist 3:14–19, 1995.

75. Endo S, Ohkusa T, Saito Y, et al: Detection of *Helicobacter pylori* infection in early stage gastric cancer: A comparison between intestinal- and diffuse-type gastric adenocarcinomas. Cancer 75:2203–2208, 1995.

76. Eidt S, Eidt H, Stolte M: Analysis of inflammatory reaction and epithelial proliferation in corpus mucosa of the stomach: A contribution to carcinogenesis. Pathologe 16:192–196, 1995.

77. Craanen ME, Blok P, Dekker W, et al: *Helicobacter pylori* and early gastric cancer. Gut 35:1372–1374, 1994.

78. De-Koster E, Buset M, Fernandes E, et al: *Helicobacter pylori*: The link with gastric cancer. Eur J Cancer Prev 3:247–257, 1994.

79. Blaser M J, Perez-Perez GI, Kleanthous H, et al: Infection with *Helicobacter pylori* strains possessing cagA is associated with an increased risk of developing adenocarcinoma of the stomach. Cancer Res 55:2111–2115, 1995.

80. Lin JT, Lee WC, Wu MS, et al: Diagnosis of gastric adenocarcinoma using a scoring system: Combined assay of serological markers of *Helicobacter pylori* infection, pepsinogen I and gastrin. J Gastroenterol 30:156–61, 1995.

81. Eidt S, Stolte M: The significance of *Helicobacter pylori* in relation to gastric cancer and lymphoma. Eur J Gastroenterol Hepatol 7:318–321, 1995.

82. Soll AH, Weinstein WM, Kurata J, et al: Nonsteroidal anti-inflammatory drugs and peptic ulcer disease. Ann Intern Med 114:307–319, 1991.

83. Graham DY, Smith JL, Spjut HJ, et al: Gastric adaptation: Studies in human during continuous aspirin administration. Gastroenterology 95:327–333, 1988.

84. Kuo YJ, Shanbour LL: Mechanism of action of aspirin on canine mucosa. Am J Physiol 230:762–767, 1976.

85. Ivey KJ: Mechanisms of nonsteroidal anti-inflammatory drug-induced gastric damage: Actions of therapeutic agents. Am J Med 84:41–48, 1988.

86. Publig W, Wustinger C, Zandl C: Non-steroidal anti-inflammatory drugs (NSAID) cause gastrointestinal ulcers mainly in *Helicobacter pylori* carriers. Wien Klin Wochenschr 106:276–279, 1994.

87. Laine L, Cominelli F, Sloan R, et al: Interaction of NSAIDs and *Helicobacter pylori* on gastrointestinal injury and prostaglandin production: A controlled double-blind trial. Aliment Pharmacol Ther 9:127–135, 1995.

88. Taha AS, Sturrock RD, Russell RI: Mucosal erosions in longterm non-steroidal anti-inflammatory drug users: Predisposition to ulceration and relation to *Helicobacter pylori*. Gut 36:334–336, 1995.

89. Wolfe MM, Alexander RW, McGuigan JE: Extrapancreatic, extraintestinal gastrinoma. Effective treatment of surgery. N Engl J Med 306:1533–1536, 1982.

90. Stabile BE, Morrow DJ, Passaro E: The gastrinoma triangle: Operative implications. Am J Surg 147:25–31, 1984.

91. Hofman JW, Fox PS, Wilson SD: Duodenal wall tumors of the Zollinger-Ellison syndrome: Surgical management. Arch Surg 107:334–339, 1973.

92. Mandujano UG, Angeles AA, de la Cruz HJ, et al: Gastrinoma of the common bile duct: Immunohistochemical and ultrastructural study of a case. J Clin Gastroenterol 20:321–324, 1995.

93. Soll AH: Review: Antisecretory drugs cellular mechanism of action. Aliment Pharmacol Ther 1:77–89, 1987.

94. Chuang C, Tanner M, Chen MCY, et al: Gastrin induction of histamine release from primary cultures of canine oxyntic mucosal cells. Am J Physiol 263:G460–465, 1992.

95. Ballard HS, Frame B, Hartsock RJ: Familial multiple endocrine adenoma-peptic ulcer complex. Medicine (Baltimore) 70:281–285, 1991.

96. Tarnawski A, Grzozowski T, Sarfeh IF, et al: Prostaglandin protection of human isolated gastric glands against endomethacin and ethanol injury: Evidence for direct cellular action of prostaglandin. J Clin Invest 81:1081–1089, 1988.

97. Hogan DL, Ainsworth MA, Isenberg JI: Review article: Gastroduodenal bicarbonate secretion. Aliment Pharmacol Ther 8:475–488, 1994.

98. Iwata F, Zhang XY, Leung FW: Aggravation of gastric mucosal lesions in rat stomach by tobacco cigarette smoke. Dig Dis Sci 40:1118–1124, 1995.

99. Holland EG, Taylor AT: Practical management of stress-related gastric ulcers. J Fam Pract 33:625–632, 1991.

100. Glavin GB, Murison R, Overmier JB, et al: The neurobiology of stress ulcers. Brain Res Brain Res Rev 16:301–343, 1991.

101. Boren T, Normark S, Falk P: *Helicobacter pylori*: Molecular basis for host recognition and bacterial adherence. Trends Microbiol 2:221–228, 1994.

102. Horrocks JC, DeDombal FT: Clinical presentation of patients with "dyspepsia": Detailed symptomatic study of 360 patients. Gut 19:19–26, 1978.

103. Plebani M, Vianello F, DiMario F: Laboratory medicine in ulcer disease. Clin Biochem 27:141–150, 1994.

104. Isenberg JI, McQuaid KR, Laine L, et al: Acid-peptic disorders. *In* Yamada T, Alpers DH, Woyang C, et al (eds): Textbook of Gastroenterology. Philadelphia, JB Lippincott, 1995, p 1347.

105. Jerris RC: Helicobacter. *In* Murray PR, Baron EJ, Pfaller MA, et al. (eds): Manual of Clinical Microbiolgy. Washington, ASM Press, 1995.

106. Yang DH, Bom HS, Joo YE, et al: Gastric juice ammonia vs CLO test for diagnosis of *Helicobacter pylori* infection. Dig Dis Sci 40:1083–1086, 1995.

107. Fabre R, Sobhami I, Laurent-Puig P, et al: Polymerase chain reaction assay for the detection of *Helicobacter pylori* in gastric biopsy specimens: Comparison with culture, rapid urease test, and histopathological tests. Gut 35:905–908, 1994.

108. Van-Swet AA, Thijs JC, Kooistra-Smid AM, et al: Use of PCR with feces for detection of *Helicobacter pylori* infections in patients. J Clin Microbiol 32:1346–1348, 1994.

109. Koletzko S, Haisch M, Seeboth I, et al: Isotope-selective non-dispersive infrared spectrometry for detection of *Helicobacter pylori* infection with 13C-urea breath test. Lancet 345:196–202, 1995.

110. Fallone CA, Mitchell A, Paterson WG: Determination of the test performance of less costly methods of *Helicobacter pylori* detection. Clin Invest Med 18:177–185, 1995.

111. Cutler AF, Havstad S, Ma CK, et al: Accuracy of invasive and noninvasive tests to diagnose *Helicobacter pylori* infection. Gastroenterology 109:136–141, 1995.

112. Yamashiro Y, Oguchi S, Otsuka Y, et al: *Helicobacter pylori* colonization in children with peptic ulcer disease. III. Diagnostic value of the 13C-urea breath test to detect gastric *H. Pylori* colonization. Acta Paediatr Jpn 37:12–16, 1995.

113. Nell B: FDA considers breath test for *Helicobacter pylori*. Clin Chem News 22:1, 1996.

114. Best LM, Veldhuyzen van Zanten SJ, Sherman PM, et al: Serological detection of *Helicobacter pylori* antibodies in children and their parents. J Clin Microbiol 32:1193–1196, 1994.

115. Edelman R: Blood, breath tests abound for *H. pylori* infection, ulcers. Clin Lab News 21:1, 19, 1995.

116. Xiang Z, Bugnoli M, Ponzelto A, et al: Detection in an enzyme immunoassay of an immune response to a recombinant fragment of the 128 kilodalton protein (CagA) of *Helicobacter pylori*. Eur J Clin Microbiol Infect Dis 12:739–745, 1993.

117. Luzza F, Maletta M, Imeneo M, et al: Salivary specific IgG is a sensitive indicator of the humoral immune response to *Helicobacter pylori*. FEMS Immunol Med Microbiol 10:281–283, 1995.

118. Tietz NW: Clinical Guide to Laboratory Tests. Philadelphia, WB Saunders, 1995.

119. Friesen SR, Tonita T: Pseudo Zollinger-Ellison syndrome: Hypergastrinemia, hyperchlorhydria without tumor. Ann Surg 194:489, 1981.

120. Kiefer ED, Sedgewich CE: Marginal ulcer following partial or subtotalgastrectomy. Surg Clin North Am 44:641, 1964.

121. Kao YS, Liu FJ, Alexander DR: Laboratory diagnosis of gastrointestinal tract and exocrine pancreatic disorders. *In* Henry JB (ed): Clinical Diagnosis and Management by Laboratory Methods. Philadelphia, WB Saunders, 1996, p 515.

122. DelValle J, Yamada T: Zollinger-Ellison syndrome. *In* Yamada T, Alpers DH, Owyang C, et al (eds): Textbook of Gastroenterology. Philadelphia, JB Lippincott, 1995, p 1430.

123. Hentschel E, Brandstätter G, Dragosics B, et al: Effect of ranitidine and amoxicillin plus metronidazole on the eradication of *Helicobacter pylori* and the recurrence of duodenal ulcer. N Engl J Med 328:308–312, 1993.

124. Karita M, Morshed MG, Ouchi K, et al: Bismuth-free triple therapy for eradicating *Helicobacter pylori* and reducing the gastric ulcer recurrence rate. Am J Gastroenterol 89:1032–1035, 1994.

125. Meko JB, Norton JA: Management of patients with Zollinger-Ellison syndrome. Annu Rev Med 46:395–411, 1995.

126. Moore NR, Rogers CE, Britton BJ: Magnetic resonance imaging of endocrine tumors of the pancreas. Br J Radiol 68:341–347, 1995.

127. Weber HC, Orbuch M, Jensen RT: Diagnosis and management of Zollinger-Ellison syndrome. Semin Gastrointest Dis 6:79–89, 1995.

128. Ruszniewski P, Amouyal P, Amouyal G, et al: Localization of gastrinomas by endoscopic ultrasonography in patients with Zollinger-Ellison syndrome. Surgery 117:629–635, 1995.

129. Orloff SL, Debas HT: Advances in the management of patients with Zollinger-Ellison syndrome. Surg Clin North Am 75:511–24, 1995.

Chapter 21

Malignancies and Bleeding of the Gastrointestinal Tract

David P. Thorne and Douglas W. Estry

MALIGNANCIES OF THE GASTROINTESTINAL TRACT

The gastrointestinal (GI) tract is a complex system consisting of many different tissue and cell types. Because malignancies that originate from most cell types within the GI tract have been reported,[1] the correct diagnosis and classification of a GI tumor is a complicated process with many possibilities. The correct classification of a neoplasm is important because it often dictates the type of therapeutic intervention and regimen to be followed. Even though many potential tumor types can exist within the GI tract, this chapter is a cursory overview of the major malignancies found in the GI tract with an emphasis on the primary pathologic mechanism and the role of the laboratory in their detection and diagnosis.

The detection and diagnosis of GI malignancies is commonly accomplished by the integration of information provided by clinical presentation, imaging techniques, and laboratory testing. The clinical laboratory plays many roles in this process. Histologic evaluation of tumors by microscopic assessment of cellular features is the most common method used for the diagnosis and classification of malignancies. In conjunction with this, the use of immunocytochemistry to identify constituents of a specific cell type has proven very useful in the classification of tumors consisting of undifferentiated cells.[2] Although not a primary means of cancer diagnosis, the evaluation of tumor markers is in many cases an important addendum to the diagnosis. Tumor markers are also important in monitoring the effectiveness of a therapeutic regimen and detecting the onset of relapse. The analysis of DNA content and composition using cytogenetic techniques, flow cytometry, and DNA probes has become an important factor used to classify tumors, generate prognostic indices, and stage the progression of cancer development.[3, 4]

Etiology

The mechanisms associated with the onset and progression of all types of cancer remain one of the enigmas of science.[5] Current evidence supports the concept of tumorigenesis as a multifactorial process that occurs in stages. Multiple factors have been implicated in the initiation and progression of this disease, including genetic predisposition, diet, immunologic responsiveness, and exposure to carcinogenic agents.[6] Even though many factors may influence this process, strong correlations have been established between damage or modification of DNA and the progression of this cellular transformation. These changes result in the stimulation of transcription of some genes and the inhibition of others. The changes may occur at allelic sites or involve chromosomes. The consequences of these changes are variable; however, certain common features appear in many types of cancers.[7] An increased rate of cellular division is a common manifestation and is accompanied by excessive autonomous growth that occurs in a nonregulated, uncoordinated manner. In many instances dedifferentiation occurs, in which cells lose characteristics associated with functional, mature cells and revert to a cell type consistent with its embryonic origin. Multiple cellular changes occur in conjunction with dedifferentiation. These include the synthesis of compounds that are normally only found during embryonic development, changes in cell surface hormone receptors, and changes in metabolism due to differences in enzyme activity compared to that in normal, differentiated cells. Monitoring these changes provides a means to detect and characterize a tumor.

Tumor Markers

Tumor markers are substances synthesized by malignant cells that can be qualitatively assayed to provide information regarding the presence of malignancies. When quantitatively assayed they provide an estimate of tumor burden or mass within a patient (see Chapter 50). A tumor marker may also be defined as a host response that provides an index related to the presence of a tumor in the host. Tumor marker testing can be used to screen for the presence of tumors in the general population or to provide information relating to the prognosis and/or the development of recurrence.[8] Several tumor markers have been useful in the detection, diagnosis, and management of GI cancers.[9, 10]

Carcinoembryonic antigen (CEA) is a protein that was first characterized immunologically in embryonic tissue. Low levels of CEA (<5 μg/L) are found in a normal healthy population. Although elevations in CEA occur in a variety of cancers,[11] the strongest correlation exists between CEA and colorectal cancer, in which persistent elevations, 5 to 10 times the upper reference limit, are found in 70% of the cases.[12]

Carbohydrate-related tumor markers are epitope-defined substances that are either secreted or exist on the surface of tumor cells. Several markers within this large group have proven useful in the diagnosis and monitoring of GI malignancies. Carbohydrate antigen (CA) 19–9 is a derivative of Lewis' blood group antigen (Le[a]). Expression of this antigen requires the presence of Lewis' gene. Thus patients who are Le[a−b−] will not produce CA 19–9. Elevations in CA 19–9 occur in a variety of cancers, but the strongest positive correlation exists with pancreatic cancer. Approximately 50% of gastric and 30% of colorectal cancers also present with persistent CA 19–9 elevations. CA 19–9 is useful in the monitoring of tumor mass as it applies to the efficacy of therapy or the onset of recurrence.

Another carbohydrate antigen related to Lewis' blood group is CA–50. Again, the strongest positive correlation exists between pancreatic cancer and CA–50 (80% to 97% sensitivity). However, 50% to 75% of late colorectal, 40% to 70% of esophageal, and 40% to 80% of gastric cancers are accompanied by elevated levels of CA–50. Good correlations have been established between levels of CA–50 and CA 19–9.

Because cancer is the outcome of genetic changes that cause the transformation from normal to cancerous cells, the use of genetic markers that reflect these cellular changes is the portal to identification of future tumor markers. Two major classes of genes, oncogenes and tumor suppressor genes, have been associated with the development of cancer. Correlations have been made between several types of GI malignancies and changes in these classes of genes. Specific mutations of the *ras* oncogene have been associated with a good prognosis in colorectal carcinomas. Mutation in the tumor suppressor gene p53 has been found in 70% to 80% of all late-stage colorectal cancers. The usefulness of genetic tumor markers has yet to be well established but holds promise for the future.

Increases in serum activity of CK_1 isoenzyme (CK-BB), lactate dehydrogenase (LD), and other enzymes occur in conjunction with several GI malignancies. The use of these, and many of the other potential indicators of tumor presence or mass have not found wide clinical utility due to a lack of specificity and sensitivity.[13]

Salivary Gland Tumors

Though not very common, a wide variety of tumors can form in the salivary glands. The *mixed salivary tumor* (pleomorphic adenoma) is the most prevalent. This usually benign tumor presents histologically with many different cell types arranged in duct-like structures. Increases in serum amylase (S-type) are common in this and in salivary malignancies.[14]

Esophageal Carcinoma

Cancer of the esophagus accounts for about 10% of all malignancies of the GI tract.[15] Carcinomas (tumors capable of invasion and metastasis) represent 90% of all esophageal cancers. The worldwide prevalence is about 4 times greater in blacks than in other races. Esophageal cancer appears to progress from normal epithelium to dysplasia to carcinoma. Factors influencing the onset and progression are unclear[16]; however, cigarette smoke and ethanol consumption are thought to act synergistically and may play a major role in its etiology. Several dietary factors have also been positively correlated with esophageal cancer, such as zinc deficiency and high total body iron content.

A disproportionally high mortality is seen with esophageal carcinoma. This may be because of the lack of symptoms in the early stages of the disease. Dysphagia (difficulty in swallowing) is usually the first symptom, but it initially presents intermittently. From this point, rapid progression to obstruction and metastasis commonly occurs. About 35% of patients initially seen already have evidence of metastatic disease, and only 20% display dysplasia or localized disease.[17]

Diagnosis is usually based on endoscopic appearance, biopsy results, and histologic evaluation. Endoscopic sonography or other imaging techniques allow assessment of the shape and degree of involvement with surrounding tissue. Tumor markers may be useful to screen for esophageal carcinoma or to monitor the efficacy of therapy. About 34% of the cases of esophageal carcinoma present with an elevated serum CA 19–9 level and about 60% with elevated CA–50 levels. Flow cytometric DNA analysis of esophageal carcinoma tissue has demonstrated that approximately 88% present with aneuploidy (less than a normal number of chromosomes).[18] Even though aneuploidy has been associated with a poor prognostic outlook, its value has yet to be well established.[6]

Gastric Carcinoma

The stomach is the second most common site of malignancy in the GI tract.[14] Many types of malignant cancers have been described as originating in the stomach. Of the four basic categories, carcinoma is the most common (90% to 95%), and far less common are lymphomas (4%), sarcomas (2%), and carcinoid tumors (3%).

Gastric carcinoma (adenocarcinoma) arises from the mucosal cells in the stomach and can be subdivided into two types, *intestinal* and *diffuse*. The diffuse type is characterized by a general thickening of the stomach wall without the formation of a discrete mass. The intestinal type forms tubular structures that are usually ulcerative. The ulcerative intestinal type is the predominant form, but both forms have a poor prognosis. The overall 5-year survival rate, with treatment, is less than 10%.

Progression of gastric carcinoma is insidious, primarily because of a lack of symptoms until the onset of advanced stages,[19] although early stages may present with vague pain and epigastric fullness. Gastric acid production varies with the stage of the disease. Early stages are commonly associated with hyperacidity resulting from stomach distention and subsequent gastrin release. Late stages are characterized by a loss of functional tissue due to displacement by nonfunctional malignant cells. Achlorhydria occurs, which results in iron deficiency and/or pernicious anemia. Secondary malabsorption of other nutrients leads to diarrhea and subsequent weight loss. Severe bleeding occurs with late stages of the ulcerative type of gastric carcinoma, and anemia secondary to the blood loss is common in advanced disease.

A variety of risk factors for gastric carcinoma have been identified. Much evidence supports the role of a heritable factor in the pathogenesis of gastric carcinoma. A notable example is the greater risk in persons of blood type A for the diffuse type than the intestinal type. Even though heritable patterns have been described, their expression appears to involve other factors. These include a wide variety of environmental factors and several precursor conditions that may transform to the malignant state.[20] Consumption of salted, smoked, or nitrate-/nitrite-preserved foods appears to be a primary environmental factor. Gastric infection with *Helicobacter pylori* has been implicated as a precursor condition[21] (see Chapter 20).

The diagnosis of gastric carcinoma is made by endoscopic evaluation, biopsy, and histologic characterization. Imaging techniques provide information regarding the location, size, and degree of tumor involvement in surrounding tissue.[22] The use of tumor markers has not proven beneficial in the diagnosis of gastric carcinoma, although elevations in serum CEA and CA 19–9 can be seen after metastasis. Gastric fluid analysis of pentagastrin-stimulated acid output supports the degree of involvement. Gastric fluid analysis is also useful to determine if obstruction exists. More than 60 different chromosomal abnormalities have been reported in gastric carcinoma. Karyotypes have demonstrated monosomic and polysomic states in several chromosomes. Numerous chromosomal rearrangements have also been observed, but the prognostic value of these has yet to be established.[6]

Malignancies of the Small Intestine

Even though the small intestine constitutes 75% of the length of the GI tract, less than 6% of GI malignancies arise from it. The most common malignancies in the small intestine are endocrine cell tumors (carcinoid) and lymphomas.[23, 24]

Lymphoma is a generic term used to characterize the unregulated proliferation of lymphocytes, histiocytes, and their derivatives or precursors within a cohesive tumorous lesion. All lymphomas are of monoclonal origin and present with similar morphologic and pathogenic characteristics. Lymphomas can arise anywhere within the GI tract; however, they are most frequently found in the stomach or small intestine.[25] In general, the growth of this tumor type is slow. Late stages of development are associated with a diffuse infiltration of muscle fibers that may cause motility problems and secondary obstruction. Large tumors commonly ulcerate, which may lead to perforation.[26]

The term *carcinoid* is a general term used to classify tumors that have arisen from endocrine cells[27] and that may arise from many different locations within the body. Within the GI tract, carcinoid tumors have been described in the esophagus, colon, stomach, and small intestine. A general characteristic of carcinoid tumors is their ability to produce and secrete bioactive substances. In many cases these substances reflect the endocrine products normally released by the cell line from which the tumor originated, such as gastrin, somatostatin, and serotonin; however, in many cases additional products normally not produced by the gut are released, including insulin, glucagon, adrenocorticotropic hormone (ACTH), calcitonin, histamine, and substance P. The relative content and quantity of endocrine products released from these tumors are variable. Thus, a wide variety of endocrine syndromes, which are the result of inappropriate tumor hormone production, are possible, including Zollinger-Ellison syndrome, Cushing's syndrome, and carcinoid syndrome.[28]

Carcinoid syndrome is most commonly associated with endocrine cell tumors of the small intestine that produce excessive amounts of serotonin or its precursor. Serotonin is a potent stimulator of smooth muscle contraction. It is derived from the amino acid tryptophan in a two-step enzymatic process.[29] The first step involves the hydroxylation of tryptophan to form 5-hydroxytryptophan (5-HTP). 5-HTP is then decarboxylated to form serotonin, or 5-hydroxytryptamine (5-HT). In normal serotonin-producing cells, the conversion of 5-HTP to 5-HT limits the availability of the active hormone. In carcinoid tumors, however, the conversion rate is very high. The half-life of extracellular serotonin is very short because of active cellular uptake and conversion to the nonactive substance 5-hydroxyindoleacetic acid (5-HIAA). Most of the 5-HIAA is cleared from the body by renal filtration.

The production and metabolism of serotonin by carcinoid tumors varies in relation to the location of the tumor within the small intestine. Patients with ileal carcinoid tumors typically produce and release large quantities of 5-HT, resulting in very high levels of urinary 5-HIAA. Patients with foregut tumors, duodenal or gastric, typically produce and secrete large quantities of the precursor 5-HTP, a portion of which is converted to serotonin after release. In these cases, urinary 5-HIAA levels may be only moderately elevated. In patients with suspected carcinoid syndrome that show borderline increases in urinary 5-HIAA, measurement of serum 5-HTP may aid in establishing the diagnosis.

The early detection and diagnosis of carcinoid tumors is critical because of the high potential for metastasis. Cancer that progresses to this stage is usually considered incurable. Diagnosis involves the correlation of clinical symptoms with an endocrinopathy and indicators of GI tract involvement. The use of urinary 5-HIAA as a screening procedure is useful in the majority of cases. Subsequent imaging techniques aid in the localization and establishment of a presumptive diagnosis.[30] Surgical biopsy results and histologic evaluation confirm the diagnosis. However, the utility of cytogenetic techniques has not been established in this disease.[31]

Malignancies of the Large Intestine

Many different tumor types, both benign and malignant, can arise within the large intestine. Of these, the most significant is colorectal cancer, which is the second leading cause of cancer deaths in the United States.[14] Approximately 4% of the population will develop a form of this cancer by the age of 75 years. The cure rate for this form of cancer has remained at about 50% for several decades. The primary factor that determines the prognosis of a given case is the stage at which this cancer exists at initial diagnosis. The mean survival time for patients with metastasis at initial diagnosis is 6 months; however with early detection, colorectal carcinoma is considered one of the most curable forms of GI malignancies. The development of colorectal cancer is a multistage process that is believed to occur over many years. Even though colorectal cancer has a slow rate of progression, the onset of overt symptoms does not occur until the late stages of the disease. Sporadic bleeding in conjunction with a change in bowel habits may precede the onset of symptoms and the establishment of incurable disease by several years. Thus, early detection currently involves the use of the fecal occult blood test (FOBT) as the screening mechanism applied to the at-risk population.

Due to the ease of accessibility, the multistage progression of colon tissue from normal to the malignant state has been very well documented. The development of colorectal cancer is a stepwise process involving morphologic and molecular changes. Colorectal cancer originates from the normal epithelium lining the large intestine. Initially, a localized hyperplasia occurs that develops into an adenomatous polyp. These are space-filling growths that protrude into the lumen of the colon. Polyps of this type are present in the colon of many older adults, but the majority of these are benign with no malignant potential,[32] although a portion may transform into a neoplastic adenoma. This stage is characterized by localized foci of dysplasia, which is confined within the polyp with no propensity for metastasis. Central or peripheral necrosis of the polyp occurs at this stage with subsequent bleeding. Conversion to an invasive carcinomatous state from neoplastic adenoma involves an increase in size, a loss of cellular differentiation, and the acquisition of cellular invasive properties. Localized spreading may involve an initial direct extension into the muscular layers of the large intestine. Subsequent penetration through the basement membrane and involvement of regional lymph nodes precedes metastasis. The final stage of distant metastatic spread occurs through lymphatic and blood vessels. Systemic deposition of cancerous cells from primary colorectal tumors favors liver, lung, and bones.

The progression of the tumorigenic process in colorectal cancer has been well correlated with abnormal gene expression and histologic presentation.[33] Monitoring specific genetic changes as a tumor marker may provide a mechanism for screening and the accurate classification of the stage of tumor progression.[34] Point mutations of the *ras* proto-oncogene occur in about 50% of neoplastic adenomas. This event appears to be an important step in the development of neoplasia and tumor development.[35] Deletion of a portion of the long arm of chromosome 18 is found in 70% of colorectal carcinomas. This loss is referred to as DCC (deleted in colorectal carcinoma). Loss of the DCC sequence is associated with a decrease in the number of cell adhesion proteins on the cell surface. Invasive neoplasia is often associated with alterations in cell–cell interactions mediated by these proteins.[36] Nearly 75% of colorectal carcinomas have detectable deletions (allelic loss) from chromosome 17. Mapping studies have shown that this loss corresponds to the loss of the p53 gene, the product of which is an important tumor suppressor. Point mutations in the remaining allele correspond to late events in the transition from neoplastic adenoma to carcinoma.

Cellular changes also accompany the transition for normal to carcinogenic states.[37] Noteworthy is the expression and synthesis of proteins associated with the loss of differentiation. CA 19–9 is an oncofetal protein secreted by 50% to 80% of neoplastic polyps and carcinomas of the colon. Sialylated Tn antigen, or TAG 72, is a mucin glycoprotein not expressed in normal tissue that appears in 50% of neoplastic adenomas and 90% of colonic carcinomas.[38] The most widely used tumor marker for colorectal cancer is CEA. The stimulation of synthesis of this glycoprotein appears to occur late in the conversion from neoplastic adenoma to carcinoma. The serum concentration of CEA is directly related to the size and extent of spread of the primary tumor. Thus, nearly 100% of metastatic colorectal carcinomas display high serum concentrations of CEA, whereas increases are only noted in 19% to 40% of neoplastic polyps. Because CEA can be produced by other cancers and a number of non-neoplastic disorders, the use of CEA as a screening test for colorectal cancer is inappropriate. The primary clinical utility of serum CEA is in the monitoring of a therapeutic regimen. If a CEA-secreting tumor is completely removed, serum levels should rapidly decrease to within the normal reference range. Return of high serum CEA is a reliable indicator of recurrence.

Correlations have been established between the incidence of colorectal cancer and the many contributing factors. The prevalence of colorectal cancer shows marked geographic variation; in addition,[39] its incidence closely parallels socioeconomic standards. It appears to be a disease of the affluent. A strong argument has been made for a hereditary basis or predisposition for the disease.[40] It has also been noted that many cases of chronic inflammatory bowel disease, such as ulcerative colitis and Crohn's disease, progress to colorectal cancer.[41, 42] Diets low in fiber, high in fat, and high in total caloric intake appear to augment its development, whereas diets high in fruits and vegetables appear to be preventive.[43] Support exists for a direct relationship between ethanol consumption and colorectal cancer.[44]

The diagnosis of colorectal cancer is based on the histologic evaluation of biopsy material acquired from surgical procedures. Colonoscopy is a relevant procedure that precedes surgical intervention. It provides information regarding the location and type of polyp or tumor. Other imaging techniques that have found utility in the diagnosis, characterization, and monitoring of colorectal cancer include the following: barium radiology, ultrasonography, computed tomography (CT), magnetic resonance imaging (MRI), and immunoscintigraphy.[45] The value of cytogenetic analysis has yet to be firmly established.[46, 47]

Treatment of Gastrointestinal Malignancies

The treatment of GI malignancies is similar to that of malignancies in other anatomic locations.[48] Curative or palliative resection of tumor is a common procedure. Excision of regional lymph nodes is indicated many times. The use of radiation therapy may be limited to cases in which the location of the tumor prevents selective exposure. The selection and utilization of a chemotherapeutic agent is dependent on an accurate classification of the tumor type and the staging or grade of the neoplasia.

GASTROINTESTINAL BLEEDING

Because only trace quantities of hemoglobin can be found in any portion of a normal GI tract, the presence of blood is an important indicator of a pathologic lesion and requires further investigation. Some possible causes of GI bleeding may be seen in Figure 21–1.

Upper Gastrointestinal Tract Bleeding

The presence of blood in gastric residue after 12 hours of fasting may be the result of peptic ulcer, gastric carcinoma, esophageal cancer or varices, Mallory-Weiss syndrome, severe gastritis, or excessive gum bleeding from periodontal disease. The gross appearance of blood in a gastric aspirate is dependent on the pH of the stomach. At the normal pH of the stomach, which is strongly acidic, blood forms acid hematin, which is dark brown. A coffee ground appearance is common with a high volume of blood loss in the stomach. Bleeding lesions within the stomach are subject to very high rates of blood loss, primarily resulting from the inhibition of coagulation and platelet function at the low pH of the stomach. The presence of overt blood (bright red) in a gastric aspirate is most commonly due to trauma, such as that which may occur during intubation. A rapid rate of blood loss from the upper GI tract commonly results in *hematemesis*, the vomiting or spitting up of blood. In these conditions, blood is usually simultaneously detectable in feces. The reporting of blood from gastric specimens or emesis should always be confirmed by chemical testing.

Peptic ulceration accounts for the majority of cases of upper GI tract bleeding. *H. pylori* is the infectious etiologic agent responsible for the majority of cases of peptic ulceration. The pathologic mechanisms and consequences of these GI lesions are discussed in Chapter 20.

Mallory-Weiss syndrome is associated with the presence of lacerations in either the gastric or esophageal mucosa.[49] It is primarily caused by an increase in intragastric pressure secondary to protracted retching, excessive vomiting, or coughing. Mallory-Weiss syndrome accounts for 2% to 7% of all cases of upper GI tract bleeding. Higher rates are seen in individuals who consume excessive amounts of ethanol. Factors characterizing this increased incidence or predisposition have yet to be adequately addressed.

Variceal vessels are dilations within the venous blood system that result from an increase in venous blood pressure. The most common cause of this condition is an increase in hepatic portal tension due to obstruction of hepatic blood flow, which can occur in several conditions, such as hepatic thrombosis, tumors, or abscesses. The most common condition associated with hepatic portal hyperten-

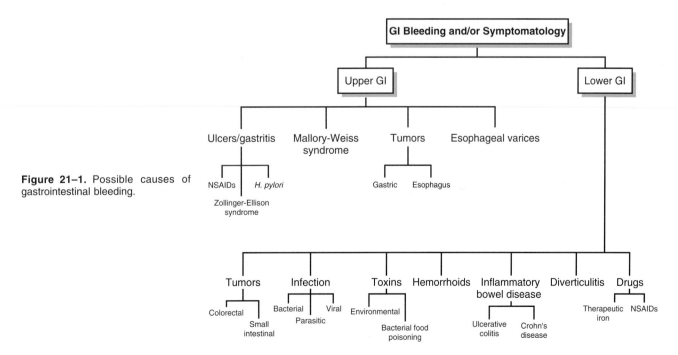

Figure 21–1. Possible causes of gastrointestinal bleeding.

sion, and thus variceal vessels, however, is alcoholic cirrhosis. Variceal vessels can form in many sites. Esophageal varices are particularly important because of their ease of rupture and subsequent bleeding. Large losses of blood can occur with hemorrhagic esophageal varices that usually result in massive hematemesis.

Lower Gastrointestinal Tract Bleeding

Blood that appears within feces may originate anywhere from the mouth to the rectum. The diagnosis of bleeding from the lower GI tract can be made by ruling out upper GI tract bleeding and by the presence of blood in feces. In most instances *overt blood* (bright red) in stool, identified by visual inspection, originates from rectal, anal, or perianal regions. Hemorrhoids or anal fissures account for the majority of overt blood in stool. In cases with simultaneous high GI motility, blood that originates from other colon lesions may also present with an overt appearance. Visually identified blood must be confirmed by chemical testing because bright red pigments, visually indistinguishable from blood, may present in stool with ingestion of several dietary substances or therapeutic agents. With normal motility, blood from nonanal regions of the GI tract presents as oxidized hemoglobin products, which appear dark brown or black. Thus, depending on the concentration of hemoglobin and the color of the stool, blood may not be visually apparent and is referred to as *occult blood*. Stools with a high content of hemoglobin present with a black tarry appearance. Blood loss of small quantities from the lower GI tract can be easily detected by chemical testing. Blood loss from the upper GI tract requires significantly higher quantities to be detected. Chemically detected occult blood may persist in stool for 5 to 12 days after a single episode of large loss. The length of persistence is dependent on the quantity lost and location of the lesion.[50]

Lower GI tract bleeding may be a result of many conditions other than GI malignancies. As previously mentioned, hemorrhoids and anal fissures are a common source of bleeding. Bacterial, parasitic, or viral infections of the GI tract may present with either overt or occult blood in feces. Diverticular disease accounts for a significant number of positive fecal occult blood tests.[51] A common clinical manifestation of inflammatory bowel disorders, such as ulcerative colitis and Crohn's disease, is the presence of blood in stool. Severe diarrhea due to ingested environmental or bacterial toxins may also result in the presence of blood in stool.[52] The presence of blood in the GI tract may also occur in conjunction with lesions in organs associated with the GI tract. Hemorrhagic pancreatitis may be a source of entry for blood into the GI tract. A variety of drugs have been associated with chemically detectable blood loss from GI tract in normal persons and an increase in loss from individuals with preexisting GI pathologic lesions. Notable is the use of nonsteroidal anti-inflammatory agents.[53] Following discontinuation of these agents, it may require up to 3 weeks for detectable blood to clear. Oral intake of iron supplements at supratherapeutic dosages may cause a positive chemically detected occult blood. This may be a direct effect of excess iron in the stool or a secondary effect of GI irritation from some iron-containing compounds.

Clinical Laboratory Tests and Gastrointestinal Bleeding

The clinical laboratory plays several roles in the diagnosis and management of GI bleeding. The detection and confirmation of blood by chemical methods in feces, vomitus, or gastric aspirates are in many cases the initial indicators that bleeding is occurring. Variation in whole blood hemoglobin content, hematocrit, and reticulocyte count are good indicators of the rate and extent of blood loss. Chronic blood loss is commonly associated with microcytic, hypochromic anemia due to iron deficiency. Changes in whole blood hemoglobin and hematocrit levels may not be immediately seen with acute loss of a high volume of blood, as may be seen with peptic ulcers. In these cases, autoregulation to maintain blood volume may require up to 24 hours before a hemodilution effect is seen. This regulatory mechanism involves the renin-angiotensin system and reflex hormonal responses. Changes in acid/base status also occurs in conjunction with acute blood loss. Rapid compensation to low peripheral arterial partial pressure of oxygen (Pao_2) due to blood loss results in hyperventilation, causing respiratory alkalosis. Metabolic alterations also occur in response to hemorrhagic shock. A conversion to anaerobic metabolism of glucose induces lactic acidosis.

Blood loss in the GI tract may influence a wide range of other laboratory tests. An increase in white blood cell and platelet counts is commonly seen with high-volume acute blood loss. Elevation of serum urea level is a very common finding in upper GI tract bleeding. This results from degradation of hemoglobin by intestinal proteases and subsequent deamination of excess amino acids by intestinal bacteria. Consistent with prerenal azotemia, the serum urea level is high, whereas the serum creatinine concentration is normal. The degree of elevation corresponds to the degree of blood loss. A serum urea level of 40 mg/dL or greater in conjunction with a normal serum creatinine level corresponds to a blood loss of at least 1 L from the upper GI tract over the previous 24 hours. Many times, transfusion is required when high volume blood loss from the GI tract occurs.[54] Replacement therapy with fresh frozen plasma, cryoprecipitate, or platelets may be necessary to maintain homeostatic integrity following extensive bleeding.

Detection of Blood in Feces

The presence of blood in stool can be evaluated by several analytic methods.[55] Most are based on chemical reactions that generate a visually detectable colored product. The Hemoccult test (Smith-Kline Diagnostics, San Jose, Calif) is currently the most common method used, and it is based on the oxidation of guaiac by peroxide. Heme iron within stool is a catalyst for this reaction. A positive reaction produces a visually detectable, soluble blue chromophore. The analytic sensitivity of this test is generally considered to be low. The lower limit of detection by this method is dependent on the variable presence of endogenous inhibitors and the prowess of the individual performing the assay. Although fecal specimen is typically smeared onto a guaiac-containing filter paper, a higher analytic sensitivity has been reported with the use of dried fecal material on the filter paper. The Hematest (Miles Inc, Elkhart, Ind.) has greater analytic sensitivity for the detection of fecal occult blood. It is based on the heme-catalyzed oxidation of *ortho*-toluidine, which produces a blue color. This test is sensitive enough to detect as little as 100 mg of hemoglobin in 100 g of stool. False-positive results may be seen with therapeutic dosages of medicinal iron and diets high in red meat. A sensitive, quantitative method for the determination of blood in fecal material is available, which evaluates heme-derived porphyrins fluorometrically after extraction from stool. This method is largely manual, and its utility in clinical practice is limited. An immunochemical method is currently being evaluated for clinical use.[56] This method is highly specific for GI bleeding and results in very few false-positive findings.

Several factors must be taken into consideration when testing for blood in feces using the guaiac-based method. The specimen should not be acquired from the toilet bowl because of the presence of peroxidase in some detergents and toilet bowl cleaners that will produce a false-positive result. Appropriate selection of sample from the stool specimen to be applied to the filter paper is important. Blood originating in the upper GI tract is usually uniformly distributed within the stool, but blood originating from the lower GI tract may only be present in a segment of the stool or only coat its surface. Thus, the final sample on the filter paper should reflect an attempt to test representative aliquots from all significant portions of the stool, including the center. Due to the fact that many sources of GI bleeding do so intermittently, relevant evaluation for GI bleeding requires testing on at least 3 specimens. Testing should be completed within 3 days after sample application to filter paper because an extended delay may produce a false-negative result.

Screening for Colorectal Cancer With the Fecal Occult Blood Test

The fecal occult blood test (FOBT), which uses the guaiac-based method, has been extensively used as a screening test for the detection of colorectal cancer. The World Health Organization has established guidelines for screening.[57] Persons with symptoms of GI abnormality are not candidates for colorectal cancer screening by FOBT but should have other diagnostic tests performed. Currently, it is recommended that the FOBT be done annually on all persons older than 50 years. High-risk populations should be monitored on a regular basis, which include individuals with a family history of colorectal cancer, those with ulcerative colitis or Crohn's disease, and those with a history of adenomas of the large intestine. Several factors must be taken into consideration with a positive result.[58] Within the recommended screening population just described, the diagnostic sensitivity of the FOBT for the detection of colorectal cancer is in the range of 50% to 70%. Current evidence indicates that within the recommended screening population only 5% to 8% of individuals who have tested positive will have colorectal cancer. The low prevalence of colorectal cancer in this population (approximately 1%) indicates a low positive predictive value. Thus, between 92% to 95% of all positive results are falsely positive for colorectal cancer, although the false-positive rate drops to

about 70% if the presence of neoplastic adenomas are also considered a positive finding. Currently in most institutions, the follow-up to a positive FOBT is sigmoidoscopy with barium enema or colonoscopy.[59] Both of these procedures are labor intensive and invasive as well as costly. Thus the low cost and ease of testing provided by the FOBT may be misleading in terms of the true cost and benefit of this screening procedure.[60] It is important to note that the FOBT is a test for the presence of blood in stool, which is a significant finding even if it does not directly relate to colorectal cancer. With some methods the analytic specificity of this test can be very high, 90% to 98%, for the presence of blood in feces. In the absence of colorectal cancer and in the absence of false-positive results from exogenous peroxidase activity, a positive result on the FOBT indicates that some other condition should be addressed.

Case Study

As part of a screening test for colorectal cancer using a guaiac-based method for the evaluation of fecal occult blood, a specimen produced a positive result. Duplicate tests on different specimens also produced positive results. Follow-up colonoscopy was unremarkable. Routine complete blood cell count (CBC) and urinalysis were also preformed. All parameters were within the normal reference range. Serum chemistry results were normal for amylase, lipase, creatinine, bilirubin, and liver enzyme; however, a slight increase in serum urea was present. Evaluation of stool appearance, pH, lipid, and starch content were all normal, but the FOBT was still positive. Ova and parasite analysis as well as bacterial culture for pathogens in stool were negative. Evaluation of upper GI tract by barium imaging produced no significant findings. In a similar manner, endoscopic evaluation of upper GI tract with biopsy was unremarkable. Gastric aspiration indicated normal acidity and no blood present. *H. pylori* infection was ruled out by culture of biopsy material and the campylobacter-like organism (CLO) test. Subsequent FOBTs continued to produce positive results despite dietary precautions that eliminated exogenous peroxidase activity.

Question

1. What is the cause of the persistent positive FOBTs?

Discussion

1. The analytic specificity of the FOBT by the guaiac method is high. The repeated positive results with other causes ruled out provide evidence that GI bleeding is occurring. The CBC is normal, which indicates that the rate and degree of blood loss are insufficient to cause anemia. Nonetheless, blood is present in feces, and exhaustive testing has failed to identify the source of the bleeding in this situation.

What choices are left? A positive occult blood test finding is common with the use of certain drugs. Oral iron supplements, whether taken alone or in combination with vitamins, can be the cause of GI bleeding. Recommended dosage regimens do not cause GI bleeding or produce a positive FOBT in the majority of the population. However high doses, whether short-term or long-term, may cause GI irritation that results in bleeding. The use of nonsteroidal anti-inflammatory drugs can also cause GI bleeding. In most of these cases observable gastric erosion and possible ulceration can be found; however, in many cases these lesions may not be apparent or may be transient.

References

1. Robbins SL, Cotran RS, Kumar V: Pathologic Basis of Disease, ed 3. Philadelphia, WB Saunders, 1984.
2. Yazdi H, Dardick I: Diagnostic Immunocytochemistry and Electron Microscopy. New York, Igaku-Shoin, 1994.
3. Garrett CT, Sell S (eds): Cellular Cancer Markers. Totowa, NJ, Humana Press, 1995.
4. Williams NN, Daly JM: Flow cytometry and the prognostic implications in patients with solid tumors. Surg Gynecol Obstet 171:257–266, 1990.
5. Brugge J (ed): Origins of Human Cancer: A Comprehensive Review. Plainview, NY, Cold Water Springs Laboratory Press, 1991.
6. Cannon-Albright LA, Bishop DT, Goldgar C: Genetic predisposition to cancer. Important Adv Oncol 1:39–55, 1991.
7. Heim S, Mitelman F (eds): Cancer Cytogenetics, ed 2. New York, Wiley–Liss, 1987.
8. Mercer DW: Use of multiple markers to enhance clinical utility. Immunol Ser 53:39–54, 1990.
9. Wahren B, Harmenberg U: Tumor markers in gastrointestinal cancer. Scand J Clin Lab Invest Suppl 206:21–27, 1991.
10. Chan DW, Sell S: Tumor markers. In Burtis C, Ashwod ER (eds): Tietz Textbook of Clinical Chemistry, ed 2. Philadelphia, WB Saunders, 1994, pp 897–927.
11. Chevinsky AH: CEA in tumors of other than colorectal origin. Semin Surg Oncol 7:162–166, 1991.
12. Woolfson K: Tumor Markers in Cancer of the Colon and Rectum. Dis Colon Rectum 34:506–511, 1991.
13. Schwartz MK: Enzymes used in predicting high risk to colon cancer. Clin Biochem 23:395–398, 1990.
14. Salt WB, Schnenker S: Amylase—Its clinical significance: A review of the literature. Medicine 155:269–289, 1976.
15. Wingo PA, Tong T, Bolden S: Cancer statistics. J Clin Cancer 45:8–30, 1995.
16. Tytgat KM, Tytgat GN: Esophageal carcinoma. Heptatogastroenterology 37:353–357, 1990.
17. Kuwano H, Baba K, Ikebe M, et al: Histopathology of early esophageal carcinoma and squamous epithelial dysplasia. Hepatogastroenterology 40:212–216, 1993.
18. Kaketani K, Saito T, Kuwahara A, et al: DNA stem line heterogenicity in esophageal cancer accurately identified by flow cytometric analysis. Cancer 72:3564–3570, 1993.
19. Fuchs CS, Mayer RJ: Gastric carcinoma. N Engl J Med 333:32–40, 1995.
20. World Health Organization: The evaluation of carcinogenic risks to humans, Monograph 61. Lyon, France, International Agency for Research on Cancer, 1994.
21. Correa P: Helicobacter pylori and gastric carcinogenesis. Am J Surg Pathol 19(suppl 1):S37–S43, 1995.
22. Halpert RD, Feczko PJ: Role of radiology in the diagnosis and staging of gastric malignancy. Endoscopy 25:39–45, 1993.
23. Haller DG: Endocrine tumors of the gastrointestinal tract. Curr Opin Oncol 6:72–76, 1994.
24. Moertel C: An odyssey in the land of small intestine tumors. J Clin Oncol 10:1503–1522, 1987.
25. Thomas CR: Update on gastric lymphoma. J Natl Med Assoc 83:713–718, 1991.
26. Isaacson PG: Primary gastric lymphoma. Br J Biomed Sci 52:291–296, 1995.
27. Creutzfeld W: Historical background and natural history of carcinoids. Digestion 55(suppl 3):3–10, 1994.
28. Marshall JB, Bodnarchuk G: Carcinoid tumors of the gut: Our experience over thirty years and review of the literature. J Clin Gastroenterol 16:123–129, 1993.
29. Whitley RJ, Meikle AW, Watts NB: Endocrinology. In Burtis C, Ashwood E (eds): Tietz Textbook of Clinical Chemistry, ed 2. Philadelphia, WB Saunders, 1994, pp 1765–1770.
30. Lappas JC: Small bowel imaging. Curr Opin Radiol 4:32–38, 1992.
31. Scappaticci S, Brandi M, Capra E: Cytogenetics of multiple endocrine neoplasia syndrome. Cancer Genet Cytogenet 63:17–21, 1992.
32. Itzkowitz SH, Kim YS: Polyps and benign neoplasm. In Sleisenger MH, Fordtran JS (eds): Gastrointestinal Disease: Pathophysiology/Diagnosis/Management, 5 ed, vol 2, Philadelphia, WB Saunders, 1993, 1402–1430.
33. Smyrk TC: Colon cancer connections: Cancer syndrome meets molecular biology meets histopathology. Am J Pathol 145:1–6, 1994.
34. Jass JR: Prognostic factors colorectal cancer. Curr Top Pathol 81:295–322, 1990.
35. Sidransky D, Tokino T, Hamilton SR, et al: Identification of ras oncogene mutations in the stool of patients with curable colorectal cancer. Science 256:102–105, 1992.
36. Johnson JP: Cell adhesion molecules of the immunoglobulin supergene family and their role in malignant transformation and progression of metastatic disease. Cancer Metastasis Rev 10:11–22, 1991.
37. Rothenberger DA: Relevant clinical information and tumor markers. Cancer 71(suppl 12): 4193–4197, 1993.
38. Itzkowitz SH: Blood group-related carbohydrate antigen expression in malignant and premalignant colonic neoplasms. J Cell Biochem (suppl 16)G:97–101, 1992.
39. Waterhouse J, Muir CS, Wagner G, et al: Cancer incidence in five continents. Lyon, France, International Agency for Research on Cancer, Vol 4:N42, 1982.
40. Winawer SJ, Zauber AG, O'Brien MJ, et al: Family history of colorectal cancer as a predictor of adenomas at follow-up colonoscopy: A study based on segregation analysis. Gastroenterology 104(suppl A):3099–3103, 1992.
41. Bernard L: Ulcerative colitis and colon cancer: Biology and surveillance. Br J Cell Biochem 16(suppl G):47–50, 1992.
42. Petras RE, Mir-Madjlessi SH, Farmer RG: Crohn's disease and intestinal carcinoma. Gastroenterology 93:1307–1314, 1987.
43. Burnstein MJ: Dietary factors related to colorectal neoplasms. Surg Clin North Am 73:13–29, 1993.
44. Klasky AL, Armstrong MA, Friedman GD, et al: The relations of alcoholic beverage use to colon and rectal cancer. Am J Epidemiol 128:1007–1013, 1988.
45. Dodd GD: The role of the barium enema in the detection of colonic neoplasms. Cancer 70(suppl 5):1272–1275, 1992.
46. Bottger TC, Potratz D, Stockle M, et al: Prognostic value of DNA analysis in colorectal cancer. Cancer 72:3579–3587, 1993.
47. Bauer KD, Bagwell CB, Giaretti W, et al: Consensus review of the clinical utility of DNA flow cytometry in colorectal cancer. Cytometry 14:486–491, 1993.
48. Geoffroy F, Grem JL: Chemotherapy of advanced gastrointestinal cancer. Curr Opin Oncol 6:427–434, 1994.
49. Grahm DY, Schwartz JF: The spectrum of the Mallory-Weiss tear. Medicine 57:301–311, 1978.
50. Beeler MF, Kao Y, Scheer WD: Malabsorption, diarrhea and examination of feces. In Henry JB (ed): Clinical Diagnosis and Management by Laboratory Methods, ed. 16. Philadelphia, WB Saunders, 1979, pp 795–798.
51. Balson R, Gibson PR: Lower gastrointestinal tract: 2. Diarrhea and diverticular disease. Med J Aust 162:217–219, 1995.
52. Afgani B, Stutman HR: Toxin-related diarrheas. Pediatr Ann 23:549–555, 1994.
53. Dajani EZ, Agrawal NM: Prevention and treatment of ulcers induced by nonsteroidal anti-inflammatory drugs. J Physiol Pharmacol 46:3–16, 1995.
54. Faenza A, Cunsolo A, Selleri S, et al: Correlation between plasma or blood transfusion and survival after curative surgery for colorectal cancer. Int Surg 77:264–269, 1992.
55. Gopalswamy N, Stelling HP: A comparative study of eight fecal blood tests and hemoquant in patients in whom colonoscopy is indicated. Am Fam Med 3:1043–1048, 1994.

56. Allison JE, Tekawa IS, Ransom LJ, et al: A comparison of fecal occult blood tests for colorectal cancer screening. N Engl J Med 334:155–159, 1996.

57. Winawer SJ, St. John J, Bond J, et al: Screening of average-risk individuals for colorectal cancer. Bull World Health Organ 68:505–513, 1990.

58. Sapir M: Hidden assumptions in the critique of occult blood testing. Comp Therap 21:172–176, 1995.

59. Metzen RN: Fecal occult blood testing: Guidelines for follow-up after a positive finding. Postgrad Med 90:181–184, 1991.

60. Liberman D: Screening/Early detection model for colorectal cancer. Cancer 74(suppl):2023–2027, 1994.

Bowel Disorders

Connie R. Mahon

ACUTE DIARRHEA

Diarrheal diseases are among the most common disorders that afflict humans. Because the disease is usually self-limiting, in most cases individuals do not seek medical attention during the first 3 to 5 days of illness. Even so, costs of diarrhea exceed millions of dollars yearly owing to loss of productivity, medical expenses, lost compensation, and financial losses suffered by the food industry.[1]

Diarrheal illnesses have a wide variety of etiologies, and may be infectious (food poisoning, *Shigella*, *Salmonella*) or noninfectious (stress, effects of antibiotic). Evaluating every possible cause of a diarrheal illness becomes costly and restrictive,[2] challenging both clinicians and laboratorians to use a practical approach that is cost effective but provides meaningful results and appropriate care for the patient.

Because diarrheal pathogens are acquired primarily through the ingestion of contaminated food or drink, the interaction between organism and host defense mechanisms in the gastrointestinal tract plays a major role in the establishment of disease. Figure 22–1 shows the anatomy of the gastrointestinal tract.[3]

When organisms associated with diarrhea are ingested and reach the stomach, they are immediately exposed to the gastric acid and enzymes there. Except for cysts of protozoans and spore-forming bacterial species, most organisms are susceptible to the acid pH of the stomach, and only a few resist this protective mechanism and reach the small intestine. Organisms that reach the small intestine are challenged with peristaltic movement, and organisms such as *Giardia lamblia*, which require attachment to initiate an infection, are at a disadvantage. In the large intestine, antibody, such as secretory IgA, is secreted locally and is effective against some of these organisms. Additionally, organisms that reach the colon must compete for nutrients and space with huge numbers of other organisms, such as the normal microbial flora, present at this site.[4]

Etiology

Acute diarrhea is an illness of short duration (usually less than 2 weeks) either because it is self-limited with spontaneous recovery or because it is easily diagnosed and treated. A patient history should comprise travel, eating and drinking patterns, including establishments frequented, toxic and allergic reactions, and medications. The frequency and nature of the stools as well as the presence of symptoms among other family members and groups of friends, are also helpful.[4] A history of travel to areas where sewage and sanitary facilities are less than ideal increases the patient's risk of having acquired an enteric pathogen. Knowledge of food recently ingested is also useful. As shown in Table 22–1, certain pathogens are strongly associated with specific food as vehicles. Information about medication intake and the immune status of the patient may also be helpful. Physical examination reveals the patient's state of hydration. Dehydration is a serious condition causing mortality and morbidity, particularly in young children and the elderly. The presence or absence of fever may also help determine whether the diarrheal illness is due to a food poisoning type of condition or by an invasive organism. The presence or absence of leukocytes in the stool may provide direction for additional laboratory testing.[3]

Because diarrheal illnesses can be caused by a wide variety of agents, a practical approach to evaluating the etiology of acute diarrhea is to divide organisms into those that cause enterotoxin-mediated diarrhea and those that are invasive. A compendium of common food-borne diseases is shown in Table 22–2.

Enterotoxin-Mediated Diarrhea

The incubation period for enterotoxin-mediated diarrhea (sometimes referred to as food poisoning) is short. Symptoms occur usually within 6 to 12 hours of ingestion of the toxin contained in the food or of the toxin-producing bacteria that multiply in the gut. In enterotoxin-mediated diarrhea, patients experience sudden onset of nausea and vomiting, often accompanied by abdominal pain. Fever is absent, and because the organisms involved in enterotoxin-mediated diarrhea do not invade the intestinal mucosa, there is no inflammatory response; hence, leukocytes are absent from the stool. Bacteremia and metastatic infections are rare.[5]

The three organisms most commonly associated with the food poisoning type of acute diarrheal illness are *Staphylococcus aureus, Clostridium perfringens,* and *Bacillus cereus. S. aureus* produces a heat-stable enterotoxin that is the most common cause of food poisoning in the western world. If food contaminated with *S. aureus* is allowed to remain at an optimal temperature, the bacteria multiply and elaborate toxin into the food. Within 6 hours of ingesting

Vehicle	Pathogen or Toxin
Undercooked chicken	*Salmonella* species, *Campylobacter* species
Eggs	*Salmonella* species (especially *Salmonella enteritidis*)
Unpasteurized milk	*Salmonella, Campylobacter,* and *Yersinia* species
Water	*Giardia lamblia,* Norwalk virus, *Campylobacter* species, *Cryptosporidium* species, *Cyclospora*
Fried rice	*Bacillus cereus*
Fish	
Shellfish	*Vibrio cholerae, Vibrio parahaemolyticus, Vibrio vulnificus,* other *Vibrio* species, neurotoxic shellfish poisoning, paralytic shellfish poisoning, Norwalk virus
Tuna, mackerel, mahi-mahi	Scombroid poisoning
Grouper, amberjack, snapper	Ciguatera
Sushi	*Anisakis* species (anisakiasis)
Beef, gravy	*Salmonella* species, *Campylobacter* species, *Clostridium perfringens*

Table 22–1. Common Food Vehicles for Specific Pathogens or Toxins

Adapted from Goodman LJ: Diagnosis, management, and prevention of diarrheal diseases. Curr Opinion Infect Dis 6:88, 1993.

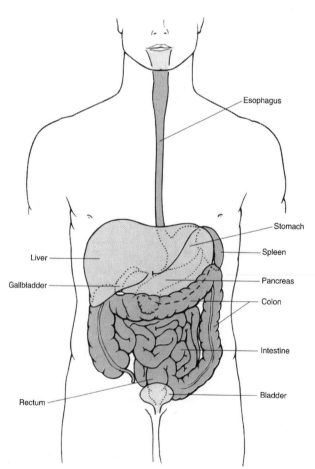

Figure 22–1. Anatomy of gastrointestinal tract. (From Mahon CR, Manuselis G: Textbook of Diagnostic Microbiology. Philadelphia, WB Saunders, 1995, p 895.)

the toxin, the patient experiences sudden nausea and abdominal cramps, with subsequent vomiting and diarrhea. This can be very serious in children and the elderly because of potential dehydration and electrolyte imbalance.[3] In this population, intravenous fluids may be needed to restore liquid and electrolyte balance. Usually, symptoms last less than 24 hours, and recovery is spontaneous. Foods commonly implicated in staphylococcal food poisoning are cream-filled pastries, custards, cheese, milk, ham, and cold meats. Sources of contamination are the skin and nasopharynx of food handlers. Treatment may range from fluid replacement to the use of antiemetics and antispasmodics to relieve the symptoms.[6]

Clostridium perfringens food poisoning usually results from ingestion of meat that has not been cooked sufficiently to kill the spores of the organism and that has then been allowed to sit at room temperature for several hours before being eaten. The spores germinate into vegetative cells that are ingested with the food. In the alkaline intestinal environment, spores are formed from the vegetative cells, and an enterotoxin is given off in the process. This enterotoxin causes abdominal cramping and diarrhea 7 to 15 hours after ingestion of the contaminated food. Most patients are afebrile, and nausea and vomiting occur in fewer than one third. Patients usually recover 2 to 3 days after onset of symptoms.[7]

Bacillus cereus food poisoning is associated with the ingestion of meats, sauces, and rice contaminated with the spores of the organism. Two types of disease are caused by the enterotoxins produced by *B. cereus:* an emetic type associated with rice, and a diarrheal type associated with meats and sauces.[8] The latter type is more common and has an incubation period of 6 to 24 hours. The symptoms

Table 22–2. Compendium of Common Food-Borne Diseases

Average Incubation Period (hr)	Organism	Average Duration	Implicated Foods	Typical Symptoms	Comments
2–16	*Bacillus cereus*	1 day	Boiled and fried rice, meats, vegetables	Nausea, vomiting (emetic); abdominal cramping, watery diarrhea	Produces two toxins; one emetic form that causes nausea and vomiting within hours, and one diarrheic form. Common year round. Isolation of large numbers from implicated foods and patient stool.
6–72	*Vibrio parahaemolyticus*	3 days	Shellfish	Pain, vomiting, fever, watery diarrhea	Blood sometimes in stool. Common spring, summer, fall in coastal United States. Stool culture using TCBS media is recommended.
6–72	*Vibrio cholerae*	3–7 days	Seafood, water	"Rice water" stools, severe diarrhea, no fever	No blood or mucus in stool; mechanism of action in vivo enterotoxin production; no tissue invasion. Stool culture using TCBS media is recommended.
<8	*Staphylococcus aureus*	<1 day	Egg salads, meat, poultry, pastries	Abrupt onset of nausea, pain, and projectile vomiting; infrequent diarrhea	Mechanism of action is preformed enterotoxin in foods. Common in summer. ELISA or reverse passive latex agglutination enterotoxin test; gel electrophoresis in lieu of phage typing.
8–22	*Clostridium perfringens*	1 day	Beef, poultry, gravy, fish	Abdominal cramping, watery diarrhea; vomiting and fever uncommon	In vivo enterotoxin production; unlike *Staphylococcus aureus*, viable organism must be ingested for disease to occur. Common in fall, winter, spring.
12–48	*Salmonella* species	3 days	Eggs, dairy products, fowl, beef	Fever, abdominal cramping, diarrhea, mild vomiting	WBCs in stool. Common in summer. Culture and serologic identification.
16–48	*Yersinia enterocolitica*	1 day–4 weeks	Milk, pork	Fever, severe abdominal pain, diarrhea	WBCs and RBCs in stool. Common in winter.
18–36	*Clostridium botulinum*	Weeks–months	Vegetables, fruits (canned foods), fish, honey (infants)	Nausea, vomiting, diarrhea, paralysis	Mechanism of action is a preformed neurotoxin. Common in summer and fall.
24–72	*Shigella* species	3 days	Egg and tuna salads, lettuce, milk	Fever, abdominal cramping, diarrhea, occasional vomiting	WBCs, RBCs and mucus in stools; tissue invasion common mechanism of action. Common in summer. Culture and serologic identification.
24–72	Enterotoxigenic *E. coli* (ETEC)	3 days	Fruits, meats, pastries, salads	Abdominal cramping, watery diarrhea, no vomiting or fever	In vivo enterotoxin, major cause of "traveler's" diarrhea, year-round distribution, patient history includes travel to Mexico and other developing countries.
24–72	Enterohemorrhagic *E. coli* (EHEC)	3 days	Undercooked ground beef, cider	Watery diarrhea progressing to bloody diarrhea, abdominal cramping, no fever or vomiting	Implicated serotype O157:H7; organisms disappear rapidly from stool. Culture of sorbitol-negative *E. coli* from stool using SMAC (sorbitol-negative MAC) plate recommended.

Abbreviations: ELISA, enzyme-linked immunosorbent assay; MAC, MacConkey's agar; RBCs, red blood cells; TCBS, thiosulfate citrate bile salts sucrose (agar); WBCs, white blood cells.

From Goodman L, Manuselis G, Mahon CR: Gastrointestinal infections and food poisoning. *In* Mahon CR, Manuselis G (eds): Textbook of Diagnostic Microbiology. Philadelphia, WB Saunders, 1995, p 909.

include watery diarrhea, abdominal cramps, and fever. Because the organism may be found in the stool of healthy individuals, its isolation from stool is not sufficient evidence for diagnosis.[8] The disease is usually mild and self limited.

The diagnosis of individual cases of food poisoning caused by any one of these three organisms is best made on the basis of a history of food ingestion and the symptoms. Because the organisms may occur in small numbers as part of the normal fecal flora, simple recovery of any of the organisms in a stool culture is not diagnostic. When a large number of people become ill after eating a common food, epidemiologic studies may be carried out that involve recovery of the organism from clinical specimens as well as from suspected food. A protocol has been established by the American Public Health Association for carrying out testing in large outbreaks of food-borne illness.[9, 10]

Other enterotoxigenic bacteria that cause diarrheal disease are *Vibrio cholerae* and enterotoxigenic *Escherichia coli* (ETEC).[11] Both bacterial species secrete an exotoxin that causes a rapid, profuse secretion of fluid across the mucosal surface of the small intestine, resulting in profuse, watery diarrhea. This in turn leads to sodium depletion, acidosis, and potassium deficiency. There is no associated inflammation or fever.[11, 12]

Cholera can be the most severe of all diarrheal diseases, but only 1% to 10% of persons infected develop the severe clinical syndrome.[13] Humans have been known to be the natural hosts of *V. cholerae,* and the most common route of transmission is via food or water contaminated by human feces, especially for the classic biotype. There have been reports, however, of detection of a free-living stage of *V. cholerae* in the environment that can support the growth and multiplication of these organisms on water plants and crustaceans. Hence, crustaceans and other shellfish have been implicated as a means of transmission, particularly for the El Tor biotype.[14] Although the disease is not endemic in the United States, cases of cholera have been reported along the Gulf Coast of Texas and Louisiana as well as from travelers in countries where the disease is endemic.[15, 16]

Symptoms begin abruptly a few days after the organism is ingested. Onset of painless, massive watery diarrhea with vomiting then follows. The stools are liquid and are often referred to as "rice water" stools. Fluid loss in an adult may reach a rate of 1 liter of isotonic fluid per hour at its peak.[17]

The organism colonizes the small intestine, where it produces an enterotoxic exotoxin. The toxin acts on the epithelial mucosal surfaces of the small intestine to make it secrete the voluminous amount of isotonic fluid. The toxin is made up of two components, an active toxic unit (A) and several binding units (B). The B units allow attachment to the mucosal receptor sites on the cell membrane. Once attached, the A unit is inserted into the cell. The A unit activates adenyl cyclase and induces the conversion of adenosine triphosphate (ATP) to cyclic adenosine 3'5'-monophosphate (cAMP), the end result of which is hypersecretion of electrolytes and water out of the cell.[4]

Enterotoxigenic *E. coli* (ETEC) produces an enterotoxin that behaves in the same manner. ETEC causes approximately 40% to 60% of "traveler's diarrhea."[1, 18] The patient suffering from ETEC gastroenteritis is usually afebrile and has moderate abdominal cramping and water stools with no inflammatory exudate. Usually, such a patient is not as ill as the patient with cholera.[18]

A newly recognized hemorrhagic diarrhea has been associated with *E. coli* serotype O157:H7, also referred to as enterohemorrhagic *E. coli* (EHEC). In 1992, there were two outbreaks of acute hemorrhagic gastroenteritis associated with eating beef. Patients experienced severe abdominal cramps and watery diarrhea that progressed to a bloody diarrhea. EHEC O157:H7 has since been associated with hemorrhagic diarrhea, colitis, and hemolytic-uremic syndrome (HUS). A feature differentiating EHEC diarrhea from *Shigella* dysentery or enteroinvasive *E. coli* (EIEC) diarrhea is the absence of leukocytes in the stool during an EHEC infection. Foods implicated in most infections are undercooked hamburgers, especially those served at fast food restaurants, unpasteurized milk, and apple cider. Young children and the elderly are at greatest risk for the severe, sometimes fatal form of this infection.[19]

Diarrhea Mediated by Invasive Organisms

Bacterial species that utilize invasive properties to produce diarrheal illnesses include *Shigella, Salmonella,* *Campylobacter, Yersinia,* and enteroinvasive *E. coli.* These organisms invade the intestinal epithelium, where they multiply and cause mucosal cell death. Inflammatory response is evidenced by the presence of blood and polymorphonuclear leukocytes (PMNs) in the stool. Patients are usually febrile and present with a bloody diarrhea, characterized by gross blood and pus. The incubation period is usually longer than that observed in enterotoxin-mediated illnesses—about 1 to 3 days—because the organisms must cross the stomach and small bowel, then multiply and invade.[20]

Shigellosis, or bacillary dysentery, is transmitted via fecal-oral route. As few as 200 bacilli are capable of causing disease.[12] There are four species of *Shigella,* the most virulent of which is *Shigella dysenteriae,* or Shiga bacillus. *S. dysenteriae* is rare in the United States but may be suspected in travelers who have visited less developed areas of the world. *Shigella boydii* is also a rare isolate. In the United States, the species that is most commonly isolated and that accounts for about 65% of all clinical isolates is *Shigella sonnei. Shigella flexneri* accounts for nearly all the rest. Populations at high risk are children in day care centers and residents of prisons and other types of custodial institutions. Sexual transmission among homosexual men has also been documented.[21]

The incubation period for shigellosis is approximately 36 to 72 hours. Symptoms consist of fever, abdominal cramps, and watery diarrhea. Within the next 24 to 72 hours, clinical dysentery appears, which is characterized by tenesmus, rectal urgency, and frequent loose bowel movements containing blood, mucus, pus, and unformed fecal material. Symptoms last less than a week in otherwise healthy individuals; however, morbidity and mortality are high in young children, who may become dehydrated and develop severe electrolyte imbalance. Shigellosis is usually limited to the lining of epithelial cells and submucosa of the colon, and the organisms do not penetrate beyond the submucosa. As a result, extraintestinal infections and septicemia are rare.[12]

Salmonellosis occurs in three different forms of infection in humans: enteric fever, gastroenteritis, and extraintestinal infection. Typhoid fever caused by *Salmonella typhi* represents the classic enteric fever spread by contaminated food and water. *S. typhi* causes prolonged fever and bacteremia. Localization of infection in the submucosal lymphoid tissue of the small intestine takes place before gastrointestinal symptoms appear. In *S. typhi* infection, constipation occurs early in the disease, and diarrhea may not appear until later on.[4]

Salmonella gastroenteritis varies from mild to severe. Sporadic cases and outbreaks are associated with contaminated foods, particularly powdered milk, meat products, powdered eggs, and poultry. Contact with infected animals and with natural reservoirs, such as reptiles and amphibians, may initiate infection.[4]

The incubation period for *Salmonella* gastroenteritis is usually 8 to 48 hours. Symptoms are nausea and vomiting followed by abdominal cramps and diarrhea. Diarrhea usually persists for 3 to 4 days. Temperature is elevated in about half of cases and usually returns to normal in 1 to 2 days.[4, 17]

Extraintestinal infections such as bacteremia with *Sal-*

monella species may occur, particularly among the elderly and the immunocompromised. This type of infection may or may not be accompanied by a gastrointestinal disease.[22]

Other bacterial species that may cause invasive intestinal disease are *Yersinia enterocolitica, Yersinia pseudotuberculosis,* and *Campylobacter* species. *Y. enterocolitica* causes a diarrheal disease, *Y. pseudotuberculosis* causes a purulent mesenteric adenitis with little or no diarrhea,[12] whereas *Campylobacter jejuni* is the most common cause of bacterial diarrhea.[23]

Yersinia enterocolitica occurs widely in the environment, and has been recovered from raw milk and water supplies as well as from wild and domestic animals. Outbreaks have been associated with consumption of infected meat and other foods. The incubation period is 4 to 10 days.[24] Yersiniosis is an intense inflammation of the terminal ileum that mimics appendicitis. Symptoms vary greatly in different age groups. Children younger than 5 years usually present with diarrhea, fever, and abdominal cramps and frequently have vomiting and bloody diarrhea. On the other hand, older children and adults present with less severe diarrhea and colicky abdominal pain that localizes in the right lower quadrant. Many patients exhibit joint pain, an arthritic form of yersiniosis, following a gastrointestinal episode.[17, 25] Septicemia is rare except in patients with underlying diseases such as acquired immunodeficiency syndrome (AIDS), diabetes, liver cirrhosis, leukemia, and other chronic illnesses.[26, 27]

The source of *Campylobacter* infections appears to be either food of animal origin or contaminated water supply. Person-to-person transmission of *C. jejuni* has been documented between mothers and neonates as well as in day care centers. Because of the invasive mechanism employed by the organism, blood and leukocytes are present in the stool. The incubation period is 2 to 4 days. Onset is sudden, and the patient exhibits abdominal pain, nausea, anorexia, fever, malaise, headache, and watery diarrhea. Most patients recover in 3 to 5 days, but there have been reports of cases in which recurrent or relapsing diarrhea occurred repeatedly, and carrier states may persist for several months. Bacteremia has been known to occur. Other enteric *Campylobacter* species that may produce similar clinical manifestations are *C. coli* and *C. lari*.[23]

Other Agents of Diarrheal Illnesses

ANTIBIOTIC-ASSOCIATED COLITIS

Antibiotic therapy may alter the intestinal flora and cause diarrhea. Often this condition is mild and disappears when the therapy is discontinued. In some patients, however, severe diarrhea occurs, with the development of a thick mucosal exudate that resembles a membrane—hence the term *pseudomembranous colitis* (PMC). The most common, but not the only, cause of antibiotic-associated diarrhea is *Clostridium difficile,* and the toxins it produces have been associated with PMC.[28] The two toxins, called A and B, mediate the clinical manifestations; toxin A is an enterotoxin, and toxin B is a cytotoxin. A wide spectrum of symptoms are associated with PMC, ranging from an asymptomatic form in carriers to bowel perforation and death.

Patients with PMC have a rapid onset of watery diarrhea with up to 10 to 20 stools per day. Abdominal tenderness, fever, and leukocytosis are also usually present. Sigmoidoscopic findings include edema, hyperemia, and friability. In fully developed cases, raised yellow plaques of exudate can be seen, which coalesce to form the pseudomembrane. Microscopic examination of the membrane reveals leukocytes, mucus, and sloughed epithelial cells.[29]

Nosocomial infections due to *C. difficile* have been known to occur. They often have been transmitted among hospitalized patients by their health care personnel.[30]

VIRAL DIARRHEA

Viral gastroenteritis due to Rotavirus and the Norwalk family of viruses is believed to be one of the most common viral illnesses in the United States, second only to the common cold. Rotaviral gastroenteritis is most prevalent among infants, young children, and the elderly,[31, 32] whereas diarrheal illness due to the Norwalk group of viruses involves predominantly older children and adults in industrialized countries.[33]

Transmitted by the fecal-oral route, rotaviral gastroenteritis usually occurs in the winter months. It has an incubation period of 1 to 2 days, with sudden onset of nausea, vomiting, and diarrhea. Vomiting and diarrhea may result in dehydration and electrolyte imbalance, requiring treatment for infants and young children. Fever occurs in the majority of the cases. Upper respiratory tract symptoms also commonly occur. The virus directly infects and damages the intestinal epithelial cells, and the diarrhea is the result of repopulation of the intestinal epithelium with immature cells that cannot absorb well. Diarrhea may last for 5 to 8 days.[34]

Named after a public school epidemic in Norwalk, Ohio,[35] Norwalk viruses cause approximately half of the gastroenteritis epidemics worldwide. The virus is spread by contaminated water and food such as shellfish. Abrupt onset of severe nausea, vomiting, diarrhea, and low-grade fever occurs after an incubation period of 24 to 48 hours. Clinical manifestations subside quickly, usually within 72 hours.[33]

PARASITIC DIARRHEA

Parasitic diarrhea may be caused by heavy infection with protozoa, roundworms, and flatworms (tapeworms). The two most common causes of parasitic diarrhea are *Entamoeba histolytica* and *Giardia lamblia*.[12] Two additional protozoans, *Blastomyces hominis*[36] and *Cryptosporidium,* have been reported increasingly over the past several years.[37] See Chapter 53 for a detailed discussion of parasitic infections.

Pathophysiology

Diarrhea occurs when there is an interference with the transport of water and electrolytes through the intestinal wall, increasing the liquidity of the stool. Diarrhea is an abnormal increase in stool liquidity and in daily stool weight to more than 200 g. There is often an increase in stool frequency to more than three per day with accompanying urgency, perianal discomfort, incontinence, or a combination of the three.[38]

Classification

The four major pathophysiologic categories of diarrhea are osmotic diarrhea, secretory diarrhea, impaired absorption, and altered bowel motility. Many cases of diarrhea involve more than one of the four mechanisms.

OSMOTIC DIARRHEA

Osmotic diarrhea occurs when excess water is pulled into the lumen from the extracellular fluid compartment. This occurs in order to maintain the iso-osmolality between the plasma and intestinal contents. For example, accumulation of hypertonic solutes in the intestine causes excess water to be pulled into the lumen. Laxatives such as citrate of magnesia cause this phenomenon. Another cause of osmotic diarrhea is ingestion of large amounts of mannitol and sorbitol; this is known as "chewing gum diarrhea" because of the use of mannitol and sorbitol as sweeteners in sugar-free gum.[39]

The ingestion of lactose in lactase-deficient individuals also may cause osmotic diarrhea. Fairly common in adults, lactase deficiency reduces lactose hydrolysis and impairs lactose absorption. Lactose remaining in the lumen causes retention of water in the small intestine. The colon flora ferment the unabsorbed lactose, producing hydrogen and small organic molecules such as lactate and butyrate. These organic molecules increase the osmotic load and cause additional water to accumulate in the colon, producing diarrhea.

In general, osmotic diarrhea is related to food ingestion and stops when the patient fasts or stops ingesting the poorly absorbed solute.[40]

SECRETORY DIARRHEA

Secretory diarrhea is caused by a malfunction of the secretory cells lining the small intestine. These cells normally secrete, as well as absorb, electrolytes and water.[38] If these cells are stimulated to secrete large amounts of fluid, secretory diarrhea occurs. Often, an increase in secretion causes a decrease in ion absorption. In this form of diarrhea, the intestinal lumen and stool contain an excess of monovalent cations and water. The water osmolality of the feces is essentially the same as that of plasma, in contrast to a higher fecal water osmolality in osmotic diarrhea.[38]

Secretory diarrhea may be caused by bacterial enterotoxins such as those of *V. cholerae* and enterotoxigenic *E. coli,* as well as by viral agents, parasites, neoplasms, and cathartics such as castor oil. Other causes are ulcerative colitis, various drugs, hyperthyroidism, and diabetes.[41] Because secretory diarrhea is independent of ingestion, it persists even when the patient fasts.

IMPAIRED ABSORPTION

Impaired absorption decreases electrolyte and water absorption and may be the cause of diarrhea. Reasons for impaired absorption include celiac and tropical sprue, exu-

dation from inflammation and ulceration of the intestinal mucosa, congenital chloridorrhea, excess bile salts resulting from ileac resection, and the presence of lumen-dwelling parasites.[6]

ALTERED MOTILITY

Altered motility is another mechanism of diarrhea. Hypomotility may allow bacterial overgrowth in the small intestine, resulting in diarrhea. This occurs because the metabolic products of bacterial activity inhibit water absorption or cause excessive water excretion.[42] Hypermotility in the small intestine may lead to delivery to the colon of large amounts of fluid containing unabsorbed nutrients. This load may exceed the colon's absorptive capabilities. Diarrhea results from premature emptying of the colon either because of the abnormality of its contents or because of irritability or inflammation in addition to the greater fluid volume.

Clinical Manifestations

The nature and duration of the diarrhea, a history of vomiting, the presence or absence of fever, and the presence of abdominal cramps all give clues to the etiology of acute diarrhea. The clinical manifestations seen depend on the pathogenic mechanism employed by the diarrheal agent, whether the disease is mediated by enterotoxins or by the invasive properties of the organism. The patient should be examined for dry mucous membranes, weak, thready, or rapid pulse, and low blood pressure—(all signs of dehydration), which is the major cause of mortality and morbidity in diarrheal illnesses. Poor skin turgor and a weak cry in infants are signs of serious dehydration.[43]

Lactase deficiency is characterized by abdominal distention, audible bowel sounds, and diarrhea after the ingestion of 50 g of lactose. Passage of blood signifies an inflammatory infection or neoplastic disease. Passage of pus or white cells indicates inflammation or invasion. Passage of nonbloody mucus suggests irritable bowel syndrome, whereas frothy stools or oil-containing stools suggest malabsorption.[38]

Laboratory Analyses and Diagnosis

Because the laboratory effort to detect all possible pathogens can be extremely costly and time consuming, the clinician should use a selective approach in requesting laboratory tests. Most acute diarrhea is self limited and does not cause extreme mortality and morbidity. Patients with a history that reveals a common source, such as seen in food poisoning, usually need no further evaluation.

Patients whose diarrhea is not profuse and who do not have dehydration, bloody stools, severe pain, or fever usually do not need further diagnostic tests if the symptoms resolve in 1 to 2 weeks. These patients do not benefit substantially from therapy. On the other hand, debilitated patients and patients with fever and severe or persistent symptoms require prompt diagnosis so that specific therapy can be initiated.[44]

Examination of stool for leukocytes helps distinguish invasive from noninvasive infection. Diagnosis of cases of food poisoning caused by enterotoxin-producing *S. aureus,* *C. perfringens,* and *B. cereus* is best confirmed by a history of food ingestion and symptoms. Because they may occur in small numbers as part of the normal colon flora, recovery of these organisms in a stool culture is not diagnostic. When a large number of people become ill after eating a common food, epidemiologic studies may be carried out that involve recovery of organisms from clinical specimens as well as from the suspected food. A protocol has been established by the American Public Health Association for carrying out testing in large outbreaks of food-borne illness.[9]

A diagnosis of cholera should be considered in the patient with appropriate history or geographic exposure who has acute, afebrile, watery diarrhea. Specimens must be transported to the laboratory immediately or must be placed on a transport medium such as Cary-Blair or in buffered salt medium in alkaline peptone water.[45] Although Gram staining of the stool may reveal short, comma-shaped, gram-negative bacilli, this characteristic morphology is not limited to *V. cholerae.*[45]

Vibrio cholerae does grow on culture media used routinely to isolate other enteric pathogens; however, a highly selective medium such as thiosulfate citrate bile salts sucrose (TCBS) agar may be added to enhance the recovery of cholera vibrio. Once they are identified, an agglutination test for serogroup 01 is performed. A latex agglutination assay and an enzyme-linked immunosorbent assay (ELISA) have been developed to detect cholera toxin in vitro.[46] These assays are performed primarily in reference laboratories.

Enterotoxigenic strains of *E. coli* are indistinguishable from other *E. coli* on routine culture techniques. Demonstration of toxin production is not routinely performed in the clinical laboratory, as it requires animal testing or cell culture techniques. Like ETEC, enteroinvasive *E. coli* (EIEC) diarrhea must be diagnosed primarily from clinical and epidemiologic data, because EIEC do not differ in their appearance, on culture or in biochemical reactions, from normal intestinal flora.[18] As for other invasive diarrheas, Gram staining or methylene blue staining of a stool smear may reveal many PMNs. Although specific serotypes have been associated with EIEC, antisera are not currently available for routine testing. The state health department may be able to serotype for EIEC in nursery or other outbreaks of diarrheal disease; however, in sporadic cases of diarrhea, it is not recommended that routine serotyping be performed. *E. coli* 0157:H7 may be screened with MacConkey-sorbitol agar, in which *E. coli* 0157:H7 appears colorless because this strain is sorbitol negative. Serotyping with 0157:H7 antisera may then be performed.[47, 48]

Stool culture for invasive diarrheal agents should include media to recover *Salmonella, Shigella,* and *Campylobacter.* For maximum recovery of *Shigella* from stool samples, a fresh stool specimen must be submitted, and it must not be allowed to stand at room temperature for more than 2 to 3 hours; otherwise, the organism, which is quite sensitive to acid products, may die before culture is performed.[49] Mucosal exudate obtained from proctoscopic examination usually produces a higher yield of organisms than a routine stool specimen. A stained stool smear may show several PMNs, a finding common in infections by enteroinvasive organisms.[17]

Diagnosis of salmonellosis can be made by recovering the organism in a stool culture. If typhoid fever is suspected, recovery of the organisms from blood cultures is more likely during the first week of the disease, whereas stool cultures may not produce the organisms until the third or fourth week of infection. Culture media such as sheep blood agar and MacConkey agar, as well as highly selective enteric media such as Hektoen enteric (HE) agar and xylose-lysine-deoxycholate (XLD) agar, are used for isolation.

Although there are more than 2000 *Salmonella* serotypes, only a few have been associated with human diseases. Clinical laboratories must determine, however, whether an isolate belongs to serogroups A through E, which are the most common groups recovered in the United States. Complete serotyping is important for public health reasons and is usually available through state health department laboratories. Widal's test, which detects antibodies against *Salmonella* O and H antigens, is helpful in invasive conditions, such as enteric fever and extraintestinal infection, but is not indicated for the diagnosis of *Salmonella* gastroenteritis.[17]

Yersinia enterocolitica may be recovered from stool, lymph nodes, and blood in cases of bacteremia. If *Yersinia* infection is suspected, the laboratory should be notified, because special culture techniques must be used for isolation and identification of this organism. Increased PMNs will be found on a stool smear because of the invasiveness of the organism.[25]

In cases of *Campylobacter* infections, the organism may be cultured from the stool. The stool specimen either should be cultured within 2 hours of collection or should be placed in transport medium and refrigerated. Special enriched media, such as Campy BAP, are used for isolation of *Campylobacter* species and are incubated at 42 °C. Because *Campylobacter* species grow slowly, cultures must be kept as long as 72 hours before being reported as negative. Tests for blood in the stool and for increased fecal PMNs are usually positive.[23]

Diagnosis of pseudomembranous colitis can be made by observing the pseudomembrane during sigmoidoscopy. This finding in a patient who recently took antibiotics is usually diagnostic; however, the absence of a pseudomembrane does not exclude the diagnosis of *C. difficile.* Taking into account that *C. difficile* may also be found as part of the normal intestinal flora, detection of toxin production by the organism is more diagnostic than the isolation of the organism in stool culture, which has been shown to be difficult and inconsistent.

Latex agglutination tests for direct detection of *C. difficile* in stool samples are available, although this method does not distinguish toxin-producing isolates from nontoxigenic strains. Nevertheless, latex agglutination tests are easy to use, and results are available within several minutes. Positive results of these tests, however, should be confirmed by testing for *C. difficile* toxin using cell culture assays or by ELISA methods. Toxin B is detected primarily by cell culture assays, which show cytotoxicity in the stool sample and neutralization activity with *C. difficile* antitoxin. The ELISAs use specific *C. difficile* toxin antibodies. Most of the available toxin detection assays detect toxin A.[50]

In viral diarrhea, because the virus is shed in the stool for up to 8 days, the laboratory diagnosis is based on the detection of virus in the stool. Stool specimens to be submitted to another laboratory for identification or to be stored should be frozen at −70 °C and shipped on dry ice.[33] Rotavirus may be identified by electron microscopy (EM), but this method is not practical, and not all clinical laboratories have the capability. Latex agglutination (LA) and enzyme immunoassay (EIA) kits are commercially available for diagnostic use in laboratories.[51] The test is most useful in diagnosing gastroenteritis in children 6 months to 2 years old and in epidemiologic studies. Because children younger than 6 months are often asymptomatic but still shed rotavirus, a positive test in this age group should not preclude searching for other pathogens.[52]

Norwalk virus is shed in the stool for only a brief period. It can be detected by electron microscopy and by radioimmunoassay (RIA), although these procedures are not widely used. Several cell culture techniques have been tried for growing Norwalk virus; none has been successful.[33]

Laboratory diagnosis of diarrheal illnesses may also include examination for parasitic agents and is discussed in Chapter 53.

Treatment

The treatment of acute diarrhea first involves fluid replacement if the patient is dehydrated. Depending on the cause of the diarrhea, antimicrobial or antidiarrheal medications may be administered.

Agents available for treating diarrhea can be grouped into four categories: antiperistaltic agents such as loperamide and diphenoxylate HCl; absorbants such as kaolin and aluminum hydroxide; inhibitors of intestinal secretion such as bismuth subsalicylate; and antimicrobial agents. The use of antiperistaltic agents is not recommended in patients with high fever, dysentery, or antibiotic-associated diarrhea, because slowing peristalsis allows organisms to stay in contact with the mucosal surface longer. This may actually lead to potentiation of the infection. Antimicrobial agents are not recommended for treatment of food poisoning, rotavirus, Norwalk agent, or *Vibrio* infections.[3, 5]

In both cholera and ETEC secretory diarrhea, replacement of fluid losses and electrolytes is the primary element of therapy. In addition to intravenous therapy, oral glucose-electrolyte preparations are available. Oral therapy may be given as the sole treatment in mild cholera cases and ETEC cases. If an antibiotic is needed, tetracycline is the agent of choice. A cholera vaccine is available.[11, 17]

Antimicrobial treatment for shigellosis is controversial, because most patients recover spontaneously; however, the duration of bacterial shedding is shortened by the administration of antimicrobials.[53] It is recommended that children and adults with severe symptoms be treated with antimicrobials. Plasmid-mediated resistance is common, and susceptibility testing should be performed on all isolates. Antidiarrheal agents such as diphenoxylate HCl prolong the symptoms and the duration of fecal excretion, and for this

reason, they are not recommended.[17] No vaccine is available to prevent *Shigella* infection.

For mild cases of *Salmonella* gastroenteritis, antimicrobials are not recommended unless diarrhea is severe or complications such as bacteremia occur.[12] It seems that antimicrobial therapy may result in a prolonged carrier state.[4]

In uncomplicated *Yersinia* gastroenteritis, the infection is usually self-limited and requires no antimicrobial treatment. In chronic or extraintestinal infection, antibiotic treatment is indicated.[27]

Campylobacter enteritis is usually self limited and does not require antimicrobial therapy, but in severe illness, fluid replacement and antibiotic treatment may be necessary.[54] For treatment of *C. difficile* colitis, vancomycin is the drug of choice. The use of antidiarrheal agents may prolong or worsen the symptoms of PMC.[29]

Treatment of parasitic infections is discussed in Chapter 53.

CHRONIC INFLAMMATORY BOWEL DISORDERS

The cause of inflammatory bowel diseases (IBD)—ulcerative colitis and Crohn's disease—remains unknown, although progress has been made in recognizing the mechanisms that initiate inflammatory changes. The role of the immune system in the destruction of cells of the intestinal tract is being established.[55] Nevertheless, the diagnosis of these diseases has been limited to radiologic, endoscopic, and histologic evaluations, in addition to clinical symptoms and signs, and after exclusion of other disorders.[56] Certain serologic markers have been evaluated, but their value in the differential diagnosis of Crohn's disease and ulcerative colitis is limited.[57] Because the causative agent or agents remain undetermined, there are few established standards for management of care and modalities of treatment for IBD.

Etiology and Pathophysiology

Classification

Inflammatory bowel disease is classified as one of two important chronic disorders, Crohn's disease (CD) or ulcerative colitis (UC). Both of these disorders progress from acute to chronic stages, with the majority of the symptoms appearing in the chronic stage. These diseases are classified and differentiated macroscopically, as summarized in Table 22–3. Crohn's disease, first described in 1932, is a form of regional enteritis, characterized as transmural inflammation of the gastrointestinal tract in any location from the mouth to the anus.[58] Anal lesions are very common in CD. Ulcerative colitis involves the colon primarily, often manifesting as pseudopolyps, which are not common in CD. The clinical severity of UC depends largely on the degree and extent of the mucosal involvement, in which bloody diarrhea is the hallmark of mucosal inflammation.[59]

Etiology

The cause of IBD is not known. A number of observations and speculations have generated causative hypothe-

Table 22–3. Macroscopic Differences Between Ulcerative Colitis and Crohn's Disease

Ulcerative Colitis	Crohn's Disease
Colonic involvement only	Mouth to anus at risk
Continuous disease	Discontinuous lesions
Rectum usually involved	Rectal sparing common (50%)
"Backwash" ileitis (2%–5%)	Terminal ileum involved (30%)
Rectal ulceration rare	Rectal ulceration common
Fistulae rare	Fistulae common (10%–20%)
Pseudopolyps common	Pseudopolyps rare
Anal lesions fairly common (20%)	Anal lesions very common (75%)

ses. Among the possibilities suggested are abnormal immunologic responses and infection, as well as dietary, psychosomatic, and genetic factors.[59–63] Additionally, there may be interaction between any or all of these factors and responses.

Epidemiology

The incidence of the two diseases ranges from 1.0 to 6.0 per 100,000 for Crohn's disease, and from 3.2 to 7.6 per 100,000 for ulcerative colitis.[64] The incidence of ulcerative colitis in the elderly is one to three times that of Crohn's disease; similar observations are made in younger populations. It also seems that UC occurs more among older men than older women, whereas sex distribution in CD remains controversial.[65] White populations are much more prone to both diseases than are other races, with American Jews having the highest incidence.[64] The age of onset peaks at approximately 20 years for both types of IBD.[63] It remains to be seen whether there is a greater predisposition to the disorders in Western than in Eastern societies.

Clinical Manifestations

Intestinal

The major intestinal manifestations of IBD are listed in Table 22–4. The onset of symptoms may be more subtle in Crohn's disease than in ulcerative colitis, with the type of symptoms often dependent on the site of the lesion.[64] The signs that appear in the two disorders are compared in Table 22–3. Crohn's disease commonly manifests as diarrhea, abdominal pain and mass, perianal disease, malabsorption, weight loss, and, less commonly, fever and rectal bleeding. In ulcerative colitis, bloody diarrhea is the major clinical manifestation, with only rare occurrences of the other signs seen in Crohn's disease.

Extraintestinal

Extraintestinal clinical manifestations are seen in both Crohn's disease and ulcerative colitis. Table 22–4 lists many of these findings, none of which alone is pathognomonic for IBD. For example, although sclerosing cholangitis seems to be clinically associated more with ulcerative colitis, other signs and symptoms, such as arthralgias, ar-

thritis, and problems with coagulation, are present in both disorders and fail to differentiate them.[56]

Laboratory Analyses and Diagnosis

At present, there is no single specific test to diagnose IBD. The differential diagnosis of IBD, not to mention the subclassifications, is based primarily on exclusion. Ruling out virtually all of the disorders that might manifest as IBD is an exhaustive undertaking, in terms of both time and cost. Nevertheless, laboratory tests may play a role in ascertaining which patients require more expanded evaluation, and in monitoring disease activity and nutritional status.[65]

Diagnostic evaluation of the patient, regardless of age, consists of a detailed history and physical examination as well as laboratory studies and appropriate radiologic and endoscopic examinations.[66] Histologic information is necessary to exclude other etiologies of intestinal inflammation. The diagnosis is generally based on visualization of the colonic mucosa and biopsy of affected areas, colon and ileum radiography, and microorganism culture or microscopy.[56]

A number of laboratory tests, however, are being studied for their correlation to the presence or severity of IBD. Because infectious diseases such as those caused by *Campylobacter, Salmonella, Shigella,* and enterohemorrhagic *E. coli* may look like IBD, stool cultures to exclude these diseases are important.[56] Other tests show promise in differentiating IBD from other disorders. Serum orosomucoid,[67, 68] C-reactive protein (CRP), and α_1-antitrypsin[69] from blood and fecal samples have been found to correlate well with IBD activity, especially in Crohn's disease. These analytes may be useful markers of endoscopic activity in the two diseases.[70]

Unfortunately, laboratory studies are of no help in the differential diagnosis except in the exclusion of disorders. The major disorders that must be excluded are listed in

Table 22–4. Clinical Manifestations of Inflammatory Bowel Disease

Symptoms	Signs
GASTROINTESTINAL	
Abdominal pain	Occult or overt stool blood
Weight loss	Abdominal mass palpitation
Nausea and vomiting	Diarrhea
EXTRAINTESTINAL	
Nutritional abnormalities: hypoalbuminemia, deficiencies (vitamins, calcium, zinc, magnesium, phosphate)	Skin and mucous membrane abnormalities
Hematologic abnormalities: anemia, leukocytosis, thrombocytosis	Arthritis: ankylosing spondylitis and sacroileitis, large-bone involvement
Hepatic and biliary abnormalities: fatty liver, pericholangitis, gallstones, carcinoma of bile ducts	Eye abnormalities: iritis, conjunctivitis, episcleritis
Renal abnormalities: kidney stones, obstructive uropathy, fistulae to urinary tract	Psychological changes Fever, increased thrombophlebitis

Table 22–5. Disorders to Be Considered in the Differential Diagnosis of Inflammatory Bowel Disease

Acute bacillary dysentery
Amebiasis
Pseudomembranous colitis
Ischemic colitis
Colonic neoplasms
Angiodysplasia
Acute appendicitis
Small intestine disease (lymphoma or tuberculosis)
Duodenal ulceration
General malabsorption
Infections
Radiation proctitis
Familial polyposis

Table 22–5, and laboratory studies appropriate to the conditions listed there remain very important. At this time, however, none of these tests possesses the diagnostic specificity to differentiate Crohn's disease from ulcerative colitis.

Treatment

The treatment of IBD is primarily medical and is similar regardless of which form of the disease is present. The principal drugs used are anti-inflammatory agents. Following the indices of nutritional status and hematologic, renal, and hepatic function is at this time the only tool available from the laboratory to assist in monitoring patients being treated for IBD. The resolution of histologic and macroscopic abnormalities listed in Table 22–2 is also used in the assessment of successful treatment and recovery of the IBD patient. Further, there are indications that disease activity may be monitored by following the orosomucoid levels and the erythrocyte sedimentation rate (ESR) with disease relapse as well as assessing activity by the level of C-reactive protein.[68] Finally, it is important for the nutritional status of the patient to be maintained. Indicators such as albumin[68] have been useful to monitor nutritional status. Failure to respond to medical management, however, may necessitate surgical intervention.

Case Study 1

A well-nourished 30-year-old woman presented with abdominal cramps, fever of 102 °F, and bloody diarrhea that had persisted for 36 hours. The symptoms appeared approximately 1 week after the patient had returned from a Caribbean cruise. She had no signs of dehydration and had not been taking any medication.

Because the patient was febrile, a "routine" stool culture was ordered as well as microscopic examination for fecal leukocytes. The culture report was "No pathogens," and the fecal leukocyte report, "12 leukocytes per high-power field." Because the fecal leukocyte examination was positive, indicating an invasive process,

and the culture revealed no pathogens, an ova and parasites examination was requested. A repeat stool culture was also performed, specifically for *Yersinia* and *Campylobacter* as well as *Salmonella* and *Shigella*. No parasites were found, but the cultures revealed *C. jejuni.*

Questions

1. Why did the report of the routine stool culture indicate no pathogens?
2. What was the consequence of the lack of information regarding laboratory protocol?
3. What steps could this laboratory have taken to avoid delay in diagnosis?

Discussion

1. The protocol for a "routine" stool culture in this particular laboratory included checking for *Salmonella* and *Shigella* only. Cultures for *Campylobacter* and *Yersinia* are performed only on special request and require special culture media and techniques for isolation. The clinician should be made aware of tests designated "routine" by the laboratory where services are obtained, because they may vary from laboratory to laboratory.
2. Because the patient presented with bloody diarrhea, the request for *Campylobacter* culture on the initial stool specimen would have speeded the diagnosis and specific treatment. The patient was started on erythromycin therapy, and the symptoms subsided within 48 hours.
3. Because *Campylobacter* infections are the most common, routine stool culture protocol should include isolation of this organism.

Case Study 2

A total of 17 students and instructors from a group of 33 became ill with diarrhea, nausea, and vomiting after a graduation banquet. Ten had severe abdominal cramps as well. All were afebrile. They all presented to a local emergency room within 2 to 6 hours after the banquet. No stool cultures were ordered. The patients were given symptomatic treatment. Five were hospitalized because of dehydration, and the other 12 were sent home.

Questions

1. What is the most likely cause of these clinical symptoms, and what history and physical findings support this conclusion?
2. Why were no stool cultures ordered?

Discussion

1. Because all the patients had similar symptoms, all had attended the banquet, and all were afebrile, the diarrhea was thought to be a form of "food poisoning." Histories revealed that all had eaten deviled eggs that had been prepared in a private home and had been stored approximately 6 hours at room temperature before being served. Because the symptoms began within 2 to 6 hours, the most probable cause was *S. aureus.*

2. Culturing for the suspected agent, *S. aureus,* would contribute nothing to the diagnosis. The pathogenic mechanism of *S. aureus* food poisoning is enterotoxin mediated; therefore, isolation of the organism from the stool would provide no meaningful information. The patients all made an uneventful recovery with symptomatic treatment.

Case Study 3

A 20-year-old man was admitted for evaluation of an eating disorder and abdominal pain. The patient's recent history included reports of chronic sore throat and dysphagia over the past 6 years. About 2 years after those began, the patient developed mild epigastric pain accompanied by vomiting after solid-food meals. At that time, the patient began a liquid diet only, which relieved most of the symptoms. He had diarrhea and abdominal pain intermittently over the course of the next 4 years. There was no history of smoking, drinking, or homosexual contacts and no fever or chills.

The patient was a light-complected man who presented as thin for his size (weight 65 kg, height 190 cm). His temperature was 37.4 °C, blood pressure was 140/70 mm Hg, pulse was 108 beats/min, and respirations were 18 per minute. Bowel sounds were elevated, without hardness or palpable masses. Cardiac and pulmonary examinations were unremarkable. Rectal examination, however, obtained a maroon stool that gave a 4+ result in the test for occult blood; otherwise, the examination was unremarkable.

Upon questioning, both of the patient's parents were found to have experienced undiagnosed ulcerative colitis. This was deduced through histories of their problems of chronic mild diarrhea, intermittent bloody stools, and cramping pain. The mother had a 20-year history of diabetes mellitus.

Laboratory analysis revealed a hematocrit of 45%; a white blood cell count of $9.5 \times 10^9/L$, with 57% neutrophils, 25% lymphocytes, 9% monocytes, 7% eosinophils, and 2% basophils. The ESR was within reference limits at 2 mm/hour. Other tests, such as liver and pancreatic function tests, were unremarkable. A biopsy specimen was taken of the duodenum via endoscopy, with negative results upon microscopic examination, and a fiberoptic esophagogastroduodenoscopic examination was also negative. Stool examination was negative for parasites and ova. Upper gastrointestinal and small bowel radiographic studies showed an abnormal jejunum with normal esophagus, stomach, duodenum, and ileum.

A diagnosis of Crohn's disease of the jejunum was made, on the basis of the results of a laparotomy that examined the small bowel and surrounding lymph nodes. Biopsy samples taken from the bowel and lymph nodes were found, on microscopic examination, to include an acute inflammation, with noncaseous granulomas adjacent to the lesions.

The patient was treated with high-dose corticosteroids initially, followed by tapering of the dose over several months. During this time, the patient gained 17 kg. The daily stools only rarely showed hematochezia. The patient continued to have occasional abdominal pain, and remained on a liquid diet.

Question

1. What assistance did the laboratory provide in making this diagnosis?

Discussion

1. The laboratory results, except for the occult blood test, were essentially within normal limits. These findings proved to exclude many disorders with symptoms similar to those of IBD. Because the diagnosis of IBD is primarily one of exclusion, the negative laboratory findings were important.

References

1. Abbott S, Janda M: Bacterial gastroenteritis. I: Incidence and etiologic agents. Clin Microbiol News 14:17, 1992.
2. Guerrant RL, Shields DS, Thorson SM, et al: Evaluation and diagnosis of acute infectious diarrhea, Am J Med 78 (suppl 6B):91, 1985.
3. Goodman LJ: Diagnosis, management, and prevention of diarrheal diseases. Curr Opin Infect Dis 6:88, 1993.
4. Ryan KJ: Enterobacteriaceae. *In* Sherris JC (ed): Medical Microbiology: An Introduction to Infectious Diseases, ed 2. New York, Elsevier, 1990.
5. Goodman L, Manuselis G, Mahon CR: Gastrointestinal diseases and food poisoning. *In* Mahon CR, Manuselis G (eds): Textbook of Diagnostic Microbiology. Philadelphia, WB Saunders, 1995.
6. Jinich H, Hersh T, Swartz H: Physician's Guide to the Etiology and Treatment of Diarrhea. Oradell, NJ, Medical Economics Books, 1982.
7. Allen SD: *Clostridium. In* Lennette EH (ed): Manual of Clinical Microbiology, ed 4. Washington, DC, American Society for Microbiology, 1985.
8. Doyle RJ, Keller KF, Wezzell JW: *Bacillus. In* Lennette EH (ed): Manual of Clinical Microbiology, ed 4. Washington, DC, American Society for Microbiology, 1985.
9. Speck ML (ed): Compendium of Methods for the Microbiological Examinations of Foods, ed 2. Washington, DC, American Public Health Association, 1984.
10. Gradus MS: Public health criteria for the diagnosis of foodborne illness. Clin Microbiol Newsl 8:85–90, 1986.
11. Carpenter CJ, Sack RB: Infectious diarrheal syndromes. *In* Isselbacher KJ, Adams RD, Braunwald E, et al (eds): Harrison's Principles of Internal Medicine: Update I. New York, McGraw-Hill, 1981.
12. Sommers HM, Shuman ST: Infectious diarrhea. *In* Shulman ST, Phair JP, Sommers HM (eds): The Biologic and Clinical Basis of Infectious Diseases, ed 4. Philadelphia, WB Saunders, 1992.
13. Sack RB, Tilton RC, Weissfeld AS: Laboratory diagnosis of bacterial

diarrhea. (Cumitech 12.) Washington, DC, American Society for Microbiology, 1980.

14. World Health Organization: Programme for control of diarrheal disease: Guidelines for cholera control. Geneva, World Health Organization, 1991.

15. Lowry P, Pavia AT, McFarland LM, et al: Cholera in Louisiana. Arch Intern Med 149:2079–2084, 1989.

16. Weissman JB, DeWitt WE, Thompson J, et al: A case of cholera in Texas, 1973. Am J Epidemiol 100:487–498, 1974.

17. Said B, Draser BS: *Vibrio cholerae. In* Draser BS, Forrest BD (eds): Cholera and the ecology of *Vibrio cholerae.* London, Chapman and Hall, 1996.

18. Levine MM: *Escherichia coli* that cause diarrhea: Enterotoxigenic, enteropathogenic, enteroinvasive, enterohemorrhagic, and enteroadherent. J Infect Dis 155:377, 1987.

19. Raj P: Pathogenesis and laboratory diagnosis of *Escherichia coli*–associated enteritis. Clin Microbiol Newsl 15:89, 1993.

20. Gianella RA: Pathogenesis of acute bacterial diarrheal disorders. Ann Rev Med 32:341–357, 1981.

21. Keusch GT, Bennish M: *Shigella. In* Farthing MJ, Keusch GT (eds): Enteric Infection: Mechanisms, Manifestations, and Management. New York, Raven Press, 1988.

22. Candy DCA, Stephen J: *Salmonella. In* Farthing MJ, Keusch GT (eds): Enteric Infection: Mechanisms, Manifestations, and Management. New York, Raven Press, 1988.

23. Kaplan R, Carnahan A: *Aeromonas, Campylobacter. In* Mahon CR, Manuselis G (eds): Textbook of Diagnostic Microbiology. Philadelphia, WB Saunders, 1995.

24. Vantrappen G, Geboes K, Ponette E: *Yersinia* enteritis. Med Clin North Am 66:639, 1982.

25. Robins-Browne RM: *Yersinia enterocolitica. In* Farthing MJ, Keusch GT (eds): Enteric Infection: Mechanisms, Manifestations, and Management. New York, Raven Press, 1988.

26. Cohen JI, Rodday P: *Yersinia enterocolitica* bacteremia in a patient with the acquired immunodeficiency syndrome. Am J Med 86:254, 1989.

27. Cover TL, Aber RC: *Yersinia enterocolitica.* N Engl J Med 321:16–21, 1989.

28. Bartlett JG, Chang TW, Gurwith M, et al: Antibiotic-associated pseudomembranous colitis due to toxin-producing *Clostridia.* N Engl J Med 298:531, 1978.

29. Trnka YM, Lamont JT: *Clostridium difficile* colitis. *In* Tollerman GHS (ed): Advances in Internal Medicine. Chicago, Year Book Medical, 1984, p 85.

30. Drapkin M: Nosocomial infection with *C. difficile.* Infect Dis Clin Pract 1:138, 1992.

31. Hara M, Mukoyama J, Tsurukara T, et al: Acute gastroenteritis among school children associated with reovirus-like agent. Am J Epidemiol 107:161, 1978.

32. Marrie TJ, Lee SHS, et al: Rotavirus infection in a geriatric population. Arch Intern Med 142:313, 1982.

33. Blacklow N, Greenberg H, Faulkner RS, et al: Viral gastroenteritis. N Engl J Med 325:252, 1991.

34. Davidson GP, Gall DG, Petric M, et al: Human rotavirus enteritis induced in conventional piglets. J Clin Invest 60:1402, 1977.

35. Barnett B: Viral gastroenteritis. Med Clin North Am 67:1031–1058, 1983.

36. Zierdt CH. *Blastocystis hominis*—past and future. Clin Microbiol Rev 4:61, 1991.

37. Current WL, Reese NC, Ernst JV, et al: Human cryptosporidiosis in immunocompetent and immunodeficient persons. N Engl J Med 308:1252, 1983.

38. Krejs GJ, Fordtran JS: Diarrhea. *In* Sleisenger MH, Fordtran JS (eds): Gastrointestinal Disease. Philadelphia, WB Saunders, 1983.

39. Hyams JS: Sorbitol intolerance. Gastroenterology 84:30, 1983.

40. Phillips SF: Diarrhea. Postgrad Med 57:65, 1975.

41. Grody WW: Stool disorders. *In* Peter JB (ed): Gastroenterology. Santa Monica, CA, Specialty Laboratories, 1997.

42. Haubrich WS: Diarrhea and constipation. *In* Buckus HL (ed): Gastroenterology, vol 2. Philadelphia, WB Saunders, 1976.

43. Woodward WE, Woodward TE: Management of dehydrating diarrhea. Hosp Pract 21:60, 1986.

44. Griner PF, Panzer RJ, Greenland P: Clinical Diagnosis in the Laboratory. Chicago, Year Book Medical, 1986.

45. Kelly, MT, Hickman-Brenner FW, Farmer JJ III: *Vibrio. In* Balows A, Hausler WJ (eds): Manual of Clinical Microbiology, ed 5. Washington, DC, American Society for Microbiology, 1991.

46. Almeida RJ, Hickman-Brenner FW, Sowers EG, et al: Comparison of a latex agglutination assay and an ELISA for detecting cholera toxin. J Clin Microbiol 28:128–30, 1990.

47. Hayes P, Wells JG, Griffin PM: Isolation and identification of *Escherichia coli* 0157:H7. BACTinews vol 2, no. 2, (published by REMEL, Lenexa, Kan), April 1994.

48. Harris AA: Hemorrhagic colitis and *Escherichia coli* 0157:H7—identifying a messenger while pursuing the message. Mayo Clin Proc 65:884, 1990.

49. Isenberg HD, Washington JJ III, Doern GV, Amsterdam D: Specimen collection and handling. *In* Balows A, Hausler WJ (eds): Manual of Clinical Microbiology, ed 5. Washington, DC, American Society for Microbiology, 1991.

50. Lyerly DM: *Clostridium difficile* testing. Clin Microbiol Newsl 17:17–22, 1995.

51. Davison V, Aldersen G: Clinical virology. *In* Mahon CR, Manuselis G. Textbook of Diagnostic Microbiology. Philadelphia, WB Saunders, 1995.

52. Bishop RF, Barnes GL, Cipriani J, et al: Clinical immunity after neonatal rotavirus infection. N Engl J Med 309:72, 1983.

53. Satterwhite TK, Dupont HL: Infectious diarrhea in office practice. Med Clin North Am 67:203, 1983.

54. Blaser MJ, Reller LB: *Campylobacter* enteritis. N Engl J Med 305:1444, 1981.

55. Shanahan F: Current concepts of the pathogenesis of inflammatory bowel disease. Ir J Med Sci 163:544–549, 1994.

56. Ogorek CP, Fisher RS: Differentiation between Crohn's disease and ulcerative colitis. Med Clin North Am 78:1249–1258, 1994.

57. Oudkerk PM, Bouma G, Meuwissen SG, et al: Serological markers to differentiate between ulcerative colitis and Crohn's Disease. J Clin Pathol 48:346–350, 1995.

58. Crohn BB, Ginsgurg L, Oppenheimer GD: Regional ileitis: A pathologic and clinical entity. JAMA 99:1323–1329, 1932.

59. Katz J: The course of inflammatory bowel disease. Med Clin North Am 78:1275–1280, 1994.

60. Mowat NAG: Inflammatory bowel disease. Practitioner 228:803–810, 1984.

61. Wright R: Crohn's disease: Diagnosis and management. Compr Ther 11:38–44, 1985.

62. Andreoli TE, Carpenter CCJ, Plum F, et al: Essentials of Medicine. Philadelphia, WB Saunders, 1986.

63. Shearman DJC, Finlayson NDC: Diseases of the Gastrointestinal Tract and Liver. Edinburgh, Churchill Livingstone, 1982.

64. Steinhardt HJ, Loeschke K, Kasper H, et al: European Cooperative Crohn's Disease Study (ECCDS): Clinical features and natural history. Digestion 31:97–108, 1985.

65. Fleischer DE, Grimm IS, Friedman LS: Inflammatory bowel disease in older patients. Med Clin North Am 78:1303–1319, 1994.

66. Hofley PM, Piccoli DA: Inflammatory bowel disease in children. Med Clin North Am 78:1281–1302, 1994.

67. Shine B, Berghouse L, Jones JEL, et al: C-reactive protein as an aid in the differentiation of functional and inflammatory bowel disorders. Clin Chim Acta 148:105–109, 1985.

68. Andre C, Descos L, Andre F, et al: Biological measurements of Crohn's activity—a reassessment. Hepatogastroenterology 32:135–137, 1985.

69. Meyers S, Wolke A, Field SP, et al: Fecal alpha$_1$-antitrypsin measurement: An indicator of Crohn's disease activity. Gastroenterology 89:13–18, 1985.

70. Moran A, Jones A, Asquith P: Laboratory markers of colonoscopic activity in ulcerative colitis and Crohn's colitis. Scand J Gastroenterol 30:356–360, 1995.

Pancreatitis

Eileen Carreiro-Lewandowski

Pancreatitis, or inflammation of the pancreas, should be considered in the differential diagnosis of abdominal pain. Approximately 5000 new cases of acute pancreatitis with a 10% mortality rate per year have been estimated to occur in the United States. Data for chronic and recurrent acute pancreatitis are not as well defined, but an incidence of 8.2 new cases per 100,000 has been reported.[1] The nonspecificity of the abdominal pain associated with pancreatitis and the relative inaccessibility of the pancreas to direct examination make the diagnosis of pancreatitis difficult. In addition, many studies reporting the incidence of pancreatitis rely on elevation of total amylase as the primary indicator. Many patients with chronic pancreatitis do not, however, have elevated amylase levels, so the occurrence of pancreatitis may be underestimated.

Pancreatitis was originally classified as acute, relapsing acute, chronic relapsing (chronic pancreatitis with acute episodes) or chronic.[2] Now it is classified as acute or chronic.[3] Pancreatitis is considered *acute* when the disorder resolves both clinically and histologically. *Chronic pancreatitis* describes irreversible and progressive inflammatory injury to pancreatic tissue. The difficulty with this classification is that chronic inflammatory disease of the pancreas may present as acute episodes, described clinically as "acute," even though the episodes are the result of "chronic" pancreatic damage. This also contributes to confusion regarding the incidence of acute and chronic pancreatitis.

ETIOLOGY AND PATHOGENESIS
Acute Pancreatitis

Box 23–1 lists the causes of acute pancreatitis.[4] In the United States, the most common causes (~80%) are alco-

hol related, followed by obstructive biliary tract disease, notably gallstones. The remaining 20% of cases are caused by drugs, infection, hyperlipidemia (particularly types I and V), structural abnormalities of the pancreatic or common bile duct, surgery, vascular disease (e.g., hypotension), trauma (particularly blunt and penetrating), hyperparathyroidism and the related hypercalcemia, renal transplantation, or hereditary pancreatitis, or have unknown etiologies.

Although the exact mechanisms in pancreatitis are unknown, the disease is postulated to be caused by autodigestion of the pancreas, which occurs because of premature activation of proteolytic enzymes within the pancreas. This is due to a pooling or reflux of the enzymes from increased duodenal pressure occurring with blockage, inflammation, or toxic changes. Ordinarily, these enzymes are produced in the pancreas as inactive zymogens that are later activated in the intestinal lumen. Activated proteolytic enzymes, particularly trypsin, are capable of digesting pancreatic tissue,

---

Box 23–1. Causes Associated with Acute Pancreatitis

- Acute and chronic alcoholism
- Biliary tract disease (gallstones, obstructive diseases of the bile ducts and duodenum)
- Pancreatic disease (pancreatic cancer, cystic fibrosis, hereditary pancreatitis, pancreas divisum)
- Trauma (blunt abdominal type, postoperative, post–endoscopic retrograde cholangiopancreatography)
- Metabolic (hypertriglyceridemia, apolipoprotein C-II deficiency, hypercalcemia/hyperparathyroidism, renal failure, acute fatty liver of pregnancy)
- Infections (mumps, viral hepatitis)
- Drug related (in order of probable association with pancreatitis: azathioprine, sulfonamides, thiazide diuretics, furosemide, estrogens, tetracycline, valproic acid, pentamidine, dideoxyinosine, acetaminophen, procainamide, erythromycin, nonsteroidal anti-inflammatory drugs, and angiotensin-converting enzyme inhibitors)
- Collagen vascular disease (systemic lupus erythematosus, thrombocytic thrombocytopenic purpura)
- Idiopathic

Data from Agarwal N, Pitchumoni CS: Acute pancreatitis: A multisystem disease. Gastroenterology 1:115–128, 1993.

causing necrosis, and the damaged cellular membrane releases more proteolytic enzyme. Trypsin release not only causes tissue damage but also rapidly activates other enzymes, such as chymotrypsinogen to chymotrypsins, proelastases to elastase, procarboxypeptidase to carboxypeptidase, and prophospholipase A_2 to phospholipase A_2. Elastase causes hemorrhage by dissolving the elastic fibers (elastin) of blood vessels. Phospholipase A_2 uses cell membrane lecithin as a substrate, causing further membrane destruction and release of more enzymes, and thereby perpetuating the pancreatitis. These enzymes can be released into the circulation, leading to systemic and metabolic disturbances.

In the approximately 5% of the cases of acute pancreatitis that are drug related, it is thought that the pancreatitis arises either through a hypersensitivity reaction or through generation of a toxic metabolite followed by autodigestion. More than 85 drugs have been implicated in acute pancreatitis.

Complications of acute pancreatitis are listed in Box 23–2.[5, 6] Cellular necrosis allows release of substances such as bradykinin peptides and vasoactive substances (e.g., histamine), which may increase vascular permeability, contributing to edema and vasodilation. In addition, interstitial hemorrhage, coagulation abnormalities, and fat cell necrosis may also be present. These events collectively not only may lead to a necrotizing pancreatitis but also may cause a multisystem disease. Systemic complications of pancreatitis include adult respiratory distress syndrome, due in part to digestion by phospholipase A of lecithin in the lung;

Box 23–2. Complications of Acute Pancreatitis

- Pulmonary (pleural effusion, atelectasis, adult respiratory distress syndrome)
- Cardiovascular (hypotension, hypovolemia, hypoalbuminemia, ST-T changes, pericardial effusion)
- Metabolic (hyperglycemia, hypertriglyceridemia, hypocalcemia, sudden blindness—Purtscher's retinopathy, encephalopathy)
- Coagulation abnormalities (disseminated intravascular coagulation)
- Renal (oliguria, azotemia—increased blood urea nitrogen and creatinine, renal artery or vein thrombosis)
- Hemorrhage (pancreatic, necrosis with erosion into major blood vessels, massive intraperitoneal, thrombosis of the major blood vessels, variceal)
- Pancreatic changes (pancreatic ascites, pseudocyst, phlegmon, abscess, interruption of the main pancreatic duct)
- Obstruction (stomach, duodenum, colon, bile ducts, obstructive jaundice)
- Bowel infarction
- Fat necrosis (fat emboli)
- Central nervous system (psychosis)

Data from Calleja G, Barkin J: Acute pancreatitis. Med Clin North Am 77:1037–1056, 1993; Krumberger JM: Acute Pancreatitis. Crit Care Nurs Clin North Am 5:185–202, 1993.

---

myocardial depression and shock, secondary to vasoactive peptides and a myocardial depressant factor; and acute renal failure, caused by related hypovolemia and hypotension. Metabolic complications include hypocalcemia, hyperlipidemia, hyperglycemia, and diabetic ketoacidosis.

In edematous pancreatitis, the inflammatory response is confined to the pancreas and mortality is low (less than 5%). In pancreatitis characterized by severe necrosis and hemorrhage, the mortality approaches 20% to 50%. Early diagnosis is crucial to avoid premature death, which is usually caused by cardiovascular insufficiency with refractory shock and renal failure; respiratory failure, with hypoxemia and possibly adult respiratory distress syndrome; and, occasionally, heart failure, which has been attributed to a myocardial depressant factor. After the first week, death is usually due to complications of pancreatic necrosis such as secondary infections, abscess formation, duodenal obstruction caused by ulcerations, and, in 15% of patients with acute pancreatitis, development of a pancreatic pseudocyst.

A *pseudocyst* is a collection of pancreatic tissue and enzyme-rich fluid encapsulated by fibrous and vascular tissue. It is differentiated from a *phlegmon*, which is a solid mass of inflamed pancreatic tissue, by sonography. In many patients, the pseudocyst resolves itself; if not, it may cause complications. As the pseudocyst expands, it presses on the adjacent tissue, resulting in pain, compression of the common bile duct, and thrombosis of the portal or splenic vein. Ruptures of the pseudocyst into the peritoneal cavity can cause severe shock or pancreatic ascites. Cysts that erode into the thorax or arterial vessel wall can cause lung problems or severe hemorrhage, respectively. Some patients develop jaundice owing to obstruction of the common bile duct, stones, or swelling of the head of the pancreas. In the patient with acute pancreatitis due to gallstone disease, the stones must be removed to avoid recurrences of the acute pancreatitis. Any abscesses arising within or around the pancreas are infected by bowel organisms, and once infection is established, aggressive antibiotic treatment is important.

Chronic Pancreatitis

Causes of chronic pancreatitis are similar to those listed in Box 23–1 for acute pancreatitis. Rarely does an episode of acute pancreatitis lead to chronic pancreatitis. In the United States, alcoholism is the most common cause of chronic pancreatitis in adults, whereas cystic fibrosis is the most common cause in children. Also, there is a higher incidence (~25%) in adults of chronic pancreatitis with an idiopathic etiology. In other parts of the world, severe malnutrition is a common cause of this disorder. Rare causes are hereditary pancreatitis, hyperparathyroidism, or obstruction by stenosis, stones, or carcinoma. Patients with marked pancreatic disease who have less than 10% of exocrine function demonstrate steatorrhea.

Although the autodigestion theory is applicable in alcohol-induced pancreatitis, it has been suggested that the primary defect is the precipitation of protein within the ducts, resulting in atrophy of the acinar cells, fibrosis, and eventual calcification of some of the protein plugs. Direct toxic effects on the pancreas are also plausible. It is also thought that although pancreatitis may be associated with alcoholism and the consumption of large quantities of alcohol, the disorder has developed in patients who regularly consume small, that is, "socially acceptable," amounts of alcohol. Many of the complications secondary to acute pancreatitis can also occur in chronic pancreatitis. In some instances, patients with noncalculus obstruction of the bile duct cannot be diagnosed preoperatively as having pancreatitis or cancer.

CLINICAL MANIFESTATIONS
Acute Pancreatitis

The dominant feature in acute pancreatitis is severe abdominal pain that, in about half of the cases, radiates straight through to the back and may persist for several hours or days without relief. The pain is described as steady and boring. Most patients also experience nausea and vomiting.

Physical examination commonly reveals an acutely ill patient who is sweating. Low-grade fever, tachycardia, and hypotension are also common findings. Jaundice is occasionally present. If metabolic and systemic disturbances have occurred, the patient may present with altered pulmonary function, increased pulse rate, variable blood pressure but significant postural hypotension, symptoms of shock, cardiac disturbances, and, often, elevated temperature. Abdominal tenderness and muscle rigidity are present to a variable extent but more marked in the upper abdomen. Abdominal distention and ascites may be found. Bowel sounds are diminished or absent. A faint blue discoloration around the umbilicus, known as Cullen's sign, and a blue-red-purple or green-brown discoloration in the flank (Grey Turner's sign), although rare, indicates the presence of subcutaneous hemorrhage from necrotizing pancreatitis.

Chronic Pancreatitis

Chronic pancreatitis may manifest like an episode of acute pancreatitis. The pain can be continuous or intermittent. Patients may seek medical attention because of the complications of pancreatitis. When acinar cell damage is extensive and pancreatic enzyme secretion is considerably diminished, the abdominal pain may subside or may be absent entirely. Ingestion of alcohol or a meal containing fat-rich foods can exacerbate the pain. Weight loss, abnormal stools, and other signs of malabsorption may also be evident.

LABORATORY ANALYSIS AND DIAGNOSIS

Pancreatitis must be considered in the differential diagnosis in any patient with abdominal pain. Unfortunately, a 100% reliable biochemical test for pancreatitis is not available. Indirect measures such as chest x-rays, abdominal x-rays, ultrasound, computed tomography (CT), which better visualizes the pancreas, and, when indicated, endoscopic retrograde cholangiopancreatography (ERCP) are helpful in assessment of acute pancreatitis.

A chest x-ray may indicate lung complications, whereas an abdominal x-ray may reveal the presence of gallstones,

dilated loops of the bowel, or calculi within the pancreatic ducts from prior inflammation. Ultrasound examination might indicate the presence of gallstones, dilation of the common hepatic duct, or edema of the pancreas, and is also useful in the diagnosing or tracking the development of a pseudocyst. The biochemical markers commonly used for acute pancreatitis assessment are amylase and lipase.

An elevated amylase value to more than three times normal is highly suggestive of acute pancreatitis. The relative enzyme elevation does not correlate with the severity of the disease, however, and it has many limitations. Amylase is cleared by the kidneys and decreases to within its reference range in 2 to 4 days. Amylase is not specific for pancreatitis and is elevated in many nonpancreatic disorders, such as renal insufficiency, salivary gland lesions, ectopic production (e.g., from lung, esophageal, breast, or ovarian carcinoma), macroamylasemia, burns, diabetic ketoacidosis, pregnancy, cerebral trauma, biliary tract disease, and intra-abdominal disease (e.g., ruptured ectopic pregnancy, perforated peptic ulcer, intestinal obstruction or infarct, peritonitis, chronic liver disease, postoperative hyperamylasemia).

Amylase isoenzymes are either of the S (salivary) or P (pancreatic) type. In pancreatitis, the elevation of P isoenzyme persists longer than the total amylase, but is not specific for pancreatitis. Evaluation of isoenzymes may be helpful in distinguishing nonpancreatic causes of elevated amylase, except in renal failure. An amylase-to-creatinine clearance ratio (ACCR) is increased in acute pancreatitis, owing to decreased tubular reabsorption of amylase; this evaluation may be helpful in ruling out elevated amylase from macroamylasemia, in which the ratio is reduced. Increased amylase levels in peritoneal or pleural fluid may also be diagnostic.

Amylase values that are reduced or are within the reference range are expected in chronic pancreatitis because of the extensive tissue damage to the pancreas. Normal or decreased serum amylase may coexist with hypertriglyceridemia. A serial dilution or use of an ultracentrifuge reveals the amylase elevation, if present. Pancreatitis, hypertriglyceridemia, and alcoholism constitute a triad for which the association mechanism is not well understood. It is known that hypertriglyceridemia and hyperchylomicronemia can precede and apparently cause pancreatitis. Although the vast majority of patients with acute pancreatitis do not have hypertriglyceridemia, almost all patients with pancreatitis and hypertriglyceridemia are either alcoholics, who had been drinking prior to the attack, or patients with pre-existing hypertriglyceridemia. Any factor that causes an abrupt and severe increase in triglycerides (e.g., alcohol, drugs) can precipitate a bout of pancreatitis. Patients with a deficiency of apolipoprotein (apo) C-II have an increased incidence of pancreatitis; apo C-II activates lipoprotein lipase. Individuals with very elevated triglyceride values (>1000 mg/dL) are at greater risk for pancreatitis. Once the triglyceride levels decrease to 500 mg/dL or less, the risk of pancreatitis is essentially eliminated.

Serum lipase measurement may be the single best biochemical test for diagnosis of acute pancreatitis. Elevations of lipase usually parallel those of amylase, but lipase activity may occur sooner and persist longer than amylase elevation. As with amylase, the increase in lipase is not proportional to the severity of the disease, and in chronic pancreatitis, lipase values may be either decreased or within the reference range. Unlike with amylase, the tissue distribution of pancreatic lipase is almost entirely pancreatic. Nonpancreatic diseases, such as inflammatory bowel disease, cholecystitis, bowel perforation, hepatitis, gallstones, and acute alcoholism, as well as abdominal trauma can elevate lipase value, but not as high as pancreatic disease. Lipase measurement has not been readily used in the past because of testing difficulties and detection of nonspecific lipolytic activities in serum. The use of improved substrates (long-chain fatty acid triglycerides) and the incorporation of bile salts, calcium, and colipase in lipase testing result in higher lipase enzymatic activity.[7] Poor specificity (increased lipase values in patients with nonpancreatic disease) has been reported with the use of the Ektachem technique,[8] even though it is rapid and contains all of the appropriate substrates. It has been suggested that the clinical specificity can be improved by increasing the cutoff (upper reference limit) for lipase values.[9, 10] There has been a report of false lipase elevations with use of the Ektachem technique, in specimens from patients who coincidentally ingested glycerol (>14 mmol/L), which was part of the formulation of their medication.[11] Glycerol is an intermediate in this assay and certainly a source of interference.

Assays for trypsin in duodenal fluid and immunoreactive trypsin in serum are available. Trysinogen I (free, unbound) is the major form ($\geq$ 80%) found in serum from healthy persons and in acute pancreatitis. It rises in parallel with amylase and lipase. It has some diagnostic utility in the assessment of severe attacks associated with increased mortality rates, in which there is a decrease in proportion of the free trypsinogen. This substance is also excreted by the kidneys and is elevated in renal failure, as are amylase and lipase. Patients with renal failure and abdominal pain remain a difficult clinical problem because no blood test is reliable for the diagnosis of acute pancreatitis.

For purposes of treatment, it is often useful to distinguish gallstone from non-gallstone acute pancreatitis. Radiographic techniques may suffice, and routine films of the abdomen, ultrasonagraphy, and CT may indicate the presence of gallstones. ERCP is indicated if impaction of a gallstone in the ampullary region is suspected and the patient's condition requires urgent confirmation; however, ERCP is associated with certain pancreatic risks and may itself cause acute pancreatitis. A 1992 report indicates that an alanine transaminase (ALT) value more than three times above the upper reference limit increases the probability of gallstone pancreatitis to 95%.[12] Aspartate transaminase (AST) values usually mimic ALT values in pancreatitis. Total bilirubin and alkaline phosphatase values were not considered to be as useful in this study.

Other laboratory findings related to the underlying cause or to complications and severity of the pancreatitis are dehydration and hypochloremia, due to vomiting; elevated white blood cell (WBC) count (12.0–20.0 × 10⁹/L); increased glucose, due to multiple factors, including reduced insulin release, increased glucagon release, and greater output of glucocorticoids and catecholamines; and hypocalcemia, probably because of its utilization in the formation of fatty acid "soaps" due to tissue necrosis and also related

to the decrease in albumin because of third-space volume losses. The hematocrit may be quite high (50%–55%), also because of hypovolemia. The presence of C-reactive protein is a reliable indicator of acute inflammation and hyperbilirubinemia is present in approximately 5% to 10% of cases. Hypertriglyceridemia, acidosis, and hypoxia—associated with the onset of adult respiratory distress syndrome—may be present. In children, a positive sweat test is diagnostic for cystic fibrosis.

In chronic pancreatitis, as has been noted earlier, the lipase and amylase values may not be elevated. Other parameters that indicate the presence of cholestasis (increased bilirubin, alkaline phosphatase, and cholesterol) or malabsorption (impaired glucose and vitamin B_{12} absorption) may be evident. Tests of exocrine function (e.g., secretin test) may be helpful. Duodenal samples of normal volume and low bicarbonate are indicative of chronic pancreatitis. Testing for tumor markers (e.g., carcinoembryonic antigen, CA19-9) may be helpful in distinguishing pancreatic cancer from pancreatitis.

It is important to identify quickly those patients with a higher risk of death. Two systems are often used to evaluate the severity of the pancreatic disease, but other systems are also becoming available. The first such system is the Ranson/Imrie criteria, based on the presence of three or more risk factors at admission or during the initial 48 hours of hospitalization; presence of such criteria raises the mortality rate. The criteria are: (1) age more than 55 years, (2) serum glucose level above 200 mg/dL, (3) increased serum lactate dehydrogenase (LD) to more than 350 IU/L, (4) AST value greater than 250 IU/L, and (5) leukocytosis, with a WBC count above 16.0 × 10⁹/L. Forty-eight hours after admission, the risk factors are (1) a decrease in hematocrit of more than 10%, (2) increase in blood urea nitrogen (BUN) above 5 mg/dL after IV fluid administration, (3) decreased total serum calcium to less than 8 mg/dL, (4) hypoxemia with a PaO_2 of more than 60 mm Hg, (5) estimated fluid sequestration of more than 4 to 6 L, and (6) hypoalbuminemia, with albumin value of 3.2 g/dL or less. Part of the problem in applying the criteria is the use of cutoff values, like those for calcium, LD, and AST, which are not standardized among laboratories. If the criteria are used by physicians in a given institution, they might find it helpful to have the laboratory verify or establish its own cutoff values for these analytes.

A second assessment system is known as the acute physiology and chronic health evaluation scoring system (APACHE II). This system provides a description of illness severity for a wide range of diseases on the basis of the worst values of 12 physiologic measurements, age, and previous health status. Key indicators are (1) hypotension (blood pressure less than 90 mm Hg) or tachycardia greater than 130 beats per minute, (2) PaO_2 less than 60 mm Hg, (3) oliguria (output less than 50 mL/hr) or increasing BUN and creatinine, and (4) metabolic (serum calcium less than 8.0 mg/dL or serum albumin less than 3.2 g/dL). The APACHE II system is fairly complex, requiring a computer program, and it has met with mixed reaction by physicians. Another risk factor relating to the severity of the disease, introduced by McMahon and colleagues,[1] is the presence of a dark or hemorrhagic peritoneal fluid. These factors or systems, considered collectively, aid in diagnosing the severity of pancreatitis and course of treatment.

TREATMENT

Patients with a tentative diagnosis of acute pancreatitis should be carefully observed for 24 to 48 hours. Dehydration is corrected with intravenous (IV) fluids. Treatment of mild cases concentrates on quieting the pancreas. Nothing is given by mouth until pain and epigastric tenderness are absent and the bowel is functioning properly. Oral feedings are resumed initially with a liquid diet low in fat and secretagogues (e.g., caffeine). The use of a nasogastric tube is variable but is often recommended to relieve vomiting and nausea if present. Supportive care includes pain management. Antibiotic therapy is usually used only for those patients who remain febrile.

Severe pancreatitis must be closely monitored, and patients are usually admitted to an intensive care unit. Life-threatening complications may develop, and invasive monitoring is often required. If hemorrhage is present, transfusions may be needed. Further treatment involves minimizing the effects of the complications from acute pancreatitis. Hyperglycemia may require insulin therapy. Hypocalcemia can often be corrected by administration of albumin-containing solutions. If there is coexisting hypomagnesemia, magnesium sulfate is also included. Patients begin parenteral nutrition early and abstain from eating for 2 to 3 weeks or longer. Surgical intervention is dictated by the severity of the pancreatitis and the cause. Pseudocyst that persists for 4 to 6 weeks and is greater than 5 cm in diameter and therefore causing abdominal symptoms requires surgical decompression. If biliary calculi are present or if gallstones are impacted in the ampulla of Vater, surgery may be beneficial.

Chronic pancreatitis may require treatment appropriate for an episode of acute pancreatitis. The patient must abstain from alcohol and heavy fatty meals, and malabsorption must be addressed. Small meals restricted in fat and protein to reduce secretion of pancreatic enzymes plus histamine H_2 receptor blockers and use of antacids to reduce acid-stimulated release of secretin and the flow of pancreatic juice have uncertain benefit.[13] Oral pancreatic enzymes or narcotics are used to ameliorate the pain. Surgery is often required, depending on the underlying organ changes. Steatorrhea may be improved by the use of pancreatic enzyme tablets with meals; if this practice proves unsatisfactory, antacids and histamine H_2 blockers can be tried. Supplementation using medium-chain triglycerides as a source of fat and administration of fat-soluble vitamins may be required.

Case Study 1

A 78-year-old man was admitted to the hospital because of severe abdominal pain and nausea. His history showed that 30 years before, he had had a cholecystectomy. The patient was in acute distress with marked epigastric tenderness and hypoactive bowel sounds. His pulse was 90 beats/min, blood pressure 150/90 mm Hg. Laboratory results were normal for urinalysis, complete blood count, blood glucose, BUN, electrolytes, calcium and bilirubin. Remarkable laboratory values (with reference ranges) were as follows: alkaline phosphatase was 118 U/L (30–110 U/L); AST 81 U/L (7–40 U/L); ALT 191 U/L (3–36 U/L); and amylase 1515 U/L (23–85 U/L). Subsequent daily amylase values were as follows: 490, 341, 116, and 80 U/L. The patient responded very well to IV treatment, analgesics, and a clear liquid diet followed by a diet low in fat. His pain completely subsided, and he was discharged.

Questions

1. Given the patient's history, clinical findings, and laboratory results, what condition probably contributed to the acute pancreatitis?
2. What follow-up procedures might be likely for this patient?

Discussion

1. The patient had had a cholecystectomy 30 years earlier. The acute pancreatitis is unlikely to be the result of gallstones but most likely secondary to biliary disease, as indicated by the increase in alkaline phosphatase, AST, and ALT. He presented with a relatively mild acute pancreatitis episode and responded well to treatment.
2. Further investigation of biliary tract disease using radiographic methods is needed. Ultrasound demonstrated a dilated common bile duct without obvious gallstones. Radionuclide excretion was delayed, supporting this diagnosis. Further episodes might indicate sludge or tumor, either pancreatic or biliary.

Case Study 2

A 30-year-old white male was admitted to the hospital with complaints of crampy severe left-sided back pain that radiated to his left flank. He also had marked nausea and vomiting, a slight fever, and chills. He stated that he consumed three to four six-packs of beer per day and that his diet contained primarily "fatty" foods. He indicated that he was taking indomethacin (Indocin) for treatment of gout.

Physical examination revealed a well-developed, obese male in discomfort. Temperature was 40 °C; pulse was 136 beats/min; icterus was minimal; heart sounds were normal; blood pressure was 120/94 mm Hg; and there were decreased bowel sounds. An electrocardiogram showed a sinus tachycardia with some ST elevation. An x-ray of the abdomen revealed an ileus or sentinel loop. Ultrasound demonstrated the possible presence of a pseudocyst.

Remarkable laboratory results (and reference ranges) were as follows: WBC $= 22.6 \times 10^9$/L $(3.5–11 \times 10^9$/L); hematocrit 50% (38 to 51%); sodium (Na) 102 mEq/L (135–145 mEq/L); potassium (K) 2.9 (3.8–5.0 mEq/L); chloride (Cl) 77 mEq/L (98–109 mEq/L); total CO_2 14 mEq/L (26–31 mEq/L). It was noted that the sample was grossly lipemic. LD was 247 U/L (118–263 U/L); total bilirubin 1.4 mg/dL (0.1–1.0 mg/dL); cholesterol 1470 mg/dL (140–240 mg/dL); albumin 2.5 g/dL (3.5–5.0 g/dL); calcium 7.4 mg/dL (8.5–10.5 mg/dL); uric acid 8.0 mg/dL (3.0–8.5 mg/dL); triglycerides 1574 mg/day (<250 mg/day); and fasting glucose 138 mg/dL (70–100 mg/dL).

Urinalysis showed albumin, acetone, and some WBCs. Because of the marked lipemia, serum amylase and lipase determinations were not performed. Urine amylase performed the following day revealed values of 4000 U. A blood gas analysis was performed, and the values were pH 7.49 (7.35–7.45), $PaCO_2$ 26 mm Hg (34–45 mm Hg), and PaO_2 70 mm Hg (80–90 mm Hg).

A nasogastric tube was placed, and the patient was put on "nothing by mouth" (NPO) status at this time. A surgical consultation revealed the presence of a pseudocyst, and a decision was made to drain it. The pseudocyst drained a dark brown, thick material. Streptodornase was administered. Once the cyst had completed draining, all laboratory values, except glucose and triglycerides, returned to within reference limits.

Questions

1. According to the criteria given for assessing the severity of the disease, would this patient be considered as experiencing an attack associated with high mortality at the time of admission?
2. List at least two causes of acute pancreatitis likely for this patient.
3. Explain the calcium and albumin abnormalities.

Discussion

1. According to the criteria and the cutoff levels given here, this case would not be classified as high mortality. According to the Ranson/Imrie classification, only the leukocytosis was greater than the cutoff of $16.0 \times 10^9/L$. The patient did have hyperglycemia and elevated LD, but not above the cutoff levels given. The hyperglycemia may be due to decreased insulin production or secondary to the patient's alcoholism and obesity. According to the APACHE II scoring system, the risk factors present were only metabolic (calcium and albumin). The anemia present was either related to the alcoholism, to hyperglyceridemia, or to some hemorrhage from the pseudocyst. A decreasing PaO_2 may further aggravate the anemia. If the PaO_2 continues dropping, the level may be due to a fat embolus or shunting of blood and can have fatal consequences. During ultrasonography, it was discovered that the pseudocyst measured approximately 16 cm and had displaced the stomach. Because of its size, drainage was indicated.

2. The two causes of acute pancreatitis most likely for this patient were his alcoholism and the hyperlipidemia. Acute pancreatitis is associated with sharp increases in triglycerides above 1000 mg/dL and in alcoholic patients. Further evaluation revealed a type V hyperlipidemia. Once the pseudocyst was drained and the pancreatitis was responding well to treatment, the cholesterol decreased to 202 mg/dL, and the triglyceride level dropped to 317 mg/dL.

3. The decreases in calcium and albumin are consistent with the other metabolic findings in an edematous type ("third space loss") pancreatitis. The urinalysis showed protein loss, which would consist mostly of albumin. Total calcium determination would have shown decreased levels with a decrease in albumin. However, with the amount of fats present, calcium is utilized in micelle formation as part of the fatty acid soaps, resulting in a real decrease in calcium. The edema most likely contributed to a dilutional hyponatremia coupled with a pseudohyponatremia because of the marked lipemia. A mild respiratory alkalosis was evidenced by the decreased $PaCO_2$ and compensation by a decreasing bicarbonate. The bicarbonate loss might be associated with loss through vomiting and, to some extent, the pseudocyst. In an alkalotic state, potassium may be exchanged preferentially for hydrogen as a compensation for the pH.

References

1. Toskes P, Greenberger N: Disorders of the pancreas. *In* Isselbacher KJ, Braunwald E, Wilson JD, et al (eds): Harrison's Principles of Internal Medicine, ed 13. New York, McGraw-Hill, 1994.
2. Searles H: Pancreatitis: Symposium at Marseilles, 1963. Basel, Karger, 1965.
3. Singer, M, Gyr, K, Sarles H: Revised classification of pancreatitis; report of the Second International Symposium on Classification of Pancreatitis in Marseilles, France. Gastroenterology 89:683–690, 1985.
4. Agarwal N, Pitchumoni CS: Acute pancreatitis: A multisystem disease. Gastroenterologist 1:115–128, 1993.
5. Calleja G, Barkin J: Acute pancreatitis. Med Clin North Am 77:1037–1056, 1993.
6. Krumberger JM: Acute pancreatitis. Crit Care Nurs Clin North Am 5:185–202, 1993.
7. Lott JA, Patel ST, Sawhney AK, et al: Assays of serum lipase: Analytical and clinical considerations. Clin Chem 32:1290–302, 1986.
8. Toskes P, Greenberger N: Disorders of the pancreas. *In* Isselbacher KJ, Braunwald E, Wilson JD, et al (eds): Harrison's Principles of Internal Medicine. ed 13. New York, McGraw-Hill, 1994.
9. Tietz N, Shuey D: Lipase in serum—the elusive enzyme: An overview. Clin Chem 39:746–56, 1993.
10. Wong E, Butch A, Rosenblum J, et al: The clinical chemistry laboratory and acute pancreatitis. Clin Chem 39:243, 1993.
11. Bilodeau L, Grotte D, Preese L, et al: Glycerol interference in serum lipase assay falsely indicates pancreas injury. Gastroenterology 103:1066–1067, 1992.
12. Tenner S, Dubner H, Steinberg W: Predicting gallstone pancreatitis with laboratory parameters: A meta-analysis. Am J Gastroenterol 89:1863–1866,1994.
13. Acute pancreatitis. *In* Berkow R (ed): The Merck Manual, ed 16. Rahway, NJ, Merck Research Laboratories, 1992.

Chapter 24

Malabsorption

Larry Schoeff

NORMAL ASSIMILATION

Normal assimilation of food into the body occurs in three phases. The first two, the *cephalic* and *gastric* phases, are purely digestive processes that break down the food for subsequent absorption. The *intestinal* phase begins as these partially digested food substances traverse the duodenum, where gastrointestinal hormones and pancreatic enzymes effect further degradation. The digestive products then enter the jejunum and ileum for absorption. Carbohydrate, fat, and protein assimilation occur in three stages within the small intestine: the intraluminal phase, the brush border phase, and, finally, intracellular absorption. Each day, the gut absorbs approximately 1.5 liters of ingested liquids and 7.5 liters of gastrointestinal secretions.[1, 2]

Carbohydrate absorption begins with the action of salivary amylase on starch and proceeds quickly to the duodenum, where pancreatic amylase essentially completes the hydrolysis of starch into disaccharides and oligosaccharides. Hydrolases of the mucosal brush border further split these sugars into monosaccharides, which are absorbed intracellularly for delivery to the liver.[3]

Fat is assimilated less efficiently than a carbohydrates and protein, requiring more time for lipolysis in the duodenum and a greater surface area in the jejunum for absorption. Although dietary triglycerides are first hydrolyzed in the stomach by pharyngeal and gastric lipases, most hydrolysis occurs in the duodenum with pancreatic lipase.[4] A pancreatic factor, colipase, is also secreted to facilitate more efficient lipolysis by binding to lipid–bile salt surfaces.[5] Moreover, cholecystokinin release from the duodenal mucosa stimulates the pancreas and gallbladder to synchronize the secretion of optimal mixtures of lipid, lipase, and bile salts for efficient lipolysis.[6] Liberated fatty acids and monoglycerides then solubilize with bile acids, forming micelles in the lumen. At the mucosal cell surface, bile salts dissociate and the lipids are absorbed, with the aid of a cytosol fatty acid–binding protein, into the jejunal mucosa. Within the cell, they reassemble into triglycerides, which stimulate specific apolipoproteins and form chylomicrons. The chylomicrons are transported out of the cell in the systemic circulation via the lymphatic pathway.

Digestion of dietary protein begins in the stomach as the acidity and pepsin denature the protein, producing polypeptides. Protein digestion is more significant in the duodenum, where proteolytic proenzymes from the pancreas, including trypsinogen and chymotrypsinogen, are secreted to hydrolyze protein into small peptides and amino acids. Once in the duodenum, these proenzyme forms are activated by a brush border enzyme, enterokinase, which selectively acts on trypsinogen to form trypsin. Traces of trypsin in turn promote activation of the other proenzymes. Some of the resulting small peptides are hydrolyzed to amino acids at the brush border membrane by aminopeptidases. Amino acids, as well as dipeptides and tripeptides, are absorbed intact into the mucosal cell, aided by several stereospecific transport systems.[7–9] The peptides are rapidly hydrolyzed in the mucosa so that only amino acids are found in portal blood.

The water-insoluble vitamins A, D, E, and K depend on the formation of soluble lipid micelles in the intestinal lumen for adequate absorption. The water-soluble vitamins folic acid and vitamin B_{12} require specialized digestive and transport mechanisms for absorption. Dietary folate in the intestinal lumen must be hydrolyzed to free folate by a brush border enzyme before absorption occurs. It is then absorbed by diffusion and carrier-mediated transport. Cobalamin (B_{12}) competes with two different substances in the stomach for binding, intrinsic factor and a binding protein called R protein. The latter has a greater affinity for B_{12}. The difficulty with intestinal absorption is that only B_{12} bound to intrinsic factor can be absorbed. Because neither free B_{12} nor R protein–bound B_{12} is absorbable, a pancreatic protease is required to alter the R protein attached to B_{12} in such a way that intrinsic factor can bind to the B_{12}. Ultimately, intrinsic factor–bound B_{12} attaches to membrane receptors of the ileal mucosa for absorption.[10]

Sodium is absorbed by active transport involving the absorption of glucose and amino acids. Calcium uptake by the jejunal mucosa is facilitated by a calcium-binding protein, synthesis of which is regulated by vitamin D and parathyroid hormone. Iron absorption is regulated by ferritin and transferrin, working together in the mucosal cells to trap and transport ferrous iron into body stores. When body iron stores are too high, mucosal cells with iron still inside are sloughed into the lumen.

ETIOLOGY AND PATHOPHYSIOLOGY OF MALASSIMILATION DISORDERS

Maldigestion vs. Malabsorption

It is important to distinguish between maldigestion and malabsorption for etiologic reasons. Although the absorptive process itself may be impaired, malabsorption may also be caused by inadequate digestion of the various nutrients before they reach the mucosal lining for assimilation. Maldigestion of nutrients may occur anywhere along the gastrointestinal tract after ingestion, but most commonly, it is the result of some form of pancreatic insufficiency.

Disease Classification[8, 11, 12]

Diseases that cause malabsorption syndrome are classified according to the stages of digestion and absorption where the pathophysiologic processes occur in the gastrointestinal tract (Box 24–1).

In the digestive, or intraluminal, stage, a deficiency of pancreatic enzymes or bile acids leads to malabsorption, because nutrients in the lumen are not digested into an absorbable state. Defective secretion of pancreatic enzymes as a result of the conditions listed Box 24–1 causes maldigestion of carbohydrates, fat, and protein. Also, duodenal hyperacidity can inactivate pancreatic enzymes. Deficiency of bile acid secretion or activity in the intestinal lumen prevents digestion of lipids. This diminution may result from biliary obstruction, liver disease, or terminal ileitis (Crohn's disease).[13] Overgrowth of bacteria in the small intestine can inactivate bile acids, leading to lipid malabsorption.[14]

In the absorptive, or intestinal mucosal, stage, defects at the brush border or impairment of the epithelium causes inadequate absorption. Genetic and biochemical abnormalities, such as deficiencies of brush border enzymes and defects in amino acid transport, and loss of absorptive surface area, as in short bowel syndrome, are examples of conditions that involve the absorptive phase.[15] Short bowel syndrome is a condition of malabsorption and malnutrition following a major resection of the small intestine.[7, 16–18] An example of infiltrative disease is Whipple's disease,[19] a rare condition of intestinal lipodystrophy associated with systemic bacterial illness. Two chronic inflammatory disorders of malabsorption with unknown etiologies and potentially severe complications are ulcerative colitis[20] and extensive regional enteritis (Crohn's disease)[13] (see Chapter 22).

Malabsorption may also result from disturbances of the mucosal immune system.[21] These include immunodefi-

---

Box 24–1. Classification of Malabsorption Syndromes

Maldigestion—Intraluminal Stage

Deficiency of Pancreatic Enzymes
    Chronic pancreatitis
    Pancreatic carcinoma
    Cystic fibrosis
    Pancreatic resection
    Duodenal hyperacidity states
    Postgastrectomy syndrome
Deficiency of Bile Acids
    Bile duct obstruction
    Intrahepatic disease
    Terminal ileitis (Crohn's disease)
    Ileal resection
    Bacterial overgrowth

Malabsorption—Intestinal Mucosal Stage

Defects at Brush Border
    Deficiencies of oligosaccharidases
    Deficiency of enteropeptidase
Impairment of Epithelium
    Celiac disease (gluten-sensitive enteropathy)
    Tropical sprue
    Whipple's disease
    Ulcerative colitis
    Short bowel syndrome
    Extensive regional enteritis (Crohn's disease)
    Primary intestinal lymphoma
    Radiation enteritis
    Amino acid transport defects
    Immunodeficiency states
    Pernicious anemia
    Food allergy
    Parasitic infections
    Amyloidosis
    Lymphangiectasia
    Abetalipoproteinemia

---

ciency states, the most common of which is selective immunoglobulin (Ig)A deficiency, proliferation or malignant expansion of immune-related cells, as in primary intestinal lymphoma, and hypersensitivity reactions, such as celiac disease.[22–25] Celiac disease, or gluten-sensitive enteropathy, is characterized by a severe allergy of the intestinal mucosa to the glycoprotein gluten found in wheat and other cereal grains.[26–28] It is the water-insoluble gliadin fraction (single polypeptide) of gluten in wheat and other cereal grains that leads to the mucosal damage. The damage characteristically manifests as a flattened surface with no villi and infiltration of the lamina propria with lymphocytes and plasma cells.

Carbohydrate Malabsorption[3, 12]

Malabsorption of various ingested sugars can occur following mucosal injury caused by a number of diseases, including celiac disease, tropical sprue,[29, 30] and gastroenteritis. Structural damage to or physiologic dysfunction of the mucosa may decrease hydrolase enzymes along the brush border,[31] may alter the active transport mechanism for monosaccharide absorption, or both. Disorders of intraluminal starch digestion are rare because of the excessive amylase normally secreted and the fact that total pancreatic insufficiency is required before the effect is significant. A normal exception to this is the transient physiologic deficiency of amylase in the neonate. Although abnormal digestion of starch in the lumen is rare, abnormal digestion of oligosaccharides at the brush border is common.

The most common disorder of carbohydrate malabsorption is lactose intolerance, caused by a deficiency at the brush border of lactase, which normally hydrolyzes the milk sugar into glucose and galactose. There are two distinct types of lactase deficiency—congenital and acquired.[32, 33] Congenital lactase deficiency is rare, with mucosal levels low or absent at birth. The disease exhibits autosomal recessive inheritance, involving a structural mutation that prevents lactase synthesis. When suspected, it must be distinguished from glucose-galactose malabsorption and from developmental lactose intolerance in the newborn. Acquired or late-onset lactase deficiency occurs in many ethnic groups around the world. In fact, most adults in the world are lactase deficient. In population groups that consume dairy products all their lives, the lactase mechanism typically persists into adulthood. In nondairy cultures, such as African and Asian groups, however, lactase levels tend to decline steadily through childhood and adolescence, and there is a high prevalence of lactose malabsorption (>65%).[33]

Two other oligosaccharidase deficiencies are sucrase-isomaltase deficiency and trehalase deficiency. Sucrase-isomaltase, a major disaccharidase in the microvillus membrane, hydrolyzes sucrose and isomaltose. Its deficiency is inherited as an autosomal recessive trait, with symptoms appearing when sucrose-sweetened foods are consumed. Trehalase deficiency, a rare genetic disorder, is caused by ingestion of mushrooms that have a high content of the sugar trehalose.

Glucose-galactose malabsorption is a rare transport defect in which poor mucosal binding of glucose and galactose occurs. Fructose malabsorption occurs rarely, following the ingestion of fruit.

Fat Malabsorption[6]

Conditions that are associated with malabsorption of lipids are classified as impaired lipolysis, impaired micelle formation, or defective mucosal absorption. Defects in lipolysis may occur in postgastrectomy patients when rapid gastric emptying of fat into the small intestine is too excessive for the lipase available. The fat may be delivered normally, but pancreatic insufficiency may prevent adequate secretion of lipase into the lumen. Diminished lipase secretion may also result if there is decreased release of cholecystokinin from a damaged duodenal mucosa, caused by celiac sprue or Crohn's disease. If none of these conditions exists, lipolysis may still be impaired by an altered luminal environment, such as a low pH from hypersecretion of gastric acid that spills into the duodenum; lipase is not effective in an acid environment. Colipase may be

deficient from the lumen, which would limit lipolysis by preventing activation of lipase.

Defects in micellar solubilization of lipolytic products with bile salts involve synthesis, conjugation, delivery, or loss of bile salts. Without micellarization, lipids do not efficiently penetrate the microvillus membrane nor diffuse into the mucosal cell. Intrahepatic cholestasis from cirrhosis or hepatitis decreases synthesis of bile salts, whereas bile duct obstruction decreases delivery to the lumen. The bile salt–binding drug cholestyramine and excess intestinal bacteria, which deconjugate bile salts, both decrease the effective concentration of conjugated bile salts already in the lumen. Deconjugation renders them less capable of solubilizing the lipids. Ileal disease or resection causes a significant defect in the enterohepatic circulation of bile salts that can result in large fecal losses.

Mucosal diseases, such as celiac and tropical sprue or regional enteritis, cause a decrease in absorption of lipids. If lipids are absorbed into the mucosa, they become dependent on the formation of chylomicrons for transport out of the cell and uptake by the lymphatic system. In the rare disorder abetalipoproteinemia, no synthesis of chylomicrons occurs because its major apolipoprotein B is absent. In Whipple's disease, transport of chylomicrons through the lamina propria to the lymphatics decreases because of "foamy" macrophages in the lamina propria that hinder the movement of chylomicrons. Finally, uptake by the lymphatics may be impaired by lymphatic obstruction, as in lymphoma or lymphangiectasia.

Protein Malabsorption[34]

Although significant protein digestion by pepsin occurs in the stomach, it is not essential, and even total gastrectomy does not alter protein metabolism significantly. There are no known malabsorption disorders from decreased pepsin. The only maldigestive disorder of protein to be considered is trypsin deficiency, which may result from any cause of pancreatic insufficiency or from a deficiency of enterokinase. Without enterokinase in the duodenum, pancreatic trypsinogen is not activated to trypsin. Enterokinase deficiency may manifest as a rare primary disorder or secondarily from congenital exocrine pancreatic insufficiency, in which a dependence of pancreatic secretions (trypsinogen) on enterokinase activity has been demonstrated.[15]

Reductions in carrier-mediated transport of amino acids in mucosal cells may occur through a number of mechanisms. Mucosal diseases may lower brush-border enteropeptidase activity as well as absorptive capability for amino acids. Segments of intestine that are specialized for absorption of certain amino acids or vitamins may be removed by surgical resection. Exudative loss of plasma proteins through inflamed or ulcerated mucosa may be a dramatic cause of protein malassimilation in protein-losing enteropathy.

Vitamin and Mineral Malabsorption[1, 35]

The fat-soluble vitamins A, D, E, and K depend on micellar solubilization for absorption; therefore, deficiencies of these vitamins may be caused by similar disorders of fat malabsorption in which formation of bile salt micelles is impaired. Folate and cobalamin (B$_{12}$) deficiencies are common in intestinal disease. Patients most susceptible to folate deficiency are those who have a poor diet and those with malabsorption secondary to jejunal mucosal disease or drugs that interfere with the metabolism of folate.[36, 37] Ileal resection is a common cause of cobalamin deficiency, because the ileal segment that absorbs the vitamin B$_{12}$–intrinsic factor complex by active transport is removed. Iron malabsorption is most significant in diseases that cause long-term blood loss, such as extensive Crohn's disease. Because calcium absorption is under the influence of vitamin D, which in turn is regulated by dietary fat and plasma parathyroid hormone levels, a decrease in calcium absorption can occur through several mechanisms. Fat malabsorption leads to decreased vitamin D absorption; unabsorbed intestinal fat and certain drugs, such as steroids, can bind calcium and prevent absorption; any disruption of absorptive surface area decreases calcium absorption; hypoparathyroidism also decreases intestinal calcium absorption.

CLINICAL MANIFESTATIONS[8, 11, 12]

The classic symptoms common to all diseases of malabsorption regardless of etiology are weight loss and diarrhea[38] (Fig. 24–1). An increase in appetite following weight loss may be the only manifestation in early or mild cases. Anorexia may also be seen, as in celiac disease, although hyperphagia typifies pancreatic insufficiency. Weight loss is primarily due to the wasting of dietary calories, and is accompanied by malnutrition as the disorder progresses. The diarrhea of malabsorption disorders reflects the stimulus effect of unabsorbed bile acids and fatty acids on the colon, resulting in water and electrolyte secretion in the stools.

The clinical hallmark, from the laboratory perspective, is *steatorrhea*, or pathologic increase in stool fat. Steatorrhea tends to be a manifestation of almost all major causes of malabsorption, because the pancreas, bile, and mucosal integrity are all important in lipid digestion and absorption. The physical findings in the malabsorption syndrome relate both to the underlying disease process and to malnutrition.

Malnutritional and abdominal symptoms are more specific in nature, reflective of the malabsorbed or deficient substance involved. Clinically, malabsorption of fat from pancreatic or mucosal disease occurs before carbohydrate or protein malabsorption, because of less efficient metabolism and dependence on intraluminal bile salt levels. In addition to steatorrhea, specific symptoms of fat malabsorption include those caused by subsequent deficiencies of the fat-soluble vitamins. Osteomalacia results from vitamin D and calcium malabsorption, susceptibility to hemorrhage from vitamin K malabsorption, xerophthalmia from lack of vitamin A, and myopathy and red blood cell fragility from lack of vitamin E.

Symptoms of carbohydrate malabsorption are abdominal distention and cramps, flatulence, and watery diarrhea. Usually, no steatorrhea is present. Unabsorbed sugars in the intestinal lumen enter the colon, where bacteria ferment them into monosaccharides, short-chain fatty acids, hydrogen, and carbon dioxide. The watery diarrhea results from

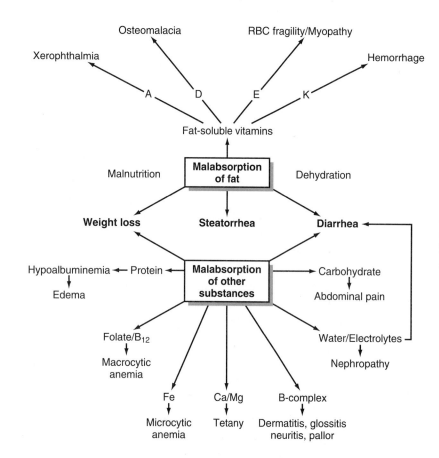

Figure 24–1. Symptoms of malabsorption. Abbreviation: RBC, red blood cell. (Reproduced with permission from Cerda J, Artnak E: Nutritional aspects of malabsorption syndromes. Compr Ther 9:35–46, 1983. © American Society of Contemporary Medicine & Surgery.)

osmotic retention of water in the colon by the fatty acids and monosaccharides. The production of hydrogen and carbon dioxide gases and the colonic fluid accumulation cause the abdominal symptoms. Symptoms of sugar malabsorption may vary, depending on the ingested sugar load, the colonic bacterial flora, and the compensatory capacity of the colon to absorb excess water and fatty acids.[3]

Dietary protein malabsorption or excessive intestinal protein loss leads to hypoalbuminemia, which in turn causes peripheral edema in association with proximal muscle wasting. If the protein deficiency or loss is severe enough, there may be some endocrine dysfunction of gastrointestinal and other hormones, as well as osteoporosis from lack of protein-bound calcium. Folate or vitamin B_{12} malabsorption manifests as a megaloblastic (macrocytic) anemia, whereas iron deficiency produces a microcytic anemia. The symptoms of dermatitis, neuritis, glossitis, and pallor are seen as a result of deficiency of vitamin B complex. In addition to osteomalacia, symptoms of tetany are also produced by calcium deficiency, with or without diminished magnesium levels. Dehydration may be present in some malabsorption patients because of electrolyte imbalance and water loss.

LABORATORY ANALYSES AND DIAGNOSIS[8, 9, 11, 12, 39-42]

The laboratory evaluation of malabsorption usually begins with screening tests for malnutrition and steatorrhea to investigate the symptoms of diarrhea and weight loss, and for symptoms related to nutritional deficiency, such as anemia and osteomalacia (Fig. 24–2). A variety of common laboratory tests can be used to screen for nutritional deficiency. They include a complete blood count (CBC) with peripheral smear, serum levels of albumin, phosphorus, calcium, and cholesterol, and prothrombin time. Follow-up studies from the CBC might include serum iron, vitamin B_{12}, and red cell folate. Other follow-up studies are protein electrophoresis, bone studies, and liver function tests. The simplest test used to detect steatorrhea is the Sudan III stain for fecal fat. This qualitative test may suffice as an alternative to the definitive test for fat malabsorption, which is a quantitative measurement of fat from a 72-hour collection of feces. Examination for parasites may also be done at this time. Because of the difficulty of collection and the unpleasantness of handling the specimen, other alternatives have been promoted. Among them are serum carotene or vitamin A assays and ^{14}C-triolein breath tests. Low carotene (<50 μg/dL) and vitamin A levels (<25 μg/ dL) are seen in 86% of patients with fat malabsorption. Serum carotene is more popular as a screening test, because vitamin A assays are more difficult to perform and the diagnostic abilities of the two tests are not significantly different. Another screening procedure is a survey x-ray of the abdomen to detect pancreatic calcification. Invasive small bowel x-rays and other visualization techniques are not initial studies.

Breath analyses are becoming the best laboratory tests to evaluate malabsorption as their availability becomes more widespread.[43-45] These tests offer the advantages of simplicity, convenience, and, in most cases, sensitivity and specificity. Specific uses of breath tests include direct detec-

tion of fat malabsorption (^{14}C-triolein), carbohydrate malabsorption (H_2-lactose and H_2-sucrose), bile salt malabsorption (^{14}C-glycocholate), and bacterial overgrowth (^{14}C-xylose). In the ^{14}C-triolein breath test, the ^{14}C-labeled triglyceride is administered orally, with the absorbed fat ultimately metabolized to carbon dioxide and water. The radioactivity of $^{14}CO_2$ is measured in specimens of expired air with scintillation counters. Results are usually expressed as a percentage of the administered dose; low results indicate impaired fat absorption. A sensitivity of 100% and a specificity of 96%, with a predictive value of approximately 90%, have been reported with this test.[46] Both the quantitative fecal fat test and the ^{14}C-triolein breath test assess the extent of lipid malabsorption.

Once the suspicion of malabsorption raised by the presenting symptoms is confirmed by the screening tests, specific tests are employed to differentiate the diagnostic possibilities. Differential diagnosis should be directed toward three major organ systems: pancreatic insufficiency, liver disease, and impairment of the small intestine itself. Surgical alteration of the stomach and intestine should also be kept in mind for absorption problems. If the diagnosis has been narrowed to the small intestine, further investigation is required to differentiate jejunal disease, ileal disease, bacterial overgrowth, or lactose intolerance.

The D-xylose absorption test continues to be widely used to distinguish malabsorption from maldigestion.[9, 47] Oral D-xylose does not require digestion and is normally absorbed directly by the jejunum only; therefore, ileal malabsorptisn is not detected by this test. After absorption into the blood stream, the amount of D-xylose excreted into the urine over a 5-hour period is closely correlated with the amount of D-xylose absorbed in the jejunum. Low urinary excretion of D-xylose (<25%) suggests jejunal disease, whereas normal results point to maldigestion, as in pancreatic disease. Low valves may also be seen in ascites, delayed gastric emptying, and kidney disease.

If D-xylose absorption is normal in the presence of steatorrhea, then pancreatic function should be evaluated. Testing for pancreatic disease may begin with serum levels of amylase, lipase, and trypsin. Intubation tests are more precise, although they are more difficult to perform. Pancreatic and duodenal secretions are aspirated, after stimulation of the pancreas with secretin or a Lundh meal, and tested for volume, bicarbonate concentration, and trypsin activity. Low results in all three parameters are highly indicative of pancreatic insufficiency. A tubeless stimulation test utilizes N-benzoyl-L-tyrosyl-p-aminobenzoic acid, which is hydrolyzed after ingestion by chymotrypsin.[9] The hydrolysis product, p-aminobenzoic acid (PABA), is absorbed and ultimately excreted in the urine. Low urinary excretion of PABA suggests pancreatic disease; however, the test depends on normal absorption and normal liver function. A glucose tolerance test assesses the endocrine function of the pancreas. Finally, if an initial abdominal film showed pancreatic calcification, more sophisticated visualization techniques might be indicated (e.g., computed tomography scan, magnetic resonance imaging, ultrasound).

If D-xylose absorption is abnormal in the presence of steatorrhea, confirmatory tests tor jejunal disease are warranted. The diagnosis of celiac disease and other abnormal-

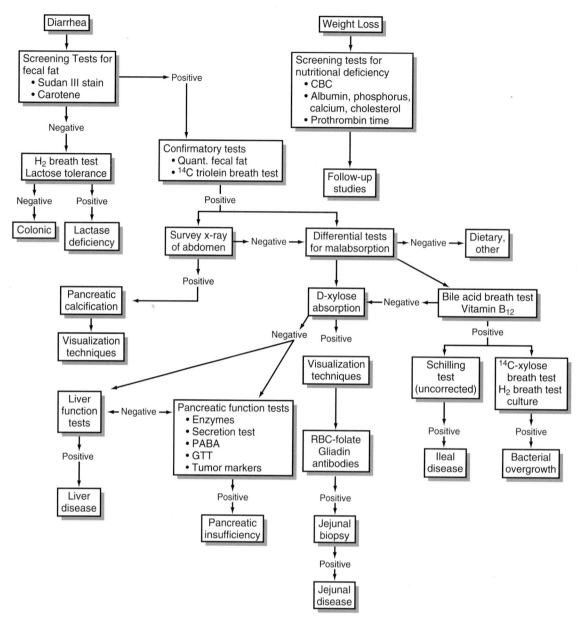

Figure 24–2. Laboratory evaluation of malabsorption. Visualization techniques include angiography, computerized tomography (CT), endoscopic retrograde cholangiopancreatography (ERCP), ultrasound, magnetic resonance imaging (MRI), and radiologic examination of intestine with contrast media. Abbreviations: H_2, hydrogen; PABA, *p*-aminobenzoic acid; GTT, glucose tolerance test; CBC, complete blood count; RBC, red blood cell.

ities of the jejunal mucosa is almost always confirmed by jejunal biopsy. The morphologic examination of the intestinal tissue and histochemical tests for enzymes may be necessary to evaluate the nature and extent of mucosal damage. Radiography with contrast media and other visualization techniques may be required to demonstrate abnormal anatomic features or motility of the small bowel. The only definitive laboratory tests worthy of investigation are red blood cell folate levels and serum levels of gliadin antibodies. Folate deficiency is commonplace in celiac disease and tropical sprue. Laboratory tests for serum antibodies to dietary wheat gluten antigens by enzyme-linked immunosorbent assay (ELISA) techniques[48] and fluorescent immunosorbent techniques[49] are highly sensitive and specific for adult and childhood celiac disease. Gliadin anti-

body titers can be used to screen for celiac disease, which must then be confirmed by biopsy. The titers are also a valuable adjunct in the follow-up of celiac disease, particularly in monitoring the clinical response to a gluten-free diet.

Ileal disease may be evaluated with tests for vitamin B_{12} and bile salts, because the ileum is the only small bowel segment capable of absorbing both substances. The test of choice is the bile acid breath test, in which radiolabeled ^{14}C-glycocholic acid is administered orally. If the terminal ileum is diseased, the unabsorbed glycocholate passes into the colon, where bacteria hydrolyze it to deconjugated bile salt and glycine. The ^{14}C-glycine is absorbed and metabolized to $^{14}CO_2$, which is measured in expired air as in the ^{14}C-triolein breath test for fat absorption. Positive results are also observed in bacterial overgrowth syndrome. The Schilling test for vitamin B_{12} absorption is the next best test for ileal dysfunction. Radioactive B_{12} is given orally with and without intrinsic factor, pancreatic enzyme extract, and antibiotics. B_{12} is normally absorbed and excreted in the urine. Low urinary B_{12} excretion implies one of four conditions, which are then differentiated by administering each of the substances previously listed to test for correction of the abnormal urine levels. Correction with intrinsic factor indicates pernicious anemia; correction with pancreatic extract suggests pancreatic insufficiency; correction with tetracycline for several days before the next B_{12} dose points to bacterial overgrowth (bacteria metabolize the B_{12}). If B_{12} absorption is not corrected by any of these substances, the patient has damaged ileal receptors or has undergone an ileal resection. Biopsy and radiography may not be necessary for ileal dysfunction.

Culture of jejunal or duodenal contents is the definitive test for bacterial overgrowth syndrome, although it is not commonly performed. The bacteria are usually anaerobes, and they multiply because of stasis of bowel contents in blind loops. Because the resulting malabsorption syndrome is very similar to that seen with ileal dysfunction, the bile acid breath test is also utilized to detect bacterial overgrowth. This test will not differentiate between the two conditions. A newer and more specific test for bacterial overgrowth is the ^{14}C-xylose breath test. When ^{14}C-xylose is given orally, subsequent measurement of $^{14}CO_2$ in the breath indicates that overgrown flora catabolized xylose to CO_2 prior to absorption.[44] This test is reported to be even more sensitive and specific than intestinal culture.[42] An alternative to laboratory testing may be a therapeutic trial of various antibiotics. The breath hydrogen test (described later) can also be used to assess bacterial overgrowth. A positive result (a combination of high fasting breath hydrogen *and* an abnormal rise in breath hydrogen after glucose) has a sensitivity of 93% and a specificity of 78%.[9, 50]

The diagnosis of lactose malabsorption has traditionally been made with the lactose tolerance test, in which oral lactose is given, and timed blood specimens are measured for glucose to confirm conversion of lactose to glucose by the patient's lactase. Currently, the most reliable and widely used test for lactose malabsorption is the breath hydrogen test.[51] Breath hydrogen testing has repeatedly been demonstrated to be the most accurate indirect indicator of lactase deficiency. Lactase-deficient patients do not absorb an oral dose of lactose, which is metabolized to hydrogen by bacteria in the colon, absorbed into the blood stream, and eliminated in exhaled breath. The breath hydrogen is measured with gas chromatography. Patients may also be tested with a milk-free diet for a specified time. Peroral mucosal biopsy may be indicated to rule out secondary causes of lactose malabsorption. The breath hydrogen test is also useful in screening for several other disaccharidase deficiencies.[52, 53]

TREATMENT[54]

In the general management of malabsorption syndromes, the first steps are treating the two most common symptoms, steatorrhea and diarrhea. Patients with steatorrhea are put on a low-fat diet. Reducing fat intake will most likely reduce steatorrhea, regardless of origin. Complex carbohydrates consumed as replacement calories for fat have less osmotic effect in the intestine. Vitamins and minerals are also important in nutrient replacement in the patient with malabsorption. More aggressive nutrient replacement may be indicated in patients with severe steatorrhea. These patients require fat replacement with short-chain and medium-chain fatty acids, which are absorbed directly into the portal circulation without requiring bile acids for absorption.

Symptomatic treatment includes volume and electrolyte replacement, correction of any acid-base imbalance, and the use of antibiotics and/or antidiarrheal agents, such as opiates, propantheline, cholestyramine, bismuth subsalicylate (Pepto-Bismol), psyllium hydrophilic mucilloid (Metamucil), octreotide, and clonidine. Beyond that the physician must find the underlying cause and treat it to obtain more permanent responsiveness and control of the diarrhea. Usually, maldigestion or malabsorption is associated with chronic diarrhea (>4 weeks), which excludes many infectious and self-limited causes.

The next level of treatment involves targeting the organ system that is causing the malabsorption syndrome. The organs responsible for causing malabsorption are the stomach, liver, pancreas, and the small intestine. Specific causes and treatment for malabsorption involving the stomach, liver, and the pancreas are discussed elsewhere.

Gluten-sensitive enteropathy, or celiac sprue, is treated with a gluten-free diet. Occasionally, patients with celiac sprue may develop refractory sprue or intestinal lymphoma when they show no response to the gluten-free diet. Prednisone may be beneficial in up to half of patients with refractory sprue.

The prevalence of primary lactase deficiency varies from 15% in whites to nearly 90% Asians and blacks. Secondary lactase deficiency can result from mucosal damage due to other processes, such as celiac sprue. The treatment is simply to minimize lactose intake. Over-the-counter lactase replacement preparations are also helpful when lactose-containing foods are consumed.

Regional enteritis, or Crohn's disease, is treated with 5-aminosalicylic acid products, corticosteroids, metronidazole, and immunosuppressant therapy. Cholestyramine, a bile salt–binding drug, may be useful in controlling choleraic diarrhea; however, this drug may exacerbate steatorrhea because of impending bile salt deficiency.

Patients with bacterial growth syndrome respond well to broad-spectrum antibiotics, such as metronidazole and tetracycline, given for 2 weeks.

Whipple's disease can usually be successfully treated with parenteral penicillin and streptomycin for 10 days, followed by a 1-year course of trimethoprim-sulfamethoxazole (Bactrim).

Tropical sprue is thought to be a bacterial-mediated disease and can be treated with tetracycline and folate for up to 6 months.

Patients with short bowel syndrome from massive resection respond well to low-fat diets, antidiarrhea agents, histamine blockers, omeprazole, octreotide, vitamin B_{12}, and, in severe cases, total parenteral nutrition.

Lymphangiectasia results from lymphatics obstruction, and affected patients are treated with a low-fat diet containing medium-chain fatty acids. Also, any underlying disease causing the obstruction, such as tuberculosis, pericarditis, or lymphoma, must be treated.

Finally, abetalipoproteinemia causing fat malabsorption is treated with fat-soluble vitamins and medium-chain triglycerides.

Other secondary causes of malabsorption include diabetes mellitus, intestinal ischemia, and radiation enteritis. They are treated primarily with antidiarrheal agents, as well as treatment of the underlying cause.

Case Study

A thin 35-year-old man was admitted to the hospital with persistent diarrhea. His medical history from childhood revealed intermittent episodes of diarrhea and failure to thrive during the first decade of life. Gradual weight loss over several months was observed. He also reported an increasing sensitivity to milk, which had never previously affected him. He had foul-smelling, bulky stools, and slight edema was observed.

His admission CBC revealed a macrocytic anemia. A vitamin B_{12} assay was normal. A screening test for fecal fat was positive. A chemistry profile revealed below-normal levels of albumin, calcium, phosphorus, and cholesterol. His prothrombin time was prolonged. A breath hydrogen test was elevated. A D-xylose absorption test was then ordered, and showed reduced urinary excretion (19%).

At this point, the presumptive diagnosis of celiac sprue was entertained. To confirm this, a peroral jejunal biopsy and radiography of the small bowel with contrast media were performed. The biopsy showed a subtotal villous atrophy. The x-ray showed thickening of mucosal folds but was otherwise unremarkable. The diagnosis of adult celiac disease was confirmed. The patient was treated symptomatically for the diarrhea and anemia, and was started on a gluten-free diet. Significant improvement with steady weight gain was observed within 6 weeks.

Questions

1. How do you account for an apparent reemergence of sprue in adulthood?

2. What is the most likely explanation for the lactose intolerance?

3. What additional laboratory findings are significant, and what follow-up is recommended?

Discussion

1. It is not uncommon for patients with childhood celiac sprue to have a clinical remission as adolescents and to tolerate gluten ingestion without symptoms until the third decade of life.

2. Secondary lactose intolerance may develop as a result of the chronic irritation and subsequent injury to the brush border.

3. Additional laboratory studies to consider are red blood cell folate and serum gliadin antibodies. Because folate is absorbed by the jejunum, deficiency is common in celiac sprue. Assessment of serum antibodies to wheat gliadin is potentially useful in the follow-up of celiac disease, particularly with the clinical response to a gluten-free diet. Treatment requires lifelong restriction of gluten from the diet.

References

1. Hopfer U: Digestion and absorption of basic nutritional constituents. *In* Devlin TM (ed): Textbook of Biochemistry with Clinical Correlations, ed 3. New York, Wiley-Liss, 1992.

2. Turnberg L, Riley S: Digestion and absorption of nutrients and vitamins. *In* Sleisinger MH, Fordtran JS (eds): Gastrointestinal Disease: Pathophysiology, Diagnosis, Management, ed 5. Philadelphia, WB Saunders 1993.

3. Ravich W, Bayliss T: Carbohydrate absorption and malabsorption. Clin Gastroenterol 12:335–356, 1983.

4. Hamash M, Klaeveman H, Wolf R, et al: Pharyngeal lipase and digestion of dietary triglyceride in man. J Clin Invest 55:908–913, 1975.

5. Borgstrom B: On the interaction between pancreatic lipase and colipase and substrate, and the importance of bile salts. J Lipid Res 16:411–414, 1975.

6. Glickman R: Fat absorption and malabsorption. Clin Gastroenterol 12:323–334, 1983.

7. Newsholme E, Leech A: Biochemistry for the Medical Sciences. New York, John Wiley & Sons, 1983.

8. Henderson A, Tietz N, Rinker A: Gastric, pancreatic and intestinal function. *In* Burtis CA, Ashwood ER (eds): Tietz Textbook of Clinical Chemistry, ed 2. Philadelphia, WB Saunders, 1994.

9. Henderson A, Tietz N, Rinker A: Gastric, pancreatic and intestinal function. *In* Burtis CA, Ashwood ER (eds): Tietz Fundamentals of Clinical Chemistry. ed 4. Philadelphia, WB Saunders, 1996.

10. Ryan M, Olsen W: A diagnostic approach to malabsorption syndromes: A pathophysiological approach. Clin Gastroenterol 12:533–550, 1983.

11. Romano T, Dobbins J: Evaluation of the patient with suspected malabsorption. Gastroenterol Clin North Am 18:467–483, 1989.

12. Riley S, Turnberg L: Maldigestion and malabsorption. *In* Sleisinger MH, Fordtran JS (eds): Gastrointestinal Disease: Pathophysiology, Diagnosis, Management, ed 5. Philadelphia, WB Saunders, 1993.

13. Kornbluth A, Salomom P, Sachar D: Crohn's disease. *In* Sleisinger MH, Fordtran JS (eds): Gastrointestinal Disease: Pathophysiology, Diagnosis, Management, ed 5. Philadelphia, WB Saunders, 1993.

14. King C, Toskes P: Small intestine bacterial overgrowth. Gastroenterology 76:1035–1055, 1979.

15. Rossi E, Lentze M: Clinical significance of enzymatic deficiencies in the gastrointestinal tract with particular reference to lactase deficiency. Ann Allergy 53:649–656, 1984.

16. Gray D: Short bowel syndrome. Am Fam Physician 30:227–323, 1984.

17. Morris J, Selwanov V, Sheldon G: Nutritional management of patients with malabsorption syndrome. Clin Gastroenterol 12:463–474, 1983.

18. Weser E: Nutritional aspects of malabsorption: Short gut adaptation. Clin Gastroenterol 12:443–461, 1983.

19. Tyor M: Whipple's disease. The Duke Connection. N C Med J 55:237–240, 1994.

20. Jewell D: Ulcerative colitis. *In* Sleisenger M, Fordtran J (eds): Gastrointestinal Disease: Pathophysiology, Diagnosis, Management, ed 5. Philadelphia, WB Saunders, 1993.

21. Doe W, Hapel A: Intestinal immunity and malabsorption. Clin Gastroenterol 12:415–435, 1983.

22. Marsh M: Gluten, major histocompatibility complex, and the small intestine: A molecular and immunobiologic approach to the spectrum of gluten sensitivity (celiac sprue). Gastroenterology 102:330–354, 1992.

23. Trier J: Celiac sprue. *In* Sleisenger M, Fordtran J (eds): Gastrointestinal Disease: Pathophysiology, Diagnosis, Management, ed 5. Philadelphia, WB Saunders, 1993.

24. Misra S, Ament M: Diagnosis of coeliac sprue in 1994. Gastroenterol Clin North Am 24:133–143, 1995.

25. Michalski J, McCombs C: Celiac disease: Clinical features and pathogenesis. Am J Med Sci 307:204–211, 1994.
26. Cole S, Kognoff M: Celiac Disease. Ann Rev Nutr 5:241–266, 1985.
27. Falchuk Z: Gluten-sensitive enteropathy. Clin Gastroenterol 12:475–493, 1983.
28. Ferguson A, Ziegler K, Strobel S: Gluten intolerance (coeliac disease) Ann Allergy 53:637–642, 1984.
29. Tomkins A: Tropical malabsorption: Recent concepts in pathogenesis and nutritional significance. Clin Sci 60:131–187, 1981.
30. Klipstein F: Tropical sprue. *In* Sleisenger M, Fordtran J (eds): Gastrointestinal Disease: Pathophysiology, Diagnosis, Management, ed 5. Philadelphia, WB Saunders, 1993.
31. Holmes R, Lobley R: Intestinal brush border revisited. Gut 30:1667–1678, 1989.
32. Flatz G: The genetic polymorphism of intestinal lactase activity in adult humans. *In* Scriver CR, Beaudet AL, Sly WS, Valle D (eds): The Metabolic Basis of Inherited Disease, ed 6. New York, McGraw-Hill, 1989.
33. Semenza G, Auricchio S: Small intestinal disaccharidases. *In* Scriver CR, Beaudet AL, Sly WS, Valle D (eds): The Metabolic Basis of Inherited Disease, ed 6. New York, McGraw-Hill, 1989.
34. Freeman H, Sleisenger M, Kim Y: Human protein digestion and absorption. Clin Gastroenterol 12:357–378, 1983.
35. Cerda J, Artnak E: Nutritional aspects of malabsorption syndromes. Compr Ther 9:35–46, 1983.
36. Gallagher N: Importance of vitamin B_{12} and folate metabolism in malabsorption. Clin Gastroenterol 12:437–441, 1983.
37. Gueant J, Champigneule B, Gaucher P, Nicolas J: Malabsorption of vitamin B_{12} in pancreatic insufficiency of the adult and of the child. Pancreas 5:559–567, 1990.
38. Fine K, Guenter J, Fordtran J: Diarrhea. *In* Sleisenger M, Fordtran J (eds): Gastrointestinal Disease: Pathophysiology, Diagnosis, Management, ed 5. Philadelphia, WB Saunders, 1993.
39. Cerda J, Dobbins W, Rider J: Simplifying diagnosis of malabsorption. Patient Care 15:128–178, 1981.
40. Theodozzi A, Gazzard B: Have chemical tests a role in diagnosing malabsorption? Am Clin Biochem 21:153–165, 1984.
41. Goldberg D, Durie P: Biochemical tests in the diagnosis of chronic pancreatitis and in the evaluation of pancreatic insufficiency. Clin Biochem 26:253–275, 1993.
42. Tietz N (ed): Clinical Guide to Laboratory Tests, ed 3. Philadelphia, WB Saunders, 1995.
43. King C, Toskes P: The use of breath tests in the study of malabsorption. Clin Gastroenterol 12:591–610, 1983.
44. West P, Levin G, Griffen G, et al: Comparison of simple screening tests for fat malabsorption. Br Med J 282:1501–1504, 1981.
45. Vantrappen G, Ghoos Y, Andriulli A: CO_2 and H_2 breath tests in the diagnosis of intestinal malabsorption. Ital J Gastroenterol 24:212–217, 1992.
46. Newcomer A, Hofmann A, DeMagno E: Triolein breath test: A sensitive and specific test for fat malabsorption. Gastroenterology 76:6–13, 1979.
47. Craig R, Atkinson A: D-Xylose testing: A review. Gastroenterology 95:223–231, 1988.
48. Scott H, Fausa O, Ek J, Brandtzaeg P: Immune response patterns in coeliac disease: Serum antibodies to dietary antigens measured by an enzyme linked immunosorbent assay (ELISA). Clin Exp Immunol 57:25–32, 1984.
49. Burgin-Wolff A, Bertele R, Berger R, et el: A reliable screening test for childhood celiac disease: Fluorescent immunosorbent test for gliadin antibodies. J Pediatr 102:655–660, 1983.
50. Kerlin P, Wong L: Breath hydrogen testing in bacterial overgrowth of the small intestine. Gastroenterology 95:982–988, 1988.
51. Rosado J, Solomons N: Sensitivity and specificity of the hydrogen breath-analysis test for detecting malabsorption of physiological doses of lactose. Clin Chem 29:545–548, 1983.
52. Newcomer A: Screening tests for carbohydrate malabsorption. J Pediatr Gastroenterol 3:6–8, 1984.
53. Perman J: Clinical application of breath hydrogen measurements. Can J Physiol Pharmacol 69:111–115, 1991.
54. Uhl M, Cooke A: Malabsorption syndromes. *In* Snape W(ed): Consultations in Gastroenterology. Philadelphia, WB Saunders, 1996.

Bibliography

Jeejeebhoy K: Gastrointestinal Diseases: Focus on Clinical Diagnosis, ed 2. New Hyde Park, NY, Medical Examination Publishing, 1985.
Yamada T: Textbook of Gastroenterology, ed 2. Philadelphia, JB Lippincott, 1995.
Haubrich W, Schafner F, Berk J: Bockus Gastroenterology, ed 5, vol 1. Philadelphia, WB Saunders, 1995.
Bayliss T: Current Therapy in Gastroenterology and Liver Disease, ed 4. St Louis, Mosby–Year Book, 1994.
Nurse's Clinical Library: Gastrointestinal Disorders. Springhouse, PA, Springhouse Corp, 1985.

Chapter 25

Liver Disease: Jaundice, Cirrhosis

Lynn Ingram

Etiology and Pathophysiology
    Prehepatic Jaundice
    Hepatic Jaundice
    Posthepatic Jaundice
    Other Causes of Jaundice
Clinical Manifestations
Laboratory Analyses and Diagnosis
Treatment
Case Studies

Jaundice is a yellow pigmentation of the tissues most often caused by an increase in the level of bilirubin in the serum. Jaundice is a symptom, not a disease in itself. The first evidence of clinical jaundice may be seen in the sclera, as this tissue has a special affinity for bilirubin. Concentrations of bilirubin above 3 mg/dL will cause the skin to take on a yellow color.

The clinical finding of jaundice can indicate several different diseases. A careful medical history, including family history, and data from various laboratory tests assist in identifying the cause of jaundice.

ETIOLOGY AND PATHOPHYSIOLOGY

The high levels of serum bilirubin that lead to jaundice occur by mechanisms that are classified as prehepatic, hepatic, and posthepatic.

Prehepatic Jaundice

Prehepatic jaundice results from an increased breakdown of hemoglobin in the absence of active liver disease.

The increased breakdown of hemoglobin to bilirubin may occur because of increased hemolysis of erythrocytes or because of ineffective hematopoiesis. Hemolysis may occur because of an abnormality within the red blood cell, such as a vitamin B_{12} or folic acid deficiency; a defective cell membrane; an enzyme deficiency, such as the lack of glucose-6-phosphate dehydrogenase (G6PD); or a hemoglobinopathy. Hemolysis may also occur due to chemical agents, disease states such as cancer, or because of antibodies or drugs coating the red blood cells. Trauma, surgery, multiple blood transfusions, and red cell destruction due to artificial heart valves can also cause an overproduction of bilirubin that a healthy liver cannot metabolize adequately. Hemolytic disease of the newborn is hemolytic anemia due to maternal antibodies coating fetal red cells, causing lysis. Danger to the neonate occurs when bilirubin levels exceed 20 mg/dL, causing *kernicterus*, or bilirubin encephalopathy, and brain damage. Box 25–1 lists various causes of prehepatic jaundice.

The major laboratory test abnormality in patients with prehepatic jaundice is an increased total bilirubin level, with the greatest part being unconjugated. All other liver function tests remain normal.

Hepatic Jaundice

Hepatic or hepatocellular jaundice develops because of an abnormality in liver function. Hepatocellular jaundice can be further classified as the result of diffuse hepatocellular failure, conjugation failure, or bilirubin transport problems. The latter two types refer, respectively, to the inability of the liver to conjugate bilirubin for excretion and to a problem with the transport of the conjugated bilirubin from the liver to the intestine. Box 25–2 lists various causes of hepatic jaundice.

229

Box 25–1. Causes of Prehepatic Jaundice

Hereditary Hemolytic Processes

Hereditary spherocytosis
G6PD deficiency
Sickle cell disease
Thalassemia
Hemoglobin C disease

Acquired Hemolytic Processes

Hemolytic disease of the newborn
Hemolytic transfusion reactions
Drug-induced hemolytic anemia
Autoimmune hemolytic anemia
Paroxysmal nocturnal hemoglobinuria

Ineffective Erythropoiesis

Megaloblastic anemia
Sideroblastic anemia
Erythroleukemia
Lead poisoning

Physiologic Jaundice of the Newborn

Prematurity

Impaired Delivery of Bilirubin to the Liver

Congestive heart failure

From Anderson SC, Cockayne S: Clinical Chemistry: Concepts and Applications. Philadelphia, WB Saunders, 1993, p 295. Reprinted with permission.

Two hepatocellular diseases causing jaundice are hepatitis and cirrhosis. Hepatitis is characterized by necrosis and inflammation of hepatic cells, regardless of its etiology. Because excretion of conjugated bilirubin by these injured cells is impaired, it reenters the systemic circulation, eventually causing jaundice. Unconjugated bilirubin concentrations may also increase, due to both impaired uptake and impaired conjugation of bilirubin. Viral hepatitis is a common cause of jaundice (see Chapter 26). Cirrhosis is a chronic liver disease characterized by diffuse liver cell destruction with fibrosis and nodular regeneration of liver cells. Because of progressive loss of liver cells, both conjugated and unconjugated bilirubin levels increase, with the conjugated bilirubin fraction dominating.

Among the important functions of the liver is the transformation of bilirubin into a water-soluble substance, bilirubin diglucuronide, by the enzyme uridine diphosphoglucuronyl transferase (UDPGT). Only this form of bilirubin can be excreted by the kidney. Crigler-Najjar syndrome is a rare, inherited disorder affecting the enzyme UDPGT. The more severe form is type I Crigler-Najjar syndrome, involving the complete absence of the enzyme, which usually results in death of an affected child by the age of 18 months. Type II Crigler-Najjar syndrome is a less severe disorder and involves reduced levels of the enzyme. Patients with this disease rarely develop kernicterus and live

to adulthood, although they are usually moderately jaundiced.[1] Both forms of Crigler-Najjar syndrome involve an elevation of bilirubin—primarily, unconjugated bilirubin.

Several diseases involving jaundice are caused by the inability of the liver to properly transport conjugated or unconjugated bilirubin within or from the liver. They are inherited chronic diseases and include Gilbert's syndrome, Dubin-Johnson syndrome, and Rotor's syndrome.

Gilbert's syndrome is a mild, chronic, unconjugated hyperbilirubinemia found in patients who do not have structural liver disease or overt hemolysis. It is an inherited disorder found in approximately 7% of the population and occurs predominantly in males.[1] It is usually detected in adolescence coincidentally with other diseases or incidentally associated with stressful conditions such as surgery or trauma. It results from impaired ability of the liver to excrete bilirubin and a 20% to 50% decrease in the enzyme UDPGT.[2] A distinctive diagnostic feature of Gilbert's syndrome is that bilirubin levels rise after prolonged fasting or calorie deprivation.[1]

Dubin-Johnson syndrome is a benign hyperbilirubinemia characterized by dark pigmentation in the liver cells, and it is inherited as an autosomal recessive trait. The uptake, processing, and storage of bilirubin by the liver is normal, and only the action of removal of bilirubin from the hepatocyte and its excretion into bile is defective.[2] Because this condition is an obstructive liver disease, much of the conjugated bilirubin circulates as δ-bilirubin, or conjugated bilirubin bound to albumin. The gallbladder or other parts of the biliary tract are not usually visualized with x-ray studies in this syndrome. The patient has few, if any, symptoms, but laboratory results are significantly more abnormal in

Box 25–2. Causes of Hepatic Jaundice

Retention Jaundice

Physiologic jaundice of the newborn
Gilbert's syndrome
Crigler-Najjar syndrome; types I and II

Regurgitation Jaundice

Dubin-Johnson syndrome
Rotor's syndrome
Recurrent benign intrahepatic cholestasis
Cholestatic jaundice of pregnancy
Cirrhosis
Viral hepatitis
Alcoholic liver disease
Drug-induced liver disease
Primary biliary cirrhosis
Postoperative jaundice
Hepatocellular carcinoma
Toxic liver injury
Autoimmune liver disease
Inborn errors of metabolism

From Anderson SC, Cockayne S: Clinical Chemistry: Concepts and Applications. Philadelphia, WB Saunders, 1993, p 296. Reprinted with permission.

patients using anabolic steroids, women using oral contraceptives, and pregnant women, due to the increased excretory load on the liver.

Rotor's syndrome is very similar to Dubin-Johnson syndrome in that it is a chronic, conjugated hyperbilirubinemia without evidence of hemolysis. The major distinction between the two syndromes is that a liver biopsy from patients with Rotor's syndrome fails to exhibit the dark pigment found in patients with Dubin-Johnson syndrome. Jaundice may increase when the patients develop an infection. Unlike Dubin-Johnson syndrome, with Rotor's syndrome the gallbladder can be visualized during x-ray studies in patients.[3]

Approximately 50% of full-term newborns become jaundiced in the first week of life. Unconjugated bilirubin concentrations usually peak between the third and fifth day of life and diminish over a period of several weeks to adult bilirubin concentrations.[4] This type of jaundice in the neonate has been termed *physiologic jaundice of the newborn* and occurs because the production of the enzyme UDPGT is often not fully developed at birth. A complicating factor in neonates is the increased hemolysis of red blood cells caused by the birth process, adding an additional bilirubin load for conjugation by an immature liver. Affected infants develop a rapid buildup of unconjugated bilirubin levels that can pass into the brain and nerve cells and result in kernicterus if serum levels become sufficiently high. Most newborn's bilirubin concentrations return to a safe range within a few days, as the liver stimulates the production of the required conjugating enzyme. Bilirubin concentrations performed on heel-stick specimens are used to monitor the course of physiologic jaundice and to assure the clinician that normal bilirubin metabolism is developing.

Cirrhosis is another common cause of hepatic jaundice. It is believed that diffuse liver cell death is the precursor of cirrhosis, a condition in which there is extensive, permanent structural damage to the liver. Morphologically, cirrhosis presents with two features; increased fibrous tissue and nodular regeneration.[3]

Although alcoholic cirrhosis is the most common, there are many causes of cirrhosis in North America (Box 25–3). Consumption of a pint or more of whiskey (or its equivalent) per day for at least 10 years results in cirrhosis. The effects on the liver include uniform liver cell loss, small islands of regenerating or preserved parenchyma, and diffuse, fine scarring.[5] Ethanol is metabolized to acetaldehyde by the enzyme alcohol dehydrogenase. Acetaldehyde is a highly reactive substance that interferes with cell function and cell wall integrity. A patient with alcoholic cirrhosis may be totally asymptomatic, but many exhibit nonspecific symptoms, including weight loss, weakness, jaundice, ascites, malnutrition, edema, hepatomegaly, and splenomegaly. A definite diagnosis of alcoholic cirrhosis can be made only by liver biopsy. The patient with alcoholic cirrhosis has at least a 30% risk of developing hepatocellular carcinoma.[6]

Postnecrotic cirrhosis is the most common type of cirrhosis worldwide. The cause is unknown, but viral hepatitis is a precursor in many cases. The pathology of the disease includes irregular, large nodules of regenerating hepatocytes that vary in size from microscopic to visible; exten-

---

Box 25–3. Causes of Cirrhosis

Chronic Hepatitis

Chronic hepatitis B, C, D
Autoimmune chronic active hepatitis
Chronic drug-induced hepatitis

Ethanol

Metabolic Causes

Hemochromatosis
Wilson's disease
α_1-Antitrypsin deficiency
Tyrosinemia
Galactosemia
Diabetes mellitus
Glycogen storage disease

Diseases of Prolonged Cholestasis

Primary biliary cirrhosis
Primary sclerosing cholangitis
Biliary atresia
Chronic bile duct obstruction
Cystic fibrosis
Hyperalimentation-induced cholestasis

Toxic Exposure

Carbon tetrachloride
Hypervitaminosis A
Methotrexate

Vascular/Congestive

Budd-Chiari syndrome
Veno-occlusive disease
    Idiopathic
    Drug-induced
    Toxin-induced
    Ethanol?
Cardiac cirrhosis

Miscellaneous

Jejunoileal bypass-induced liver disease
Indian childhood cirrhosis
Cryptogenic

From Gitnick, G: Diseases of the Liver and Biliary Tract. St Louis, Mosby–Year Book, 1992, p 448. Reprinted with permission.

---

sive liver cell loss; and stromal collapse and fibrosis, which produce broad bands of connective tissue.[6]

The etiology is also unknown for a third major kind of cirrhosis: primary biliary cirrhosis. Primary biliary cirrhosis is a chronic, progressive, obstructive liver disease characterized by destruction of intrahepatic bile ducts, the presence of inflammation and scarring, and the eventual development of cirrhosis.[2] Because 90% of the cases occur in middle-aged women, it is believed that the cause may have an endocrine origin, but evidence also indicates that viral destruction of the liver or drug hypersensitivity initiates the disease. Primary biliary cirrhosis often occurs in the presence of some immunologic abnormality. About 80% of patients with biliary cirrhosis exhibit elevated immunoglobulin M (IgM) serum levels, and more than 95% of patients exhibit a circulating immunoglobulin G (IgG) mitochondrial antibody.

A type of biliary cirrhosis also occurs that is secondary to an obstruction of the bile duct or its major branches. Gallstones, tumors, or postoperative strictures may cause the obstruction. Whatever the cause of biliary cirrhosis, however, the disease is characterized by inflammation, impaired bile excretion, progressive destruction of the intrahepatic bile ducts, and fibrosis.[5]

Hemochromatosis, Wilson's disease, and α_1-antitrypsin deficiencies can also cause hepatic cirrhosis, although by completely different processes. Hemochromatosis is a condition in which there is excessive deposition of iron in many organs, including the liver. It can be a result of an inherited condition, whereby an inappropriately high concentration of iron is absorbed, or because of abnormal or ineffective erythropoiesis, leading to excessive iron metabolism. The liver is the major recipient of the excess iron, and after several years of high tissue iron levels, fibrosis and, eventually, cirrhosis develop.[7] *Wilson's disease*, or progressive lenticular degeneration, is the result of excessive accumulation of copper. It is a familial condition and can result in both hepatic and neurologic symptoms that are direct results of copper toxicity. The primary defect appears to be an increased absorption of copper from the gastrointestinal tract and decreased copper excretion. Hereditary deficiency of the serum protease inhibitor α_1-antitrypsin is associated with both hepatic cirrhosis and pulmonary emphysema. α_1-Antitrypsin inhibits the action of trypsin and other hydrolytic enzymes. Without its preventive activity, hydrolytic damage occurs to many organs, most frequently the lungs and liver.

Posthepatic Jaundice

Posthepatic jaundice is not the result of liver disease but rather of an obstruction blocking the flow of bile from a normally functioning organ. The obstruction can be caused by gallstones in the common bile duct, a severe stricture, or tumor. *Extrahepatic bile duct atresia* is a condition defined as the lack of a lumen in part or all of the extrahepatic bile ducts, causing a complete obstruction of the flow of bile from the liver. Continuing controversy exists over whether the etiology and pathogenesis are developmental or viral in origin.[8] Whatever the cause, the condition is a progressive inflammatory lesion of the bile ducts that often leads to death in affected infants by the age of 2 years. Various causes of posthepatic jaundice are listed in Box 25–4.

The most common obstructive jaundice occurs when gallstones block the flow of bile in the common bile duct. Stones usually form in the gallbladder but cause blockage if they drop into the common bile duct. Gallstones may be present for years without causing symptoms.

A stricture in the extrahepatic bile ducts can be caused by trauma during abdominal surgery or by a congenital defect causing complete or partial blockage. Jaundice may appear early or may be delayed for several months or

---

Box 25–4.	**Causes of Posthepatic Jaundice**

Common bile duct stone
Cancer of the bile ducts, pancreas, ampulla of Vater
Bile duct stricture or stenosis
Sclerosing cholangitis
Choledochal cysts
Biliary atresia in infants

From Anderson SC, Cockayne S: Clinical Chemistry: Concepts and Applications. Philadelphia, WB Saunders, 1993, p 297. Reprinted with permission.

---

years. Cancerous obstructions of the extrahepatic bile ducts are also causes of posthepatic jaundice.

Other Causes of Jaundice

Jaundice that occurs during pregnancy is rare and can be caused by any of the processes described earlier or by specific conditions resulting from the pregnancy. One such condition is intrahepatic cholestasis of pregnancy. Although very uncomfortable, it is generally not serious. The actual cause of this condition is not known, but it may be related to a patient's unusual response to estrogen.[9]

Acute fatty metamorphosis is a second type of jaundice of pregnancy. It is a much more serious disease and most often occurs in a first pregnancy. The condition is often difficult to differentiate from acute viral hepatitis. Mortality rates for the mother and baby are high, and about half of all patients with this condition develop renal failure. Premature labor is common, often with the delivery of a stillborn child.

Other causes of jaundice of pregnancy include megaloblastic anemia (vitamin B_{12} deficiency), hyperemesis gravidarum (excessive vomiting during pregnancy), and pregnancy-induced hypertension. It is important to keep in mind when evaluating jaundice in pregnant women that the cause may not be related to the pregnancy.

Jaundice is a fairly common symptom after surgery and can be due to a variety of causes. The use of anesthesia, especially halothane anesthesia, is known to affect liver function in some patients. Patients who have undergone a cholecystectomy may become jaundiced because of a stone remaining in the common bile duct or a stricture in the duct, requiring additional surgery. It is also possible for the surgeon to accidentally cut the common bile duct during abdominal surgery, resulting in jaundice. A number of drugs often given to postoperative patients are hepatotoxic. Certain antibiotics, phenothiazines, and anabolic steroids are among the drugs known to cause jaundice. Because stored blood may contain older red blood cells, which are more likely to hemolyze and cause an increased bilirubin load, surgical patients who have received several units of blood may also become jaundiced. When large amounts of blood are lost into tissues during surgery, resorption from the extravascular spaces may cause postoperative elevations of conjugated bilirubin up to 20 to 40 mg/dL.[10] This is generally a self-limited condition if recovery from the surgery progresses well.

CLINICAL MANIFESTATIONS

The clinical manifestations of diseases associated with jaundice are varied and nonspecific but include malaise, pruritus, weight loss, fever and/or chills, right upper quadrant pain, anorexia, nausea, arthralgia, rash, bleeding and bruising, hepatomegaly, splenomegaly, dark urine, pale stools, edema, or ascites.

Most of the clinical manifestations of cirrhosis are common to all types. Jaundice, fluid accumulation in the peritoneal cavity (ascites), central nervous system dysfunction, and increased interstitial fluid volume (edema) are common. Additionally, the fibrosis results in distorted intrahepatic vasculature, which causes portal venous hypertension with splenomegaly and esophageal and gastric varices. The shape of the liver may also become distorted, and the intrahepatic venous and lymphatic radicals may become compressed, contributing to the ascites and portal hypertension.[5]

There are, however, some differentiating clinical features among the types of cirrhosis. In addition to the symptoms of fluid retention, portal hypertension, and liver dysfunction, an individual with alcoholic cirrhosis may experience weakness, fatigue, anorexia, and weight loss. The liver may be firm and enlarged, and muscle wasting, gynecomastia, and testicular atrophy or amenorrhea may also be present. These features are generally secondary to the large intake of ethanol.

Postnecrotic cirrhosis presents somewhat differently than alcoholic cirrhosis. The clinical manifestations are the result of the initial disease process causing the cirrhosis. Usual symptoms are related to portal hypertension, ascites, splenomegaly, encephalopathy, and bleeding esophageal varices.[5]

Some of the clinical signs of biliary cirrhosis are different than the signs for alcoholic or postnecrotic cirrhosis. A patient with biliary cirrhosis, typically female, may complain of itching, jaundice, pale stools, and dark urine. Steatorrhea, diarrhea, osteomalacia, backache, bone pain, and yellowish plaques or nodules (xanthomas) in the subcutaneous tissues that result from lipid deposits may also be present.

Clinical symptoms of hemochromatosis begin with an iron overload of 24 to 50 g and typically become apparent at about 50 years of age. These symptoms are weakness, abdominal pain, hepatomegaly, splenomegaly, edema, ascites, loss of libido or potency in men, and jaundice. Overt diabetes or mild glucose intolerance may also be present. Wilson's disease begins with mild symptoms and progresses to malaise, fatigue, anorexia, jaundice, hepatomegaly, splenomegaly, portal hypertension, ascites, and, eventually, hepatic failure. Neurologic symptoms of Wilson's disease are frequently found, and the presence of Kayser-Fleischer rings in the patient's cornea is a strong indication of the disease. Other neurologic symptoms include lack of coordination, clumsiness, tremors, dysarthria, excessive salivation, dysphagia, and deteriorating academic performance. Psychiatric problems such as aggressive behavior, psychoneurosis, manic-depressive or schizophrenic psychosis, and dementia are also common. All symptoms seen in patients with Wilson's disease are the result of deposition of copper in the liver, cerebrum, and nervous tissue. Patients with α_1-antitrypsin deficiencies demonstrate cholestatic jaundice and pulmonary symptoms early in life.

Posthepatic jaundice, particularly if it is due to gallstones, can be associated with acute attacks often involving nausea, vomiting, fever, right upper quadrant guarding, and severe pain. Symptoms may follow a heavy, fatty meal. Bilirubinuria may also be present within 24 hours of acute pain. Patients often present with a markedly elevated bilirubin concentration and jaundice. They may have an enlarged liver and a palpable gallbladder, and the stools are usually pale. Chills and fever may accompany the jaundice. A newborn with extrahepatic bile duct atresia exhibits deep jaundice, beyond the time expected in physiologic jaundice of the newborn, pale stools, and hepatomegaly.

Symptoms of intrahepatic cholestasis of pregnancy are mild, except for severe pruritis. In acute fatty metamorphosis, however, patients are often overweight, have a bloated face, and often have pregnancy-induced hypertension. Symptoms occur after the 30th week of gestation and include severe and persistent vomiting, abdominal pain, and headache. Tachycardia is present without fever, and jaundice develops within a few days.

LABORATORY ANALYSES AND DIAGNOSIS

The determination of the concentrations of conjugated and total serum bilirubin, urine urobilinogen, and urine bilirubin is necessary to identify the type of jaundice. In addition, a routine blood smear will be helpful in evaluating a prehepatic jaundice. Morphologic evidence, including the presence of spherocytes, target cells, schistocytes, and moderate anisocytosis, serves to identify the jaundice as hemolytic in nature. Special procedures, such as the direct antiglobulin test, G6PD assay, osmotic fragility test, and reticulocyte count, can also be helpful. In prehepatic jaundice serum bilirubin levels are usually lower than 10 mg/dL, with the unconjugated fraction predominating.

In addition to bilirubin levels, other analytes may aid the evaluation of liver function. These include alkaline phosphatase (ALP), alanine aminotransferase (ALT), aspartate aminotransferase (AST), γ-glutamyltransferase (GGT), albumin, and 5'-nucleotidase (5'-NT). Expected results of these tests related to jaundiced states can be seen in Table 25–1.

Patients with type I Crigler-Najjar syndrome have no bilirubin in their urine, have normal colored stools with a decrease in fecal urobilinogen, and show no evidence of hemolysis. Unconjugated bilirubin levels range from 20 to 45 mg/dL. Patients with type II Crigler-Najjar syndrome may be free of jaundice until adolescence, when unconjugated bilirubin levels rise to 6 to 18 mg/dL. Patients with type II Crigler-Najjar have few neurologic complications and a moderate decrease in fecal urobilinogen.

Patients with the Dubin-Johnson and Rotor's syndromes are often indistinguishable and usually have a normal complete blood cell count (CBC) and prothrombin time and normal levels of albumin, cholesterol, AST, ALT, and ALP. Serum bilirubin levels are most often between 2.0 and 5.0 mg/dL, but they are occasionally increased to 20 to 25 mg/dL. Fifty percent or more of the bilirubin is conjugated, and bilirubin is also present in the urine.

Table 25–1. Expected Laboratory Results in Conditions Accompanied by Jaundice

Liver Function Test	Condition			
	Prehepatic	*Acute Hepatocellular*	*Chronic Hepatocellular*	*Posthepatic*
Total bilirubin	Normal to increased	Increased	Increased	Increased
Conjugated bilirubin	Normal to increased	Increased	Increased	Increased
Unconjugated bilirubin	Increased	Increased	Increased	Increased
Urine urobilinogen	Increased	Increased	Increased	Decreased
Urine bilirubin	Normal	Increased	Increased	Increased
Albumin	Normal	Normal	Decreased	Normal
Globulin	Normal	Normal	Increased	Normal
Aminotransferases	Normal	Increased AST and ALT	Increased AST and ALT	Normal to slight increase in AST and ALT
Alkaline phosphatase	Normal	Normal to 3× ULN	Normal to 3× ULN	Increased to 10× ULN
Lactate dehydrogenase	Increased when hemolysis is present	Increased	Increased	Normal
BSP dye test	Normal	Increased	Increased	Increased
Prothrombin time	Normal	Normal	Prolonged	Normal

Abbreviations: AST, aspartate transaminase; ALT, alanine aminotransferase; BSP, bromsulphalein; ULN, upper limits of normal.
From Anderson SC, Cockayne S: Clinical Chemistry: Concepts and Applications. Philadelphia, WB Saunders, 1993, p 296. Reprinted with permission.

In posthepatic jaundice, serum bilirubin levels rise as high as 15 to 25 mg/dL, but vary greatly with the degree of blockage. Patients usually have pale stools, no urine urobilinogen, a normal AST level, and an elevated ALP level. Bilirubin elevations are predominantly of the conjugated type.

Laboratory results must be interpreted carefully in the jaundiced pregnant patient. The most valuable laboratory tests to use include AST, ALT, prothrombin time, GGT, and lactate dehydrogenase (LD) isoenzyme measurements. These concentrations remain normal in patients with uncomplicated pregnancies but are elevated in patients with liver disease. Serum ALP levels are not very useful because they rise slowly in the first half of pregnancy and then sharply during the seventh month, peaking at term. This elevation has been shown to be caused by the placental isoenzyme of ALP. Laboratory features of acute fatty metamorphosis include white blood cell (WBC) counts elevated up to 46.0 × 10⁹/L, and bilirubin levels ranging from 2 to 36 mg/dL. Coagulation disorders and hypoglycemia are common. AST and ALP levels are elevated, and renal function tests such as blood urea nitrogen (BUN) and creatinine show elevated levels as well. Women who survive the disease show complete recovery of liver function after delivery.[9]

The most definitive means of diagnosing cirrhosis is a liver biopsy. Abnormalities in analytes that are useful in diagnosing alcoholic cirrhosis are summarized in Table 25–2. Because analyte level is to some degree reflective of the degree of liver function impairment, some variation may be seen in analyte increases, depending on the course and extent of the disease process. For example, cholestasis, a lack of flow of bile from the liver cells into the common bile duct, is responsible for transient increases in bilirubin, GGT, and ALP levels. Increases in AST, ALT, and LD levels are transient with liver cell injury, and metabolic abnormalities are the reasons for changes in levels of albumin, globulin, and cholesterol, and prothrombin time. Anemia is usually caused by folic acid deficiency, gastroin-

testinal blood loss, or toxic effects of alcohol on bone marrow, and may be accompanied by thrombocytopenia and leukopenia.

The results of laboratory tests in postnecrotic cirrhosis resemble those of alcoholic cirrhosis. The increase in bilirubin, however, is usually higher, and increases in AST and ALT levels are usually more persistent.

In primary biliary cirrhosis, serum ALP concentration is the earliest abnormal result, with an elevation of 2 to 5 times the reference range. The bilirubin, AST, and ALT levels are initially only slightly elevated. Later in the disease the levels of bilirubin increase further, but AST and ALT remain only slightly elevated. A laboratory finding unique to primary biliary cirrhosis is the presence of specific antibodies in the serum. They may be anti–smooth muscle antibodies, antimitochondrial antibodies, antinuclear antibodies, or antibodies directed against one or more liver antigens. One or more of these antibodies are present in 80% to 95% of persons with biliary cirrhosis, if the cirrhosis is not secondary to obstruction of the bile ducts.

In addition to the laboratory results already discussed, other abnormal results may occur in certain types of cirrhosis. In alcoholic cirrhosis, respiratory alkalosis, resulting from an increased depth of breathing, may be observed and magnesium levels, because of dietary deficiencies and urine loss, may be decreased. Ascites and edema may result in decreased sodium and potassium concentrations. Impaired liver function also results in elevated levels of ammonia in the blood. Through successful treatment the physician may note improvement in these analyte levels, but permanent damage to the liver may still result.

Serum bile salts are increased in biliary cirrhosis and a unique low-density lipoprotein, called *lipoprotein X*, containing 65% lecithin, 30% cholesterol, and 5% protein, is present. The presence of this atypical lipoprotein is a strong indication of an obstructive process. Another finding is an increased level of serum bile salts. Serum copper levels are elevated in primary biliary cirrhosis because of interruption of the enterohepatic circulation of copper; however, studies

Table 25–2. Disease States and Levels of Several Constituents

	ALP	GGT	AST	ALT	Albumin	5'-NT
Acute hepatitis	↑	↑	↑ ↑ ↑	↑ ↑	N	↑
Alcoholic or drug hepatitis	N to SL ↑	↑ ↑ ↑	↑	↑	N to ↓	↑
Cirrhosis	N to SL ↑	N to SL ↑	N to SL ↑	N to SL ↑	↓	N to SL ↑
Cholestatic disease	↑	↑ ↑	↑	↑	N	↑ ↑ ↑
Chronic hepatocellular disease	N to SL ↑	N to SL ↑	↑	↑	↓	N to SL ↑

Abbreviations: N, normal; SL, slight.

indicate that the copper retention is not pathogenic.[6] Treatment with D-penicillamine does not reduce copper concentrations in primary biliary cirrhosis.

The most striking laboratory abnormalities in hemochromatosis are the serum iron, transferrin, and ferritin concentrations and transferrin saturation. Serum iron and ferritin concentrations and transferrin saturation are significantly increased, whereas the transferrin concentration is usually decreased. Serum bilirubin concentration, hepatic enzyme (AST, ALT, and GGT) levels, and the prothrombin time are elevated. Serum albumin may be decreased in advanced cirrhosis due to hemochromatosis. In addition to the laboratory abnormalities associated with cirrhosis, a decreased serum ceruloplasmin and increased serum copper concentration are frequently found in Wilson's disease. Urinary excretion of copper and hepatic deposits of copper are also increased. α_1-Antitrypsin deficiency is characterized by a decrease in the α_1-globulin fraction of serum proteins on serum protein electrophoresis. Isoelectric focusing techniques identify the specific protein deficiency, and liver biopsy is necessary for a definitive diagnosis.[2]

Increased conjugated bilirubin concentrations are seen in extrahepatic bile duct atresia, but liver enzymes are often normal or only slightly elevated.

TREATMENT

Conditions that cause prehepatic and posthepatic jaundice do not originate in the liver, so specific treatment for those conditions alleviates any abnormalities in liver function. Prehepatic and posthepatic jaundice resolve when the cause of the bilirubin overproduction or bile duct obstruction is corrected. Extrahepatic bile duct atresia in severely affected infants is effectively treated only by orthotopic liver transplantation.

Gilbert's, Rotor's, and Dubin-Johnson syndromes do not require treatment as they are benign conditions with few, if any, symptoms and excellent prognoses. No effective treatment is available for type I Crigler-Najjar syndrome short of orthotopic liver transplantation, which has been shown to correct the condition. Type II Crigler-Najjar syndrome does respond to enzyme-inducing drug therapy, such as phenobarbital, but type I does not.

Physiologic jaundice of the newborn requires monitoring of the child's serum bilirubin concentration to ensure that the levels begin to drop after 2 to 3 days. Phototherapy, exchange transfusions, and the administration of phenobarbital may be required in severe cases to reduce the bilirubin deposited in the tissues and to prevent kernicterus.

The course of alcoholic cirrhosis is long and extensive. By the time the liver is damaged to the extent that cirrhosis has occurred, the prognosis is poor. If the patient abstains from alcohol and maintains good nutrition, and if liver damage is not too severe, enzyme levels may return to normal, as may some of the other values. Liver damage resulting from cirrhosis, however, is often advanced and irreversible by the time the disease is detected.

Postnecrotic cirrhosis tends to progress with the majority of cases terminating within 1 to 5 years in death from complications despite supportive therapy.[5]

No medical treatment is known to alter the course of primary biliary cirrhosis other than liver transplantation. Secondary biliary cirrhosis may be treated early by correcting the obstruction. Any abnormal laboratory results subsequently return to normal.

Regular therapeutic phlebotomy is an effective long-term treatment of hemochromatosis as it reduces the iron overload by using the stored iron to produce new erythrocytes. Treatment of Wilson's disease with daily D-penicillamine reduces the copper load and generally alleviates hepatic and neurologic abnormalities. Development of α_1-antitrypsin products to replace the missing inhibitor are under investigation, but currently the only available therapy for α_1-antitrypsin deficiency is orthotopic liver transplantation.[8]

Disorders that cause jaundice associated with pregnancy usually subside when the pregnancy is terminated or completed.

Case Study 1

A 40-year-old man was admitted with weakness, lethargy, abdominal pain, slight jaundice, hepatomegaly, and signs of carbohydrate intolerance. Significant laboratory data include the following:

	Values	Reference Ranges
Total bilirubin (mg/dL)	2.3	(0.2–1.2)
Direct bilirubin (mg/dL)	1.1	(0–0.4)
ALP (IU/L)	141	(30–115)
LD (IU/L)	217	(60–200)
Random glucose (mg/dL)	302	(65–120)

Glycated hemoglobin (%)	9.7	(5.5–8.5)

After investigation of the family history, iron studies were ordered, with the following results:

Serum iron (μg/dL)	200	(4–150)
Total iron-binding capacity (μg/dL)	273	(250–350)
Serum ferritin (ng/mL)	275	(20–250)

A bone marrow examination revealed erythroid hyperplasia with a slightly increased storage iron content. Liver biopsy results showed micronodular cirrhosis with a marked increase of iron. Iron stains showed marked increase of iron-positive material throughout the liver biopsy specimen.

Questions

1. What is the most likely diagnosis?
2. What is the mechanism of damage to the liver?
3. What is the standard treatment for persons with this condition?
4. Is the glucose intolerance related to this condition or to a separate disease entity?

Discussion

1. Hereditary hemochromatosis is the likely diagnosis.
2. Iron overload caused by increased intestinal absorption of iron and deposition of iron in many organs. Iron deposits in the liver will eventually lead to cirrhosis.
3. Regular therapeutic phlebotomy is the treatment of choice, which will reduce the stored iron by forcing accelerated erythrocyte production.
4. Glucose intolerance is a common symptom of hemochromatosis and is caused by iron deposits in the pancreas, leading to a decrease in islet cells and, thus, in insulin release.

Case Study 2

A 28-year-old woman, 7 months pregnant with her first child, is being evaluated for asymptomatic jaundice. She has no known exposure to hepatitis and no history of liver disease or transfusions. Biochemical and hepatitis profiles show the following results:

	Values	Reference Ranges
Total bilirubin (mg/dL)	6.3	(0.2–1.0)
Conjugated bilirubin (mg/dL)	4.1	(0–0.4)
ALT (IU/L)	22	(8–30)
AST (IU/L)	12	(8–22)

GGT (IU/L)	14	(2–33)
Antibody to hepatitis A virus, IgM		negative
Hepatitis B surface antigen		negative
Hepatitis B early antigen		negative
Antibody to hepatitis B surface antigen		negative
Antibody to hepatitis C virus		negative

A routine CBC was normal. Cholecystography was performed to rule out gallstones, and the gallbladder was not visualized.

Questions

1. What is the most probable diagnosis?
2. How can hemolytic conditions be ruled out as a cause of the jaundice?
3. What additional information would be helpful in making this diagnosis?
4. Why is it important to obtain a definite diagnosis since this condition is benign?

Discussion

1. The most probable diagnosis would be Dubin-Johnson syndrome.
2. The CBC is normal.
3. A distinctive feature of Dubin-Johnson syndrome is the dark pigmentation of the liver. A liver biopsy would demonstrate this pigmentation, but a liver biopsy will not be scheduled until after the baby is born because of the risks involved to the patient and the baby.
4. Establishing a definite diagnosis is necessary to differentiate this benign condition from more serious disorders that might require specific treatments. This diagnosis should also prevent unnecessary anxiety or further medical and/or surgical intervention.

References

1. Berk PD: The familial unconjugated hyperbilirubinemias. Semin Liver Dis 14:321–322, 1994.
2. Ingram LR: Liver function. *In* Anderson SC, Cockayne S (eds): Clinical Chemistry: Concepts and Applications. Philadelphia, WB Saunders, 1993, pp 280–321.
3. Sherlock S, Dooley J: Diseases of the Liver and Biliary System, ed 9. Oxford, Blackwell Scientific Publications, 1993, pp 199–213.
4. Blanckaert N, Fevery J: Physiology and pathophysiology of bilirubin metabolism. *In* Zakim TD, Boyer D (eds): Hepatology: A Textbook of Liver Diseases, ed 2. Philadelphia, WB Saunders, 1990, pp 254–291.
5. Podolsky DK, Isselbacher KJ: Alcohol-related liver disease and cirrhosis. *In* Isselbacher KJ, Martin JB, Braunwald E, et al (eds): Harrison's Principles of Internal Medicine, vol 2, ed 13. New York, McGraw-Hill, 1994, pp 1483–1495.
6. Zetterman RK: Cirrhosis of the liver. *In* Gitnick, G (ed): Diseases of the Liver and Biliary Tract. St Louis, Mosby–Year Book, 1992, pp 447–466.
7. Tavill AS, Bacon BR: Hemachromatosis: Iron metabolism and the iron overload syndromes. *In* Zakim TD, Boyer D (eds): Hepatology:

A Textbook of Liver Diseases, ed 2. Philadelphia, WB Saunders, 1990, pp 1273–1294.

8. Ghishan FK, Greene HL: Alpha-1-Antitrypsin deficiency. *In* Zakim TD, Boyer D (eds): Hepatology: A Textbook of Liver Diseases, ed 2. Philadelphia, WB Saunders, 1990, pp 1273–1294.

9. Van Dyke RW: The liver in pregnancy. *In* Zakim TD, Boyer D (eds): Hepatology: A Textbook of Liver Diseases, ed 2, Philadelphia, WB Saunders, 1990, pp 1438–1453.

10. Isselbacher KJ: Bilirubin metabolism and hyperbilirubinemia. *In* Isselbacher KJ, Martin JB, Braunwald E, et al (eds): Harrison's Principles of Internal Medicine, vol 2, ed 13. McGraw-Hill, New York, 1994, pp 1453–1458.

Chapter 26

Hepatitis

Lynn Ingram

Hepatitis is a general term describing nonspecific inflammation of the liver; it is associated with a broad range of diseases and with liver injuries that are caused by infectious and noninfectious agents. Patient history, physical examination, and laboratory data are required for obtaining a differential diagnosis of the many types of hepatitis because they cannot be distinguished based on clinical symptoms alone.

Anicteric, typical acute (icteric), *chronic*, and *fulminant* are terms used to describe the different stages of hepatitis. Anicteric hepatitis is usually a mild form of the disease and is often subclinical, because no jaundice is evident. The patient may not seek medical attention, and the only evidence of hepatitis may be the presence of serologic markers in cases of infectious hepatitis. Icteric hepatitis is the most readily recognized type of hepatitis because the patient exhibits jaundice as well as other symptoms such as fatigue, anorexia, malaise, nausea, and myalgia. Chronic hepatitis occurs in 1% to 10% of patients with icteric hepatitis B and in up to 50% of patients infected with hepatitis C virus (HCV).[1] Chronic hepatitis is defined as persistent hepatic inflammation for 6 months to a year. Patients with chronic hepatitis, especially those infected with hepatitis B or non-A, non-B hepatitis (NANBH), may be clinically asymptomatic but serve as reservoirs of infection. Two types of chronic hepatitis may be identified: chronic persistent and chronic active. In chronic persistent hepatitis, jaundice and other symptoms may continue intermittently for 10 years or more, but the patient usually recovers and has a favorable long-term prognosis because cirrhosis or fulminant hepatic failure does not occur.[2] Chronic active hepatitis, however, is a progressive disease that often results in cirrhosis and/or liver failure. It is a much more serious condition with both hepatic and extrahepatic involvement and is often associated with an autoimmune process. Both chronic persistent and chronic active hepatitis can be diagnosed only through examination of liver biopsy tissue. Fulminant hepatitis results in acute liver failure due to massive hepatic necrosis and is characterized by rapid onset and high mortality. This severe form of hepatitis occurs in less than 1% of patients with acute hepatitis caused by hepatitis B virus (HBV); however, it occurs more frequently in NANBH patients.[3] It has also been known to occur in toxic and alcoholic hepatitis and in hepatitis of unknown origin.

ETIOLOGY AND PATHOPHYSIOLOGY

Infectious Causes

The infectious causes of hepatitis are primarily viral; however, bacterial and parasitic organisms have been linked to individual cases of hepatitis. Box 26–1 shows the most common viral agents reported to cause hepatitis. At least the following five hepatitis viruses are primary causes of the disease: hepatitis A (HAV), HBV, HCV, hepatitis D (HDV), and hepatitis E (HEV). NANBH is also of viral origin, although the specific virus(es) have not been fully identified at this time. Efforts using recombinant technology to identify and isolate the non A through E hepatitis viruses are ongoing, and evidence shows that hepatitis F and G viruses have been provisionally identified. Even though viral hepatitis is known to be under-reported, the Centers for Disease Control and Prevention have calculated

---

Box 26–1. Viral Agents of Hepatitis

RNA Viruses	DNA Viruses
HAV	HBV
Coxsackie viruses	Cytomegalovirus
Echoviruses	Epstein-Barr virus
Yellow fever virus	Herpes simplex virus
Rubella virus	Varicella zoster virus
Junin virus	Adenoviruses (?)
Machupo virus	
Lassa virus	**Unidentified Virus**
Rift Valley fever virus	
Marburg virus	NANBH
Ebola virus	
Measles virus	

---

that of the reported cases of acute viral hepatitis in the United States in 1994, 61% are attributable to hepatitis A, 28% to hepatitis B, 10% to hepatitis C, and 1% to nonspecified viral hepatitis.[4] Yellow fever virus, Ebola virus disease, Marburg disease, Lassa fever virus, and Rift Valley fever virus invariably cause liver damage.[5] Other viruses such as cytomegalovirus and Epstein-Barr virus may produce hepatitis as a complication of the primary disease.

HAV, a member of the family Picornaviridae, is transmitted primarily by fecal-oral route from contaminated food or water, and causes the type of hepatitis formerly known as infectious hepatitis. Exposure to the virus is linked to point sources as well as to poor sanitation and crowded living conditions. Parenteral transmission is rare, although a transient viremia of 7 to 10 days occurs before the clinical symptoms appear.[6] The virus is a nonenveloped RNA virus that replicates in the liver cells and is excreted in the stool. Stool specimens are infectious for 3 to 10 days before and up to 8 days after the onset of symptoms. The incubation period is approximately 30 days, with a range of 20 to 45 days. Symptoms, if present, have an abrupt onset. However, the disease is usually mild, with 25% to 50% of cases being subclinical. No documented cases indicate that chronic hepatitis, carrier states, or end-stage liver disease have developed from infection with HAV.[7]

HBV, a member of the family Hepadnaviridae, is an antigenically complex virus that causes serum hepatitis. It is a DNA virus composed of an inner core of DNA and DNA polymerase and an outer protein layer. The entire molecule is referred to as the *Dane particle*. Core material is produced in the nucleus of the hepatocyte, and the protein is produced in the cytoplasm. Coating of the core material with protein occurs before the molecule is excreted into the blood. Excess protein coat, known as the hepatitis B surface antigen (HB$_s$Ag), is also excreted into the blood. Although usually determined only for epidemiologic studies, the following are four antigenic subtypes of the surface antigen: adw, adr, ayw, ayr. The incubation period for HBV is 6 to 20 weeks, and clinical symptoms may last for 4 to 12 weeks. The most common route of infection is parenteral, although the virus may also be transmitted through intimate contact. HBV is easily transmitted, and currently, the most common route of transmission is through shared needles

by intravenous (IV) drug users. Eighty-five percent to 90% of acutely infected persons will recover completely, between 5% and 10% will develop chronic disease, and 1% to 2% will progress to cirrhosis and/or death.

HCV was first identified in 1989, although the existence of at least one hepatitis virus other than HAV and HBV was presumed from the mid-1970s when diagnostic tests for hepatitis A and hepatitis B became widely available. At this time it was discovered that 90% of post-transfusion hepatitis was caused by an infectious agent other than hepatitis A or hepatitis B.[8] To indicate exclusion of the presence of these two viruses, the term *non-A, non-B* was used to describe these cases of viral hepatitis. Serologic tests for the presence of hepatitis C antibodies have now shown that at least 85% of all cases of NANBH post-transfusion hepatitis are due to hepatitis C.

HCV is a small, lipid-encapsulated RNA virus related to the flaviviruses, with a worldwide distribution. It is transmitted predominantly by blood and blood products and is a major threat to IV drug users, health care workers, and transfusion and hemodialysis patients. Minor routes of transmission have also been reported by sexual contact, from mother to infant, and by saliva and other body fluids. The incubation period for HCV is intermediate between that for HAV and HBV, approximately 3 to 8 weeks. Most patients are asymptomatic or have only mild nonspecific symptoms, and therefore many infections are not diagnosed. Only 25% of hepatitis C infections cause jaundice, and mortality with hepatitis C infection is less than 1%. Approximately 80% of the acute cases progress to a chronic state, however, which involves a much greater risk for cirrhosis and/or hepatocellular carcinoma. HCV appears to mutate rapidly, which contributes to its tendency to chronicity and explains the recurrent bouts of hepatitis C documented in some individuals.

Approximately 10% of transfusion-associated hepatitis and 4% of community-acquired hepatitis in the United States cannot be ascribed to any of the five recognized hepatitis viruses.[6] Because the viral agent or agents responsible for these cases have yet to be identified, the diagnosis of NANBH is based on exclusion of the known viral etiologies.[9] Although 85% of the previously designated NANBH cases can be linked to infection with hepatitis C, approximately 15% of hepatitis cases can be placed into a category of non-A, non-B, and non-C hepatitis. Negative tests for antibody to hepatitis A virus (anti-HAV) IgM, HB$_s$Ag, antibody to hepatitis B core antigen (anti-HB$_c$) IgM, and antibody to hepatitis C virus (anti-HCV) in the presence of clinical symptoms suggestive of hepatitis indicate an unknown viral etiology. Generally this type of hepatitis causes a milder clinical form of disease, with approximately 50% of the cases being anicteric.[9]

HDV, formerly known as the delta agent, was described by Rizzetto in 1977.[6] The unique property of this virus is that it requires the presence of HBV, in particular HB$_s$Ag, for replication. Transmission, like that of HBV, is primarily parenteral in nonendemic areas. In areas where the virus is endemic, it may also be spread through body fluids or intimate contact. The following three patterns typify HDV infection: (1) simultaneous infection of HBV and HDV, causing an acute hepatitis that is usually self-limited but has a higher mortality rate than HBV infection alone,[10]

(2) acute HDV infection in a chronic HBV carrier, and (3) chronic HBV-HDV infection. In any of these patterns, HDV infection is usually severe and associated with fulminant hepatitis and a rapidly progressive course leading to subacute or chronic hepatitis in many cases. The mortality rate is 2% to 20%.[6]

HEV is a nonenveloped RNA virus that produces hepatitis that is similar to hepatitis A in many respects. Recognized in the early 1980s, it is an enterically transmitted virus with a 40-day incubation period. Although rarely the cause of hepatitis outbreaks in the United States, it has caused widespread outbreaks of disease in Asia, Africa, the former Soviet Union, and Mexico.[7] It is a mild to moderate disease and has a mortality rate of 0.2% to 1% in the general population. Hepatitis E infections in pregnant women are much more severe, however, and can cause death in up to 20% of individuals.[6]

Comparison of the etiologic forms of viral hepatitis is shown in Table 26–1.

Bacterial agents of hepatitis are usually associated with septicemia. Parasites that may cause hepatitis include *Toxoplasma gondii, Entamoeba histolytica, Echinococcus granulosus, Schistosoma* species, and the hepatic flukes.

Noninfectious Causes

Noninfectious causes of hepatitis include chemicals, metabolic disorders, and idiopathic agents. The role of the liver in detoxification renders it especially susceptible to chemical damage. The chemical most frequently cited as a cause of hepatitis is ethanol, and the resulting condition is typically referred to as *alcoholic hepatitis*. One theory often used to describe liver damage by alcohol suggests that the accumulation of acetaldehyde, a highly toxic chemical waste product of ethanol metabolism, and the increased production of nicotinamide adenine dinucleotide-reduced form (NADH) cause hepatocellular damage.[11] A second theory suggests that the presence of either ethanol or one of its metabolites causes antigenic components to be expressed in the hepatocytes, and these components stimulate lymphocyte activity, resulting in an autoimmune disorder.

Nitrofurantoin is commonly used to treat urinary tract infections and on rare occasions has been linked to hepatic damage. It has been known to result in chronic active hepatitis that is similar to an autoimmune hepatitis. Halothane hepatitis has also been well documented.[12] Other chemicals known to cause hepatic damage are listed in Box 26–2.

Several metabolic disorders are known to result in hepatitis. Although clinical symptoms may resemble viral hepatitis, treatment should be directed at the primary defect rather than at being strictly supportive in nature. Wilson's disease is a hereditary disorder of copper metabolism that may present initially as fulminant hepatitis. Other metabolic disorders that may present with a clinical picture of hepatitis include galactosemia, fructosuria, tyrosinosis, and α_1-antitrypsin deficiency. Ischemic hepatitis has been described in cardiac patients who suffer a decrease in cardiac output. This condition can be differentiated from other types of hepatitis based on patient history and on lack of persistence of the elevation of enzymes. In addition, it is usually demonstrated for only 1 to 2 days in the serum.

Autoimmune hepatitis is an unresolving inflammation of the liver characterized by hypergammaglobulinemia, autoantibodies in serum, and the presence of piecemeal necrosis on histologic examination.[13] A list of autoantibodies associated with autoimmune hepatitis is shown in Box 26–3.

Table 26–1. Differentiation of the Etiologic Forms of Viral Hepatitis

Feature	Hepatitis Viruses				
	A	B	C	D	E
Viral characteristic					
Size of the virus (nm)	27	42	30–60	35–37	32
Nucleic acid	RNA	DNA	RNA	RNA	RNA
Incubation period (days)					
Range	15–49	28–160	15–160	21–140	15–65
Mean	30	70–80	50	?35	42
Patterns of immunity					
Heterologous immunity	No	No	No	No	No
Homologous immunity	Yes	Yes	Second attacks may indicate another distinct agent or weak immunity	Yes	Unknown
Epidemiologic features					
Viral excretion in feces	Yes	No	No	No	Yes
Fecal-oral transmission	Yes	No	No	No	Yes
Percutaneous transmission	Rare	Yes	Yes	Yes	?No
Carrier state	No	Yes	Yes	Yes	No
Clinical features					
Risk of chronic hepatitis	No	Yes	Yes	Yes	No
Risk of cirrhosis	No	Yes	Yes	Yes	No
Risk of primary hepatocellular carcinoma	No	Yes	Yes	?No	No

From Koff RS: Viral hepatitis: *In* Schiff L, Schiff ER: Diseases of the Liver, ed 7. Philadelphia, JB Lippincott, 1993, p 494.

Box 26–2. Chemicals and Toxins Known to Cause Hepatic Damage

Chlorinated Hydrocarbons

Carbon tetrachloride
Tetrachlorethane
Chloroform
Trichloroethane
Dichloroethane

Yellow Phosphorus

Acetaminophen (Paracetamol)

Psychotropic Drugs

Tricyclic antidepressants
Neuroleptics
Phenothiazines
Thioxanthenes
Butyrophenonones
Anxiolytics
Antidepressants
Monoamine oxidase inhibitors
Hydrazines

Foods or Food Contaminants

Amanita phalloides
Cycad nut
Nutmeg
Aflatoxins
Ochratoxin
Luteoskyrin

Anesthestic Drugs

Halothane
Methoxyflurane
Enflurane

Oral Hypoglycemics

Antithyroid Drugs

Antineoplastic Agents

Methotrexate
Antipyrimidines
Antipurines

Anti-Inflammatory Agents

Phenylbutazone
Indomethacin
Sulindac
Ibuprofen
Diclofenac
Naproxen
Piroxicam
Benoxaprofen
Clometacine
Gold
Propoxyphene
Salicylates
Allopurinol
Probenecid

Steroids and Associated Agents

Anabolic-androgenic (C-17)
Oral contraceptives
Tamoxifen
Danazol
Glucocorticoids

Antimicrobial Agents

Tetracyclines
Erythromycins
Penicillins
Chloramphenicol
Cephalosporins
Clindamycin
Sulfonamides
Nitrofurantoin
Amphotericin
Flucytosine
Aminosalicylic acid
Isoniazid
Rifampin

CLINICAL MANIFESTATIONS

When a patient presents with jaundice, complaints of nausea or vomiting, abdominal pain, and general malaise or fatigue, hepatitis should be suspected.

Infectious hepatitis exhibits four phases in a typical acute infection: incubation, prodromal (pre-icteric), icteric, and convalescent. During the incubation period, the patient rarely exhibits symptoms, and the duration varies depending on the etiologic agent. In the prodromal period, which may persist for 4 to 7 days before the onset of jaundice, the patient exhibits generalized symptoms including malaise, anorexia, slight fever, weight loss, and upper right quadrant pain or tenderness. In addition, the patient may experience nausea and vomiting, headache, and myalgia. Onset of jaundice marks the beginning of the icteric phase, which may last 4 to 6 weeks in uncomplicated cases. The patient may also experience dark urine or pale stools; however, up to 50% of infections may be anicteric.[14] The disappearance of jaundice and other major symptoms marks the beginning of the convalescent period. Noninfectious hepatitis may present with these same phases, except that the incubation phase is absent.

The clinical manifestations of hepatitis syndromes can vary greatly, from the mild gastrointestinal and systemic complaints of anicteric hepatitis to the fever, deep jaundice, coma, and seizures of fulminant hepatitis.

LABORATORY ANALYSES AND DIAGNOSIS

Chemistry Tests

Chemical test results that are typically abnormal in patients with hepatitis include the enzyme measurements of aspartate aminotransferase (AST) and alanine aminotransferase (ALT). Both enzyme levels are typically elevated during the final weeks of the incubation phase in viral hepatitis and are usually the first abnormal biochemical test results regardless of the causative agent.[15] In viral hepatitis the values may be 10 to 100 times those of normal, although values of less than 10 times normal may suggest a nonviral etiology.[15] There is no specific test to diagnose alcoholic hepatitis; however, AST levels are generally more elevated in this condition than are ALT levels. Levels of alkaline phosphatase and the hepatic fraction of lactate dehydrogenase may also be elevated, although not elevated to the same degree as the transaminases. Urine bilirubin is usually detected before the appearance of jaundice. Serum bilirubin begins to rise during the prodromal phase. As

Box 26–3. Autoantibodies Associated With Autoimmune Hepatitis

Antinuclear antibody (ANA)
Smooth muscle antibody (SMA)
Antimitochondrial antibody (AMA)
Antibodies to liver/kidney microsome type I (Anti-LKM1)
Antibodies to P-450 IID6*
Antibodies to P-450 IA2*
Antibodies to liver cytosol type I (anti-LC1)
Antibodies to liver-pancreas (anti-LP)
Antibodies to asialoglycoprotein receptor (anti-ASGPR)
Perinuclear antineutrophil cytoplasmic antibodies (pANCA)

*Cytochrome oxidase enzymes found in the liver.

the disease progresses, the prothrombin time may become prolonged and the erythrocyte sedimentation rate may be increased. Hypoalbuminemia typically is present only in chronic hepatitis due to the longer half-life of albumin (approximately 21 days).

Serology Tests

Identification of the causative agent of hepatitis is greatly dependent on the immunology laboratory. Patients with suspected hepatitis should be tested for antibodies and/or antigens to HAV, HBV, and HCV.

Diagnostic serologic markers for HAV are anti-HAV IgM and anti-HAV IgG. Anti-HAV IgM, which develops about 4 weeks after exposure and continues to rise for 4 to 6 weeks before dropping to undetectable levels, is used to confirm acute HAV infection. The anti-HAV IgG develops after anti-HAV IgM and may persist for years. The presence of anti-HAV IgG confirms previous HAV exposure and usually indicates immunity to the virus (Fig. 26–1).

Although hepatitis B viral particles have been isolated in saliva, semen, and other body fluids, serologic methods are used to detect infection. Three antigens are associated with HBV: HB_sAg, hepatitis B early antigen (HB_eAg), and hepatitis B core antigen (HB_cAg). HB_sAg and HB_eAg serve as antigenic serologic markers. HB_cAg is not usually found free in the serum but may be detected in hepatocyte nuclei. Recently, another antigen-antibody combination has been discovered, the HB_xAg and antibody. HB_xAg can be found after the peak of virus replication and may be the only detectable antigen in the blood of some chronically infected patients.[16]

HB_sAg is the first detectable antigen, and is a useful marker for HBV infection. It usually appears 4 to 6 weeks after infection. It is not only present in patients with acute infections but also persists in patients who are carriers. HB_eAg, which is detected shortly after HB_sAg, is a distinct component of the core, and its presence indicates infectivity.[14] Persistence of this antigen and lack of conversion to antibody to hepatitis B early antigen (anti-HB_e) indicate possible chronic HBV infection (Fig. 26–2).

There are three antibodies that serve as serologic markers for infection with HBV; antibody to hepatitis B surface antigen (anti-HB_s), anti-HB_e, and anti-HB_c. Anti-HB_c is the first antibody produced, usually 4 weeks after exposure or at the time clinical symptoms become evident. The anti-HB_c IgM lasts about 60 days but may persist for up to 6 months, and the anti-HB_c IgG may persist for years. Presence of the anti-HB_c IgM is indicative of acute HBV infection, and may be used to distinguish persons who are chronic HB_sAg carriers from those with acute infections. Anti-HB_e production usually begins during the first 10 weeks of the illness and its presence indicates the beginning of the recovery period. Anti-HB_s is the last antibody to be produced, usually 3 to 6 months after development of clinical symptoms. Production of this antibody indicates probable immunity to HBV. Thus, the sequential order of serologic markers of HBV is usually HB_sAg, HB_eAg, anti-HB_c, anti-HB_e, and anti-HB_s (see Fig. 26–2).[14] In acute HBV infection, there is a period of time, referred to as the *core window*, during which HB_sAg is below detectable levels and only anti-HB_c IgM is detectable to indicate a recent infection. Anti-HB_e may also be present. Recovery from HBV is indicated by the presence of anti-HB_c and anti-HB_s in the patient's serum.

Diagnosis of chronic hepatitis may be made by persistence of HB_sAg and HB_eAg in the serum, presence of anti-HB_c, and lack of production of anti-HB_e. The presence of HB_eAg indicates active viral replication; its conversion to anti-HB_e indicates termination of active replication. However, HB_sAg will persist. In fulminant hepatitis due to HBV infection, HB_sAg and HB_eAg may be of lower concentration and cleared more rapidly than in an acute infection. In

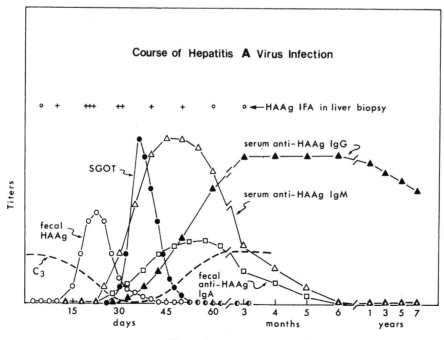

Figure 26–1. Schematic representation of viral markers in the blood, liver, and feces throughout the course of primary HAV infection. (From Zakim TD, Boyer D: Hepatology: A Textbook of Liver Diseases, vol 2, ed 2. Philadelphia, WB Saunders, 1996, p 923.)

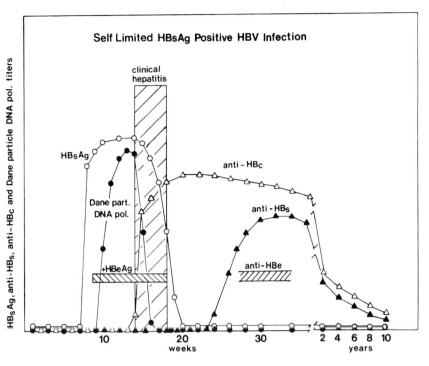

Figure 26–2. Schematic representation of viral markers in the blood throughout the course of self-limited HB$_s$Ag-positive primary HBV infection. (From Zakim TD, Boyer D: Hepatology: A Textbook of Liver Diseases, vol 2, ed 2. WB Saunders, Philadelphia, 1996, p 904.)

addition, there is an enhanced antibody response to these antigens.[17]

In hepatitis D infections, in which simultaneous HBV-HDV infection occur, tests for HB$_s$Ag, anti-HB$_c$ IgM, and antibody to hepatitis D virus (anti-HDV) are positive. In acute hepatitis in a chronic HBV carrier, the presence of anti-HB$_c$ IgM helps to differentiate acute HBV infection from HDV superinfection, in which anti-HB$_c$ IgM is absent. In chronic HBV-HDV infection, the virus can be detected in hepatocyte nuclei by use of immunofluorescent techniques. Serologic kits for detection of anti-HDV have recently become available. Anti-HDV IgM occurs in the early acute phase of the infection. Anti-HDV IgG may occur in the late phase and persists for only a few months if the infection is self-limited.[14]

Hepatitis C is diagnosed by the presence of anti-HCV in the serum. The fact that 80% or more of HCV-infected individuals have persistent infection despite the presence of multiple HCV-directed antibodies suggests that such antibodies have a minimal role in viral clearance.[18] Figure 26–3 depicts biochemical, serologic, and molecular biologic profiles seen in acute and chronic hepatitis C. NANBH is characterized by negative tests for anti-HAV IgM, HB$_s$Ag, anti-HB$_c$ IgM, and anti-HCV. Demonstration of antibody to hepatitis E virus (anti-HEV) in a patient's serum is diagnostic for hepatitis E infections.

The usual panel for diagnosing acute hepatitis consists of testing for anti-HAV (IgM), HB$_s$Ag, anti-HB$_c$ IgM, and anti-HCV. Results of these tests may indicate the need for additional testing of serologic markers, including HB$_e$Ag, anti-HB$_e$, and anti-HB$_s$. Combinations of these tests may be used to monitor chronic hepatitis patients, follow infants who have been treated for perinatal exposure, or track sexual contacts of persons with HBV infection.

Additional Tests

Biochemical tests are not specific for different types of hepatitis and only indicate the presence of hepatocyte injury. Serum protein levels may be decreased, especially albumin. The presence of increased α-fetoprotein and immunoglobulin levels may offset any decrease in albumin, and the patient may demonstrate a normal total protein concentration. Alcoholic hepatitis may be diagnosed based on patient history, liver biopsy, and failure to detect a viral cause. Drug-induced hepatitis follows the same protocol. Nitrofurantoin hepatitis may present with a positive antinuclear antibody and anti–smooth muscle antibody. The lupus erythematosus preparation (LE$_{prep}$) may also indicate a positive result.

Hematologic changes may be seen in hepatitis. Most commonly seen is mild anemia, low reticulocyte count, leukopenia, atypical lymphocytosis, and mild to moderate thrombocytopenia.[15]

Due to the treatability or possible severity of metabolic disorders, it is important that they be ruled out in the differential diagnosis. In Wilson's disease, serum, urine, and liver levels of copper are elevated, and serum ceruloplasmin levels are decreased. Kayser-Fleischer rings may be present in the cornea of the eyes. A$_1$-Antitrypsin deficiency may be detected by serum protein electrophoresis and is characterized by an absence, or a greatly reduced level, of the α_1-globulin fraction. The phenotype may be identified by isoelectric focusing.[19] Tyrosinosis may be initially diagnosed by metabolic screening spot tests using urine. Definitive diagnosis can be made by specific enzyme assays. Galactosemia and fructosuria may also be screened for in urine, using nonspecific tests for reducing substances with confirmations made by specific enzyme assays.

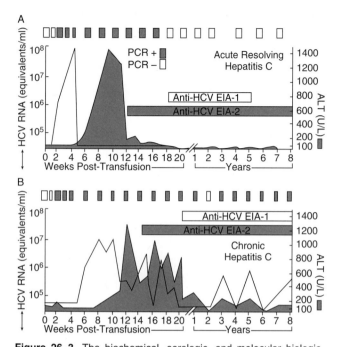

Figure 26–3. The biochemical, serologic, and molecular biologic profile of acute and chronic TAH C virus infection is shown. Acute, resolving hepatitis C is shown in *A* and chronic hepatitis C in *B*. Resolving disease cannot be distinguished from progressive disease based on the time of onset of detectable HCV RNA by PCR, the magnitude of HCV RNA elevation as measured by branched DNA assay, the interval to the first ALT elevation, the magnitude of ALT elevation in the acute phase, or the interval between exposure and the first appearance of antibody. Hence, progression to chronic disease cannot be predicted in the acute phase and the only distinguishing features in these patterns are the persistence of ALT elevation and the persistence of HCV RNA in those who develop chronic hepatitis C. The acute, resolving pattern *(A)* may be seen in 10% to 15% of patients with TAH C and the chronic pattern *(B)* in 85% to 90%. Other points of note are as follows: (1) HCV RNA is detectable very early after exposure. In the cases shown, PCR was positive in the 2-week postexposure sample, but it may become positive even sooner. (2) Detectable HCV RNA by the branched DNA assay may appear coincident with PCR reactivity, but it may be delayed as in these cases. (3) The major peak of viral replication, as assessed by HCV RNA level, occurs before the first rise in ALT and hence, before any clinical or biochemical evidence of hepatitis. It is presumed that persons might be most infectious in this pre-acute-phase interval. (4) In acute resolving infection, HCV RNA decrease rapidly and the decrease precedes the decline in serum ALT. (5) In chronic infection, the level of HCV RNA diminishes and may either persist at low level, fluctuate, or become nondetectable. As shown in B, sometimes HCV RNA levels show a periodicity that parallels the fluctuations in ALT. In this case, the increase in HCV RNA shortly precedes the decrease in ALT. (6) Second-generation anti-HCV assays considerably diminish the seronegative window in HCV infection as compared with first-generation assays. Nonetheless, anti-HCV was not detectable for 12 to 15 weeks after exposure and for 6 to 7 weeks after the first significant increase in ALT. (7) Antibody to HCV, as detected by second-generation assays, almost always persists in chronic cases and, generally, even in acute resolving cases; antibodies detected in the first-generation assay (anti-c100, anti-5-1-1) generally disappear in resolving cases. (From Alter HJ: To C or Not to C: These are the questions. Blood 85:1681–1695.)

TREATMENT AND PROPHYLAXIS
Nonspecific Treatments

Specific treatment for hepatitis is not available, but supportive measures are usually instituted once the symp-toms have begun. Bedrest and a high-protein diet are recommended during the acute phase of hepatitis. Drugs should be avoided because drug metabolism is compromised in hepatitis. Corticosteroids were once thought to hasten recovery from acute hepatitis, but no beneficial effects have been proven, and their use is now contraindicated. Antiviral agents such as ribavirin or inosine pranobex (Isoprinosine) have generally not been shown to be effective as routine treatment for hepatitis.

Immune Globulin

The decision to use immune prophylaxis often depends on the type of hepatitis, type of exposure, and immune status of the patient. In hepatitis A infections, the use of immune serum globulin may prevent or decrease the clinical symptoms if given within 2 weeks of exposure. However, because exposure to HAV is often not known until symptoms are evident, the immune serum globulin is often not used. Pregnant women rarely transmit HAV to the fetus because of the short viremic phase, but the infant may be given immune serum globulin at birth as a precaution.[20] For HBV exposure, the current immune prophylaxis is hepatitis B immunoglobulin (HBIG), which contains high levels of anti-HB$_s$, usually greater than 1:100,000.[15] HBIG should be given within 7 days after exposure to the virus to be effective in decreasing the attack rate.[5] The patient should be tested for immune status before HBIG is given. Tests used may include anti-HB$_c$, anti-HB$_s$, and HB$_s$Ag. A positive result for any test contraindicates HBIG administration. No current prophylaxis is recommended against NANBH or hepatitis D infection, although infants born to mothers with NANBH may also be given immune serum globulin at birth and at 28 days.[20]

Vaccination

Hepatitis B vaccine is recommended as pre-exposure prophylaxis in persons at high risk of infection by HBV. These include health care workers, IV drug users, male homosexuals, and hemodialysis patients. The vaccine contains purified HB$_s$Ag and requires a three-dose regimen. Anti-HB$_s$ develops in nearly 100% of persons who receive the vaccine.[1] A second vaccine, developed by recombinant DNA methods using the S gene encoded into *Saccharomyces cerevisiae*, has been developed. This vaccine appears to stimulate an antibody similar in titer, affinity, and specificity to that produced by the plasma-based vaccine.[15] Pre-vaccination serologic screening using anti-HB$_s$ tests may be recommended, depending on prevalence of HBV serologic markers in the population and cost.

Pregnant women who are HBV carriers present a problem because they may transmit the virus to the infant, especially during birth. Approximately 90% of infected infants become chronic HBV carriers, with 25% of these dying due to HBV-related complications such as cirrhosis and primary hepatocellular carcinoma.[1] If prophylaxis is started at delivery, infections with HBV can be prevented in more than 90% of the infants born to HB$_s$Ag positive women.[18] A combination of active and passive immunization is used. The child is protected passively by HBIG during the time it takes to mount an immune response to the vaccine. HBIG is administered to the infant at birth, followed by doses of HBV vaccine within 24 hours, at 1 month, and at 6 months.

There is no vaccine for hepatitis C, E, or D, although individuals are protected from infection with HDV if they are also protected from HBV infection.

Sequelae of viral hepatitis infections are outlined in Table 26–2.

Treatment of Noninfectious Hepatitis

Alcoholic hepatitis has sometimes been treated with corticosteroids, but this has not proven very helpful in the majority of cases. Propylthiouracil has also been administered but has not proven effective in all cases. Drug-induced hepatitis can usually be reversed by removing the precipitating drug before the hepatitis proceeds to liver failure.

Wilson's disease can be managed through life-long administration of a chelating agent such as penicillamine, but treatment must begin early in its course.[21] α_1-Antitrypsin deficiency, which results in hepatitis and/or cirrhosis, does not lend itself well to treatment. Experimental treatment using IV administration of concentrates of α_1-antitrypsin and oral use of the androgen danazol to raise serum levels has been attempted.[22] Tyrosinosis, fructosuria, and galactosemia have been treated primarily by diet control. Foods that contain phenylalanine, tyrosine, and methionine are restricted for patients with tyrosinosis, and foods or medicines that contain fructose or sucrose must be withheld from patients with fructosuria. Foods or medicines that contain galactose must be restricted for patients with a diagnosis of galactosemia.

Table 26–2. Estimated Frequency of Outcomes or Sequelae of Hepatitis Infections in Adults

Outcomes or Sequelae	Estimated Frequency (%)				
	HAV	HBV	HCV	HEV	HBV-HDV Co-infection
Complete recovery	95–99	85–95	50	99	90
Fulminant hepatitis	<1	1	<1	<1	<1
Confluent hepatic necrosis	<1	1–4	?1–5	<1	<1
Carrier state	0	1–10	50	0	5
Chronic hepatitis	0	1–10	50	0	1–5
Cirrhosis	0	<4	10–20	0	1–5
Primary hepatocellular carcinoma	0	<1	<1	0	<1
Aplastic anemia	<1	<1	<1	0	?<1
Glomerulonephritis	0	<1	?	0	?<1
Necrotizing vasculitis	0	<1	?	0	?<1

From Koff RS: Viral hepatitis: *In* Schiff L, Schiff ER: Diseases of the Liver, ed 7. Philadelphia, JB Lippincott, 1993, p 541.

Case Study 1

A 52-year-old female with symptoms of anorexia, nausea, diarrhea, dysarthria, weakness, and lethargy during the past month was seen by her physician. She was slightly jaundiced and reported light colored stools and dark urine. She has no history of jaundice, hepatitis, liver disease, or exposure to persons with known hepatitis. The following are significant laboratory results on admission:

	Values	Reference Ranges
ALT(IU/L)	3900	(0–41)
AST(IU/L)	2210	(0–45)
ALP(IU/L)	265	(30–115)
LD(IU/L)	560	(100–250)
GGT(IU/L)	152	(2–33)
Total bilirubin (mg/dL)	14.6	(0.2–1.0)
Conjugated bilirubin (mg/dL)	8.5	(0–0.4)

Routine urinalysis revealed an amber, hazy urine with 3+ bile and a positive Ictotest. Hepatitis profile results were the following:

Anti-HAV, IgM	Negative
HB$_s$Ag	Positive
HB$_c$Ab	Positive
Anti-HB$_s$	Negative
Anti-HCV	Negative

The patient's total bilirubin and ALT activity were monitored over a period of 6 weeks. Measurement of total bilirubin rose to 21.0 mg/dL 10 days after her admission, and ALT activity peaked at 8800 IU/L 7 days after admission. Both laboratory results were approaching normal at the end of the 6-week period. During the evaluation for the need for prophylactic treatment, it was found that both HB$_e$Ag and Anti-HB$_s$ were positive in the patient's husband.

Questions

1. What is the patient's probable diagnosis?
2. Did the patient infect her husband or did her husband infect her?
3. Should the patient's husband be treated for this condition?
4. What is the preferred treatment for this condition?

Discussion

1. This patient has a current hepatitis B infection. This is determined by the presence of HB$_s$Ag and HB$_c$Ag along with the fact that HB$_s$Ab has not yet appeared.
2. The patient's husband has been infected with HBV for a longer period of time than this patient, as

indicated by the presence of HB$_s$Ab in the husband. HB$_s$Ab is the last of the hepatitis B antibodies to appear, usually 3 to 6 months after clinical symptoms have developed.

3. No, the presence of HB$_s$Ab usually indicates immunity to HBV.

4. No specific treatment is available, but bedrest and a high-protein diet are helpful in minimizing the symptoms of hepatitis B infection.

Case Study 2*

A 24-year-old male presented to the hospital emergency department with jaundice, dark urine, and fatigue. The previous week he had moved from New Delhi, India to the United States for graduate studies. He denied IV drug usage, homosexual or recent heterosexual activity, or history of blood transfusions. He had no known family history of liver disease but reported jaundice with an unknown illness as a child. Significant laboratory data on admission:

	Values	Reference Ranges
AST(IU/L)	1543	(5–40)
ALT(IU/L)	1230	(7–56)
ALP(IU/L)	209	(36–126)
LD(IU/L)	1592	(313–618)
Total bilirubin (mg/dL)	16.1	(0.2–1.3)
Conjugated bilirubin (mg/dL)	11.1	(0.1–0.3)
Anti-HAV	Negative	
HB$_s$Ag	Negative	
Anti-HB$_s$	Negative	
Anti-HB$_c$	Negative	
Anti-HCV	Negative	

Because of the acute illness and the origin of this patient, HEV infection was considered. Enzyme-linked immunosorbent assays based on clonal recombinant HEV antigens have been developed to detect anti-HEV IgM and IgG antibodies. The results of these tests were:

Anti-HEV, IgM(EU/mL)	7.82 (Positive >0.348)
Anti-HEV, IgG(EU/mL)	9.66 (Positive >0.386)

The patient was treated with supportive therapies and monitored for several weeks. There was continual improvement in his health and in laboratory results, and no further complications were noted.

Questions

1. What is the most probable diagnosis in this patient?

2. What is the likely source of his infection?

3. Why is it important that an infection of this type be accurately diagnosed?

4. Should this patient have any long-term effects of this infection?

Discussion

1. The most probable diagnosis in this patient is acute hepatitis E infection.

2. Outbreaks of hepatitis E are common in Asia and the incubation period is approximately 40 days. This indicates that this patient was infected in India, probably as the result of a contaminated water source.

3. Until recently HEV infection was not considered a significant infection problem in the United States. HEV infection should also be considered as a possible etiologic agent in international travelers and foreign visitors to the United States. If it is not, the patient could be diagnosed with a more serious condition such as NANBH.

4. No, HEV is a relatively mild condition with no reports of chronicity and only rare incidence of fulminant hepatitis in nonpregnant patients.

*Appreciation is expressed to David Smalley, PhD, University of Tennessee, Memphis, Department of Pathology, for sharing this case.

References

1. Koff RS: Viral hepatitis. *In* Schiff L, Schiff ER (eds): Diseases of the Liver, ed 7. Philadelphia, JB Lippincott, 1993.
2. Ockner RK: Chronic hepatitis. *In* Wyngaarden JB, Smith LH (eds): Cecil's Textbook of Medicine, ed 17. Philadelphia, WB Saunders, 1985.
3. Riegler JL, Lake JR: Fulminant hepatic failure. Med Clin North Am 77:1057–1083, 1993.
4. US Department of Health and Human Services: Summary of notifiable diseases, United States, 1994. MMWR Morb Mortal Wkly Rep 43:3, 1995.
5. Schiff G: Hepatitis caused by viruses other than hepatitis A, hepatitis B and non-A, non-B hepatitis viruses. *In* Schiff L, Schiff ER (eds): Diseases of the Liver, ed 7. Philadelphia, JB Lippincott, 1993, p 578.
6. Purcell RH: Hepatitis viruses: Changing patterns of human disease. Proc Natl Acad Sci U S A 91:2401–2406, 1994.
7. Gurevich I: Hepatitis Part I: Enterically transmitted viral hepatitis: Etiology, epidemiology, and prevention. Heart Lung 22:370–2, 1993.
8. Alter JH, Purcell RH, Holland PV: Clinical and serological analysis of transfusion-associated hepatitis. Lancet 2:838–841, 1975.
9. Alter HJ, Bradley DW: Non-A, non-B hepatitis unrelated to the hepatitis C virus (Non-ABC), Semin Liver Dis 15:110–120, 1995.
10. Craxi A, Dimarco V, Iacono OL, et al: The natural history of chronic HDV infection. Prog Clin Biol Res 382:301–310, 1993.
11. Weiner FR, Esposti SD, Zern MA: Ethanol and the liver. *In* Arias IM, Boyer JL, Fausto MD, et al (eds): The Liver: Biology and Pathobiology, ed 3. New York, Raven Press, 1994, pp 1383–1412.
12. Zimmerman HJ, Maddrey WC: Toxic and Drug-Induced Hepatitis. *In* Schiff L, Schiff ER (eds): Diseases of the Liver, ed 7. Philadelphia, JB Lippincott, 1993.
13. Czaja AJ: Autoimmune hepatitis: Evolving concepts and treatment strategies. Dig Dis Sci 40:435–456, 1995.
14. Gurevich I: Hepatitis Part II: Viral hepatitis B, C and D. Heart Lung 22:450–458, 1993.
15. Seeff LB: Diagnosis, therapy, and prognosis of viral hepatitis. *In* Zakim TD, Boyer D (eds): Hepatology: A Textbook of Liver Diseases, vol I, ed 2. Philadelphia, WB Saunders Co, 1990.

16. Feitelson MA, Clayton MM: X antigen polypeptides in the sera of hepatitis B virus infected patients. Virology 177:367–371, 1990.

17. Kirsh BM, Lam N, Layden TJ, et al: Diagnosis and management of fulminant hepatic failure. Comp Ther 21:166–171, 1995.

18. Alter HJ: To C or not to C: These are the questions. Blood 85:1681–1695, 1995.

19. Kaplan LA, Pesce AJ: Clinical Chemistry: Theory, Analysis, Correlation. St Louis, CV Mosby, 1984, p 433.

20. Snydham DR: Hepatitis in pregnancy. N Engl J Med 313:1398–1401, 1985.

21. Sternlieb I, Scheinberg IH: Wilson's disease. *In* Schiff L, Schiff ER (eds): Diseases of the Liver, ed 7. Philadelphia, JB Lippincott, 1993.

22. Schwarzenberg SJ, Sharp HL: Alpha-1-antitrypsin deficiency. *In* Schiff L, Schiff ER (eds): Diseases of the Liver, ed 7. Philadelphia, JB Lippincott, 1993.

Chapter 27

Hepatic Failure

Lynn Ingram

Hepatic failure is a condition in which the liver fails to function adequately, leading to many abnormalities, including faulty metabolism and excretion of bilirubin, decreased synthesis of coagulation factors, diminished glucose synthesis, and increased lactate generation (Box 27–1). These abnormalities result in jaundice, coagulopathy, hypoglycemia, and metabolic acidosis, respectively.[1] Failure occurs when liver cells cannot perform their functions because of severe injury to the hepatocytes or massive necrosis.[2]

Hepatic failure is a rare condition, occurring in approximately 2000 patients per year in the United States,[3] but it is a frequently lethal condition with a mortality rate ranging from 78% to 95%, depending on the specific cause of the failure.[4] Due to its life-threatening nature, it is imperative that liver failure be detected as early in its course as possible. The degree and duration of the failure determines the prognosis for survival.

Hepatic failure may be the result of long-term liver disease, called a *chronic* (or subacute) course, or it may be of sudden onset caused by massive liver cell destruction,[5] described as a *fulminant* (or acute) course. Chronic liver failure develops over a long period, with a progressive decrease in liver function due to a particular disease process. For a condition to be diagnosed as fulminant hepatic failure, the following three criteria must be met: (1) a lack of pre-existing liver disease, (2) the presence of encephalopathy, and (3) the development of the condition over a period of less than 8 weeks.

ETIOLOGY AND PATHOPHYSIOLOGY

Causes of liver failure can be placed into one of four categories: (1) infections; (2) poisons, chemicals, and drugs; (3) hepatic ischemia and hypoxia; and (4) metabolic anomalies[6] (Box 27–2). Infectious diseases and drugs or poisons account for the vast majority of cases of hepatic failure.

Viral hepatitis is the most common cause of hepatic failure. Hepatitis types A, B, C, D, E, and non-A, non-B have been implicated with varying degrees of frequency. Although hepatic failure is an uncommon complication of hepatitis A, 30% to 60% of patients with fulminant liver failure are positive for hepatitis B surface antigen.[6] Non-A, non-B hepatitis is the predominant cause of late-onset hepatic failure, accounting for more than 90% of cases in one study.[7] Hepatitis C is not a common cause of hepatic failure, despite the high incidence of this condition with non-A, non-B hepatitis infections. In a recent summary of four studies using tests for antibody to hepatitis C virus (anti-HCV) and hepatitis C virus (HCV) RNA, hepatitis C accounted for only 2% of cases of fulminant hepatic failure.[8] Hepatitis E infection appears to induce hepatic failure, especially in pregnant women. Rare viral causes of hepatic failure include cytomegalovirus, varicella, herpes simplex virus, and Epstein-Barr virus.

Drugs, medications, and toxins make up a second group of related causes of liver failure. Intentional acetaminophen overdose in suicide attempts is a relatively common cause of hepatic failure in Great Britain. Accidental acetaminophen toxicity is seen when therapeutic doses of acetaminophen are taken with alcohol. The synergistic effect of these two drugs is devastating to hepatocytes. Induction of hepatic failure by tetracycline, valproate, methyldopa, isoniazid, and various monoamine oxidase inhibitors is also seen. Ingestion of the poisonous mushroom, *Amanita phalloides*, is a rare example of accidental food poisoning that causes liver failure. Liver failure has also been seen in patients as a result of several exposures to halothane anesthesia and poisoning with industrial solvents, such as chlorinated hydrocarbons.

Hepatic ischemia is often caused by heat stroke; decreased blood flow to the liver, due to cardiac decompensation during surgery; drug-induced veno-occlusive disease; and Budd-Chiari syndrome. Loss of function of hepatocytes caused by a loss of blood flow, for whatever reason, may lead to hepatic failure.

Box 27–1. Functions of the Liver Affected by Hepatic Failure

Metabolic Functions

Carbohydrate metabolism
  Glycogenesis
  Glycogenolysis
  Gluconeogenesis
Lipid metabolism
  Lipoproteins
  Phospholipids
  Cholesterol
  Endogenous triglycerides
Protein metabolism
  Albumin
  Transferrin
  Haptoglobin
  Amino acids
  Coagulation factors
Vitamins
  Vitamin A from carotene

Circulatory Functions

Transfer of blood from portal to systemic circulation
Reticuloendothelial system involvement in immune responses
Regulation of blood volume

Protective, Detoxifying, Excretory Functions

Phagocytosis by Kupffer's cells
Humoral defenses
Secretion of IgA
Removal of ammonia as urea
Detoxification of drugs and steroids by conjugation, methylation, oxidation, and/or reduction
Bile formation and excretion

Hematologic Functions

Cell formation
Coagulation factor production
Production of fibrinogen, heparin, and prothrombin
Blood formation in the embryo

Storage Functions

Glycogen
Iron
Vitamins A, D, E, K, and B_{12}
Lipids
Copper

Box 27–2. Etiology of Hepatic Failure

Infections

Viral hepatitis: Types A, B, C, D, E, non-A, non-B
Cytomegalovirus
Herpes simplex virus
Yellow fever virus
Dengue fever virus
Varicella-zoster virus
Epstein-Barr virus
Coxiella burnetii bacteria
Rift Valley fever virus

Poisons, Chemicals, Drugs

Acetaminophen
Tetracycline
Methyldopa
Rifampin
Nonsteroidal anti-inflammatory drugs
Carbon tetrachloride
Tricyclic antidepressants
Sodium valproate
Allopurinol
Propylthiouracil
Amanita phalloides mushrooms
Alcohol
Phosphorus
Halothane anesthesia
Aflatoxin
Isoniazid
Monoamine oxidase inhibitors
Sulfonamides
Phenytoin

Hepatic Ischemia and Hypoxia

Heat stroke/hyperthermia
Budd-Chiari syndrome
Congestive heart failure
Pericardial tamponade
Loss of blood flow to liver
Postsurgical liver disease
Acute circulatory failure
Sepsis
Ischemic liver cell necrosis

Metabolic Anomalies

Wilson's disease
Fructosemia
Tyrosinosis
Sickle cell disease
Malignant infiltration of the liver
Primary graft nonfunction following liver transplantation
α_1-Antitrypsin deficiency
Galactosemia
Reye's syndrome
Fatty liver of pregnancy
Autoimmune chronic hepatitis

Several metabolic anomalies can lead to hepatic failure. Some of the more common disorders include Wilson's disease, Reye's syndrome, and fatty liver of pregnancy. In many such cases, the only effective treatment is liver transplantation.

CLINICAL MANIFESTATIONS

Edema

Regardless of the cause of hepatic failure, one of the more typical manifestations is edema, or fluid accumulation. Fluid, typically a transudate, may accumulate in the extremities or in the abdominal area as *ascites*. This is caused by the low oncotic pressure that results from the decrease in protein synthesis and transport (of albumin, in particular) when liver cells fail to function. Edema and ascites are reflections of both fluid and electrolyte imbalances and may predispose an individual to infection and septicemia.

Jaundice

Jaundice is frequently a presenting feature and should be looked for in the sclera and skin. Bilirubin accumulation may arise from several causes but is due primarily to the liver's failure to conjugate this substance for elimination.

Encephalopathy

As the severity of hepatic failure progresses, encephalopathy may occur. The symptoms that are associated with this condition are dependent on the grade of encephalopathy that occurs; they may range from slight tremors, to drowsiness and forgetfulness, to coma and, finally, death. Hepatic encephalopathy is a required clinical manifestation for the diagnosis of fulminant hepatic failure and is classified as one of four stages of encephalopathy.[9] Patients with stage I encephalopathy are described as generally alert with mainly neuropsychiatric disturbances and mild speech impairments. Stage II patients are drowsy and eventually respond to commands, but they are apathetic and forgetful. Marked sleepiness and mental confusion is characteristic of stage III encephalopathy, and stage IV patients are in full coma and may or may not respond to noxious stimuli. Hepatic fetor of the breath is attributed to accumulation of toxic substances and is typically associated with liver failure. Some individuals experience itching caused by the accumulation of bile salts under the skin.

Other

Other clinical manifestations of liver failure include coagulopathy and hypertension. Because several important clotting factors are synthesized in the liver, bleeding is not uncommon. Prolonged bleeding from puncture sites may occur, as may gastrointestinal hemorrhage, often resulting in death. Portal hypertension may result from bypass shunting and lowered renal function.

Hepatorenal syndrome is a condition in which renal failure results as a sequela to hepatic failure and occurs in 30% to 70% of patients.[9] The renal failure results in both oliguria and azotemia.

Pulmonary and circulatory involvement are seen in the form of hyperventilation, resulting in hypocapnia and in increased cardiac output due to a low systemic vascular resistance.[10] Table 27–1 summarizes the clinical indications of hepatic failure and the major causes of each.

Table 27–1. Clinical Indications of Hepatic Failure and Their Causes

Condition	Cause(s)
Hypoglycemia	Faulty gluconeogenesis and increased circulating insulin concentrations
Jaundice	Accumulation of bilirubin
Infection	Neutrophil adherence is decreased, contributing to the high infection rate
Electrolyte imbalance	Hyponatremia is a reflection of the fluid imbalance that occurs due to lowered oncotic pressure, and hypokalemia results from intestinal loss of fluid
Acid/base abnormalities	Massive hepatic necrosis complicated by hypotension and hypoxemia causes lactic acid to accumulate, causing metabolic acidosis; inadequate ventilation adds a respiratory component; hypokalemia and hyperventilation cause alkalosis
Edema/ascites	Hypoalbuminemia causes low oncotic pressure that leads to fluid imbalance and the formation of a transudate
Coagulopathy	Factors I, II, V, VII, IX, and X are not being synthesized at an effective rate by the liver; platelets are being destroyed by the spleen or production is reduced due to bone marrow suppression
Encephalopathy	Toxic accumulation of ammonia, amines, bile salts, and other wastes leads to central nervous system involvement
Cerebral edema	Cellular alterations allow increased uptake of water into brain cells
Hypotension	Hypovolemia from inadequate fluid therapy or hemorrhage; sepsis and cardiopulmonary dysfunction also contribute

Infections

Neutrophil adherence is decreased in hepatic failure, and it has been suggested that this is a contributing factor to the high infection rate. Infection develops in as many as 80% of patients with hepatic failure.[1] Pulmonary, kidney, and blood infections are common, and they must be monitored carefully, with repeated cultures, for early diagnosis and appropriate treatment. *Staphylococcus aureus* is the most common bacterial isolate, but streptococci and gram-negative bacilli are also seen. Fungal infections are also common, with most cases being attributed to *Candida albicans*.

LABORATORY ANALYSES AND DIAGNOSIS

Because of the severe and complex nature of hepatic failure, the laboratory plays a comprehensive and vital role in its diagnosis and treatment. Although individuals do not always respond alike to similar disease processes, particular laboratory findings are representative of hepatic failure. Generally, the degree of the laboratory test abnormality will reflect the degree of liver failure (Box 27–3).

Bilirubin Assays

Plasma and urine bilirubin levels are frequently elevated and may be the presenting features. An elevated bilirubin

Box 27–3. Expected Laboratory Results in Hepatic Failure

Clinical Chemistry

Routine Testing
Increased total bilirubin
Increased conjugated bilirubin
Increased unconjugated bilirubin
Decreased glucose
Decreased cholesterol
Decreased albumin
Increased creatinine
Increased uric acid
Decreased sodium
Decreased potassium
Decreased calcium
Decreased magnesium
Increased lactic acid
Increased plasma bile acids
Increased ammonia
Increased or decreased pH
Decreased PaO_2
Enzyme Testing
Increased alanine aminotransferase
Increased aspartate aminotransferase
Increased γ-glutamyl transferase
Increased alkaline phosphatase
Increased lactate dehydrogenase
Increased 5′-nucleotidase

Hematology

Decreased fibrinogen
Decreased prothrombin
Decreased factors V, VII, IX, X
Decreased antithrombin III
Decreased platelet count
Decreased platelet aggregation

Microbiology

Increased incidence of bacterial and fungal infections, especially of the blood, lungs, and kidney

Immunology

The presence of viral hepatitis markers depends on a viral source, such as the following:
Hepatitis A virus (HAV)
Antibody to hepatitis A virus (anti-HAV), immunoglobulin M (IgM)
Hepatitis B surface antigen (HB_sAg)
Hepatitis B core antigen (HB_cAg)
Hepatitis B early antigen (HB_eAg)
Antibody to hepatitis B surface antigen (anti-HB_s)
Antibody to hepatitis B core antigen (anti-HB_c) IgM
Antibody to hepatitis B early antigen (anti-HB_e)
Hepatitis C virus (HCV)
Antibody to hepatitis C virus (anti-HCV)
Antibody to hepatitis D virus (anti-HDV)
Hepatitis E virus (HEV)

---

concentration is not in itself diagnostic of liver failure, but it is strong evidence that the hepatocytes are not functioning normally. Typically, the unconjugated fraction of bilirubin is elevated to a greater degree than is the conjugated fraction. Urine bilirubin often becomes detectable before the appearance of jaundice.[11] Initially, urine urobilinogen levels may be decreased or normal because less conjugated bilirubin is available for conversion in the intestinal tract; however, as the disease progresses, the levels of urobilinogen may become elevated.

Enzymes

Several enzymes have been used as liver disease markers. These enzymes are normally present in the liver, and their levels of activity are affected by the presence of disease. Four enzymes frequently monitored in liver disease include alkaline phosphatase (ALP), aspartate aminotransferase (AST), alanine aminotransferase (ALT), and γ-glutamyl-transferase (GGT). ALP levels show a greater degree of elevation in obstruction and liver metastasis than with intrinsic liver diseases, whereas AST and ALT levels show greater elevation in hepatocyte injury than in obstruction. In the presence of hepatic failure, all three serum enzyme levels are elevated during the early course of the disease, although ALP levels may be elevated only moderately. Each of these enzymes will eventually return to normal levels, either as the condition improves or as the liver cell injury becomes massive and virtually complete. GGT is a very sensitive indicator of hepatocyte toxicity and is elevated in alcohol and drug abusers. It is also significantly elevated in liver failure.

Miscellaneous Laboratory Assays

Plasma levels of bile acids have been found elevated in hepatic failure, and it is believed that measuring the rate of clearance of free bile acids, such as cholic acid, can be helpful in predicting the likelihood of survival for individuals who have reached stage IV encephalopathy.[12] In one study, it was found that a higher survival rate was likely for persons who had a faster clearance rate of injected carbon-14 (^{14}C) cholic acid from plasma than for those with a prolonged rate of clearance.[13]

Because its half-life is 21 days, the concentration of serum albumin may be slow to fall in a patient with liver failure; therefore, albumin is not a reliable indicator of hepatic protein synthesis in acute liver disease.[14] Cholesterol, which is synthesized in the liver, may also be found in decreased amounts in the plasma.

Typically, hypoglycemia is present, and hyponatremia and hypokalemia are often observed. Defective gluconeogenesis in a diseased liver and increased concentrations of circulating insulin may lead to hypoglycemia. It is believed that hyponatremia is a reflection of hemodilution and failure of the sodium pump, and hypokalemia results from intestinal loss of fluid.[6]

The single most important diagnostic hematologic test for hepatic failure is the prothrombin time. Unlike enzyme and albumin levels, results of the prothrombin time can be used to judge the progress of the hepatic failure because the degree of liver failure parallels the degree of prolongation of the prothrombin time.[14] It is for this reason that serial measurements of prothrombin time are usually recommended. The half-life of the coagulation factors is relatively short (about 7 days), and a decrease in synthesis manifests early in the course of the disease. The partial thromboplastin time may also be prolonged.

Miscellaneous Diagnostic Tests

An additional aid in the diagnosis of hepatic failure is the use of nuclear medicine technology. Colloid liver scans can aid in the confirmation and detection of abnormal liver and spleen size and in the location of abnormal growths or abscesses. Ultrasounds can serve a similar purpose, with the added benefit of avoiding radiation exposure to the patient. Because interpretations of the results of these two procedures can be difficult, a more costly, but perhaps more informative, procedure is computed tomography (CT). Liver biopsy may be necessary to ascertain the exact etiology of liver failure, but it must be approached with caution in a patient with severe bleeding problems.

Brain involvement in hepatic failure may be assessed by electroencephalography (EEG), and serial measurements can aid in monitoring the progress of encephalopathy.

Follow-Up Testing

Once the presence of hepatic failure has been established, it will be of the utmost importance to monitor the life-threatening complications that may follow. Hypokalemia should be monitored closely and corrected as soon as possible because it could be a precipitating factor for coma if allowed to fall to critical concentrations. If sodium is only being measured in plasma, the results should be interpreted with the understanding that the values attained may be a reflection of hemodilution. In this condition, urinary sodium is typically decreased below normal levels, and a 24-hour collection for analysis is recommended. Increased creatinine levels and decreased urinary output are associated with hepatorenal syndrome and should be monitored to aid in its detection. Urea production by the liver may be decreased, so the urea nitrogen concentration may not be pronounced in patients with liver failure.[4]

Ascitic fluid may be withdrawn for its identification as a transudate or exudate; however, this procedure may compromise the patient's condition and should be done only if necessary.

Although ammonia levels are difficult to interpret because of problems with standardization and collection, they may be helpful as a measure of toxic waste accumulation.

Blood gas analyses are helpful in assessing the presence of alkalosis or acidosis, which are common findings in hepatic failure. Alkalosis has been associated with reduced cerebral perfusion and lowered oxygen consumption, which may contribute to encephalopathy in the patient.[5]

Because bleeding is a frequent complication, it may be necessary to monitor the hemoglobin and hematocrit levels to determine whether blood replacement therapy is needed, and whether a hemorrhagic protein overload, which can in turn contribute to hepatic encephalopathy, has occurred. Laboratory tests that assess coagulation factors should be closely monitored because all clotting factor concentra-

tions, except for factor VIII, are decreased in patients with hepatic failure.[10]

TREATMENT

The ultimate goal of treatment is to cure the hepatic failure and to return the liver function to normal, although with conventional medical treatment alone only about 20% of patients can be expected to survive.[9] Few effective treatments are available for hepatic failure. Most specific treatments have been aimed at reducing the toxic load or at promoting hepatocyte regeneration (Box 27–4).[7] Insulin and glucagon have been used to promote regeneration of the liver and in one study showed an increase in survival from 14.4% to 22.6%.[7] Prostaglandin administration and charcoal hemoperfusion have been used to reduce circulating hepatotoxins.

Due to the high mortality rate of hepatic failure, treatment plans usually follow three basic strategies. The first is to correct or remove the primary cause of the hepatic failure. Drugs or other toxic agents can be removed by the use of antidotes, when they are available; by perfusion; or, less commonly, by repeated plasmapheresis. To be success-

---

Box 27–4. Therapies for Hepatic Failure

Used to Promote Hepatocyte Regeneration

Insulin and glucagon infusions
Balanced amino acid infusions
Putrescine administration

Reduction of Toxic Load

Charcoal hemoperfusion
Hemodialysis
Antidotes to specific drugs or toxins, if available
Use of appropriate antibiotics for infections
Prostacyclin hemoperfusion
Prostaglandin administration
Plasmapheresis
Exchange transfusions

Treatments for Specific Conditions

Penicillamine chelation for Wilson's disease
Use of concentrates for α_1-antitrypsin deficiencies
N-acetylcysteine treatment for acetaminophen toxicity
Administration of cimetidine/vitamin K for gastrointestinal bleeding

Artificial Hepatic Supports*

Hepatocyte transplantation
Enzyme therapy
Artificial liver of cultured liver cells
Liver cytosol infusion
Extracorporeal perfusion devices

Liver Transplantation

*Currently experimental therapies.

ful, measures aimed at removing the toxic substances should be instigated shortly after their identification. Infection, a primary cause of hepatic failure, may respond to specific treatment. Antibiotics should be used only when needed to treat an infection and should not be used prophylactically. However, neomycin may be given prophylactically to reduce the urea-splitting bacteria of the gut. It is believed by some investigators, although it has not been proven, that reducing the numbers of these bacteria aids in the prevention of coma. Specific treatments for α_1-antitrypsin deficiency and Wilson's disease may also reverse hepatic failure caused by these conditions. An acetaminophen overdose can be treated with *N*-acetylcysteine. Although the mechanism for its action is not entirely known, it is postulated that *N*-acetylcysteine either detoxifies acetaminophen directly or increases the levels of hepatic glutathione, which indirectly detoxifies acetaminophen.[15] Patients who exhibit renal and liver dysfunction may require hemodialysis to prevent irreversible renal failure.

In viral hepatitis, which has no specific treatment, the second strategy of liver failure treatment, supportive care, is important. The goal of supportive care is to gain time for the liver to regenerate. Because a common feature of hepatic failure is hypokalemia and fluid imbalance, potassium-sparing diuretics are often administered. Potassium supplements may also be given when laboratory data indicate that this is necessary. Sodium intake should be restricted in the presence of edema or ascites to avoid aggravating these conditions. A diet low in protein has been recommended as a further measure against precipitating encephalopathy.[16]

Gastrointestinal bleeding may be prevented by the prophylactic administration of cimetidine, which may be given orally or by intravenous infusion. Vitamin K administration has also proven useful. In the event that disseminated intravascular coagulation develops, subcutaneous heparin may be given, or plasmapheresis with replacement fresh-frozen plasma may be attempted.[4] Temporary relief can be attained by transfusing platelet concentrates.

In persons with the potential for liver regeneration, several measures have been suggested to enhance the process. Infusions that have been suggested to increase hepatocyte regeneration include glucose, insulin, and glucagon.[9] Regeneration can be monitored by serial α-fetoprotein levels and by other liver function tests, such as prothrombin time and transaminase levels.

Any or all of these supportive measures may be used until the liver regenerates or transplantation, the third treatment strategy, can be undertaken. In persons who fail to improve with time, liver transplantation may be the ultimate recourse. The successful use of orthotopic liver transplantation in fulminant hepatic failure has had the single greatest impact on the management of this condition, with survival rates ranging from 50% to 72%.[7] The success rate of this treatment is dependent on the appropriate selection of suitable candidates. Unfortunately, one third to one half of liver failure patients die awaiting a donor liver for transplantation.[9]

Currently available therapies for hepatic failure are not entirely satisfactory, as mortality rates remain high. Artificial liver support mechanisms have attracted much interest as a means of supporting and maintaining patients until

hepatic recovery or a donor organ becomes available.[17] Hepatocyte transplantation (creation of an artificial liver using cultured liver cells) liver cytosol infusion, enzyme therapies, and improved extracorporeal perfusion devices are being investigated as possible treatments, but until the mechanisms of liver failure and hepatocyte regeneration are better understood, it is likely that liver transplantation will continue to be the only effective treatment.[18] Hepatotrophic factors such as epidermal growth factor, transforming growth factor α, and human hepatocyte growth factor are also being considered as potential therapeutic agents.

Complete restoration of normal hepatic function usually occurs in survivors of hepatic failure, even if they have been in deep coma and have had massive hepatocellular necrosis. Typically, with survival, the results of liver function tests and the histologic features of the liver return to normal 45 to 75 days after the onset of the process.[6] Figure 27–1 presents one algorithm used to manage fulminant hepatic failure.

Case Study

A 43-year-old man, exhibiting disorientation and agitation, was brought to the emergency room after complaining of severe abdominal pain, diarrhea, and vomiting. The patient had been on a camping trip 3 days prior to becoming ill. Physical examination revealed slight hepatomegaly. Admission laboratory results were as follows:

	Values	Reference Ranges
Hemoglobin (g/dL)	12.9	(14–17.7)
Hematocrit (%)	36	(42–53)
Prothrombin time (sec)	34.2	(16–18)
Partial thromboplastin time (sec)	42	(30–50)
Blood urea nitrogen (BUN) (mg/dL)	6	(8–26)
Creatinine (mg/dL)	0.9	(0.6–1.2)
Glucose (mg/dL)	161	(70–105)
Albumin (g/dL)	3.2	(3.4–5.0)
AST (IU/L)	16,648	(8–22)
ALT (IU/L)	9844	(8–30)
Total bilirubin (mg/dL)	2.3	(<1.0)
Arterial pH	7.15	(7.35–7.45)
Arterial carbon dioxide partial pressure (Paco$_2$) (mm Hg)	30	(35–45)
Serum bicarbonate (mEq/L)	12	(22–28)
Arterial oxygen partial pressure (Pao$_2$) (mm Hg)	124	(80–90)

The patient's condition deteriorated over the next 48 hours. Renal function was greatly reduced with creatinine values rising to 5.3 mg/dL. The hematocrit dropped to 30% as a result of gastrointestinal bleeding. Liver function progressively worsened as the total bilirubin concentrations increased to 11.3 mg/dL and ALT activ-

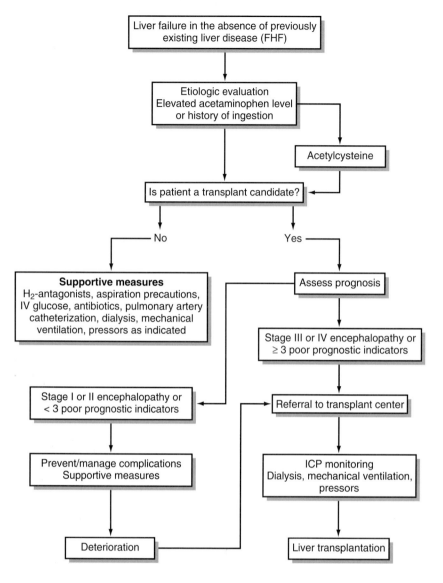

Figure 27–1. Algorithm for managing patients with fulminant hepatic failure. Abbreviations: ICP, intracranial pressure; IV, intravenous. (Adapted from Reigler JL, Lake JR: Fulminant hepatic failure. Med Clin North Am 77:1070, 1993.)

ity increased to 14,365 IU/L. The patient fell into a stage III coma, and mechanical ventilation and peritoneal dialysis were undertaken. The extent of the liver failure prompted a decision to perform transplant as soon as possible. Orthotopic liver transplantation was performed 5 days after admission. Histologic examination of the patient's liver showed virtually no viable hepatocytes and massive intraparenchymal hemorrhage. Extensive interviews with the patient's camping partners revealed that he had eaten several wild mushrooms consistent with photographs of the *Amanita* species.

Questions

1. Is *Amanita* mushroom poisoning a reasonable diagnosis for this patient?

2. Is there a specific laboratory result that would confirm this diagnosis?

3. Is there an alternative therapy to liver transplantation for this patient's condition?

4. Do you expect the renal failure and encephalopathy to resolve after transplantation?

Discussion

1. Yes, the patient's history revealed the opportunity for ingestion of these mushrooms, and the *Amanita* species is a potent hepatorenal toxin. It is known for being a most toxic mushroom and is responsible for the majority of the fatal mushroom poisonings in the United States. His symptoms, laboratory results, and clinical course are consistent with this diagnosis.

2. No, there are no chemical or serologic tests for myxotoxins that detect these substances. Diagnostic spores from the mushroom may be present in the gastric and intestinal contents early in the course of illness, but severe diarrhea and vomiting will make the likelihood of finding them remote.

3. No, orthotopic liver transplantation is the only effective treatment for *Amanita* poisoning. The mush-

rooms cause such severe liver and other organ damage that the patient cannot recover with other treatments.

4. Yes, this patient's mental condition improved significantly after transplantation, and renal function returned to normal after 2 weeks of continued peritoneal renal dialysis.

References

1. Lidofsky SD: Fulminant hepatic failure. Crit Care Clin 11:415–430, 1995.
2. Lee WM: Acute liver failure. N Engl J Med 329:1862–1872, 1993.
3. Hoofnagle JH, Carithers RL Jr, Shapiro C, et al: Fulminant hepatic failure: Summary of a workshop. Hepatology 21:240–252, 1995.
4. Fingerote RJ, Bain VG: Fulminant hepatic failure. Am J Gastroenterol 88:1000–1010, 1993.
5. Hetzel DJ: Fulminant hepatic failure. Anaesth Intensive Care 13:272–282, 1985.
6. Jones EA, Schafer DF: Fulminant hepatic failure. *In* Zakim TD, Boyer D (eds): Hepatology: A Textbook of Liver Disease, vol 1, ed 2. Philadelphia, WB Saunders, 1990.
7. O'Grady JG, Portmann B, Williams R: Fulminant hepatic failure. *In* Schiff L, Schiff ER (eds): Diseases of the Liver, ed 7. Philadelphia, JB Lippincott, 1993, pp 1077–1090.
8. Wright TL: Etiology of fulminant hepatic failure: Is another virus involved? Gastroenterology 104:648–653, 1993.
9. Reigler JL, Lake JR: Fulminant hepatic failure. Med Clin North Am 77:1057–1083, 1993.
10. Yanda RJ: Fulminant hepatic failure: Medical staff conference. West J Med 149:586–591, 1988.
11. Petersdorf RG, Adams RD, Braunwald E, et al (eds): Harrison's Principles of Internal Medicine, ed 10. New York, McGraw-Hill, 1983, pp 1771–1789.
12. Bremmelgaard A, Ranek L, Bahnsen M, et al: Cholic acid conjugation test and quantitative liver function in acute liver failure. Scand J Gastroenterol 18:797–802, 1983.
13. Horak W, Waldran R, Murray-Lyon IM, et al: Kinetics of [^{14}C] cholic acid in fulminant hepatic failure: A prognostic test. Gastroenterology 71:809–813, 1976.
14. Stolz A, Kaplowitz N: Biochemical tests for liver disease. *In* Zakim TD, Boyer D (eds): Hepatology: A Textbook of Liver Disease, vol I, ed 2. Philadelphia, WB Saunders, 1990, pp 637–667.
15. Hinson JA, Pohl LR, Monks TJ, et al: Minireview: Acetaminophen-induced hepatotoxicity. Life Sci 29:107–116, 1981.
16. Barber JR, Teasley KM: Nutritional support of patients with severe hepatic failure. Clin Pharmacol 3:245–251, 1984.
17. Kirsh BM, Lam N, Layden TJ, et al: Diagnosis and management of fulminant hepatic failure. Compr Ther 21:166–171, 1995.
18. Katelaris PH, Jones DB: Fulminant hepatic failure. Med Clin North Am 73:955–970, 1989.

Chapter 28

Cholestasis

James A. Jackson

Cholestasis is a clinical and biochemical syndrome that occurs whenever bile salts and bilirubin accumulate in the blood because of failure to reach the intestinal tract. The impairment of bile flow or blockage may occur at any point from the liver cell canaliculus to the entrance of the common bile duct (Fig. 28–1).

ETIOLOGY AND PATHOPHYSIOLOGY

As Box 28–1 indicates, the etiology of cholestasis can be either intrahepatic or extrahepatic. The more common causes of *intrahepatic* cholestasis are viral hepatitis and drug- or alcohol-induced liver disease. A stone in the bile

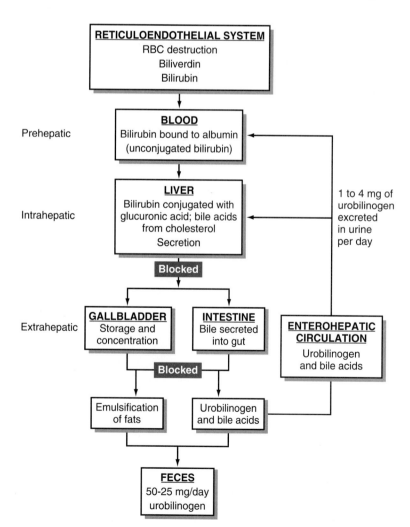

Figure 28–1. Formation and flow of bilirubin and bile acids. Intrahepatic and extrahepatic cholestasis formed at sites shown as blocked. Abbreviation: RBC, red blood cell.

Box 28–1. Etiology of Cholestasis

Intrahepatic—Liver Cell Damage and/or Blockage of Bile Canaliculi

- Drugs or chemical toxins
- Dubin-Johnson syndrome
- Estrogens or pregnancy
- Hepatitis—viral, chemical
- Infiltrative tumors
- Intrahepatic biliary hypoplasia or atresia
- Primary biliary cirrhosis

Extrahepatic—Obstruction of Bile Ducts

- Compression obstruction from tumors
- Congenital choledochal cyst
- Extrahepatic·biliary atresia
- Intraluminal gallstones
- Stenosis—postoperative or inflammatory

duct and pancreatic cancer are more common causes of the *extrahepatic* type. In addition, cholestasis may occur in the third trimester of pregnancy in patients who have an idiosyncratic response to estrogens that causes a slight disruption in bile transport. The condition disappears after delivery.

When normal draining of bile into the intestine is completely blocked or substantially reduced, bile backs up into the liver as cholestasis progresses. As the bile canaliculi become congested with bile, they tend to enlarge and eventually rupture.[1] This results in escape of bilirubin and bile salts directly into the blood (Fig. 28–1). The initial influx of bilirubin is of the conjugated type, which will start to appear in the urine. Eventually, as uptake of bilirubin by the hepatic cells declines, unconjugated bilirubin also increases in the blood, giving a mixed hyperbilirubinemia. About 75% of hyperbilirubinemia results from conjugated bilirubin.[1] If the obstruction is complete, the feces will be gray (the so-called clay-colored stools), as a result both of the lack of bile pigment (urobilinogen) and of increased fat content in the feces.

Fat malabsorption results from the lack of bile's emulsifying action in the intestine. Fat emulsification and adsorption may be diminished to about half of normal levels, causing *steatorrhea* (fat in the stools) and interference with the absorption of fat-soluble vitamins (A, D, E, K) and calcium. Vitamin K, which depends on bile salts for its absorption, is required for normal liver synthesis of various clotting factors. If cholestasis persists, bleeding problems may occur, with an increase in the prothrombin time. Malabsorption of vitamin D and calcium may lead to osteoporosis and bone pain.[1]

CLINICAL MANIFESTATIONS

A patient with jaundice, pruritus (itching), persistently pale stools, positive urine bilirubin, and negative urobilinogen should be evaluated for cholestasis. The onset of jaundice in patients with cholestasis is slow, occurring over days rather than hours.[2] Although the exact etiology of pruritus is unknown, it is thought to be associated with the high levels of bile acids in the blood moving to the peripheral tissues. Unrelieved pruritus of cholestasis can interfere with normal activities and may lead to sleep deprivation and even suicidal ideation.[3] Pain and fever, if present, may indicate an extrahepatic cause, usually gallstones.[2] Another characteristic of prolonged cholestasis is hypercholesterolemia, which may result in fatty tumors or *xanthomas*.

LABORATORY ANALYSES AND DIAGNOSIS

Procedures for determining the etiology of cholestasis are performed in the nuclear medicine and radiology departments as well as by the clinical laboratory. Some of the imaging modalities available are intravenous cholangiography, infusion tomography, ultrasound, and cholescintigraphy with technetium Tc 99m iminodiacetic acid (^{99m}Tc-IDA) or its analog, technetium Tc 99m hepatoiminodiacetic acid (^{99m}Tc-HIDA). In cholestasis, the best initial diagnostic imaging procedure for evaluating the jaundiced patient is ultrasound, which can pinpoint ductal dilation with a high degree of accuracy and can often determine the level and cause of obstruction.[4]

The clinical laboratory is involved early in the diagnosis of cholestasis with tests listed in Table 28–1. In biliary obstruction, jaundice is present when the serum bilirubin exceeds approximately 4 mg/dL.[4] The enzymes alkaline phosphatase (ALP) and γ-glutamyl transferase (GGT) are both helpful in identifying cholestasis, because they are located on the surface of cell membranes bordering bile canaliculi and liver sinusoids (ALP)[1, 5] and membranes of the bile canaliculi and epithelial cells of the bile ducts (GGT).[1, 6]

γ-Glutamyl transferase is usually most significantly elevated (more than five times the reference range) by obstructive or biliary diseases, has good specificity for the liver, and is not elevated in bone disease or pregnancy (as is ALP) or in skeletal muscle disease (as is aspartate transaminase [AST]). GGT can also help to differentiate mechanical and viral from drug-induced cholestasis. In mechanical and viral cholestasis, GGT and ALP are about equally elevated, whereas in drug-induced cholestasis, GGT is increased more significantly than ALP.[1, 6] GGT is an induc-

Table 28–1. Diagnostic Hepatic Panel

Component	Reference Ranges*
ALP	35–100 U/L
ALT	8–30 U/L 30°C
AST	8–22 U/L 30°C
GGT	5–45 U/L
Total bilirubin	0.2–1 mg/dL
Conjugated (direct) bilirubin	0–0.2 mg/dL
Prothrombin time	11–15 sec
Total protein	6.4–8.3 g/dL
Albumin	3.5–5 g/dL
Urine bilirubin	Negative
Urobilinogen	0.2–1 EU

*May vary depending on methodology used, patient population, etc.
Abbreviations: ALP, alkaline phosphatase; ALT, alanine aminotransferase; AST, aspartate transaminase; GGT, γ-glutamyl transferase.

ible liver enzyme, however, and elevated serum GGT may be found in patients who take such medications as phenobarbital and phenytoin on a long-term basis (e.g., for treatment of epilepsy) or who abuse alcohol. A patient's overall history must be considered in the evaluation of elevated GGT values.

The alkaline phosphatase value, although increased in conditions other than cholestasis, is still one of the tools of choice for evaluating cholestasis and obstructive jaundice. ALP is only modestly increased in parenchymal damage—such as in hepatitis (intrahepatic) with cholestasis, in which ALP levels are rarely higher than twice the upper reference limits for adults. In disease or damage to the ducts (extrahepatic) with cholestasis, ALP levels may be two to four times the normal reference range for adults.[5]

A simple but important diagnostic procedure that is often overlooked is the urinalysis test. The urine color may range from dark amber to brown-orange. A fresh urine specimen (less than a half-hour old) should be analyzed for bilirubin. A fresh specimen is necessary, because prolonged exposure to light and water converts the conjugated bilirubuin to free bilirubin and/or biliverdin, both of which are nonreactive to urine dipsticks.[7] Urine bilirubin testing should be positive owing to the presence of conjugated bilirubin. Urine urobilinogen testing should be negative. It is important to remember that urine dipsticks cannot detect the absence of urobilinogen, they can only detect normal or elevated levels.[7] Only by using a quantitative chemical test (2-hour or 24-hour collection) is it possible to determine true absence of urobilinogen.

Prothrombin times are increased and the patient exhibits bleeding tendencies if cholestasis is prolonged, mainly because of malabsorption of fats and vitamin K.

Markedly increased serum transaminase levels suggest an intrahepatic or hepatocellular cholestasis but may also be seen in extrahepatic cholestasis with acute obstruction due to common bile duct stones. Elevated serum amylase levels usually indicate extrahepatic obstruction from the head of the pancreas. If the diagnosis is still in doubt, a liver biopsy may be necessary.

TREATMENT

Because cholestasis is a syndrome of blockage of the flow of bilirubin and bile acids, treatment of the underlying disease(s) will resolve the cholestasis. A gallstone, for example, generally requires surgical intervention. The practical problem in cholestasis is to determine at what level in the hepatobiliary system the block has occurred,[8] because the location determines the type of treatment. If the block is in the hepatic ducts (usually distal to the bifurcation), surgical intervention may be necessary. If the block is at the level of the liver cell or the canaliculi, surgical intervention is not possible.

Pruritus may respond to cholestyramine, a resin-like substance given orally that binds bile salts in the intestine. Opiate antagonists, such as naloxone have also been shown to relieve pruritus. The best treatment is to remove the cause of the cholestasis. Intractable pruritus associated with liver disease may be an indication for liver transplant.[3]

Supplements of calcium and the fat-soluble vitamins (A, D, E, and K) supplements may be given as needed.

Malabsorption and steatorrhea should disappear as bile flow to the intestine is restored. Urobilinogen also reappears in the urine, bilirubin disappears, and stool color returns to normal.

Case Study 1

A 68-year-old white male was admitted to the hospital with jaundice, stomach pain, "dark urine," itching of the skin, and a rapid weight loss of 21 lb. There was no history of alcohol or drug abuse.

Laboratory studies revealed the following data (with reference ranges):

CBC:	"Within normal limits"
Total bilirubin:	14 mg/dL (0.2–1.0 mg/dL)
GGT:	300 U/L (5–45 U/L)
ALP:	360 U/L (35–100 U/L)
AST:	80 U/L (8–22 U/L)
ALT:	75 U/L (8–30 U/L)
Urinalysis:	Positive bilirubin; "normal urobilinogen" on dipstick (negative bilirubin)
Serum amylase:	Elevated

Ultrasonography and computed tomography of the liver revealed a blocked bile duct and a pancreatic mass.

Questions

1. What is the most probable diagnosis for this patient? Why?
2. Which laboratory tests provided the most information, and which provided the least?

Discussion

1. The most probable diagnosis in this patient is cholestasis caused by a blockage of the common bile duct by some type of tumor, because of imaging tests showing a pancreatic mass, the patient's symptoms, and laboratory tests indicating a biliary obstruction. At surgery, a large tumor mass involving the head of the pancreas, bile duct, stomach, and duodenum was observed. The pathology report showed a grade 1 adenocarcinoma of the pancreas with metastasis.
2. All the laboratory tests, with the exception of the CBC, were helpful. The GGT was elevated more than five times the upper reference limit, which is a sensitive indicator of biliary tract disease (sensitivity of 85% to 93% for cholestasis). The ALP level was four times the upper reference, also indicating disease of the biliary system; levels two to four times normal would indicate intrahepatic parenchymal damage. The results of the total bilirubin and urine bilirubin tests and the presence of jaundice also help in the diagnosis of cholestasis. The elevated amylase value indicated pancreatic involvement.

Case History 2

A 38-year-old white female was seen in the emergency department and admitted to the hospital with jaundice, right upper quadrant abdominal pain, nausea, vomiting, and itching skin. She had a history of intravenous drug use and alcohol abuse. Laboratory data showed an elevated total bilirubin (8.0 mg/dL) with a conjugated bilirubin (direct reading) of 6.0 mg/dL. The urine was orange-brown with a 3+ bilirubin reading and "normal" urobilinogen using Ames N-Multistix. The serum ALP was one and one-half times the upper reference range, and the GGT was three times the upper reference range. Serum transaminase levels were markedly increased, at five times the upper reference range. There were modest increases in serum cholesterol and triglyceride levels.

Questions

1. What is the probable diagnosis for this patient? Why?
2. What other laboratory test would you recommend to confirm this diagnosis?
3. Which laboratory tests ordered provided the most information? Why?

Discussion

1. The patient probably has cholestasis of the intrahepatic type, caused by a viral hepatitis. The jaundice and itching of the skin indicate cholestasis. The GGT level was less than five times normal and the ALP less than two times normal, and the transaminases were markedly increased. All of these findings suggest parenchymal cell damage or intrahepatic disease. The positive urine bilirubin reading confirmed liver disease with jaundice due to conjugated bilirubin.
2. The history of intravenous drug use suggests that the hepatitis is of the viral type. A test for the hepatitis B surface antigen (Hb$_s$Ag) and other tests for hepatitis B and C should be performed.
3. All tests were of value in identifying the cholestasis in this patient as the intrahepatic type. In intrahepatic cholestasis, the GGT is less than five times the upper reference range, the ALP is less than two to four times the upper reference range, and the transaminases are greatly elevated. The elevated total and direct bilirubin values and urine bilirubin reading confirmed jaundice and liver disease.

References

1. Ingram LR: Liver function. *In* Anderson SC, Cockayne S (eds): Clinical Chemistry: Concepts and Applications. Philadelphia, WB Saunders, 1993.
2. Sherlock S: Jaundice—the first 48 hours. Practitioner 266:1017, 1992.
3. Bergasa NV, Jones EA: The pruritus of cholestasis: Potential pathogenic and therapeutic implications of opioids. Gastroenterology 108:1582, 1995.
4. Hulse PA, Nicholson DA: Investigation of biliary obstruction. Br J Hosp Med 52:103, 1994.
5. Batsakis JG: Serum alkaline phosphatase: Refining an old test for the future. Diagn Med 5:25, 1982.
6. Shaw LM: Keeping pace with a popular enzyme. Diagn Med 5:59, 1982.
7. Jackson JA, Conrad ME: Technical aspects of urine dipstick reagent areas. Am Clin Prod Rev 12:10, 1985.
8. Pasanen P, Pikkarainen E, Alhava E, et al: Value of serum alkaline phosphatase, aminotransferases, gammaglutamyl transferase, leucine aminopeptidase, and bilirubin in the distinction between benign and malignant diseases causing jaundice and cholestasis: Result from a prospective study. Scand J Clin Lab Invest 53:35, 1993.

Endocrine Disorders

Chapter 29

Thyroid Disorders

Shauna C. Anderson

The thyroid is a large, bilobed gland, weighing between 15 and 25 grams, and located in the lower portion of the neck lying over the trachea just below the larynx. The two lobes of the thyroid are connected by a narrow area known as the *isthmus*. A normal thyroid gland may be somewhat asymmetric, with the right lobe slightly larger than the left.

Two types of cells are found in the thyroid: the follicular cells and the parafollicular or C cells. The follicular cells are components of the functional unit of the thyroid, called a *follicle*. Follicular cells are cuboidal cells arranged in a sphere situated on a basement membrane and enclosing an inner lumen filled with a material called *colloid*. Colloid is an amorphous material composed of an iodinated glycoprotein, thyroglobulin, and small amounts of an iodinated albumin, thyroalbumin. The colloid serves as an extracellular storage site for the thyroid hormones, and the follicular cells are responsible for the manufacture and secretion of the thyroid hormones. The parafollicular cells are situated among the follicles. They are responsible for the secretion of calcitonin, which is involved in the regulation of serum calcium levels.

It is essential to understand the regulatory mechanism of the thyroid gland secretion in order to interpret thyroid function test results properly. The regulation of thyroid hormone production begins with the hypothalamus. The hypothalamus releases a tripeptide known as thyroid-releasing hormone (TRH). This hormone travels along the hypothalamic stalk to the thyrotropic cells of the anterior pituitary, where it stimulates the synthesis and release of thyroid-stimulating hormone (TSH).

TSH is a glycoprotein consisting of two subunits, alpha and beta, which are linked. The specificity of the hormone activity is conveyed by the beta subunit, which is unique. The alpha subunit provides the shape of the molecule and is identical to the alpha subunit found in luteinizing hormone (LH), follicle-stimulating hormone (FSH), and human chorionic gonadotropin (hCG). The overall shape of the molecule allows it to bind to a receptor on the outer membrane of the thyroid follicular cells. When TSH binds to this receptor, adenylate cyclase is activated through a G protein. Adenylate cyclase in turn catalyzes a reaction that produces cyclic adenosine monophosphate (cAMP), the second messenger responsible for cell action. TSH is the main stimulus for the uptake of iodide from the blood by the thyroid gland. It also stimulates the activation of the protease enzymes, which in turn catalyze the hydrolysis of the thyroglobulins. The secretion of TSH is regulated not only by TRH but also by the levels of circulating free thyroxine (T_4) and triiodothyronine (T_3). Free T_3 levels appear to be primarily responsible for decreasing the TSH release and also reducing the responsiveness of the thyrotropic cells of the pituitary to TRH. Higher levels of norepinephrine, estrogens, and stress may actually raise TRH levels. On the contrary, increased levels of somatostatin, growth hormone, dopamine, glucocorticoids, and opiates inhibit either the release of TRH or the response of TSH to TRH. Refer to Figure 29–1 for a summary of thyroid regulation.

The main components needed for the synthesis of the thyroid hormones are tyrosine and iodide. Both of these substances are taken up from the blood by the follicular cells. The iodide is trapped at the base of the follicular cells and is then actively transported into the cell. This step is competitively opposed by inorganic ions such as thiocyanate and perchlorate. The inorganic iodide molecule is oxidized to a more reactive organic form. This reaction is mediated by a peroxidase that resides at the interface of the cell and the lumen. The reactive oxidized iodide finally reaches the colloid. All steps of thyroid hormone synthesis take place on the thyroglobulin molecules within the colloid. The iodide ion is incorporated into the hydroxyl residues of tyrosine to form monoiodotyrosine (MIT) and diiodotyrosine (DIT). Utilizing the same peroxidase, enzymatic coupling of iodinate tyrosine molecules occurs to form T_4 and T_3. Propylthiouracil and methimazole inhibit the peroxidase enzymes and thus the oxidation of the iodide molecule and subsequently its incorporation into the tyrosine molecule.

The thyroid gland has the unique features of being able to store large quantities of thyroid hormones and releasing them at a relatively slow rate. In order for hormones to be released into the blood stream, the thyroglobulin molecules must enter into the follicular cell through an endocytosis process. The engulfed colloid droplets fuse with lysosomes and are hydrolyzed, splitting off molecules of T_4, T_3, MIT, and DIT. The thyroid hormones are very lipophilic and pass freely through the outer membranes of the follicular cells and into the blood stream. The MIT and DIT molecules are deiodinated by iodotyrosine deiodinase and the free iodine molecules can be recycled for synthesis of more thyroid hormones. This proteolytic step is stimulated by TSH and inhibited by iodine and lithium. The synthesis of the thyroid hormones is summarized in Figure 29–2.

Approximately 90% of the secretory product released from the thyroid gland is in the form of T_4. T_4 is actually a prohormone of T_3. About 20% of the circulating T_3 is produced within the thyroid from the coupling of MIT and DIT. The remaining 80% is produced by the monodeiodination of T_4. This process takes place in the peripheral tissues, especially in the liver and kidneys. The monodeiodination can produce either T_3 or reverse T_3 (rT_3), depending on which iodide is removed. Only T_3 is biologically active.

The circulating thyroid hormones bind to serum proteins as they are released into the blood stream. Approximately 75% of T_4 and 70% of T_3 are bound to thyroxine-binding globulin (TBG). Smaller amounts of both hormones are bound to thyroxine-binding prealbumin and albumin. Approximately 0.03% of T_4 and 0.3% of T_3 and rT_3 are not bound to serum proteins. These free hormones are physiologically active, because they are able to diffuse into the target tissues and bring about their actions by the method used by other steroid hormones. T_3 is about 3 to 4 times more biologically active than T_4, for at least two reasons. First, there is a greater amount of T_3 in the free state, and second, the receptor protein in the cell nucleus has a higher affinity for T_3 than for T_4.

Every tissue in the body is affected either directly or indirectly by the thyroid hormones. First, the thyroid hormones increase the body's overall basal metabolism. Second, because they increase metabolic activity, heat production is also increased. Third, the thyroid hormones raise target cell responsiveness to the catecholamines (mainly epinephrine and norepinephrine). Fourth, because of the greater responsiveness of the heart to the catecholamines, thyroid hormones increase both heart rate and the force of

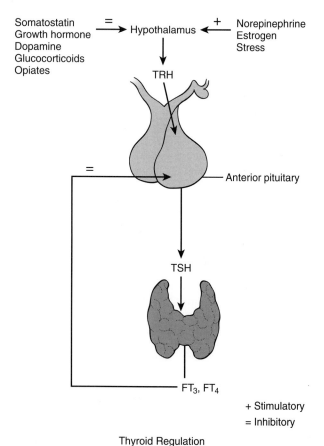

Figure 29–1. Thyroid regulation. Abbreviations: +, stimulatory; =, inhibitory; TRH, thyroid-releasing hormone; TSH, thyroid-stimulating hormone; FT_3, free triiodothyronine; FT_4, free thyroxine.

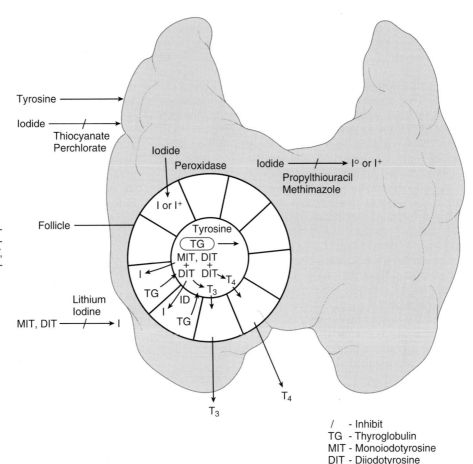

Figure 29–2. Thyroid hormone synthesis. Abbreviations: /, inhibit; TG, thyroglobulin; MIT, monoiodotyrosine; DIT, diiodotyrosine; ID, iodotyrosine deiodinase.

/ - Inhibit
TG - Thyroglobulin
MIT - Monoiodotyrosine
DIT - Diiodotyrosine
ID - Iodotyrosine deiodinase

heart contraction and, thus, cardiac output. Lastly, thyroid hormones are essential for the normal growth and central nervous system (CNS) development in children and CNS function in adults. This function seems to be secondary to the effect of the thyroid hormones on growth hormone.

ETIOLOGY AND PATHOPHYSIOLOGY

Hyperthyroidism

Hyperthyroidism is a disorder manifested as excessive circulating levels of thyroid hormones. *Thyrotoxicosis* is applied to a group of syndromes caused by the high levels of thyroid hormones.

The most common cause of hyperthyroidism in the United States is Graves' disease, which is also known as diffuse toxic goiter. This condition occurs in about 85% of all hyperthyroid cases. It occurs most often in young women and is characterized by hyperthyroidism and diffuse goiter enlargement. Graves' disease is one of a group of autoimmune diseases caused by circulating antibodies against functional cell surface receptors. The pathogenesis of Graves' disease appears to be related to the production of thyroid-stimulating antibody (TSAb), which interacts with the TSH receptor of the follicular cell membrane to stimulate the uptake of iodide, the synthesis of thyroid hormones, and the release of the hormones into the circulation. Unlike TSH, TSAb is not subject to negative feedback inhibition by the thyroid hormone levels. Other types of

antibodies to the TSH receptor may also be produced in these patients. One particular antibody that occurs does not activate thyroid cell function. Because of the diverse activities of these antibodies, clinical expressions of the disorder are various.

Other etiologies of hyperthyroidism are toxic nodular goiter, thyroiditis, hCG-secreting tumors, pituitary tumors, thyroid carcinomas, excessive ingestion of inorganic iodine, and factitious use of T_3 or T_4.

Toxic nodular goiter is associated with single or multiple, autonomously functioning nodules. The goiter may have been present for years and the thyroid function parameters normal. Gradually, nodules can produce excessive hormones but are not associated with the production of thyroid antibodies. The gland itself may show hyperplasia, fibrosis, and calcification. Plummer's nodule is only sometimes seen in toxic nodular goiter, in which a single adenoma may overproduce the thyroid hormones.

Thyroiditis may produce hyperthyroidism at some time in the course of the disorder. In subacute and painless thyroiditis, the increase in the thyroid hormones presumably results from the release of stored hormone from damaged thyroid follicular cells. The mechanism may be similar in chronic thyroiditis, but it is possible that thyroid-stimulating immunoglobulins (TSIs) are elaborated as part of this immunologic disorder.

The alpha subunit in hCG is identical to that in TSH. Excessive amounts of hCG can be produced by hydatidiform mole, choriocarcinoma, or embryonal carcinoma of the testes. The excessive amounts of hCG can have thyroid-stimulating ability because of the molecular similarity of hCG to TSH.

Hyperthyrotropic hyperthyroidism may occur from excessive TSH secretion by a pituitary adenoma, although excessive TSH secretion without evidence of a pituitary tumor has also been described. This condition results from either the hypersecretion of TRH or the loss of the inhibition of TSH secretion normally produced by excessive levels of thyroid hormones.

Thyroid carcinoma can cause thyrotoxicosis as a result of the secretion of thyroid hormone by a large mass of well-differentiated metastatic follicular tumors.

Hyperthyroidism can result from the excessive ingestion of inorganic iodide (Jod-Basedow phenomenon). It was first described when patients were given iodide for endemic goiter. Most of these patients, however, have a multinodular goiter, an autonomous functioning thyroid, or history of Graves' disease.

Factitious use of thyroxine is also a significant cause of hyperthyroidism. Factitious thyroxine use can be due to overmedication of a patient under a physician's care (iatrogenic) or unprescribed abuse (surreptitious).

Hypothyroidism

Hypothyroidism results when there are insufficient levels of thyroid hormones to fulfill the metabolic needs at the cellular level. The condition can be classified as either congenital or acquired.

Defects in the development of function of the thyroid gland itself, known as *primary hypothyroidism*, constitute most cases of congenital hypothyroidism. The frequency of congenital primary hypothyroidism is approximately 1 in 3500 to 1 in 4000 live births.[1]

Rarely, congenital hypothyroidism may be caused by dyshormonogenesis. These rare disorders are inherited as autosomal recessive traits. The dysgenesis is due to impaired thyroid hormone synthesis because of enzymatic defects.

Secondary hypothyroidism exists when there is a failure of the pituitary gland to produce sufficient TSH, and *tertiary hypothyroidism* exist when the hypothalamus fails to produce enough TRH. As congenital conditions, they occur only rarely—1 in 80,000 live births.[2]

Acquired hypothyroidism most often results from inadequate secretion of the thyroid hormones by a damaged thyroid gland. Causes associated with acquired primary hypothyroidism are (1) chronic thyroiditis, (2) surgical or radioactive iodine treatment of hyperthyroidism, goiter, or cancer, (3) idiopathic atrophy, and (4) metastatic cancer or other infiltrative disorders.

Chronic thyroiditis, also called Hashimoto's disease, is the most common cause of acquired primary hypothyroidism. This is an autoimmune disease that results in a massive diffuse infiltration of lymphocytes, abundant numbers of plasma cells, and increased amounts of connective tissue into the thyroid gland. The condition may be genetically determined and leads to the production of sensitized lymphocytes and antibodies to thyroid antigens. This may eventually lead to the destruction of the thyroid tissue. The

peak incidence of Hashimoto's thyroiditis occurs during the sixth decade of life. It is estimated to occur in 2% to 4% of the population in the United States[2]; however, over the last 50 years, the number of newly diagnosed cases has increased exponentially.[3] The disease is often asymptomatic, and the patients may be euthyroid, hypothyroid, or hyperthyroid.

Acquired hypothyroidism may also result from a lack of TSH or TRH. In secondary hypothyroidism, the patient usually has a pituitary tumor. With tertiary hypothyroidism, the hypothalamic failure may be the result of tumor, vascular insufficiency, infectious or infiltrative processes, or trauma.

Thyroid Inflammation

Thyroiditis has been classified as acute, subacute, chronic, and fibrous. Acute thyroiditis is characterized by abscess and suppuration of the thyroid gland. The onset is sudden and is associated with fever, chills, and malaise. The disorder usually results from a bacterial infection, in particular a staphylococcal, streptococcal, or pneumococcal infection.

Subacute thyroiditis, also known as de Quervain's thyroiditis, is most likely caused by a virus. No autoimmune mechanism has been established for this disease, which appears in the second to fifth decade of life and is more common in females.

Chronic thyroiditis, also known as lymphocytic thyroiditis or Hashimoto's disease, is caused by an unidentified abnormality in the immune system and extensive infiltration of the gland with chronic inflammatory cells. This leads to the production of antibodies and eventually the destruction of the thyroid tissue.

Fibrous or Riedel's thyroiditis is an uncommon disorder. The condition appears rapidly, and the etiology is unknown. It affects individuals in the fourth to seventh decades of life. A fibrous reaction annihilates the thyroid gland and extends into the surrounding structures of the neck.

Thyroid Neoplasms

Irregular, localized, or nodular enlargement of the thyroid gland may indicate the presence of a neoplasm. Thyroid neoplasms may occur singly or as portions of benign nodular goiters. Their cause is unknown. Some of the adenomas function as normal tissue, but some are more active and produce thyroid hormones. Follicular adenomas are the most common benign tumors. These tumors occur most commonly in young adults but can be found in any age group. Adenomas are encapsulated and may compress the adjacent parenchymal tissue.

Carcinoma of the thyroid is relatively uncommon compared with benign adenomas.[4] Typically, these tumors have a slow growth pattern and stay within the confines of the thyroid gland. Patients who have undergone irradiation to the neck in childhood have a higher risk of thyroid cancer. The malignant tumors are classified as papillary, follicular, undifferentiated, medullary, and epidermoid. The papillary carcinomas make up the majority of the thyroid cancers in the United States. The peak incidence of these tumors is the third to fourth decade of life, and they occur most commonly in females.

Medullary thyroid cancer (MTC), which accounts for only about 5% of the thyroid cancers,[2] derives from the parafollicular cells of the thyroid. This tumor may occur sporadically or may demonstrate a familial occurrence in association with other endocrine neoplasms. The peak incidence for this tumor is in the fourth to sixth decade, with a slight female preponderance.

Goiters

Goiter is applied to diffuse enlargement of the thyroid gland. The disorder may develop from chronic iodine deficiency, ingestion of goitrogens, or in genetic deficiencies involving thyroglobulin production or enzymes needed for hormone synthesis.

Euthyroid Sick Syndrome

Critically ill hospitalized patients may have abnormal thyroid function parameters and are referred to as being euthyroid sick. Various types of illness can cause changes in thyroid hormone secretion, distribution, and metabolism. In addition, these conditions may decrease levels of thyroxine-binding proteins or may induce the presence of circulating inhibitors to the binding of T_4 and T_3. In general, the more severe the illness, the greater the abnormality of thyroid function values. Examples of conditions that can cause the euthyroid sick syndrome are malnutrition, neoplasms, congestive heart failure, febrile illnesses, kidney failure, and liver disease.

CLINICAL MANIFESTATIONS

Hyperthyroidism

The clinical symptoms of thyrotoxicosis are related to the catabolic, hypermetabolic effects caused by increased activity in the various tissues and the greater sensitivity to catecholamines. The increased catabolic effects may be reflected as weight loss, loss of muscle mass, dyspnea, loss of fat stores, exercise intolerance, and easy fatigability. Nervousness, irritability, insomnia, pruritus, tremor, heat intolerance, excessive sweating, tachycardia, palpitations, increased cardiac output, frequent bowel movements, and the tendency of the skin to be warm and moist are all manifestations of greater sensitivity to catecholamines. Mobilization of bone mineral leads to osteoporosis, and about 10% of the patients have a hypercalcemia.[2] Acropachy may be present; in this condition, the free margin of the nail is lifted up from its base.

Almost all patients with active thyrotoxicosis have some manifestation of noninfiltrative ophthalmopathy, usually in the form of a prominent stare and lid lag. Infiltrative ophthalmopathy is potentially a more serious condition. It manifests in a mild form with puffy lids and protrusion of the globes due to infiltration of the retro-orbital space with lymphocytes, mast cells, and mucopolysaccharides. The bulging of the eyes is known as *exophthalmos*. Besides proptosis, ophthalmic symptoms include increased lacrimation, gritty sensation in the eyes, diplopia, and reduction of vision.

Pretibial myxedema is less common than infiltrative ophthalmopathy. The infiltrative dermopathy usually involves the pretibial region of the legs, where the skin is thickened and shiny. The dermis is infiltrated with mucopolysaccharides and cells of chronic inflammation.

There may also be changes associated with the reproductive system, such as oligomenorrhea or amenorrhea in females and gynecomastia and impotence in males.

An endocrine emergency associated with thyroid dysfunction is known as a *thyroid storm*. It is characterized by accentuated signs and symptoms of thyrotoxicosis plus fever. Such readily recognizable signs and symptoms of thyrotoxicosis as tremor, tachycardia, exophthalmos, and heat intolerance are usually present in young and middle-aged patients with this disorder but seldom occur in the elderly. Elderly patients tend to have more substantial weight loss than that noted in younger patients and often have congestive heart failure; they may not have fever. Progression to coma, shock, and death can occur in all age groups. The proximate cause of thyroid storm is not known, but it can occur in any patient with uncontrolled thyrotoxicosis who is subjected to stress. Infection, especially pneumonitis, is a common precipitating event.

Hypothyroidism

Cretinism, or congenital primary hypothyroidism, is associated with numerous clinical manifestations: puffy face; open mouth with enlarged protruding tongue; short, thick neck; narrow forehead; pug nose; short legs; distended abdomen; hoarse voice or cry; dry, mottled skin; yellowish skin discoloration; hirsutism; lethargy; and mental retardation. These symptoms manifest if treatment is not begun in early infancy.

With acquired deficiency of thyroid hormones comes the slowing of many metabolic processes. The symptoms found include fatigue, slowing of mental and physical performance, change in personality, impaired memory, cold intolerance, exertional dyspnea, hoarseness, constipation, muscle cramps, and paresthesia.

The classic features of severe hypothyroidism are referred to as *myxedema*, a term used to describe the peculiar nonpitting swelling of the skin. The skin becomes infiltrated by mucopolysaccharides so that the face is puffy, especially around the eyes. The features become coarse and the eyebrows thinned. The tongue may become enlarged and the vocal cords thickened, leading to the hoarseness. The speech slows, and there is usually a weight gain. The skin tends to be dry and has a yellowish color. Myocardial contractility is reduced, and the pulse slows.

Anemia may be present. The anemia may be due to hypometabolism, reduced oxygen requirement, and a decreased erythropoietin.

Myxedema coma is a severe presentation of hypothyroidism. The clinical symptoms are coma, hypothermia, hypoglycemia, hypotension, hyponatremia, and respiratory failure. Even though the condition is rare, the mortality rate is high.

Thyroid Inflammation

The clinical manifestations of thyroiditis vary according to the classification of the thyroiditis. Acute thyroiditis is usually secondary to a penetrating injury of the neck and is only rarely found.

Subacute thyroiditis is accompanied by symptoms of upper respiratory tract infection in addition to pain in the thyroid region and fever. Pain may not be a universal symptom, however. Upon palpation, tenderness is commonly manifest, and the gland itself is usually diffusely enlarged. At early onset of the condition, only one side of the gland may be tender and palpable.

The manifestations of chronic thyroiditis are extremely variable. The major symptom is a painless goiter. During the late stages of chronic thyroiditis, in which fibrosis of the gland is the prominent feature, the patient may not have a goiter.

Thyroid Neoplasms

Localized, irregular, or nodular enlargements of the thyroid gland may be a manifestation of neoplasm. A localized nodular enlargement of the gland usually represents an adenoma. Even though cancer of the thyroid is rare, it must be considered whenever a nodule is found, especially if a nodule is enlarging disproportionately.

Goiters

Symptoms of simple nontoxic goiter are related to the size and position of the mass in the throat area. Compression of the trachea or esophagus may cause difficulty in swallowing.

LABORATORY ANALYSES AND DIAGNOSIS

Tests of thyroid function can be divided into two major groups. First are tests that establish thyroid dysfunction; this group includes determinations of TSH, total T_3 (TT_3), and total T_4 (TT_4). The second group of tests is performed

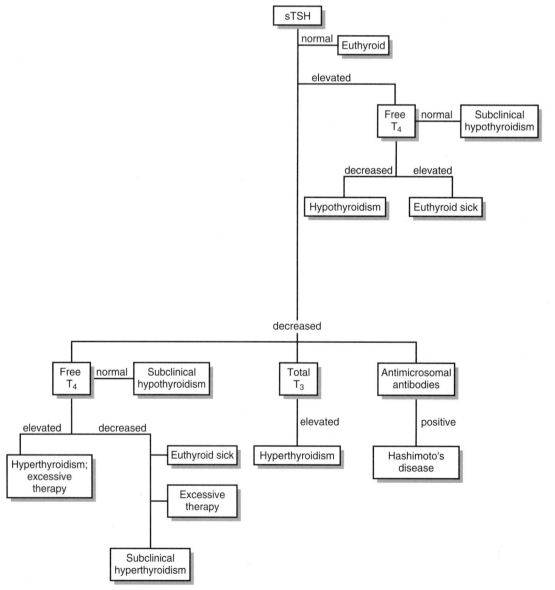

Figure 29–3. One approach to laboratory investigation of thyroid status. Abbreviations: T_3, triiodothyronine; T_4, thyroxine; sTSH, sensitive (second generation) thyrotropin.

to elucidate the cause of the thyroid dysfunction; procedures such as tests for thyroid antibodies, TBG measurements, ultrasonography, and biopsy are included in this group.

Historically, the principal serum thyroid function tests that establish thyroid dysfunction have been TT_4; free T_4 (FT_4) estimate or index (FT_4I); TT_3; free T_3 (FT_3) estimate or index (FT_3I); resin T_3 uptake (RT_3U); or the indirect estimate of the TBG concentration or thyroid hormone–binding ratio (THBR) and TSH. Many physicians and laboratories continue to utilize these tests and the algorithms discussed here. Advocates for a somewhat different approach, however, based on a second-generation TSH assay as the starting point, are urging its adoption as a more cost-effective means of determining thyroid status.[5] Figure 29–3 illustrates this alternative approach.

Hyperthyroidism

In hyperthyroidism, the serum TT_4, TT_3, FT_4I, and RT_3U values are elevated. The second-generation TSH level is reduced. Approximately 90% of patients with hyperthyroidism have an increased TT_4.[6] However, the serum TT_3 level may be the most sensitive indicator of hyperthyroidism and is elevated in the other 10% of patients with this disorder.

Other laboratory values may be abnormal in hyperthyroid patients. The creatine kinase (CK) level may be half of normal. The alkaline phosphatase (ALP) level may be about 2.5 times normal owing to increased bone turnover. The bone turnover may also raise the serum calcium and urinary hydroxyproline levels. The elevated metabolic rate may elevate serum free fatty acid levels and reduce total cholesterol levels. A glucose tolerance test may demonstrate a diabetic curve, because thyroxine increases the gastric absorption of glucose and also glycogenolysis.

Hematologic manifestations include a decreased white blood cell (WBC) count because of decreased number of neutrophils, a lymphocytosis, anemia, and an greater red cell mass due to excess demand for oxygen. Serum estrogen, testosterone, and sex hormone–binding globulins (SHBG) may be elevated.

A hyperthyroidism panel should include an FT_4 estimate and possibly an FT_3 estimate. Confirmation of hyperthyroidism is made with a second-generation TSH assay. This TSH assay is sensitive enough to distinguish low from normal TSH value (Fig. 29–4).

The FT_4 estimate may be falsely elevated in cases of familial dysalbuminemia and other serum protein–binding abnormalities. Inappropriate TSH secretion, found in secondary hyperthyroidism, may also elevate the FT_4 estimate. In other instances, a second-generation TSH assay confirms the diagnosis of hyperthyroidism, because the TSH is low. In secondary hyperthyroidism, the TSH level should be elevated but may be normal and therefore misleading. A free T_4 assay may be of value in detecting the elevated level of T_4 in cases of secondary hyperthyroidism.

Some laboratories may use the second-generation TSH assay as the initial test. If the result is decreased, confirmation of hyperthyroidism may be made with an FT_4 estimate. FT_4 estimates are less costly and have a quicker turnaround time. The second-generation TSH measurements are more sensitive but may be misleading in the rare cases of secondary hyperthyroidism.

Once hyperthyroidism has been established, the cause

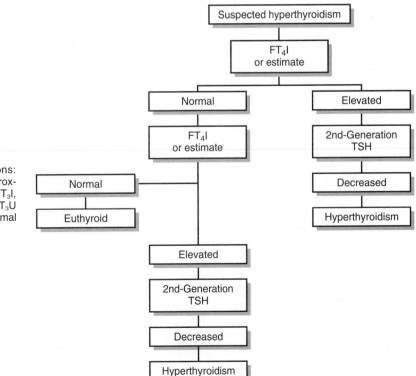

Figure 29–4. Hyperthyroid panel. Abbreviations: TSH, thyroid-stimulating hormone; FT_4I, free thyroxine index (total thyroxine [TT_4] × RT_3U ratio*); FT_3I, free T_3 index (total triiodothyronine [TT_3] × RT_3U ratio*). *RT_3U ratio = RT_3U patient ÷ RT_3U normal serum pool.

must be established. The presence of TSAb would establish the diagnosis of Graves' disease.

Hypothyroidism

The laboratory abnormalities found in hypothyroidism include decreases in TT_4, TT_3, FT_4I, and FT_4. The most sensitive indicator of primary hypothyroidism is the TSH value, which is increased. With secondary or tertiary hypothyroidism, the TSH value is decreased. Because the metabolic rate is reduced in patients with hypothyroidism, other abnormal laboratory results may be observed. The total cholesterol level is high because the rates of degradation and excretion are decreased. There is a rise in the CK level because of increased release of enzyme through greater permeability of muscle membranes or diminished catabolism of circulating enzyme. The glucose tolerance test shows a flat curve because of reduced absorption of glucose by the gut.

Anemia may be present. It can be normocytic; normochromic because of the hypometabolism and reductions in oxygen requirement and erythropoietin; microcytic in the presence of menorrhagia resulting in iron deficiency; or macrocytic if there is a folate deficiency due to malabsorption.

A hypothyroidism panel may begin with an FT_4 estimate. Confirmation is made by an elevated serum TSH. Some hypothyroidism panels actually begin with the TSH assay and use the FT_4 estimate as the confirmatory test. There are advantages to both approaches. As previously mentioned, the FT_4 estimate may be less expensive and has a quicker turnaround time, but the TSH assay has a greater sensitivity (Fig. 29–5).

In a patient with suspected secondary hypothyroidism, the TSH level can be low or normal, which may be misleading. The FT_4 estimate revealing a low level confirms the secondary hypothyroidism. Some patients with subclinical hypothyroidism have elevated TSH levels and normal FT_4 estimates. The hypothyroidism in these patients would not be detected if the FT_4 estimate were the initial test. However, the clinical significance of this condition is uncertain.

The diagnosis of Hashimoto's disease, the most common cause of hypothyroidism, is confirmed by the demonstration of antibodies to thyroid tissue components. Traditionally, the antibody procedures have involved antimicrosomal or antithyroglobulin antibody detection. A newer technique has been developed for the detection of thyroid peroxidase (TPO) autoantibodies. This procedure may provide greater sensitivity and specificity for the diagnosis of Hashimoto's disease than the demonstration of microsomal antibodies.

Thyroid Inflammation

In acute thyroiditis, the TT_4 and TT_3 levels are usually normal. Acute thyroiditis may produce hyperthyroidism at some time during the course of the disorder. Thyroiditis antibodies are not usually present. Because this condition is commonly associated with a bacterial infection, fever, an elevated WBC count, and accelerated erythrocyte sedimentation rate (ESR) are characteristic. Fine-needle aspiration biopsy of the thyroid may be used to make the identification of the causative organism possible.

In subacute and painless thyroiditis, the increase in thyroid hormones and TT_4 presumably results from the release of stored hormone from damaged thyroid follicular cells. In addition to hyperthyroidism, radioactive uptake of iodine by the thyroid gland is low. This feature can distinguish thyroiditis from Graves' disease.

The presence of a goiter is important in the diagnosis of chronic thyroiditis or Hashimoto's disease. Some patients present with symptoms of hypothyroidism and do not have thyroid enlargement. Antithyroid antibodies are positive in 95% of patients.[3] Fine-needle aspiration biopsy may be needed to confirm the diagnosis in some patients and also to rule out thyroid carcinoma. The biopsy reveals the presence of lymphocytic infiltration.

Thyroid Neoplasms

The annual incidence of thyroid nodules in the United States is about 0.1%, or approximately 250,000 nodules per year.[7] Nodules are manifestations of goiters and thyroid tumors. The challenge to physicians is to detect the malignant tumors that actually occur in a small number of cases.

Certain risk factors accompany thyroid cancer. One risk factor is age; the risk is higher if the patient is young. Another risk factor is gender; the risk is increased in males. Characteristics of the nodule itself may also be important. The risk of malignancy is higher if the nodule has progressively increased in size or if it is firm and fixed and there is a regional lymphadenopathy. A history of prior neck irradiation is also associated with greater risk of malignancy.

TT_4, TT_3, and TSH determinations may be performed. Usually, all values are within reference ranges unless the nodule is hyperfunctioning, in which case the TT_4 and/or TT_3 will be elevated, and the TSH level decreased. Further evaluation can be provided by thyroid scans, ultrasonography, and fine-needle aspiration biopsy.

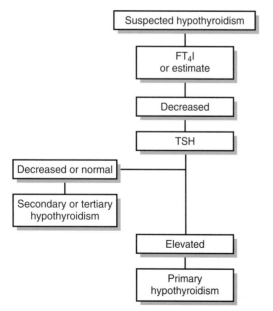

Figure 29–5. Hypothyroid panel. Abbreviations: FT_4I, free thyroxine index; TSH, thyroid-stimulating hormone.

Thyroid scan utilizing radioactive iodine or technetium Tc 99m pertechnetate may assess the anatomy of the thyroid gland and aid in classifying the nodule as functioning or nonfunctioning. Ultrasonography can locate the nodule and characterize it as either solid or cystic.

Fine-needle aspiration biopsy is safe and a very valuable procedure because it enables the cytology of the nodule to be assessed. Cytologic review classifies the aspirate as one of three categories: benign, malignant, or suspicious.

Euthyroid Sick Syndrome

As previously mentioned, thyroid function tests may be abnormal in critically ill hospitalized patients. Levels of serum thyroid binding protein concentrations or of circulating inhibitors of thyroid hormone binding, and conversion of T_4 to T_3 in the peripheral blood may be decreased, or qualitative abnormalities may be found in serum TSH glycosylation. Laboratory data may indicate low levels of TT_4 and TT_3, but the TSH level is seldom elevated. The FT_4I or FT_4 estimate may not provide reliable information, and therefore, direct measurements of free T_4 provide the most information for the diagnosis of hypothyroidism.

In this clinical situation, a third-generation assay for serum TSH (chemiluminescent technology) is the most dependable test for hyperthyroidism. If a third-generation assay is not performed, the FT_4 estimate is more likely to reflect true hyperthyroidism than an undetectable TSH level using a second-generation TSH assay. Even in such cases, an elevated TSH value along with a decreased FT_4I or FT_4 estimate usually indicates true hypothyroidism. Nevertheless, all patients with nonthyroidal acute illnesses should be reevaluated after recovery for the most accurate diagnosis (Fig. 29–6).

TREATMENT

Hyperthyroidism

The treatment for hyperthyroidism involves radioactive iodine, antithyroid drugs, and subtotal thyroidectomy. The thyroid gland traps the ^{131}I isotope, enabling delivery of high-dose irradiation to the diseased tissue. If the dose is adequate, almost all patients with Graves' disease and most of the patients with toxic nodular goiter can be rendered euthyroid. The use of radioactive iodine eliminates any surgical complications; however, there is a risk of hypothyroidism in such a patient after treatment.

Antithyroid drugs are generally effective and safe. These drugs block the oxidation of iodine as well as the incorporation of the iodide molecules into the tyrosyl ring. Propylthiouracil and methimazole are the most widely utilized antithyroid drugs. Allergic reactions and agranulocytosis may occur as serious complications. In addition, if the patient continues to take the medication after being rendered euthyroid, hypothyroidism may result.

Subtotal thyroidectomy may be the treatment of choice for patients who are pregnant or who are apprehensive about radioactive iodine and are not candidates for drug therapy. Complications of surgery include hemorrhage, hypoparathyroidism, and laryngeal nerve damage. Regardless of the choice of treatment, the patient must be followed for the development of hypothyroidism or the recurrence of hyperthyroidism.

Hypothyroidism

The treatment of hypothyroidism is levothyroxine therapy. Patients who are receiving thyroid hormone replacement should be monitored with second-generation TSH measurements rather than FT_4 estimates.

Thyroid Inflammation

No specific treatment exists for thyroiditis. Symptomatic therapy utilizing aspirin or glucocorticoids is common. If the patient with chronic thyroiditis becomes hypothyroid, the hypothyroidism is treated.

Thyroid Neoplasms

Thyroid nodules may be categorized through fine-needle aspiration biopsy as neoplastic, inflammatory, or hyperplastic. Confirmed neoplastic lesions as well as inflammatory

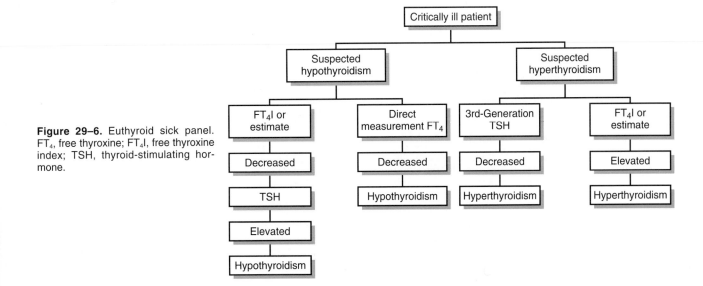

Figure 29–6. Euthyroid sick panel. FT_4, free thyroxine; FT_4I, free thyroxine index; TSH, thyroid-stimulating hormone.

or hyperplastic nodules for which neoplasm cannot be ruled out are excised. In the past, suppressive therapy with levothyroxine was utilized. Owing to the low percentage of tumors reduced in size and the complications of thyrotoxicosis, this treatment of thyroid nodules is no longer used as commonly.[7]

Case Study 1

A 45-year-old woman complained of extreme fatigue for the past year, during which time her neck gradually enlarged. She had never experienced any neck pain. She also complained of constipation and long menstrual periods. On physical examination, her physician found a diffuse goiter; the cervical lymph nodes were not enlarged.

The laboratory findings (with reference ranges) were as follows:

TT_4:	3.0 µg/dL (4.5–13.0 µg/dL)
TT_3:	120 ng/dL (60–220 ng/dL)
RT_3U ratio:	0.6 (0.8–1.35)
TSH:	15 µU/mL (0.4–4.0 µU/mL)
ESR:	40 mm/hr (0–20 mm/hr)
Thyroid peroxidase autoantibodies:	22 IU/mL (<2 IU/mL)
Antimicrosomal antibodies titer:	1:128 (<1:40)

Questions

1. What is the probable diagnosis as indicated by the clinical and laboratory findings?
2. Calculate the FT_4I for this patient.
3. What additional procedure would confirm the diagnosis?

Discussion

1. The thyroid laboratory tests, particularly TT_4 and TSH, strongly support the clinical diagnosis of hypothyroidism. Hashimoto's chronic lymphocytic thyroiditis is implicated as the cause of the hypothyroidism for the following reasons: A painless goiter with nodules is present along with the high titer of antimicrosomal antibodies and the elevated level of thyroid peroxidase autoantibodies. Elevated ESR can be observed in patients with this disorder.
2. $FT_4I = TT_4 \times RT_3U$ ratio
   $FT_4I = 3.0 \times 0.6$
   $FT_4I = 1.8$ (reference range: 4.5–12.5).
3. Pathologic examination of a fine-needle aspirate of the thyroid gland would confirm the diagnosis.

Case Study 2

A 23-year-old woman visited her physician complaining of protruding eyes and serious vision problems. She had also experienced excessive sweating, extreme nervousness, and weight loss (20 lb in 2 months). Her pulse rate was 105 beats/minute; blood pressure was 140/88 mm Hg; and temperature was 98.4 °F. No goiter was observed.

The laboratory findings (with reference ranges) were as follows:

TT_4:	10.5 µg/dL (4.5–13.0 µg/dL)
TT_3:	250 ng/dL (60–220 ng/dL)
RT_3U ratio:	1.50 (0.8–1.35)
TSH:	0.4 µU/mL (0.4–4.0 µU/mL)

Questions

1. On the basis of the laboratory findings, what is the probable diagnosis?
2. Calculate the FT_3I.
3. Explain the TT_4 findings.
4. What other procedure could be used to determine the etiology of the diagnosis?

Discussion

1. The TT_3 indicates hyperthyroidism.
2. $FT_3I = TT_3 \times RT_3U$ ratio
   $FT_3I = 250 \times 1.50$
   $FT_3I = 375$ (reference range: 85–205).
3. The TT_4 result is within the reference range; however, the TT_3 level is a more sensitive test, and it is elevated. The FT_3I confirms the diagnosis of hyperthyroidism.
4. A test to detect the presence of TSAb would confirm the diagnosis of Graves' disease.

References

1. Whitley RJ, Meikle AW, Watts NB: Thyroid function. *In* Burtis CA, Ashwood ER (eds): Tietz Textbook of Clinical Chemistry. Philadelphia, WB Saunders, 1994.
2. Hershman JM: Endocrine Pathophysiology: A Patient-Oriented Approach. Philadelphia, Lea & Febiger, 1988.
3. Schubert MF, Kountz DS: Thyroiditis—a disease with many faces. Postgrad Med 98:101–112, 1995.
4. National Cancer Institute (Division of Cancer Prevention and Control). Annual Cancer Statistics Review. (NIH publication No. 87-2789). Bethesda, MD, Dept of Health and Human Services, 1986.
5. Check W: Polishing thyroid testing practices. CAP Today 11:1–3, 1997.
6. Federman DD: Thyroid. *In* Rubenstein E, Federman DD (eds): Scientific American Medicine, vol III. New York, Scientific American, 1994.
7. Gharib, H, Mazzaferri, E: Strategy for the solitary thyroid nodule. Hosp Prac Sept 30:53-60, 1992.

Chapter 30

Disorders of the Parathyroid Glands

Shauna C. Anderson

Most individuals possess two pairs of parathyroid glands. The superior glands are generally located close to the upper posterior aspect of the thyroid. The location of the inferior glands is far more variable, ranging from the lower pole of the thyroid caudally to the thymus. Although 90% of individuals possess four parathyroid glands, as many as six or as few as two may be present.

Two types of cells are identified in the glandular parenchyma, oxyphil cells and chief cells. Oxyphil cells increase in number with age and may be mature, nonfunctional, or degenerative chief cells. It is the active chief cells that synthesize and secrete the polypeptide hormone, parathyroid hormone (PTH).

PTH synthesis begins on rough endoplasmic reticulum of the chief cells with the formation of a large molecule. This precursor molecule is known as pre-pro-PTH. It is immediately cleaved to form pre-PTH. Although the half-life of this molecule is longer than that of the previous molecule, pre-PTH is not secreted by the parathyroid glands, and neither molecule is biologically active. Enzymatic cleavage of the pre-PTH molecule produces PTH, which can be stored within secretory vesicles of the chief cells, cleaved again to produce amino-terminal and carboxyl-terminal fragments, or released into the circulation. Once in the circulation, the whole intact molecule is further degraded in the peripheral tissues, especially the liver and the kidney, producing the amino-terminal and carboxyl-terminal fragments. The amino-terminal fragment has a shorter half-life than the carboxyl-terminal fragment, but only the intact molecule and the amino-terminal fragments possess biologic activity.

Synthesis and release of PTH are controlled primarily by the extracellular fluid calcium ion concentration. A negative feedback regulation exists between ionized calcium levels and hormone release; that is, hypercalcemia reduces and hypocalcemia enhances the basal rate of PTH secretion. The calcium ion binds to an extracellular receptor that is coupled to an intracellular portion by membrane-spanning segments. Calcium consequently acts as a first messenger in this circumstance. Other factors may also regulate the rate of PTH synthesis and release. Higher levels of serum phosphorus lower the levels of serum calcium, in turn causing the release of PTH. This mechanism is important in renal insufficiency. Decreased levels of magnesium can impair the release of PTH and also the responsiveness of the tissues to it. Other substances, such as catecholamines, cortisol, prostaglandins, and vitamin D, have effects on PTH but are not normally regulators.

Upon binding to the target tissues, mainly the kidney tubular cells and bone, PTH works by stimulating adenylate cyclase, which produces cyclic adenosine monophosphate (cAMP) and facilitates a cellular influx of calcium in the target tissues. Because magnesium is required for the binding of PTH to the target tissue, severe magnesium deficiency leads to decreased PTH secretion and an impairment of hormone action. PTH indirectly causes the absorption of calcium from the intestines by effecting the change of 25-hydroxyvitamin D (25-OHD) to 1,25-dihydroxyvitamin D (1,25-dihydroxycholecalciferol [DHCC]) in the kidneys, the dihydroxyvitamin D metabolite that directly stimulates intestinal uptake of calcium.

PTH also engenders the release of calcium from bone. In the bone, PTH stimulates the osteoclasts, the principal bone resorption cells, which is followed by osteoblastic activity. The osteoclasts cause a release of phosphate from bone mineral. Simultaneously, phosphaturia occurs through the hormone's inhibition of renal tubular reabsorption of phosphate.

In the kidney, PTH increases calcium reabsorption and reduces calcium excretion. It also causes the excretion of cAMP, hydroxyproline, sodium, potassium, and bicarbonate. In turn, PTH promotes the reabsorption of hydrogen ions, magnesium, and ammonia. PTH also acts on the kidney by inhibiting reabsorption of phosphate, increasing the phosphate in urine and decreasing the phosphate in serum. Figure 30–1 contains a summary of the effects of PTH.

Calcium in the plasma circulates in three forms: free or ionized, protein-bound (mainly albumin), and diffusible but non-ionized complexes. Only the free, ionized fraction, which accounts for approximately 50% of the total calcium, is physiologically active. It is this fraction that serves as the negative feedback for PTH.

Binding of calcium by plasma proteins varies with the pH of the blood. By inhibiting both bicarbonate reabsorption and exchange of hydrogen ions for sodium ions in the proximal tubules of the kidney, PTH generates a metabolic acidosis. This condition favors displacement of calcium from the plasma proteins and bone, with a resulting increase in ionized calcium.

The main functions of calcium are as follows:

1. Maintaining the electrical gradient across cell membranes. Cell membranes bear an electrical gradient or potential difference, such that the extracellular compartment bears a relatively positive charge and the intracellular compartment a relatively negative charge. Calcium is primarily an extracellular cation and contributes to the net extracellular positive charge. As calcium levels rise, neurons and muscle cells become refractory and cease to function. As calcium levels fall, the opposite sequence of events occurs, and when extracellular positivity falls and the cell-membrane potential difference is reduced the cell membrane becomes "hyperexcitable."
2. Serving as a structural component. The skeleton derives most of its strength from the mineral hydroxyapatite, the crystals of which are composed largely of calcium.

3. Functioning as an intracellular messenger.

Abnormalities in parathyroid gland structure or function come to the attention of the physician when a patient presents with symptoms resulting from calcium "imbalance." Pathologic consequences of this alteration in mineral metabolism range from minimal to profound.

Increased circulating levels of PTH lead to clinical manifestations of hypercalcemia. If mild, this condition may warrant only continued observation by the physician and periodic laboratory monitoring of blood and urine to ensure early detection of further changes. If hypercalcemia is progressive, differential diagnosis must be undertaken. When disruption is severe, immediate medical intervention to promptly restore and maintain normal calcium levels is mandatory for the preservation of life. In such an endocrine emergency, the laboratory's role often expands to include provision of data that will assist the medical team in localization and quantitation of PTH-secreting tissue for subsequent surgical removal.

Inadequate secretion of the parathyroids is reflected in lowered serum ionized calcium levels. Laboratory results are vital for early diagnosis and effective management. Preservation of calcium balance is achieved through numerous complex enzymatic and hormonal interactions.

ETIOLOGY AND PATHOPHYSIOLOGY
Hyperparathyroidism

Hyperparathyroidism (HPT) and therefore the excessive production of PTH, may be caused by increased total mass

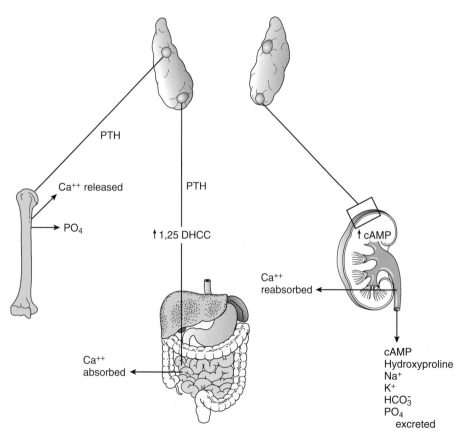

Figure 30–1. Effects of parathyroid hormone (PTH). Abbreviations: DHHC, dihydroxycholecalciferol; cAMP, cyclic adenosine monophosphate.

of secretory tissue, chief cell hyperfunctioning, or change in set point for calcium suppression of hormone release. Hyperparathyroid states have been classified as primary, secondary, and tertiary. Hypercalcemia that accompanies cancers and the familial multiple endocrine neoplasia syndromes (MENS) are also associated with hyperparathyroidism.[1]

The most common parathyroid disorder, *primary HPT,* is characterized by an increased concentration of serum calcium and an inappropriately high level of PTH. On the basis of the frequency with which hypercalcemia is detected during routine blood analyses, it is estimated that one in every 900 adults in the United States has some degree of HPT.[2] This disorder can be due to parathyroid hyperplasia, adenoma, or carcinomas. In more than 80% of cases, neoplastic transformation in the form of a single benign adenoma is the cause of hyperparathyroidism. Multiple-gland hyperplasia occurs in approximately 20% of patients, and all four glands are usually affected. Carcinomas are found in fewer than 1% of patients.[3] The cancers seem to grow slowly and usually metastasize locally. Primary HPT occurs more commonly in the elderly and is at least twice as common in females as in males. A disease incidence of 0.18% for females more than 60 years of age has been reported.[4] Although an idiopathic etiology is common for primary HPT, the medical history of approximately one-quarter of such patients reveals previous head and neck irradiation.[3] Dose-dependent, radiation-induced HPT may arise as long as 30 years after initial exposure.[5]

Hyperparathyroidism may arise as a compensatory response to prolonged hypocalcemia. In long-standing impairment of kidney function, there is an accompanying reduction in renal production of 1,25-DHCC. Intestinal calcium absorption is sharply reduced, and hypocalcemia develops. Continual stimulation of PTH release through feedback regulation induces glandular hyperplasia and hypersecretion, which are thus secondary to chronic renal disease or vitamin D deficiency; this condition is called *secondary HPT.* Classic chemical manifestations of secondary HPT due to chronic renal failure include hypocalcemia, hyperphosphatemia, and increased levels of PTH. The mass of parathyroid tissue present in patients with secondary HPT is generally far greater than that found in patients with primary HPT.[6] Studies indicate that there is a decreased sensitivity to the suppressive effects of ionized calcium on PTH release in both primary and secondary HPT.[7] In conclusion, *secondary PTH* refers to parathyroid hyperplasia stimulated by hypocalcemia or hyperphosphatemia. Secondary parathyroid hyperplasia developing into an autonomous tertiary parathyroid neoplasia has been postulated.

In *tertiary HPT,* hypercalcemia results when the parathyroid glands develop "autonomous" or nonsuppressible PTH secretion following an extended period of secondary HPT. Parathyroid hyperplasia may also occur when there is target-organ resistance to hormone action. In the condition of pseudohypoparathyroidism, low serum calcium triggers increased PTH secretion, but the kidneys and bone are unresponsive. This unresponsiveness is presumably due to defective hormone receptors or an inherited deficiency in regulatory protein within the cell membrane.[8] Hypocalcemia persists despite increased PTH secretion.

The production of a molecule that closely resembles PTH at the amino-terminal end by nonparathyroid neoplasms is rare. Solid tumors such as squamous cell carcinomas of the lung may produce this PTH-related protein (PTHrP). Excessive amounts of PTHrP are actually the cause of humoral hypercalcemia of malignancy (HHM).[9] The hypercalcemia that accompanies many of these malignancies was formerly called "ectopic hyperparathyroidism" or "pseudohyperparathyroidism." Severe hypercalcemia accompanied by low or undetectable levels of PTH may indicate malignancy. Oncogenic hypercalcemia is attributable to development of osteolytic metastases, as in breast cancer, or to the secretion of humoral, but non-PTH, bone-mobilizing factors such as osteoclast-activating factor (OAF) in multiple myeloma and other hematologic malignancies.[10]

It is critical that the hypercalcemias of malignancy and primary HPT be differentiated as early as possible, so that appropriate therapy may be initiated. It has generally been observed that primary HPT is associated with lower serum calcium levels than are seen in malignancies and with normal to slightly elevated 1,25-DHCC. The duration of the hypercalcemia is typically longer than 6 months. In contrast, serum calcium levels are higher and serum 1,25-DHCC levels are usually decreased in patients with tumor-associated malignancy. The onset of the hypercalcemia is rapid. Unfortunately, clear separation of these conditions on the basis of laboratory findings is not always possible.

Elevated serum PTH levels also occur in 80% to 90% of patients with familial multiple endocrine neoplasia syndrome type I.[11] Type I or Werner's syndrome is inherited as an autosomal dominant trait. Affected individuals exhibit parathyroid hyperplasia or adenoma as well as pituitary and pancreatic tumors. The presentation of hyperparathyroidism is often the most common symptom in MENS type I.

Hypoparathyroidism

Inadequacies in glandular secretion of PTH often are limited in duration and are associated with a specific traumatic event. Acute PTH deficiency may be encountered among patients who have experienced a temporary disruption of blood flow to the neck, as from an injury, surgery, or infarction. A period of hormone insufficiency, the so-called hungry bones phenomenon, may also occur in patients with significant preoperative bone disease. Following removal of adenomatous or hyperplastic parathyroid tissue, hypocalcemia and recalcification tetany are often observed. The remaining glandular tissue, which is capable of normal functioning, temporarily remains suppressed in response to the preexisting, long-standing hypercalcemia. In addition, rapid remineralization of bone through increased osteoblastic activity quickly depletes circulating ionized calcium. Such a hypoparathyroid condition is usually transient.

A number of drugs have been reported to alter parathyroid function. Patients with acute leukemia who are treated with doxorubicin or cytarabine may experience a temporary hypocalcemia, hypomagnesemia, and lowered levels of PTH.[3] The organic thiophosphate compound WR-2721, employed to protect healthy tissue during irradiation and chemotherapy, inhibits PTH secretion. Aminoglycosides and cisplatin may suppress serum magnesium levels. Severe hypomagnesemia, in turn, causes hypocalcemia through suppression of PTH secretion and diminished end-organ responsiveness to the hormone.[3, 4]

Permanent primary hypoparathyroidism may occur following removal of or damage to the glands. Thyroid surgery is the most common cause of hypoparathyroidism.[1] In the immediate postoperative period, a serum ionized calcium value of 8.0 mg/dL has been interpreted as suggestive of partial hypoparathyroidism, and levels of 5.0 to 6.0 mg/dL as suggestive of functional aparathyroidism.[4] Damage to the glands may also result from autoimmune responses.

It is unusual to encounter a person with missing or rudimentary parathyroid glands. DiGeorge's syndrome is a rare congenital disorder in which neonatal PTH deficiency is caused by aplasia of the parathyroids and thymus. Patients die in early childhood of severe hypocalcemia and persistent infections.[1]

Functional hypoparathyroidism and hypocalcemia are often seen in pediatric patients, particularly preterm, low-birth-weight infants. This is attributed to a temporary "immaturity" or unresponsiveness of the glands to low circulating levels of calcium for several hours after birth.[12, 13] Fetal PTH secretion may be inhibited in utero in response to maternal hypercalcemia.[14] Serum calcium levels below 3.0 mg/dL should be considered an emergency and treated aggressively. Plasma phosphate levels usually exceed 6.0 mg/dL in children who are hypoparathyroid.

Pseudohypoparathyroidism was a term applied to a condition in which there is a resistance to PTH action in the target tissues. Abnormalities in sensitivity or numbers of membrane receptors or regulatory proteins appear to be the basis for the decrease in end-organ response.[1, 11] The resultant hypocalcemia, hyperphosphatemia, and parathyroid hyperplasia were associated with a characteristic appearance in these patients. The characteristics noted were short stature, obesity, round face, short metacarpals, and basal ganglia calcification. Some patients, however, have the same defect in the nucleotide regulatory units but are not hypocalcemic. These patients were described as having "pseudopseudohypoparathyroidism." Both syndromes are now known as Albright's hereditary osteodystrophy (AHO).[15]

Idiopathic hypoparathyroidism refers to a broad category of disorders. Onset of symptoms may occur in early childhood or late in life. Although circulating glandular antibodies have been reported in some cases, the etiology of parathyroid destruction in these patients is unclear.

Acquired defects of PTH release and PTH activity are not uncommon. A decreased magnesium level impairs PTH release and also blunts its hypercalemic effect. Once the magnesium deficiency has been corrected, PTH secretion is promptly restored, but the PTH effect is resolved more slowly. Persons prone to malnutrition, such as alcoholics, may have a tendency to develop hypomagnesemia.

CLINICAL MANIFESTATIONS

Abnormalities in parathyroid structure or function come to the attention of the physician when a patient presents with symptoms resulting from calcium "imbalance" or when an abnormal calcium level is detected during routine laboratory screening in conjunction with a regular or routine physical examination.

Hyperparathyroidism

Increased levels of PTH lead to elevations of serum calcium. The severity of the hypercalcemia may be either life-threatening or of no apparent consequence to the patient. The clinical manifestations reflect both the severity and duration of the hypercalcemia, and the most serious organ damage involves the kidneys, heart, and brain.

The clinical manifestations of hypercalcemia are diverse. The central nervous system (CNS) manifestations are depression, coma, and seizures. With a sustained hypercalcemia, glomerular filtration declines, and polyuria, nocturia, polydipsia, and mild azotemia are seen. Nephrolithiasis is a common manifestation of hypercalcemia.

Hypercalcemia has an effect on the contractility of smooth and skeletal muscle. Fatigue, weakness, and hyporeflexia or hyperreflexia are manifest. The gastrointestinal (GI) tract is affected, and anorexia, nausea, abdominal pain, and constipation may be seen in some patients. Occasionally, increased gastrin secretion leads to greater gastric acid production and the formation of peptic ulcers. The pancreatic enzymes can be activated, resulting in overt pancreatitis.

The skeletal system may be affected. Bone pain, fractures, bone cysts, and pseudogout may be observed. If the hypercalcemia continues over a long time, calcium may be precipitated in the soft tissues, including the lung, kidney, blood vessels, and joints. Calcium salts may also be deposited in the cornea of the eye, resulting in band keratopathy.

Clinical presentation of primary HPT ranges from asymptomatic to severe. About one-half of patients report no symptoms, and the only evidence of the condition is laboratory-identified hypercalcemia, hypophosphatemia, and hypercalciuria detected during routine analysis. When the condition was first described, a combination of symptoms were described, including severe bone disease, loss of stature, weakness and wasting, anemia, and renal impairment.[1] The hypercalcemic state can produce a constellation of symptoms. Common nonspecific mild complaints are malaise, general fatigue, anorexia, muscle weakness, aching, and excessive thirst and urination. Constipation due to decreased smooth muscle activity in the GI tract is seen in approximately one-third of patients. Peptic ulcers and associated abdominal pain are also commonly reported. It has been reported that up to 50% of primary HPT patients have hypertension.[3, 4] Bone pain and arthralgia may occur without radiographic evidence of skeletal lesions. Significant bone disease, such as osteitis fibrosa cystica, characterized by generalized patchy demineralization, bone cysts, brown tumors, and excessive bone resorption, have also been described in some patients. Renal damage may occur. There may be evidence of renal stone disease, nephrocalcinosis, and reduced glomerular filtration. Mental disturbances are common. The affected patient may exhibit somnolence, coma, paranoia, or even hallucinations.

Secondary HPT results from hypersecretion of PTH in response to another disease. This response seldom produces hypercalcemia. Patients with secondary HPT have the signs and symptoms of the underlying disease. Advanced chronic renal failure is often associated with secondary HPT. When glomerular filtration declines, serum levels of phosphorus rise, resulting in reduced calcium levels. The net effect of the imbalance is the production of bone disease and the condition of renal osteodystrophy. Only if the secondary HPT is severe does renal osteodystrophy occur. This disease manifests predominantly as osteomalacia and, in very severe cases, osteitis fibrosa cystica. With osteomalacia, the disorder is manifest clinically by bone pain, fracture, and radiographic evidence of demineralization of the bones. Radiographs showing a "ground-glass" appearance of the skull, subperiosteal resorption in the hand, or resorption of the distal ends of the clavicles are characteristics of osteitis fibrosa.

If the patient develops tertiary HPT, any of the clinical manifestations of primary HPT can be seen in addition to those seen in secondary HPT. Even if the symptoms accompanying the secondary HPT are alleviated, adenoma or hyperplastic glands continue to secrete excessive quantities of PTH, and thus, the symptoms of primary HPT persist.

Hypoparathyroidism

A lowered serum ionized calcium level is the chemical basis for the signs and symptoms associated with hypoparathyroidism. It is the rapidity with which calcium deficiency develops, more than the absolute value of the serum ionized calcium, that determines the clinical manifestations of hypocalcemia.[1] Influenced by the extent and duration of calcium deficiency, a wide diversity of signs and symptoms are encountered. For example, patients with chronic hypocalcemia may be asymptomatic, may develop cataracts at an early age, or may have such dermatologic diseases as moniliasis or psoriasis. Most often, there is evidence of neuromuscular irritability and tetany, ranging from weakness and muscle cramps to seizures.[6] Indications of latent tetany include the ability to elicit contractions in response to specific stimuli of facial or wrist muscles. These spasmodic muscular contractions are known respectively as Chvostek's and Trousseau's signs. If respiratory muscles become involved, laryngospasm, bronchospasm, and respiratory arrest may follow.[4] Psychiatric manifestations range from anxiety and irritability to dementia. Cardiovascular difficulties include arrhythmias, digitalis insensitivity, hypotension, and congestive heart failure.[3, 4]

Symptoms of primary hypoparathyroidism resulting from surgical intervention are usually transient. The remaining parathyroid tissue only remains suppressed temporarily, and normal function returns within a short time. Paresthesia, restlessness, and Chvostek's or Trousseau's sign may be present during the interim. If the hypocalcemia has developed over a longer period, changes in the skin, development of cataracts, fatigue, and muscle aches or cramps may be the prominent clinical manifestations.

In classic cases of AHO or pseudohypoparathyroidism, individuals are characterized by physical as well as biochemical abnormalities. They are short (less than 5 feet), of stocky build or obese, and moon faced. Most show some mental impairment. Skeletal abnormalities include shortening of the phalanges as well as the fourth and fifth metacarpals and metatarsals. Ectopic ossifications are common. Most patients will also show signs of chronic hypocalcemia.[6,15,17]

LABORATORY ANALYSES AND DIAGNOSIS

Hyperparathyroidism

Assessment of parathyroid function is one of the ways in which the clinical laboratory scientist can assist the physician in the identification and management of diseases of bone and calcium metabolism. Gland activity may be evaluated by means of either direct or indirect methodologies. Selection of a particular assay or group of tests is made with the goal of clearly distinguishing normoparathyroid from hypoparathyroid individuals and differentiating patients with primary hyperparathyroidism either from those with hyperparathyroidism secondary to chronic renal failure or from those with hypercalcemia of nonparathyroid origin as seen in malignancy. The clinical laboratory scientist's responsibility must be to provide recommendations to the clinician as to procedures most likely to provide data eliminating, or at least minimizing, overlap among patient populations. The most effective and efficient diagnostic protocols are most likely to be cost-effective as well.

Establishment and confirmation of hypercalcemia remains the pivotal event in the laboratory diagnosis of parathyroid dysfunction. Although serum calcium level alone is an insufficient discriminator of parathyroid function, evaluation of this analyte offers a readily obtainable, inexpensive means of identifying individuals with possible gland disorders.[12] The total serum calcium level is elevated at some time in 96% or more of patients with primary hyperparathyroidism.[1]

To evaluate total serum calcium results, correction must be applied for the serum protein status. For each change in serum albumin of 1.0 g/dL, total serum calcium changes in parallel by approximately 0.8 mg/dL. The serum calcium can be adjusted to correct for a decreased albumin by using the following formula:

$$\text{Adjusted calcium (mg/dL)} = \text{total calcium (mg/dL)} - \text{albumin (g/dL)} + 4.0$$

In hypercalcemia, serum calcium is often in the range of 10.2 to 11.0 mg/dL. Hypercalcemic crisis is reached when values exceed 14.0 to 15.0 mg/dL.

Among hospital patients, the most common cause of hypercalcemia is malignancy with bone metastases.[18] Other conditions characterized by hypercalcemia are hyperthyroidism, renal disease, adrenal insufficiency, sarcoidosis, myeloma, milk-alkali syndrome, hypervitaminosis A or D, long-term immobilization, and therapy with thiazide diuretics.[16] Persistent hypercalcemia in the absence of other identifiable causes is often the basis for a diagnosis of primary HPT. In secondary HPT, serum calcium levels are generally normal or decreased.

Measurements by the clinical laboratory that have proved relevant, but not conclusive, in the diagnosis of disorders of the parathyroid include serum levels of inorganic phosphorus, chloride, bicarbonate, and alkaline phosphatase, and urine levels of calcium and cAMP. In primary

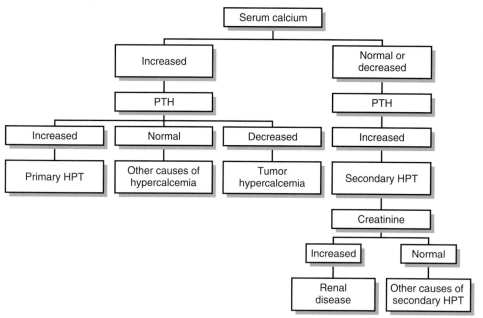

Figure 30–2. Hyperparathyroid panel. Abbreviations: HPT, hyperparathyroidism.

HPT, the serum phosphorus level is usually low. The serum chloride level is usually greater than 102 mmol/L, and the bicarbonate slightly decreased. The elevated chloride and decreased bicarbonate levels reflect the influence of excess PTH on renal bicarbonate excretion. A mild metabolic acidosis is commonly the result. Patients with hypercalcemia due to causes other than primary HPT tend to develop metabolic alkalosis and have chloride levels less than 102 mmol/L. In some patients, there is evidence of bone disease. With the marked bone resorption and osteoblastic activity, there is a release of alkaline phosphatase, causing an increase in the serum alkaline phosphatase level. Urine levels of calcium, phosphorus, and cAMP are elevated.

The definitive assessment of parathyroid dysfunction is the measurement of circulating PTH levels. Until recently, the techniques utilized made the interpretation of PTH levels difficult; however, the double-antibody immunoradiometric assay (IRMA) method has made the PTH assay a very useful assay. An elevated value confirms the hyperparathyroidism but does not delineate the etiology.

As described previously, the parathyroid gland secretes a mixture of PTH molecules. Intact PTH (PTH$_i$) represents a small portion of the total circulating PTH, and its half-life can be measured in minutes. Primary HPT, secondary HPT, and tumor hypercalcemia can be differentiated by utilizing serum calcium measurement and IRMA PTH assay (Fig. 30–2).

If the calcium level is decreased and the PTH level is increased, the condition is secondary HPT. This condition is most often caused by chronic renal failure and can be confirmed with a renal function test such as a serum creatinine measurement. In patients with impaired renal function, an elevated PTH may mean inadequate clearance. The assay should be repeated when the patient is rehydrated and renal function has improved.

If the calcium level is increased and the PTH level is decreased, the results are usually due to a malignancy. The calcium elevation is caused by the release of PTHrP. The high calcium levels then suppress the PTH levels. This condition, also called tumor hypercalcemia, is seen in 10% to 20% of patients with malignancy.[19]

If the calcium level and the PTH level are both increased, the cause is most likely primary HPT.

Hypoparathyroidism

If both the calcium levels and the PTH$_i$ levels are below normal, the condition is hypoparathyroidism (Fig. 30–3). This is caused by deficient secretion of PTH, which can be due to autoimmune destruction or to unintentional removal of or damage to the glands during thyroidectomy. Because PTH secretion is low, calcium absorption from the gut is decreased. As a consequence, calcium is not mobilized from the bone, and renal absorption of phosphorus is maximized. In addition to the elevated serum calcium level, serum phosphorus and urine calcium and phosphorus levels are decreased.

Laboratory findings are identical with regard to serum and urine calcium and phosphorus levels in pseudohypoparathyroidism. The main exception is the increased PTH$_i$ found in pseudohypoparathyroidism and also the elevated level of serum alkaline phosphatase that may be present.

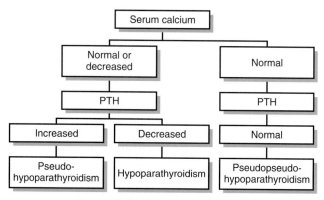

Figure 30–3. Hypoparathyroid panel.

The alkaline phosphatase level is normal in hypoparathyroidism.

TREATMENT

Hyperparathyroidism

Rapid correction of moderate to severe hypercalcemia involves restoration of intravascular volume with normal saline infusion and acceleration of calcium excretion by forcing saline diuresis. In some patients with primary HPT, no treatment is necessary. This is true if the patient is elderly and the hypercalcemia is mild. In those cases, hydration may restore the calcium level to normal.

In most patients, however, surgery is usually recommended and is the only curative therapy. If an adenomatous lesion is found, only one gland is removed. If no tumor is found and biopsies show changes consistent with HPT, three glands are removed completely, and part of the fourth is removed. Other surgeons remove all four glands and then implant some of the glandular tissue in a muscle that is accessible to maintain homeostasis. After surgery, most patients who do not have severe osteitis have some degree of hypocalcemia. This finding usually reflects transient suppression of the other glands, and temporary calcium replacement maintains the patient until PTH secretion resumes.

The treatment for secondary HPT is to control the underlying disease. Pharmacologic manipulation may help if control is not possible. If the secondary HPT is due to chronic renal failure, serum phosphorus levels may be controlled with oral phosphate binders.

Hypoparathyroidism

PTH is not used for the treatment of hypoparathyroidism. The actions of vitamin D are so similar to those of PTH that new analogues of vitamin D in combination with calcium are used in the treatment of the hypocalcemia. Dihydroxyvitamin D_3 or $1-(OH)D_3$ can be used in the treatment of hypoparathyroidism, because the hepatic enzyme, 25-hydroxylase, can utilize this compound as a substrate. Calcitriol is also available for treatment. If the patient has liver disease or malabsorption problems, calcifediol is used, with the expectation that the kidney will add the $1-\alpha$-OH group. Treatment with all vitamin D or vitamin D analogues must be monitored with serum calcium levels. Doses decrease with normalization of serum calcium levels and healing of bone lesions.

Case Study 1

During a routine preemployment physical examination conducted by her family physician, a 37-year-old woman was found to have a blood pressure of 148/95 mm Hg. The patient was of average height and weight. She stated that although she had tired somewhat more easily over the past few months, she had no specific physical complaints. Both the patient and her physician considered her to be in good health. At the time of her last physical examination (18 months previously), her blood pressure was 130/80 mm Hg, and all laboratory test results were within reference ranges.

The laboratory findings (with reference ranges) are as follows:

Calcium	11.8 mg/dL (8.5–10.5)
Phosphorus	1.6 mg/dL (2.5–4.5)
Sodium	137 mmol/L (135–145)
Potassium	4.2 mmol/L (3.5–4.5)
Chloride	107 mmol/L (96–106)
Bicarbonate	24 mmol/L (23–27)

The complete blood count and urinalysis were normal. A chest x-ray taken at the time was unremarkable. The patient reported that the only medications she was taking were an over-the-counter multiple-vitamin supplement once a day and a calcium supplement that she believed would minimize her risk of developing osteoporosis later in life.

The patient was instructed by her physician to return to the clinic later in the week for additional laboratory tests.

Questions

1. What element(s) of the physical examination and initial laboratory findings support a preliminary diagnosis of primary hyperparathyroidism?
2. In addition to a disorder of the parathyroids, what other etiologies of hypercalcemia would the physician be likely to consider?
3. What laboratory tests will the physician order to assess parathyroid function in follow-up testing of the patient?

Discussion

1. A diagnosis of primary hyperparathyroidism is suggested by the patient's hypertension, hypercalcemia, hypophosphatemia, and elevated serum chloride.
2. In most clinical circumstances, hypercalcemia suggests either hyperparathyroidism or malignancy. Other causes of hypercalcemia that would need to be excluded are nonparathyroid endocrine disorders such as hyperthyroidism and MENS; drug usage with vitamin A or D, thiazide diuretics, or a combination of calcium and antacids; or the presence of a granulomatous disease such as tuberculosis, sarcoidosis, histoplasmosis, or coccidioidomycosis.
3. The physician will require an additional serum calcium evaluation to verify the existence of hypercalcemia. Parathyroid profiles provided by most laboratories include measurements of serum calcium, phosphorus, creatinine, and PTH_i.

Case Study 2

A 9-year-old boy was seen by his physician. He was 4 feet 7 inches tall and weighed 100 lb. He had not been in good health since age 6, when he began to experience seizures. His seizures have been controlled by medication. He underwent bilateral cataract surgery at age 8. He recently experienced fatigue and muscle cramps.

The laboratory findings (with reference ranges) were as follows:

Calcium	7.2 mg/dL (8.5–10.5)
Phosphorus	5.0 mg/dL (2.5–4.5)
Alkaline phosphatase	120 U/L (35–100)
Urine calcium	75 mg/day (100–400)
Total protein	5.6 g/dL (6.0–8.0)
Albumin	3.2 g/dL (3.4–5.0)

Questions

1. What is the serum calcium level when corrected for the decreased albumin?
2. From the laboratory findings and the patient's history, what disease state is present?
3. Describe the pathophysiology of this disease state.
4. What laboratory test would confirm the proposed condition, and what results would be expected?

Discussion

1. The formula that can be used to correct the calcium level is as follows:

   Adjusted calcium = Total calcium − Albumin + 4.0
   8.0 = 7.2 − 3.2 + 4.0
2. The findings are consistent with pseudohypoparathyroidism.
3. Pseudohypoparathyroidism is caused by abnormalities in sensitivity or numbers of membrane receptors or regulatory proteins.
4. PTH assay should be performed; the level should be increased.

References

1. Federman DD: Parathyroid. *In* Dale DC, Federman DD (eds): Scientific American Medicine 3(VI). New York, Scientific American, Inc, 1995, pp 1–17.
2. Boonstra CE, Jackson CE: Hyperparathyroidism detected by routine serum calcium analysis—prevalence in a clinical population. Ann Intern Med 6:468–474, 1965.
3. Jubiz W: Endocrinology: A Logical Approach for Clinicians, ed 2. New York, McGraw-Hill, 1985.
4. Zaloga GP, Chernow B: Calcium metabolism. *In* Geelhoed GW, Chernow B (eds): Endocrine Aspects of Acute Illness. New York, Churchill Livingstone, 1975.
5. Rao SD, Frame B, Miller MJ, et al: Hyperparathyroidism following head and neck irradiation. Arch Intern Med 140:205–207, 1980.
6. Rabin D, McKenna TJ (eds): Clinical Endocrinology and Metabolism: Principles and Practice. New York, Grune & Stratton, 1982.
7. LeBoff MS, Shoback D, Brown EM, et al: Regulation of parathyroid hormone release and cytosolic calcium by extracellular calcium in dispersed and cultured bovine and pathological human parathyroid cells. J Clin Invest 75:49–57, 1985.
8. Teitelbaum AP, Arnaud CD: Parathyroid hormone receptors: An assay for circulating PTH? Diagn Med 5:69–74, 1982.
9. Seymour JF: Malignancy-associated hypercalcemia. Sci Med 2:48–57, 1995.
10. Mundy GR, Ibbotson KJ, D'Souza SM: Tumor products and the hypercalcemia of malignancy. J Clin Invest 76:391–394, 1985.
11. Williams TF, Streck WF: Multiple endocrine neoplasia (MEN) syndromes. *In* Streck WF, Lockwood DH (eds): Endocrine Diagnosis: Clinical and Laboratory Approach. Boston, Little, Brown, 1983.
12. Bower GN Jr, Brassard C, Sena SF: Measure of ionized calcium in serum with ion-selective electrodes: A mature technology that can meet the daily service needs. Clin Chem 32:1437–1447, 1986.
13. Pena A: Hormonal and metabolic concerns in younger patients. *In* Geelhoed GW, Chernow B (eds): Endocrine Aspects of Acute Illness. New York, Churchill Livingstone, 1985.
14. Tasan RC, Steichen JJ, Chan GM: Neonatal hypocalcemia: Mechanisms of occurrence and management. Crit Care Med 5:56–61, 1977.
15. Schwindinger WF, Levine MA: Albright hereditary osteodystrophy. Endocrinologist 4:17, 1994.
16. Licata AA, Streck WF: Hypocalcemia. *In* Streck WF, Lockwood DG (eds): Endocrine Diagnosis: Clinical and Laboratory Approach. Boston, Little, Brown, 1983.
17. Arnaud CD, Kolb FO: The calciotropic hormones and metabolic bone disease. *In* Greenspan FS, Forsham PH (eds): Basic and Clinical Endocrinology. Los Altos, CA, Lange Medical, 1983.
18. Fisken RA, Heath DA, Somers S, et al: Hypercalcemia in hospital patients. Lancet 1:202–207, 1981.
19. Fraser D, Jones G, Kooh SW, Radde IL: Calcium and phosphate metabolism. *In* Tietz N (ed): Textbook of Clinical Chemistry. Philadelphia, WB Saunders, 1986.

Chapter 31

Disorders of the Adrenal Cortex

Shauna C. Anderson

A pair of adrenal glands cap the superior borders of the kidneys. Each adrenal gland consists of an outer portion and an inner portion, the cortex and the medulla, respectively. The adrenal cortex is derived from embryonic tissue known as mesoderm, and the medulla from neural crest ectoderm. Consequently, these tissues function as separate glands. The medulla secretes catecholamine hormones, mainly epinephrine, into the blood in response to stimulation by preganglionic sympathetic nerve fibers. The cortex consists of three zones: an outer zona glomerulosa, a middle zona fasciculata, and an inner zona reticularis. The cortex produces and secretes steroid hormones called corticosteroids. Depending on the functions of the steroids, they are classified as (1) mineralocorticoids, (2) glucocorticoids, and (3) sex steroids. The mineralocorticoids are produced by the zona glomerulosa, whereas the glucocorticoids and sex hormones are produced by the zona fasciculata and zona reticularis, respectively.

The glucocorticoids regulate the metabolism of carbohydrates, proteins, and fats. Cortisol is the principal glucocorticoid. Adrenocorticotropic hormone (ACTH) is the main regulator of cortisol production and secretion. ACTH is synthesized by the corticotropic cells in the anterior pituitary in response to corticotropin-releasing hormone (CRH), a peptide released by the hypothalamus. Although CRH is the principal regulator of ACTH synthesis, antidiuretic hormone (ADH), oxytocin and catecholamines may influence the diurnal rhythm of ACTH.[1] In addition, fever, hypoglycemia, stress, and psychological disturbances may trigger the release of ACTH.

ACTH is actually synthesized as a small segment of the complex molecule called pro-opiomelanocortin (POMC).[2] ACTH is secreted in a pulsatile fashion, with one to three pulses occurring each hour and clustering in the morning hours.[3] ACTH acts like other polypeptide hormones by activating adenylate cyclase in the target cell membrane and increasing levels of cyclic adenosine monophosphate (cAMP) and eventually the synthesis of cortisol. As cortisol is released from the adrenal gland into the blood stream, most of it is bound to an α-globulin called transcortin or cortisol-binding globulin (CBG). Only a small percentage of the cortisol circulates in the free state and is thus biologically active. The half-life of cortisol is longer than that of ACTH, and the pulses of ACTH produce an accumulation of cortisol levels that result in higher levels during the morning hours and lower levels in the evening, yielding a diurnal rhythm. Cortisol acts as a negative feedback product to the hypothalamus and the anterior pituitary, decreasing the release of CRH and ACTH. Figure 31–1 summarizes the regulation of cortisol levels.

Circulating steroid hormones can be metabolized in many organs, but the great majority are metabolized in the liver. After reduction and a number of other biotransformations, the molecules are conjugated with glucuronide or sulfate and excreted in the urine. Cortisol is metabolized and excreted as tetrahydrocortisol, tetrahydrocortisone, cortols, and cortolones. The metabolites are commonly known as 17-hydroxycorticosteroids (17-OH steroids).

The sex hormones are produced in varying amounts at different stages of life. The weak androgens that are produced by the adrenal glands may serve as precursors for the production of more potent androgens and estrogens in

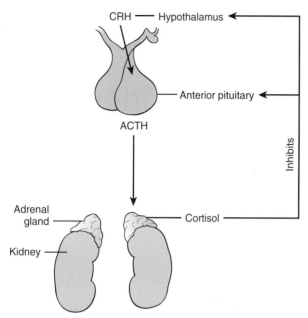

Figure 31–1. Regulation of cortisol. Abbreviations: CRH, corticotropin-releasing hormone; ACTH, adrenocorticotropic hormone.

other tissues. ACTH has been described as the regulator of adrenal androgen synthesis. Because ACTH levels do not vary in different age groups, another pituitary hormone called adrenal androgen-stimulating hormone has been proposed as an additional stimulator in order to explain the age-related levels of androgen production.[1] The sex hormones circulate bound to plasma proteins, the main one being steroid hormone–binding globulin (SHBG). Only a small percentage of the hormones circulate in the free state, and they are responsible for the biologic activity.

The sex hormones are metabolized in the liver. The androgens are excreted in the urine as 17-ketosteroids (17-KSs), and the estrogens are converted to estriol and then excreted in the urine.

Aldosterone, the main mineralocorticoid, is regulated by several control mechanisms. The renin-angiotensin system, the most important regulator, operates via changes in extracellular fluid volume. Under conditions of volume depletion, renin is released from the juxtaglomerular cells of the renal afferent arterioles. Renin acts enzymatically on a circulating α-globulin known as angiotensinogen. The action of renin produces angiotensin I. Angiotensin-converting enzyme (ACE), a peptidase found in the membrane of vascular endothelium, converts angiotensin I to angiotensin II. Angiotensin II is converted to angiotensin III by an aminopeptidase. Both angiotensin II and angiotensin III can bind to the receptor on the target cell. The binding of the angiotensin to the receptor activates the phosphatidylinositol cycle, which eventually stimulates the release of intracellular calcium and the secretion of aldosterone. Other stimuli to aldosterone secretion include increases in serum potassium and estrogen and reductions in blood volume and serum sodium.[1]

Aldosterone's action can be blocked by atrial natriuretic peptide (ANP), which is released from the atrium of the heart. ANP can also reduce the production of renin and inhibit the production of aldosterone by interfering with

the action of angiotensin II. Figure 31–2 summarizes the regulation of aldosterone levels.

After aldosterone is secreted by the zona glomerulosa cells, it circulates weakly bound to albumin, CBG, and other plasma proteins. Aldosterone is mainly metabolized in the liver and is excreted in the urine as glucuronic acid conjugates of aldosterone and tetrahydroaldosterone.

ETIOLOGY AND PATHOLOGY

Hypercortisolism

Hypercortisolism is characterized by elevated levels of plasma cortisol and loss of its diurnal variation. All causes of cortisol excess are classified under the generic name *Cushing's syndrome*. This syndrome is due to one of five factors: (1) exogenous administration of cortisol or ACTH, (2) excessive ACTH secretion by the anterior pituitary with resultant hyperplasia of the adrenal cortex and an increase in cortisol secretion (Cushing's disease), (3) ectopic ACTH or CRH secretion by a nonpituitary tumor, (4) autonomous hypersecretion of cortisol by an adrenal adenoma or carcinoma, or (5) adrenocortical nodular dysplasia.

By far the most common cause of Cushing's syndrome is prolonged glucocorticoid therapy. This condition is known as *iatrogenic Cushing's syndrome.*

It is estimated that two-thirds of all patients with endogenous Cushing's syndrome have Cushing's disease, which is caused by a pituitary adenoma that secretes ACTH.[1] Some of these patients do not actually have a discrete pituitary tumor, but the hypersecretion of the ACTH may be the result of hypothalamic disease.

Cushing's syndrome due to ectopic production of ACTH by malignant nonpituitary tumors is caused by an oat cell carcinoma of the lung in about one-half of cases.[1] Other types of tumors, such as islet cell tumors, renal tumors, thymomas, and bronchial adenomas, may also produce the ACTH. In addition to ectopic production of ACTH, some tumors can elaborate CRH. A bronchial carcinoma is the most common type of tumor to secrete both ACTH and CRH.[5]

Less than one-third of the causes of Cushing's syndrome are adrenal neoplasms.[1] Benign adrenal adenomas produce cortisol very efficiently. Adrenal carcinomas do not produce cortisol as efficiently and may also secrete large amounts of androgens.

A rare cause of Cushing's syndrome is primary adrenocortical nodular dysplasia. Patients with this condition have an autonomous production of glucocorticoids and low or normal levels of ACTH.[6] Histologically, the adrenal cortex contains brown-black nodules with atrophy of the rest of the cortex. This may be a familial disorder.[1]

Adrenal Insufficiency

Adrenal insufficiency may be primary or secondary. In primary adrenal insufficiency, there is a marked increase in ACTH. In secondary adrenal insufficiency, the ACTH level is decreased. Secondary adrenal insufficiency is commonly the result of prolonged therapeutic use of glucocorticoids, such as cortisone and prednisone. Less commonly, it may be due to a decrease in ACTH formation caused by a pituitary tumor. For patients experiencing hypopituitarism,

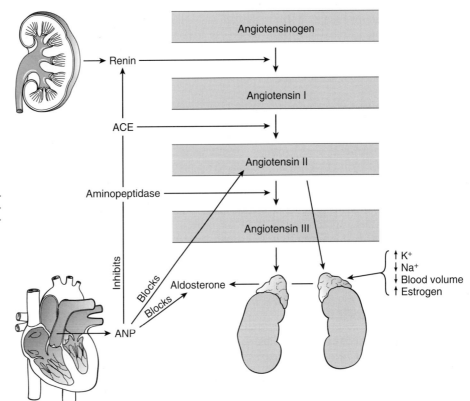

Figure 31–2. Regulation of aldosterone. Abbreviations: ACE, angiotensin-converting enzyme; ANP, atrial natriuretic peptide.

concurrent decreases in other pituitary hormones, such as growth hormone, thyroid-stimulating hormone, and gonadotropin-releasing hormone, may lead to symptoms associated with these deficiencies.

There are two manifestations of primary adrenal insufficiency, acute and chronic. Acute adrenal insufficiency is a rare condition. The most common cause is adrenal hemorrhage in patients who are undergoing anticoagulant therapy.[7, 8] Overwhelming sepsis (especially fulminant meningococcal sepsis, which may produce Waterhouse-Friderichsen syndrome)[9], surgery, trauma, myocardial infarction, and pregnancy have also been implicated as causes.

Chronic adrenal insufficiency has also been called Addison's disease. The most common cause is an autoimmune process. Initially, the adrenal cortex is infiltrated with lymphocytes and plasma cells, and then gradually, the cortical cells are destroyed. Granulomatous infections such as tuberculosis and histoplasmosis, amyloidosis, and infiltration by other pathogens, such as cytomegalovirus, and by Kaposi's sarcoma are also causes of Addison's disease. For all primary adrenal insufficiencies, the dysfunction results in decreased cortisol production, causing an elevation in ACTH from the removal of negative feedback.

Adrenogenital Syndrome

The adrenogenital syndrome encompasses a group of disorders characterized by the excessive production of adrenal corticosteroids. In most cases, the patients have increased production and secretion of androgens, resulting in virilization. Disorders causing this syndrome are (1) congenital adrenal hyperplasia (CAH), (2) "postpubertal"

or late-onset adrenal hyperplasia (LOCAH), (3) adrenal adenoma, and (4) adrenal carcinoma.[10]

Congenital adrenal hyperplasia comprises a group of genetically transmitted inborn errors of the enzyme systems involved in cortisol synthesis by the adrenal glands. Deficient synthesis leads to increased ACTH release, followed by hyperplasia of the adrenal glands and increased production of a number of intermediate steroid hormones up to the point of the enzyme deficiency.

The most common enzyme deficiency is 21-hydroxylase deficiency. If the deficiency is complete, the patient suffers severe salt loss from the low production of aldosterone and adrenal insufficiency because of the low production of glucocorticoids. Other causes of CAH are deficiencies of 17-hydroxylase, 11-hydroxylase, 3β-hydroxysteroid dehydrogenase, and cholesterol desmolase.

Virilization may not appear until after puberty. These individuals may have a very mild enzyme deficiency, which is either congenital or acquired, but adrenal hyperplasia is present. Tumors producing excess androgens are very rare. These tumors may occur in persons at any age, but they are more common in adults.

Aldosterone Excess

Aldosterone is secreted in response to ACTH, intravascular volume contraction, or sodium deprivation. A chronic increase in aldosterone secretion can also occur in the presence of normal or enhanced dietary sodium intake and normal intravascular volume. In these instances, a state of mineralocorticoid excess or hyperaldosteronism occurs.[11] *Primary aldosteronism* exists when there is an excessive amount of aldosterone coming from the adrenal gland. When a reduction in renal perfusion occurs as a consequence of conditions such as heart failure or renal artery stenosis and elevated plasma renin levels increase the aldosterone levels, the condition is called *secondary hyperaldosteronism.*

The sites of action of aldosterone are the distal convoluted tubules and collecting tubules of the kidney nephron. At these sites, sodium and water are retained at the expense of potassium, magnesium, and hydrogen, resulting in increased total body sodium and hypervolemia. At a certain point, however, sodium retention halts and sodium excretion increases. Because of this phenomenon, patients rarely exhibit volume expansion or edema but do have arterial hypertension. Primary aldosteronism may be caused by unilateral adenoma (Conn's syndrome), bilateral hyperplasia, and, rarely, carcinoma. Most cases of primary aldosteronism are due to a single aldosterone-producing adrenal adenoma.[12]

Aldosterone Deficiency

Isolated defects of aldosterone synthesis are rare.[13] Partial defects are seen in CAH caused by 21-hydroxylase deficiency, which has been discussed previously. There are two forms of isolated aldosterone deficiency, idiopathic hypoaldosteronism and hyporeninemic hypoaldosteronism.

Idiopathic hypoaldosteronism is a rare condition. Hyporeninemic hypoaldosteronism is much more common. Typically, patients with hyporeninemic hypoaldosteronism are older than 45 years and have chronic renal disease. The kidney tubules and interstitial tissue are affected rather than the glomeruli. Because of the aldosterone deficiency, hyperkalemia and metabolic acidosis are seen. Renal excretion of potassium and hydrogen ions is impaired. The aldosterone appears to be diminished because of decreased renin release by defective juxtaglomerular cells; however, the condition has been shown to occur in indomethacin-induced prostaglandin deficiency. The condition is aggravated by heparin, calcium channel blockers, or β-adrenergic blockers.[1]

CLINICAL MANIFESTATIONS

Hypercortisolism

Regardless of the etiology, the clinical manifestations of Cushing's syndrome are similar with some slight variations. Because of the catabolic action of cortisol, amino acids are diverted from muscle tissue, leading to marked muscle wasting and muscle weakness. The amino acids that are diverted into the liver are deaminated, gluconeogenesis results, and blood glucose levels are raised. Glucose intolerance is common, but ketosis is uncommon.

Patients have a peculiar distribution of body fat. There is a tendency toward central obesity with the presence of a supraclavicular "buffalo hump." The face is rounded, being described as a "moon face."

The catabolic effects of cortisol also cause a loss of elastic fiber in the skin, giving it a thin, fine texture. Because of the thin nature of the skin, the underlying vasculature is more visible. Purple striae appear over the abdomen, thighs, arms, and chest. Capillary fragility results in easy bruisability. Wounds heal poorly.

Increased levels of glucocorticoids inhibit osteoblasts. As a consequence, osteoporosis and kyphosis occur in adults, and there is a retardation of growth in children.

One of the most common symptoms in hypercortisolism is hypertension. The hypertension appears to be the direct result of the weak mineralocorticoid activity of cortisol or of the increased secretion of deoxycorticosterone, which is a mineralocorticoid. In addition, glucocorticoids inhibit the synthesis of prostacyclin, a potent vasodilator, resulting in an imbalance between vasodilation and vasoconstriction.[14]

Psychiatric disturbances are common. Symptoms range from mild irritability or excitability to frank psychosis.

If androgen secretion is excessive, female patients may have oligomenorrhea, amenorrhea, or hirsutism. If excessive estrogens are produced, females may have a suppression of the luteinizing hormone (LH) surge and ovulation, whereas males may have decreased libido, testicular softening, or gynecomastia.

Cushing's syndrome due to ectopic production of ACTH or CRH by malignant nonpituitary tumors progresses so quickly that many patients do not have the classic features. Commonly, these patients actually have weight loss.

Patients in whom adrenal carcinoma is the etiology of the Cushing's syndrome may have very large tumors before they show the typical characteristics, because such tumors do not manufacture cortisol very efficiently. These patients often have metastatic tumors by the time the symptoms appear.

Adrenal Insufficiency

Acute primary adrenal insufficiency is characterized by profound asthenia, severe pains in the abdomen, lower back, and legs, peripheral vascular collapse, and, finally, renal shutdown. Body temperature may be subnormal, or it may be elevated if the cause is sepsis.

Patients who have had chronic adrenal insufficiency for a long period have a marked hyperpigmentation of the skin. Because of the decreased production of cortisol, the anterior pituitary gland is stimulated to synthesize large quantities of ACTH. ACTH is a product of the larger molecule POMC, which also produces melanocyte-stimulating hormone (MSH). The hyperpigmentation is accentuated in skin creases, scars, and buccal mucosa.

A number of symptoms, such as weakness, malaise, weight loss, fever, myalgia, and hypotension, are common complaints. Unless adrenal collapse occurs, the laboratory findings are not impressive. With adrenal collapse, hyponatremia, hyperkalemia, hypoglycemia, hemoconcentration, and elevations of blood urea nitrogen (BUN) levels are seen. The changes in the electrolytes and BUN are related to a volume deficiency and prerenal azotemia.

Patients with secondary adrenal insufficiency due to ACTH hyposecretion have a syndrome similar to that in patients with Addison's disease; however, because aldosterone is not primarily under ACTH control, electrolyte and volume regulation are less affected in patients with hypopituitarism than in patients with Addison's disease. Hyperpigmentation is also absent in secondary adrenal insufficiency, because the ACTH levels are low.

Adrenogenital Syndrome

The clinical manifestations of adrenogenital syndrome depend on the age and gender of the patient as well as the underlying pathology. Excessive circulating androgens produce virilization, which manifests as clitoral hypertrophy, deepening of the voice, temporal hair recession, and balding.[15] Inappropriate heavy hair growth in androgen-sensitive areas such as the beard and mustache areas (hirsutism) is also present.

In CAH, in which there is a deficiency in enzymes, the fetus is exposed to excessive quantities of circulating androgens and continued virilization after birth. The female has ambiguous external genitalia at birth. In the male, abnormalities at birth are difficult to detect. If the condition is not treated, the female does not show signs of puberty, and amenorrhea and hirsutism are common findings. In the male, virilization continues, producing increased somatic growth, advancement of epiphyseal maturation, and premature development of pubic, axillary, and facial hair.

In about one-half of patients with complete 21-hydroxylase deficiency, a salt-losing crisis and the tendency to be hypotensive occurs because of the decreased synthesis of aldosterone. Some patients actually have greater production of aldosterone but do not have signs of hyperaldosteronism. The external genitalia of females are abnormal, and hirsutism develops. In mild deficiencies, females may have abnormal external genitalia, but signs of virilization may not appear until later in life.

With 11-hydroxylase deficiency, the clinical manifestations of virilization are similar; however, the absence of 11-hydroxylation leads to the formation of 11-deoxycorticosterone, a potent retainer of sodium. Hypertension is a result.

Aldosterone Excess

Primary aldosteronism occurs most commonly between the ages of 30 and 50 years and is more common in females than in males.[16] The main clinical manifestation of primary aldosteronism is arterial hypertension. It is estimated that 0.05% to 2.0% of hypertension may be due to primary aldosteronism.[1] In addition, affected patients may have borderline-low or low levels of potassium. Potassium depletion results in muscle weakness and fatigue, which is usually more pronounced in the lower extremities but can progress to transient paralysis. Another consequence of hypokalemia is a defect in urinary concentration. Patients may have nocturnal polyuria sometimes in association with polydipsia. The potassium depletion may also be related to a diminished glucose tolerance, which may manifest as diabetes mellitus in some patients. Hydrogen ions may be excreted in the urine as well as potassium. The loss of hydrogen ions may lead to a metabolic alkalosis in some patients.

Secondary aldosteronism occurs when there is an elevation of aldosterone due to increases in renin levels. Some patients have hypertension, and some do not. Most of the cases of secondary aldosteronism are the edematous disorders without hypertension, including nephrotic syndrome, cirrhosis with ascites, and congestive heart failure. With these conditions, there is a disturbance of circulating blood volume, which stimulates the renin-angiotensin-aldosterone axis. Patients with secondary aldosteronism and hypertension commonly have malignant or accelerated hypertension. This condition is associated with high levels of renin and aldosterone owing to decreased renal perfusion.

Aldosterone Deficiency

The main symptom of aldosterone deficiency is hypotension. With idiopathic hypoaldosteronism, the patient may present with heart block, which is secondary to hyperkalemia, or with postural hypotension, which is secondary to hypovolemia. Diabetes mellitus is a common finding in patients with hyporeninemic hypoaldosteronism. These patients have a mild to marked chronic hyperkalemia and a tendency to develop a hyperchloremic metabolic acidosis with a normal or low sodium level. Sodium restriction aggravates the clinical manifestations.

LABORATORY ANALYSES AND DIAGNOSIS

Hypercortisolism

Routine laboratory data in Cushing's syndrome may not reveal any abnormalities. Leukocytosis, in particular neutrophilia, may be seen because of the demargination of the neutrophils in hypercortisolism. Because there is increased gluconeogenesis and glycogenolysis, a glucose tolerance test (GTT) may reveal the glucose intolerance. Some patients may have hypernatremia and hypokalemia.

A diagnosis of hypercortisolism must be established first, and then the cause is elucidated. The best screening test is the measurement of urinary free cortisol (UFC) in a 24-hour urine sample. This should be performed on three different collection samples.[17] The screening test should be followed by measurements of plasma ACTH and cortisol and 17-OH steroids, which are used to evaluate adrenal function. Normally, cortisol levels show a diurnal variation, with levels higher in the morning than in the evening. There is a loss of the normal diurnal pattern in Cushing's syndrome. The plasma cortisol level is influenced by the CBG levels. This fact should be kept in mind during evaluation of results. If the UFC is elevated, an overnight dexamethasone suppression test is recommended.

Dexamethasone is a potent analogue of cortisol, and in a normal subject, 1 mg given at 11:00 PM suppresses plasma cortisol levels to below 140 nmol/L at 8:00 or 9:00 AM the following day. Suppression occurs in normal subjects and in some with stress and depression, hypercortisolism ensues. If the cortisol level is not suppressed, a low-dose dexamethasone suppression (LDDS) test may be indicated.

For the LDDS test, dexamethasone (0.5 mg) is administered every 6 hours for 2 days. If a 24-hour urinary 17-OH steroid level is less than 3.5 mg/24 hours on the second day or the plasma cortisol is less than 140 nmol/L on the third morning, Cushing's syndrome is ruled out. The next step is to identify the etiology of the hypercortisolism.

To establish whether the hypercortisolism is ACTH dependent or not, simultaneous plasma assays of cortisol and

ACTH should be performed. If the cortisol level is increased and the ACTH level is decreased, the patient has non–ACTH-dependent hypercortisolism. If the cortisol level is increased and the ACTH level is normal or elevated, the patient has ACTH-dependent hypercortisolism.

Evaluation using a high-dose dexamethasone suppression (HDDS) test may further define the pathology. Dexamethasone (2 mg) is administered every 6 hours for 2 days. Usually, if the urinary 17-OH steroid level is less than 35% of the baseline level, or if the plasma cortisol is less than 280 nmol/L, the patient has Cushing's disease.[1] If the urinary 17-OH steroid and the plasma cortisol levels are not suppressed, adrenal tumors producing high levels of cortisol or ectopic ACTH-producing tumors are most likely present. The previously performed plasma ACTH test is valuable in separating these conditions; ACTH level is low with an adrenal tumor and high with an ACTH-producing tumor. Computed tomography (CT) or magnetic resonance imaging (MRI) can pinpoint the location of the tumor. Figure 31–3 summarizes a diagnostic approach to hypercortisolism.

Adrenal Insufficiency

The finding of a low cortisol value with a high ACTH value in plasma or serum is diagnostic of primary adrenal insufficiency. If the condition is acute, the electrolyte changes and hypoglycemia may indicate that urgent treatment is required.

A short ACTH stimulation test is performed to assess adrenal reserve and, thereby, chronic adrenal insufficiency. A standard dose of Synacthen, a synthetic ACTH, is administered intramuscularly or intravenously. Plasma cortisol levels are determined at 0, 30, and 60 minutes. A normal person responds with a rise in plasma cortisol above 500 nmol/L. Failure of response suggests adrenal failure, which is confirmed by an elevated plasma ACTH value.

A long ACTH stimulation test may be indicated if ACTH levels cannot be assessed. A higher dose of Synacthen than the standard is given intramuscularly, and cortisol levels are assessed at 0, 1, 2, 8, 12 and 24 hours. Normally, the cortisol level peaks by 8 hours with a value of 900 nmol/L. If primary adrenal insufficiency is present, the response is impaired throughout the test. The presence of circulating antibodies to the adrenal cortex indicates an autoimmune process.

The diagnosis of secondary adrenal insufficiency requires the long ACTH stimulation test. In this condition, the cortisol levels rise slowly and do not peak until about 24 hours after Synacthen is injected. If the condition is of long standing, it may be necessary to give Synacthen for 3 days prior to a short ACTH stimulation test, which is performed on day 4 in order to demonstrate the response. Patients with secondary adrenal insufficiency may have normal, low, or undetectable levels of ACTH. These pa-

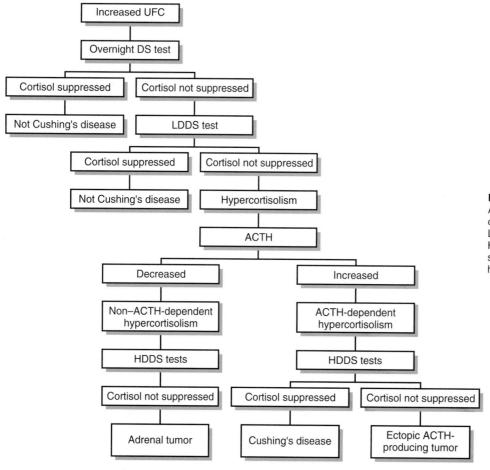

Figure 31–3. Hypercortisol panel. Abbreviations: UFC, urinary free cortisol; DS, dexamethasone; LDDS, low-dose dexamethasone; HDDS, high-dose dexamethasone; ACTH, adrenocorticotropic hormone.

tients commonly have deficiencies of other pituitary hormones.

CRH is available to distinguish between hypothalamic and pituitary etiologies of secondary adrenal insufficiency. If the ACTH level increases after a CRH stimulation test, the disease is of a hypothalamic origin. If there is no ACTH response, the pituitary is the origin of the ACTH deficiency. Figure 31–4 summarizes the laboratory diagnosis of adrenal insufficiency.

Adrenogenital Syndrome

Regardless of the pathology of the adrenogenital syndrome, the levels of androgens are increased, and virilization is a common clinical manifestation. Excessive levels of circulating androgens can be confirmed by measuring plasma levels of total and free testosterone and dehydroepiandrosterone sulfate (DHEAS). All patients with CAH have decreased plasma cortisol levels and increased ACTH levels.

The steroid elevated in direct response to a 21-hydroxylase deficiency is 17-hydroxyprogesterone (17-OHP). In severe cases, prompt evaluation of fluid and electrolyte status is crucial to avoid vascular collapse. Elevated serum potassium and low serum sodium values reflect the deficiency of the mineralocorticoid synthesis. In milder cases

of LOCAH, the simplest approach is to measure 17-OHP before and 1 hour after administration of intravenous cosyntropin. Sometimes basal levels are not elevated, but a post-ACTH value of 350 ng/dL or greater is diagnostic. Care should be exercised in interpreting 17-OHP levels, because timing of the blood sampling is very important.[17]

Patients with an 11-hydroxylase deficiency, in addition to increased levels of androgens and ACTH and decreased levels of cortisol, have elevation of serum sodium and a low serum potassium level. The main steroid increased is plasma 11-deoxycortisol.

The other enzyme defects are identified biochemically by demonstrating high plasma levels or urine metabolites of the respective enzyme substrates. However, ACTH is raised in all cases of CAH. Figure 31–5 summarizes the laboratory approach to the diagnosis of adrenogenital syndrome.

When an adenoma or a carcinoma is the cause of increases in DHEAS or testosterone levels, glucocorticoid suppression does not lower the levels. This suppression test can be used to differentiate hyperplasia from tumor. Clinical signs of glucocorticoid excess generally suggest adrenal carcinoma rather than adenoma. In addition, carcinomas are often palpable.[10]

Aldosterone Excess

The laboratory diagnosis of primary aldosteronism is made by demonstrating elevated aldosterone levels and the suppression of plasma renin activity (PRA). Aldosterone and other mineralocorticoids decrease urinary sodium excretion and increase potassium excretion and urinary acidification. Typical laboratory findings are decreases in serum potassium and magnesium, increases in urinary potassium and serum sodium, abnormal GTT, normal BUN, and a tendency toward metabolic alkalosis.

The patient who has clinical manifestations of primary aldosteronism should discontinue medication that can interfere with the renin-angiotensin-aldosterone axis before the laboratory investigation begins. Screening tests are serum and urine potassium measurements. If the serum potassium level is less than 3.5 mmol/L and the urine potassium level is greater than 30 mmol/24 hours, the next step is to measure plasma and urinary aldosterone and PRA.[1] The patient must be on a diet that provides at least 100 mEq of salt a day before the test is performed. After overnight recumbency, plasma aldosterone and renin levels are measured at 8:00 AM and again on a sample drawn 4 hours after the patient has been upright. A 24-hour urine sample is collected during that time, for which the aldosterone level is determined. In patients with primary aldosteronism, the plasma renin level is less than 1 ng/mL/hour and the plasma aldosterone level is greater than 15 ng/dL. The urinary aldosterone level is also increased.[1]

In some patients, it may be necessary to exclude other causes of hypokalemia or hypertension. This can be accomplished by demonstrating inappropriate and nonsuppressible aldosterone secretion with a suppression test. Methods to achieve suppression are (1) normal saline infusion, (2) fludrocortisone, and (3) captopril. The captopril suppression test may be the most cost-effective and the most reliable suppression test.[18]

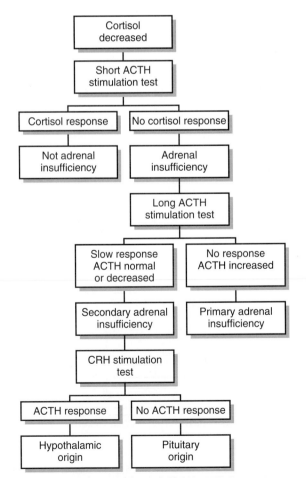

Figure 31–4. Adrenal insufficiency panel. Abbreviations: ACTH, adrenocorticotropic hormone; CRH, corticotropin-releasing hormone.

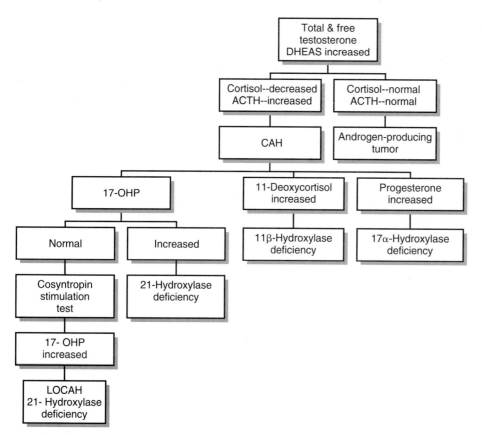

Figure 31–5. Adrenogenital syndrome panel. Abbreviations: DHEAS, dehydroepiandrosterone sulfate; ACTH, adrenocorticotropic hormone; CAH, congenital adrenal hyperplasia; 17-OHP, 17-hydroxyprogesterone; LOCAH, late-onset adrenal hyperplasia.

The presence of a tumor may be detected by CT or MRI or through selective sampling of blood from both adrenal veins and determination of aldosterone levels. If the patient has bilateral elevation of aldosterone levels, the condition is known as *idiopathic hyperaldosteronism.*

If the patient is suspected of having secondary aldosteronism, renal function tests are valuable to detect hypertension related to renal disease. A simple urinalysis demonstrating proteinuria and hematuria confirmed by elevated serum creatinine or elevated BUN may indicate renal disease. Other causes of secondary aldosteronism can be detected when the PRA is measured. PRA is elevated in cases of secondary aldosteronism. Figure 31–6 summarizes the laboratory diagnosis of aldosterone excess.

Aldosterone Deficiency

Even though the number of cases of idiopathic hypoaldosteronism is extremely low, one would expect to see low plasma and urinary aldosterone levels combined with increased PRA. In addition, the patient may have an increased serum potassium level and/or decreased serum sodium level.

In patients with hyporeninemic hypoaldosteronism, both the PRA and plasma aldosterone levels are decreased. In addition, these patients have decreased serum sodium levels, increased serum potassium and chloride levels, and acidosis. Figure 31–7 summarizes the laboratory diagnosis of aldosterone deficiency.

TREATMENT

Hypercortisolism

The treatment of choice for Cushing's disease is transsphenoidal microadenomectomy.[19] When the treatment is successful, plasma ACTH and cortisol levels are normal or low soon after surgery. Some of the patients may require adrenal replacement therapy postoperatively.

Removal of the tumor is the treatment of choice for adrenal adenoma or carcinoma. Successful removal results in adrenal insufficiency, and the patient requires adrenal replacement therapy.

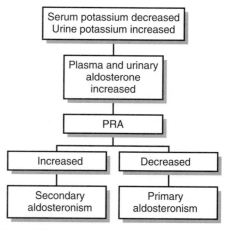

Figure 31–6. Aldosterone excess panel. Abbreviation: PRA, plasma renin activity.

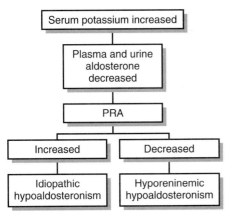

Figure 31–7. Aldosterone deficiency panel. Abbreviation: PRA, plasma renin activity.

Adrenal Insufficiency

If a patient is suspected of having an acute adrenal insufficiency, replacement therapy using intravenous hydrocortisone is urgent. In addition, glucose and plasma expanders may be required. If the insufficiency is chronic, oral glucocorticoid replacement is the treatment of choice.

Secondary adrenal insufficiency also requires glucocorticoid replacement therapy. Electrolyte and volume regulation are not usually necessary, because the aldosterone level in patients with this disorder is not commonly affected.

Adrenogenital Syndrome

The treatment of adrenogenital syndrome is aimed at reducing elevated androgen levels to normal with amounts of glucocorticoids that do not cause Cushing's syndrome, further growth impairment, or any of the other effects of excess glucocorticoids. When glucocorticoids are administered in physiologic amounts, the abnormal steroid levels fall. The severity of the disease and the age of the patient dictate the treatment required. Closely monitoring therapy, especially in children, leads to normal growth, sexual development, and fertility.[20] Abnormal blood and urine steroid levels return to their respective age and gender reference intervals when the appropriate metabolic end-product is supplied. Patients with treated hypocortisolism must be monitored during times of stress for the possibility of acute vascular collapse. For patients with LOCAH therapy commonly consists of glucocorticoid suppression, but if the clinical manifestations are mild, only hair removal is necessary.[10]

When an adenoma or carcinoma is responsible for the androgen elevations, surgical removal is the treatment of choice.

Aldosterone Excess

Excessive secretion of aldosterone due to a simple adenoma is best treated by surgical removal of the neoplasm. Patients with idiopathic hyperaldosteronism are better managed medically with oral spironolactone; this substance blocks aldosterone's action, lowering the blood pressure and returning potassium levels to normal. Secondary aldosteronism is corrected by treatment of the underlying cause.

Aldosterone Deficiency

The treatment for idiopathic hypoaldosteronism is the administration of fludrocortisone combined with liberal salt intake. Correction of the acidosis and control of the potassium level with fludrocortisone in addition to the liberal salt intake are used in treating hyporeninemic hypoaldosteronism.

Case Study 1

A 32-year-old white female had been well until 8 months previous to her medical visit, when she had noticed herself bruising easily and gaining weight that seemed to be "localized" to her face, neck, and abdomen. She also had increased hair growth, acne, and generalized weakness. Physical examination revealed an anxious patient who was slightly hypertensive. The enlarged abdomen was characterized by reddish purple streaks. She denied the use of any drugs other than aspirin during the past year. Initial laboratory tests revealed the following data (with reference ranges):

Red blood cell count (10^{12}/L)	7.3 (4.2–5.4)
White blood cell count (10^9/L)	16.2 (4.5–11.0)
White blood cell differential counts (%)	
Neutrophils	86 (33–66)
Lymphocytes	11 (22–40)
Eosinophils	0 (1–4)
Monocytes	1 (4–8)
Basophils	0 (0–1)
Plasma cortisol (nmol/L)	
0800	1120 (140–644)
1600	115 (84–420)
Serum potassium (mmol/L)	2.9 (3.5–4.4)
Serum total protein (mg/dL)	7.4 (6.4–8.3)
Serum glucose (mg/dL)	
Fasting	110 (70–105)
2 h postprandial	138 (<120)
Plasma aldosterone (ng/dL)	42 (5–30)
Urine calcium (mg/24 hr)	420 (100–300)

The urinary free cortisol value was elevated. An LDDS test showed a continued elevation of urinary cortisol. An HDDS test did not suppress the cortisol production. Plasma ACTH values at 8 and 160 hours both were 0 μg/dL.

Questions

1. What diagnosis should be suspected at this point?

2. What is the most likely source of the elevated cortisol, on the basis of the laboratory findings?

3. What treatments are available?

Discussion

1. Cushing's syndrome should be suspected.

2. Because the cortisol is not suppressed by dexamethasone and ACTH levels are low, an adrenal tumor should be suspected.

3. Localization and excision of the adrenal tumor and antisteroidogenesis drugs will alleviate some of the cushingoid symptoms, but the prognosis is not good.

Case Study 2

A 42-year-old female was admitted to the hospital because of refractory hypertension. The duration of the hypertension was about 1 year prior to admission. Despite various trials with antihypertensive regimens, the patient's systolic pressure remained above 160 mm Hg.

The patient revealed that she had frequent headaches and muscle cramps, and she had to urinate three to four times during the night. The laboratory findings (with reference ranges) were as follows:

Serum sodium (mmol/L)	140 (136–145)
Serum potassium (mmol/L)	2.8 (3.5–4.4)
Serum chloride (mmol/L)	94 (99–109)
Serum bicarbonate (mmol/L)	36 (22–28)
Serum creatinine (mg/dL)	1.0 (0.5–1.0)
BUN (mg/dL)	17 (10–20)

Questions

1. On the basis of clinical manifestations and laboratory findings, what disease might this patient have?

2. What laboratory tests should be performed next?

3. Using these laboratory results, how does one differentiate primary from secondary aldosteronism?

4. What would one expect to find about the acid-base status for this patient? Why?

5. Can a patient with Cushing's syndrome present with hypertension? Why?

6. What is another name for primary aldosteronism that is caused by an adrenocortical adenoma?

Discussion

1. Aldosterone excess.

2. Urinary and plasma aldosterone evaluations, followed by PRA.

3. In primary aldosteronism, aldosterone levels are increased, suppressing renin levels, whereas in secondary aldosteronism, aldosterone levels are increased because of increased renin levels.

4. One would expect to see a metabolic alkalosis. Aldosterone acts on the renal tubules to cause the increased reabsorption of sodium. In turn, hydrogen and potassium ions are excreted, leading to hypokalemia and alkalosis.

5. A patient with Cushing's syndrome can present with hypertension. The hypertension appears to be the direct result of the weak mineralocorticoid activity of cortisol or the increased secretion of desoxycorticosterone, which is a mineralocorticoid.

6. Conn's syndrome.

References

1. Federman DD: The adrenal. Sci Am Med 9:1–17, 1994.
2. Imura H: Control of biosynthesis and secretion of ACTH: A review. Horm Metab Res (Suppl) 16:1, 1987.
3. Iranmanesh A, Lizarralde G, Short D, et al: Intensive venous sampling paradigms disclose high frequency adrenocorticotropin release episodes in normal men. J Clin Endocrinol Metab 71:1276, 1990.
4. Felicetta JV: Cushing's syndrome: How to pinpoint and treat the underlying cause. Postgrad Med 86:79, 1989.
5. Orth DN, Kovaks WJ, DeBold CR: The adrenal cortex. In Wilson JD, Foster DW (eds): Williams' Textbook of Endocrinology, ed 8. Philadelphia, WB Saunders, 1992.
6. Berner JJ: Effects of Diseases on Laboratory Tests. Philadelphia, JB Lippincott, 1983.
7. McCroskey RD, Phillips A, Mott F, et al: Antiphospholipid antibodies and adrenal hemorrhage. Am J Hematol 36:60, 1991.
8. Asherson RA, Hughes GR: Hypoadrenalism, Addison's disease and antiphospholipid antibodies [editorial]. J Rheumatol 18:1, 1991.
9. Kaplan LA, Pesce AJ: Clinical Chemistry: Theory, Analysis, and Correlation. St Louis, CV Mosby, 1984.
10. Longcope C: Adrenogenital syndrome. Hosp Med Apr: 79–85, 1984.
11. Weber KT, Villarreal D: Role of aldosterone in congestive heart failure. Postgrad Med 93:203–221, 1993.
12. Hershman JM: Endocrine Pathophysiology: A Patient-Oriented Approach. Philadelphia, Lea & Febiger, 1988.
13. Ulick S, Wang JZ, Morton DH: The biochemical phenotypes of two inborn errors in the biosynthesis of aldosterone. J Clin Endocrinol Metab 72:145, 1992.
14. Jeremy JY, Dandona P: Inhibition by hydrocortisone of prostacyclin synthesis by rat aorta and its reversal with RU 486. Endocrinology 119:661–665, 1986.
15. Lipsett M, Wessler S, Alvioli LV: The differential diagnosis of hirsutism and virilism. Arch Intern Med 132:616–619, 1973.
16. Maxell MH, Waks AU: Secondary hypertension: Treatable entities. Hosp Med Jan: 47–76, 1987.
17. Honour JW: The investigation of adrenocortical disorders. Journal of the International Federation of Clinical Chemists 6:154–158, 1994.
18. Baylis PH, Phillips EMG: The endocrine investigation of disorders of sodium and water homeostasis. Journal of the International Federation of Clinical Chemists 6:158–163, 1994.
19. Jeffcoate WJ: Treating Cushing's disease. Br Med J 296:227, 1988.
20. Gornall AG: Applied Biochemistry of Clinical Disorders. Hagerstown, MD, Harper & Row, 1980.

Impaired Glucose Metabolism

Susan Cockayne

Carbohydrates are the most abundant compounds found in nature. One carbohydrate in particular, glucose, is the major energy source necessary to sustain life. Alterations in glucose metabolism result in a number of metabolic derangements with very serious consequences to the body's state of health. It is estimated that as many as 200 million people suffer one type of glucose metabolic disorder known as diabetes mellitus.[1] Despite major advances in both the diagnosis and treatment of diabetes mellitus, it remains a disorder of major medical concern.

GLUCOSE METABOLISM AND REGULATION

A knowledge of normal glucose metabolism helps one better understand the events that occur when this metabolism is disturbed. Figure 32–1 presents a summary of the biochemical pathways of normal carbohydrate metabolism. Preliminary digestion of carbohydrates occurs in the oral cavity with the action of salivary amylase; however, the principal digestive process occurs in the small intestine through the action of pancreatic amylase. Additional disaccharidases continue the hydrolysis until all carbohydrates exist as monosaccharides. These monosaccharides, glucose, galactose, and fructose, are then actively reabsorbed into the portal circulation, where they are taken to the liver to undergo further metabolic processes for either energy production or storage, depending on the states and needs of the body. Galactose and fructose are further metabolized to glucose. The pathway of *glycolysis* promotes the production of energy in the form of adenosine triphosphate (ATP), if needed, or it provides an intermediate product for the production of glycogen by the process of glycogenesis. Glycogen is the main storage form of carbohydrates and is found primarily in the liver and skeletal muscle of animals. *Glycogenolysis* is the biochemical pathway by which glycogen is metabolized to glucose when additional energy is needed. Another pathway, *gluconeogenesis*, results in the formation of glucose from noncarbohydrate sources, such as amino acids, glycerol, fatty acids, and lactic acid. Gluconeogenesis is an important source of glucose for energy production when glucose is not otherwise available.

Glucose Utilization

The biochemical regulation of carbohydrate metabolism is a tightly controlled process that involves the integrated action of several hormones. Only one hormone, insulin, is significantly involved in lowering the glucose level in the extracellular fluid. Insulin is a peptide hormone produced by the β-cells of the pancreas. Its production and secretion are stimulated by an increase in level of plasma glucose, such as occurs following ingestion of carbohydrate. Insulin's main action is to bind to receptors on target cells, increasing the permeability of cells to glucose. Once inside the cells, glucose can then undergo various metabolic processes as previously described. The end result is the lowering of the plasma glucose concentration. The extent of response to insulin depends on the number of receptors and the binding affinity of these receptors for insulin. Insulin promotes lipogenesis and protein synthesis in addition to glucose utilization.

Glucose Mobilization

Carbohydrate metabolism is also regulated by other hormonal actions that result in increases in plasma glucose levels by the pathways of glycogenolysis or gluconeogenesis. Glucagon, produced by the α-cells of the pancreas, mobilizes glucose by inducing glycogenolysis in the liver. It helps control glucose levels during periods of fasting. Epinephrine also mobilizes glucose by stimulating glycoge-

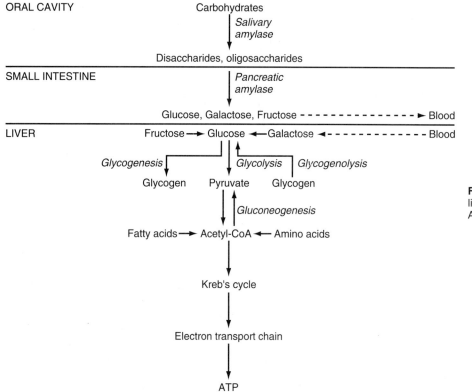

ORAL CAVITY

SMALL INTESTINE

LIVER

Figure 32–1. Carbohydrate metabolism. Abbreviations: CoA, coenzyme A; ATP, adenosine triphosphate.

nolysis. Cortisol stimulates gluconeogenesis. Secretion of cortisol is stimulated by adrenocorticotropic hormone (ACTH) from the anterior pituitary. ACTH, therefore, has an effect similar to that of cortisol. The thyroid hormone thyroxine shows a twofold action when present in abnormally high amounts; it stimulates both rapid uptake of dietary glucose and glycogenolysis. Growth hormone also has a dual effect; it stimulates glycogenolysis in the liver and inhibits insulin in its promotion of cellular glucose uptake. Finally, somatostatin, secreted from the δ-cells of the pancreas as well as the hypothalamus, has an inhibitory effect on the release of three of the regulating hormones, insulin, glucagon, and growth hormone. The effect of somatostatin is most likely one of fine tuning the glucose supply.

ETIOLOGY AND PATHOPHYSIOLOGY

Hyperglycemia

Disorders of glucose metabolism are generally referred to as hyperglycemia and hypoglycemia. Hyperglycemia has been commonly known as diabetes mellitus and characterized as juvenile-onset diabetes and maturity-onset diabetes. The existence of these two forms of diabetes was first documented in 1936.[2] Considerable research has been conducted since then by the National Diabetes Data Group (NDDG) and the World Health Organization (WHO), leading to a more complete and comprehensive classification of the different clinical forms of diabetes. The new classification, which was proposed by the NDDG in 1979, consists of five categories of hyperglycemia and two statistical risk categories (Box 32–1).[3]

The two major categories of diabetes mellitus are known as insulin-dependent diabetes mellitus (IDDM), or type I diabetes, and non–insulin-dependent diabetes mellitus (NIDDM), or type II diabetes. IDDM is a relatively rare disease, affecting 1 in 250 individuals in the United States.[2] Ten percent of known diabetics have type I disease. Although age is no longer a valid criterion for classification, the majority of type I diabetics are younger than 20 years at the time of diagnosis. It is now quite clear that IDDM results from an autoimmune attack on the β-cells of the pancreas.[4] Certain individuals are genetically predisposed to the development of IDDM, owing to the presence of certain human leukocyte antigens (HLAs) (D3/D4). Upon exposure to a foreign viral antigen, the immune system mounts an immune response characterized by both antibodies and cytotoxic T cells. The immune system begins destroying the foreign antigen as well as the β-cells of the pancreas, because the cell membrane of the β-cell contains a protein, called 64-kilodalton (64-kD) protein, that closely resembles the foreign antigen. This type of autoimmune destruction, known as *molecular mimicry*, is similar to the autoimmune destruction in rheumatic heart disease following a streptococcal infection. It appears that the immune system slowly eliminates the β-cells over a period of several years and that the classic symptoms of diabetes manifest only after about 80% of the β-cells have been destroyed, resulting in little or no insulin production.

Type II diabetes mellitus, or NIDDM, has two subcategories: obese and nonobese. The majority of cases (60% to 90%) are obese NIDDM. Both genetic susceptibility and environmental factors are associated with the development of NIDDM. There is no evidence of any particular HLA antigen or viral involvement in the development of

Box 32-1. Classification of Diabetes Mellitus and Other Categories of Glucose Intolerance

Diabetes mellitus
   Type I: Insulin-dependent diabetes mellitus (IDDM)
   Type II: Non–insulin-dependent diabetes mellitus (NIDDM)
   Other types associated with certain conditions and syndromes
      Pancreatic disease
      Hormonal
      Drug-induced
      Insulin receptor abnormalities
      Certain genetic syndromes
      Other types
Impaired glucose tolerance (IGT)
Gestational diabetes (GDM)
Statistical risk classes
   Previous abnormality of glucose tolerance (PrevAGT)
   Potential abnormality of glucose tolerance (PotAGT)

Data from National Diabetes Data Group: Classification and diagnosis of diabetes mellitus and other categories of glucose intolerance. Diabetes 28:1039–1057, 1979.

NIDDM. The majority (90%) of known diabetics have NIDDM, which generally occurs after age 40 years.

NIDDM is characterized by impaired insulin secretion or insulin resistance. The impairment of insulin secretion may be due to reduced β-cell mass or to a dysfunction of a normal number of β-cells or both. Tissue resistance to insulin is caused by a reduction in number either of insulin receptors on target cells or of glucose transporters. The end result is decreased permeability of the target cells to glucose with a resultant hyperglycemia. Depending on the exact cause, insulin levels may be low, normal, or high in NIDDM.

A third category of diabetes is associated with other conditions, such as pancreatic disease, endocrine disease that upsets the intricate hormonal regulation of glucose, and certain medications that may interfere with insulin secretion or function.

Impaired glucose tolerance (IGT) is an asymptomatic condition which may simply represent the normal variation of glucose in the population. It may also represent a temporary condition of abnormal glucose levels following a stressful event, such as a myocardial infarct. Statistics reveal that 30% of people categorized as having IGT may eventually develop NIDDM.[2]

Gestational diabetes mellitus (GDM) is characterized as glucose intolerance occurring during pregnancy, usually at 24 to 30 weeks' gestation. It affects approximately 2% to 3% of the obstetric population.[5] GDM most often develops in conjunction with elevated human placental lactogen (HPL), which has been found to increase insulin resistance.[2] Diagnosis of GDM is important because the disor-

der is associated with significant perinatal and maternal morbidity (see also Chapter 34).

Two categories represent statistical risk classes for the development of diabetes. These are classified as previous abnormality of glucose intolerance (PrevAGT) and potential abnormality of glucose intolerance (PotAGT).

Hypoglycemia

When endogenous glucose production is inadequate, abnormally low plasma glucose levels develop, possibly leading to clinical hypoglycemia. Because the signs and symptoms of hypoglycemia occur at varying levels in different individuals, it is difficult to establish a specific glucose level at which clinical hypoglycemia is present. Generally, a cutoff value of less than 50 mg/dL is used to define hypoglycemia; however, low glucose values can exist without characteristic signs or symptoms of hypoglycemia, particularly after a prolonged fast. Accurate diagnosis, therefore, depends on the concurrent existence of low plasma glucose values and hypoglycemic symptoms that are relieved by the administration of glucose.

Hypoglycemia can be classified into three categories: (1) insulin-or drug-related in the treatment of diabetic patients, (2) fasting, and (3) reactive.[6] Diabetic patients requiring insulin or sulfonylurea therapy—particularly, intensive insulin therapy—have a higher risk of hypoglycemic episodes. Fasting hypoglycemia is defined as low plasma glucose levels occurring in the fasting state, generally 6 or more hours after eating. Reactive hypoglycemia occurs in response to a meal, with symptoms occurring in the postabsorptive state, generally 2 to 4 hours after eating.

Causes of fasting hypoglycemia are listed in Box 32-2. Insulinoma is a tumor of the β-cells of the pancreas that results in inappropriate insulin secretion. Normally, insulin secretion declines as plasma glucose levels decline, but insulinoma is characterized by continuous insulin secretion concurrent with low plasma glucose levels. This type of fasting hypoglycemia can result in very severe hypoglycemia with symptoms that are generally neuroglycopenic. Factitious hypoglycemia is caused by self-administration of insulin. It can result when a diabetic inadvertently administers too much insulin, or it can be seen in some

Box 32-2. Classification of Hypoglycemia

Insulin- or drug-related
Fasting
   Insulinoma
   Factitious (self-administration)
   Endocrine tumors
   Hepatic disease
   Drug induced
Reactive
   Idiopathic (spontaneous reactive hypoglycemia)
      Hypersecretion of insulin after eating
      Hypersensitivity of peripheral tissues
      Deficiency of counterregulatory mechanisms
   Alimentary

emotionally unstable people who have access to insulin and inject themselves surreptitiously.[7] Various endocrine tumors can cause a deficiency of counterregulatory hormones that leads to defective glycogenolysis or gluconeogenesis with insufficient hepatic glucose output. Hepatic disease can also impair hepatic glucose output. Drug-induced hypoglycemia also results in insufficient hepatic output through various mechanisms, depending on the specific drug or medication.

Causes of reactive hypoglycemia are also listed in Box 32–2. Idiopathic reactive hypoglycemia is a poorly defined entity. Some people may experience hypersecretion of insulin after eating, whereas others may experience a hypersensitivity of peripheral tissues to insulin secretion. An excessive affinity of the insulin receptor for insulin could also be a mechanism leading to hypoglycemic symptoms. Another explanation may be a deficiency of counterregulatory mechanisms.

Alimentary hypoglycemia results from rapid gastric emptying of food contents into the small intestine. Accelerated absorption of glucose results, with excessive insulin release and a consequent lowering of plasma glucose values. Alimentary hypoglycemia can occur following gastrectomy.

CLINICAL MANIFESTATIONS

Hyperglycemia

The clinical manifestations that are regarded as classic symptoms of diabetes mellitus are polyuria, polydipsia, and polyphagia. As plasma glucose levels become elevated, the body attempts to rid itself of the excess glucose by excreting it in the urine. Because glucose is an osmotically active substance, its excretion in the urine necessitates the loss of large amounts of water. This excessive urination results in *polyuria*. The water loss, in turn, stimulates the thirst mechanism, so that larger amounts of water are ingested in an attempt to balance the urinary water loss and prevent dehydration. Increased ingestion of water is termed *polydipsia*. *Polyphagia* is an increased sensation of hunger caused by the inability of the cells to properly utilize glucose for energy production and the resultant greater breakdown of fats and proteins. As a result, weight loss may also be a common presenting clinical manifestation.

Patients with uncontrolled diabetes mellitus, particularly IDDM, are prone to the development of diabetic ketoacidosis (DKA); refer to Figure 32–2 for a summary of ketoacidosis. With severe insulin deficiency, DKA develops because the body is unable to utilize glucose as an energy source. Plasma glucose levels rise, and the body resorts to the metabolism of proteins and fats for its energy needs. The clinical hallmarks of DKA include electrolyte depletion, dehydration, and acidosis. Increased lipolysis results in elevated concentrations of glycerol and free fatty acids (FFAs) in the plasma. Because glycerol is a gluconeogenic precursor, its higher concentration, together with the amino acids from accelerated protein breakdown, enhances gluconeogenesis, which in turn compounds the developing hyperglycemia.

Some of the elevated FFAs can be converted to cholesterol, leading to the higher risk of atherosclerosis; however, the majority of the FFAs are converted to ketone bodies. The ketone bodies are weak acids that must be buffered. Eventually, the buffer bases become depleted, and acidosis develops. In an attempt to compensate for the developing acidosis, the respiratory center is stimulated, resulting in shallow, rapid breathing known as Kussmaul's respiration. The ketone bodies also contribute to electrolyte depletion. Available cations, primarily sodium, must be combined with ketone anions to promote their urinary excretion. Dehydration is a consequence of the developing osmotic diuresis as the kidneys attempt to excrete excess glucose. These are the general mechanisms by which insulin deficiency affects carbohydrate, protein, and fat metabolism, leading to the symptoms that characterize DKA.

Patients with both IDDM and NIDDM suffer serious complications after some years, even with the best of control of the glucose level. The complications are generally more severe in patients with IDDM. The major complications are classified as microangiopathies and macroangiopathies. *Microangiopathies* are lesions of vascular tissue characterized by increased thickness of the capillary basement membrane. This thickness is due, in part, to excess glycated protein, which is a result of hyperglycemia. The most severely affected sites are the retina, kidneys, and nervous system, causing disorders known, respectively, as retinopathy, nephropathy, and neuropathy.

Retinopathy is the leading cause of new blindness in the United States, with an estimated 12,000 new cases per year. Severe visual loss results from capillary basement membrane thickness due to protein glycation. This damage to the vascular walls predisposes to retinal and vitreous hemorrhages and subsequent scar tissue. Risk factors for the development of diabetic retinopathy include the duration of diabetes and the severity of hyperglycemia. It is estimated that 50% of patients have some degree of retinopathy after 7 years of IDDM, whereas 90% are affected after 17 to 25 years.[8]

Nephropathy results from a thickening of the capillary basement membrane in the glomeruli of the kidney due to protein glycosylation. Eventually, glomerular permeability is altered, with a resultant loss of protein in the urine. Diabetic nephropathy is typically characterized by persistent proteinuria of greater than 0.3 g/24 hours, hypertension, and deterioration of renal function. From 30% to 45% of type I diabetics and about 30% of type II diabetics develop diabetic nephropathy. With severe proteinuria and azotemia, the disease may progress to end-stage renal disease.[9]

Diabetic neuropathy is the least well-researched major complication of diabetes. The effects become quite pervasive after some years, displaying loss of nerve function while possibly causing pain elsewhere. Diabetic neuropathy is also apparently unrelated to the severity of the glucose abnormality. The neuropathy, together with atherosclerosis in the lower extremities and a high concentration of glucose, which favors growth of microorganisms, predisposes the patient to serious infections with the possibility of gangrene and eventual amputation.

Another complication of diabetes mellitus is macroangiopathy due to the abnormal lipid metabolism, which may lead to the development of atherosclerosis. Patients have a

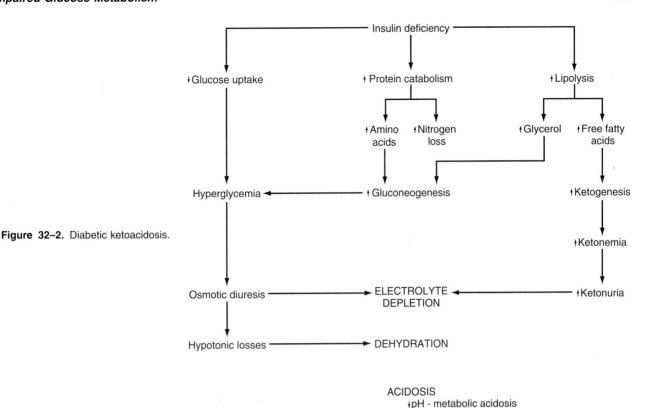

Figure 32–2. Diabetic ketoacidosis.

ACIDOSIS
↓pH - metabolic acidosis
↓PaCO₂ - Kussmaul respiration
↓HCO₃⁻ - buffer action

twofold to sixfold higher risk for the development of stroke and a twofold to fourfold higher risk for the development of heart disease.[2]

Hypoglycemia

The clinical manifestations of hypoglycemia can be classified as adrenergic or neuroglycopenic. Adrenergic symptoms are induced by an excessive secretion of counterregulatory hormones, particularly epinephrine and glucagon. When plasma glucose levels approach the hypoglycemic range, the counterregulatory hormones are released, which then stimulate glycogenolysis and gluconeogenesis in an attempt to restore plasma glucose levels to normal. Rapid epinephrine release causes symptoms such as sweating, tremor, anxiety, tachycardia, and hunger due to stimulation of the adrenergic nervous system.

Neuroglycopenic symptoms result from a lack of adequate glucose supply to the brain and are characterized by dizziness, headache, and confusion that may progress to seizures and coma. Neuroglycopenic symptoms predominate when the drop in plasma glucose levels is gradual rather than rapid.

LABORATORY ANALYSES AND DIAGNOSIS

Hyperglycemia

The diagnosis of diabetes mellitus has historically been based on a combination of clinical symptoms, urine, and blood glucose values. The research findings of the NDDG,

however, have recommended certain guidelines allowing more consistent and accurate interpretation of laboratory data and thus facilitate a more accurate diagnosis. These guidelines are presented in this discussion and are summarized in Figure 32–3.[3]

When a patient presents with a clinical impression of diabetes, the following criteria can be used to confirm the diagnosis: If the classic symptoms of diabetes are present (polyuria, polydipsia, ketonuria, and rapid weight loss) and there is an unequivocal elevation of the plasma glucose, a clinical diagnosis of diabetes mellitus can be made. In the absence of these signs and symptoms, a fasting plasma glucose test (FPG) is indicated for making a clinical diagnosis. The blood sample must be drawn after a fast of 10 to 16 hours. Values of 140 mg/dL or higher for plasma or of 120 mg/dL or higher for capillary whole blood obtained on more than one occasion are diagnostic of diabetes mellitus.

If these FPG values are not obtained, an oral glucose tolerance test (OGTT) is indicated. A 2-hour OGTT is recommended, in which an oral dose of 75 grams of glucose (1.75 g/kg of ideal body weight for children) is administered, and the blood sample is drawn every 30 minutes. Tests of both the 2-hour blood sample and some other sample taken between the administration of the oral dose and 2 hours later must meet the following criteria: Both the plasma value and the capillary whole blood value must be 200 mg/dL or higher on more than one occasion. The recommendation that a patient must demonstrate these abnormal glucose values for both the FPG and the OGTT on more than one occasion attempts to lessen the diagnostic

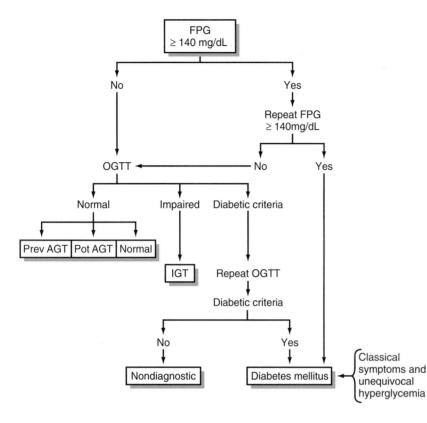

Figure 32–3. Procedure for classifying adult research subjects or clinical patients. Abbreviations: FPG, fasting plasma glucose; OGTT, oral glucose tolerance test; AGT, abnormal glucose tolerance; IGT, impaired glucose tolerance.

challenge presented by other well-recognized problems and limitations of the procedures.

A 2-hour postprandial (2-h pp) screening test has commonly been used as an alternative method for detecting glucose abnormalities. Although it may be useful as a preliminary screening test, the 2-h pp value is not included in the criteria proposed by the NDDG, because it does not allow a definitive diagnosis. Measurement of FPG or OGTT is necessary to reach a definitive diagnosis in the absence of classic symptoms and unequivocal glucose elevation.

The glycated hemoglobin (G-Hb) test is a significant laboratory test for use in the management of diabetes mellitus, but not for diagnosis. Glycated hemoglobins are minor components of the hemoglobin A molecule of the blood. Three minor components actually exist—HbA$_{1a}$, HbA$_{1b}$, and HbA$_{1c}$. The test is often referred to as the HgbA$_{1c}$test, because this is the major component. Glycated hemoglobin is identical to Hb A, with the exception of a glucose molecule attached to one of the beta chains. The glycated hemoglobin level is proportional to the average concentration of glucose within the cell and reflects the glucose concentration over the previous 2-month time frame. Normal adult hemoglobin contains less than 6% HbA$_{1c}$. The extent of elevation in diabetics is proportional to the average plasma glucose concentration over the 2 months preceding the sampling. The G-Hb test is, thus, an indication of the state of glucose control over this period and is useful in the management of diabetic patients.

Glycation of other proteins also occurs. Fructosamine measurement is a test that determines the amount of glycated albumin. Because albumin has a shorter half-life than hemoglobin, the fructosamine value provides an index of

plasma glucose levels over a 3-week period prior to sampling.

The urine albumin assay, also known as the microalbuminuria test, is used to detect albumin concentrations in the urine that are greater than normal but are not detectable with urine reagent strip tests for protein. The primary intent of urine albumin assays in diabetes is to detect and treat patients with early diabetic nephropathy, a practice that has been found to be extremely cost effective as well as beneficial to life expectancy.[10] Different assay methods, disagreement of the best diagnostic method of urine collection, and the different units of expression of urine albumin concentrations lend confusion to the interpretation of this assay, however.

Hypoglycemia

An important consideration for the diagnosis of fasting hypoglycemia is to demonstrate the presence or absence of hyperinsulinism. To do so, simultaneous measurements of plasma glucose and insulin levels are performed; refer to Figure 32–4 for a summary of hypoglycemic test strategies. Because there is no definitive lower limit of plasma glucose diagnostic of hypoglycemia, it is of much more value to interpret the insulin value in reference to the glucose value. A normal or elevated insulin value concurrent with a low plasma glucose value is inappropriate and is suggestive of hypoglycemia due to hyperinsulinemia.

If a patient has a previous history of hypoglycemia but symptoms are not readily apparent in the fasting state, hospitalization may be required to conduct an extended fast. The fast is usually extended for 72 hours unless symptoms appear earlier. Blood is drawn every 6 hours to

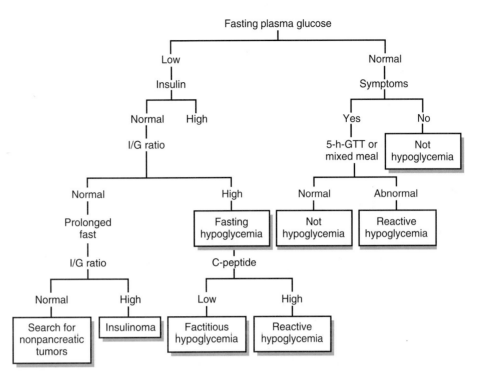

Figure 32–4. Hypoglycemia test strategies. Abbreviations: I/G ratio, insulin/glucose ratio; 5-h GTT, 5-hour glucose tolerance test.

monitor the plasma glucose and insulin levels. A presumptive diagnosis may be made if the plasma glucose falls below 50 mg/dL with the appearance of typical hypoglycemic symptoms; however, it is more helpful to determine the insulin-glucose ratio (I/G ratio) rather than merely to measure absolute values. The following formula is commonly used to determine the I/G ratio:

$$\frac{\text{Plasma insulin } (\mu U/mL)}{\text{Plasma glucose } (mg/dL)}$$

A normal ratio is less than 0.3, but patients with insulinoma generally have ratios greater than 0.3 and often as high as 1.0, indicating inappropriate insulin secretion concurrent with low plasma glucose.[6]

It may be necessary, on occasion, to differentiate fasting hypoglycemia due to insulinoma from factitious hypoglycemia. In factitious hypoglycemia, the I/G ratio may be elevated owing to self-administration of insulin. An additional test, the C peptide assay, can differentiate the two conditions. C peptide is released into the circulation in equimolar amounts with insulin, because both substances are cleaved from the proinsulin molecule. C peptide has no biologic activity, but its presence is an indication of pancreatic secretory activity. A person with insulinoma has an elevated C peptide value, which indicates hyperinsulinemia due to pancreatic secretory activity. A person with factitious hypoglycemia, however, has decreased pancreatic secretory activity owing to the exogenous insulin administration, and therefore, has a low C peptide value.

Reactive hypoglycemia has been widely diagnosed with the 5-hour glucose tolerance test (5-h GTT), in which a low plasma glucose value may be demonstrated only during the last 2 hours; however, normal people may have low plasma glucose levels after 5 hours in the absence of hypoglycemic symptoms. The 5-h GTT is thus not suffi-

ciently diagnostic. An alternative to the 5-h GTT is to measure plasma glucose levels after ingestion of a mixed meal, which may be a better physiologic stimulus.[6]

Perhaps a better approach to diagnosis of reactive hypoglycemia is to demonstrate low glucose values concurrent with hypoglycemic symptoms. The use of glucose self-monitoring devices allows immediate glucose measurement when symptoms appear. Relatively normal glucose levels concurrent with hypoglycemic symptoms can rule out reactive hypoglycemia.[6] Low plasma glucose values accompanied by characteristic symptoms in a patient who has undergone gastrointestinal surgery is suggestive of alimentary hypoglycemia.

TREATMENT

Type I Diabetes Mellitus

IDDM requires daily insulin injections to minimize elevations in plasma glucose. Other crucial components of diabetes care are dietary therapy and exercise. The results of a long-range study, the Diabetes Control and Complications Trial (DCCT), have revealed that intensive therapy rather than conventional insulin therapy has a large and beneficial effect on the development and progression of long-term diabetic complications.[11] Intensive insulin treatment consists of three or more daily insulin injections and frequent blood glucose monitoring. The goals of intensive insulin therapy are to maintain preprandial glucose concentrations between 70 and 120 mg/dL; postprandial concentrations of less than 180 mg/dL; a weekly 3 AM glucose concentration of more than 65 mg/dL; and a HbA$_{1c}$ value within the normal range, or less than 6.05%. If these values can be maintained, the onset and progression of the major diabetic complications—retinopathy, nephropathy, and neuropathy—can be significantly delayed. Studies have also indicated that early antihypertensive treatment with angiotensin-converting enzyme inhibitors retards the development of nephropathy.

The main adverse event of intensive insulin therapy is the higher incidence of severe hypoglycemia. Nevertheless, the researchers believe that the risk of severe hypoglycemia is greatly outweighed by the reduction in the microvascular complications. It is recommended that most patients with IDDM be treated with closely monitored intensive insulin therapy to maintain their glucose levels as close to normal as safely possible.

Type II Diabetes Mellitus

The major component of therapy in NIDDM is diet. Weight loss is the primary goal of diet therapy, because the majority of patients with NIDDM are obese. Some patients are also treated with sulfonylureas when dietary therapy alone is unsuccessful in lowering the plasma glucose. Sulfonylureas are oral hypoglycemic agents that stimulate the pancreas to produce higher amounts of insulin. Additionally, some patients with NIDDM require insulin treatment.

Two other classes of medication are now available for treating type II diabetes. The biguanines decrease insulin resistance and have also been found to lower low-density lipoprotein (LDL) cholesterol levels and increase high-density lipoprotein (HDL) cholesterol levels, an advantage for many obese patients with elevated cholesterol levels. The second class of medications include acarbose, an α-glucosidase inhibitor, which slows absorption of sugars from the gut.

Hypoglycemia

The treatment of serious hypoglycemia involves the immediate infusion of glucose, either by oral or intravenous administration, which temporarily relieves the hypoglycemic symptoms until the patient is able to eat a meal. The meal is necessary to restore hepatic glycogen.

Surgery is required for insulinoma and for a number of hormone-secreting tumors of the pancreas. Hormonal replacement is necessary for pituitary or adrenal insufficiency, but therapy for other forms of hypoglycemia is primarily dietary.

Case Study 1

A 24-year-old male college student was referred to the student health center by a laboratory instructor following the finding of a 3 + urine glucose value during a laboratory exercise. When questioned about any unusual symptoms, the patient expressed feelings of fatigue and excessive thirst.

A fasting plasma glucose (FPG) test was performed; the result was 131 mg/dL.

Questions

1. How would one evaluate the FPG using NDDG criteria?

2. What should the next diagnostic procedure be? A 2-h GTT was performed, with the following results:

   FPG: 139 mg/dL
   30′: 183 mg/dL
   60′: 231 mg/dL
   90′: 225 mg/dL
   120′: 218 mg/dL

3. Should the FPG test be repeated?
4. Do these glucose results indicate diabetes mellitus?
5. How would one categorize the condition?
6. Of what value would the G-Hb test be for this patient?

Discussion

1. The FPG value should be > 140 mg/dL on more than one occasion to be diagnostic of diabetes mellitus.
2. The next diagnostic procedure should be a 2-h GTT.
3. Abnormal FPG values should be demonstrated on more than one occasion.
4. If the 2-hour value and one other value between 0 and 2 hours are > 200 mg/dL on more than one occasion, the results are diagnostic of diabetes mellitus. The test was repeated, with essentially the same results.
5. The condition can be categorized as type I diabetes mellitus.
6. The G-Hb test is useful to monitor the state of glucose control over a previous 2-month period following initiation of insulin therapy. It is not used for diagnosis.

Case Study 2

A 32-year-old female was seen for evaluation of recurrent hypoglycemic episodes. She had experienced weakness and dizziness periodically for 5 years and had experienced a seizure 2 years previous to this evaluation. There is no history of drug abuse or other organ dysfunction. A fasting plasma glucose value was 66 mg/dL, with no accompanying symptoms.

Questions

1. What type of hypoglycemia is most consistent with the patient's glucose value and symptoms?
2. What diagnostic procedure should be performed next?

The patient was hospitalized, and an extended fast was conducted that was terminated at 48 hours. The following values were obtained:

	12 hr	24 hr	36 hr	48 hr	Normal Range
Glucose (mg/dL)	60	55	48	38	65–105
Insulin (μU/mL)	8	12	17	35	5–22

3. Is inappropriate hyperinsulinism demonstrated by these values?

4. What additional laboratory test would be helpful in the differential diagnosis of this patient?

5. The C peptide value at 48 hours was 5 ng/mL (normal, 1–4.2 ng/mL). On the basis of these laboratory values, what is the most probable diagnosis?

Discussion

1. Because the symptoms appear to be more neuroglycopenic than adrenergic and do not appear in the postabsorptive state (2–4 hours after a meal), the most probable diagnosis would be fasting hypoglycemia versus reactive hypoglycemia.

2. The diagnosis of fasting hypoglycemia, especially due to insulinoma, often needs to be made by means of a fast extended to 72 hours and concurrent measurements of glucose and insulin values.

3. Inappropriate hyperinsulinism is demonstrated at 36 and 48 hours by calculation of the I/G ratio. At 36 hours, the I/G ratio is 0.35, and at 48 hours, it is 0.92. A ratio greater than 0.3 is abnormal.

4. Measurement of the C peptide level would be helpful in differentiating hypoglycemia due to insulinoma from factitious hypoglycemia.

5. An elevated C peptide value indicates pancreatic secretory activity, which is most consistent with the diagnosis of insulinoma.

References

1. WHO Expert Committee on Diabetes Mellitus: Second report. WHO Tech Rep Ser 646, 1980.

2. Nathan DM: Diabetes Mellitus. *In* Dale DC, Federman DD (eds): Scientific American Medicine 9(VI). New York, Scientific American, Inc, 1997, pp 1–24.

3. National Diabetes Data Group: Classification and diagnosis of diabetes mellitus and other categories of glucose intolerance. Diabetes 28:1039–1057, 1979.

4. Atkinson MA, Maclaren NK: What causes diabetes? Sci Am 263:62–63, 66–71, 1990.

5. Landon MB: Gestational diabetes mellitus: Screening and diagnosis. Lab Med 21:527–531, 1990.

6. Nathan DM: Hypoglycemia. *In* Dale DC, Federman DD (eds): Scientific American Medicine 9(I). New York, Scientific American, Inc, 1996, pp 1–8.

7. Field JB: Hypoglycemia: A systematic approach to specific diagnosis. Hosp Pract 21:187–194, 1986.

8. Goyal AK, Gamel JW: Diabetic retinopathy: Current concepts. Hosp Med August:67–76, 1993.

9. American Diabetes Association: Consensus Development Conference on the Diagnosis and Management of Nephropathy in Patients with Diabetes Mellitus. Diabetes Care 17:1357–1361, 1994.

10. Siegel JE, Krolewski AS, Warram JH, et al: Cost effectiveness of screening and early treatment of nephropathy in patients with insulin-dependent diabetes mellitus. J Am Soc Nephrol 3(4 suppl):S111–S119, 1992.

11. The Diabetes Control and Complications Trial Research Group: The effect of intensive treatment of diabetes on the development and progression of long-term complications in insulin-dependent diabetes mellitus. N Engl J Med 329:977–985, 1993.

Chapter 33

Pituitary Disorders

Susan Cockayne

The pituitary gland lies at the base of the skull in a bony depression called the *sella turcica*. The pituitary is a small gland with multiple endocrine functions. It has been called the "master gland," because many of its hormones regulate other endocrine functions. The pituitary itself, however, is regulated by secretions from the hypothalamus. The pituitary has two separate and distinct lobes. The posterior pituitary, or *neurohypophysis*, stores and secretes two peptide hormones that are synthesized by the neurosecretory cells of the hypothalamus. The posterior pituitary is connected to the hypothalamus by a pituitary stalk. The anterior pituitary, or *adenohypophysis*, synthesizes and secretes its own hormones in response to hypothalamic hormones. Releasing hormones from the hypothalamus stimulate the anterior pituitary to secrete its hormones, whereas inhibiting hormones inhibit anterior pituitary hormone secretion.

Figure 33–1 illustrates the structural relationship between the hypothalamus and the pituitary gland and the controls involved in the production of anterior pituitary hormones. Different cells within the anterior pituitary secrete different hormones. These cells were formerly differentiated on the basis of histologic staining reactions. Those that stained with acidic dyes were categorized as acidophils (40%), those that stained with basic dyes were known as basophils (10%), and chromophobes resisted staining (50%). These cells are now categorized into the following five cell types according to more advanced techniques of immunohistochemistry and electron microscopy:

- Somatotropes secrete growth hormone (GH, somatotropin).
- Mammotropes secrete prolactin (PRL).
- Thyrotropes secrete thyroid-stimulating hormone (TSH).
- Gonadotropes secrete both luteinizing hormone (LH) and follicle-stimulating hormone (FSH).
- Corticotropes secrete adrenocorticotropic hormone (ACTH) and β-lipoprotein hormone (β-LPH).[1]

Because of the intimate contact of the hypothalamus and pituitary gland and the small concentrations of hormones secreted from them, it is often difficult to determine which of these two glands is the primary source of endocrine dysfunction. Symptoms of pituitary dysfunction ultimately reflect derangement of the final target hormone concentration, the reader is therefore referred to the following chapters for discussions of the hypothalamic-pituitary hormones: Chapter 31, for the adrenal cortex (CRH, ACTH); Chapter 29 for the thyroid (TRH, TSH); and Chapters 36 and 37 for reproduction (GnRH, FSH, LH). This chapter focuses on the following four hormones that are stored or synthesized in the pituitary: antidiuretic hormone (ADH), oxytocin, GH, and PRL. This chapter also contains a discussion of panhypopituitarism, which affects more than one pituitary hormone.

ETIOLOGY AND PATHOPHYSIOLOGY
Antidiuretic Hormone

The posterior pituitary (neurohypophysis) is a storehouse for hormones produced by the neurons of the hypothalamus. Antidiuretic hormone (ADH), or vasopressin, is a small peptide synthesized by the supraoptic nuclei of the hypothalamus. These neurons produce a carrier protein specific for ADH and then package the hormone and carrier in granules that travel down the axons to the posterior

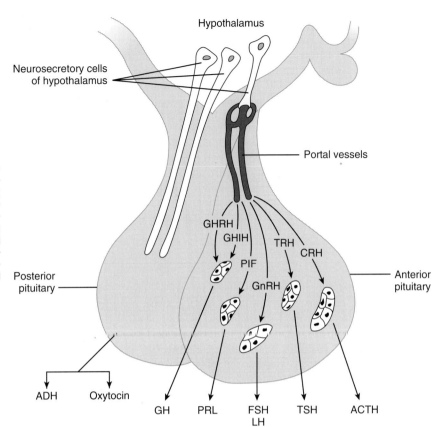

Figure 33–1. Structure and hormones of hypothalamus and pituitary glands. Abbreviations: ACTH, adrenocorticotropic hormone; ADH, antidiuretic hormone; CRH, corticotropin releasing hormone; FSH, follicle-stimulating hormone; GnRH, gonadotropin-releasing hormone; GHIH, growth hormone–inhibiting hormone; LH, luteinizing hormone; PIF, prolactin inhibiting factor; TRH, thyrotropin-releasing hormone; TSH, thyroid-stimulating hormone.

pituitary for storage and subsequent release upon appropriate stimuli.

The main function of ADH is to help regulate the osmolality of the blood. A group of nerve cells known as *osmoreceptors* in the hypothalamus monitor blood osmolality. The osmoreceptors respond to increased plasma osmolality by shrinking owing to an osmotic effect and then transmit impulses to neurosecretory cells in the hypothalamus. This action ultimately results in the release of ADH from the posterior pituitary into the general circulation. ADH acts on the cells of the kidney to increase the water permeability of the collecting ducts. As water is reabsorbed by the collecting ducts and returned to the general circulation, the plasma osmolality returns to normal. The osmoreceptors respond to the reduced osmolality by slowing the release of ADH, thereby maintaining a very tightly controlled regulatory mechanism. ADH is secreted in response to a change in the plasma osmolality of as little as 1% to 2%.[1] Baroreceptors in the thorax, in response to a 5% to 10% drop in blood volume or blood pressure, also stimulate the release of ADH. The baroreceptor response is thought to override the osmoreceptors in instances of significant blood loss. Overriding leads to generalized vasoconstriction and elevated arterial blood pressure. The combined hormonal and renal responses maintain the plasma osmolality in states of health within a narrow range of approximately 284 to 295 mOsm/kg.[1]

Hypofunctioning of ADH (Production and Action)

A physiologic decrease in ADH production may be seen in response to hypo-osmolality, to exposure to cold, and to the ingestion of certain drugs, such as alcohol, phenytoin,

and glucocorticoids.[2] Pathologic hyposecretion most commonly occurs following neurosurgery. If the destruction of the hypothalamus or posterior pituitary leaves enough axons intact, the hyposecretion may be transient. Less commonly, infection, head trauma, or degenerative or infiltrative lesions of the pituitary or hypothalamus cause hyposecretion. Pathologic hyposecretion that results from these conditions when the hypothalamus or posterior pituitary does not respond normally to appropriate stimuli is known as *central, or hypothalamic, diabetes insipidus* (DI). *Nephrogenic DI* results from the inability of the kidney to respond to ADH secretion. In this instance, the kidney is unable to maximally concentrate the urine despite a higher plasma ADH concentration. Congenital nephrogenic DI is an inherited autosomal recessive trait in which a genetic defect renders the cells of the collecting ducts unresponsive to the action of ADH.[3] Acquired factors affecting the kidney's response to ADH include amyloidosis, multiple myeloma, and association with drugs, including lithium, colchicine, and propoxyphene.[1] Additionally, hypokalemia and hypercalcemia can cause nephrogenic DI by unknown mechanisms that reduce the kidney's responsiveness to ADH.[3] Use of lithium appears to be the most common cause of acquired nephrogenic DI.[3]

Another condition that resembles diabetes insipidus and may be difficult to differentiate is psychogenic polydipsia. It is a psychiatric illness characterized by compulsive drinking of water, which suppresses ADH secretion and results in polyuria.

Hypersecretion of ADH

Physiologic elevation of ADH may occur in response to nausea, pain, stress, exercise, sleep, and certain drugs, such as nicotine, morphine, and barbiturates.[2] Pathologic increases may be relative or absolute. Relative increases reflect the normal baroreceptor response to a decrease in blood volume resulting from fluid or electrolyte loss. Paradoxically, this increase in ADH may cause fluid retention in spite of low plasma osmolality, indicating the overriding effect of the thorax baroreceptors on the hypothalamic osmoreceptors. Absolute hypersecretion of ADH is called the *syndrome of inappropriate ADH secretion* (SIADH). It may be associated with normal or increased blood volume. Forty percent of patients with oat-cell carcinoma may produce an ADH-like substance (ectopic tumor). Trauma to the central nervous system, some infections, pulmonary diseases, meningitis, and encephalitis may also result in SIADH.[4]

Oxytocin

Oxytocin is the second hormone stored in and secreted by the posterior pituitary. It is similar to ADH in structure and site of synthesis in the hypothalamus. It functions to cause milk ejection from the breast and contraction of the pregnant uterus at parturition. The major stimuli for its release are suckling and stretching of the uterus.[1] Progestins and stress are believed to inhibit its action. Hyperoxytocin and hypooxytocin states are not characterized at present; therefore, laboratory assays are not routinely performed.

Growth Hormone

Growth hormone, the most abundant hormone of the anterior pituitary, is synthesized in the somatotropic cells. Growth hormone acts directly on a wide spectrum of tissues, such as soft tissue, cartilage, and bone. Its main action is to promote growth in these tissues by promoting protein synthesis, and GH is the major hormone involved in controlling postnatal growth. Additional actions are increased uptake of nonesterified fatty acids by muscle, mobilization of fat by adipose tissue, and greater intestinal absorption of calcium.

Chronic GH excess increases blood glucose concentrations by stimulating hepatic glycogenolysis and antagonizing the effects of insulin.[1] Most significant is its induction of hepatic synthesis of peptides known as somatomedins or insulin-like growth factors (IGFs); these hormones mediate the action of GH on cartilage and bone. IGF-I shows insulin-like activity in some tissues as well as having growth-promoting effects on cartilage.[1] Growth hormone release is stimulated by growth hormone–releasing hormone (GHRH) and is inhibited by growth hormone–inhibiting hormone (GHIH) secreted from the hypothalamus.

Hypersecretion

Hypersecretion of GH occurs in association with pituitary adenomas.[1] The effects of hypersecretion of GH are age-dependent. If prolonged exposure of skeleton and soft tissues to hypersecretion of GH occurs early in life, before growth of long bones is completed, the patient will be disproportionate in size for age, a condition known as *gigantism*. Affected children may eventually exceed 8 feet

in height.[5] If the hormone elevation occurs following puberty, the resulting condition is known as *acromegaly*; it is characterized by a gradual enlargement primarily of the bones of the face, jaw, and extremities.

Hyposecretion

Symptoms of GH hyposecretion, like those of GH hypersecretion, vary with age. It is rarely clinically significant in adults but may result in pituitary dwarfism in children. An affected child is small, but proportionally built.[2] Growth hormone deficiency diseases can be primarily grouped into two categories; primary pituitary disease and hypothalamic dysfunction. Primary pituitary failure can result from such genetic disorders as pituitary hypoplasia, pituitary aplasia, familial panhypopituitarism, and familial isolated GH deficiency.[6] Pituitary destruction may also result from trauma, tumors, granulomatous disease, or therapeutic radiation of the central nervous system.[6] Most cases of GH deficiency are due to a hypothalamic defect. These defects may be associated with birth trauma due to breech delivery, hypothalamic tumors, or infections.[7] Causes of GH hyposecretion secondary to hypothalamic dysfunction include hypothalamic damage, disease, and tumors.

Prolactin

Prolactin is an anterior pituitary hormone secreted from the lactotropes that acts directly on target tissues. Its only known function in humans is initiation and maintenance of postpartum lactation. It is found, however, in males and nonpregnant females.[8] Unlike other pituitary hormones, PRL is regulated by inhibition rather than by stimulation. Dopamine, a hypothalamic neurotransmitter, controls the synthesis of PRL through inhibition and, hence, is named *prolactin inhibition factor* (PIF).

Prolactin secretion rises during pregnancy. Lactation becomes possible when estrogen levels, which also rise during pregnancy, begin to fall. As nursing continues, levels of PRL fall toward nonpregnant levels. Lactation can continue at normal resting levels of PRL.[8]

Hypoprolactinemia

Hypoprolactinemia occurs in panhypopituitarism. The only known clinical significance of low PRL levels is the inability of affected females to breast-feed after giving birth.

Hyperprolactinemia

Hyperprolactinemia is a much more common problem than PRL deficiency. The hypersecreting lactotrope adenoma (prolactinoma) is the most frequently occurring cause of anterior pituitary dysfunction.[9] The tumors may be either microadenomas or macroadenomas, slow or rapid growers, and producers of only PRL or of both PRL and somatotropin.[10] Elevated PRL may also result from removal of dopamine's inhibition of the lactotropes by a craniopharyngioma, by compression of the pituitary stalk due to an adenoma, or by granuloma formation after pituitary stalk section.[11] All of these conditions cause problems with dopamine's movement from the hypothalamus down the pituitary stalk to the anterior pituitary. Drugs such as phenothiazines block dopamine's action, and some, such as methyldopa, prevent its synthesis.[1] Patients who are receiving estrogen therapy or have primary hypothyroidism may experience hyperprolactinemia owing to the stimulatory effect of estrogen and TRH. Other causes of PRL elevation are stress, chronic renal failure, pregnancy, breast stimulation, and chest wall trauma, as well as idiopathic etiology.[1]

Panhypopituitarism

Panhypopituitarism is a generalized insufficiency of pituitary hormones. It may be total, in which all pituitary hormones are involved, or selective, in which only some hormones are deficient. Causes of panhypopituitarism are conditions that destroy the pituitary gland, hypothalamus, or both. These conditions include pituitary adenomas; infections such as tuberculosis, encephalitis, syphilis, and meningitis; pituitary surgery or irradiation; head injuries; and vascular conditions such as postpartum hemorrhage (Sheehan's syndrome), hypertensive hemorrhage, and aneurysms.

CLINICAL MANIFESTATIONS

Antidiuretic Hormone Disorders

Diabetes Insipidus

Diabetes insipidus (DI), due to deficient production or action of ADH, results in a polyuric state accompanied by thirst and polydipsia. Hypothalamic DI may be partial or complete. With partial hormone deficiency, the volume of urine excreted per day may only be a few liters, and patients experience little inconvenience or clinical symptoms. Complete hormone deficiency, however, may result in the excretion of up to 18 liters of urine per day.[6] The most obvious clinical manifestations occur if the patient is deprived of access to water: Hypertonic volume depletion results; it is characterized by central nervous system (CNS) disturbances ranging from irritability to mental dullness progressing to coma.

Nephrogenic DI results in polyuria when the collecting ducts of the kidney are unable to conserve water in response to ADH production. Characteristically, large volumes of hypotonic urine are excreted. Patients become dehydrated and experience symptoms of volume contraction and electrolyte imbalance, such as hypernatremia and hyperchloremia.[3, 6] In infants with congenital nephrogenic DI, additional clinical manifestations are failure to thrive, growth and mental retardations (due to recurrent bouts of severe hypernatremia), and early death.[3]

Psychogenic or primary polydipsia results from excessive ingestion of water over an extended period. The excess water suppresses ADH secretion, resulting in a hypotonic polyuria.

Syndrome of Inappropriate ADH Secretion

SIADH results from excessive secretion of ADH in the absence of appropriate osmotic or nonosmotic stimuli. Patients typically retain water and become hyponatremic. A modest volume expansion occurs, and body weight increases by 5% to 10% owing to the fluid retention. Symptoms are not specific for SIADH but mainly reflect the degree of hyponatremia, with CNS disturbances ranging from weakness and apathy in mild cases to lethargy, coma, and seizures in more severe cases.[1]

Growth Hormone Disorders

Gigantism

Gigantism occurs when there is hypersecretion of GH before growth of the long bones is complete. Clinical manifestations include overgrowth of the bone and soft tissues of the face and extremities and a marked acceleration of linear growth. Affected individuals may eventually exceed 8 feet in height.[5]

Acromegaly

Hypersecretion of GH in the adult results in acromegaly. Signs and symptoms occur as a gradual progression over a number of years. These manifestations include a thickening and coarsening of the facial skin, scalp, and vocal chords, enlargement of the hands and feet, and an increase in head size. Joint pain due to accelerated osteoarthrosis is also a common feature.[6] All of these findings reflect proliferation of cartilage, bone, and soft tissue. A concurrent elevation of PRL results in menstrual disorders and galactorrhea in a majority of acromegalic females.

Dwarfism

Hypopituitary dwarfism is characterized by *short stature*, which is typically defined as height below the third percentile on growth charts for children. Abnormally slow growth velocity and delayed skeletal maturation that are more than two standard deviations below the mean compared with chronologic age are also clinical manifestations of dwarfism.[12]

Hyperprolactinemia

The main direct consequence of hyperprolactinemia is galactorrhea, or lactation that is not associated with childbirth or nursing. Indirect consequences may be more common as initial clinical manifestations of hyperprolactinemia. These indirect consequences usually are erectile dysfunction in the male and menstrual abnormalities in the female.[8]

Panhypopituitarism

Panhypopituitarism can occur in children or adults. Symptoms are related to the cells affected and usually do not occur until 75% of the cells have been destroyed.[2] Prepubertal panhypopituitarism is a rare disorder characterized by dwarfism with normal body proportions. There is usually subnormal sexual development owing to cessation of gonadal function and insufficient thyroid and adrenal function. DI is also common. The signs and symptoms of postpubertal panhypopituitarism reflect the sequential loss of pituitary hormones. The presenting signs, therefore, in order of occurrence, are as follows: thin, pale, finely wrinkled skin, which reflects decreased GH; hypogonadism, which reflects decreases in LH or FSH and may be compounded if compression causes hyperprolactinemia; disproportionate pallor, apathy, lethargy, weakness, irritability, and hypothermia, which reflect decreased TSH and ACTH; and headache and visual complaints proportional to the tumor size.

LABORATORY ANALYSES AND DIAGNOSIS

Antidiuretic Hormone Disorders

Diabetes Insipidus

The laboratory finding considered the hallmark of DI is persistent hyposthenuria with a urine specific gravity of 1.005 or less and a urine osmolality less than 200 mOsm/kg.[6] Additional laboratory findings include hypernatremia resulting in elevated plasma osmolality, prerenal azotemia, and metabolic acidosis.[3] Psychogenic polydipsia, in contrast, is characterized by a mild dilutional hyponatremia due to the excessive water ingestion.

Laboratory evaluation of DI relies on the demonstration of the inability of the patient to concentrate urine. This is usually done with an overnight (8-hour) water deprivation test. The patient should avoid the use of nicotine, alcohol, and caffeine during the test because of their inhibitory actions on ADH function. Plasma and urine osmolalities are measured numerous times during the procedure. Table 33–1 lists the expected results of this test for each disorder.[1, 2, 5]

If serum ADH can be measured, a hypertonic saline infusion test may be performed. Normally, patients should experience a rise in ADH as the plasma osmolality rises, with a concurrent increase in urine osmolality and decrease in urine volume. The patient with hypothalamic DI has a low or normal serum ADH level that does not change in the presence of hyperosmolality. In the patient with nephrogenic DI, the basal ADH level is elevated initially and does not change after the saline infusion. The major disadvantage of this procedure is the unavailability of serum ADH assays owing to method complexity and lack of sensitivity and specificity. The use of osmolality measurements, however, seems to be sufficient for a differential diagnosis. Specimens for osmolality may be serum, heparinized plasma, or unpreserved urine. All particulate matter must be removed from the specimen. If analysis is delayed, the specimen should be refrigerated (serum, plasma, urine) or frozen (serum, plasma). Urine samples should be brought to room temperature before analysis.

Syndrome of Inappropriate ADH Secretion

Differential diagnosis of excessive ADH secretion requires evidence of plasma hyponatremia and hypoosmolality. After any adrenal, thyroid, or renal disease is ruled out, a urine sodium measurement differentiates between total body sodium depletion (urine sodium decreased) and dilutional hyponatremia (urine sodium elevated). Comparison of the ratio of urine and plasma osmolalities shows a ratio of less than 1 in hyponatremia from excessive fluid intake, whereas a ratio greater than 1 suggests SIADH. In fact, the classic finding in SIADH is an inappropriately elevated urine osmolality concurrent with a low plasma osmolality, indicating the inability of the kidney to excrete water.

If needed, a water loading test may be performed. In this test, a comparison is made of plasma and urine osmolalities before and after ingestion of a standard amount of water. A urine osmolality higher than 100 mOsm/kg with less than 90% of the water load excreted confirms a diagnosis of SIADH. As with diabetes insipidus, plasma ADH levels may be measured but are usually not needed (Fig. 33–2).

Growth Hormone Disorders

Acromegaly

A single random serum GH measurement is usually not helpful in the diagnosis of acromegaly, because of the episodic GH secretion in this disorder. The laboratory diagnosis of acromegaly more appropriately involves determining whether GH is suppressed by glucose. Normally, GH levels are quite low after glucose ingestion. In acromegaly, however, the main hormonal feature is the absence of the normal suppressibility of GH by glucose.[8] Growth hormone is released at a higher level in acromegaly than in healthy individuals.

For this test, the patient ingests 75 to 100 g of glucose. If the serum GH value is greater than 3 ng/mL 1 or 2 hours after glucose ingestion, acromegaly should be strongly suspected. Normal serum GH levels should be less than 2 ng/mL. An alternative method is to assay the level of serum IGF-I, the level of which correlates with the clinical activity of acromegaly better than serum GH level. Repeated measurements of both serum GH and IGF-I are useful ways to evaluate the effectiveness of therapy.[8] Additionally,

Table 33–1. Response to 8-Hour Water Deprivation Test for Evaluation of Diabetes Insipidus (DI)

Assay	Result			
	Normal	*Hypothalamic DI*	*Nephrogenic DI*	*Psychogenic Polydipsia*
Prestimulation				
Plasma osmolality (mOsm/kg)	<300	>300	>300	<300
Urine osmolality (mOsm/kg)	>600	<270	<270	<270
Urine volume (mL/min)	~1	>2	>2	>2
Urine/plasma osmolality ratio	>1	<1	<1	<1
Poststimulation				
Urine osmolality	<5% increase	>5% increase	No change	<5% increase
Urine volume (mL/min)	<0.5	<2	No change	<0.5

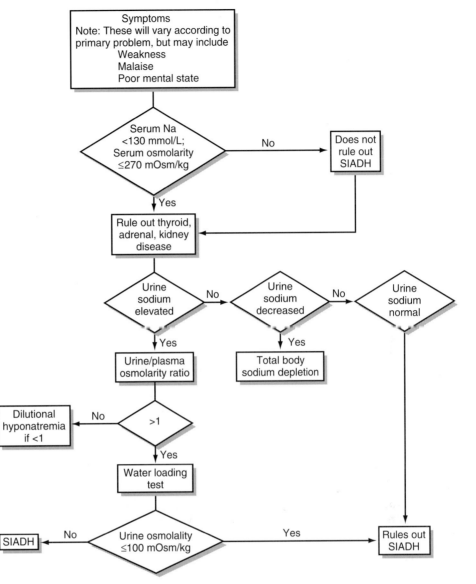

Figure 33–2. Diagnosis of syndrome of inappropriate ADH (antidiuretic hormone) production (SIADH).

serum PRL levels should also be measured. PRL is elevated in about 30% of patients, usually owing to secretion from the adenoma (Fig. 33–3).

Dwarfism

Because GH levels are usually low in the basal state, a deficiency of GH is typically determined by stimulation tests. Before such tests are undertaken, it must be ensured that conditions that may cause falsely low GH levels are not present and that the patient is euthyroid. Hypothyroidism may cause a subnormal response of GH to stimulation.[12] Additionally, Turner's syndrome must be eliminated in females.

The stimulation tests are used to test the capacity of the somatotrope cells of the pituitary to secrete GH. Pharmacologic stimuli, such as insulin, arginine, clonidine, glucagon, levodopa, and propranolol, are most commonly used. Serum growth hormone levels are measured at two 20-minute intervals following stimulus administration. Because the administration of insulin induces hypoglycemia, glucose

levels should also be monitored. No universally accepted level of GH establishes GH deficiency; generally, a peak GH concentration less than 5 ng/mL indicates GH deficiency.[7] Because of the wide variation in results and the 15% false-negative rate, however, two tests using different stimuli are usually employed.[7] Children with milder forms of the deficiency may respond normally to the stimulation tests. IGF-I may also be assayed as an aid to diagnosis; the likelihood of GH deficiency is reduced if the IGF-I level is normal.

Hyperprolactinemia

Assessment of hyperprolactinemia should begin with patient history and a physical examination. A history of stress or ingestion of dopamine antagonist, along with thyroid and renal function evaluations, usually help determine nonpituitary causes. Computed tomography (CT) scan of the head with contrast agent or magnetic resonance imaging (MRI) is very highly recommended.

Suppression and stimulation tests have been used to

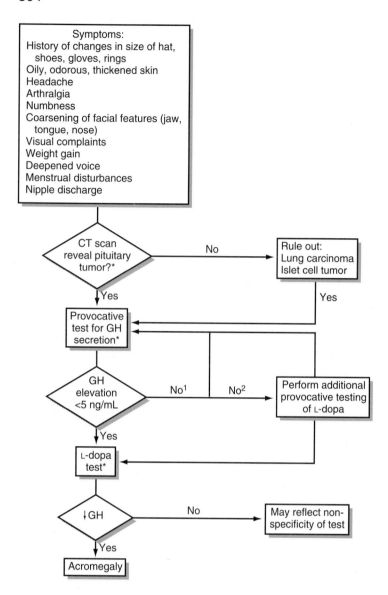

Figure 33–3. Diagnosis of acromegaly. *Note: If clinical signs clearly show evidence of elevated GH, additional confirmatory testing may be unnecessary. Abbreviations: CT, computerized tomography; GH, growth hormone; L-dopa, levodopa.

differentiate hypothalamic from pituitary origin of hyper-prolactinemia, but these are not consistently reliable. Basal levels of PRL in excess of 200 μg/L (reference interval less than 20 μg/L) are highly suggestive of an adenoma. PRL levels of 50 to 300 μg/L found with a large tumor may indicate compression of the pituitary stalk by the tumor with blockage of dopamine inhibition of PRL release instead of an adenoma[8] (Fig. 33–4).

Panhypopituitarism

Because hyposecretion of pituitary hormones may be secondary to other endocrine disorders, excluding any primary disease of the thyroid, adrenals, or gonads first is important. Skull x-rays with tomography and CT scans may reveal masses in the sella, with the associated structural changes.

A triple-bolus hormone test may also be used, although the test itself is costly, and interpretation may be difficult. Intravenous insulin, gonadotropin-releasing hormone (GnRH), and TRH are administered to the patient, and timed blood samples are taken for measurements of GH,

cortisol, LH, FSH, TSH, PRL, and glucose. The result is valid only if glucose levels are suppressed below 40 mg/dL. A physician must be in attendance throughout the testing. Table 33–2 lists the normal and disease responses to the triple-bolus hormone test[9] (see also Fig. 33–5).

TREATMENT
Antidiuretic Hormone Disorders
Diabetes Insipidus

Therapy for DI is directed toward reducing polyuria. Nasal sprays with an analog of arginine vasopressin, injectable ADH, or drugs that stimulate the release of or potentiate ADH action are effective for patients with hypothalamic DI. Patients with nephrogenic DI respond to diuretics and dietary restrictions of protein and sodium to lower the plasma osmolality. Patients with psychogenic polydipsia usually require psychiatric intervention.[9]

Syndrome of Inappropriate ADH Secretion

Therapy for SIADH consists of eliminating the stimulus of the excessive ADH secretion such by as tumor excision

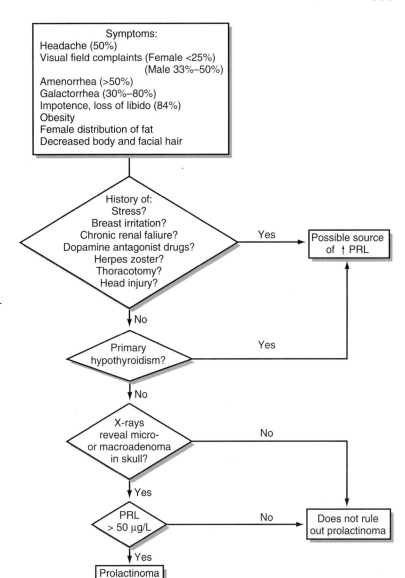

Figure 33–4. Diagnosis of hyperprolactinemia. Abbreviation: PRL, prolactin.

or correction of hypovolemia. Water restriction or drug therapy may effectively lower ADH and return plasma sodium levels to normal.

Growth Hormone Disorders

Acromegaly

Therapy for acromegaly is aimed at tumor elimination, normalization of GH secretion, and reversal of the acromegalic signs. The initial treatment is trans-sphenoidal resection. Massive tumors may require craniotomy. Approximately 70% to 75% of patients achieve reduction in GH secretion levels through surgery. Bromocriptine and octreotide are used in the medical management of acromegaly. Early treatment reverses many of the abnormalities associated with acromegaly. If left untreated, however, acromegaly may cause severe disability and death from cardiac or neurologic complications.[1]

Dwarfism

Children with GH deficiency can now be treated with synthetic preparations of GH derived from recombinant DNA techniques. Several studies of children treated with GH for 6 to 12 months show significantly accelerated growth rates in more than half of the patients.[3] Many questions still remain, however, concerning GH replacement therapy, including the most appropriate treatment regimen and the potential risks of such therapy. The effects of GH on adult height may not be known for many years.[3]

Hyperprolactinemia

Therapeutic success in hyperprolactinemia depends on the size of the adenoma causing the PRL elevation. Trans-sphenoidal adenectomy is usually successful for microadenomas, but not for large tumors. Dopaminergic antagonists, such as bromocriptine, cause the disappearance or marked reduction of most tumors and force PRL levels down.

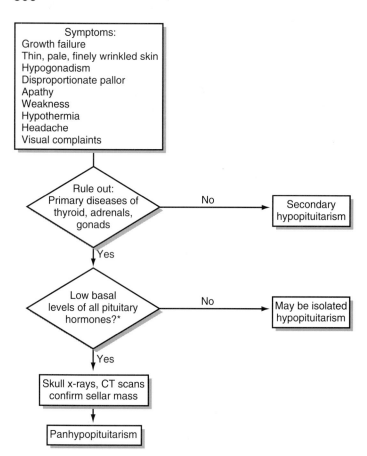

Figure 33–5. Diagnosis of panhypopituitarism. *Prolactin (PRL) may be elevated if tumor is compressing pituitary stalk. Abbreviation: CT, computerized tomography.

After cessation of drug therapy, PRL rises again with a microadenoma but not with a macroadenoma.[11]

Panhypopituitarism

In panhypopituitarism, surgical excision of a causative tumor may actually result in the destruction of healthy pituitary tissues. Chronic anterior pituitary deficiency is usually irreversible and requires long-term replacement of all target gland hormones. As in isolated pituitary dysfunction, stimulation or suppression testing of individual hormones may be required to evaluate the success of therapy. To the extent that target gland hormones are successfully replaced, laboratory results return to normal and typical symptoms disappear.

Case Study 1

A 45-year-old man entered a fertility clinic for evaluation of erectile dysfunction. He and his wife had tried to have a third child without success for the previous 3 years. Physical examination revealed a moderately obese patient with a history of frequent headaches and numerous problems with vision. He spoke of having to shave less frequently, and on further examination, his pubic and axillary hair were found to be reduced. There were no other remarkable findings. He denied the use of any drugs except aspirin for his headaches.

Skull x-rays revealed a mass in the sella turcica.

Results of the laboratory studies performed are as follows:

Analyte	Result	Reference Range
GH(ng/mL)	Undetectable	<2
FSH(U/day)	Undetectable	4–18
LH(mU/mL)	Undetectable	6–23
TSH(μU/mL)	8	<10
ACTH (0800 h)(pg/mL)	83	25–100
PRL(ng/mL)	376	<20
Testosterone(ng/dL)	93	437–707

Table 33–2.	**Responses to the Triple-Bolus Hormone Test: Normal vs. Hypopituitarism**

Assay	Normal Response	Hypopituitarism
Glucose	Decreased to 50% of baseline	Decreased to 50% of baseline
GH	Increased >8 ng/mL (8 μg/L)	No response
Cortisol	Increased >70 μg/dL (2.0 μmol/L)	No response
PRL	2-fold increase	No response
TSH	Increased >5 μU/mL (5 mIU/L)	No response
FSH	Increased >3 mU/mL (3 IU/L)	No response
LH	Increased >3 mU/mL (3 IU/L)	No response

Abbreviations: GH, growth hormone; PRL, prolactin; TSH, thyroid-stimulating hormone; FSH, follicle-stimulating hormone; LH, luteinizing hormone.

From Gornall AG: Applied Biochemistry of Clinical Disorders. Hagerstown, MD, Harper & Row, 1980.

Questions

1. What is the most probable diagnosis?
2. Which therapy will most effectively reduce the pro-lactin level?

Discussion

1. The probable diagnosis is macroprolactinoma caus-ing a hypopituitarism by compression, as evidenced by decreased GH and gonadotropins.
2. Use of a dopamine antagonist, such as bromocriptine, will decrease the size of the adenoma. There is a good chance that cessation of the drug will not result in a return of the hyperprolactinemia.

Case Study 2

A 42-year-old female complained of excessive thirst and having to drink 6 to 8 L of water per day. Labora-tory data were as follows (with reference ranges):

Serum

Sodium:	135 mmol/L (136–145)
Potassium:	3.8 mmol/L (3.5–5.0)
Chloride:	98 mmol/L (99–109)
Bicarbonate:	23 mmol/L (2–28)
Blood urea nitrogen:	10 mg/dL (8–26)
Glucose:	80 mg/dL (70–105)
Osmolality:	285 mOsm/kg (284–295)
ADH:	Decreased

Urine

Sodium:	Normal
Potassium:	Normal
Osmolality:	150 mOsm/kg (300–900)

Questions

1. What is the most probable diagnosis?
2. How can the abnormalities in sodium, ADH, and urine osmolality be explained?

Discussion

1. The most probable diagnosis is psychogenic polydip-sia.
2. The sodium level is slightly low owing to the exces-sive water intake causing a mild hyponatremia. The ADH level is decreased because the excessive water intake causes inhibition of ADH secretion. The urine osmolality is decreased owing to polyuria from ex-cessive water intake and insufficient ADH to con-serve water.

References

1. Burtis CA, Ashwood ER (eds): Tietz Textbook of Clinical Chemistry ed 2. Philadelphia, WB Saunders, 1994.
2. Kaplan LA, Pesce AJ: Clinical Chemistry: Theory, Analysis, and Correlation. St Louis, CV Mosby, 1984.
3. Holtzman EJ, Ausiello DA: Nephrogenic diabetes insipidus: Causes revealed. Hosp Prac 29:89–93, 97–98, 103–104, 1994.
4. Bennett BD, Wells DJ: Endocrinology. *In* Bishop ML, Duben-Von Laufen JL, Fody EP (eds): Clinical Chemistry. Philadelphia, JB Lip-pincott, 1985.
5. Berner JJ: Effects of Diseases on Laboratory Tests. Philadelphia, JB Lippincott, 1983.
6. Wilson JD, Foster DW (eds): Williams Textbook of Endocrinology. Philadelphia, WB Saunders, 1992.
7. Feld RD: Growth hormone deficiency. Clin Chem News July: 1993.
8. Dale DC: Pituitary. Scientific American Medicine 5(I). New York, Scientific American, Inc, 1992, pp 1–17.
9. Gornall AG: Applied Biochemistry of Clinical Disorders. Hagers-town, MD, Harper & Row, 1980.
10. Kovacs K, Horvath E: Morphology of adenohypophyseal cells and pituitary adenomas. *In* Imura H (ed): The Pituitary Gland. New York, Raven Press, 1985.
11. Von Werder K: Recent advances in the diagnosis and therapy of hyperprolactinemia. *In* Imura H (ed): The Pituitary Gland. New York, Raven Press, 1985.
12. LaFranchi S: Human growth hormone. Postgrad Med 91:367–388, 1992.

Reproduction

Chapter 34

Pregnancy

Denise L. Uettwiller-Geiger

Pregnancy is a special condition that induces both obvious and subtle changes in maternal metabolism and biochemistry. These changes are natural responses of maternal organs to the increasing demands of the growing fetus and placenta. As a result, many pregestational reference intervals are of limited use during pregnancy. Knowledge of these naturally occurring changes is necessary for correct interpretation of analytical results and for differentiation of normal from pathologic conditions.

DIAGNOSIS OF PREGNANCY

The diagnosis of pregnancy may be made on the basis of information obtained from physical examination and results of laboratory tests. The signs and symptoms of pregnancy revealed during an examination are classified into three categories of evidence: presumptive, probable, and positive. *Presumptive* evidence consists of amenorrhea in women of childbearing age and should be regarded with caution, because lack of menses maybe due to other factors. *Probable* findings are uterine enlargement, softening of uteric and isthmus, as well as vaginal and cervical cyanosis. *Positive* findings include fetal heart tones, fetal movements, and intrauterine gestational sac at 5 to 6 weeks on ultrasound.

Laboratory assays for pregnancy measure human chorionic gonadotropin (hCG), a glycoprotein derived from the placental trophoblast. hCG is composed of two dissimilar alpha and beta subunits, which are synthesized separately and are subsequently joined noncovalently.[1] Immunohistochemical studies have shown that alpha hCG messenger RNA (mRNA) is localized in differentiating cytotrophoblast and syncytial regions, whereas beta hCG mRNA is localized primarily in the syncytiotrophoblast.[2] The rate of differentiation of cytotrophoblast into syncytiotrophoblast appears to be the main factor that leads to hCG production.[3] The function of hCG is to provide hormonal stimulation to continue and maintain the corpus luteum beyond its normal postovulatory life span, thereby allowing synthesis of progesterone and estrogens that support the endometrium. The alpha subunit of the placental hormone hCG has biologic and immunologic similarities to luteinizing hormone (LH), follicle-stimulating hormone (FSH), and human thyroid-stimulating hormone (TSH). The beta subunit confers unique specificity to hCG. Neither subunit is active by itself; only the intact molecule exerts a hormonal effect. Bioassays, receptor assays, and agglutination inhibition assays have all been replaced by modern enzyme immunoassays, which utilize monoclonal antibodies specific for the two subunits of hCG. This approach permits immunochemical differentiation between hCG and the other glycoproteins.

Secretion of hCG in maternal serum is detectable 7 to

9 days after fertilization and increases to maximum levels at about 8 to 10 weeks of gestation. By the 20th week, serum hCG levels fall slightly to a plateau that is maintained throughout the pregnancy. Urinary concentrations of hCG are similar to those found in serum. In women with uncomplicated pregnancy, hCG levels rise so rapidly during the 2 to 4 weeks following ovulation that hCG concentrations double every 2 days. Absolute hCG levels may vary, however, depending on the calibrators used in the assay kit. The First International Reference Preparation (1st IRP) succeeded the Second International Standard (2nd IS) in 1974; 2 units of the 1st IRP are equivalent to 1 unit of the 2nd IS, so levels would be double in absolute value. Today, the 1st IRP is being replaced with the newer 3rd International Standard, and absolute values are equivalent. It should be noted that the intermethod calibration differences will produce different absolute numerical results, and care must be taken in comparing values obtained with different assays because of different standards.

With quantitative laboratory determinations on serum and urine, hCG levels of 25 mIU/mL or greater are interpreted as positive for pregnancy. Levels less than 5 mIU/mL are interpreted as negative, whereas levels between 5 and 25 mIU/mL are considered indeterminate and require further investigation and monitoring. The sensitivity of these assays, defined as the lowest detectable concentration that can be distinguished from zero, is 2.0 mIU/mL or less. It is this sensitivity that allows early pregnancy detection and monitoring.

Qualitative laboratory determinations utilize either serum or urine on a single-use reaction unit or disk. These assays have built-in procedural controls to ensure that reagents are functioning properly and that test results are accurate. The primary limitation of qualitative analysis is the inability to confirm early pregnancy or to diagnosis abnormal pregnancy.

Home-use "self-testing" qualitative pregnancy tests are capable of detecting urine levels of hCG at 50 mIU/mL. They are very popular, because they can be performed in the privacy of the patient's home. It should be noted that the reliability of home pregnancy test kits depends, to a great extent, on strict compliance with written instructions. A higher rate of false negatives has been demonstrated when instructions are not followed exactly.[4]

It should also be noted that the results of laboratory tests for hCG do not positively confirm or rule out the diagnosis of pregnancy. A positive test or elevated hCG levels has been associated with other clinical conditions, such as hCG-producing tumors and trophoblastic disease. Likewise, sharply reduced or falling hCG levels may indicate an ectopic or abnormal intrauterine pregnancy. For diagnostic purposes, hCG levels should be used in conjunction with other data, symptoms, clinical impressions, sequential hCG monitoring, and results of other tests (e.g., ultrasound).

The differences between the wide variety of commercially available intact and total beta hCG assays should be noted. Results of hCG assays represent the intact hCG, meaning that such an assay is measuring the alpha and beta subunits but not the free beta subunit component. Although normal trophoblast produces both intact hormone and free beta chains, production of free beta chain declines early in the first trimester, and these hCG fragments represent only 1% to 4% of the total hCG production. Total beta hCG assays measure both the intact molecule and the free beta chain. The production of free beta chain is higher in trophoblastic disease or germ cell tumors and in males with testicular tumors; therefore, a total beta hCG assay capable of measuring free beta hCG plus intact hCG is preferable for detecting and monitoring these disease states.

Once pregnancy has been recognized clinically, a maternal and fetal assessment should be performed. This prenatal workup should include the following: a complete history and physical examination, complete blood count (CBC), Papanicolaou (Pap) smear, Rh compatibility testing, blood typing, urinalysis, plasma reagin test, gonococcal culture, and hepatitis B surface antigen (HBsAg) testing. Additionally, at 16 to 18 weeks of gestation, a screen for neural tube defects and Down syndrome can be performed.

UNCOMPLICATED PREGNANCY

Biochemical Changes

Biochemical changes associated with pregnancy may occur during the first, second, and third trimesters, often becoming more pronounced as the pregnancy progresses and returning to pregestational levels within weeks of parturition. Table 34–1 summarizes the biochemical changes that normally occur in uncomplicated pregnancies.

As shown in Tables 34–1 and 34–2, hormones that appear in the maternal circulation may be derived from both placental and maternal endocrine glands. Generally, the concentration of placental hormones increases with placental mass. Human chorionic gonadotropin is the exception to the rule. The increases seen in the hormones of maternal origin—cortisol, thyroxine (T_4), triiodothyronine (T_3)—may be explained by the estrogen-associated rise in serum concentrations of their respective binding proteins. These hormonal increases are primarily in the bound, not the free fraction.

The concentrations of many plasma proteins are altered as a result of pregnancy. Rising estrogen levels may partly explain the increases seen in ceruloplasmin, thyroxine, and cortisol-binding globulins. Albumin decreases, whereas α_1-antitrypsin, fibrinogen, several complement components, and C reactive protein all increase. The decrease in albumin coupled with a slight increase in globulins results in an albumin/globulin (A/G) ratio similar to that seen in certain hepatic disorders. Although the A/G ratio has been largely replaced by assays for specific protein fractions, the reduced ratio coupled with changes in enzyme activities, discussed later, illustrates the importance of careful evaluation of liver function tests if hepatic dysfunction is also suspected. Serum alkaline phosphatase (ALP) activity may rise as much as twofold to fourfold over nonpregnancy levels during the third trimester. This total ALP increase is primarily due to an increase in heat-stable ALP of placental origin. ALP activity in leukocytes also increases during pregnancy, a response similar to that seen in inflammatory conditions. Significant elevations of the hepatic enzymes—serum transaminases, bilirubin, and γ-glutamyl transpeptidase (GGTP)—do not occur in pregnancy and, if present, should be investigated.

Table 34-1. Biochemical Changes in Uncomplicated Pregnancy

Analyte	Alteration from Nonpregnant Reference Interval
Hormones	
Total T$_4$	Increased
Free T$_4$	Slight increase first trimester, then slight decrease
Total T$_3$	Increased by 50%
TSH	No change
Free T$_3$	No change
Thyroxine-binding globulin	Increased
Serum cortisol	Increased
Cortisol-binding globulin	Increased
Aldosterone	Increased twofold to threefold
Renin	Increased
Angiotensin II	Increased
Parathyroid hormone	Increased by 50%
Prolactin	Increased threefold to fourfold
Proteins	
Serum total protein	Slight decrease
Serum albumin	Decreased
Fibrinogen	Increased by 50%
α_1-antitrypsin	Increased
C reactive protein	Increased
Enzymes	
Alkaline phosphate	Increased twofold to fourfold
Cholinesterase	Decreased
Leucine aminopeptidase	Increased
Lipids	
Total lipids	Increased 46%
Total cholesterol	Increased 40%
Triglycerides	Increased
Phospholipids	Increased 37%
Free fatty acids	Increased 60%
Lipoproteins	Increased
Glucose	Normal (fasting levels slightly decreased)
Electrolytes, Minerals	
Sodium	Normal to slightly decreased
Potassium	Normal to slightly decreased
Calcium, total	Decreased
Iron	Decreased if not supplemented
Renal Function Tests	
GFR	Increased
Serum urea nitrogen	Decreased
Creatinine	Slight increase
Creatinine clearance	Increased (150–170 mL/min)
Blood Gas/Acid-Base Parameters	
Pa$_{CO_2}$	Decreased
HCO$_3$	Decreased

Plasma cholinesterase (ChE) activity decreases during pregnancy, whereas leucine aminopeptidase (LAP) activity increases. The changes seen in ALP, ChE, and LAP may also be seen in certain hepatobiliary diseases.

A relative hyperlipidemia (compared with values in nonpregnancy) exists during the latter half of pregnancy. Levels of total lipids, total cholesterol (esterified and nonesterified), triglycerides, free fatty acids, phosholipids, and lipoproteins rise appreciably, with increases ranging from 37% for phospholipids to 60% for free fatty acids.[5] This hyperlipidemia may be the result of greater lipid metabolism, storage, and utilization of lipids.

Even though pregnancy is potentially diabetogenic, fasting glucose levels in healthy pregnant women decline slightly. Randomly measured glucose levels are usually euglycemic. The finding of glycosuria, which is common during pregnancy, can be attributed to higher glomerular filtration rate and a lowered renal threshold; however, the possibility of impaired carbohydrate metabolism should not be ignored when glycosuria is found.

In addition to larger fetal and placental demand, the changes seen in electrolyte and mineral concentration during pregnancy may result from hemodilution, lowered plasma protein concentration, or increased excretion. In fact, hemodilution may explain the slight decrease in sodium and potassium levels seen during pregnancy even though aldosterone levels are higher.

Changes in calcium levels during pregnancy do not appear to be significantly related to the changes in concentration of either circulating parathyroid hormone or calcitonin.[6] Thus, the reduced total calcium concentration found during pregnancy is quite probably due to two factors: larger fetal and placental demand and the decrease in albumin-bound calcium (45% to 50% of total calcium) caused by the lower albumin concentration. Ionized calcium remains within nonpregnant ranges. During pregnancy, maternal need for iron rises secondary to greater perfusion needs of the fetal/placental unit and increased maternal erythropoiesis. Iron supplements are therefore needed during pregnancy.

Hematologic Changes

Table 34–3 summarizes the hematologic changes that occur during uncomplicated pregnancy. The life span of the red cells is normal, with higher production of red cells leading to greater red cell mass.[7] Although accelerated erythropoiesis raises the total red cell volume during pregnancy, the erythrocyte count typically is slightly lower than nonpregnant levels, because plasma volume expands to three times the red cell volume. Because plasma volume expands more rapidly than red cell mass, hemoglobin and hematocrit are decreased, resulting in a physiologic anemia of pregnancy. The anemia is moderate in severity, with hemoglobin concentrations seldom going below 10g/dL.[8] The hemoglobin level is rarely less than 10 g/dL in a normal pregnancy; therefore, a lower reading should be considered abnormal requiring further evaluation. The expansion of total blood volume may be a physiologic protective mechanism against the effects of excessive blood loss at the time of delivery and in the immediate postpartum period.

Table 34-2. Hormonal Changes in Maternal Circulation of Placental Orgin

Hormone	Peak Concentration	Trimester
Human chorionic gonadotropin	500,000–1,000,000 mIU/mL	1st
Human placental lactogen	3.6–8.2 µg/mL	3rd
Progesterone	100–200 ng/mL	3rd
Estrogens		
Estradiol, total	127–281 pg/mL	3rd
Estriol, total	80–350 ng/mL	3rd
Estriol, free	10–34 µg/mL	3rd

Table 34–3. Hematologic Changes in Uncomplicated Pregnancy

Analyte	Alteration from Nonpregnant Reference Interval
Blood volume	Increased by 45%
RBCs	Decreased
Hemoglobin	Decreased
Hematocrit	Decreased
Reticulocytes	Increased
Platelets	Normal to slightly decreased
Erythrocyte sedimentation rate	Markedly increased
Coagulation Parameters	
Fibrinogen (factor I)	Increased up to 200%
Factor VIII (antihemophilic factor, AHF)	Increased up to 300%
Factor IX (plasma thromboplastin component, PTC)	Increased
Factor X (Stuart factor)	Increased up to 200%
Activated partial thromboplastin time	Slightly decreased
Prothrombin time	Slightly decreased
Fibrin split products	Slightly increased
Factor XI (plasma thromboplastin antecedent)	Decreased
Factor XIII (fibrin-stabilizing factor)	Decreased
Antithrombin III	Decreased
Proteins S and C	Slightly decreased at term

Coagulation Factors

The clotting factors that increase during pregnancy are fibrinogen and factors VIII, IX, and X. As a result of these increases, the activated partial thromboplastin time (APTT) and the prothrombin time (PT) are both prolonged as the pregnancy progresses. Fibrinogen levels can rise as high as 400 mg/dL. The presence of these activated clotting factors during pregnancy suggests activation of the coagulation system. Fibrinolytic activity is decreased. Fibrin/fibrinogen split products (FSPs) rise slightly during pregnancy, possibly as a result of increased fibrinogen and plasminogen and a reduction in the coagulation inhibitor antithrombin III (AT III).

COMPLICATIONS OF PREGNANCY
Etiology and Pathophysiology
Abruptio Placentae

Abruptio placentae (premature separation of a normally implanted placenta) is a relatively common complication of pregnancy that is especially dangerous to the mother and can cause fetal or newborn death. With a frequency of about 1 in every 100 pregnancies, this complication accounts for approximately 30% of all cases of antepartum bleeding. The primary cause of abruptio placentae is unknown; however, certain predisposing factors have been suggested, including vascular injury or stasis, renal disease, pregnancy-induced or chronic hypertension, malnutrition, shortness of the umbilical cord, vasodilation, trauma, cocaine abuse, and smoking.

The sequence of events leading to the detachment of the placenta from the uterine wall begins with bleeding into the inner lining of the uterine mucosa, the decidua basalis. The hemorrhage may be concealed and without an avenue of escape, as in retroplacental bleeding, or it may drain through the cervix, causing an external hemorrhage (Fig. 34–1). The developing hematoma ultimately results in compression and destruction of the adjacent placental function. The severity of abruptio placentae is directly related to the extent of detachment that occurs.

Because the placenta is rich in thromboplastic agents, disseminated intravascular coagulation (DIC), a consumptive coagulopathy, often results. The thromboplastic agents enter the maternal circulation and activate the coagulation cascade to fibrin formation. This leads to the accelerated consumption and severe depletion of all the coagulation factors (especially factors VIII and X), fibrinogen, and platelets. Fibrinolysis is also initiated with the conversion of plasminogen to plasmin, which exerts a lytic effect on the already depleted coagulation proteins. FSPs increase in concentration and inhibit fibrin formation. This series of events results in a greatly reduced capacity for coagulation and repair of the initial insult, leading to severe hemorrhage. Laboratory evidence that DIC is in progress is prolongations of thrombin-clotting time (TCT), prothrombin time (PT), and activated partial thromboplastin time (APTT), decreases in platelets, fibrinogen, and antithrombin III levels, and elevations of FSPs and fibrin monomers.[9] D-Dimer, a major component of the breakdown of cross-linked fibrin clot by plasmin, can now be measured and is positive in almost all patients with DIC.

Gestational Diabetes

Pregnancy is potentially diabetogenic, as evidenced by the development of gestational diabetes, the aggravation of diabetes mellitus (DM), and the development of ketoacidotic states during pregnancy. The induction and intensification of the condition, however, may be reversible following delivery. Gestational diabetes is the primary subject of this discusssion.

Gestational diabetes is defined as carbohydrate intolerance of variable severity with onset or recognition during pregnancy.[10] This condition may disappear following deliv-

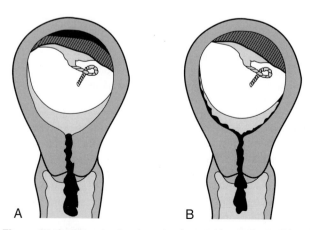

Figure 34–1. Placenta showing retroplacental hemorrhage *(A)* and external hemorrhage *(B)*.

ery and complicates about 2% to 3% of all pregnancies. Diabetes mellitus results from deficiency of insulin secretion or from resistance to the peripheral action of insulin. Although screening should be performed in any pregnant woman between the 24th and 28th week of gestation, women who are at high risk, that is, who have a family history of DM, are overweight, or have a previous newborn weighing more than 10 lb, should be screened early in the pregnancy.

The diabetogenic nature of pregnancy may be explained by the presence of increased levels of glucogenic hormones, namely human placental lactogen, estrogen, progesterone, cortisol, and thyroxine. Human placental lactogen causes a relative peripheral insulin resistance, whereas cortisol and thyroxine stimulate gluconeogenesis and glycogenolysis. The glucogenic effects of estrogen may be indirectly related to the estrogen-associated rise in thyroxine and cortisol-binding proteins, and therefore in higher total thyroxine and cortisol concentrations. Additionally, placental insulinase may contribute to the overall diabetogenic state by accelerating insulin degradation.

Ectopic Pregnancy

Implantation of a fertilized ovum anywhere other than in the endometrial lining of the uterine cavity is referred to as an *ectopic pregnancy*. In order of decreasing frequency, the locations of ectopic pregnancy are tubal (90% to 95%), ovarian, cervical, abdominal, and combined (intrauterine and extrauterine). The frequency of ectopic gestation is 1 in every 75 to 100 pregnancies. Because tubal pregnancy is the most common type of ectopic gestation, the remainder of this discussion is limited to it.

Factors or conditions that delay or prevent the passage of a fertilized ovum through the uterine tube and into the uterine cavity have been implicated as causes of ectopic pregnancy. Examples are salpingitis, pelvic inflammatory disease (PID), endometriosis, peritubal adhesions, use of intrauterine contraceptive devices, increasing maternal age, and assisted reproductive techniques. Additionally, previous ectopic pregnancy has been associated with a high recurrence rate.[11] The problem in ectopic pregnancy occurs because nonuterine organs cannot adapt to pregnancy. The trophoblast does not remain on the surface, but rather, penetrates the epithelium and rapidly invades the muscle. Maternal blood vessels are opened, with a resultant internal hemorrhage. As the trophoblast continues to grow, the tubal wall becomes distended and weakened and eventually ruptures.

Pregnancy-Induced Hypertension

Hypertensive disorders are among the most common medical complications of pregnancy. *Pregnancy-induced hypertension* (PIH), which often is incorrectly used interchangeably with the term *preeclampsia*, is the most common hypertensive disorder of pregnancy and is the focus of this discussion. PIH includes hypertension without proteinuria and edema. Preeclampsia is characterized by PIH, edema, and proteinuria, and eclampsia by hypertension with proteinuria, edema, and convulsions.

PIH develops in the latter half of pregnancy, usually after 20 weeks of gestation; however, there is growing acceptance of the concept that preeclampsia is a chronic problem throughout pregnancy, rather than an acute disease arising at the time of the development of hypertension.[12] Evidence to support this concept includes decreased clearance rate of dehydroepiandrosterone sulfate (DHEAS), Doppler blood flow studies, and routine measurements of blood pressure. Preeclampsia occurs in 6% to 10% of pregnancies but is severe in less than 1%. It is the leading cause of fetal growth retardation, premature delivery, and maternal death. Preeclampsia only occurs in the presence of the placenta or placental tissue, and its symptoms disappear shortly after delivery.

Preeclampsia is characterized by intense vasospasm, hypertension, and increased surface-mediated platelet activation and consumption. Serotonin, transported in the blood by platelets, is released when platelets are triggered to aggregate.[13] One of the triggers is dysfunctional endothelium.[14, 15] Sera from preeclamptic patients contain cytotoxic factors that damage endothelial cells. The identity of these cytotoxic factors is not currently known, but the placenta is a likely source.

Endothelial cell dysfunction is the major pathophysiologic mechanism in the development of clinical preeclampsia. The intense vasospasm of peripheral arterioles leads to ischemia, especially in renal, cerebral, and uteroplacental vascular beds. Additional contributing pathophysiology of preeclampsia includes increased vasoconstrictor action due to a greater responsiveness to the pressor effects of vasoactive agents such as angiotensin II and an imbalance between the vasodilator and vasocontrictor members of the prostaglandin family, prostacyclin and thromboxane. The extent of the vasospasm appears to be directly proportional to the severity of the disease. Hypertension that occurs prior to 20 weeks of gestation is considered to be preexisting or chronic hypertension.

Clinical Manifestations

Abruptio Placentae

The signs and symptoms of abruptio placentae may vary considerably (Table 34–4). Women with milder, more common forms pose additional difficulties for diagnosis, because their symptoms may be subclinical. Physical symptoms in severe abruption are uterine pain, tenderness at the site of abruption, and petechiae of the uterus. External bleeding may or may not be present and may not correlate with the amount of separation. Hypertonic, painful, and dysrhythmic uterine contractions, maternal anemia, fetal

Table 34–4. **Signs and Symptoms Associated with Severe Abruptio Placentae**

Sign or Symptom	Frequency (%)
Vaginal bleeding	78
Uterine tenderness or back pain	66
Fetal distress	60
High-frequency contractions	34
Idiopathic premature labor	22
Dead fetus	15

distress as evidenced by fetal heart sounds, shock, DIC, and coagulation defects may also be present.

Gestational Diabetes

The clinical symptoms of gestational diabetes are similar to the classic symptoms of diabetes mellitus. They are persistent hyperglycemia, glycosuria, polyuria, and polydipsia.

Ectopic Pregnancy

Unfortunately, no specific signs or symptoms are diagnostic for ectopic pregnancy prior to tubal rupture, and the clinical picture is variable at best. Patients commonly are asymptomatic or are mildly symptomatic prior to distention and rupture of the fallopian tube. Amenorrhea and vaginal spotting may be present. After distention and rupture, the symptoms are severe abdominal pain, abnormal uterine bleeding, and an adnexal mass. Ninety-five percent to 100% of patients present with abdominal pain (usually on the side of the ectopic implantation), 55% to 84% with abnormal uterine bleeding, and 68% to 86% with amenorrhea.[16]

Preeclampsia

The classic triad of symptoms in preeclampsia are hypertension, edema, and proteinuria. These symptoms manifest in varying intensity, leading to their classification as mild or severe. In addition to the symptoms of preeclampsia, eclampsia is characterized by convulsions. Physical symptoms are headaches and visual disturbances, epigastric or right upper quadrant pain, nausea, vomiting, and oliguria.

Laboratory Analyses and Diagnosis

Abruptio Placentae

In abruptio placentae, thromplastic agents released from the separated placenta may cause a consumptive coagulopathy; therefore, coagulation studies are critical. In suggested order, these are (1) APTT, PT, and fibrinogen measurements, (2) platelet count, (3) FSP determination, or (4) D-dimer assay, if available. In extreme emergencies, thrombin time, which is unaffected by deficiencies in either the intrinsic or the extrinsic systems, may be more useful as an indication of relative fibrinogen concentration than fibrinogen quantitation.

For both the APTT and the PT, sufficient amounts of factors V and X as well as fibrinogen must be present in order to have normal results. More specifically, the APTT enables evaluation of the intrinsic clotting factors (VIII, IX, XI, and XII), whereas the PT enables evaluation of the extrinsic clotting factors (VII). Both the APTT and PT may be markedly elevated in severe abruptio placentae. Generally, when the APTT and PT are abnormal, other indices of coagulative abilities are usually abnormal.

Fibrinogen levels are markedly abnormal, with a concentration of less than 100 mg/dL indicative of severe placental abruption. However, because the fibrinogen concentration may be elevated as a result of the pregnancy itself, "normal" concentrations of fibrinogen may be encountered in less severe cases of placental abruption. Many quantitative methods for the measurement of fibrinogen are currently available, and it is important to realize that there may be discrepancies in fibrinogen concentration as measured by the various methods on the same specimen. Semi-automated and automated instruments routinely perform quantitative fibrinogen analyses today, thereby reducing the turnaround time for the result. Fibrinogen/fibrin split products are typically increased because plasmin acts on both the fibrin formed from fibrinogen and the unconverted fibrinogen. If available, the D-dimer assay would replace the fibrin split product assay, because the D-dimer assay measures the degraded fibrinogen and is a specific indicator that activation of both plasmin and thrombin has occurred. The presence of the D-dimer fragment of fibrin at levels exceeding 500 mg/dL indicates DIC. Additionally, a reduced platelet count and a normocytic anemia may also be present. It should be emphasized that all of the laboratory abnormalities mentioned occur more commonly in classic, severe placental abruption, in which fetal death occurs, and are less common in cases in which the fetus survives.

Gestational Diabetes

Diagnosis of gestational diabetes mellitus depends on the results of laboratory tests for carbohydrate metabolism. These include a fasting blood glucose, 1-hour postprandial (PP) glucose or 1-hour tolerance test, and the glucose tolerance test (GTT), including both serum or plasma and urine. Box 34–1 shows criteria for screening diabetes in

---

Box 34–1. Screening and Diagnosis Criteria for Gestational Diabetes Mellitus

Screening Criteria

- All pregnant women without a diagnosis of gestational DM prior to 24 weeks.
- 50-g oral glucose load, between 24 and 28 weeks of gestation, and plasma glucose measured 1 hour later.
- Value of 140 mg/dL or greater indicates need for 3-hour glucose tolerance test.

Diagnosis Criteria

- Plasma glucose is measured at fasting.
- 100-g glucose load, administered in morning after 8- to 14-hour fast; drink is administered, and glucose is measured at 1, 2, and 3 hours after glucose load (subject should remain seated and should not smoke).
- Two or more of the following venous plasma concentrations (mg/dL) must be met or exceeded for positive diagnosis:

    Fasting: 105
    1 hour: 190
    2 hours: 165
    3 hours: 145

pregnancy during the second trimester. The most widely used screening test is the measurement of serum or plasma glucose 1 hour after the administration of a 50-g oral glucose load. This test is generally performed at 24 to 28 weeks of gestation. A 3-hour, 100-g oral glucose tolerance test should be performed for any patient whose screening test value exceeds 140 mg/dL. Normal values for the glucose test differ during pregnancy from those in the nonpregnant state. The demonstration of any two values meeting or exceeding the threshold confirms the diagnosis of gestational diabetes.

Because urine contains both carbohydrate and noncarbohydrate reducing substances, reduction tests for glycosuria are not recommended. Glycosuria is better evaluated by reagent dipsticks specific for glucose (glucose oxidase or other glucose-specific enzymes). The finding of glycosuria alone is not diagnostic of diabetes mellitus in pregnancy, because pregnant females often have a lowered renal threshold for glucose. The reliability of the glucose tolerance test depends on correct patient preparation and proper specimen collection (e.g., timing, preservation).

Ectopic Pregnancy

The most important biochemical finding in an ectopic pregnancy is the presence of hCG at concentrations lower than anticipated for a normal pregnancy of equal gestation. The rate of increase of hCG over time is lower in ectopic pregnancy than in normal intrauterine pregnancy. The mean doubling time of hCG in normal pregnancies is 2 days. Serial serum hCG testing aids in the identification of abnormal pregnancies, ectopic pregnancy, and pregnancies destined to be aborted in 85% of cases if the rate of increase is less than 66% within 2 days.

Central to the diagnosis of ectopic pregnancy is the concept of the *discriminatory zone*, which is the hCG concentration corrresponding with an identifiable uterine gestational sac. An hCG concentration of 6,500 mIU/mL or higher indicates an embryo of sufficient size to be seen reliably with transabdominal ultrasonography; lack of a gestational sac in a patient with that hCG result is highly suggestive of an ectopic pregnancy. Only about 20% of ectopic pregnancies manifest present initially as hCG greater than 6,500 mIU/mL. The improved resolution of transvaginal ultrasound transducers decreases the dicriminatory zone to approximately 1,500 mIU/mL, allowing physicians to diagnose an additional 39% of cases.[17] For those patients presenting with hCG values below 1,500 mIU/mL, diagnosis relies on clinical judgment, expectant management, and serial paired hCG values from the laboratory. Serial measurements of progesterone may also be used to evaluate an ectopic pregnancy. Low progesterone levels (less than 10 ng/mL) do occur in problem pregnancies; however, the clinical utility of progesterone as an indicator of ectopic pregnancy is still under investigation. Hematologic parameters may support the diagnosis of ruptured ectopic pregnancy. Following an acute hemorrhage, possible findings are a normochronic, normocytic anemia, slightly reduced hemoglobin level or hematocrit, normal to slightly high leukocyte count, and slightly increased erythrocyte sedimentation rate. The hCG values gradually decrease to less than 5 mIU/mL within 4 weeks of successful treatment, and hematologic alterations return to normal within 2 weeks.

Several conditions have presenting symptoms similiar to those of a ruptured ectopic pregnancy; they are salpingitis, appendicitis, and abortion of an intrauterine pregnancy. Laboratory data can be useful in the differential diagnosis of these conditions; however, caution should be exercised in interpreting the results of laboratory tests. Although hCG values are absent in salpingitis and appendicitis, negative results may also be obtained in patients with ectopic pregnancy, depending on the sensitivity of the assay method. Detectable hCG values are found in both ectopic pregnancy and abortion of an intrauterine pregnancy. Moderately elevated amylase activity and moderate leukocytosis, found in acute appendicitis, may also be seen in some cases of ruptured ectopic pregnancy. Thus, for differential diagnosis, laboratory tests must be augmented by other diagnostic aids, such as laparoscopy, sonography, patient history, and physical symptoms.

Preeclampsia

Preeclampsia is a progressive disease in which the pathophysiology precedes the recognition and diagnosis by weeks to months. It is diagnosed when two of the three following conditions are present during the second half of pregnancy:

- Blood pressure (BP) higher than 140/90 mm Hg on at least two occasions 6 or more hours apart, or a rise in systolic pressure of 30 mm Hg and/or in diastolic pressure of 15 mm Hg over baseline BP
- Edema of more than 1 kg/week
- Proteinuria (>1 + by dipstick consistently or >300 mg/ 24 hours)

Although the concentrations of several laboratory analytes may be altered as a result of preeclampsia (see Table 34–5), there are inherent problems in using these results alone either to establish or to rule out the diagnosis of preeclampsia. First, such results are not specific for preeclampsia. Elevations in blood urea nitrogen (BUN), creatinine, and uric acid along with a decrease in creatinine clearance may be caused by an underlying renal disease. In a patient in whom epigastric or right upper quadrant pain, nausea, vomiting, and abnormal liver function values—bilirubin, aspartate transaminase (AST), alanine transaminase (ALT), ALP, GGTP—exist, preeclampsia may be confused with hepatobiliary dysfunction. Second, these tests are not sufficiently sensitive to detect preeclampsia in its early stages. For example, proteinuria, described previously, is the most useful laboratory test in the diagnosis of the condition; however, proteinuria is usually a late sign. Cases have been documented in which convulsions have occurred without significant proteinuria. Additionally, proteinuria is a common finding in pregnancy. Third, biochemical and hematologic changes that occur normally during pregnancy may mask the often subtle changes in concentration listed in Table 34–5. The glomerular filtration rate (GFR) normally rises in pregnancy. Thus the GFR, as measured by the creatinine clearance, may be misleading, because the 25% to 50% decrease observed during preeclampsia may still result in a value above nonpregnant

Table 34–5. Biochemical Changes Associated With Preeclampsia-Eclampsia

Analyte	Alteration
Albumin	Decreased
Uric acid	Increased
Blood urea nitrogen	Increased
Creatinine	Increased
Sodium	Increased
AST/ALT	Increased
GFR	Decreased
Urine protein	Increased
Hematocrit	Increased
Platelets	Decreased

Abbreviations: AST, aspartate transaminase; ALT, alanine transaminase; GFR, glomerular filtration rate.

levels. Hematologic changes such as intravascular hemolysis and coagulation abnormalities can be associated with preeclampsia. Hypofibrinogenemia, thrombocytopenia, and increases in FSPs may or may not be present. These findings are more often seen in the more severe form of the disorder.

No one laboratory test or profile is consistently accurate in the diagnosis of preeclampsia-eclampsia; however, the laboratory tests commonly performed certainly may be used to help support the diagnosis of preeclampsia-eclampsia in the appropiate clinical setting.

Treatment

Abruptio Placentae

Treatment of abruptio placentae depends on the status of the mother and fetus. In severe abruption with fetal distress, and bleeding, prompt delivery is indicated. Transfusions of packed red cells, cryoprecipitate, fresh-frozen plasma, platelets, and electrolyte solution may be indicated for severe maternal hemorrhage, anemia, and depleted coagulation factors. Following transfusion, coagulation studies may return to within normal reference ranges. Coagulation factors return to within reference ranges spontaneously within 24 hours after delivery, with the exception of platelets, which take 2 to 4 days to reach normal levels.[5]

Gestational Diabetes

In the treatment of gestational diabetes, usually by diet alone, measurement of the glycated hemoglobin level (HbA$_{1C}$) and at-home measurements of blood glucose are most useful for monitoring the effectiveness of glycemia control. When exposed to high plasma glucose concentrations, the beta chain of the hemoglobin molecule binds irreversibly with glucose. The glycated hemoglobin remains in circulation for the life span of the erythrocyte, and therefore reflects inadequate control weeks to months preceding the test. The normal value for glycated hemoglobin ranges from 3% to 6% but may rise as high as 18% to 20% with prolonged hyperglycemia.

Blood glucose values should be obtained at least four times a day, in both fasting and postprandial states, with a blood glucose reflectance meter; reference intervals are 60 to 90 mg/dL for fasting, less than 140 mg/dL for 1-hour postprandial, and less than 120 mg/dL for 2-hour postprandial measurements.[18] Those women whose blood glucose values exceed the reference intervals should be started on insulin therapy to achieve euglycemia. Women with gestational diabetes should be evaluated in the postpartum period with a 2-hour 75-g oral glucose tolerance test.

Ectopic Pregnancy

Ectopic pregnancy is usually treated surgically (laparoscopy or laparotomy); however, methotrexate therapy is becoming an increasingly popular treatment option for the patient without rupture and when the mass is less than 3.5 cm. Rh immunization is possible after ectopic pregnancy, and a dose of Rh$_0$(D) immune globulin (RhoGAM) should be given to any Rh-negative, unsensitized patient. Quantitative serum hCG values should be followed and maintained at levels less than 5 mIU/mL, because patients with rising or persistently high levels of hCG require repeat surgery or additional methotrexate therapy.

Pregnancy-Induced Hypertension

Treatment of pregnancy-induced hypertension varies according to the severity of the process. In mild cases, antihypertensives alone may be used, whereas severe cases may require hospitalization and induction of labor or cesarean delivery if central nervous system involvement occurs. Proteinuria usually disappears within a few weeks after termination of pregnancy.

Case Study

A 33-year-old, gravida 1, para 1 white woman was brought to the antepartum unit of labor and delivery with a twin gestation of 36 weeks. Physical examination at her physician's office immediately prior to admission revealed a blood pressure of 154/92 mm Hg (baseline blood pressure on first prenatal visit: 110/58 mm Hg), and notable pitting edema of the lower extremities. The remainder of the physical examination was normal. The patient's prenatal history was otherwise unremarkable. Initial laboratory data upon admission and data obtained 8 hours after admission are shown in the second and third columns of the following table.

As the day progressed, the patient's antepartum course worsened, with the baseline blood pressure increasing to 180/110 mm Hg. The patient began to complain of headaches, dizziness, and seeing spots before her eyes. She was delivered by cesarean section. Laboratory data immediately following the C-section are shown in the fourth column of the table:

Anaiyte	Initial	8 hours	Post–C-Section
Na (mmol/L)	136	137	134
K (mmol/L)	3.6	3.6	3.5
Glucose (mg/dL)	88	85	86
Blood urea nitrogen (mg/dL)	20	21	23

Serum creatinine (mg/dL)	1.2	1.2	1.3
Uric acid (mg/dL)	8.4	8.4	8.4
Total protein (g/dL)	4.7	3.2	3.2
Albumin (g/dL)	3.0	2.4	2.4
Bilirubin (mg/dL)	1.3	1.3	1.3
AST (IU/L)	19	20	20
ALT (IU/L)	18	20	20
ALP (IU/L)	419		
Lactate dehydrogenase (IU/L)	254		
24-hour urine protein (g/24 hr)	2.08		
Creatinine clearance (mL/min)	88		
PT (seconds; control, 12)	12	12	14
APTT (seconds; control <40)	41	42	50
Fibrinogen (mg/dL)	500	450	90
Platelet count (cells/mm³)	150,000	90,000	25,000
Fibrin split products (µg/mL)	Normal		40

Questions

1. What was the most likely provisional diagnosis upon admission of the patient?

2. What is the significance of the elevations in serum creatinine, blood urea nitrogen (BUN), and uric acid?

3. Are the results of the creatinine clearance compatible with those for serum creatinine, BUN, and uric acid?

4. What is the significance of the change in coagulation studies?

Discussion

1. The presence of hypertension (BP, 154/92 mm Hg), proteinuria, and edema is strongly suggestive of preeclampsia.

2. The elevations in BUN, serum creatinine, and uric acid suggest renal dysfunction, that is, decreased glomerular filtration secondary to preeclampsia.

3. The normal range for creatinine clearance in non-pregnant women is 88 to 128 mL/min. However, the creatinine clearance normally increases in pregnancy to 120 to 150 mL/min. Thus, this creatinine clearance value, 88 mL/min, is abnormal (decreased) and is therefore compatible with the other indices of decreasing renal function secondary to preeclampsia.

4. The decreases in platelet count and fibrinogen level, prolonged PT and APTT, and elevated fibrin split products indicate that the preeclampsia is being further complicated by disseminated intravascular coagulation.

References

1. Lapthorn AJ, Harris DC, Littlejohn A, et al: Crystal structure of human chorionic gonadotropin. Nature 369:455–461, 1994.
2. Hoshina M, Boothby M, Hussa R, et al: Linkage of human chorionic gonadotropin and placental lactogen biosynthesis to trophoblast differentiation and tumorogensis. Placenta 6:163–172, 1985.
3. Hay DL: Placental histology and the production of human chorionic gonadotropin and its subunits in pregnancy. Br J Obstet Gynaecol 95:1268–1275, 1988.
4. Valanis BG, Perlman CS: Home pregnancy testing kits: Prevalence of use, false-negative rates, and compliance with instructions. Am J Public Health 72:1034–1036, 1982.
5. Pritchart JA, Mac Donald PC, Gant NF: Williams Obstetrics, ed 17. Norwalk, CT, Appleton-Century-Crofts, 1985.
6. Pedersen EB, Johannesen P, Kristensen S, et al: Calcium, parathyroid hormone, and calcitonin in normal pregnancy and preeclampsia. Gynecol Obstet Invest 18:156–164, 1984.
7. Pritchard JA, Adams RH: Erythrocyte production and destruction during pregnancy. Am J Obstet Gynecol 79:750, 1960.
8. Lotspeich-Steininger CA: Anemia of abnormal nuclear development. *In* Lotspeich-Steininger CA, Stiene-Martin EA, Koepke JA: Clinical Hematology: Principles, Procedures, Correlations. Philadelphia, JB Lippincott, 1992.
9. Schmidt MC: Disorders of coagulation and fibrinolysis. *In* Clinical Hematology: Principles, Procedures, Correlations. Philadelphia, JB Lippincott, 1992.
10. Metzger BE: Summary and Recommendations of the Third International Workshop-Conference on Gestational Diabetes Mellitus. Diabetes 40(suppl 4): 197, 1991.
11. DeCherney AH, Jones EE: Ectopic pregnancy. Clin Obstet Gynecol 28:365–374, 1985.
12. Sperof L, Glass RH, Kase G: Clinical Gynecologic Endocrinology and Infertility, 5 ed. Baltimore, Williams & Wilkins, 1995.
13. Rand M, Reid G: Source of "serotonin" in serum [letter]. Nature 168:385, 1951.
14. Weiner CP: The role of serotonin in the preeclampsia-eclampsia syndrome [review]. Cardiovasc Drugs Ther 4:37–43, 1990.
15. Zeeman GG, Dekker GA: Endothelial function in normal and preeclamptic pregnancy: A hypothesis. Eur J Obst Gynecol Reprod Biol 43:113–22, 1992.
16. Gordon JD: Obstetrics, Gynecology, and Infertility: Handbook for Clinicans, ed 4. Menlo Park, CA, Scrub Hill Press, 1995.
17. Barnhart K, Mennutim T, Benjamin I, et al: Prompt diagnosis of ectopic pregnancy in an emergency department setting. Obstet Gynecol 84:1010–1015, 1994.
18. National Diabetes Data Group: Classification and Diagnosis of Diabetes Mellitus. Washington, DC, National Institutes of Health, 1986.

Bibliography

Brizot ML, Jauniaux E, McKie AT, et al: Placental expression of α and β subunits of human chorionic gonadotrophin in early pregnancies with Down's syndrome. Molecular Human Reprod 10:2506–2509, 1995.

Carson SA, Buster JE: Ectopic pregnancy. N Engl J Med 329:1174–1181, 1993.

Kadar N, Devore G, Romero R: Discriminatory hCG zone: Its use in the sonographic evaluation for ectopic pregnancy. Obstet Gynecol 58:156–161, 1981.

Kadar N: The gestational sac and hcg levels [letter]. Am J Radiol 146:1098–1099, 1986.

Klee G: Serum hCG assays: Wide across-method differences. 1993 Ligand Assay Survey Set K-C. Northfield, IL: College of American Pathologists, 1994.

Middelkoop CM, Dekker GA, Kraayenbrink AA, et al: Platelet-poor plasma serotonin in normal and preeclamptic pregnancy. Clin Chem 39:1675–1678, 1993.

Mishalani SH, Seliktar J, Braunstein GD: Four rapid serum-urine combination assays of choriogonadotropin compared and assessed for their utility in quantitative determinations of hCG. Clin Chem 50:1944–1949, 1994.

Reece EA, Homko CJ, Sivan E, et al: When the pregnancy is complicated by diabetes. Contemporary OB/GYN, July:43–61, 1995.

Reece EA, Homko CJ, Wiznitzer A: Hypoglycemia in pregnancies complicated by diabetes mellitus: Maternal and fetal considerations. Clin Obstet Gynecol 37:50–58, 1994.

Saller B: Testicular cancer secretes intact hCG and its free subunits: Evidence that hCG (plus hCG-beta) assays are the most reliable in diagnosis and follow-up. Clin Chem 36:234–239, 1990.

Sokolove PJ: Agreement of intact and beta chain-specific hCG assays in abnormal pregnancy. J Clin Lab Anal 14:196–200, 1991.

Stewart BK, Nazar-Stewart V, Toivola B: Biochemical discrimination of pathologic pregnancy from early, normal intrauterine gestation in symptomatic patients. Am J Clin Pathol 103:386–390, 1995.

Tietz NW (ed). Clinical Guide to Laboratory Tests, ed 3. Philadelphia, WB Saunders, 1995.

Tietz NW: Textbook of Clinical Chemistry, ed 2. Philadelphia, WB Saunders, 1994.

Young DS: Effects of Preanalytical Variables on Clinical Laboratory Tests. Washington, DC, AACC Press, 1993.

Walsh SW, Yuping W: Trophoblast and placental villous core production of lipid peroxides, thromboxane, and prostacyclin in preeclampsia. J Clin Endocrinol Metab 80:1888–1892, 1995.

Fetal Monitoring

Timothy G. McManamon

The laboratory plays an important role in monitoring the progress of fetal development. Table 35–1 lists laboratory tests that are used in fetal monitoring. Some of the tests are routine to all pregnancies, and others are used only when problems are suspected. This chapter reviews a number of gestational conditions for which the laboratory can provide the physician valuable information.

Rh DISEASE

Rh-negative mothers who have been exposed to Rh-positive blood may develop the anti-D antibody. Subsequently, Rh disease develops when anti-D antibody passes from the mother to the fetus, destroying the fetal red blood cells. Rh disease is associated with severe fetal anemia developing into hydrops fetalis and fetal death as early as 20 to 24 weeks of gestation. *Hydrops fetalis* is a combination of anemia, hepatosplenomegaly, ascites, and edema.[1] As gestation progresses, a larger amount of antibody is passed to the fetus, increasing the risk of Rh disease as the pregnancy proceeds. A detailed discussion of Rh disease in the fetus and newborn may be found in Chapter 67.

NEURAL TUBE DEFECTS AND DOWN SYNDROME

Etiology and Pathophysiology

Neural tube defects (NTDs) are among the most common birth defects resulting in infant mortality and serious disability.[2] Neural tube defects are caused by failure of the neural tube to close during early fetal development. They include anencephaly, spina bifida, encephalocele, omphalocele, gastroschisis, and multiple vertebral defects.[3] Anencephaly is a lethal condition. Spina bifida varies in severity but is often severely disabling. Anencephaly and about 90% of cases of spina bifida are "open" defects, in which there is either complete exposure of the neural tissue to amniotic fluid or separation by only a thin, transparent membrane.

The incidence of NTDs varies by ethnic group and location. The incidence of anencephaly and spina bifida in

Weeks of Gestation	Offered to or Performed on All Patients	Offered or Performed If Clinically Indicated
2–12	ABO, Rh typing Direct Coombs' test Hepatitis B surface antibody Qualitative urine protein	—
9–13	—	Chromosome analysis by chorionic villus sampling
16–18	Maternal serum screening for: AFP hCG Estriol	Chromosome analysis α-Fetoprotein testing Acetylcholinesterase by amniocentesis Anti-D titer in Rh disease
20–40	—	Urine protein Uric acid Antithrombin III Urine calcium Liver enzymes Platelet count Magnesium in preeclampsia Anti-D titer ΔOD450 Percutaneous umbilical blood sampling in Rh disease
24–28	Gestational diabetes screen	3-hour glucose tolerance
33–39	—	Fetal lung maturity testing

Table 35–1. **Laboratory Tests Used for Fetal Monitoring**

the US is approximately 1 per 2000 live births. The incidence of ventral wall defects, omphalocele and gastroschisis, is about 1 in 5000 births. In uncomplicated cases, ventral wall defects have a relatively favorable prognosis. The incidence of NTDs has been declining over the past 20 years.

Neural tube defects have been associated with certain drugs taken during pregnancy, including valproic acid, thalidomide, and carbamazepine.[4] Studies have shown that a deficiency of folic acid can increase the risk of an NTD; the Centers for Disease Control and Prevention recommend that all women of childbearing age who have the potential for becoming pregnant consume 0.4 mg of folic acid per day.[2, 5] Studies have also demonstrated a relationship between maternal heat exposure and NTDs. Women exposed to heat from hot tubs, saunas, or fever during early pregnancy are at higher risk of having offspring affected by an NTD.[6]

Fetuses with NTDs who are delivered by cesarean section before the onset of labor have better motor function than those delivered vaginally or by cesarean section after labor has started.[3] For this reason, early detection of NTDs is very important.

α-Fetoprotein Testing

Maternal serum α-fetoprotein (MSAFP) screening during the second trimester is effective in detecting neural tube defects prenatally.[7] α-Fetoprotein (AFP) is the predominant serum protein in the fetus during embryonic development. During pregnancy, AFP passes into the maternal circulation in one of two ways: by diffusion across the placenta and by leakage across the fetal kidney into the amniotic fluid and then diffusion across the amnion. During the second trimester, MSAFP increases approximately 15% per week.[4] In fetuses with NTDs, the close contact between the neural tube and the amniotic fluid allows AFP to easily diffuse into the fluid. The AFP then diffuses into the maternal circulation, raising the MSAFP concentration.

A serum sample is collected between the 14th and 20th weeks of gestation, preferably between the 16th and 18th weeks, and the AFP concentration is quantitated using an immunoassay.[4] In 80% to 90% of cases of NTD, the AFP is elevated in the mother's serum and in the amniotic fluid.[3] Closed defects, such as hydrocephalus, are not associated with abnormal AFP concentrations.

AFP results are reported as *multiples of the median (MoM)*, which relates the result to the median in normal pregnancies at the same gestational age. The reporting laboratory determines the median AFP concentration for its population for each gestational week. The MoM is calculated with the following formula[4]:

$$\frac{\text{Measured AFP } (\mu g/L)}{\text{Median AFP for gestational age } (\mu g/L) \times \text{adjustments}}$$

The adjustments in the formula are to correct for variables that affect the MSAFP concentration but not the risk of NTD. The most significant factor is maternal weight. Heavier mothers tend to have lower AFP concentrations, probably because the AFP is diluted by a larger blood volume. Black women with normal pregnancies have MSAFP concentrations 10% to 15% higher than white women. Multiple pregnancies increase the MSAFP.[4] In mothers with preexisting insulin-dependent diabetes mellitus, the MSAFP concentration is 20% to 40% lower, but the risk of NTD and other malformations is significantly higher.[8]

Follow-Up for Elevated α-Fetoprotein

Multiples of the median greater than 2 indicate that the fetus is at increased risk for NTD. Approximately 1.65% of pregnant women screened have elevated MoMs, but only 2% to 3% of their fetuses have NTDs.[3] These statistics should be communicated to the mother so that proper follow-up and decisions can be made.

Figure 35–1 outlines the steps to be followed when an elevated MSAFP is detected. If gestation has not passed the 20th week, the MSAFP can be repeated. The most common reason for an elevated MoM is improper calculation of the gestational age; therefore, the first step is to use ultrasound to determine whether the gestational age is correct. If the gestational age is determined to be different from that used to calculate the MoM, the MoM should be recalculated using the correct gestational age.

If the gestational age is correct, a level 2 ultrasound should be performed to determine the presence of an NTD. Depending on the ultrasound equipment and how well the fetal spine can be visualized, ultrasound can detect 70% to 90% of the moderate-sized spinal defects. Small defects are more difficult to detect.[3] If the ultrasound detects a malformation, the parents should be counseled concerning their options. If the pregnancy continues, delivery by cesarean section prior to labor may decrease the disability. If the ultrasound does not detect a malformation, amniocentesis to measure the amniotic fluid levels of AFP and cholinesterase can be considered.

Patients with normal ultrasound examinations and elevated MSAFP values should be followed more closely than other patients. These patients have an increased risk of stillbirth, neonatal death, preeclampsia, low birth weight, and premature delivery.[3, 9, 10]

Down Syndrome Testing

Low MoMs indicate an elevated risk of Down syndrome (trisomy 13 syndrome). MSAFP concentrations in pregnancies affected by Down syndrome are approximately 25% lower than in unaffected pregnancies. This difference is believed to be caused by slower development of the fetal liver whereby the rate of AFP production may be approximately 2 weeks behind.

The use of MSAFP alone is not nearly as sensitive for Down syndrome as when it is used for NTD detection. Use of the MSAFP in combination with age detects only 20% of Down syndrome cases.[11] Two other markers are routinely measured, however, to screen for Down syndrome. The unconjugated estriol level is decreased in the serum of mothers carrying fetuses affected by Down syndrome, whereas the human chorionic gonadotropin (hCG) level is elevated.[3] When the three tests are performed together and the relative risk is calculated with the appropriate algorithm, the detection rate rises to 67% with a false-positive rate of 7.2%.[11]

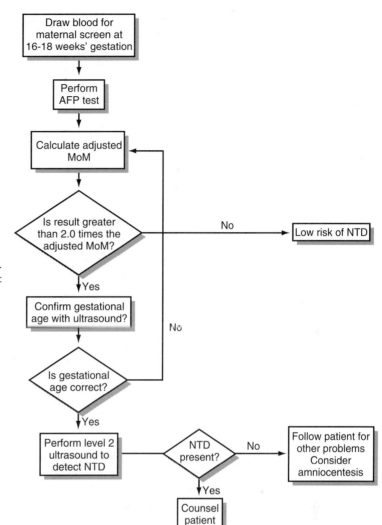

Figure 35–1. Flow chart for the determination of increased risk of neural tube defect (NTD). Abbreviations: AFP, α-fetoprotein; MoM, multiples of the median.

Mothers with higher risk of Down syndrome should be counseled and followed with amniocentesis because of the false-positive rate. Because one third of the Down syndrome cases are not detected by maternal serum screening, any patient with a family history of Down syndrome or who will be 35 years or older on her due date should be offered amniocentesis.

AMNIOCENTESIS AND CHORIONIC VILLUS SAMPLING

Indications for Testing

The indications for invasive prenatal diagnosis are listed in Box 35–1. Three techniques can be used to obtain samples. The traditional and most common procedure is transabdominal amniocentesis, in which a sample of amniotic fluid is obtained during the midtrimester. Another option is chorionic villus sampling (CVS), which has become popular with the increasing demand for results during the first trimester. During CVS, a sample of placenta is obtained either transabdominally, transvaginally, or transcervically. Chorionic villus sampling is usually performed between the 9th and 13th weeks of gestation. The third

invasive procedure to obtain fetal cells is percutaneous umbilical blood sampling (PUBS).[12]

Laboratory Analysis

Cultured cells from amniotic fluid obtained during an amniocentesis can be analyzed cytogenetically, enzymatically, or with DNA analysis. Furthermore, the fluid can be analyzed for cholinesterase or α-fetoprotein. Because CVS

Box 35–1. Indications for Offering Invasive Prenatal Diagnosis

- Maternal age greater than 35 years at the time of delivery
- Positive maternal serum screening for neural tube defects or Down syndrome
- Previous family history of or offspring with chromosome abnormalities
- More than three previous miscarriages
- Increased risk of sickle cell anemia, cystic fibrosis, or Tay-Sachs disease

specimens come from actively proliferating cells, it is possible to perform a direct chromosome preparation, results of which are available within 2 days. These preparations have higher false-positive rates than results from cell cultures; therefore, results from direct analysis should be considered preliminary and should not be released until confirmed by cell culture. The chromosome analysis performed on lymphocytes obtained via PUBS is similar to the procedure used for postnatal chromosome analysis.[16] α-Fetoprotein and acetylcholinesterase analysis can be performed only on amniotic fluid; therefore, patients for whom testing for NTDs is of interest should wait for an amniocentesis rather than an early CVS.

Risks Involved

There is 0.5% increased risk of fetal mortality associated with amniocentesis and CVS. In addition, CVS is also associated with a higher risk of limb defects. These defects involve tissue loss from at least one extremity and often result in an amputation-like defect. The incidence of limb defects is estimated at 6 per 10,000 samplings.[12] PUBS has a higher risk than amniocentesis or CVS.[13]

Several analytical risks are involved in cytogenetic analysis.[1] The cells obtained in any of the procedures may not grow; thus, no diagnosis will be possible.[14] The culture may be contaminated by maternal cells, leading to an incorrect diagnosis; this is more of a problem with CVS or PUBS than with amniocentesis.[15] Chromosome abnormalities may occur during the growth process of the culture that do not represent abnormalities in the fetus.[16] Some identified chromosomal abnormalities are not phenotypically evident and are of little consequence.[2] Finally, the abnormality may not be cytogenetically apparent but may be phenotypically apparent after birth. All patients undergoing invasive prenatal diagnostic procedures must be counseled about the clinical risks and limitations of the procedure.[12]

GESTATIONAL DIABETES

During the second half of pregnancy, the placenta produces increasing amounts of the hormones estrogen, progesterone, and human placental lactogen. All of these hormones have an antagonistic effect on insulin. In mothers who cannot compensate by increasing insulin production, gestational diabetes develops.[17, 18] *Gestational diabetes* is glucose intolerance that develops or is first noted during pregnancy but disappears following delivery.

If the diabetes is untreated, the developing fetus is in a hyperglycemic environment, which leads to increased insulin output from the fetal pancreas. In addition to lowering the blood glucose concentration, insulin also promotes fat and protein synthesis, possibly resulting in macrosomia.[17] *Macrosomia* is a condition in which the fetus is significantly larger than expected for the gestational age. During delivery, macrosomia can lead to major complications if vaginal delivery is attempted, and in most cases of macrosomia, cesarean section is required.[19]

Following birth, babies of mothers with gestational diabetes often become hypoglycemic, because the pancreas continues to produce insulin at the rate it did in utero, although the baby is no longer in a hyperglycemic environment. For the mother, gestational diabetes is clearly a risk factor for the development of diabetes later in life.[18]

There are various recommendations for diagnosing gestational diabetes. The conservative approach is to screen all pregnant women at 24 to 28 weeks of gestation.[20] A less conservative approach, screening only those women who are identified as having risk factors for gestational diabetes, would miss 50% of the cases.[18] This disorder is discussed in detail in Chapter 34.

HYPERTENSION IN PREGNANCY

About 10% of pregnancies are complicated by hypertension. The incidence is higher in first pregnancies and in women carrying multiple fetuses. The National High Blood Pressure Education Working Group recommends the use of the American College of Obstetrics and Gynecologists classification of hypertension during pregnancy. Hypertension in pregnancy is divided into four categories: (1) chronic hypertension, (2) preeclampsia, (3) preeclampsia superimposed on chronic hypertension, and (4) transient hypertension.[21] The most dangerous of these to the fetus is preeclampsia, either by itself or superimposed. This disorder is discussed in Chapter 34.

FETAL LUNG MATURITY
Etiology and Pathophysiology

Complications of pregnancy as well as premature labor require the obstetrician to decide whether it is better to deliver the baby immediately or to support the mother so that the fetus can mature. Of the organs required to sustain life, the lungs are the last to develop. One of the major complications of premature birth is respiratory distress syndrome (RDS), which results from a lack of surfactant in the alveoli.

Mature alveoli consist of two types of cells. Type I cells, which make up 95% of the alveolar surface, function in gas exchange. Type II cells, which produce and store pulmonary surfactant, proliferate during the last stages of fetal development. Surfactant is made up primarily of the phospholipids lecithin, phosphatidylglycerol (PG), and phosphatidylinositol. These molecules, which are made up of a hydrophobic region and a hydrophilic region, form a monolayer between the lining of the alveoli and the air.

The presence of surfactant stabilizes the alveoli by lowering the surface tension at the air-alveolar interface, decreasing the air pressure required to maintain an inflated alveolus. Because alveoli are spherical, the physical laws related to spheres apply. According to the LaPlace relationship, the smaller the sphere or alveolus, the greater the interior pressure. The pressure differences between different alveoli would cause the gases to move from areas of higher pressure to areas of lower pressure, leading to the collapse of smaller alveoli. The surfactant reduces the surface tension within the alveoli, allowing all of the alveoli to remain open and capable of exchanging gases.

Surfactant begins to develop between the 26th and 30th weeks of gestation. When insufficient surfactant is present at birth, alveoli collapse, and RDS develops. The signs of RDS are tachypnea, expiratory grunting, nasal flaring, and costal retractions.[22] RDS is a life-threatening condition requiring aggressive treatment. A small percentage of infants subsequently develop chronic lung conditions.[23–25]

Tests of Fetal Lung Maturity

Several tests are available to determine fetal lung maturity, but before they are used, the physician must decide whether they are necessary. The American College of Obstetricians and Gynecologists guidelines state that if one of the following criteria is met, fetal lung maturity may be assumed and no invasive testing is needed.

1. Fetal heart tones have been heard for 20 weeks by nonelectronic fetoscope or for 30 weeks by Doppler transducer.
2. It has been 36 weeks since a positive pregnancy test was performed by a reliable laboratory.
3. An ultrasound measurement during the pregnancy supports a current gestational age of at least 39 weeks.[26]

If delivery is imminent, fetal lung maturity testing may have little influence on the obstetrician's decisions but may provide valuable information for the neonatologist.

The specimen of choice for fetal lung maturity testing is amniotic fluid that has been obtained by a transabdominal tap. Fluid can also be obtained vaginally after the membranes have ruptured. Vaginal specimens are problematic, because the sample may not be amniotic fluid but other secretions that can yield erroneous results. The laboratory should insist that all vaginal specimens be obtained from freely flowing fluid rather than standing pool fluids. Treatment of the sample in the laboratory is critical. Different tests require different sample preparation, and centrifugation speed is important. Each laboratory must determine its sample preparation guidelines according to the tests being conducted.

Available tests range from the simple and inexpensive to the labor intensive. They include the foam stability or shake test, the lamellar body number density count, the absorbance at 650 nm, amniotic fluid creatinine, the surfactant/albumin ratio, slide agglutination for the presence of PG, and the thin-layer chromatographic (TLC) determination of the lecithin/sphingomyelin (L/S) ratio with PG. The approach discussed in this chapter is a strategy using a combination of the surfactant/albumin ratio and the L/S ratio.

The surfactant/albumin ratio is available on the Abbott

TDx analyzer as the fetal lung maturity (FLM) test. A ratio is used to correct for differences in amniotic fluid volume. As the fetal lungs mature and surfactant is produced, it diffuses from the lungs into the amniotic fluid. The albumin concentration remains relatively constant throughout the latter portion of gestation; therefore, expressing the concentrations as a ratio eliminates the volume effect. Abbott FLM results are reported as mg/g. This test serves as an excellent screening test. Values less than 44 mg/g can be interpreted as indicating immature lungs, whereas those higher than 55 mg/g can be interpreted as indicating mature lungs. Values between 44 and 55 mg/g are considered borderline, and an L/S ratio should be performed.

The L/S ratio, like the FLM, utilizes the measurement of a changing marker, lecithin, and a constant, sphingomyelin, to determine fetal maturity and correct for fluid volume differences.[27] The L/S ratio is considered by many authorities to be the standard of fetal lung maturity testing, but it is analytically less precise than the FLM; therefore, some authorities believe that it may become obsolete in the near future. The L/S ratio is a TLC method requiring 3 to 4 hours to complete. Each laboratory must determine the appropriate cutoff for maturity on the basis of its procedure. Generally, the cutoff is between 2.0 and 2.5.

In addition to obtaining the L/S ratio, the presence or absence of PG can also be determined from the TLC plate. Caution must be exercised in reporting PG results because of pseudo-PG, which can give false-positive results if a single migration in one dimension is used.[28] The pseudo-PG can be eliminated by using a double migration system or by performing a two-dimensional chromatographic technique, either of which adds significant time to the procedure.[29] Another option is to perform the PG test by slide agglutination using the AmnioStat-FLM procedure. PG results are usually reported as absent, trace, or present. Another advantage of offering the slide agglutination PG test is that specimens contaminated with meconium or blood can be analyzed with this technique but not by the Abbott FLM test or the L/S ratio.[30]

As Table 35–2 indicates, all three tests are very reliable when a mature value is obtained. Immature values do not guarantee that RDS will develop. When fetal lung maturity testing indicates immaturity, the obstetrician must weigh the "false-immature" rate with the risk to the mother and fetus when deciding to wait or deliver the baby. Many babies with test results indicating lung immaturity do not develop RDS. If a baby is at increased risk of developing

Table 35–2. Diagnostic Performance Statistics for Fetal Lung Maturity Testing

Test	Cutoff	Sensitivity (%)	Specificity (%)	Predictive Value (%) In Mature Lungs	In Immature Lungs
FLM-II	39 for immature 55 for mature	93	76	100	42
AmnioStat PG	Trace	91.6	58.7	99.4	24.1
	Positive	95.7	80.9	99.2	39.3
L/S ratio	>2 Helena Method	81.1	84.5	98	47

Abbreviations: FLM-II, method of determining the surfactant-albumin ratio; PG, phosphotidylglycerol; L/S, lecithin-sphingomyelin ratio.
Data from Strassner HT, Nochimson DJ: Determination of fetal lung maturity. Clin Perinatol 9:297, 1982; Abbott Laboratories: Fetal Lung Maturity II TDx Assays Manual. Abbott Park, IL, Abbott Laboratories, 1994.

RDS, synthetic surfactant can be given as an aerosol shortly after birth in hopes of preventing RDS, which usually develops approximately 8 hours after birth. Once RDS has developed, it is too late to give the surfactant; therefore, it is important to know whether the baby is at increased risk so the surfactant can be given early.

The effect of diabetes on fetal lung maturity remains controversial. The long-held belief has been that fetal lung maturation is delayed in fetuses of diabetic mothers and that the L/S ratio is not a reliable indicator of maturation. If possible, delivery should be postponed until the PG test is positive.[30] Other authorities conclude that if the diabetes is well managed during pregnancy, there is no difference in infant fetal lung maturity between diabetic and nondiabetic mothers.[22] Until this issue is resolved, caution should be exercised in interpreting fetal lung maturity test results in diabetic mothers.

Case Study

A 22-year-old gravida 1 woman had a maternal serum screening at 18 weeks of gestation. The hCG and estriol levels were normal but the AFP level was 3.1 multiples of the median. The result was received from the laboratory at 21 weeks of gestation; therefore, it was not possible to repeat the screening. An ultrasound was performed to verify gestational age. The result was consistent with the calculated age. No neural tube defects were observed on ultrasound. The mother opted not to undergo amniocentesis for AFP or cholinesterase.

Question

1. What risks would be associated with such findings?

Discussion

1. The mother would be at increased risk for stillbirth, neonatal death, preeclampsia, low birth weight, and premature delivery. This patient was followed closely by her obstetrician, but no further complications developed.

References

1. Bussel JB, McFarland JG, Berkowitz RL: Antenatal management of fetal alloimmune and autoimmune thrombocytopenia: Transfus Med Rev 4:191–207, 1990.
2. American Academy of Pediatrics Committee on Genetics: Folic acid for the prevention of neural tube defects. Pediatrics 92:493–494, 1993.
3. Carroll JC: Maternal serum screening. Can Fam Physician 40:1756–1764, 1994.
4. Bock JL: Current issues in maternal serum alpha-fetoprotein screening. Am J Clin Pathol 97:541–554, 1992.
5. Recommendations for the use of folic acid to reduce the number of cases of spina bifida and other neural tube defects. MMWR Morb Mortal Wkly Rep 41:1–7, 1992.
6. Milunsky A, Ulcickas M, Rothman KJ: Maternal heat exposure and neural tube defects. JAMA 268:882–885, 1992.
7. Saller DN, Carnick JA, Palomaki GE, et al: Second-trimester maternal serum alpha-fetoprotein, unconjugated estriol, and hCG levels in pregnancies with ventral wall defects. Obstet Gynecol 84:852–855, 1994.
8. Martin AO, Dempsy LM, Minogue J, et al: Maternal serum alpha-fetoprotein levels in pregnancies complicated by diabetes: Implications for screening programs. Am J Obstet Gynecol 163:1209–1216, 1990.
9. Silver RM, Draper ML, Byrne JL, et al: Unexplained elevations of maternal serum alpha-fetoprotein in women with antiphospholipid antibodies: A harbinger of fetal death. Obstet Gynecol 83:150–155, 1994.
10. Maher JF, Davis RO, Goldenberg RL, et al: Unexplained elevation in maternal serum alpha-fetoprotein and subsequent fetal loss. Obstet Gynecol 83:138–141, 1994.
11. MacDonald ML, Wagner RM, Slotnick RN: Sensitivity and specificity of screening for Down syndrome with alpha-fetoprotein, hCG, unconjugated estriol, and maternal age. Obstet Gynecol 80:353–358, 1992.
12. Shulman LP, Elias S: Amniocentesis and chorionic villus sampling. West J Med 159:260–268, 1993.
13. Schonberg SA: Cytogenetic analysis in prenatal diagnosis. West J Med 159:360–365, 1993.
14. Kaufman GE, Paidas MJ: Rhesus sensitization and alloimmune thrombocytopenia. Semin Perinatol 18:333–349, 1994.
15. Ryan G, Morrow RJ: Fetal blood transfusion. Clin Perinatol 21:573–589, 1994.
16. Meagher SE, Fisk NM: Intrauterine transfusion in Rh alloimmunisation. Med J Austr 156:302–304, 1992.
17. Narayanan S: Laboratory monitoring of gestational diabetes. Ann Clin Lab Sci 21:392–401, 1991.
18. Coustan DR: Screening and diagnosis of gestational diabetes. Semin Perinatol 18:407–413, 1994.
19. Sacks DA: Fetal macrosomia and gestational diabetes: What's the problem? Obstet Gynecol 81:775–781, 1993.
20. American Diabetes Association: Position statement: Gestational diabetes mellitus. Diabetes Care 9:430, 1986.
21. National High Blood Pressure Education Program Working Group Report on High Blood Pressure in Pregnancy. Am J Obstet Gynecol 163:1691–1712, 1990.
22. Kjos SI, Walther FJ, Montoro M, et al: Prevalence and etiology of respiratory distress in infants of diabetic mothers: Predictive value of fetal lung maturation tests. Am J Obstet Gynecol 163:898–903, 1990.
23. Avery ME, Mead J: Surface properties in relation to atelectasis and hyaline membrane disease. Am J Dis Child 97:517, 1959.
24. Strassner HT, Nochimson DJ: Determination of fetal lung maturity. Clin Perinatol 9:297, 1982.
25. Chapman JF, Herbert WNP: Fetal Lung Maturity Testing: Practical Clinical and Laboratory Considerations. Workshop, 47th National Meeting of the American Association for Clinical Chemistry, Pasadena, CA, July 16, 1995.
26. Fetal Maturity Assessment Prior to Elective Repeat Cesarean Delivery. ACOG Committee Opinion 98. Washington, DC, 1991.
27. Gluck L, Kulovich MV, Borer RC, et al: Diagnosis of the respiratory distress syndrome by amniocentesis. Am J Obstet Gynecol 109:440–445, 1971.
28. Helena Laboratories: Fetal-Tek 200 Method Package Insert. Beaumont, TX, Helena Laboratories, 1985.
29. Spillmann T, Cotton DB, Lynn SC: Removal of a component interfering with phosphatidylglycerol estimation in the Helena system for amniotic phospholipids. Clin Chem 30:737–740, 1984.
30. Ojomo EO, Coustan DR: Absence of evidence of pulmonary maturity at amniocentesis in term infants of diabetic mothers. Am J Obstet Gynecol September 163:954–957, 1990.
31. Abbott Laboratories: Fetal Lung Maturity II TDx Assays Manual. Abbott Park, IL, Abbott Laboratories, 1994.

Chapter 36

Female Reproductive Disorders

Denise L. Uettwiller-Geiger

A complex system involving neural stimuli, hypothalamus, pituitary, and ovaries regulates sexual maturation and reproduction in women. The system is modulated by several areas of the brain that contain neurons, the axons of which relay neurotransmitters to alter hypothalamus activity. Neurotransmitters involved include dopamine, epineph-

rine, norepinephrine, serotonin, acetylcholine, and histamine.[1] In response, the neurons in the hypothalamus synthesize and secrete a 10–amino acid peptide known as gonadotropin-releasing hormone (GnRH). This neurohormone, which is secreted in discrete pulses, controls the production and release of the gonadotropins follicle-stimulating hormone (FSH) and luteinizing hormone (LH) from the anterior pituitary via the hypothalamic pituitary portal capillary plexus system.

FSH is considered the gonadotropin responsible for ovarian follicular growth and maturation. LH stimulates ovarian production of the steroids estrogen, progesterone, and androgens. Three naturally occurring estrogens are involved in the menstrual cycle. Estradiol-17β, (E2), the major secreted estrogen, is in equilibrium in the circulation with estrone. Estrone is further metabolized in the liver to estriol. Estradiol is the most potent estrogen, and estriol the least. Almost all of the estrogens during the menstrual cycle are derived from the ovary.

Progesterone, a C21 steroid, is secreted along with estrogens from the ovarian follicles. It is converted to pregnanediol in the liver, conjugated to glucuronic acid, and excreted in the urine. The androgens, testosterone and androstenedione, are also released by the ovarian follicles under the stimulus of LH and FSH.

A negative feedback mechanism is responsible for the interaction of these hormones. The primary stimulus for LH and FSH release is the concentration of estrogens in the peripheral circulation; that is, when the level of estradiol falls below a set point, the gonadotropins are released. Alternatively, when the level of estradiol is above a set point, release of the gonadotropins is reduced. Feedback actions of estrogen seem to occur at the hypothalamus, where GnRH secretion is stimulated, and at the pituitary, where the glycoprotein hormones LH and FSH are released. Inhibin, a nonsteroid FSH inhibitor, has been demonstrated in ovarian follicles and plays a role in the differential suppression of FSH secretions.

PUBERTY AND THE MENSTRUAL PHASES

Puberty

The changes in the body that constitute puberty have been classified according to skeletal growth patterns, fat distribution, and the development of the gonads, reproductive organs, and secondary sex characteristics. In the female, they include the development of the breast tissue and the sprouting of pubic and axillary hair. The precise signal that initiates these events involves a complex set of neuromechanisms interacting with the hypothalamus, pituitary, gonads, and adrenal cortex.[2] Prior to puberty, this system is functional but is inhibited by low levels of circulating gonadal steroids. At puberty, for a reason yet unknown, the hypothalamic hormone receptor sites become less sensitive to the steroid hormones. Consequently, the hypothalamic release of pulsatile GnRH prompts production by the pituitary of large amounts of the gonadotropins LH and FSH, which in turn stimulate gonadal production of estradiol and progesterone. In early puberty, episodic secretions of LH are associated with sleep. The FSH levels seem to plateau by midpuberty, whereas LH and estradiol levels continue to rise until late puberty. By midpuberty, the ovary is ready to secrete estrogen in irregular cycles of 28 to 40 days. The estrogens promote the proliferation of the uterine endometrium. By mid- to late puberty, the decrease in E2 brings menarche. Approximately 6 to 12 months later, the increase in circulating estrogens near midcycle induces a surge of LH and FSH, resulting in ovulation. The length of time involved in this evolution is usually 2 to 4 years.

Although the system follows an orderly progression, the age of onset of puberty is variable. Factors involved include genetic makeup, socioeconomic conditions, nutrition, and general health. There has been a progressive decrease in the mean age of menarche in the United States for the last 100 years, believed to be due to improvement in nutrition. Now, puberty generally begins some time between 8 and 14 years of age, with menarche occurring between 9 and 18 years (mean, 12.8 years).

Owing to the wide variance in sexual maturation, abnormal conditions can be difficult to diagnose. In general, a young woman with menarche before the age of 9 or failure to menstruate after the age of 16 warrants evaluation.

Menstrual Phases

Menstrual Cycle

The complex changes in hormonal levels during the menstrual cycle are regulated by the estradiol gonadotropin feedback mechanism. The length of the cycle is variable but averages 28 days from the start of one menstrual period to the start of the next. The days of the cycle are often identified by number, starting with the first day of menstruation. The cycle can be divided into three primary stages: the follicular phase, ovulation, and the luteal phase.

The *follicular phase* is initiated by a rise in FSH that occurs in response to the decline in estradiol in the preceding cycle (Fig. 36–1).[3] This initial phase lasts 10 to 14 days and results in one surviving mature follicle. Low levels of LH early in the cycle are the result of the negative feedback from estradiol. During the late follicular phase, under FSH stimulation, the maturing follicle begins estrogen production from its granulosa cells. Estrogen levels, specifically estradiol, rise slowly at first and then rapidly reach a peak just before ovulation. The estradiol peak varies from 500 to 1000 pg/mL and triggers a midcycle surge of LH and FSH. In order for the LH and FSH surge to occur, estradiol levels of more than 200 pg/mL for a critical period of 50 hours or more are required.[4] Ovulation of the mature follicle into the abdominal cavity occurs about 12 hours after gonadotropin peak, or about days 14 to 16 of the menstrual cycle.[4] The ovum is picked up by the oviducts and transported to the uterus. Unless fertilization occurs, the ovum passes through the uterus and out the vagina.

In the majority of menstrual cycles, the system allows only one follicle to mature and reach the point of *ovulation.* However, multiple fraternal births may be due in part to the random maturation of more than one follicle per cycle, the rupture of the follicle, and release of the ovum. The follicle accumulates a yellow pigment, lutein, which lends its name to the third and final phase of the cycle, the *luteal phase.* The time from ovulation to menses is consistently close to 14 days in length. The variability in cycle lengths among women is due to the varying number of days required for follicular growth.

The mature follicle, known as the *corpus luteum,* begins synthesizing estrogens, progestin, and androgen steroids and by day 8 or 9 after ovulation, peak levels of progesterone occur in the blood. Even though progesterone levels of 20 to 30 ng/mL are not uncommon during the luteal phase, a level of 3 ng/mL is considered a reliable indicator of ovulation and corpus luteum activity.[5] From 10% to 20% of the progesterone is excreted in the urine as the metabolite pregnanedione, which peaks at 3 to 6 mg/day and is maintained until 2 days prior to menses. Owing to the steroid negative feedback process, LH and FSH are now at their lowest levels in the cycle.

Ten to 12 days after ovulation, the corpus luteum enters a stage of regression in which progesterone and estradiol levels decrease, leading to menses and a new cycle. The corpus luteum is eventually replaced by fibrous tissue, forming a *corpus albicans.*

Pregnancy

The menstrual cycle renewal is inevitable unless pregnancy occurs. With pregnancy, the life span of the corpus luteum is prolonged by the emergence of a new stimulus, human chorionic gonadotropin (hCG). This gonadotropin appears at the peak of corpus luteum development (9 to 13 days after ovulation). It serves to maintain progesterone and estradiol levels until approximately the ninth to tenth week of gestation, by which time placental steroidogenesis is well established.

Menopause

At approximately 40 years of age, women enter a period known as the *climacteric.* This stage lasts as long as 20 years and carries women through decreased fertility, menopause, and manifestations of progressive tissue atrophy and aging. Menopause, or the ceasing of cyclic menses, occurs in the United States between ages 48 and 55, with the median age being 51.4 years. Because this age range is so long, menopause may be presumed or misdiagnosed, and the presence of other conditions may be missed. As a woman reaches menopause, residual follicles are least sensitive to gonadotropin stimulation and less likely to achieve

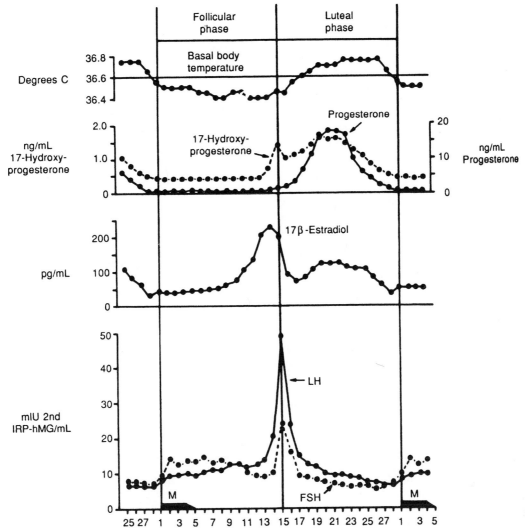

Figure 36–1. Typical basal body temperatures and plasma hormone concentrations during a normal 28-day human menstrual cycle. (From Midgely AR: Human Reproduction. Hagerstown, Md, Harper & Row, 1973.)

complete maturation and estrogen production; therefore, FSH and LH rise to their highest levels to stimulate the aging ovary. Levels of FSH greater than 40 mIU/mL may be seen despite continued menstrual bleeding, although LH levels usually remain in the normal range. Eventually, there is a 10- to 20-fold increase in FSH and a 3-fold increase in LH, reaching a maximum level 1 to 3 years after menopause, after which there is a gradual and slight decline. The circulating estradiol level after menopause is approximately 10 to 20 pg/mL, most of which is probably derived from peripheral conversion of testosterone and estrone. Interestingly, estrone levels are higher than estradiol levels at this point, with a mean of approximately 30 pg/mL.

PRECOCIOUS PUBERTY

Etiology and Clinical Manifestations

In precocious puberty, increased growth is often the first noted change, followed by breast development and pubic hair growth. Precocity occurs in girls 5 times more frequently than in boys. If the child has cyclic ovarian activity resulting in menarche and ovulation, the syndrome is termed *GnRH-dependent precocious puberty,* or true precocious puberty, indicating early activation of the hypothalamic-pituitary-gonadal axis. If a similar increase in steroid hormones occurs without gonadotropin stimulation and ovulation, *GnRH-independent precocious puberty,* or precocious pseudopuberty, exists. Sexual maturation in these instances may be due to extrapituitary secretion of hCG or sex steroid secretion independent of hypothalamic-pituitary gonadotropin stimulation.[4] Distinguishing the syndromes can be difficult and of little practical use. Because both conditions can be due to serious disease, particular attention should be given to obtaining careful histories, with dating of events and detailing of behavioral changes, and performing a thorough physical examination in order to rule out the possibility of central nervous system (CNS) problems such as tumor, cranial trauma or encephalitis, retarded growth with symptoms of hypothyroidism, and pelvic or abdominal mass.

Laboratory Analyses and Diagnosis

When the cause of precocious puberty is not obvious from physical examination or history, diagnostic radioisotopic and automated nonisotopic assays can be helpful in differential diagnosis. These methods utilize new technologies, such as monoclonal antibodies, solid-phase separations, sandwich techniques, nonradioactive labeling reagents, and human serum calibrators to improve analytical sensitivities; however, differences in chosen monoclonal antibodies and in assay standardization can affect the clinical use of the assay kits. Values obtained on serum for specific hormones may vary widely, even in the same sample from technique to technique and depending on the assay system used; therefore, results and the resulting ratios should be interpreted and compared cautiously. Because many hormone levels are affected by diurnal rhythm, samples should be consistently collected in the morning. A comprehensive evaluation should include: thyroid function tests (TSH, thyroxine [T_4] and free T_4), steroids (serum estradiol, testosterone, progesterone, dehydroepiandrosterone sulfate [DHAS], and 17-hydroxyprogesterone), FSH, LH, hCG, and GnRH testing. Blood estrogens and FSH and LH values compatible with those in sexually mature women are found in true precocious puberty. In contrast, low levels of FSH and LH with increased estrogens are often seen with tumors. Elevated hCG may also indicate a teratoma or an ovarian dysgerminoma. High blood levels of 17-hydroxycorticosteroid (17-OH) progesterone and adrenal androgens confirm the diagnosis of 21-hydroxylase–deficient adrenal hyperplasia, whereas an increase in 11-deoxycortisol indicates an 11-hydoxylase–deficient adrenal hyperplasia. An adrenal cortical adenoma or carcinoma is suspected when the two hormones are normal and serum DHAS or androstenedione is increased. An increase in testosterone suggests an ovarian cause of precocity.

Other tests useful in diagnosing sexual precocity are ultrasound scanning of the adrenals and ovaries, or magnetic resonance imaging (MRI) or computed tomography (CT) scanning of the adrenals, and skull and bone age determinations.

Treatment

The treatment of precocious puberty is designed to suppress menstruation, ovulation, and fertility and to prevent excessively short stature. Both administration of GnRH analogues in true precocious puberty and appropriate replacement of thyroid hormone have been shown to cause regression and suppression of secondary sexual changes. Treatment of GnRH-independent precocity uses medroxyprogesterone to suppress LH secretion and gonadal steroidogenesis. The treatment of choice for ovarian tumors causing precocious pseudopuberty is surgical removal. In cases of adrenalocortical hyperplasia, glucocorticoid replacement therapy is indicated.

AMENORRHEA
Etiology

Amenorrhea is defined as either *primary* (no menses by the age of 16 years, despite the presence of normal growth and development and secondary sex characteristics) or *secondary* (absence of menses for 6 months or for the equivalent of three previous cycle intervals after onset of regular menses). As suggested by Speroff and colleagues,[4] disor-

ders producing amenorrhea can be classified into the following four compartments:

Compartment I: Outflow tract (uterus, cervix, vagina).
Compartment II: Ovary (follicular development and response).
Compartment III: Anterior pituitary (gonadotropin production and release).
Compartment IV: CNS and hypothalamus (gonadotropin-releasing hormone, production and release).

Once the compartment has been identified, the physician can usually determine a cause and formulate a treatment plan (Fig. 36–2).

Because a minimal change in thyroid function can alter pituitary function, amenorrhea and infertility may be the first clinical symptoms of thyroid dysfunction. Increased thyrotropin-releasing hormone (TRH) and TSH in primary hypothyroidism have been shown to induce hyperprolactinemia. Normal ovulatory function, however, usually returns after approximately 3 months of hormone replacement therapy.[6]

Outflow Tract Abnormalities (Compartment I)

Outflow tract defects can be congenital abnormalities, such as müllerian agenesis or testicular feminization, or can represent destruction of the endometrium, as seen in Asherman's syndrome.

In the patient with a competent outflow tract who fails to bleed after progestational medication, inadequate levels of endogenous estrogen needed to stimulate endometrial growth are usually found. This fault may be due to ovarian unresponsiveness (compartment II) or inadequate FSH gonadal stimulation (compartment III or IV).

Ovarian Dysfunction (Compartment II)

Ovarian dysfunction is almost always irreversible; however, cases do exist in which estrogen therapy has triggered only temporary return to ovarian activity. The perimenopausal woman's gonadotropins may rise before bleeding actually ceases. Usually these women present with increased FSH and a normal LH value. It is likely that the elevated FSH levels are needed to stimulate the few remaining follicles that have diminished estrogen-producing ability. Once LH and FSH are elevated, total ovarian failure is likely.

Resistant ovarian syndrome is suggested in the patient with increased gonadotropins and functioning ovarian follicles. Large amounts of gonadotropins are needed to produce follicular growth in this rare syndrome. Achieving pregnancy is unlikely even with high doses of exogenous gonadotropins.

Premature ovarian failure is characterized by the cessation of ovarian function before the age of 40 years. It occurs secondary to increased atresia of the ovarian follicles, resulting from infection, radiation, chemotherapy, or autoantibody exposure. Sex chromosome abnormalities, such as Turner's syndrome, silent Y chromosome, and a variety of other anomalies, are also associated with premature ovarian failure.

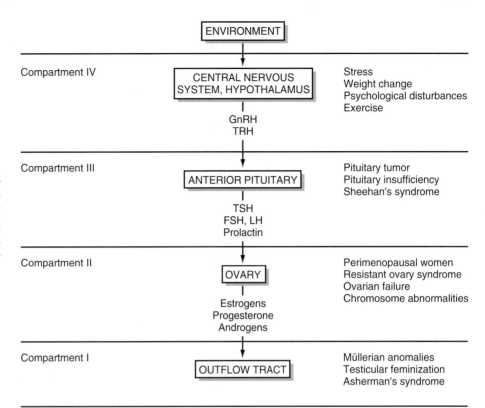

Figure 36–2. Classification of common etiologies of amenorrhea by compartments and associated hormones. Abbreviations: GnRH, gonadotropin-releasing hormone; TRH, thyroid-releasing hormone; TSH, thyroid-stimulating hormone; FSH, follicle-stimulating hormone; LH, luteinizing hormone.

Turner's syndrome, a gonadal dysgenesis in females, is the result of any of several defects of the X chromosome. About half of patients with this syndrome have a 45,X karyotype; the cytogenetic findings in the remainder vary. The 45,X defect may result from chromosome loss during gametogenesis in the parents or from an error in mitosis during an early division of the zygote. This disorder must be distinguished clinically from Noonan's syndrome, which can occur in both males and females; however, patients with the latter disorder have a normal karyotype.[7]

The presence of a Y chromosome leading to mosaicism occurs, and testicular tissue may predispose the patient to malignancy or virilization. Approximately one-third of the patients carrying a Y chromosome do not exhibit signs of virilization. Thus, a normal phenotypic female with amenorrhea and increased gonadotropins should be karyotyped, evaluated, and diagnosed accordingly. In the case of "testicular feminization," in which a genotypic male appears phenotypically female, a complete end-organ resistance to androgens is present.

Pituitary Disorders (Compartment III)

With greater sensitivity of radiologic examinations along with increased utilization of prolactin assays, pituitary tumors are more commonly associated with amenorrhea. As many as one-third of patients with secondary amenorrhea have a pituitary tumor.[8]

Pituitary insufficiency leading to amenorrhea may also be due to nearby lesions, carotid artery aneurysms, or an obstruction of the aqueduct of Sylvius or ischemia, as seen in Sheehan's syndrome. This last disorder is caused by a postpartum vascular infarction of the pituitary. In affected patients, the necrosis is due to extensive thrombosis of the

pituitary circulation during or following delivery and is usually associated with excessive blood loss and hypotension. Characteristically, patients with Sheehan's syndrome are able to lactate and menstruate. The association of these signs with low circulating levels of prolactin suggests the diagnosis. Some patients appear quite healthy, but others gradually lapse into severe anterior, pituitary insufficiency involving gonadal, thyroid, and adrenal function. The pituitary gland has a large reserve, however, and substantial amounts of pituitary tissue must be damaged before significant hormone deficiency develops.

Hypothalamic Amenorrhea (Compartment IV)

Amenorrhea stems from an impaired release of GnRH with low levels of LH, FSH, and estrogens leading to anovulation.[9] It is postulated that the impaired release of GnRH is due to abnormal metabolism of dopamine and norepinephrine in the central nervous system; however, bromocriptine, a dopamine antagonist, has no effect on the abnormalities.[10]

Strenuous physical activity, as seen in avid marathon runners, ballet dancers, and swimmers, has been shown to have detrimental effects on reproductive functions, such as producing exercise-induced amenorrhea. It has been estimated that there are 4.4 million oligomenorrheic athletes.[11] In one study, more than 35% of the females running 60 miles per week experienced amenorrhea.[12] This chronic anovulation is influenced by a combination of physical, hormonal, and psychologic effects. Changes in weight, percentage of body fat, daily protein intake, and stress may all contribute to the problem.

Clinical Manifestations

Outflow Tract Abnormalities (Compartment I)

The clinical findings in outflow tract abnormalities depend on the nature of the anatomic or structural defect that precludes menstrual bleeding. Menstrual blood often accumulates behind the obstacle, and affected women may have cyclic episodes of abdominal pain. Surgery is the treatment.

Ovarian Dysfunction (Compartment II)

A patient with amenorrhea due to ovarian dysfunction has a variety of other symptoms, depending on the cause of dysfunction. A thorough medical history assists in ruling out some disorders. The patient with normal menses early in her history may be evaluated for previous treatments or development of an autoimmune disorder. Patients who have never achieved menses have a variety of symptoms based on etiology. Turner's syndrome (45,X) one example. It is usually recognized from the classic physical characteristics short stature, webbed neck, shield crest, and increased angle of the arms. The gonads are usually bilateral pale "streaks" of connective tissue; however, primary follicles have been described, with a rare occurrence of menarche and variable menses.[13]

Pituitary Disorders (Compartment III)

A patient with a disorder of the pituitary can have a variety of symptoms. In addition to amenorrhea, symptoms can include headaches, visual difficulties, acromegaly, cushingoid appearance, and lactation.

Hypothalamic Disorder (Compartment IV)

Patients with hypothalamic disorders often have experienced physical or emotional stress, psychologic disturbances, or drastic weight loss with a history of menstrual disorders. Many women on "crash diets" or suffering from anorexia nervosa initially have no complaints other than amenorrhea. The drastic weight loss seen in anorexia is considered a psychologic disorder, with behavioral and endocrine changes associated with malnutrition and inhibition of normal GnRH pulsatile secretion normally controlled by the hypothalamus.

Laboratory Analyses and Diagnosis

Initial Evaluation

Before an elaborate evaluation of the sexually active patient is undertaken, pregnancy should be ruled out. Today, pregnancy usually can be detected 1 week after conception with monoclonal antibody pregnancy assays.

Following pregnancy testing, evaluation of an amenorrheic patient should comprise thyroid function tests (TSH), serum prolactin levels, and the progestogen challenge test (Provera) used to assess the competency of the outflow tract (Fig. 36–3). Normal results of these studies indicate a diagnosis of anovulation. Management of these cases de-

pends on whether or not the patient would like to become pregnant. If pregnancy is desired, ovulation induction is indicated. If pregnancy is not desired, the patient can be started on oral contraceptives or a barrier method of contraception, because ovulation and fertility may return without warning.

Outflow Tract Abnormalities (Compartment I)

The lack of withdrawal flow within 2 weeks after a course of exogenous progestin treatment can establish the diagnosis of a defect in compartment I.

Ovarian Dysfunction (Compartment II)

To rule out ovarian failure (compartment II), blood LH and FSH levels should be assayed. For accuracy, these hormones should be measured no earlier than 2 weeks after any hormonal medications are administered to the patient. Elevations of LH and FSH gonadotropins occur from the loss of negative feedback, indicating ovarian unresponsiveness (compartment II), whereas low or normal levels suggest hypopituitarism, pituitary tumor, or pituitary dysfunction (compartment III).

An amenorrheic patient with FSH values higher than 20 mIU/mL and low estrogen levels is considered to have ovarian failure.

Patients in whom Turner's syndrome is suspected can be screened by determination of the X chromosome pattern on a buccal smear, but should be diagnosed definitively by a blood lymphocyte karyotype analysis. Gonadotropin levels, especially FSH, are useful in assessing the functional status of the gonads. FSH levels are usually elevated from birth to the age of 4 years, but decrease to high-normal values between 5 and 10 years of age. After 10 years, FSH levels reach their highest points. The pattern of change in LH is similar, but the concentrations are 1/3 to 1/10 those of FSH. GnRH-induced LH and FSH responses exhibit a pattern with age similar to that for basal levels; that is, patients younger than 5 years and older than 10 years exhibit a rise in gonadotropins after GnRH, whereas in those between the ages of 5 and 10 years, the response is less.

Before the age of 10 years patients with Turner's syndrome also show normal concentrations of adrenal androgens. After the age of 15, however, levels of dehydroepiandrosterone (DHEA), testosterone, and androstenedione are lower than normal owing to the lack of gonadal production.[8] Patients with silent Y syndrome (46,XY) have increased plasma LH and testosterone concentrations. Estradiol concentrations are higher than those normally seen in men, and FSH levels are often normal or slightly increased.

Pituitary Disorders (Compartment III)

The association of pituitary tumors, amenorrhea, and elevated prolactin levels is high. Hyperprolactinemia has been reported in 15% to 40% of patients with secondary amenorrhea and is the most common form of pituitary hyperfunction.[14] In addition to pituitary adenomas, the factors leading to increased prolactin release can be classified as follows:

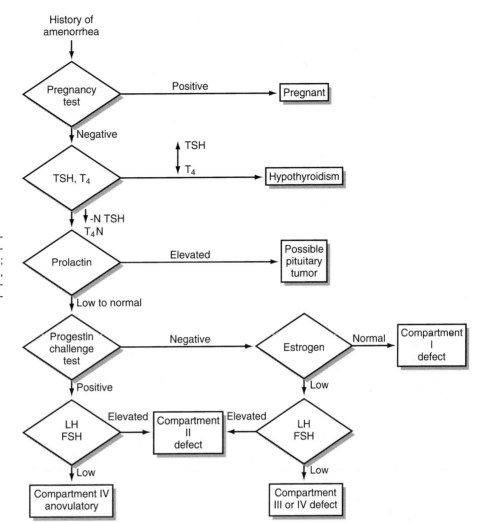

Figure 36–3. Evaluation of amenorrhea. Abbreviations: TSH, thyroid-stimulating hormone; T_4, thyroxine; T_4N, normal serum thyroxine; $-N$, below normal; LH, luteinizing hormone; FSH, follicle-stimulating hormone.

- Stress (trauma, exercise, surgery, psychologic pressures)
- Physiologic factors (breast and nipple stimulation)
- Pharmacologic (oral contraceptives, phenothiazines, tricyclic antidepressants, progestins, TRH)

Secretion of prolactin is pulsatile and variable throughout the day. Prolactin levels in patients with prolactin-secreting tumors vary from 20 ng/mL to greater than 10,000 ng/mL. In one study, all patients with levels in excess of 300 ng/mL had a demonstrable pituitary adenoma.[14] Pharmacologic agents usually do not increase serum prolactin levels above 100 ng/mL.[15] If a single prolactin determination is only slightly elevated (20 to 40 ng/mL), it is suggested that three sequential specimens obtained on different days be evaluated to establish a diagnosis of hyperprolactinemia. A CT scan of the sella turcica is warranted if hyperprolactinemia is found.

Hypothalamic Amenorrhea (Compartment IV)

A patient suffering from hypothalamic amenorrhea usually has a normal CT scan of the brain and normal prolactin levels. Patients may exhibit high growth hormone levels and plasma somatomedin activity, decreased T_4 and triiodothyrone (T_3) increased reverse T_3, and upper normal or elevated cortisol values. With the return of weight and normal hormone levels, menses usually resume also.

Schwartz and Cumming[16] found that LH levels in amenorrheic runners were significantly higher than in their normal counterparts, whereas TSH levels were lower and basal steroids did not differ; however, the ratio of estrone to estradiol was significantly higher in the runners. Increases in prolactin and β-endorphins, known LH and FSH inhibitors, have also been reported.[17]

Treatment

Turner's Syndrome

Treatment of Turner's syndrome is directed toward attempts to augment stature and correct somatic anomalies. Estrogen therapy, in patients older than 15 years, is also initiated to induce secondary sexual characteristics, to permit withdrawal bleeding, and to prevent osteoporosis. This therapy also reduces the risk of endometrial hyperplasia and possible endometrial adenocarcinoma later in life.[18]

Silent Y Syndrome

Therapy for the silent Y syndrome consists of orchidectomy with estrogen replacement therapy, vaginal dilation, and psychologic reinforcement of female gender identity.

Pituitary Disorders

Therapy for pituitary tumors is controversial at present. Neurosurgery (trans-sphenoidal adenectomy) is the preferred treatment for macroadenomas. For the patient with prolactin levels of less than 100 ng/mL and a normal CT scan, either bromocriptine therapy or surveillance can be chosen. If surveillance is chosen, CT scans and prolactin levels should be monitored to detect an emerging tumor.

Hypothalamic Disorders

Medical treatment of the amenorrheic athlete depends on her goals. Estrogen replacement may be recommended for a hypoestrogenic female to avoid osteoporosis. If pregnancy is desired, a reduction in exercise may be all that is necessary for ovulation to return. In severe cases, clomiphene gonadotropin therapy has been indicated.

INFERTILITY

Etiology

Infertility, which occurs in 15% of U.S. couples, is usually defined as 1 year of unprotected coitus without pregnancy. Women account for approximately 50% of fertility problems. Of these, 40% have failure to ovulate, 10% have an inadequate luteal phase, 40% have tubal abnormalities, and 10% have cervical factors or thryoid disease that complicates fertility.

Although a specific cause of ovulation failure is not found in the majority of women, anovulation or oligo-ovulation may result from abnormalities of the hypothalamic-pituitary axis of from ovary, thyroid, or adrenal dysfunctions.

Luteal Phase Disorder

The short or inadequate luteal phase is considered a possible cause of infertility in addition to anovulation discussed elsewhere in this chapter. This abnormality, which affects between 3.5% and 20% of women with infertility, is characterized either by a short interval (less than 11 days) between ovulation and menstruation with a normal progesterone peak, or by a normal-length luteal phase with lower than normal progesterone levels. Both result in inadequate stimulation of the endometrium, resulting in more unexplained short cycles or a history of habitual abortions. Decreased levels of FSH and estradiol during the follicular phase and a lower midcycle FSH peak suggest a subnormal stimulation prior to ovulation. Increased prolactin levels have also been associated with this abnormality.[19]

Clinical Manifestations

Clinical indicators of ovulation include mittelschmerz (abdominal pain midway between menstrual periods), ultrasound detection of preovulatory follicles and corpus luteum, and a serum progesterone level of 3 ng/mL or more.[20] Progesterone at the midluteal phase should be 10 ng/mL or more to indicate sufficient production by the corpus luteum. Biologic effects of progesterone that may be used to evaluate ovulation indirectly include basal body temperature changes, a secretory endometrium, premenstrual molimina, thick cervical mucus, and a change in vaginal cytology.

Laboratory Analyses and Diagnosis

Anovulation

Many of the abnormalities resulting in anovulation are included under the discussions of amenorrhea and hirsutism in this chapter. The history and physical examination of an anovulatory woman should include laboratory quantitation of FSH, LH, prolactin, and progesterone. Thyroid studies and DHAS and testosterone measurements should be performed if symptoms suggest thyroid disease or hyperandrogenism.

Luteal Phase Disorder

The diagnosis of a luteal phase disorder can be approached in a variety of ways. A biphasic basal body temperature chart with a duration of the temperature rise of less than 11 days may indicate a shortened luteal phase. A serum progesterone level of 10 ng/mL or more 5 to 10 days prior to the next menstrual period may rule out an inadequate luteal phase. The diagnosis of a shortened or inadequate luteal phase can be corroborated with an endometrial biopsy. A biopsy, performed 2 to 3 days prior to menstruation, in which the tissue is found to be more than 2 days out of phase is diagnostic of this abnormality. Despite the discomfort and expense involved in this procedure, it remains the classic way to diagnose an inadequate luteal phase.

Treatment

When a specific etiology for infertility can be identified, therapy is directed toward the cause; for example, thyroid replacement therapy for hypothyroidism, or prolactin suppression with bromocriptine. For patients with no known identifiable cause, treatment is tailored to the goals of the woman. Ovulation therapy with clomiphene is warranted for the woman who desires pregnancy. Anovulatory women who do not desire to conceive require treatment with a course of oral progestin to correct cycle irregularities and to protect against abnormal bleeding episodes.

In luteal phase disorder, progesterone vaginal suppositories, hCG injections, and clomiphene, as well as in vitro fertilization (IVF), have been used to lengthen the luteal phase and to achieve pregnancy.

HIRSUTISM

Etiology

Hirsutism is defined as excessive terminal hair in the body skin areas where such growth is considered a male secondary sexual characteristic. The increase in hair growth occurs with increased glandular (ovary and/or adrenal) androgen production (glandular hirsutism—functional or neoplastic) or enhanced sensitivity of the skin to circulating androgens (peripheral/idiopathic hirsutism). More than 90% of all patients who present with hirsutism are diagnosed as having polycystic ovary disease (PCO) or idiopathic hirsutism.

The ovary and adrenal glands account for a large part of androgen production in both normal and hirsute women. Serum levels of testosterone, androstenedione, and DHAS are used as markers of glandular overproduction of androgens and are often elevated in hirsute women.[21] Testosterone is not a specific marker for the ovary but best serves as a guide to abnormal ovarian androgen production. Free testosterone testing does not usually add more information in determinating an abnormal source of androgen production but the level is always increased in hirsute women. It is more difficult to find markers of skin androgen metabolism. The skin sensitivity to androgens is modulated by the 5α-reductase enzyme, which converts testosterone to dihydrotestosterone. Dihydrotestosterone is the hormone most active in increasing hair growth in such areas as the upper lip, chin, chest, and abdomen; however, because of rapid turnover, peripheral dihydrotestosterone is not a good marker of peripheral androgen activity. In fact, before entering the circulation, dihydrotestosterone is rapidly metabolized to other compounds, including androstanediols (3α, 3Ad, and 3β androstanediols), androsterone and their glucuronide and sulfate conjugates.

Polycystic ovary syndrome or disease is associated with anovulation. PCO disease is an endocrine imbalance involving the hypothalmic-pituitary–ovarian adrenal axis and often involves an increased ovarian sensitivity to gonadotropins. In women with persistent anovulation, the average daily production of estrogen and androgens is both increased and dependent on LH stimulation. This is evidenced by increased circulating levels of testosterone, androstenedione, dehydroepiandrosterone, DHAS, 17-hydroxyprogesterone, and estrone. Hirsutism in PCO disease is an expression of androgenicity, secondary both to androgen excess and to greater sensitivity of the pilosebaceous unit to androgen. Clinical symptoms include bilaterally enlarged ovaries with a smooth pearly white capsule, menstrual disturbances, infertility, and virilism.[22] Virilism, which consists of frontal balding, hirsutism, deepening of the voice, acne, and clitoromegaly, is almost always associated with increased testosterone from an ovarian source. Obesity is also commonly seen in affected women. Adrenal activity also plays a role in PCO disease.

Congenital adrenal hyperplasia (CAH) arises through 21-hydroxylase deficiency. It has similarities to PCO disease, in that it causes increased androgen levels, anovulation, and disorders in gonadotropin secretion. It is intermediate to PCO disease in many aspects of hormone secretion.[23] Evaluation of the corticosteroids assists in identification of this cause of hirsutism.

Clinical Manifestations

Most hirsute women present initially to their physician with a cosmetic problem. Common findings are beard growth, sternal and areolar hair growth, irregular menses, and obesity. Patients usually have a normal menarche and only later develop menstrual disorders.

Laboratory Analyses and Diagnosis

Hormonal testing can be very helpful in distinguishing between ovarian and adrenal abnormalities. Serum level measurements of testosterone, prolactin, 17-hydroxyprogesterone, androstenedione, dehydroepiandrosterone, LH, FSH, and thyroid hormones should be performed. An increase in dehydroepiandrosterone is highly suggestive of adrenal dysfunction. In PCO disease, normal or low levels of FSH are seen, whereas levels of LH are elevated, resulting in a LH:FSH ratio greater than 3:1. Serum prolactin levels tend to be slightly elevated. The time of sampling for hormone studies should be recorded because of circadian variations, which influence the interpretation of the values obtained.

Treatment

Hirsutism is treated either by suppression of excess androgen production (oral contraceptives or dexamethasone) or by the use of antiandrogen blocking agents (cyproterone acetate), or by surgical removal of the ovarian or adrenal tumor.

GESTATIONAL TROPHOBLASTIC DISEASE

Etiology

Gestational trophoblastic disease involves a broad spectrum of interrelated neoplasms, including hydatidiform mole, invasive mole, placental site trophoblastic tumor, and choriocarcinoma. Hydatidiform moles are the most common trophoblastic neoplasm, occurring in approximately 1 of every 1500 pregnancies in the United States. Two types of hydatidiform mole have been described, complete or classic, and partial. The complete or classic mole has no evidence of an ascertainable fetus or embryo and is androgenic in origin. Fertilization occurs by a haploid sperm, with duplication of its chromosomes without cell division, resulting in the common karyotype, 46,XX, with about 10% having a 46,XY karyotype. In the partial mole, which occurs approximately 10% of the time, there is a identifiable fetal sac or fetus exhibiting degeneration of chorionic villi and constant trophoblastic immaturity. Partial moles usually have a triploid karyotype (69,XXY) on chromosome analysis. Trophoblastic sequelae or further neoplasms (invasive mole or choriocarcinoma) follow complete hydatidiform mole in 15% to 20% of cases, whereas partial moles have neoplastic sequelae in 4% to 11% of cases.[24] Additionally, there is an increased risk of molar pregnancy for women older than 40 years. In one study, the risk for complete mole was increased twofold for women older than 35 years and 7.5 fold for women older than 40 years.

Clinical Manifestations

Approximately 95% of classic molar pregnancies manifest as vaginal bleeding, usually at 6 to 16 weeks of gestation. Additionally, about 50% of patients have uterine enlargement greater than expected for gestational dates, whereas 25% of patients may present with preeclampsia-eclampsia before 24 weeks. Hyperthyroidism and ovarian cysts (>6 cm in diameter) may also occur in a small number of patients. Partial moles usually manifest as signs and symptoms of a spontaneous or missed abortion. In more than 80% of cases, the first evidence of hydatidiform mole is the passage of vesicular tissue, and the diagnosis of partial mole may be made only after histologic review of curettage specimens.

Laboratory Analyses and Diagnosis

Hydatidiform mole is confirmed by the use of ultrasonography and sequential determinations of hCG serum levels. Trophoblastic disease is distinguished by very high hCG levels, which can be 3 to 100 times higher than normal pregnancy levels, although low or normal levels have been documented. Pelvic ultrasonography, which demonstrates multiple echoes and holes within the placental mass and no fetus, is considered a valuable diagnostic tool for the perioperative diagnosis of hydatiform mole. An immunoassay capable of measuring free β-hCG may also be helpful in detecting and monitoring trophoblastic disease, because production of intact hCG in such tumors is rare.

Treatment

When the diagnosis of hydatidiform mole is established, suction evacuation followed by gentle sharp curettage of the uterus is the treatment of choice. A hysterectomy may be performed in those women who do not desire to preserve fertility. Because trophoblastic cells express RhD factor, patients who are Rh negative should receive Rh-immune globulin at the time of evacuation. Prophylactic chemotherapy with methotrexate has been recommended for patients who have no metastases and are at high risk of developing further neoplastic sequelae. According to the National Cancer Institute, pre-evacuation hCG levels of less than 40,000 mIU/mL are considered indicative of low-risk metastatic trophoblastic disease, whereas hCG levels higher than 40,000 mIU/mL are considered indicative of high-risk metastatic trophoblastic disease.

In monitoring of the patient, weekly serum hCG measurements should be obtained after evacuation and should be continued on a weekly basis until hCG levels are less than 5 mIU/mL. The average time to achieve the first normal hCG level after evacuation is approximately 9 weeks. After hCG levels have returned to the expected range, these levels should be measured on a monthly basis for 6 months. An hCG regression curve should be plotted for each patient and compared with that of a normal molar hCG regression curve (Fig. 36–4).[25] Any patient with a titer plateau (no increase in a 3-week period) or rise (two-fold increase in a 2-week period) should be evaluated for further trophoblastic tumors (invasive or choriocarcinoma).

TROPHOBLASTIC TUMORS

Etiology

Most trophoblastic tumors follow a molar pregnancy; however, they may develop after an ectopic pregnancy, abortion, or normal-term pregnancy. Local invasive tumors, limited to the uterus, develop in 15% of molar pregnancies. Metastatic disease occurs in 3% of patients and is usually associated with choriocarcinoma. Common sites of metastases are the lungs (80%), liver (10%), vagina (30%), and

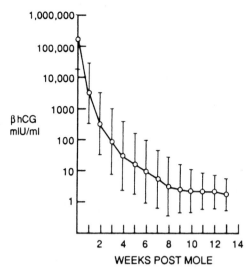

Figure 36–4. The mean value (0) and 95% confidence limits (vertical bars) describing normal postmolar serum βhCG regression curve. (From Schlaerth JB, Morrow CP, Kletzky OA, et al: Prognostic characteristics of serum hCG titer regression following molar pregnancy. Obstet Gynecol 58:478, 1981. Reprinted with permission from the American College of Obstetricians and Gynecologists.)

brain (10%). A four-stage anatomic staging system was adopted by the International Federation of Gynecology and Obstetrics (FIGO) in 1982 and amended in 1992 to aid in the objective classification and treatment of patients with trophoblastic tumors.

Clinical Manifestations

Patients usually present with irregular vaginal bleeding, ovarian cysts, size and date discrepancy, uterine subinvolution, and rising or persistently elevated hCG levels greater than expected.

Laboratory Analyses and Diagnosis

A thorough assessment of the extent of the disease prior to the initiation of treatment is essential. Complete history and physical examination, hCG measurements, complete blood count (CBC), and hepatic, thyroid, and renal function tests should be performed. To further evaluate the possibility of metastatic disease, lung CT scan, ultrasonography of abdomen and pelvis, as well as CT of the head should be performed.

Treatment

Treatment for postmolar trophoblastic tumor depends on the clinical situation, but the overall cure rate for treated patients is 90%. The treatment of choice for women who prefer infertility is a hysterectomy with adjuvant single-agent chemotherapy. Treatment with a single chemotherapy agent, such as actinomycin D or methotrexate, is recommended for patients wishing to preserve fertility, until hCG levels drop below 5 mIU/mL. Higher levels of hCG indicate the need for a more aggressive approach to testing and therapy, with brain and liver scans and a combination of multiple chemotherapeutic agents. Following treatment, hCG determinations should be performed monthly for at least 1 year, then biannually for 5 years. Additional courses of chemotherapy may need to be administered if hCG levels plateau, rise, or do not decline by 1 log within 3 weeks after completion of the first treatment.

Case Study

A 16-year-old girl with a history of diabetes was admitted to the hospital with complaints of weakness and abdominal pain. Owing to the patient's extreme obesity (277 lb), abdominal examination by the physician was difficult. On examination, the physician noted a tall, well-developed, sexually inactive teenager who had been amenorrheic for 8 months. She had slight hirsutism of the face. The rest of the examination was unremarkable.

Results of initial laboratory hormone studies (including reference values) were as follows:

T_4 (μg/dL)	0 (5–12)
TSH (mU/mL)	4.0 (2.0–6.0)
LH (mIU/mL)	36 (2–30)
FSH (mIU/mL)	7 (4–20)
Total testosterone (ng/dL)	114 (0–90)

Questions

1. What condition is most often associated with these clinical findings?
2. What other procedure may be performed to confirm this abnormality?
3. What course of treatment might be prescribed?

Discussion

1. The obesity, amenorrhea, and abnormal androgens along with the 5:1 LH/FSH ratio are most often seen in polycystic ovary disease.
2. In this case, a laparoscopy was performed. Small fallopian tubes with large ovaries of irregular dimensions were noted.
3. Typically, oral contraceptives to suppress TST levels and to induce menses are prescribed. This patient was started on contraceptives, and subsequent clinic visits were scheduled. Her insulin dose was adjusted, and she was instructed to stay on a strict 1800-calorie diet.

References

1. Yen S, Jaffe RB: Reproductive Endocrinology: Physiology, Pathophysiology, and Clinical Management, ed 3. Philadelphia, WB Saunders, 1991.
2. Badawy S: Reproductive Endocrinology and Infertility. Chicago, Year Book Medical, 1980.
3. Midgley AR: Human Reproduction, Hagerstown, Md, Harper & Row, 1973.
4. Speroff L, Glass RH, Kase NG: Clinical Gynecologic Endocrinology and Infertility, ed 5. Baltimore, Williams & Wilkins, 1994.
5. Gold JJ, Josimovich JB: Gynecologic Endocrinology, ed 4. Hagerstown, Md, Harper & Row, 1987.
6. Given JR: Endocrine Causes of Menstrual Disorders. Chicago, Year Book Medical, 1977.
7. Wilson JD, Foster DW (eds): Williams Textbook of Endocrinology, ed 7. Philadelphia, WB Saunders, 1985.
8. Wilson JD, Griffin JE: Disorders of sexual differentiation. *In* Petersdorf RG, Adams RA, Braunwald E, et al (eds): Harrison's Principles of Internal Medicine. New York City, McGraw-Hill, 1983.
9. Schwabe AD, Lippe BM, Chang RJ: Anorexia nervosa. Ann Intern Med 94:371–381, 1981.
10. Beaumont PJ, Abraham SI: Continuous IV fusion of luteinizing-hormone-releasing hormone (LHRH) in patients with anorexia nervosa. Psychol Med 11:477–484, 1981.
11. Bitner MR: Secondary amenorrhea in the female athlete. N Engl J Med 10:363, 1985.
12. Feicht CB, Johnson TS, Martin BJ, et al: Secondary amenorrhea in athletes. Lancet 2:1145, 1978.
13. Kohn G, Yarkon S, Cohen MM: Two conceptions in a 45,X woman. Am J Med Genet 5:339–343, 1980.
14. Quigley MM, Haney AI: Evaluation of hyperprolactinemia clinical profiles. Clin Obstet Gynaecol 23:337–348, 1980.
15. Malo JW, Bezdicek BJ: Secondary amenorrhea: A protocol for pinpointing the underlying cause. Postgrad Med 79:91, 1986.
16. Schwartz B, Cumming DC: Exercise-associated amenorrhea: A distinct entry. Am J Obstet Gynecol 141:662–669, 1981.
17. Colt EW, Wardlaw SJ, Frantz AG: The effect of running on plasma β-endorphin. Life Sci 28:1637–1641, 1981.
18. Gambrell RD Jr: The menopause: Benefits and risks of estrogen-progestogen replacement therapy. Fertil Steril 37:457–474, 1982.
19. Insler V, Lunenfeld B: Infertility: Male and Female. New York, Churchill Livingstone, 1986.
20. Keller DW, Strickler RC, Watten JC: Clinical Infertility. Norwalk, Conn, Appleton-Century-Crofts, 1984.
21. Hare JW: Signs and Symptoms in Endocrine and Metabolic Disorders. Philadelphia, JB Lippincott, 1986.
22. Hatch R, Rosenfield RL, Kim M: Hirsutism: Implications, etiology, and management. Am J Obstet Gynecol 140:815, 1981.
23. Edwards RG, Brody SA: Principles and Practice of Assisted Reproduction Philadelphia, WB Saunders, 1995.
24. Berek JS, Adashi EY, Hillard PA: Novak's Gynecology, ed 12. Baltimore, Williams & Wilkins, 1996.
25. Schlaerth JB, Morrow CP, Kletzky OA, et al: Prognostic characteristics of serum human chorionic gonadotropin titer regression following molar pregnancy. Obstet Gynecol 58:478, 1981.

Bibliography

Balasch J, Fabreques F, Creus M, Vanrell JA: The usefulness of endometrial biopsy for luteal phase evaluation in infertility. Hum Reprod 7:973–977, 1992.
Cooke NE: Prolactin: basic physiology. *In* DeGroot LJ (ed): Endocrinology, ed 3. Philadephia, WB Saunders, 1995.
Jones GS: Luteal phase defects. *In* Behrman SJ, Kistner RW (eds): Progress in Infertility, ed 2. Boston, Little, Brown, & Co, 1975.
Jones GS: The luteal phase defect. Fertil Steril 27:351–356, 1976.
Gordon JD, Rydors JT, Druzin ML, et al: Obstetrics, Gynecology and Infertility, ed 4. Menlo Park, Cal, Scrub Hill Press, 1995.
Nakajima ST, Gibson M: Pathophysiology of luteal-phase deficiency in human reproduction. Clin Obstet Gynecol 34:167–179, 1991.

Chapter 37

Male Reproductive Disorders

Shauna C. Anderson

STRUCTURAL COMPONENTS

The male gonads are the testes. Each of the two that are present in the normal male consists of supporting structures, interstitium, and seminiferous tubules. The seminiferous tubules consist of highly coiled tubes lined by Sertoli's cells and germ cells and are the sites of spermatogenesis. The interstitium encompasses the seminiferous tubules and contains Leydig's cells, which are responsible for production of the androgen hormones.

The testes are held outside the abdominal cavity in a fold of skin known as the *scrotum.* After spermatogenesis in the seminiferous tubules, sperm pass into coiled tubules in the epididymis. The sperm are stored in the epididymis

until final maturation; therefore, the epididymis plays an important role in sperm transport, sperm maturation (including acquisition of motility), sperm concentration, and sperm storage. During ejaculation, the sperm are moved from the epididymis through the vas deferens. The vas deferens consists of two ducts that provide a passageway from the scrotum around and behind the urinary bladder where each duct is joined to a tubule from the seminal vesicle and becomes the ejaculatory duct. The seminal vesicles contribute a thick, clear fluid containing mucus, fructose, and amino acids to the ejaculatory duct. The fluid in the ejaculatory duct is known as *semen.*

The ejaculatory duct continues through the prostate gland. This gland secretes a thin, alkaline, milky fluid containing an enzyme (acid phosphatase), citric acid, calcium, and coagulation proteins. After passage through the prostate gland, the ejaculatory duct connects to the urethra.

A pair of bulbourethral glands located along the urethra anterior to the prostate secrete a clear viscous fluid prior to ejaculation. The urethra passes out of the abdominal cavity and through the penis. The urethra is supplied with mucus derived from a large number of minute glands located along its entire structure. The penis is composed of spongy erectile tissue. The final ejaculate contains sperm cells from the seminiferous tubules as well as the secretions from the seminal vesicles, prostate gland, bulbourethral glands, and urethral glands.

HORMONAL REGULATION

Regulation of male reproductive hormones begins at the hypothalamus, which secretes a hormone known as *gonadotropin-releasing hormone* (GnRH). This decapeptide hormone reaches the anterior pituitary gland via the hypophyseal portal system. At the anterior pituitary gland, GnRH attaches to receptors on the gonadotropic cells and stimulates the production of adenylate cyclase, which in turn increases the level of cyclic adenosine monophosphate (cAMP) in these cells. This signaling component eventually stimulates the production and secretion of luteinizing hormone (LH) and of follicle-stimulating hormone (FSH).

LH and FSH are both glycoproteins. During infancy and childhood, levels of LH and FSH are low and relatively constant, but during puberty the levels increase significantly.

After LH and FSH are secreted from the anterior pituitary gland, they are carried in the blood to the testis, which is their site of action. In the testis, LH binds to receptors on Leydig's cells and activates adenylate cyclase, which in turn increases the level of cAMP. As a result of the increase in cAMP, the cells synthesize pregnenolone, which is subsequently converted to testosterone. Leydig's cells are responsible for the production of most of the androgen hormones including testosterone, which is either secreted directly into the blood or delivered to the seminiferous tubules. Approximately 97% of the testosterone that is secreted into the blood is bound to plasma proteins. Most of the testosterone is carried in the plasma by sex hormone–binding globulin (SHBG), also known as testosterone-binding globulin (TeBG). The remaining 3% of the testosterone circulates as a free hormone and is capable of entering the target cells, which are capable of forming dihydrotestosterone. Testosterone is responsible for growth of the external genitalia at puberty, lowering of the voice, and the masculine pattern of skeletal muscle development. However, dihydrotestosterone, or its metabolite, is responsible for the growth and maturation of the seminal vesicles and the prostate gland as well as the development of characteristics described as secondary male sex traits, such as occurrence of acne, development of body and facial hair, and recession of scalp hairline.[1]

Testosterone delivered to the seminiferous tubules stimulates Sertoli's cells and, eventually, spermatogenesis. The interaction of Sertoli's cells with FSH and testosterone stimulates these cells to produce androgen-binding protein (ABP). This protein is responsible for the transport of testosterone into the Sertoli cell and to the epididymis. Testosterone or its metabolites also completes the feedback control of the release of GnRH from the hypothalamus and the release of LH from the anterior pituitary gland.

FSH released from the anterior pituitary gland activates adenylate cyclase in Sertoli's cells. As a result, testosterone in these cells is converted to estradiol. This action produced by FSH occurs during puberty when the initial wave of spermatogenesis takes place. Continued action of FSH does not appear to be necessary for maintenance of the process.

Inhibin, a peptide synthesized by Sertoli's cells, appears to be the regulator of the negative feedback mechanism for FSH. It inhibits the release of GnRH from the hypothalamus and the release of FSH from the anterior pituitary gland. Figure 37–1 summarizes the regulation of the male reproductive hormones.

ETIOLOGY AND PATHOLOGY

Hypogonadism or Infertility

The testes serve two primary functions: (1) production of sperm by germ cells within the seminiferous tubules and (2) synthesis and secretion of testosterone by Leydig's cells. Male hypogonadism or infertility can be classified as *pretesticular, testicular,* or *posttesticular.*[2] Pretesticular infertility is usually associated with hypothalamic or pituitary lesions. These conditions are also referred to as *secondary causes of hypogonadism.*

Congenital gonadotropin deficiency is more commonly of hypothalamic origin than of pituitary origin. Disorders of the hypothalamus may result in simple delayed puberty or idiopathic hypogonadotropic hypogonadism (IHH). With

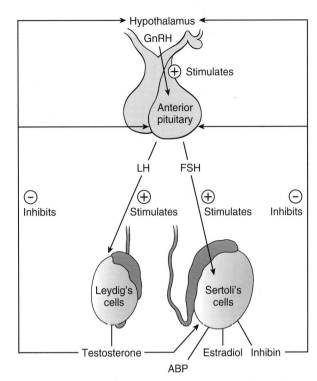

Figure 37–1. Male reproductive hormone regulation. Abbreviations: GnRH, gonadotropin-releasing hormone; LH, luteinizing hormone; FSH, follicle-stimulating hormone; ABP, androgen-binding protein.

a condition of simple delayed puberty, boys are normal upon physical examination except for their immature appearance and prepubertal genitalia.[3] If there is a family history of pubertal delay, the diagnosis is familial delay.

Patients with IHH fail to initiate or complete puberty because of abnormalities in GnRH secretion. Boys with this condition continue to grow physically but do not have a normal pubertal growth spurt or normal sexual maturation. Other abnormalities may accompany IHH, such as very small testes without signs of puberty. Some patients also have a decreased or absent sense of smell and are diagnosed as having Kallmann's syndrome.[4] Kallmann's syndrome is an X-linked disorder that leads to a deficiency in the secretion of GnRH.

Acquired gonadotropin deficiency is more often of pituitary than of hypothalamic origin. The absence of puberty due to pituitary disease is frequently caused by a tumor. Delayed skeletal growth and visual defects often accompany the pubertal delay. Pituitary disease after puberty can also result in a gonadotropin deficiency. Erectile dysfunction or impotence may be an early manifestation of pituitary insufficiency, even though growth hormone may also be decreased. Prolactin (PRL)-secreting pituitary tumors can also produce symptoms of both erectile dysfunction and infertility. Increased PRL levels act by suppressing the production of GnRH. Other causes of pretesticular hypogonadism may be due to hypothyroidism, Cushing's syndrome, or alcoholic cirrhosis.

Testicular causes of infertility or hypogonadism may be either congenital or acquired. Testicular causes of hypogonadism are referred to as *primary hypogonadism.* Congenital causes include Klinefelter's syndrome, cryptorchidism, Sertoli cell–only syndrome, and idiopathic hypospermatogenesis.

Klinefelter's syndrome is caused by a chromosomal defect when an extra X chromosome results in an XXY chromosomal pattern. In this disease, the testicular tubules remain small and collapsed or show hyalinization with only minimal spermatogenesis. *Cryptorchidism,* failure of the testes to descend, is found in approximately 3% of newborn males and 0.8% of infants by the time they reach 1 year of age.[5] Sertoli cell–only syndrome is also known as *germ cell aplasia* and is a disorder in which the seminiferous tubules contain only Sertoli's cells. These patients usually have smaller than normal testes but have a normal karyotype, and a testicular biopsy reveals the absence of germ cells. The condition is caused by a defect in the long arm of the Y chromosome.[3] The most common defect in testicular function is *idiopathic hypospermatogenesis.* This is a quantitative abnormality and is not confined to a particular stage of spermatogenesis.

The most common acquired disorder of testicular failure is *orchitis,* which may be caused by the mumps virus. Mumps that occurs after puberty produces bilateral orchitis in about 10% of male patients.[3] In one half of those patients, testicular atrophy and infertility develop.

Trauma is the second most frequently occurring cause of acquired testicular failure and may result from physical damage to the testis. Radiation in very small amounts may also cause testicular damage. Long-term effects increase as the amount of radiation exposure increases.[6]

Cyclophosphamide, an antineoplastic agent, is an increasingly important cause of testicular insufficiency. The germ cells of the testes are selectively damaged by the drug. If administration of the drug occurs for a period of less than 18 months, the damage is gradually reversible. If the administration is longer, recovery is slow and often incomplete. Other neoplastic drugs are also known to damage testicular tubules.[3]

Posttesticular causes of infertility are usually due to functional impairment or mechanical obstruction of sperm transport or to disorders of sperm function. Possible causes include scarring and occlusion of the epididymis due to epididymitis in which blockage of the epididymis occurs, which may be due to in utero exposure to diethylstilbestrol (DES), cystic fibrosis, idiopathic vasal agenesis, or ejaculatory dysfunction.

Erectile Dysfunction

Erectile dysfunction (impotence) is a common cause of male reproductive failure. This is a complex syndrome that may involve arterial, venous, sinusoidal, neurologic, hormonal, biochemical, social, or psychological factors. It is defined as the inability to achieve an erection long enough to complete satisfactory intercourse.[7] It usually consists of partial erectile dysfunction rather than complete lack of penile rigidity. Loss of erection before ejaculation is the most common complaint and may be the only presenting complaint, or it may accompany other erectile dysfunction.

Erectile dysfunction can be classified on either a physiologic or a functional basis.[8] Neurogenic dysfunction involves a failure to initiate erection because of the absence of autonomic pelvic nerve stimulation and corporal nerve release of endogenous neurotransmitter substances. Neurogenic dysfunction may be caused by diabetes, spinal cord disorders, cauda equina lesions, polyneuropathy, myelopathy, multiple sclerosis, dorsal nerve dysfunction, and radial pelvic surgery.[9] Certain medications, anxiety, or alcohol may also be the etiology of this dysfunction. Medications that affect either the central nervous system or the adrenalin surge of anxiety can cause the penile vasculature sacs to collapse, with a decreased blood flow and resultant flaccidity. Such drugs as the older antihypertensive agents, β-blockers, thiazide diuretics, methyldopa, cimetidine, and some lipid-lowering drugs are examples. Ingestion of alcohol may also reduce sexual functioning. The intrapenile nerve conduction mechanisms may be damaged, and with long-term alcoholism or cirrhosis, testicular atrophy and gynecomastia may occur.

The second classification is based on vascular disorders. The main vascular causes of erectile dysfunction are atherosclerosis, Leriche's syndrome, other vascular obstructions, microangiopathy, pelvic steal syndrome, anginal syndromes, congestive heart failure, priapism, aging, and excessive venous outflow. Vasculogenic dysfunction may be arteriogenic, venogenic, or a mixture of these. With arteriogenic dysfunction, the corpora cavernosa fail to fill because of hypogastric-cavernous arterial bed restriction of corporal arterial inflow and blood pressure. Many patients have hypertension, diabetes, elevated serum cholesterol levels, angina, or a history of cigarette smoking. With venogenic dysfunction, the corpora cavernosa fail to store blood because of excessive corporal venous outflow. This may be due to trauma, aging, or inadequate production of cavernous neurotransmitters.[9]

Prostatitis

Prostatitis can refer to a variety of conditions, including acute bacterial prostatitis, chronic bacterial prostatitis, nonbacterial prostatitis, and prostatodynia.[10] Acute bacterial prostatitis is the least common of the types. This condition results in an abrupt onset of fever accompanied by urinary tract infection; obstructive and irritative voiding symptoms; low back or perineal pain; and, often, malaise, arthralgia, and myalgia. These patients are usually younger men and the causative organism is often a gram-negative bacillus.[11]

Chronic bacterial prostatitis typically occurs in older patients who have recurrent urinary tract infections, usually caused by gram-negative organisms. Many of these patients have been found to have stones in the prostate. In some patients, the presence of stones may sequester the causative bacteria, leading to chronic refractive infection.

The most common type of prostatitis is nonbacterial.[12] Microscopic examination of expressed prostatic secretions reveals 10 to 15 white blood cells per high-power field, but no apparent evidence of any infecting organism is found. Several organisms have been suspected of causing this condition including *Chlamydia trachomatis, Ureaplasma urealyticum,* and *Trichomonas vaginalis.*

Prostatodynia is actually a symptom complex with an unknown etiology. Typically the patients are between the ages of 22 and 56 years.[13]

Neoplasms

Testicular cancer accounts for approximately 1% of malignant tumors of internal organs of males.[14] The peak incidence of these tumors is in men age 30 to 40 years. Cryptorchidism is the only known risk factor for testicular cancer. Testicular cancer occurs 10 times more often in testes that have failed to descend into the scrotum during development than in normal testes. It is not known whether the cancer develops because the testes were in an abnormal position or because they did not descend into an abnormal scrotum. More than 95% of testicular tumors originate from germ cells inside the seminiferous tubules,[15] and these tumors are usually malignant. Germ cell tumors can be subdivided according to their pathologic characteristics into seminomas and nonseminomas.[16] A uniform population of cells with clear cytoplasm along with the presence of a fibrous stroma, lymphocytic infiltration, and granulomatous reactions are characteristic of seminomas. About 5% to 7% of the seminomas contain syncytiotrophoblastic giant cells, which elaborate human chorionic gonadotropin (hCG). The most common nonseminomas are embryonal cell cancer, teratoma, and choriocarcinoma.

In addition to germ cell tumors, the testis may give rise to tumors derived from supporting intratubular Sertoli's cells or from the hormone-secreting Leydig's cells. Such tumors are generally benign.

Carcinoma of the prostate gland is diagnosed in approximately 200,000 men each year in the United States.[17] Most of the prostatic neoplasms are adenocarcinomas.[18] The nuclear morphology, cellular size, and glandular differentiation are used in assigning the histologic grade of the carcinoma and thus the prognosis. The aging American male population may be one reason for the increasing number of new cases each year. In addition, the discovery of prostate-specific antigen (PSA) as a tumor marker has led to screening programs resulting in earlier and, possibly, more frequent diagnosis.

CLINICAL MANIFESTATIONS
Hypogonadism or Infertility

Hypogonadism is usually diagnosed secondary to some other clinical complaint of the patient. Physical examination reveals the following possible manifestations of hypogonadism: (1) abnormal facial and body hair distribution, (2) decreased muscle mass with abnormal distribution, (3) abnormal fat distribution, (4) an increased ratio of arm span over height or a decreased upper body–to–lower body ratio, (5) decreased testicular size, (6) decreased or absent sense of smell, and (7) gynecomastia. A history should include questions about age of puberty and physical development, changes in libido, erectile dysfunction, infertility, and marital difficulties related to sexual dysfunction.

Kallmann's syndrome is characterized by absent or decreased sense of smell, color blindness, renal agenesis, neurosensory deafness, cleft lip and palate, decreased or absent male secondary sex characteristics, and small testes.[19] In hypogonadism due to hyperprolactinemia, patients may present with galactorrhea, erectile dysfunction, and decreased libido.[20] Typical clinical symptoms found in Klinefelter's syndrome after puberty include eunuchoid appearance, small firm testes, gynecomastia, azoospermia, and, sometimes, mental retardation.[21]

Erectile Dysfunction

The inability to achieve or maintain an erection is a symptom found in from 10 to 20 million American men.[9] Erectile dysfunction may result from testosterone deficiency from pituitary or testicular disease, estrogen excess, or hyperprolactinemia. The increase in PRL exerts an antigonadotropic effect that is manifest by erectile dysfunction. Hyperthyroidism, hypothyroidism, or Cushing's syndrome can each cause reversible erectile dysfunction.

Prostatitis

Acute bacterial prostatitis is manifest by fever, low back or perineal pain, malaise, arthralgia, and myalgia. Prostatic edema may result in acute urinary retention. Chronic prostatitis may have less dramatic, subtle, or even absent symptoms.

Nonbacterial prostatitis may produce such symptoms as perineal, suprapubic, or low back pain and irritative or obstructive urinary tract manifestations without urinary tract infection. This type of prostatitis is usually self-limiting and is not life-threatening urinary tract disease.

The symptoms of prostatodynia are similar to those of prostatitis. Pain in the perineum, pelvis, or low back or other symptoms suggest prostatitis, but there is no inflammation in the prostate gland and no infection of the urinary tract. Obstructive voiding symptoms are frequent.

Neoplasms

The presenting symptoms are varied in testicular cancer. Many patients present with a painless nodule in one or both testes. Few patients actually have swollen or painful testicles, dysuria, or other urologic complaints. Other unusual symptoms include weight loss, feminization, gynecomastia, and decreased libido.

In many instances, no symptoms are observed with prostate cancer. If a rectal examination detects a discrete nodule or diffuse induration, the physician may suspect the presence of prostate cancer. Some patients present with urinary obstruction problems or erectile dysfunction, and subsequent rectal examination may lead to the diagnosis of prostate cancer.

LABORATORY ANALYSES AND DIAGNOSIS
Hypogonadism

The diagnosis of hypogonadism can be supported by the proper selection of laboratory tests. The most important of these are measurements of serum testosterone, LH, FSH, PRL, and SHBG. Secretion of testosterone by the testes is episodic; a pattern of maximal secretion in the early morning and minimal secretion about 13 hours later has been demonstrated.[22] It is recommended that several blood specimens be collected approximately 30 minutes apart and pooled to obtain a more accurate testosterone measurement. Measurement of testosterone is best done by radioimmunoassay (RIA). To further aid the diagnosis and classify the hypogonadism, measurement of LH, FSH, and PRL should be performed on the same samples. Assays for LH and FSH present particular problems because they circulate in different forms. The immunoassay procedures use antisera directed at specific epitopes and thus measure different populations of analytes. The two-site immunometric assays (IMAs) are more specific because they use monoclonal antibodies, but IMAs may not be an advantage if the molecular species of the circulating hormone is not detected.[23]

If the serum testosterone levels are decreased and the LH and FSH levels are increased, the condition is primary hypogonadism. If the serum testosterone level is decreased and the LH and FSH levels are also decreased, the condition is secondary hypogonadism. Pituitary disease can be distinguished from hypothalamic disease through the use of dynamic function tests.[23] The GnRH stimulation test assesses the pituitary reserve of the gonadotropins. The clomiphene test is used to assess the integrity of the whole hypothalamic-pituitary axis. Clomiphene, an anti-estrogen, is given orally for 10 days and the LH and FSH levels are measured on days 0, 3, 7, and 10. If the LH and FSH levels increase after GnRH but not after clomiphene, the disorder is hypothalamic rather than pituitary. Figure 37–2 summarizes the laboratory diagnosis of hypogonadism.

Delayed Puberty

Primary gonadal disorders can be determined with the LH and FSH levels. In such cases, both values would be elevated. An abnormal karyotype with a male phenotype points to Klinefelter's syndrome. The laboratory evaluation of a patient suspected of having Klinefelter's syndrome is confirmed by a chromatin-positive buccal smear and a semen analysis that reveals a lack of spermatozoa.

Thyroid-stimulating hormone (TSH) levels should be measured to rule out hypothyroidism, and PRL levels determined to rule out hyperprolactinemia. The TSH level is elevated in primary hypothyroidism and the PRL levels are elevated in hyperprolactinemia. Both conditions delay puberty.

In cases of simple delayed puberty, idiopathic delay, hypothalamic GnRH deficiency, or pituitary disease, the LH, FSH, and testosterone levels are low. Patients with IHH fail to initiate or complete puberty because of abnormalities in GnRH. If the GnRH deficiency is accompanied by anosmia (decreased sense of smell) or color blindness, the deficiency may be due to Kallmann's syndrome. The GnRH stimulation test assesses pituitary reserve of gonadotropins by determining the LH and FSH response after the intravenous injection of GnRH. Intracranial space-occupying lesions may be suspected in the presence of other clinical symptoms and require radiologic assessment. Figure 37–3 summarizes the laboratory diagnosis of delayed puberty.

Infertility

In general, the only physical symptom of infertility is the inability to achieve a pregnancy. The patient may have a history of cryptorchidism, scrotal swelling, or genitourinary tract infection. Semen analysis remains the most valuable investigative step in the evaluation of male infertility. At least three specimens after a fixed period of abstinence are required. Care should be taken when instructing the patient to collect a complete specimen by masturbation into a sterile container. The semen analysis should include a check for coagulation liquefaction within 30 minutes, semen fructose, and viscosity. The volume of the ejaculate should be measured, and the sperm count, motility, and viability evaluated by microscopy. Sperm morphology should also be evaluated. Special tests such as antisperm antibody, cervical mucus interaction, and sperm penetration tests are usually not available at all facilities, but reference laboratories are available to do them. They should be used only after other investigations are complete.

Laboratory results of the semen analysis should direct the clinician to the proper diagnosis (Fig. 37–4). Normal semen should coagulate immediately. If it does not, then a fructose test should be done. Fructose is absent when the ejaculatory ducts or seminal vesicles are absent or obstructed. Liquefaction usually occurs within 30 minutes after collection of the ejaculate due to the presence of a prostatic enzyme. A prostatic enzyme deficiency may be suspected if it does not liquefy. Viscosity should be noted because an increase may affect fertility by trapping sperm, especially if both sperm count and motility are low. Liquefaction and viscosity problems may be seen with inflammation of the accessory glands.

Normal volume for a semen specimen is 1.5 to 5 mL. High volume may dilute the sperm and decrease motility, although very low semen volumes are seen with anatomic or functional obstruction and prostatovesiculitis.

The median sperm count of fertile patients is about 60 million sperm per milliliter of semen. Less than 20 million sperm per milliliter of semen is considered subfertile. Absence of any sperm (azoospermia) may be caused by bilateral ductal obstruction, retrograde ejaculation, or congenital absence of vas deferens or seminal vesicles. A negative fructose test and a vasogram, which gives a radiologic

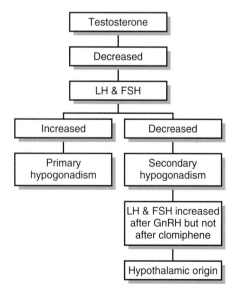

Figure 37–2. Hypogonadism panel. Abbreviations: LH, luteinizing hormone; FSH, follicle-stimulating hormone; GnRH, gonadotropin-releasing hormone.

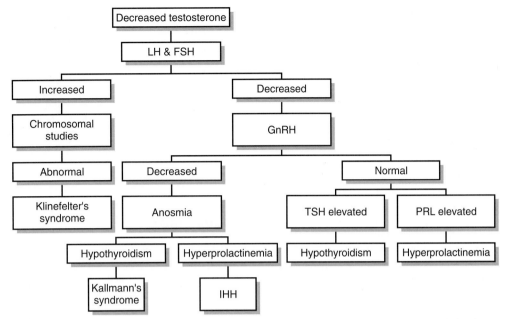

Figure 37–3. Delayed puberty panel. Abbreviations: LH, luteinizing hormone; FSH, follicle-stimulating hormone; GnRH, gonadotropin-releasing hormone; TSH, thyroid-stimulating hormone; PRL, prolactin; IHH, idiopathic hypogonadotropic hypogonadism.

picture of the vas deferens and seminal vesicles, will aid in the diagnosis. If the fructose test is positive, serum FSH should be measured. If it is elevated to twice the normal level, the patient should be evaluated for hypogonadism. If a normal FSH level is found, a testicular biopsy should be performed.

Sperm motility should be studied on all sperm counts. At least 60% of the sperm should exhibit good motility, and sperm motion should be forward and progressive. If motility is low, then endocrine dysfunction, antisperm antibody reactions, and varicocele should be considered. Via-

bility of the sperm should be more than 65% to be normal. Less than 40% viability is abnormal and may suggest poor collection of specimens or an antisperm antibody reaction. In evaluation of morphology, 60% of the sperm should appear normal. If morphology is abnormal, the patient should be further evaluated for a varicocele. Sperm autoagglutination or persistent, unexplained problems of motility may indicate a sperm antibody problem. The presence of leukocytes may indicate an infection or autoimmunity.

Normal sperm morphology in patients with a low or normal sperm count indicates that further test of sperm

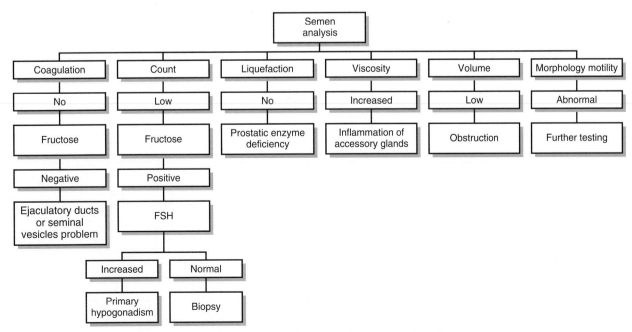

Figure 37–4. Infertility panel. Abbreviation: FSH, follicle-stimulating hormone.

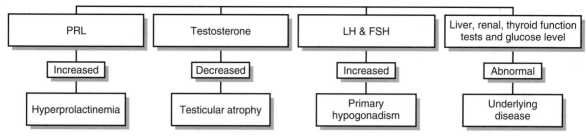

Figure 37–5. Erectile dysfunction panel. Abbreviations: PRL, prolactin; LH, luteinizing hormone; FSH, follicle-stimulating hormone.

function is necessary. A cervical mucus interaction study measures the ability of the sperm to travel through cervical mucus to the site of fertilization. Results have been shown to correlate with fertility. Sperm penetration tests assess ability of the sperm to undergo physiologic changes that make penetration of the oocyte possible.

Testis biopsy is indicated in patients with azoospermia or severe oligospermia, relatively normal-sized testes, and normal level of FSH. This helps differentiate obstruction from deficient spermatogenesis.

Erectile Dysfunction

General laboratory testing for liver, renal, and thyroid disease, in addition to fasting glucose studies, should be performed, because a large number of diseases are known to be associated with erectile dysfunction. A serum PRL level will rule out hyperprolactinemia due to pituitary adenomas, hypothalamic tumors, and dysfunction as a result of use of certain drugs. If free testosterone levels are low, testicular atrophy should be suspected. The LH and FSH levels can be measured to confirm or eliminate a diagnosis of primary gonadal failure (see Fig. 37–5).

Prostatitis

The diagnosis of acute prostatitis is generally straightforward. Examination of a urine specimen revealing white blood cells (pyuria) is indicative of a urinary tract infection rather than inflammation. Follow-up urine cultures usually produce a gram-negative organism such as *Escherichia coli*.

To confirm chronic prostatitis, a massage can be done to express the prostatic secretions onto a slide. If 10 to 15 white blood cells are seen, chronic infection is indicated, and follow-up culture usually produces a gram-negative organism.

In nonbacterial prostatitis, cultures yield no infecting organisms within the prostate fluid when cultured on media traditional for urinary tract infections; however, 10 to 15 white blood cells are seen when a prostatic massage sample is examined. Figure 37–6 summarizes the laboratory diagnosis of prostatitis.

If the condition prostatodynia is suspected, no inflammation and no urinary tract infection are involved. Cystoscopic examination of the bladder neck and prostatic urethra or urodynamic testing performed by a urologist may be necessary to detect the nature of the problem.

Neoplasms

If testicular cancer is suspected from physical examination or ultrasonography, tumor markers should be assessed (Fig. 37–7). Germinal cancers of the testis often secrete α-fetoprotein (AFP) and hCG, and these tumor markers may be detected in the peripheral blood. If AFP is elevated, the presence of nonseminomatous elements are indicated because pure seminomas do not elaborate this marker. If hCG is elevated, choriocarcinomas or embryonal cell components should be suspected. Only rarely is hCG elaborated from pure seminomas. Histologic examination of the orchiectomy specimen is needed to identify seminomas and nonseminomatous elements.

Screening for PSA has changed the way that prostatic cancer is diagnosed. The interpretation of results can be problematic, however, because of biologic variability of this analyte in serum and variability in assays among manufacturers. If the PSA levels are elevated, follow-up digital rectal examination and transrectal ultrasonography (TRUS)

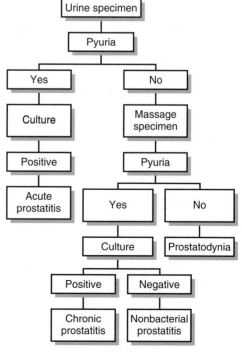

Figure 37–6. Prostatitis panel.

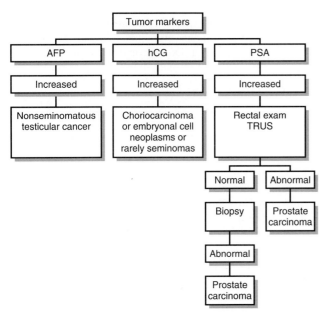

Figure 37–7. Neoplasm panel. Abbreviations; AFP, α-fetoprotein; hCG, human chorionic gonadotropin; PSA, prostate-specific antigen; TRUS, transrectal ultrasonography.

evaluations are performed. If these evaluations are normal, a biopsy of the prostate gland may then be performed to demonstrate the presence of the cancer.

Histologic examination of transurethral, transrectal, or transperineal biopsy specimens of the prostate are needed to confirm the diagnosis. Subsequent laboratory evaluations, including complete blood cell count (CBC), lactate dehydrogenase (LD) and alkaline phosphatase (ALP) measurements, and hepatic and renal function studies may be performed to determine whether the lesion is confined to the prostate gland or has spread to other areas.

TREATMENT

Hypogonadism

The treatment of hypogonadism depends on the etiology. Treatment for pituitary tumors (secondary hypogonadism) includes surgery, radiation, and medication, usually bromocriptine. Effectiveness of these treatments is closely related to the size and prolactin-secreting ability of the tumor.[24] Drug-related hyperprolactinemia may be helped by withdrawal from medication. Testosterone or gonadotropin replacement is then initiated.

The treatment for Kallmann's syndrome includes androgen therapy with testosterone esters. The aim of androgen therapy is to restore to normal such male secondary sex characteristics as beard, body hair, and external genitalia. Therapy also increases muscle mass, hemoglobin, nitrogen balance, and closure of the epiphysis. When therapy is initiated at the expected age of puberty, the normal events of male puberty take place. If therapy is delayed until later in life, results are more variable. As secondary male sex characteristics appear, serum testosterone, LH, and FSH should rise to normal adult levels.

Treatment for Klinefelter's syndrome is also best accomplished by testosterone replacement with testosterone esters. The testosterone levels rise slowly, and the LH and FSH levels decrease. Androgen therapy usually does not restore spermatogenesis in these patients.

Treatment for IHH is the pulsatile administration of synthetic GnRH. These patients can undergo normal puberty, including spermatogenesis.[25]

Infertility

Treatment for infertility is as varied as the causes of the infertility. The clinician generally looks for and treats the most obvious symptoms first, such as drug and alcohol abuse, infection, exposure to toxins, and other disease processes that may cause infertility. If endocrine dysfunctions such as hyperprolactinemia, panhypopituitarism, or primary gonadal abnormalities are suspected, several options are available for treatment, depending on the diagnosis. Androgen therapy, gonadotropin therapy, and drug therapy have been reported to restore fertility. A varicocele is the most common surgically correctable abnormality seen in infertile men. Ductal obstruction can be corrected surgically but is difficult.

Erectile Dysfunction

Treatment for erectile dysfunction is complex. In general, the clinician looks for and treats underlying disease first and then progresses to treatment for specific dysfunctions. If no specific diagnosis is made, an injection of papaverine alone or in combination with phentolamine is one of several options available as treatment.

Recently, the compound Viagra has been introduced and has been widely reported as successful in treating this condition. Serious side effects have been reported for individuals with coronary heart disease, particularly if on a regimen of nitrates. Studies continue with respect to side effects and contraindications of Viagra. Efforts are being made to develop other medications that can achieve the same effects on erectile dysfunction but without cardiac risks.

Prostatitis

Treatment of acute prostatitis is immediate empirical use of antibiotics such as trimethoprim-sulfamethoxazole (Bactrim or Septra). In more severe cases, intravenous aminoglycoside and ampicillin sodium, ofloxacin, or ciprofloxacin is indicated.

Although chronic bacterial prostatitis is also treated with antibiotics, a long-term dosage is usually necessary. If prostatic calculi are present, it may be necessary to perform a transurethral resection to remove the calculi.[26]

Patients with nonbacterial prostatitis commonly receive a 2- to 4-week trial of antibiotics such as minocycline, doxycycline, or erythromycin. In addition, nonsteroidal anti-inflammatory agents; sitz baths; normal sexual activity; and avoidance of spicy food, caffeine, and alcohol may be beneficial.

The cause of prostatodynia dictates the treatment. Symptomatic management may include the same regimen as for patients with nonbacterial prostatitis.

Neoplasms

The treatment of testicular cancer is based on whether the cancer is localized or has disseminated and the pathologic examination, which indicates pure seminoma or the presence of nonseminoma. Depending on the staging and tumor classification, orchiectomy followed by surveillance or orchiectomy followed by radiotherapy and combination chemotherapy are options.

The choice of treatment of prostate cancer depends largely on the stage of the disease. If the disease is localized, radical prostatectomy or definitive radiation therapy is used. If the disease has disseminated, the treatment depends on the staging of the disease but may include hormonal ablative therapy and orchiectomy.

Case Study 1

A 32-year-old man and his wife were seen at an infertility clinic. They had been having regular intercourse for 2 years without a resulting pregnancy. Findings of the tests of the wife were unremarkable.

Physical examination of the husband showed slightly decreased testicular size, normal muscle mass and distribution, normal male hair amount and distribution, and absence of gynecomastia. Semen analysis showed normal coagulation liquefaction, viscosity, and volume. No sperm were seen with microscopic examination. The fructose test was positive.

Other laboratory tests revealed normal liver, renal, and thyroid results. The testosterone level was low, with increased levels of LH and FSH. Because an acquired disorder was suspected, the patient was questioned about childhood disease, use of drugs, and other environmental factors that had affected him. He reported having "mumps" at age 21 years. Diagnosis was infertility due to orchitis.

Questions

1. Which result(s) in semen analysis indicated the need for endocrine evaluation?
2. Why were liver, renal, and thyroid function tests ordered?
3. Which laboratory test(s) helped pinpoint or support the diagnosis?

Discussion

1. The fact that the semen analysis was essentially normal, except for the absence of sperm, indicated that the problem may be a seminiferous tubule problem. Because testosterone is required for spermatogenesis in the seminiferous tubules, evaluation of testosterone and its feedback mechanism should have been the next step in the investigation.
2. Renal, hepatic, and thyroid function tests were ordered to rule out the presence of drug consumption, infection, tumors, and thyroid disease that may result in infertility.

3. The high concentration of LH and FSH ruled out the hypothalamic-pituitary problems. The low testosterone concentration ruled out androgen insensitivity problems. The presence of normal male secondary sex characteristics and history of mumps ruled out probable abnormal karyotype and pointed to orchitis.

Case Study 2

A 15-year-old male presented with obesity and no signs of puberty. The physician noted gynecomastia, small firm atrophic testes, and a disproportionate growth pattern.

The testosterone level was decreased and the LH and FSH levels were slightly increased.

Questions

1. What is the most likely chromosomal pattern in this patient?
2. What would be expected if a semen analysis were performed?
3. Is the hypogonadism primary or secondary?
4. What is the name of the syndrome described?
5. How could this disorder be differentiated from Kallmann's syndrome?

Discussion

1. The most likely pattern is 47 XXY.
2. Azoospermia is expected if a semen analysis is performed.
3. The hypogonadism is primary.
4. Klinefelter's syndrome is the name used to describe the syndrome.
5. In Kallmann's syndrome one would expect to see a history of anosmia and a normal chromosome pattern.

References

1. Fregly MJ, Luttage WG: Human Endocrinology: An interactive text, New York, Elsevier Science Publishing, 1982.
2. Wheatly JK: Evaluating male infertility. Hosp Pract 24:154–179, 1983.
3. Federman DD: The testis. *In* Rubenstein E, Federman DD (eds): Scientific American Medicine 3(II). New York, Scientific American Inc, 1995, pp 1–16.
4. Christensen RB, Matsumoto AM, Bremner WJ: Idiopathic hypogonadotropic hypogonadism with anosmia (Kallmann's syndrome). Endocrinology 2:332, 1992.
5. Oates RD: Male infertility: Acute or potential. Hosp Pract Sep:20–31, 1989.
6. Griffin JE, Wilson JD: Disorders of the testes and male reproductive tract. *In* Wilson JD, Foster DW (eds): Williams Textbook of Endocrinology, ed 7. Philadelphia, WB Saunders, 1985.
7. Guay AT: Erectile dysfunction. Postgrad Med 97:127–143, 1995.
8. Goldstein I: Vasculogen impotence. Probl Urol 1:547–563, 1989.
9. Whitehead ED, Lyde BJ, Zussman S, et al: Diagnostic evaluation of impotence. Postgrad Med 88:123–136, 1990.

10. Meares EM, Stamey TA: Bacteriologic localization pattern in bacterial prostatitis and urethritis. Invest Urol 5:492–518, 1968.

11. Childs SJ: Treatment of chronic bacterial prostatitis with ciprofloxacin. Infect Surg Nov:649–651, 1987.

12. Crawford ED, Davis MA: Categorizing and treating prostatitis. Infect Surg Oct:593–598, 1987.

13. Moul JW: Prostatitis: Sorting out the different causes. Postgrad Med 94:191–194, 1993.

14. Damjanov I: Testicular cancer. Sci Med Jan/Feb:48–57, 1995.

15. Garnick MB: Bladder, renal and testicular cancer: *In* Rubenstein E, Federman DD (eds): Scientific American Medicine 12(IXB). New York, Scientific American, Inc, 1995, pp 1–12.

16. Mostofi FK: Testicular tumors: Epidemiologic, etiologic, and pathologic features. Cancer 32:1186, 1973.

17. Garnick MB: Prostate cancer. *In* Rubenstein E, Federman DD (eds): Scientific American Medicine 12(IXA). New York, Scientific American, Inc, 1995, pp 1–11.

18. Benson MC: Prostate cancer: Current concepts and controversies. Semin Urol 1:323–330, 1983.

19. Lieblich JM, Rogol AD, White BJ, et al: Syndrome of anosmia with hypogonadotropic hypogonadism (Kallmann's syndrome). Am J Med 73:506, 1982.

20. Carter JN, Tyson JE, Tolis G, et al: Prolactin-secreting tumors and hypogonadism in 22 men. N Engl J Med 299:847, 1978.

21. Odell WD, Larson JL: Reproduction: The New Frontier in Occupational and Environmental Health Research. New York, Alan R Liss, 1984.

22. Kicklighter EJ, Kulkarni B: The gonads. *In* Kaplan LA, Pesce AJ (eds): Clinical Chemistry: Theory, Analysis, and Correlation. St. Louis, CV Mosby, 1984.

23. Jeffcoate W: Endocrine investigation of gonadal dysfunction. J Int Fed Clin Chem 6:177–180, 1994.

24. Wollesen F, Bendson BB: Effect rates of different modalities for treatment of prolactin adenomas. Am J Med 78:114, 1985.

25. Spratt DI, Finkelstein JS, O'Dea LS, et al: Long-term administration of gonadotropin-releasing hormone in men with idiopathic hypogonadotropic hypogonadism: A model for studies of the hormone's physiologic effects. Ann Intern Med 105:848, 1983.

26. Childs SJ: Prostatitis: Current diagnosis and treatment. Contemp Urol 4:31–40, 1992.

Chapter 38

Degenerative Processes

Kozy Corsaut

The term *degenerative disease* connotes a decline from a normal state to a lower level of functioning. In degenerative neurologic disease, the nervous system is affected, and often a gradual progressive course of decline in neurologic function occurs after a period of normalcy.[1] Symptoms depend on the segment of the nervous system affected. If the brain is involved, dementia with loss of mental faculties may be present. If only the peripheral nerves are affected, mental function remains intact, but ataxia (uncoordinated movements) may be present. Unfortunately, the arsenal of laboratory tests for the diagnosis of these diseases is small, and the physician must rely heavily on clinical features and family history to make the final diagnosis.

The diseases presented in this section may be found classified with disorders discussed in other chapters (e.g., Wilson's disease with hepatic disorders, Gaucher's disease with hematologic disorders, mucopolysaccharidosis with other genetic defects). These diseases, however, often present neurologic changes, such as mental retardation, loss of mental ability and muscle coordination, personality dis-

turbances, or behavior disorders. In the majority of the following disease states, these symptoms are due to a progressive degeneration of some portion of the nervous system. As the nervous system has limited ability for regeneration, many of these diseases are without cure.

DISEASES PRIMARILY AFFECTING ADULTS

Progressive Dementia

Dementia is defined as the loss of mental ability. The most common causes of dementia in patients older than 60 years are Alzheimer's disease (which accounts for 70% of dementias) and the toxic effects of drugs (which accounts for about 10% of dementias in elderly). Diseases that typically present with dementia as the only symptom are Alzheimer's disease, Pick's disease, and some cases of acquired immunodeficiency syndrome (AIDS). Conditions in which dementia is associated with clinical and laboratory evidence of other disease processes are hypothyroidism, hypoglycemia, hyponatremia, hyperparathyroidism, Cushing's disease, vitamin B_{12} deficiency, Wilson's disease, chronic drug intoxication, and some cases of AIDS. Miscellaneous diseases that present with dementia associated with other neurologic abnormalities are Huntington's disease, lipid storage disease, Creutzfeldt-Jakob disease, cerebral infarction, brain tumors, and brain trauma.[1, 2]

A cost-effective evaluation for patients presenting with dementia has been suggested by Larson[2]:

- Patient history with complete physical and neuropsychiatric evaluation
- Laboratory screening tests: complete blood cell count (CBC), glucose, sodium, calcium, creatinine, thyroid-

stimulating hormone (TSH), erythrocyte sedimentation rate (ESR), and VDRL
- Follow-up tests as needed: thyroxine (T$_4$), triiodothyronine uptake test (T$_3$U) in patients with increased TSH, and folate and B$_{12}$ in patients with anemia and/or macrocytosis
- Computed tomography (CT) scan of patients with specific clinical indications or high-risk patients
- An alternative is to screen all patients for folate and vitamin B$_{12}$ as the elderly population may be at increased risk for deficiencies

Dementia may be the major or even the sole manifestation of human immunodeficiency virus (HIV) infection, and in the later stages, findings of dementia are not uncommon. Some authors recommend screening dementia patients for HIV.[1]

Alzheimer's Disease

Alzheimer's disease, named for the German physician Alois Alzheimer, is a form of presenile dementia. The etiology is unknown, but theories have been advanced involving genetic (up to 10% of cases are thought to be of autosomal dominant inheritance), viral, and immunologic factors.[3–5]

The disease can affect any age group and has been reported in patients with Down syndrome, but it is mostly a disease of patients aged 50 to 60 years and older. Women are more likely to be afflicted than men. The disease may be prevalent in some families but is most often sporadic. It has been estimated that as many as 4% of the population older than 65 years is affected with Alzheimer's disease and that 10% may have the disease but are still able to function in society.[6, 7]

The cerebral cortex appears atrophied, and the frontal and temporal lobes may be more seriously affected. On microscopic examination, the brain cortex shows neuronal loss, and demyelination may also be present. Senile plaques are characteristically present, and their numbers can be correlated with the loss of intellectual ability. In some patients, presynaptic defects correlate with decreased levels of choline acetyltransferase and acetylcholinesterase in the brain.[4] Alzheimer's disease begins slowly. The initial complaints are of memory loss, difficulty in problem-solving, and depression. As the disease progresses, patients experience difficulty in walking, speech impairment, and loss of bodily functions and mental ability.[7]

In the clinical laboratory, findings of blood analyses are normal. Most often spinal fluid studies are also within normal limits, although a slight increase in total protein in cerebrospinal fluid (CSF) may be found. Tests on serum and CSF for syphilis, measles, and *Cryptococcus* are also negative. It has recently been reported that patients with Alzheimer's disease are likely to display oligoclonal banding in CSF, though this is not a routine method for diagnosis at this time.[5]

Diagnosis is made by clinical symptoms and CT. The CT scan will show enlargement of the brain ventricles and cortical sulci. An exact diagnosis is obtained at autopsy with histologic studies of brain tissues. The course of the disease is relentlessly progressive, often over a period of 8 to 10 years. Specific treatment or a cure for Alzheimer's disease is presently not available: only custodial care can be given to these patients.[4]

Dementia With Other CNS Signs

Creutzfeldt-Jakob Disease

Creutzfeldt-Jakob disease, also known as *Jakob-Creutzfeldt disease* or *subacute spongiform encephalopathy,* is a rare dementia found in about 1/1,000,000 persons. It appears to be viral in origin and affects the cortex, basal ganglia, and spinal cord. Inflammation of the brain is not apparent. At autopsy, cerebral atrophy and enlarged ventricles are seen, along with degeneration of the nerve cells.[7]

Creutzfeldt-Jakob disease generally occurs in patients more than 50 years of age. Patients complain of memory loss, personality changes, and behavioral disorders. Patients usually display a characteristic monoclonus (involuntary muscle spasm). Later in the disease pronounced mental loss, muscle atrophy, seizures, and coma occur. The disease progression is rapid, and death occurs within an average of 15 months.[4]

Creutzfeldt-Jakob disease is caused by a transmissible spongiform encephalopathy agent. Transmission has been reported in corneal transplant patients and in association with inadequately sterilized stereostatic brain electrodes. It should be considered a potential biohazard, and universal tissue precautions should be heeded. The agent can be detected in most internal organs of the patients but not in their body fluids and secretions (saliva, urine, feces, and blood). The disease has been transmitted to chimpanzees experimentally.[7]

The CSF total protein level may be slightly increased in these patients but is most often normal.[7] Blood cell counts and routine chemistry tests are normal. No signs of infection or inflammatory response is apparent. Later in the disease the electroencephalogram (EEG) is abnormal.[4] Neuron-specific enolase (NSE), a biochemical marker in the CSF, has been useful in differentiating Creutzfeldt-Jakob disease from other dementias.[8]

Central nervous system (CNS) depressants such as bromide intoxication should be ruled out. Alzheimer's disease or subacute sclerosing panencephalitis demonstrates an increased CSF immunoglobin (IgG) value. Neural syphilis, which presents with a reactive CSF VDRL, should also be ruled out. There is no treatment for Creutzfeldt-Jakob disease, and death is inevitable.

Huntington's Disease

Huntington's disease, also called *Huntington's chorea* and *Woody Guthrie's disease,* is inherited as an autosomal dominant trait, affecting both men and women equally, with an incidence of about 5/100,000. The symptoms of this disease do not begin before the age of 25 years and generally appear in the fourth or fifth decades of life—the time of life when many patients already have children. The children of these patients have a 50% chance of developing the disease.[7]

In patients affected with the disease, nerve cells that produce γ-aminobutyric acid (GABA) die and levels of glutamic acid decarboxylase (GAD) and choline acetyl-transferase decrease. The brain appears shrunken and atrophied, and on microscopic examination at autopsy, the nerve loss can be seen.

The disease begins slowly over a period of 10 to 25 years. The first symptoms are clumsiness, irritability, and forgetfulness. Later, speech and intellectual ability deteriorate. Uncontrolled movements (chorea) of arms, legs, head, and trunk worsen until the patient eventually degenerates to a state of helplessness and total disability.[7]

All laboratory findings for blood, CSF, and urine are essentially normal. The disease is usually diagnosed by clinical symptoms, magnetic resonance imaging (MRI), CT, EEG, and family history. The gene defect is on the short arm of chromosome 4, in which an expanded sequence of CAG repeats. Presently DNA linkage analysis is used to determine the gene presence.[9] Patients who have relatives with Huntington's disease may be tested with DNA linkage analysis for the marker. The test is reported to be 99% accurate when adequate numbers of family members are tested.[10] Two treatable diseases, Wilson's disease and viral encephalitis, should be ruled out before making a diagnosis of Huntington's disease.[11]

Treatment with neuroleptic medications may alleviate some of the chorea, possibly by blocking dopamine receptor sites. One hypothesis suggests that the chorea in these patients is due to a heightened receptor response to dopamine.[12] There is no cure for Huntington's disease, and patients usually die within 15 to 20 years of diagnosis.

Loss of Muscular Coordination and Control

Peripheral neuropathy can result in loss of muscle coordination and muscle control. When the peripheral nerves that supply a muscle are destroyed, the patient loses use of the muscle. The affected muscle weakens, tone is lost, and the muscle atrophies.

Amyotrophic Lateral Sclerosis

Amyotrophic lateral sclerosis (ALS), also known as *Lou Gehrig's disease,* is the most common of the motor neuron diseases. It is confined to the voluntary motor system of the skeletal muscles and involves progressive deterioration of the α-motor neurons.[7] The cause of the disease is unknown, but a chronic viral infection and immunologic factors have been suggested.

The disease usually begins in middle to late life and affects approximately 5/100,000 people.[7] Approximately 5% of the cases are hereditary, in which the genetic defect is an autosomal dominant gene on chromosome 21; the remaining cases appear sporadically. The symptoms generally begin with weakness in the arms and legs, and a progressive atrophy of the muscles, sometimes affecting the facial muscles, tongue, and respiratory muscles, occurs. Muscle mass can be reduced to 20% of original bulk in 3 months.[1] The patient's intellectual ability is not affected by this disease. ALS can have a rapid progression, with death occurring in 2 to 5 years due to respiratory muscle involvement.[7]

Results of routine blood analyses are generally normal, although some patients may display an increased concentration of serum creatine kinase (a reflection of the muscle loss), as much as 50% above normal if rapid nerve loss is occurring. In most patients the CSF total protein is within normal limits, although in a few it may be increased 20 mg/dL above normal.[7, 11]

Spinal cord compression due to tumors, chronic inflammatory disorders such as syphilitic meningomyelitis, metabolic disorders such as thyrotoxicosis, salt depletion, and lead toxicity are treatable diseases that should be ruled out.[11]

There is no cure for ALS, and only supportive therapy can be offered to these patients.[7]

Guillain-Barré Syndrome

Guillain-Barré syndrome, sometimes called *acute idiopathic polyneuritis,* is a rapidly progressive disease causing inflammation of the nerves and resulting in paralysis. Throughout the cranial and spinal nerves, infiltration of monocytic cells accompanied by demyelination of the nerve cells is seen. Guillain-Barré syndrome occurs in approximately 1/100,000 persons. Often there is a history of a recent viral illness or vaccination, and a few cases have been associated with surgery.[7] Some researchers have reported a link between development of Guillain-Barré syndrome and a preceding infection with *Campylobacter jejuni.*[7] There may be a shared antigenic site between the *Campylobacter* organism and GM_1 carbohydrate. Antibodies to GM_1 (ganglioside antibodies) can be found in Guillain-Barré patients and in the serum of patients with a variety of polyneuropathies.[13, 14] Although the syndrome can occur at any age, the incidence increases as the age of the patient increases.

Symptoms range from mild to severe enough to cause respiratory failure. Weakness is the earliest symptom, along with loss of sensation in hands and feet and slowing of the reflexes. There may be total paralysis of the limbs and/or total motor paralysis, including the muscles of respiration.[7] Usually no evidence of muscle atrophy presents, as the muscle weakness develops rapidly.[7]

There is no specific test for this disease. Electrophysiologic testing will show evidence of demyelination of the peripheral nerves. The CSF total protein is increased, often to very high levels between 100 to 400 mg/dL, whereas the CSF cell count is most often within normal limits.[7] Some patients may also display oligoclonal bands in the CSF, along with an increased IgG synthesis rate. The IgG index is usually normal, although the albumin index is increased, indicating increased blood-brain barrier (BBB) permeability.[15] A preceding viral infection may be detected by demonstrating increased serum titers of antibody to the suspected viral antigen.

Most patients recover with demyelination of the nerves, and death is uncommon. Recovery is slow, taking 6 months to 2 years, and is often incomplete. Approximately 10% of the patients experience significant long-term disability, and 40% may have mild long-term symptoms, although fewer than 5% die.

Multiple Sclerosis

Multiple sclerosis (MS) is one of most frequently seen neurologic diseases and is the most common of the demyelinating diseases. The term *sclerosis* refers to the hardened areas of scar tissue formed by the glial cells found throughout the CNS.[16]

The cause of MS remains unknown; however, immunologic processes or a virus of long incubation have been implicated.[7] T cells active against myelin in the CSF have been connected to the demyelination process.[17]

Plaques (patches of demyelination) that are macroscopic (1 to 4 cm) are found on the spinal cord, cerebellum, brain stem, cerebral hemispheres, and optic pathways. These plaques are infiltrated by macrophages, lymphocytes, and plasma cells; the macrophages may be implicated in the demyelination process. It appears that the peripheral nerves are not affected.[7]

MS often begins in early adulthood but can be found in children as well as in patients older than 40 years. The disease is rare to nonexistent in the tropics, and incidence increases north and south of the equator. The population that appears to be at most geographic risk are those at latitudes of 45 to 65 degrees, in Europe and North America. In these areas, the disease has an incidence of 30 to 80/100,000 and an even greater incidence in certain local regions. The risk factor appears to be determined by the geographic location in which the patient spent the adolescent years. Although MS is not inherited, it has a tendency to be familial, and siblings of MS patients are at greater risk than are the children of MS patients. A common link (perhaps exposure to virus) during childhood is theorized.[7]

Initial MS attacks tend to be precipitated by acute trauma, fatigue, pregnancy, emotional upsets, or vaccinations. Symptoms vary greatly and correlate with the area of CNS demyelination. Frequently the eyes are involved, causing blurring of vision, loss of vision, double vision, and loss of eye movement. Often weakness, numbness, and clumsiness in arms and legs occur. Urinary urgency and frequency are common complaints. The symptoms may last for several weeks to months, interspersed with periods of complete or almost complete remission that last for months to years. As the disease progresses, the periods of remission become shorter and less frequent, with only partial relief of symptoms. The course is variable, ranging from an acute case of only a few months with unremitting symptoms to the more common remitting and relapsing course seen in most patients and lasting for 20 to 30 years. A few patients have an attack on one occasion and are free of disease for the remainder of their lives.[18]

MS can be difficult to diagnose, as symptoms vary widely, and their occurrence is interspersed with remissions. The attempt to identify lesions in the CNS by CT may be helpful; lesions should be found on more than one occasion and at more than one site.[18]

Studies of CSF are the most useful clinical laboratory tests in making a diagnosis. About 30% of MS patients have a slightly increased CSF white blood cell (WBC) count, rarely more than 40/mm³ with lymphocytes predominating. A WBC count more than this or the presence of neutrophils indicates an alternative diagnosis. The CSF total protein level is generally normal or slightly increased in about 40% of the patients.[7]

One of the most valuable tests for the diagnosis of MS is the presence of *oligoclonal bands,* which are discrete bands of immunoglobulin detected by specialized electro-

phoresis of the CSF. At least one band is present in more than 90% of MS patients, and many patients have four or more bands present (Fig. 38–1). A serum protein electrophoresis should be ordered at the same time, to rule out paraproteinemia. If abnormal bands are seen in both serum and CSF, CSF oligoclonal bands are probably not present. If the bands are present in only the CSF and not in the serum, a diagnosis of MS is likely but not certain.

Patients with MS produce IgG in the CNS. Thus, it is necessary to prove that the presence of increased IgG in CSF is due to such de novo synthesis rather than to damage to the BBB. Several calculations attempt to correct for interfering factors such as traumatic taps:

- Expressing the CSF IgG as a percentage of the total CSF protein or albumin
- Calculation of the IgG index, in which the CSF IgG/blood IgG ratio is compared to the CSF-albumin/blood-albumin ratio
- Calculation of the IgG synthesis rate in the CSF

The calculated values will vary from laboratory to laboratory, depending on methods of protein measurement, and on normal values and ratios. Another useful calculation in assessing the origin of CSF IgG, either de novo synthesis or BBB damage, is calculation of the albumin index. This index is expressed as the ratio of CSF albumin to blood albumin. When the index is increased, damage to the BBB or traumatic tap is likely[19] (Table 38–1).

The presence of oligoclonal bands in the CSF is strong evidence for MS, if other causes are ruled out by using CT and MRI. Oligoclonal bands have a 3% false-positive rate, although about 10% of MS patients are negative for the bands.[17] Other diseases that can also present with oligoclonal bands include Alzheimer's disease, neurosyphilis, both bacterial and viral encephalitis, Guillain-Barré syndrome and some other polyneuropathies.[19] It should be noted that in addition to routine CSF electrophoresis, tests for oligoclonal bands must be ordered specifically.

Levels of myelin basic protein (MBP) more than 8 ng/mL are present in almost all MS patients with recent exacerbations (less than 1 week) of the disease. Less recent

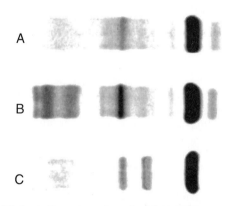

Figure 38–1. *A,* Normal cerebrospinal fluid (CSF) electrophoretogram. *B,* SPE II CSF pattern positive multiple sclerosis (MS) patient with oligoclonal bands. *C,* SPE II serum pattern from above patient negative for oligoclonal bands. (From Specialty Laboratories: Laboratory Report Form and Update: Neurooncology and Neuroimmunology Come of Age. Los Angeles, Specialty Laboratories, 1987.)

Table 38–1. CNS IgG Synthesis Indices

IgG Index	IgG Synthesis Rate/24 hr	Albumin Index	Interpretation
Normal	Normal	Normal	Normal
Increased	Increased	Normal	CNS IgG synthesis likely
S1 increased	Increased	Increased	Equivocal results, BBB damage, or traumatic tap; cannot rule out CNS IgG synthesis
Normal	Normal or increased	Increased	BBB damage likely
Increased	Normal or increased	Increased	CNS IgG synthesis likely

Data from Specialty Laboratories: Laboratory report form and update: Neurooncology and neuroimmunology come of age. Los Angeles, Specialty Laboratories, 1987.

attacks give lower values of 4 to 8 ng/mL, and fewer than 5% of patients in remission have a positive result more than 4 ng/mL. The MBP test is useful for evaluating the severity of a recent demyelinating process, but it is not specific for MS. Increased MBP levels can be found in other diseases in which primary or secondary demyelination is present.[20]

Many laboratories offer a panel of tests for diagnosis of MS. These tests often include oligoclonal bands, MBP, CSF IgG, IgG synthesis rate, and IgG and albumin indices.[15]

When attempting to make a diagnosis of MS, diseases such as disseminated lupus erythematosus, polyarteritis nodosa, brain-stem gliomas, cord neoplasms, syringomyelia, and spondylosis should be ruled out.[7] Differential diagnosis also includes ALS, Guillain-Barré syndrome, and leukodystrophy.

MS has no prevention and no cure. Treatment includes adrenocorticotropic hormone (ACTH), prednisone, or other corticosteroids to reduce severity of recurrent attacks. Interferon β-1b (Betaseron) was recently licensed for treating relapsing-remitting MS with the goal of reducing frequency of exacerbations.[21]

Parkinson's Disease

Parkinson's disease affects the brain basal ganglia. Patients lack sufficient amounts of the neurotransmitter dopamine, resulting in symptoms of the disease that are due to an inhibitory influence on the ganglia. At autopsy the brain shows a loss of nerve cells and a loss of pigmentation of the substantia nigra. The etiology of this disease is still unclear.[7]

Parkinson's disease generally begins in middle to late life, and it is a leading cause of neurologic degeneration in patients older than 60 years. It has been estimated that 1/1000 persons is affected by Parkinson's disease.

The patient generally shows a characteristic tremor, stiffness in walking, loss of dexterity, and slowed movements. In addition to other symptoms, there may be an immobile, unblinking, "frozen" facial expression and difficulty in speech. Mental ability is not affected. The disease progresses slowly over a prolonged period, ending in a state of total invalidism.

All routine blood tests and CSF tests are within normal limits. The clinical picture of Parkinson's disease is unique, but similar syndromes may occur with phenothiazine administration, carbon monoxide poisoning, heavy metal poisoning, head trauma, cerebral neoplasms, infectious encephalitis, and cerebral arteriosclerosis.

Treatment with levodopa has been reported to relieve the symptoms in some patients, and a few have responded to surgery. The disease is progressive, with no known cure.[7]

Other Peripheral Neuropathies

HIV and Peripheral Nerve Involvement

Neuromuscular disease symptoms are associated with HIV infection. In HIV, the nervous system can be invaded by the virus, and it is estimated that 15% of AIDS victims are affected by peripheral nerve involvement. These symptoms may be the only indication of HIV infection, which is otherwise asymptomatic. It has been suggested that all patients with symptoms of an inflammatory demyelinating polyneuropathy be tested for HIV.[1]

Malignancy and Peripheral Nerve Involvement

Some malignancies are accompanied by peripheral neuropathies. When a cause for a neuropathy is not found, the possibility of a monoclonal gammopathy or lung neoplasm associated with sensory loss should be considered. Antibodies to myelin-associated glycoprotein (MAG) are found in approximately 50% of the patients with signs of peripheral neuropathy suffering from monoclonal gammopathy of immunoglobulin M (IgM) type. Antineuronal nuclear antibodies of type 1(Hu) can be found in patients suffering from sensory neuropathy in small cell carcinoma of the lung. The antibody is often present before the tumor is diagnosed.[14]

DISEASES PRIMARILY AFFECTING CHILDREN

Progressive Dementia and Other CNS Signs

Wilson's Disease

Wilson's disease, also known as *hepatolenticular degeneration,* is characterized by a disturbance of the transport mechanism and storage of copper due to a defect in ceruloplasmin synthesis. Wilson's disease is relatively rare and is inherited as an autosomal recessive gene located on chromosome 13 at the position q14. Symptoms seen are a direct result of the copper deposition in nerve and other body tissues, leading to lesions in the brain, liver, eye, and kidney.[7] The symptoms of liver dysfunction, such as jaundice, usually occur after the age of 6 years. The neurologic symptoms, characterized by tremor, double vision, lack of coordination, drooling, and dysphagia (difficulty in swallowing), usually occur between the ages of 12 and 30 years. Renal tubular and neurologic involvement may appear, along with development of kidney stones.

Neurologic symptoms can be highly variable, but often tremors are present along with muscle spasms and rigidity. Often these patients move the upper extremities, especially hands and fingers, with a twisting or "flapping" movement, and facial features show a fixed "smile." Psychological changes are noticed as the ganglion cells degenerate, and mental deterioration progresses.[16] Later, liver cirrhosis is present, and many patients display the characteristic rust-colored ring (Kayser-Fleischer) on the cornea caused by copper deposits.

Routine CSF tests are within normal limits; however, some patients will have an increased CSF copper level. Other laboratory tests results may vary, but those that provide useful laboratory findings are increased aspartate transaminase (AST), increased alanine transaminase (ALT), increased bilirubin, similar total protein and electrophoresis patterns to those seen in chronic active hepatitis, and decreased uric acid.[22] Liver function tests should be performed at frequent intervals, as these results may be normal except during periods of liver involvement.

Of great diagnostic value is the ceruloplasmin level, which is usually decreased to less than 20 mg/dL. It should be kept in mind that serum ceruloplasmin levels may be normal when liver involvement is advanced; thus normal values do not rule out Wilson's disease.

Measures of 24-hour urinary copper are also very useful. Early in the disease, these levels may be normal or slightly increased. As the disease progresses, urine output of copper is markedly increased. Some physicians advocate measuring 24-hour urine copper levels before and after treatment with penicillamine. This chelating agent releases tissue-bound excess copper, resulting in dramatically increased levels of urinary copper. Liver biopsy results show increased deposits of copper, which help to confirm diagnosis.[22]

Early diagnosis is important so that treatment can be instituted before irreversible damage occurs to the brain and liver. With early diagnosis and treatment, patients have a good chance of survival with complete or almost complete remission of symptoms.[7] Patients are advised to consume low-copper diets and to take copper chelating agents, such as penicillamine, to minimize absorption of copper and facilitate its excretion.

Wilson's disease should be ruled out in any young patient displaying symptoms similar to those of chronic hepatitis accompanied by neurologic changes.[22] Other diseases to consider are primary biliary cirrhosis, heavy metal poisoning, and Huntington's disease.

Lysosomal Storage Diseases

Lysosomes are granules found in the cytoplasm of macrophages. One function of lysosomes is to catabolize lipids ingested by those cells. Large molecular substances may require a series of hydrolase enzyme activities before the products are small enough to leave the cell. Any molecule not metabolized accumulates in the macrophage.[22] A genetic deficiency in the cytoplasmic lysosomes of one of the enzymes necessary for degradation of glycosides or peptides results in the eventual buildup of these ingested materials.

Many of these enzyme defects involve the sphingolipids. Although sphingolipids have a normal rate of synthesis, they accumulate because a specific lysosomal enzyme that degrades the lipid is absent. The undegraded substrate is deposited in the tissues, eventually interfering with the function of the tissue.[1] The type of accumulated metabolite and its distribution in the tissues determines the clinical signs of each distinct disease.

The entire reticuloendothelial system is involved due to the large number of phagocytes found in the spleen, liver, and bone marrow. The skeletal system and connective tissues may also be involved, as well as the CNS (Table 38–2).[22]

The poliodystrophies (such as Tay-Sachs disease, Gaucher's disease, Niemann-Pick disease) are characterized by early onset of seizures, loss of mental ability, blindness due to retinal destruction, and indications of gray matter involvement of the brain.

Tay-Sachs Disease

Tay-Sachs disease is an autosomal recessive disease, mostly affecting the Eastern European Jewish population. The defective gene is located on chromosome 5.[23] Approximately 1/30 Ashkenazi Jews carry the Tay-Sachs gene. The symptoms begin within a month of birth. The infant is listless and irritable, has delayed development, and may have regression of previous skills. Degeneration continues, and the child develops motor seizures, blindness, and dementia. Death occurs between 3 and 5 years of age.[1] In the majority of patients a characteristic cherry-red macular spot is seen in the retina, corresponding with vision failure. The EEG is also abnormal.

The deficient enzyme is hexosaminidase A, which cleaves *N*-acetylgalactosamine from gangliosides. This defect allows GM_2 ganglioside to accumulate in the brain and spinal cord. Testing of serum, WBCs, or cultured fibroblasts from amniotic fluid displays the decreased enzyme level. Enzyme level testing is available for heterozygotes for purposes of genetic counseling. There is no specific treatment for Tay-Sachs disease, and treatment is supportive.[1] Sandhoff's disease is a form of Tay-Sachs disease but is not limited to any ethnic group.

Gaucher's Disease

Gaucher's disease is the most common of the lysosomal storage diseases and occurs more frequently in people of Jewish descent than in other populations.[24]

The defective gene is probably located on chromosome 1, q21–q31 region. The deficient lysosomal glucocerebrosidase results in the subsequent accumulation of the substrate glucocerebroside, which is a normal product of cellular breakdown. These lipids tend to build up in the reticuloendothelial system (RES), as the leukocytes are cleared from circulation.[22]

Gaucher's disease may be classified into three types:

Table 38-2. Characteristics of Lysosomal Storage Diseases

	Enzyme Deficiency	Accumulated Metabolite	Neurologic Signs	Genetics	Other	Laboratory Results
Sphingolipidosis						
Tay-Sachs disease (GM$_2$ gangliosidosis)	Hexosaminidase A	GM$_2$ ganglioside	Dementia	Recessive	Cherry-red macula	↑ AST, ↑ vacuolated lymphs, urine N, CSF N
Gaucher's disease (glucosylceramide lipidosis)	β-Glucosidase	Glucocerebroside	Spastic paralysis	Recessive	Hepatosplenomegaly	Acid phosphatase, urine N, CSF N, Gaucher cells in BM
Niemann-Pick disease (sphingomyelin lipidosis)	Sphingomyelinase	Sphingomyelin	Spastic paresis, dementia	Recessive		Serum lipids, ↑ vacuolated lymphs, urine N, CSF N, foam cells in BM
GM$_1$ gangliosidosis	GM$_1$ ganglioside β-galactosidase	GM$_1$ ganglioside, galactose-containing oligosaccharides				
Krabbe's disease (globoid cell leukodystrophy)	Galactocerebrosidase	Galactocerebroside	Spastic paresis, mental deterioration	Recessive		Blood urine N, CSF ↑ TP (150–300 mg/dL); determination of deficiency of β-galactosidase in leukocytes or serum
Metachromatic leukodystrophy (sulfatide lipidosis)	Arylsulfatase A	Galactosyl sulfatide	Loss of motor and mental functions	Recessive		CSF TP > 100 mg/dL, metachromic granules in blood leukocytes
Adrenal leukodystrophy		Very long chain fatty acids	Memory loss, dementia	X-linked or autosomal recessive	Adrenal gland involvement, symptoms of Addison's disease	
Mucopolysaccharidosis*						
Hurler-Scheie syndrome	α-Iduronidase	Dermatan sulfate, heparan sulfate	Mental retardation	Recessive	Dwarfism, skeletal deformities	
Hunter's syndrome	Iduronate sulfatase	Dermatan sulfate, heparan sulfate	Symptoms are milder, life expectancy can be normal	X-linked		
Sanfilippo's syndrome						
Type A	N-acetylgalactosamine-6-sulfate sulfatase	Heparan sulfate	Mental retardation	Recessive	Skeletal deformities	Urine contains excess of heparan sulfate
Type B	α-N-Acetylglucosaminidase	Heparan sulfate	—			
Type C	Heparan-N-acetyltransferase	Heparan sulfate				
Type D	α-N-Glucosamine-6-sulfatase	Heparan sulfate				—
Morquio syndrome						
Type A	N-Acetylgalactosamine-6-sulfate sulfatase	Keratan sulfate	No mental retardation	Recessive	Skeletal deformities, respiratory problems, corneal clouding	Urine contains dermatan sulfate
Type B	β-Galactosidase	Keratan sulfate				
Maroteaux-Lamy syndrome	Arylsulfatase B	Dermatan sulfate	No mental retardation, life expectancy normal	Recessive		
Sly's syndrome	β-Glucuronidase	Dermatan and heparan sulfate	Variable picture	Recessive		Urine dermatan and heparan sulfate

Abbreviations: AST, aspartate aminotransferase; N, normal; BM, bone marrow; TP, total protein.
*For suspected cases examine blood smear for Alder-Reilly bodies, inclusion granules (azurophilic and basophilic) in neutrophils, eosinophils, basophils, and lymphs (Gasser cell), and monocytes. Buhot's cells (large mononuclear cells) are in the bone marrow.

adult onset, juvenile onset, and *infantile onset.* The earlier the clinical symptoms appear, the more severe the disease, accompanied by a shortened life span. The infantile form of the disease shows the greatest level of CNS involvement, and death before 2 years of age is usual. Adult onset is more common, with little or no mental retardation.[25]

Because of the RES involvement, patients display an enlarged spleen and liver. There may also be bone destruction. Often there is a tendency for patients to bruise and bleed easily after a small injury. Laboratory data typically reveal a hypochromic normocytic anemia, thrombocytopenia, and leukopenia with WBCs in the range of 2.0 to 3.0×10^9/L. A marked increase in the concentration of serum acid phosphatase with increased isoenzyme 5 is found. Gaucher's cells are found occasionally in peripheral blood but more often in the bone marrow or in liver and spleen biopsies. A deficiency in the specific enzyme β-glucosidase can be demonstrated in peripheral blood leukocytes or, preferably, in cultured fibroblasts.[22]

Carrier status can be determined by identifying decreased enzyme activity in leukocytes or cultured fibroblasts. Usually carriers display approximately 50% of the enzyme activity of normal individuals; however, the "normal" level varies considerably.

Fetuses considered to be at risk can be monitored at 14 to 16 weeks by amniocentesis, and the cultured fetal cells can be tested for enzyme activity.[25]

The clinical course of Gaucher's disease varies, from the severe form of infantile onset and early death to the relatively mild chronic form of adult onset with a normal life expectancy. There is little treatment available for Gaucher's disease at this time, although trials using enzyme replacement may prove successful in the future.[25] Glucocerebrosidase/β-glucosidase (Ceredase) which is a placentally derived enzyme, may be used to treat adult onset disease.[26]

Niemann-Pick Disease

Niemann-Pick disease is also a lipid storage disease; it is caused by a deficiency of the enzyme sphingomyelinase, which results in the storage of sphingomyelin in the brain, liver, and other body organs. Niemann-Pick disease is inherited as an autosomal recessive gene and is more common in persons of Jewish descent than in other population groups.[25]

Occasionally the disease is not diagnosed until adulthood, but most commonly, infants are affected. Because of RES involvement (as in Gaucher's disease), patients display hepatomegaly and splenomegaly, accompanied by a mild jaundice due to liver damage. The nervous system is affected, leading to severe mental retardation. Approximately one-third of these patients have a characteristic cherry-red spot in the retina due to retinal degeneration.[25]

Routine laboratory tests are essentially normal. The anemia and thrombocytopenia seen in Gaucher's disease are not present or are very mild. Serum acid phosphatase concentration is also normal, helping to differentiate this disease from Gaucher's disease.[24]

The diagnosis of Niemann-Pick disease can be made by finding Niemann-Pick cells in bone marrow aspirates. These are large macrophages filled with globules of sphin-gomyelin. Enzyme studies in leukocytes are useful in identifying the disease by confirming the deficiency of the enzyme sphingomyelinase, using the substrate 2-hexadecanoylamino-4-nitrophenylphosphorylcholine, which closely resembles sphingomyelin. These tests can also be performed to identify carrier status of parents, to monitor the fetus, and to assist in genetic counseling.[25]

At present no cure for Niemann-Pick disease is available, and most of the affected children die early. This makes recognition of heterozygotes important for purposes of family planning. Investigational therapies include bone marrow transplantation and the use of drugs such as lovastatin, nicotinic acid, and cholestyramine to lower blood cholesterol levels.[27, 28]

Leukodystrophy

The leukodystrophies are a group of rare, progressive, inherited metabolic diseases that affect the CNS and sometimes the peripheral nerves. The leukodystrophies affect the white matter (myelin) of the brain and are characterized by early onset of spastic paralysis of limbs and visual impairment due to optic atrophy, although the retina is not involved. The leukodystrophies can be considered *dysmyelinating diseases,* in which an enzyme defect affects the production and maintenance of the nerve myelin sheath. Lipids accumulate in tissues, primarily affecting the CNS, causing motor disturbances, and resulting in mental retardation that can be severe.

Leukodystrophy has a high familial incidence and is inherited as an autosomal recessive gene. A number of diseases share this classification, two of which are *Krabbe's disease* and *metachromatic leukodystrophy.* In Krabbe's disease, also known as *globoid cell leukodystrophy,* widespread dysmyelination is present. Histologically, globoid cells are seen with multilobed nuclei in the white matter of the brain. Biochemically, deficiencies in two enzymes appear to be involved: β-galactase and sulfotransferase. These deficiencies account for increased deposits of cerebrosides found in globoid cells.[5]

Krabbe's disease is rare and usually appears during infancy, although occasionally it may appear in childhood. Such children often display unexplained fever, light and noise sensitivity, and a halt in psychomotor development. Later, myoclonic jerks appear in the legs and arms, followed by blindness and mental deterioration.

The CSF shows an increased level of total protein, generally more than 100 mg/dL. Determination of enzyme deficiency by the substrate galactocerebroside, in serum or leukocytes, is highly indicative of Krabbe's disease. Parents can be tested for decreased enzyme activity to determine carrier status.[25]

There is no treatment or cure for this disease, and death usually occurs within 6 to 12 months. Genetic counseling should be offered to those parents who already have an affected child. Prenatal diagnosis can be made on amniotic fluid.[25]

In *metachromatic leukodystrophy,* also referred to as *sulfatide lipoidosis,* a deficiency of arylsulfatase is found. This deficiency leads to galactosyl sulfatide (lipid) accumulation in both the central and the peripheral nervous systems and in the renal tubules. The term *metachromatic* refers to the fact that the deposits of sulfatide change the color of certain tissue stains. The excess galactosyl sulfatide is excreted in the urine, and metachromatic granules can also be found in the urine sediment and WBCs.[22]

Metachromatic leukodystrophy is relatively rare, although it is more common than Krabbe's disease, with an onset in late infancy or early childhood.[22] Affected children display a loss of motor abilities and muscle weakness, thus losing the ability to walk. Mental functions show progressive degeneration.

The CSF total protein level is elevated, often to greater than 100 mg/dL. A search for metachromatic granules in blood leukocytes or urine may be helpful. Determination of arylsulfatase A activity by the nitrocatecholsulfate test can be diagnostic. This test can be performed on urine, serum, and cultures of WBCs and fibroblasts, thus making carrier status and prenatal testing available.[4]

When clear-cut laboratory results are not available, the following conditions should be ruled out: Niemann-Pick disease, Gaucher's disease, aminoaciduria, and subacute sclerosing panencephalitis.

There is no treatment for metachromatic leukodystrophy, and death usually occurs within 5 years. Parents should receive genetic counseling when heterozygotes can be identified by discovering decreased levels of arylsulfatase in cultured fibroblasts.[25]

Adrenal leukodystrophy is characterized by the presence of very long chain fatty acids in blood and tissues, which accumulate in the brain and adrenal glands. The most common form is the X-linked childhood form that affects boys between 4 to 8 years of age. These children display behavioral changes; poor memory; loss of emotional control; dementia; and speech, hearing, and visual problems. Symptoms of decreased adrenal function can be present and include low blood pressure, generalized weakness, fatigue, dehydration, weight loss, and decreased adrenal response to ACTH stimulation. Adult onset of adrenal leukodystrophy should be suspected in men who have decreased adrenal function and have a family history of Addison's disease. The disease progresses more slowly in adults but can result in brain dysfunction.

Diagnosis is made by CT or MRI. Laboratory findings of very long chain of fatty acids (VLCFAs) are an important diagnostic clue.[29] Suspected carriers and newborns can also be tested for VLCFA, and cell cultures (amniocentesis or chorion villus sampling) can also be tested. Treatment includes use of adrenal steroids, as in Addison's disease. Neurologic symptoms can be treated with anticonvulsants.

Canavan's disease is a rare condition characterized by spongy degeneration of the CNS, due to a deficiency of aspartoaculase, which breaks down *N*-acetylaspartic acid (NAA). The defective gene is located on chromosome 17. Canavan's disease tends to affect Eastern European Jewish ethnic groups. Diagnosis is by CT scan or MRI, which may show vacuolation of the brain along with areas of demyelination. Affected infants have high levels of NAA in CSF, blood, and urine. Prenatal diagnosis can be made by measuring NAA in the amniotic fluid.

Mucopolysaccharidosis

Mucopolysaccharidosis (MPS) refers to any of a group of inherited diseases characterized by defective mucopolysaccharide metabolism due to an enzyme deficiency, subsequently resulting in an excess of dermatan sulfate, heparan sulfate, keratan sulfate, or chondroitin sulfate. These substances are stored in the body tissues and excreted in the urine. Deposits can be found in arteries, skeleton, eyes, joints, skin, liver, bone marrow, and CNS. An affected child may appear normal at birth but then begins to show signs of mental and growth retardation. The severity of the symptoms varies with the type of mucopolysaccharide present.[7]

There are a number of different classifications for the MPS diseases. All are inherited as autosomal recessive genes except Hunter's syndrome, which is inherited as an X-linked gene.

TYPE I: HURLER'S SYNDROME

The deficient enzyme is α-L-iduronidase, and the excessive mucopolysaccharides are dermatan sulfate and heparan sulfate. This disease is characterized by skeletal deformities, dwarfism, mental retardation, and heart and liver involvement. Death usually occurs before the patient reaches 10 years of age.[30, 31]

TYPE II: HUNTER'S SYNDROME

L-Iduronide sulfatase is the deficient enzyme, with an increase in urinary dermatan sulfate and heparan sulfate. This disease is similar to type I, but symptoms are milder and only males are affected. Patients may have a normal life expectancy.[30, 31]

TYPE III: SANFILIPPO'S SYNDROME A AND B

The enzyme deficiencies are, respectively, heparan *N*-sulfatase and *N*-acetyl-D-glucosaminidase, and urine contains an excess of heparan sulfate. Patients have some skeletal deformities and severe mental retardation. Death usually occurs before the third decade.[31]

TYPE IV: MORQUIO'S SYNDROME

The deficient enzyme is hexosamine-6-sulfatase, and an excess of urinary keratan sulfate is seen. Patients have severe skeletal deformities, comeal clouding, and respiratory problems. There is no mental retardation. Some patients live to age 60.[30]

TYPE V: SCHEIE'S SYNDROME

α-L-Iduronidase is deficient, causing an excess of dermatan sulfate and heparan sulfate. Symptoms may begin at age 10 with stiffness of hands and feet. Corneal clouding and heart disease are also features. Little or no mental retardation is seen in this disease, and patients often have a normal life expectancy.[30]

TYPE VI: MAROTEAUX-LAMY SYNDROME

Arylsulfatase is deficient and dermatan sulfate increased. There is no mental retardation. Life expectancy is normal.[30]

TYPE VII: SLY'S SYNDROME

The deficient enzyme is β-glucuronidase, with urinary excess of dermatan sulfate and heparan sulfate. These patients have a clinically variable picture.[30]

All suspected MPS patients should have peripheral blood smears examined for the presence of Alder-Reilly bodies, which are significant evidence for the diagnosis.[16] The inclusions are seen as azurophilic and basophilic granules in neutrophils, eosinophils, and basophils, and sometimes in lymphocytes (Gasser's cells) and monocytes. The inclusions are more likely to be found in the bone marrow as Buhot's cells (large mononuclear cells). Basophilic inclusions can be easily confused with toxic granulation.[16] In patients with MPS and other storage diseases, vacuolated lymphocytes can be seen (Mittwoch cells), and the smear may also show abnormally large platelets. It should be noted that these inclusions are most often seen in Hurler's, Hunter's, and Sanfilippo's syndromes and are not seen in Morquio's syndrome.[24]

Urine screening tests for the detection of MPS are the toluidine blue spot test, which detects dermatan sulfate and heparan sulfate, and the acid albumin turbidity test. The acetylpyridium chloride test also detects excess mucopolysaccharides in the urine. These screening tests may have false-positive and false-negative reactions and will not detect the keratan sulfate found in Morquio's syndrome. All positive reactions should be confirmed by either thin-layer chromatography or ion-exchange chromatography of the urine to determine the exact MPS present. Enzyme assays can also be performed on cultures of fibroblasts and leukocytes to identify the specific enzyme deficiency. The enzyme assays can be performed on cultured amniotic cells to make a prenatal diagnosis of MPS.[31]

The confirmatory tests are not routine in many laboratories and usually must be performed by specialized reference laboratories.

Other Etiologies

Postinfectious and Postvaccinal Encephalomyelitis

Postinfectious encephalomyelitis can occur, although rarely, following certain childhood diseases such as measles, rubella, smallpox, and mumps. Neurologic complications can occur at a rate of between 1:800 to 1:2000 cases in measles cases. Mortality occurs in about 10% to 20% of the cases. The disease is an acute demyelinating disease, and areas of demyelination can be found in the brain and the spinal cord. The patient suffers from an acute onset of confusion, convulsions, fever, and stiffness in the neck. If the spinal cord is involved, paraplegia or even quadriplegia may be present, with loss of bladder and bowel control. Among those who survive, permanent neurologic damage is likely. The exact etiology is unknown, but theories suggest that the virus or the toxin associated with the virus causes neurologic damage. Current thinking leans more to an autoimmune response in the patient that results in an immune-related complication.

The CSF generally shows an increase in the lymphocyte count and in total protein concentration. Reye's syndrome, in which the CSF is normal, should be ruled out, but the serum ammonia and liver enzyme levels are increased. Steroids are given as treatment, in an attempt to reduce the severity of the allergic encephalomyelitis.[1]

A similar disease can occur after vaccination for such diseases as rabies, smallpox, or measles. Smallpox vaccinations are no longer given and thus do not play a role in the development of the disease. With the transition from rabies vaccine grown in rabbit brain to one made in duck eggs or human cells, the incidence of rabies postvaccinal encephalomyelitis is greatly decreased.

The onset tends to be abrupt. The patient experiences drowsiness, fever, and vomiting. Stiffness of the neck and convulsions may be present. The mortality rate is between 30% to 50%. The CSF shows a moderate increase in protein and lymphocytes.[1]

Subacute Sclerosing Panencephalitis

Caused by the measles virus, subacute sclerosing panencephalitis (SSP) is considered a slow viral infection and is extremely rare today due to the routine vaccination of children for measles. The pathology of this disease is not totally understood, but current theory suggests immune complex deposits in the brain as a factor.

Case Study

A 24-year-old white woman was seen by her physician because of fatigue, weakness in arms and legs, difficulty in walking, and blurring of vision. She reported weakness in her legs during the summer, when she found she was no longer able to water-ski. After the birth of her third child, the weakness became progressively worse, to the point at which she had difficulty walking and required assistance if there was no support to lean on. The weakness also appeared in her arms, making it difficult for her to set and comb her hair. When her vision began to blur, she sought medical help.

Up to this time the patient had been healthy with only the usual childhood diseases. There was no history of recent illness or vaccinations. She had been raised in a rural area of Ohio and had not been out of the area recently.

Laboratory Findings

Analysis	Results	Interpretation
Blood		
Total protein (g/dL)	7.1	Normal
Albumin (g/dL)	5.3	Normal
IgG (mg/dL)	998	Normal
Serum electrophoresis	Normal	Normal
WBC differential	Normal	Normal
Urine		
Routine urinalysis	Normal	Normal

CSF

Gross examination	Clear and color-less	Normal
Cell count (mm^3)	26	Increased
RBC	Negative	Normal
WBC (mm^3)	26	Increased
Lymphocytes (mm^3)	26	Increased
Granulocytes (mm^3)	0	Normal
Glucose (mg/dL)	52	Normal
VDRL	Nonreactive	Normal
Culture	No organisms	Normal
Total protein (mg/dL)	55	Slight increase
Albumin (mg/dL)	21	Normal
IgG (mg/dL)	6.6	Increased
Oligoclonal bands	4	Abnormal
Myelin basic protein (ng/mL)	wk pos (4–0)	Abnormal
IgG synthesis rate (mg/24 hr)	5.7	Increased
Calculated Results		
IgG index	1.7	Increased
Albumin index	4.0	Normal

Questions

1. What do the CSF oligoclonal bands and increased IgG index and IgG synthesis rate indicate?
2. What is a likely tentative diagnosis for this patient?
3. Does patient history correlate with the diagnosis?
4. Has the patient had a recent active episode?
5. What would be another diagnostic test to help confirm the diagnosis?

Discussion

1. These test results point to de novo IgG synthesis in the CSF of the patient. Leakage in the BBB is ruled out by the CSF cell count (no RBCs), appearance of the CSF (no xanthochromia), and a normal albumin index.
2. MS may be likely.
3. The patient's history supports the diagnosis. She has been living in a geographic area where incidence of MS is high, and her symptoms worsened after the pregnancy. Her symptoms (generalized fatigue, progressive weakness in both arms and legs, blurring of vision) are common to MS.
4. The weakly positive MBP indicates an active episode more than 1 week old, consistent with recovery from a flare-up of MS or a slow demyelination.
5. A CT scan and identification of lesions consistent with MS would be helpful in diagnosis.

References

1. Adams RD, Victor M: Principles of Neurology, ed 5. New York, McGraw–Hill, 1993.
2. Larson EB, Reifler BV, Sumi SM, et al: Diagnostic tests in the evaluation of dementia: A prospective study of 200 elderly patients. Arch Intern Med 146:1917–1922, 1986.
3. National Organization of Rare Diseases Data Base 158. Fairfield, Conn, 1995.
4. Baker AB, Baker LH (eds): Clinical Neurology. New York, Harper and Row, 1984.
5. Williams A, Papadopoulos N, Chase T: Demonstration of CSF gamma-globulin banding in presenile dementia. Neurology 30:822–884, 1980.
6. Kandel ER, Swartz JH: Principles of Neural Science, ed 2. New York, Elsevier Science Publishing, 1985.
7. Merritt HH: Textbook of Neurology, ed 6. Philadelphia, Lea & Febiger, 1979.
8. Zerr I, Bodemer M, Racker S, et al: Cerebrospinal fluid concentration of neuron-specific enolase in diagnosis of Creutzfeldt-Jakob disease. Lancet 345:1609–1610, 1995.
9. Kremer B, Goldberg P, Andrew SE, et al: A worldwide study of Huntington's disease mutation: The sensitivity and specificity of measuring CAG repeats. N Engl J Med 330:1401–1406, 1994.
10. National Organization of Rare Disorders Data Base 511. Fairfield, Conn, 1995.
11. Collins DR: Illustrated Manual of Neurologic Diagnosis, ed 2. Philadelphia, JB Lippincott, 1982.
12. Price SA, Wilson LM: Pathophysiology: Clinical Concepts of Disease Processes, ed 3. New York, McGraw–Hill, 1986.
13. Simone IL, Annunziata P, Maimone D, et al: Serum and CSF anti-GMI antibodies in patients with Guillain-Barré syndrome and chronic inflammatory demyelinating polyneuropathy. J Neurol Sci 114:49–55, 1993.
14. Cohen B, Mitsumoto H: Neuropathy syndromes associated with antibodies against the peripheral nerves. Lab Med 26:459–463, 1995.
15. Specialty Laboratories: Laboratory report form and update: Neurooncology and neuroimmunology come of age. Los Angeles, Specialty Laboratories, 1987.
16. Wintrobe M (ed): Harrison's Principles of Internal Medicine, ed 6. Philadelphia, JB Lippincott, 1982.
17. Bentz J: Laboratory investigation of multiple sclerosis. Lab Med 26:393–399, 1995.
18. Stahlheber PA, Peter JB: Multiple sclerosis: A clearer path to a complex diagnosis. Diagn Med 1:43–48, 1984.
19. Bioscience Laboratories: Assay Update: Oligoclonal gammaglobulins in CSF by agarose electrophoresis. Van Nuys, Calif, Bioscience Laboratories, 1986.
20. Bioscience Laboratories: Assay Update: Myelin basic protein. Van Nuys, Calif, Bioscience Laboratories, 1986.
21. National Organization of Rare Diseases Data Base 2313. Fairfield, Conn, 1995.
22. Kaplan LA, Pesce AJ: Clinical Chemistry: Theory, Analysis, and Correlation. St Louis, CV Mosby, 1984.
23. National Organization of Rare Diseases Data Base 2214. Fairfield, Conn, 1995.
24. Miale J: Laboratory Medicine Hematology, ed 6. St Louis, CV Mosby, 1982.
25. Brady RO, Kolodney EH: Sphingolipid storage disorders: Diagnosis and detection. Lab Manage 7:27–37, 1982.
26. National Organization of Rare Diseases Data Base 444. Fairfield, Conn, 1995.
27. Bayever E, Kamari N, Ferreira P, et al: Bone marrow transplantation for Niemann-Pick type IA disease. J Inherit Metab Dis 15:919–928, 1992.
28. Paterson CC: The effect of cholesterol lowering agents on hepatic and plasma cholesterol in Niemann-Pick disease type C. Neurology 43:61–64, 1993.
29. National Organization of Rare Diseases Data Base 3018. Fairfield, Conn, 1995.
30. Bennington JL (ed): Saunders Encyclopedia and Dictionary of Laboratory Medicine and Technology. Philadelphia, WB Saunders, 1984.
31. Knight JA, Wu JY: Screening profile for detection of inherited metabolic disorders. Lab Med 13:681–687, 1982.

Bibliography

Bauer JD: Clinical Laboratory Methods, ed 9. St Louis, CV Mosby, 1982.

Graff L: Handbook of Routine Urinalysis. Philadelphia, JB Lippincott, 1983.

Henry JB (ed): Clinical Diagnosis and Management by Laboratory Methods, ed 17. Philadelphia, WB Saunders, 1984.

Robbins SH, Cotran RS: Pathologic Basis of Disease, ed 2. Philadelphia, WB Saunders, 1979.

Wintrobe M: Clinical Hematology, ed 7. Philadelphia, Lea & Febiger, 1974.

Chapter 39

Infectious Processes (Neurologic)

Maribeth L. Flaws

ACUTE MENINGITIS

Etiology and Pathophysiology

The term *meningitis* refers to an inflammation either of the leptomeninges or within the subarachnoid space, or both. Meningitis is always cerebrospinal, meaning that the disease involves both the brain and the spinal cord.

Acute meningitis has a short, relatively severe course and may be caused by a variety of infectious and noninfectious agents. When caused by bacteria, the disease is referred to as *bacterial meningitis. Aseptic meningitis* or *acute nonbacterial meningitis* is a milder form of meningitis in which routine bacteriologic culture techniques are unsuccessful. Most cases of aseptic meningitis are caused by viruses.

Bacterial Meningitis

Bacterial meningitis may be caused by a number of different pathogenic bacteria. The most common etiologic agents vary according to patient age group (Table 39–1).[1, 2] In general, the bacteria causing acute bacterial meningitis are encapsulated, with the capsule serving to protect the organisms from phagocytosis by host leukocytes.

The three most common etiologic agents of acute bacterial meningitis are *Haemophilus influenzae* (45% of reported cases), *Streptococcus pneumoniae* (18% of cases), and *Neisseria meningitidis* (14% of cases),[1] although the exact incidence of each organism varies according to the geographic location and patient population of the reported study.[3] Other organisms that may cause bacterial meningitis are *S. agalactiae* (group B streptococci), *Listeria monocytogenes*, and gram-negative bacilli.

Neonatal meningitis is most often caused by colonization of the maternal genital tract by species of bacteria at the time of birth. Neonates have the highest prevalence of meningitis and the highest mortality rate.[4]

Ninety-five percent of all cases of meningitis in the United States occur in children 1 to 6 years of age.[4] Meningitis in this age group is most often due to *H. influenzae* type b, which tends to cause meningitis during the time when the child no longer has maternal antibodies to this organism and has not yet produced antibodies to antigenically similar bacteria.[4] Meningitis caused by *H. influenzae* type b in children 1 to 6 years of age can be prevented if the children are vaccinated.

The most common causes of bacterial meningitis in previously healthy adults are pneumococci and meningococci. In young adults, outbreaks of meningococcal meningitis are commonly associated with crowded conditions, such as military barracks and college dormitories, and occur among individuals lacking antibody to *N. meningitidis*. Serogroups A and C are most often associated with epidemics of meningococcal meningitis, whereas serogroup

Table 39–1. Etiologic Agents of Acute Bacterial Meningitis

Patient Age or Clinical Group	Organism(s)	CSF Morphology on Gram Stain	Route of Entry
Newborn	*Streptococcus agalactiae* (group B streptococci)	Gram-positive cocci	Direct invasion of flora from the mother during vaginal delivery
	Enteric gram-negative bacilli (especially *Escherichia coli*)	Gram-negative bacilli	
	Listeria monocytogenes	Gram-positive coccobacilli	
Infant and young child	*Haemophilus influenzae*	Gram-negative coccobacilli or short rods with rounded ends	Associated with otitis media, pneumonia, and epiglottitis
	Neisseria meningitidis	Gram-negative diplococci	Acquired via the respiratory tract; colonizes the nasopharynx and invades the blood stream
	S. pneumoniae	"Lancet-shaped," gram-positive cocci	May spread via the blood stream or as an extension of infection from the sinuses or middle ear
Young adult	*N. meningitidis*	Gram-negative diplococci	Acquired via the respiratory tract; colonizes the nasopharynx and invades the blood stream
Middle-aged and elderly	*S. pneumoniae*	"Lancet-shaped," gram-positive cocci	May spread via the blood stream or as an extension of infection from the sinuses or middle ear
	Gram-negative bacilli (mostly *E. coli*)	Gram-negative bacilli	—
Association with head trauma or surgery	*Staphylococcus aureus*	Gram-positive cocci	Accidental or surgical penetrations of the skull
	Gram-negative bacilli	Gram-negative bacilli	

B is the principal cause of sporadic cases.[5] Conditions such as immunosuppression, alcoholism, splenectomy, sickle cell disease, diabetes mellitus, and intracranial shunts increase the risk of developing meningitis at any age.

Aseptic Meningitis

The term *aseptic meningitis* was originally used to describe a disease characterized by an acute onset, meningeal symptoms, fever, increased leukocytes in the cerebrospinal fluid (CSF), and, most important, bacteriologically sterile CSF cultures. Today, it is known that aseptic meningitis is a condition of multiple etiologies, including both infectious and noninfectious agents.

INFECTIOUS AGENTS CAUSING ASEPTIC MENINGITIS

Although the vast majority of cases of aseptic meningitis are caused by viruses, this disease may also be caused by bacteria (e.g., *Mycobacterium tuberculosis, Treponema pallidum*), protozoa (e.g., *Naegleria fowleri*), and fungi (e.g., *Candida albicans, Cryptococcus neoformans, Coccidioides immitis*). The majority of these etiologic agents are not detected when routine CSF culture protocols are used.

The list of viruses that can produce aseptic meningitis is lengthy and includes enteroviruses (echoviruses, coxsackieviruses), herpesviruses (herpes simplex I and II, cytomegalovirus, Epstein-Barr virus), mumps virus, a number of arboviruses, hepatitis viruses, measles virus, adenoviruses, and lymphocytic choriomeningitis virus.[6, 7] Free-living amebic protozoa, such as *N. fowleri* and *Acanthamoeba* species, can cause primary amebic meningoencephalitis, an inflammation of both the brain and the meninges.

Microorganisms may gain access to the central nervous system (CNS) in any of several ways. The most common means is hematogenously, by incompletely understood mechanisms. The microorganisms may also gain access via CSF shunts or by direct inoculation following trauma to the head or a neurosurgical procedure. Some viruses are capable of entering the CNS along neural pathways (e.g., herpes simplex) or via the olfactory tract (e.g., adenoviruses). Free-living amebae may enter via the nasal mucosa and olfactory nerve following swimming or diving in contaminated freshwater ponds or lakes. Meningitis can also result from a ruptured or leaking brain abscess.

When local defense and clearance mechanisms are unable to eliminate the invading microorganisms, an infectious process develops, with inflammation, tissue necrosis, and vasculitis. The resulting hypoxia, edema, and impairment of CSF flow can result in increased intracranial pressure and impaired neurologic function.

NONINFECTIOUS AGENTS CAUSING ASEPTIC MENINGITIS

Noninfectious causes of aseptic meningitis include tumors,[8] chemical agents (e.g., contrast agents for radiographic studies, chemotherapeutic agents,[9] and local anesthetics), or material released into the subarachnoid space from cutaneous or noncutaneous cysts. Aseptic meningitis may also accompany such noninfectious disorders as sarcoidosis and systemic lupus erythematosus (SLE).

Clinical Manifestations

The initial symptoms experienced by the patient with acute meningitis are chills, fever, lethargy, stiff neck, and a severe headache. Depending on the origin of the infection, the patient may also experience symptoms associated with pneumonia, sinusitis, or otitis media. With increased hypoxia and intracranial pressure, the headache may become more severe, vomiting may occur, and there is evidence of neurologic dysfunction (e.g., photophobia, confusion, drowsiness, stupor, coma, occasionally convulsions). Attempts by the physician to flex the patient's stiff neck forward causes flexion at the hips and knees (Brudzinski's sign), resulting in neck and lower back pain. Another sign of meningeal irritation is Kernig's sign, or the inability to completely extend the legs.[2]

In the elderly, debilitated, or immunosuppressed patient, the only symptom of meningitis may be a change in mental status. It may manifest as confusion, agitation, disorientation, or coma.[2]

Skin lesions (rash) occur in approximately 50% of cases of meningococcal meningitis,[10] a disease that can have a fulminant course and can cause death within a matter of hours. Rashes are also common in coxsackievirus and echovirus infections. A diagnosis of meningitis is somewhat difficult to establish in infants; therefore, a tentative diagnosis of meningitis must be considered in any infant with temperature instability, respiratory difficulties, or feeding problems.[11]

Laboratory Analyses and Diagnosis

If the physician suspects that the patient has bacterial meningitis, a CSF specimen is required for a definitive diagnosis of the etiologic agent. A CSF sample is obtained by lumbar puncture, and ideally, three to four tubes of fluid should be collected and sent promptly to the laboratory. When the CSF pressure is high, however, lumbar puncture is particularly hazardous and can result in brain herniation. Thus, a computed tomographic (CT) scan should first be performed to rule out a mass lesion such as a brain abscess.[12]

The seriousness of acute bacterial meningitis and other CNS infections cannot be overemphasized. Every effort must be made to process the CSF specimen as quickly as possible. Untreated bacterial meningitis is devastating and rapidly fatal. Ideally, it should never take longer than 1 hour for presumptive diagnosis and initiation of treatment for this disease. A detailed discussion of the differential diagnosis of acute meningitis is described by Cunha.[13]

The traditional laboratory evaluation of a CSF specimen consists of a gross examination (color and turbidity), analyses of the protein and glucose concentrations (tube 1), culture and Gram stain of the sediment following centrifugation of the specimen (tube 2), as well as a total leukocyte count of the uncentrifuged specimen and a differential count of the resuspended sediment following centrifugation (tube 3). Additional tests may be helpful, as described later. Blood specimens should also be sent to the laboratory for culture and for a complete blood count and differential count.

Results of each of the various laboratory analyses useful in the diagnosis of CNS infections must be communicated to the physician as soon as they become available, even if it is necessary to provide this information in a piecemeal manner.

Of the procedures listed in Table 39–2, culturing of CSF and blood and the microscopic examination of the gram-stained sediment are the most useful in acute bacterial meningitis. The results of the latter procedure can be available shortly after collection of the specimen. Because infected CSF usually contains only small numbers of microorganisms, some type of concentration procedure (e.g., centrifugation or filtration) must be performed prior to culturing the specimen or preparation of a smear for staining. Failure to observe bacteria in the gram-stained smear or to culture bacteria does *not* rule out bacterial etiology. The organisms may be too few in number to be observed microscopically, and prior antibiotic therapy may prevent the bacteria from being cultured from CSF or blood.

False-positive Gram stain results may be due to the presence of nonviable bacteria either in the collection tubes

Table 39–2. Results of Traditional CSF Laboratory Tests in Acute Meningitis			
Laboratory Test	**Normal Result**	**Acute Bacterial (Septic) Meningitis**	**Aseptic Meningitis**
Pressure	<140 mm H$_2$O (recumbent position)	Increased	Normal or increased
Gross examination	Clear	Usually turbid	Clear or slightly turbid (CSF may be clear and yet contain as many as 300 to 400 cells/mm^3)
Gram stain of sediment	Sterile	Bacterial commonly observed; Gram stain reaction and morphology useful in tentative identification	
Culture	Negative	Positive in 70%–80% of cases	Viral, fungal, or acid-fast bacillus cultures may be positive
Blood culture	Negative	Positive in 40%–60% of cases of meningococcal, pneumococcal, or *Haemophilus influenzae* meningitis	
Total leukocyte count	<5 cells/mm^3	Generally >1000 cells/mm^3 (av. = 5,000–20,000/mm^3)	Generally <1000/mm^3 (usually 10–100/mm^3), but can be 3000/mm^3 or even higher
Predominant leukocyte type	All lymphocytes	>90% polymorphonuclear leukocytes	Usually >75% mononuclear
Glucose concentration	50–80 mg/dL (or >50% concomitant serum glucose level)	Decreased (<50% of serum level)	Normal
Protein concentration	15–45 mg/dL	Increased (>100 mg/dL); usually 150–500 mg/dL	Normal to increased

or on the microscope slides, or of viable organisms present in the staining reagents. Thus, great care must be taken in interpretation of gram-stained CSF, and the suspected organism should be consistent with patient history and age and other laboratory findings. Whenever only a single specimen container is submitted to the laboratory, it must first be processed by the microbiology section to prevent contamination of the CSF specimen in other sections of the laboratory.

Because they can be destroyed by centrifugation, motile amebae (*Naegleria* or *Acanthamoeba*) are best observed by examining a drop of fresh, uncentrifuged CSF by wet mount, using either a phase-contrast or a bright-field microscope.[5] Whenever *C. neoformans* is suspected, a drop of CSF sediment should be examined in an India ink preparation or, alternatively, should be tested by latex agglutination for the presence of cryptococcal antigens. Because these organisms may be sparse in CSF specimens, appropriate culture media should also be inoculated. An acid-fast stain should be performed when mycobacteria are suspected, and when deemed appropriate, CSF specimens should be cultured for anaerobes, fungi, and mycobacteria in addition to nonanaerobic bacteria.

Whenever viral meningitis is suspected, a variety of specimens (e.g., stool, urine, saliva, throat washings, CSF) should be submitted to the laboratory for culture, as well as acute and convalescent serum samples for serologic studies. In most cases of viral meningitis, the agent is not isolated from CSF (exceptions include mumps virus) or blood.[14] The CSF can be examined for viral antigen using either fluorescein-labeled antibody or immunoenzymatic methods.

Other Traditional Laboratory Tests

In acute aseptic meningitis, which is usually due to viral infection, the total CSF cell count is usually less than 1000 per mm³, and mononuclear cells are the predominant cell type; however, during the first 24 to 48 hours of infection, the predominant cell type can be polymorphonuclear leukocytes (PMNs), as in bacterial meningitis.[11] It is also important to remember that one-third of the cases of tuberculosis and viral meningitis will show a predominance of PMNs, and approximately 10% of the cases of bacterial meningitis will have greater than 80% lymphocytes.[5] Thus, the often quoted distinctions between bacterial and viral meningitis are not always clear cut.

Blood leukocyte (white blood cell; WBC) counts are usually elevated in acute bacterial meningitis, with a shift to the left. Although the WBC count is usually normal in viral meningitis, leukopenia can be present in about one-third of patients.[14]

Although the CSF glucose concentration is usually normal in aseptic meningitis, certain viral meningitides can be associated with decreased values, as found in bacterial meningitis.[11, 14]

Additional Procedures of Value in the Diagnosis of Acute Meningitis

A number of additional laboratory procedures performed on CSF are available as adjuncts in the diagnosis of acute meningitis. They are agglutination procedures for the detection of bacterial and fungal antigens; lactic acid and lactate dehydrogenase (LD) determinations; and assays for the detection of endotoxin.

Latex agglutination procedures are available for the detection of *S. pneumoniae*, *H. influenzae* type b, *S. agalactiae*, and *N. meningitidis* groups A, B, C, W135, and Y in CSF, urine, and serum specimens. These procedures are commonly of greater value than the Gram stain in establishing a rapid presumptive diagnosis. A latex agglutination procedure is also available for the detection of cryptococcal antigen.

Reference values for CSF lactate are 1.1 to 2.4 mmol/L.[15] Levels of CSF lactic acid in excess of 10 mmol/L have been reported to be associated with bacterial meningitis, although both false-negative and false-positive results occur.[13] Levels lower than 3 mmol/L suggest nonbacterial meningitis.[13] Levels between 3 and 6 mmol/L are difficult to interpret, because they may have many causes, including the presence of red blood cells (RBCs).[13]

Increased levels of LD isoenzymes have been reported to occur in the majority of cases of bacterial meningitis, with mean values of 113 units for isoenzymes 4 and 5 (normal range, 2–7 units).[10] In viral meningitis, the average level is 23 units, and the isoenzymes consist mainly of fractions 1 and 2.[10]

The limulus lysate test, which involves the use of amebocytes from the horseshoe crab, is capable of detecting endotoxin in CSF, thus indicating the involvement of a gram-negative pathogen.[1] Although both false-positive and false-negative results occur,[14] this test is a sensitive adjunct in the diagnosis of meningitis caused by such agents as *Escherichia coli*, *H. influenzae*, and *N. meningitidis*.[1]

Treatment

Specific treatment of acute meningitis depends on its cause. Bacterial, fungal, and protozoal pathogens are treated with appropriate antimicrobial agents, and whenever possible and appropriate, the selection of agent is based on the results of antimicrobial susceptibility testing. Prior to the availability of susceptibility results, empirical treatment may be necessary, with the selection of agent being based on gram stain, India ink, or antigen detection results. For the empirical treatment of neonatal meningitis, a penicillin combined with an aminoglycoside or cefotaxime is commonly used.[16] In general, any drug selected must be effective against the organism, must be capable of crossing the blood-brain barrier, and must be administered in an appropriate dose and by an appropriate route (usually intravenously).

Drugs used successfully to treat bacterial meningitis include penicillin or ampicillin (*S. pneumoniae* and *N. meningitidis*), third-generation cephalosporins plus ampicillin (*H. influenzae, L. monocytogenes, E. coli*), and a third-generation cephalosporin or chloramphenicol (*H. influenzae*).[13] Because of possible infection with resistant strains of *H. influenzae*, children should be treated with both chloramphenicol and ampicillin until the results of culture and susceptibility tests are known.[13]

Supportive therapy may include intracranial pressure

monitoring, steroids, fluid replacement, and bedrest. Patients are usually monitored by direct observation rather than by laboratory analysis of any convalescent specimens. Repeat lumbar punctures are usually not necessary, unless the patient's clinical response is atypical.

CHRONIC MENINGITIS

Etiology and Pathophysiology

Chronic meningitides develop more slowly and tend to be less dramatic than the acute types. By definition, clinical or CSF abnormalities must have lasted at least 4 weeks before the diagnosis of chronic meningitis can be made.

Most cases of chronic meningitis are caused by slowly growing microorganisms such as *M. tuberculosis*, other mycobacteria, fungi (e.g., *C. neoformans, Histoplasma capsulatum*), *Nocardia* species, *Borrelia burgdorferi*, and *T. pallidum* (neurosyphilis). Other microorganisms that can cause chronic meningitis are *Leptospira, Toxoplasma gondii, Brucella*, and *Taenia solium* (cysticercosis).

Patients most apt to develop chronic meningitis are those who are immunosuppressed and those with diseases such as histoplasmosis, syphilis, tuberculosis, and brucellosis. Most of the etiologic agents of chronic meningitis gain access to the CNS by the same routes as the agents associated with acute meningitis. Exceptions are the leptospires, which apparently can penetrate tissues mechanically, and intracellular organisms that can be transported via the blood within phagocytic leukocytes.[11]

Humans acquire cysticercosis by ingesting *T. solium* eggs. After the eggs hatch in the stomach and duodenum, oncospheres penetrate the intestinal epithelium, enter the lymphatic and vascular systems, and are carried to many different locations in the body. Approximately 60% of patients with cysticercosis have cysticerci in their brains, and of these, approximately 50% develop symptoms.[17]

Clinical Manifestations

In chronic meningitis, the disease progression is slow, and the patient experiences few, if any, symptoms that give an indication of the seriousness of the disease. Personality changes, altered levels of consciousness, and headaches may occur, although they tend to be much less severe than those associated with acute bacterial meningitis. Nausea and vomiting, together with the headaches and other symptoms resulting from increased intracranial pressure, may resemble the symptoms associated with the development of a tumor. Hydrocephalus and cerebral edema may cause a sudden deterioration of neurologic function. About half of patients with neurocysticercosis have meningeal cysts and the signs and symptoms of chronic meningitis, including intense inflammation, obstructive hydrocephalus, arterial thrombosis, and stroke.[17]

Laboratory Analyses and Diagnosis

Whereas examination of CSF in acute meningitis can be diagnostic, such is usually not the case in chronic meningitis. An evaluation of CSF may be suggestive, however (Table 39–3), and rapid processing of the specimen

Table 39–3. Results of Traditional CSF Laboratory Tests in Chronic Meningitis*	
Laboratory Test	**Result**
Pressure	Normal to increased
Gross examination	Often clear; at least 200 leukocytes/mm³ are required to cause slight turbidity
Gram stain of sediment	Rare spherules of *Coccidioides immitis* may be present
Acid-fast bacillus stain of sediment	Positive in 10%–22% of cases of tuberculous meningitis
India ink preparation of sediment	Round, encapsulated, sometimes budding yeast in >50% of cases of cryptococcal meningitis
Culture	Positive in 33%–50% of cases of coccidioidal meningitis; in >75% of cases of cryptococcal meningitis; in 38%–88% of cass of tuberculous meningitis
Total leukocyte count	Generally 1000/mm³
Predominant leukocyte type	Mononuclear
Glucose concentration	Usually decreased
Protein concentration	Increased (often markedly)

*Reference values are shown in Table 39–2.

and expeditious correlation, interpretation, and reporting of results are critical.

A history of diseases such as tuberculosis and syphilis can be helpful in establishing a diagnosis and can serve to guide the clinical laboratory scientist in the selection of appropriate media, stains, and other laboratory procedures. The CSF should always be cultured and examined using appropriate staining techniques. A cytologic examination of the sediment can help rule out the possibility of a tumor.

An India ink preparation can demonstrate the presence of *C. neoformans*. Serum and CSF should be tested for the presence of cryptococcal and coccidioidal antigens and antitreponemal antibodies. Owing to the blood-brain barrier, normal serum-CSF antibody ratios are greater than 200.[11] Lower ratios usually indicate either that the blood-brain barrier has been injured or altered in some way, or that synthesis of antibody has occurred within the central nervous system (CNS). Thus a serum-CSF ratio of less than 200 for a given etiologic agent may indicate CNS infection by that agent. As with infections not involving the CNS, identification of an etiologic agent may also be made by demonstrating a rise in specific antibody titers in acute and convalescent serum specimens.

The diagnosis of neurocysticercosis may be made by a combination of CT scanning and radiography, antibody detection in CSF or serum, peripheral blood eosinophilia, and the presence of eosinophils in the CSF.

Treatment

As with acute meningitis, antimicrobial therapy for chronic meningitis depends on the specific etiologic agent involved. The same considerations with respect to effectiveness against the pathogen, ability to cross the blood-brain barrier, dosage, and route apply in the treatment of chronic meningitis. Although surgical intervention may be necessary, the investigational drug praziquantel is sometimes used successfully in the treatment of neurocysticercosis,[17, 18] either alone or in combination with albendazole or cimetidine.[18] Praziquantel crosses the blood-brain barrier and kills cysticerci but apparently does not affect calcified cysts and, thus, does not always alleviate the patient's signs and symptoms.[17] For cryptococcal meningitis, amphotericin B, usually in combination with flucytosine, is recommended.[19] In general, the prognosis for chronic meningitis depends on the specific pathogen involved, the extent of the damage, and the susceptibility of the etiologic agent to the drugs used.

FOCAL SUPPURATIVE LESIONS
Etiology and Pathophysiology

Brain abscesses, subdural empyema, and epidural abscesses are examples of focal suppurative lesions and are associated with the production of pus. All are medical and surgical emergencies that can cause death or permanent neurologic deficit. The key to their successful treatment is early diagnosis.

The dura or dura mater is the outermost of the three membranes (meninges) covering the brain and spinal cord, and is the toughest and most fibrous of the three. The term *epidural* refers to the area between the dura and the skull, whereas *subdural* refers to the potential space between the dura and the arachnoid (the membrane located between the dura mater and the pia mater). The only actual meningeal compartment within the skull under normal conditions is the subarachnoid space.[20] Of the three types of focal suppurative lesions, brain abscesses (located within the brain parenchyma) are by far the most common.

Brain Abscess

Brain abscesses can be caused by bacteria, fungi, or parasites (Tables 39–4 and 39–5). Most cases of brain abscess are secondary to infection in some other area(s) of the body. Thus, microorganisms involved in the abscess are those causing the underlying or initial infection. Such infections are commonly polymicrobial and often contain anaerobes in addition to other types of bacteria.

The microorganisms listed in Tables 39–4 and 39–5 may gain access to the brain in any of several ways. They may travel from an original site of infection to the brain either by direct extension of the infection (e.g., from the sinuses or middle ear) or by the circulatory system from virtually any body site, most commonly from lung infections such as pneumonia, bronchiectasis, and abscesses, as well as heart infections such as endocarditis. Another method by which microorganisms gain access to the brain is by direct inoculation during or following some type of trauma (e.g., neurosurgical procedure, automobile accident, gunshot wound).[21, 22]

Subdural Empyema and Epidural Abscess

Subdural empyemas and epidural abscesses are focal collections of suppurative material that differ mainly in their anatomic location.[20] A subdural empyema is located in the potential space between the dura mater and the

Table 39–4. Examples of Bacterial Etiologic Agents of Brain Abscesses

Underlying Infection or Event	Microorganisms Likely to Be Involved
Chronic sinusitis	Anaerobes (e.g., *Bacteroides fragilis*, anaerobic gram-positive cocci) *Haemophilus influenzae* *Staphylococcus aureus* *Streptococcus pneumoniae* Other streptococci Enterobacteriaceae
Ear infection (otitis media)	Anaerobes (e.g., *B. fragilis*, anaerobic gram-positive cocci) Enterobacteriaceae Streptococci
Dental sepsis	Polymicrobic, involving *Fusobacterium* and *Bacteroides* species, anaerobic gram-positive cocci
Lung infection	Streptococci *Fusobacterium* species *Bacteroides* species, occasionally *Nocardia* or *Actinomyces* species
Endocarditis	*S. aureus* Streptococci
Congenital heart problems	Streptococci (including the viridans group) Anaerobic gram-positive cocci *Haemophilus* species
Intra-abdominal infection	Enterobacteriaceae Anaerobes
Trauma to head (e.g., skull fracture, bullet wound, neurosurgery)	*S. aureus* Streptococci Enterobacteriaceae *Clostridium* species

Data from Austin TW: Infections of the central nervous system. *In* Mandell LA, Ralph ED (eds): Essentials of Infectious Disease. Boston, Blackwell Scientific, 1985; and Scheld WM, Winn HR: Brain abscess. *In* Mandell GL, Douglas RG, Bennett JE (eds): Principles and Practice of Infectious Diseases. New York, John Wiley & Sons, 1985.

arachnoid, whereas an epidural abscess is localized between the dura mater and the skull or in the epidural space of the spinal canal. The two conditions commonly coexist in the same patient.

Subdural empyemas and epidural abscesses are essentially identical with respect to etiology, epidemiology, and pathophysiology. A variety of bacteria may be associated with these conditions, including streptococci (about 35%

Table 39–5. Examples of Fungal and Parasitic Etiologic Agents of Brain Abscesses

Fungi	Parasites
Aspergillus species	*Strongyloides stercoralis*
Mucor species	*Entamoeba histolytica*
Candida species	*Schistosoma japonicum*
Cryptococcus neoformans	*Paragonimus* species
Coccidioides immitis	*Toxoplasma gondii*
Curvularia species	*Taenia solium* (cysticercosis)
Blastomyces dermatitidis	
Histoplasma capsulatum (rarely)	

Data from Scheld WM, Winn HR: Brain abscess. *In* Mandell GL, Douglas RG, Bennett JE (eds): Principles and Practice of Infectious Diseases. New York, John Wiley & Sons, 1985.

of cases of subdural empyema[23]), anaerobic gram-positive cocci, Enterobacteriaceae, *Bacteroides fragilis, Staphylococcus aureus* (17% of cases of subdural empyema[23]; 60% to 90% of cases of epidural abscess[24]), *S. pneumoniae, H. influenzae,* and *Pseudomonas aeruginosa.* Anaerobes are isolated in 33% to 100% of cases of subdural empyema.[23] *M. tuberculosis* may be a cause of epidural abscess. Polymicrobial infections are quite common in subdural empyema and occur in approximately 10% of cases of epidural abscess.[24]

As with brain abscesses, the etiologic agents gain access to the area by direct extension, hematogenous spread, or direct inoculation. Most cases of subdural empyema are secondary to infections involving the paranasal sinuses, middle ear, or mastoid.[22] Intracranial epidural abscesses almost always originate from frontal sinusitis, mastoiditis, or craniotomies.[22] Spinal epidural abscess may follow a penetrating injury, back surgery, lumbar puncture, or epidural anesthesia.

Clinical Manifestations

Brain Abscess

The signs and symptoms of brain abscess are the combined result of increased intracranial pressure and the particular site of brain tissue damage. Generalized or localized headaches occur and are often severe. Other symptoms are nausea, vomiting, changes in mental status, and, sometimes, coma. Depending on the site of tissue destruction, seizures and visual disorders may occur. Additional symptoms relate to the specific underlying infection. It is possible for a brain abscess to rupture into the subarachnoid space, producing a severe meningitis with a high mortality rate.

Subdural Empyema and Epidural Abscess

Symptoms of subdural empyema and cranial epidural abscess consist of fever and headaches, the latter being initially localized in the area of involvement. Increased intracranial pressure may cause vomiting, papilledema, seizures, focal neurologic dysfunction, and some decrease in mental status. Progression of the disease can lead to extensive neurologic damage, stupor, and coma. Additional symptomatology relates to the underlying condition, if any, such as chronic sinusitis and mastoiditis. The conditions that need to be distinguished clinically from subdural empyema are cerebral thrombophlebitis, which is a common associated finding, brain abscess, acute hemorrhagic leukoencephalitis, and acute viral (inclusion body) encephalitis.

The most common symptoms of spinal epidural abscesses are headache, fever, spinal pain and tenderness, progressive weakness of the legs, and urinary retention or incontinence. The differential diagnosis includes transverse myelitis, acute disk herniation, and compression of the spinal cord by tumor.

Laboratory Analyses and Diagnosis

Brain Abscess

Clinical laboratory techniques are of less value in the diagnosis of brain abscess than of meningitis. Routine blood and urine tests are seldom helpful. The collection of CSF is potentially dangerous in patients with brain abscess, increased intracranial pressure, and papilledema. Lumbar puncture is not routinely done, therefore, both because it may precipitate brain herniation and death, and because normal CSF findings do not exclude the diagnosis.

CT scans are of value, not only for diagnosis and to provide information about the size and site of the mass, but also for follow-up. Radionuclide brain scan or CT scan with contrast enhancement is more than 90% effective in identifying and localizing brain abscesses.[21] Cerebral arteriography may also be required to define the exact location of the lesion.

If CSF is obtained, it is processed rapidly, just as for the diagnosis of meningitis. The CSF results can be quite variable, ranging from essentially normal to quite abnormal. There may be a mild to moderate increase in pressure; some white blood cells may be present (generally fewer than 200 per mm³; predominantly mononuclear, although PMNs may also be present); protein may be mildly elevated; and glucose may be normal or reduced. Gram stains and CSF cultures are negative, unless the abscess is draining into the CSF in the subarachnoid space. Blood cultures are rarely positive. Possible hematologic findings are leukocytosis with some shift to the left, and an elevated sedimentation rate, but such findings are certainly not specific for brain abscess. As in suspected cases of meningitis, the clinical laboratory scientist should correlate and integrate the CSF results and should communicate them to the requesting physician as rapidly as possible. Material obtained from the abscess during surgery should be cultured for organisms likely to be etiologic agents.

Subdural Empyema and Epidural Abscess

As with brain abscesses, a lumbar puncture is potentially dangerous for the diagnosis of subdural empyema and epidural abscesses, because of the increased intracranial pressure. CT scanning, carotid arteriography, or angiography can delineate the involved area, and routine skull x-rays may show evidence of sinusitis or mastoiditis when either of these conditions is the predisposing cause. Blood cultures can be performed, although subdural empyema is rarely associated with bacteremia.

When examined, the CSF of a patient with subdural empyema shows increased pressure; cloudiness; an elevated WBC count (50–1000 per mm³) that includes both PMNs and lymphocytes; an elevated protein concentration (75–300 mg/dL); and a normal glucose concentration.[10] The CSF cultures are negative unless the subdural space became infected as a result of extension of bacteria from the CSF or from a brain abscess. The CSF from a patient with an epidural abscess is under normal pressure; is usually clear; may contain 20 to 100 lymphocytes and PMNs per mm³, and may have a slightly elevated protein concentration.[10] Cultures of the CSF are negative.

Treatment

Brain Abscess

Treatment for a brain abscess consists of immediate appropriate antimicrobial therapy (intravenous, high-dose).

Craniotomy may be performed to relieve the intracranial pressure and to drain as much infected material as possible.

Prior to receipt of the results of antimicrobial susceptibility testing, empirical therapy may be initiated, on the basis of knowledge of the microorganisms most likely to be involved in the underlying infection and the drugs capable of penetrating into the CNS. Because brain abscesses commonly are polymicrobic and include anaerobes, a combination of penicillin G and chloramphenicol (or metronidazole) is often used.[21] Nafcillin or methicillin may be used when staphylococci are suspected, or vancomycin if the staphylococcal organism is known to be methicillin-resistant.[21] Following treatment, the lesion can be monitored by CT scanning or radionuclide imaging.

In spite of treatment, the mortality rate for brain abscess is about 15% to 20%.[21] Furthermore, survivors commonly have residual paralysis or other equally severe CNS sequelae.

Subdural Empyema and Epidural Abscess

Treatment of subdural empyema and epidural abscess consists of surgical evacuation of the empyema, appropriate antimicrobial therapy, and steroids when intracranial pressure is elevated. *S. aureus* may be suspected in cases that occur following head trauma or surgery. These cases may be treated empirically until antimicrobial susceptibility tests are available. Samples taken at the time of surgery should be sent to the laboratory for aerobic and anaerobic culture and sensitivity testing.

The overall mortality rate for subdural empyema is approximately 14% to 18%,[23] and survivors have a high incidence of residual brain damage. If epidural abscesses are treated early, very few patients die and many have complete recovery. Delayed treatment in patients with spinal epidural abscesses may result in paraplegia.

ENCEPHALITIS

Etiology and Pathophysiology

Encephalitis is defined as inflammation of the brain parenchyma, the cells that make up the functional elements of the brain. Unlike brain abscesses, encephalitis is not confined to a specific site within the brain but, in fact, may be quite diffuse. *Meningoencephalitis* refers to inflammation of both the brain and the surrounding meninges; *encephalomyelitis* implies involvement of both the brain and the spinal cord; and *meningoencephalomyelitis* refers to inflammation of the meninges, brain, and spinal cord. Encephalitis may have a sudden onset (acute encephalitis) or there may be a slow, gradual progression of symptoms (chronic encephalitis).

Acute encephalitis may result from either infectious or noninfectious agents. The list of potential infectious agents is lengthy (Table 39–6), and includes viruses,[6] bacteria,[25, 26] fungi, protozoa, and helminths. Of these agents, arboviruses cause most cases of epidemic encephalitis.[27] Arboviral encephalitides of the United States include eastern and western equine encephalitis, St. Louis encephalitis, and California encephalitis. In each of these diseases, the viruses are transmitted to humans by mosquitoes. The most

Table 39–6. Potential Infectious Causes of Acute Encephalitis

Category	Examples
Viruses	Herpes simplex virus, arboviruses, enteroviruses, mumps virus, measles virus, rubella virus, rabies virus, varicella-zoster virus, adenoviruses
Bacteria	*Listeria, Brucella, Mycobacterium tuberculosis,* mycoplasmas, chlamydiae, rickettsiae (Rocky Mountain spotted fever; murine, epidemic, and scrub typhus), spirochetes (*Treponema pallidum, Leptospira,* and *Borrelia*)
Fungi	*Candida, Aspergillus, Cryptococcus, Histoplasma, Coccidioides*
Protozoa	*Toxoplasma, Plasmodium, Trypanosoma,* amebae (*Naegleria, Acanthamoeba*)
Helminths	*Taenia solium* (cysticercosis), *Trichinella spiralis,* schistosomes

Data from Austin TW: Infections of the central nervous system. *In* Mandell LA, Ralph ED (eds): Essentials of Infectious Diseases. Boston, Blackwell Scientific, 1985; and Mateos-Mora M, Ratzan KR: Acute viral encephalitis. *In* Schlossberg D (ed): Infections of the Nervous System. New York, Springer-Verlag, 1990.

common sporadic form of fatal encephalitis in North America is that caused by herpes simplex virus type I.[27]

Noninfectious causes of acute encephalitis include vasculitis, neoplasms, toxins, metabolic diseases, and hypersensitivity reactions. Demyelinating processes, probably representing allergic reactions, have occurred following rabies and smallpox vaccinations.

Chronic encephalitides, also called "slow" virus infections, may result from "conventional" viral diseases or may be due to "unconventional" acellular infectious agents called prions. The conventional diseases include subacute sclerosing panencephalitis (SSPE), also called inclusion body encephalitis, which is due to measles virus[28]; progressive multifocal leukoencephalopathy, due to a papovavirus; and progressive rubella encephalitis, due to a rubella virus. Mad cow disease, a spongiform encephalopathy found in cattle, is thought to be caused by *prions,* infectious agents that are smaller than traditional viruses. Prions are also thought by some authorities to cause two other "slow" virus infections, kuru and Creutzfeldt-Jakob disease.[29]

Some infectious agents gain direct access to the brain tissue via hematogenous spread or through peripheral nerves (e.g., herpes simplex virus, rabies virus).[30] Following their entry, these agents may cause focal or generalized infection. Other infectious agents are capable of causing encephalitis without actually invading the brain. For example, demyelination of nerve cells near veins occurs during certain viral infections, such as with measles, rubella, varicella-zoster and variola (smallpox) viruses. The demyelination process is thought to represent a hypersensitivity reaction, possibly being directed against myelin.[27]

The so-called slow virus diseases may result from ineffective host responses to the agents or from protection of the viruses or viral genomes from host responses by their location within host cells. No host response seems to be elicited against the prion agents that cause kuru and Creutzfeldt-Jakob disease. In these latter two diseases, the CNS lesions tend to be spongiform (vacuolation of the brain tissue, so that it resembles a sponge) rather than inflammatory or demyelinating. For this reason, these diseases are sometimes referred to as the subacute spongiform virus encephalopathies.

Clinical Manifestations

The signs and symptoms of encephalitis vary widely according to a number of factors, including the specific causative agent, the host response to the agent, and the area(s) of the brain affected. Illness can range from a mild headache and slight fever to an acute devastating disease with rapid progression to coma. Classic acute encephalitis involves sudden onset of fever, headache, stiff neck, and, frequently, changes in mental status.

Arbovirus infections are generally subclinical but can develop to clinically overt disease varying in severity. Herpes simplex infection may result in meningitis, focal encephalitis, mild diffuse encephalitis, or severe diffuse meningoencephalitis. Herpes simplex encephalitis tends to be a much more severe disease than herpes meningitis. Patients usually have headache, fever, and altered levels of consciousness. Seizures, the inability to smell (anosmia), speech defects, and hallucinations may also occur, depending on the area(s) of brain tissue involvement.

Laboratory Analyses and Diagnosis

Various radiologic and laboratory techniques are required to diagnose encephalitis definitively. Except for CSF examination, laboratory tests are of less value than procedures such as CT scanning, electroencephalography (EEG), and radionuclide (technetium) imaging. Electron microscopy of brain tissue may even be required to demonstrate the presence of viral particles.[28] Nevertheless, a lumbar puncture should be performed, because examination of CSF is an essential diagnostic procedure in encephalitis.[27]

Pressure may be normal or slightly elevated, and the CSF is clear or only slightly turbid. There is usually an increased leukocyte count ($<1000/mm^3$), with a predominance of mononuclear cells (lymphocytes). In early stages of viral encephalitis, PMNs may be the predominant cell type. In severe cases of herpes simplex or *Naegleria* encephalitis, in which tissue necrosis occurs, red blood cells ($>100/mm^3$) may be seen in addition to PMNs. It should be noted that, in all other forms of CNS infection, fewer than 100 red blood cells per mm^3 of CSF are observed, except in the event of "bloody" or traumatic spinal tap. Protein concentrations are slightly to moderately elevated, and glucose concentrations may be normal or reduced, depending on the etiologic agent. CSF glucose concentrations are usually reduced in bacterial infections and normal in viral infections; however, the glucose level can be reduced in lymphocytic choriomeningitis virus and mumps virus infections. Glucose levels are also low in tuberculosis, fungal, *Listeria*, and amebic infections. Occasional viral encephalitides show no CSF abnormalities, thus making the diagnosis more difficult.

Direct examination of the CSF by Gram stain, acid-fast stain, and India ink preparation may provide useful information, as may a wet preparation for amebae and Giemsa stain for trypanosomes. CSF and biopsy specimens should be cultured for bacteria, mycobacteria, fungi, and viruses. Because the viremia is usually brief and occurs prior to the onset of neurologic symptoms, viruses are rarely isolated from blood specimens.

Paired acute and convalescent serum samples and CSF specimens should be tested for increasing antibody titers. Most cases of epidemic viral encephalitis are diagnosed in this manner. Under normal conditions, the concentration of specific antibodies is about 200 times higher in serum than in CSF. The presence of antibodies to a particular pathogen (e.g., mumps virus, herpes virus, rubella virus, *T. pallidum*) in CSF in a concentration as high as or higher than in serum, with CSF protein only moderately elevated, indicates CNS infection due to that pathogen.[27] Microbial antigen detection procedures are often more sensitive than culture techniques.

Treatment

Supportive therapy, such as cardiorespiratory monitoring, intravenous fluids, adequate nutrition, fever control, and management of seizures, may be necessary for patients with viral encephalitis.[27]

Specific antimicrobial therapy depends on the etiologic agent. Acyclovir or vidarabine may be used to treat herpes simplex encephalitis.[27] Early administration of intravenous ribavirin has been successful in the treatment of SSPE caused by the measles virus.[28] At present, no specific treatment is available for the "slow" virus diseases.

INTRACRANIAL SHUNT INFECTIONS
Etiology and Pathophysiology

Intracranial shunts are plastic tubes that are used to drain CSF from the brain for the relief of hydrocephalus. These shunts are of two general types, ventriculoatrial and ventriculoperitoneal. The ventriculoatrial shunt drains CSF from a cerebral ventricle into a cardiac atrium, whereas the ventriculoperitoneal shunt drains the CSF into the peritoneal cavity.

Infections associated with these shunts are usually due to bacterial skin flora, such as coagulase-negative and coagulase-positive staphylococci. Other etiologic agents are Enterobacteriaceae and enterococci. In most cases of intracranial shunt infections, contamination probably occurred at the time of shunt insertion or replacement.

Clinical Manifestations

Approximately 10% to 30% of patients with shunts develop meningitis.[5] In addition to exhibiting the usual signs and symptoms of meningitis, such patients may present with extracranial symptoms that will relate to the site of CSF drainage. If the lower end of the shunt lies in a cardiac atrium, for example, the patient may show signs of endocarditis. A patient whose CSF is being drained into the peritoneal cavity may develop peritonitis. Fever is a common finding, and, if the shunt is malfunctioning, the patient may show signs of increased intracranial pressure.

Laboratory Analyses and Diagnosis

The most useful diagnostic procedure is a complete examination of the CSF, a specimen of which is collected either by lumbar puncture or percutaneously through the shunt reservoir. The CSF specimen should be processed, and results reported, as described for meningitis. Both blood and CSF should be cultured.

Treatment

Treatment consists of removal of the contaminated shunt in most cases, surgical intervention when necessary, and appropriate antimicrobial therapy. When replaced, the shunt is inserted at a site as far removed as possible from the site of infection.

NEUROLOGIC COMPLICATIONS OF ACQUIRED IMMUNODEFICIENCY SYNDROME

Etiology and Pathophysiology

The etiology and general pathophysiology of acquired immunodeficiency syndrome (AIDS) are described in Chapter 45. The etiologic agent, human immunodeficiency virus (HIV), is capable of invading T lymphocytes, resulting in adverse effects on the immunocompetence of the infected individual. Infection with HIV-1 can lead directly to neurologic damage by HIV itself or indirectly by opportunistic pathogens, neoplasms, or metabolic-nutritional disorders acquired as a result of the immunosuppression caused by HIV infection.[31–33] In fact, neurologic disease is one of the first manifestations of HIV infection and is an AIDS-defining condition.[31]

CT scanning of the brain in AIDS patients commonly shows a shrunken brain with larger than normal ventricles.[31, 32] Specimens obtained at autopsy reveal damage to both white and gray matter and vacuolar myelopathy, a vacuolization of the myelin tracts in the spinal cord.[31, 32] Immunologic staining procedures have revealed the presence of HIV antigen in neurologic tissue, the vast majority (95%) of which is located within multinucleated giant cells derived from macrophages.[31, 32] The multinucleated giant cells result from virus-induced cell fusion and are thought to be the pathologic hallmark of neurologic disease.[31, 32]

Mechanisms by which HIV-1 infection directly leads to encephalopathy are proposed to include the death or dysfunction of HIV-infected neurons; an HIV-induced alteration either in factors necessary for neuronal survival or in neurotransmitter production and release; and the release of cytokines, produced in response to HIV, that are toxic to neural cells.[31, 32] Some of the most common opportunistic pathogens causing neurologic disease in HIV-infected patients are *C. neoformans, M. tuberculosis, M. avium-intracellulare* complex, *T. pallidum, T. gondii*, cytomegalovirus, varicella-zoster virus, and progressive multifocal leukoencephalopathy due to papovavirus JC.[31–33]

Clinical Manifestations

Individuals infected with HIV may present with a variety of clinical manifestations, ranging from asymptomatic infection to severe immunodeficiency and life-threatening secondary infectious diseases or cancers. The Centers for Disease Control and Prevention (CDCP) has described a classification system that places AIDS patients with neurologic symptoms and no concurrent illness or condition that would explain the findings into Group IVB.[31] Neurologic symptoms often include dementia (a general mental deterioration), myelopathy (a disturbance or disease of the spinal cord), and peripheral neuropathy (a disorder affecting peripheral nerves).

Although the exact incidence of neurologic problems in AIDS patients is unknown, it has been estimated that as many as 60% develop dementia.[31, 32] Prior to the diagnosis of HIV infection, HIV-infected patients may present with an acute meningitis whose symptoms resemble those of infectious mononucleosis—sweats, nausea, vomiting, sore throat, fever, generalized lymphadenopathy, splenomegaly, and maculopapular rash.[31, 32] These symptoms appear approximately 3 to 6 weeks after exposure to HIV, but anti-HIV antibodies are not detectable until 8 to 12 weeks after exposure.[31, 32] Later in the progression of HIV infection, HIV encephalopathy occurs, in which patients complain of forgetfulness, inability to concentrate, mild confusion, and being mentally slow. Symptoms of HIV myelopathy, another neurologic manifestation, include leg weakness, an unsteady gait, poor coordination, and difficulty in writing, and the patient may become apathetic, withdrawn, agitated, or depressed.[31, 32]

Laboratory Analyses and Diagnosis

Many persons infected with HIV have circulating antibodies to the virus, and serologic procedures for the detection of these anti-HIV antibodies are commercially available. Seroconversion may not occur until 8 to 12 weeks after exposure to HIV, however, so tests for the detection of anti-HIV antibodies should be repeated if the initial results are negative in a patient with suspected HIV infection.[31] HIV-specific antibodies have also been detected in CSF specimens of AIDS patients, although these antibodies do not prevent neurologic disease.[31]

HIV has been isolated from CSF as well as from brain, spinal cord, and peripheral nerve tissue specimens of AIDS patients manifesting a variety of neurologic symptoms, including acute and chronic meningitis, dementia, subacute encephalitis, vacuolar myelopathy, and peripheral neuropathy.[31] In fact, the concentration of free, non–cell-associated HIV within the CSF is high.[31] It has been shown that there is intra–blood-brain barrier production of HIV-specific antibody, indicating infection by the virus within the blood-brain barrier. Thus, HIV appears to be directly involved in the pathogenesis of neurologic disease.[31]

In general, the diagnosis of neurologic disease directly due to HIV requires the exclusion of other causes of neurologic disease. Analysis of CSF from patients with acute meningitis and encephalopathy due to HIV usually reveals an increased protein level, mononuclear pleocytosis, and normal glucose levels, although these results are not diagnostic on their own.[31] HIV antigen and specific antibody are also detectable within the CSF of these patients. HIV encephalopathy is differentiated from acute meningitis on the basis of dementia, cognitive dysfunction, and depression experienced by the patient and by characteristic histology of the brain tissue, including the presence of multinucleate giant cells. Myelopathy is also diagnosed by excluding other causes, including the presence of a mass lesion or epidural abscess visualized by magnetic resonance imaging (MRI) of the spinal cord.

Diagnosis of the opportunistic pathogens causing neurologic disease in HIV-infected patients would be accomplished in the same manner as described earlier.

Treatment

The treatment of HIV infection is discussed in Chapters 45 and 58. Treatment of opportunistic pathogens causing neurologic disease in HIV-infected patients depends on the specific etiologic agent. Encephalitis caused by *T. gondii* can be treated with pyrimethamine and sulfadiazine. Fluconazole has been used for the treatment of cryptococcal meningitis. Standard antituberculosis drug regimens have been successful in treating meningitis due to *M. tuberculosis* in AIDS patients. There is some evidence that penicillin may not be sufficient for the treatment of neurosyphilis in immunocompromised patients. Finally, ganciclovir may have some efficacy against cytomegalovirus.[32]

Case Study 1[34]

A 65-year-old man suffering from confusion was brought to the emergency room by his wife. Five days earlier, he had complained of headache and malaise and had had a low-grade fever. These symptoms persisted, and the day before presentation, his wife noted intermittent confusion. The patient had a long history of recurrent sinusitis but had received no medicine during the previous month.

Physical examination revealed the patient to be stuporous and disoriented, with slight nuchal rigidity. He had a temperature of 39 °C, and a pulse rate of 110 beats/min. Respiration rate and blood pressure were normal, as were the remaining findings of the general physical examination. Neurologic examination revealed a slight drift of the left arm and leg, hemianopia (loss of vision for one-half of the visual field) of the left eye, and a left Babinski sign.[34]

Questions

1. At this point, what can be determined about the patient?

2. Is a lumbar puncture indicated at this time?

3. Is a laboratory examination of this patient's CSF likely to be helpful in establishing a diagnosis?

4. What nonlaboratory procedure might be more helpful than CSF examination in establishing a diagnosis?

5. If this patient has a brain abscess, would you expect anaerobic bacteria to be involved? Would clindamycin be a suitable choice of antimicrobial agent?

6. What treatment is necessary in addition to appropriate antimicrobial therapy?

Discussion

1. This patient has presented with signs of a CNS infection as well as focal neurologic signs. He is more likely to have a brain abscess or encephalitis than bacterial meningitis.

2. A lumbar puncture would be very risky without additional information concerning this patient's intracranial dynamics. Cerebellar tonsillar herniation may result if cranial pressure is too high at the time of lumbar puncture.

3. CSF examination is not very helpful in cases of brain abscess or encephalitis. In brain abscesses, bacteria are usually localized to the brain substance, rarely gain access to the CSF, and thus are not apt to be isolated from CSF specimens.

4. A CT scan of this patient's brain is indicated, and the results should reveal whether it is safe to perform a lumbar puncture. In this case, a CT scan with contrast medium revealed a low-density right frontotemporal lesion surrounded by a ring of high density, suggestive of a brain abscess.

5. Anaerobic bacteria are involved in 80% to 85% of brain abscesses. Although clindamycin is commonly effective in treating infections caused by anaerobes, it does not cross the blood-brain barrier well enough for treatment of CNS infections.

6. The most likely origin of infection in this patient is his recurrent sinusitis; therefore, his paranasal sinuses should be drained.

Case Study 2[35]

A 28-year-old woman gave birth to a 3500-gram male infant at term, following an uneventful labor and delivery. Physical examinations of the neonate performed at birth and at 8 hours of age were essentially normal. At 18 hours of age, however, the infant began vomiting, refused to feed, and became irritable. By 30 hours of age, the baby was lethargic, and seizure activity was noted.

Physical examination revealed a bulging of the anterior fontanelle, a supple neck, clear lungs, a regular rhythmic heart, and no enlargement of liver or spleen. A chest x-ray was negative. The infant's temperature was 37.8 °C, blood pressure was 90/70 mm Hg, pulse was 110 beats/min, and respiration rate was 36/min. A lumbar puncture was performed, and blood and urine specimens were also submitted to the laboratory. Pertinent laboratory data are as follows:[35]

Hemoglobin	14.5 g/dL
White blood cell count	13.5×10^9/L
Blood differential	60% neutrophils, 29% lymphocytes, 4% monocytes, 7% band forms
Urinalysis	Normal
Serum BUN, sugar, electrolytes	Normal
CSF appearance	Cloudy
CSF WBC count	2800/mm³

CSF differential	98% neutrophils
CSF glucose	30 mg/dL
Blood glucose	90 mg/dL
CSF protein	150 mg/dL
CSF Gram stain	Many WBCs, gram-positive cocci in chains
CSF culture	Results pending
Blood culture	Results pending

Questions

1. What prompted the physician to perform a lumbar puncture in this case?

2. Which etiologic agent(s) of meningitis would the physician be most apt to suspect in this case, prior to receipt of any laboratory results?

3. On the basis of your knowledge of this patient and the laboratory results, which etiologic agent do you suspect?

4. What additional laboratory procedures could have been performed to aid in the diagnosis of meningitis due to this particular pathogen?

Discussion

1. Because many of the usual signs of meningitis may be lacking in neonates, the diagnosis must be considered in any infant with temperature instability, respiratory difficulties, or feeding problems. In this case, the patient was also lethargic, was demonstrating seizure activity, and had a bulging fontanelle (indicating a late stage of infection in newborns). Because bacterial meningitis can be rapidly fatal, speed was essential in the processing of a CSF specimen and in the interpretation and reporting of laboratory results.

2. Although *N. meningitidis*, *S. pneumoniae*, and *H. influenzae* are common causes of bacterial meningitis in children and adults, the primary etiologic agents in neonates are group B β-hemolytic streptococci (*S. agalactiae*), *L. monocytogenes*, and *E. coli*, any of which may be colonizing the birth canal at the time of delivery.

3. The appearance of the CSF specimen, its cellular contents, and the CSF glucose and protein levels are consistent with a diagnosis of bacterial meningitis. The Gram stain results—finding of gram-positive cocci in chains—are consistent with the appearance of streptococci. Therefore, because this patient is a newborn, *S. agalactiae* is the most likely cause of the bacterial meningitis.

4. Latex agglutination and counterimmunoelectrophoresis procedures are commercially available and permit rapid detection of bacterial antigens (to include *S. agalactiae* antigen) in CSF specimens. Such procedures are often positive in cases in which the Gram stains are negative.

References

1. Mahon CR, Manuselis G (eds): Textbook of Diagnostic Microbiology. Philadelphia, WB Saunders, 1995.

2. Koneman EW, Allen SD, Janda WM, et al: Color Atlas and Textbook of Diagnostic Microbiology. Philadelphia, JB Lippincott, 1992.

3. Luby JP: Southwestern Internal Medicine Conference: Infections of the Central Nervous System. Am J Med Sci 304:379–391, 1992.

4. Baron EJ, Petersen L, Finegold SM: Bailey and Scott's Diagnostic Microbiology. St Louis, Mosby–Year Book, 1992.

5. McGee ZA, Kaiser AB: Acute meningitis. *In* Mandell GL, Douglas RG, Bennett JE (eds): Principles and Practice of Infectious Diseases. New York, John Wiley & Sons, 1985.

6. Bale JF Jr: Viral Encephalitis. Med Clin North Am 77:25–42, 1993.

7. Rotbart HA: Enteroviral infections of the central nervous system. Clin Infect Dis 20:971–981, 1995.

8. Zachariah B, Zachariah SB, Varghese R, Balducci L: Carcinomatous meningitis: Clinical manifestations and management. Int J Clin Pharmacol Ther 33:7–12, 1995.

9. River Y, Averbuch-Heller L, Weinberger M, et al: Antibiotic induced meningitis. J Neurol Neurosurg Psychiatry 57:705–708, 1994.

10. Adams RD, Petersdorf RG: Pyogenic infections of the central nervous system. *In* Petersdorf RG, Adams RD, Braunwald E, et al (eds): Harrison's Principles of Internal Medicine. New York, McGraw-Hill, 1983.

11. Austin TW: Infections of the central nervous system. *In* Mandell LA, Ralph ED (eds): Essentials of Infectious Diseases. Boston, Blackwell Scientific, 1985.

12. Adams RD, Chiappa KH, Martin JB, et al: Diagnostic methods in neurology. *In* Petersdorf RG, Adams RD, Braunwald E, et al (eds): Harrison's Principles of Internal Medicine. New York, McGraw-Hill, 1983.

13. Cunha BA: The diagnosis and therapy of acute bacterial meningitis. *In* Schlossberg D (ed): Infections of the Nervous System. New York, Springer-Verlag, 1990.

14. Harter DH, Petersdorf RG, Adams RD: Viral diseases of the central nervous system—aseptic meningitis and encephalitis. *In* Petersdorf RG, Adams RD, Braunwald E, et al (eds): Harrison's Principles of Internal Medicine. New York, McGraw-Hill, 1983.

15. Kjeldsberg CR, Krieg AF: Cerebrospinal fluid and other body fluids. *In* Henry JB (ed): Todd-Sanford-Davidson Clinical Diagnosis and Management by Laboratory Methods. Philadelphia, WB Saunders, 1984.

16. Paap CM, Bosso JA: Treatment options for the pharmacological therapy of neonatal meningitis. Drugs 43:700–712, 1992.

17. McGreevy PB, Nelson GS: Larval cestode infections. *In* Strickland GT (ed): Hunter's Tropical Medicine. Philadelphia, WB Saunders, 1984.

18. Overbosch D: Neurocysticercosis: An introduction with special emphasis on new developments in pharmacotherapy. Schweiz Med Wochenschr 122:893–898, 1992.

19. Dismukes WE: Management of cryptococcosis. Clin Infect Dis 17(Suppl 2):S507–S512, 1993.

20. Brodal P: The Central Nervous System: Structure and Function. New York, Oxford University Press, 1992.

21. Scheld WM, Winn HR: Brain abscess. *In* Mandell GL, Douglas RG, Bennett JE (eds): Principles and Practice of Infectious Diseases. New York, John Wiley & Sons, 1985.

22. Sokolov RT Jr, Meyer RD: Brain abscess and related focal intracranial suppuration. *In* Schlossberg D (ed): Infections of the Nervous System. New York, Springer-Verlag, 1990.

23. Greenlee JE: Subdural empyema. *In* Mandell GL, Douglas RG, Bennett JE (eds): Principles and Practice of Infectious Diseases. New York, John Wiley & Sons, 1985.

24. Greenlee JE: Epidural abscess. *In* Mandell GL, Douglas RG, Bennett JE (eds): Principles and Practice of Infectious Diseases. New York, John Wiley & Sons, 1985.

25. Koskiniemi M: CNS manifestations associated with *Mycoplasma pneumoniae* infections: Summary of cases at the University of Helsinki and review. Clin Infect Dis 17(Suppl 1):S52–S57, 1993.

26. Armstrong RW, Fung PC: Brainstem encephalitis (rhombencephalitis) due to *Listeria monocytogenes*: Case report and review. Clin Infect Dis 16:689–702, 1993.

27. Mateos-Mora M, Ratzan KR: Acute viral encephalitis. *In* Schlossberg D (ed): Infections of the Nervous System. New York, Springer-Verlag, 1990.

28. Mustafa MM, Weitman SD, Winick NJ, et al: Subacute measles encephalitis in the young immunocompromised host: Report of two cases diagnosed by polymerase chain reaction and treated with ribavirin and review of the literature. Clin Infect Dis 16:654–660, 1993.

29. Prusiner SB, Hsiao KK: Prions causing transmissible neurodegenerative diseases. *In* Schlossberg D (ed): Infections of the Nervous System. New York, Springer-Verlag, 1990.
30. Mrak RE, Young L: Rabies encephalitis in humans: Pathology, pathogenesis and pathophysiology. J Neuropathol Exp Neurol 53:1–10, 1994.
31. Berger JR, Levy RM, Dix R: AIDS and other immunocompromised states. *In* Schlossberg D (ed): Infections of the Nervous System. New York, Springer-Verlag, 1990.
32. Berger JR, Levy RM: The neurologic complications of human immunodeficiency virus infection. Med Clin North Am 77:1–23, 1993.
33. Wiley CA: Pathology of neurologic disease in AIDS. Psychiatr Clin North Am 17:1–15, 1994.
34. Cobb CG, Griffin FM, Avent CK: Infectious Disease Case Studies. New York, Medical Examination Publishing Company, 1986.
35. Frothingham TE, Gutman LT, Idriss ZH, et al: Pediatric Infectious Disease Case Studies. New York, Medical Examination Publishing Company, 1978.

Chapter 40

Cerebrovascular Accidents

Alexander von Laufen

A cerebrovascular accident (CVA), or stroke, in which the brain's oxygen supply is reduced or cut off, can be a life-threatening event. A stroke occurs when an artery to the brain ruptures or becomes clogged, thereby reducing or interrupting the blood flow to particular parts of the cerebral cortex. Brain tissue that is deprived of oxygen and other special nutrients dies within a matter of minutes, and consequently, the part of the body controlled by those brain cells cannot function properly.[1–4] Fortunately, there is redundancy in the complexity of cerebral vascularity, and collateral circulation can provide blood to a region of the brain if it is deprived of its normal supply.[4, 5] A stroke, therefore, can affect any of the senses, speech, behavior, thought patterns, and memory functioning. If severe, a stroke may also cause partial or complete paralysis, coma, or death.

Every year, more than 550,000 Americans experience a new or recurrent cerebrovascular accident.[6–9] Stroke is now the third leading cause of death in the United States, after heart disease and cancer. It is the number one cause of adult disability, more than 3 million Americans being permanently disabled because of a cerebrovascular accident.[8, 9]

Even though brain cells die within a matter of minutes after interruption of the blood supply, stroke specialists believe that many cells in the surrounding brain can be saved through prompt medical treatment, and certain functions can be partially or completely restored with a rehabilitative process. For patients who do recover, improvement typically follows a decelerating learning curve, with the most improvement noticed within the first 6 months. Physical disabilities typically resolve more quickly than cognitive deficits.[10–13]

Research on cerebrovascular disease and strokes indicates that prompt restoration of blood flow can help prevent further damage to brain tissue, and new drugs may help protect brain cells if they are given quickly following a stroke event. Early intervention is therefore necessary to help restore damaged brain tissue and thereby regain function.

DYNAMICS OF CEREBRAL CIRCULATION

Each hemisphere of the brain is supplied by the extensive branches of the two internal carotid arteries and the two vertebral arteries. The internal carotid arteries arise at the bifurcation of the common carotids in the neck region, just below the angle of the mandible.[1, 10, 14] The internal carotid arteries do not branch in the neck, but begin to branch off inside the cranial cavity itself. The internal carotid arterial system consists of the ophthalmic artery and the anterior choroidal artery along with the anterior and middle cerebral arteries.[1]

The vertebral arteries are branches of the subclavian artery that ascend in the neck through the foramen magnum of the skull and join to form the basilar arterial system.[1, 10, 14, 15] This is referred to as the *vertebrobasilar artery system* and includes the posterior cerebral artery, which serves the terminal branches of the basilar artery.

The circle of Willis, located at the base of the cerebral cortex,[15, 16] is formed by the anterior and posterior communicating arteries as well as portions of the anterior, middle, and posterior cerebral arteries. The primary function of the circle of Willis is to provide an adequate supply of blood to the brain, even in case of occlusion to either the carotid or vertebral arteries due to arteriosclerosis. This gradual stenosis results in progressive narrowing of the cerebral vessels, and eventually, blood flow through the arteries may become totally occluded.

ETIOLOGY AND PATHOPHYSIOLOGY

As people grow older, the cerebral circulation gradually declines because of progressive arteriosclerosis, resulting in increased hypoxia and the eventual death of brain cells. Through this constriction and gradual deterioration, areas of the brain begin to atrophy, and hemorrhage or thrombosis and embolism with infarction may occur.[3–5]

SPECIFIC RISK FACTORS

Certain conditions in an individual's lifestyle can increase the potential for a stroke to occur. These specific risk factors generally are either controllable or noncontrollable variables.[7, 8, 17]

Controllable risk factors are medical disorders and life style factors that can be modified or treated to markedly decrease the risk for stroke.[17] They include high blood pressure or hypertension, high cholesterol, carotid artery disease, heart disease, smoking, and obesity.

Noncontrollable risk factors cannot be modified. Examples are age, race, diagnosis of diabetes, heredity, and previous history of stroke. The risk of sustaining a stroke actually doubles with each decade of a person's life past the age of 55 years.[17] Blacks and Hispanics seem to have a greater risk of death and disability from an acute stroke phenomenon. Although diabetes is generally treatable in some form, this condition makes an individual more susceptible to stroke. Risk of stroke is also much greater in individuals with a family history of stroke or a personal history of stroke.[7–9, 18, 19]

CLINICAL MANIFESTATIONS

Although the process of arteriosclerosis is insidious and may go undetected or unmanaged, the following clinical symptoms can warn an individual of an impending stroke:

- Sudden weakness or numbness of the face, arm, or leg (particularly on one side of the body)
- Blurred or decreased vision (especially in one eye)
- Difficulty in talking or understanding speech
- Loss of balance or unsteadiness while walking
- Unexplained dizziness
- Sudden and severe headache

Symptoms of a stroke, or transient ischemic attacks (TIAs), require immediate emergency treatment. Prompt medical attention increases the chances for survival, successful rehabilitation, and recovery of brain function. TIAs generally do not cause permanent damage to the brain, but they are still a critical warning sign. Other clinical manifestations are discussed later. A complete physical and neurologic examination usually suggests the diagnosis of TIA or CVA. Further evaluation can be done through computed tomography (CT) scanning or magnetic resonance imaging (MRI) in order to pinpoint the area of concern and the extent of the brain damage.[7, 8, 13, 17]

LABORATORY ANALYSES AND DIAGNOSIS

The clinical laboratory may not play a major role in the diagnosis of CVA, although it may assist in distinguishing CVA from other disorders, such as severe hypothyroidism, hypoglycemic states, and drug intoxication. Table 40–1 identifies laboratory analyses useful in the differential diagnosis of infarction. Other diagnostic procedures are discussed later.

Table 40–1. Differential Diagnosis and Treatment of Infarction

Etiology	Signs and Symptoms	Laboratory	Treatment
Thrombosis			
Internal carotid	Hemiparesis, hemianesthesia, hemianopsia, aphasia (global or mixed transcortical), neglect	Serum lipids; GTT; noninvasive studies (i.e., CT)	Supportive; if hypertensive, blood pressure must be reduced gradually; ? dextran; ? glycerol
Middle cerebral	Hemiparesis (arm and face > leg), hemianopsia, cortical signs, cortical sensory defect	Same as above	Same as above
Anterior cerebral	Hemiparesis (leg > arm), grasp, callosal disconnection syndrome	Same as above	Same as above
Posterior cerebral	Hemianopsia, defective memory, alexia without agraphia	Same as above	Same as above
Vertebral basilar	Cranial nerve abnormality, cerebellar signs, weakness, sensory signs	Same as above	Same as above
Embolus	Has localization similar to thrombosis	Cardiac evaluation	Anticoagulation
Other (i.e., vasculitis and sickle cell)	Similar to above; however, there may also be systemic signs	Sedimentation rate, hematologic studies, LE prep, ANA, temporal artery biopsy, hemoglobin electrophoresis	Treat underlying disease

From Heilman KM, Watson RT, Greer M: Handbook for Differential Diagnosis of Neurologic Signs and Symptoms. New York, Appleton-Century-Crofts, 1977.
Abbreviations: GTT, glucose tolerance test; CT, computed tomography; LE, lupus erythematosus; ANA, antinuclear antibodies.

TRANSIENT ISCHEMIC ATTACKS

TIAs are brief interruptions in the cerebral blood flow during which some neurologic function is temporarily lost. Full functional capacity is usually restored within 3 to 30 minutes,[1, 2, 10] although recovery sometimes does not occur for up to 12 hours. Most TIAs are believed to originate from platelet emboli that form within arteriosclerotic extracranial arteries and subsequently travel throughout the cerebral artery distribution.[1] The importance of TIAs lies not only in the episodes of neurologic dysfunction they cause, but also in their indication of underlying arteriosclerotic cerebrovascular disease. Without appropriate medical treatment, about 25% percent of patients who have TIAs develop a permanent neurologic deficit within 1 year.[8]

Carotid Artery TIAs

Platelet emboli probably develop on the internal surface of narrowed and ulcerated plaques that travel upward into the internal carotid artery (Fig. 40–1). Each internal carotid artery provides blood directly to the majority of the ipsilateral cerebral hemisphere and, through collateral circulation, to a portion of the contralateral hemisphere.[1, 12, 20] The carotid artery also supplies the ipsilateral eye through its first branch structure, the ophthalmic artery. Consequently, TIAs of the carotid artery often temporarily obscure vision in one eye. Such an episode, referred to as amaurosis fugax, has been described as a "blanket of gray" coming down slowly in front of the visual field of one eye.[21] Other symptoms of carotid artery TIA involve periods of (contralateral) hemiparesis, hemisensory loss, paresthesias, and hemianopsia. TIAs in the dominant hemisphere of the brain cause aphasia, or language disturbance. Under specific circumstances, mental confusion and personality changes may also occur.[20, 21]

In most cases in which there is evidence of brief motor or sensory loss, the diagnosis of a carotid artery TIA can be made reliably on the basis of clinical evaluation alone. Because TIAs are considered precursors of strokes or may even be confused with other conditions, many neurologists recommend a series of laboratory tests to confirm the diagnosis and to search for arteriosclerotic lesions at the carotid bifurcation. Typically, a routine evaluation consists of an electrocardiogram, 24-hour Holter monitoring to study cardiac rhythm, a standard electroencephalogram if seizures are suspected, and a CT scan of the brain to exclude mass lesions or evidence of completed strokes.

Over the years, several noninvasive procedures have been developed to help diagnose carotid artery stenosis. The definitive test remains cerebral arteriography, however, which requires injection of radiopaque dye through a catheter directly into the carotid arteries, although this procedure itself exposes the patient to a risk of vascular accident.[18, 19]

The preferred treatment for carotid artery TIA is nonsurgical. Commonly, aspirin (1–3 tablets/day) is prescribed for use as a platelet inhibitor, or an antiplatelet medication, such as sulfinpyrazone (Anturane), ticlopidine (Ticlid), or dipyridamole (Persantine), is chosen.[12] When carotid artery stenosis is more serious, the standard surgical procedure involves a carotid endarterectomy for the removal of any atheromatous plaques.[13]

Vertebrobasilar Artery TIAs

The two vertebral arteries join to form the basilar artery (see Fig. 40–1). This group of vessels, which is usually

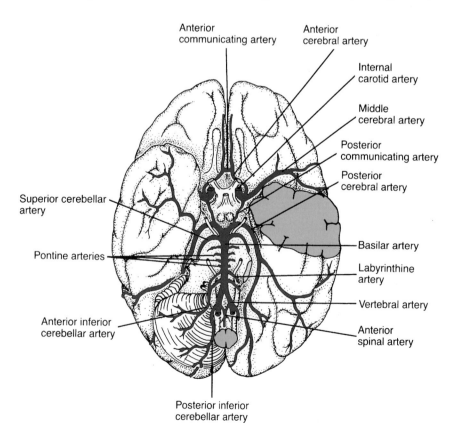

Figure 40–1. The arterial circle of Willis at the base of the brain, with the distribution of the internal carotid and vertebrobasilar systems. (From Burt AM: Textbook of Neuroanatomy. Philadelphia, WB Saunders, 1993.)

Anterior communicating artery

Anterior cerebral artery

Internal carotid artery

Middle cerebral artery

Posterior communicating artery

Posterior cerebral artery

Basilar artery

Labyrinthine artery

Vertebral artery

Anterior spinal artery

Superior cerebellar artery

Pontine arteries

Anterior inferior cerebellar artery

Posterior inferior cerebellar artery

called the vertebrobasilar system or simply the basilar artery, supplies the brain stem, cerebellum, and inferomedial portion of the temporal lobes.[10, 14, 16] The mechanism of basilar artery TIAs is probably similar to that of carotid artery TIAs, with the exception that occlusions are found at the origin of the vertebral arteries in the chest and at their junction at the undersurface of the brain. Because these locations are virtually inaccessible to surgeons, endarterectomy cannot be performed as with the carotid arteries.[1]

Signs and symptoms of basilar artery TIAs are distinctly different from those of carotid artery TIAs. Patients with basilar artery TIAs typically have vertigo, which might be accompanied by nausea and tinnitus.[22] Patients experience tingling around the mouth, dysarthria, nystagmus, or gait ataxia because of ischemia of the brain stem. On rare occasions, when all cerebral blood flow through the basilar artery is interrupted and the entire brain stem becomes ischemic, a patient experiences a drop attack, which involves a brief loss of consciousness and body tone. During a basilar artery TIA, patients are usually incapacitated to some extent because of the vertigo.[1, 10, 12, 23]

Noninvasive procedures such as ultrasonography are not as applicable to the vertebrobasilar system as to the carotid artery system. Therapy for basilar artery TIAs usually follows the same guidelines as those for carotid artery disease. Intracranial-extracranial arterial bypass surgeries are still in the experimental phases and are controversial.[13, 24]

Transient Global Amnesia

Transient global amnesia sometimes occurs in older individuals upon physical exertion and probably results from ischemia of the posterior cerebral arteries. These vessels are terminal branches of the basilar artery that supply the temporal lobes.[1] Because the temporal lobes contain portions of the limbic system, vascular attacks can result in temporary memory impairment as well as frank personality changes. While in a state of transient global amnesia, a patient demonstrates mental confusion, disorientation, amnesia, and apathy. Symptoms of transient global amnesia can mimic those of partial complex seizures, migraine attacks, metabolic abnormalities, and also a variety of psychologic aberrations. An electroencephalogram (EEG) during an attack is often helpful in making a differential diagnosis.[25]

CEREBROVASCULAR ACCIDENTS

In contrast to the brief neurologic deficits of transient ischemic attacks, cerebrovascular accidents result in permanent physical and neuropsychologic deficits. With completed strokes, the cerebral blood supply is irreversibly interrupted because of arterial thromboses, emboli, or hemorrhages. Portions of the brain are permanently damaged.

The incidence of stroke increases almost in exponential fashion after the age of 65 years, although about 20% of stroke victims are younger than 65.[6, 17] An even greater risk factor than age is hypertension. Whether it is systolic, diastolic, or systolic-diastolic, uncontrolled hypertension increases risk for CVAs in middle-aged as well as older adults.[17–19] It is also believed to be one of the primary causes of multi-infarct dementia. Cardiac valvular disease,

myocardial infarctions, and atrial fibrillations are additional risk factors, because in each of these conditions, thromboses tend to form on the endocardial surface and may embolize to the brain or elsewhere.[6, 17]

Thromboses and Emboli

In thrombotic or embolic CVAs, the area of the brain that the artery supplies becomes infarcted, and the surrounding tissue becomes edematous. Some spontaneous recovery of function does seem to occur when the edema resolves,[10, 23, 26] but the infarction itself leaves a permanent scar that in turn can become epileptogenic.[25] The majority of CVAs are caused by either a thrombosis that propagates within an arteriosclerotic cerebral artery or an embolus that originates within an internal carotid artery. Thrombotic CVAs strike rapidly and painlessly. A disproportionate number occur suddenly during sleep, and others develop in an intermittent fashion over several days. The worst deficits associated with cerebral infarction seem to occur between the third and tenth day after stroke, when the edema is the most severe.[5, 20]

Because each of the major cerebral arteries supplies a particular region in the brain, characteristic neurologic deficits are associated with each artery[2, 3, 23, 27] (Box 40–1).

Lacunar Infarcts

Lacunar infarcts, which account for nearly 20% of all strokes, are the result of gradual occlusion of small pene-

---

Box 40–1. Manifestations of Cerebrovascular Accidents (CVAs)

Carotid Artery

Anterior cerebral:

• Contralateral lower extremity paresis

Middle cerebral:

• Contralateral hemiparesis, hemianopsia, and hemisensory loss
• Aphasia
• Hemi-inattention

Posterior cerebral:

• Contralateral homonymous hemianopsia

Vertebrobasilar System

Basilar artery:

• Total occlusion: coma or locked-in syndrome
• Occlusion of branch: cranial nerve palsy with contralateral hemiparesis, internuclear ophthalmoplegia

Vertebral artery:

• Lateral medullary (Wallenberg's) syndrome

From Kaufman DM: Clinical Neurology for Psychiatrists, ed 2. New York, Grune & Stratton, 1985.

trating cerebral arteries.[1] They may be infarcts so small that they do not produce any recognizable symptoms, or they may be cause motor or sensory deficits, depending on their location. There is a strong association between lacunar infarcts and both arteriosclerosis and hypertension, suggesting that lacunar infarction is the result of the extension of the arteriosclerotic disease process into the smaller vessels.[4, 24]

Cerebral Hemorrhage

One of the most serious aspects of CVAs involves the completed stroke or cerebral hemorrhage. This occurs when blood from a ruptured cerebral artery leaks directly into the brain. Hematomas can develop anywhere in the brain but seem to occur more commonly in the cerebral hemisphere, pons, or cerebellum. Brain damage can be quite extensive and is often fatal.

Although thromboses begin in a slow or intermittent fashion and are usually painless, most cerebral hemorrhages are abrupt in onset and often accompanied by severe headaches, nausea, and vomiting. In many cases, patients may lapse into a stuporous state with profound neurologic complications[10, 21, 23, 26] (Fig. 40–2).

Most patients with acute cerebral hemorrhaging cannot be helped; however, there are two types of hemorrhage for which surgical intervention can be a remedy. Cerebellar hemorrhages result in an occipital headache, gait ataxia, dysarthria, and lethargy. Evacuation of a cerebellar hematoma is feasible and can be life saving. Subarachnoid hemorrhages are usually the result of ruptured arterial aneurysms. Patients typically have sudden onset of an extraordinarily severe headache with nuchal rigidity.[1, 23] In some cases, however, there may not be any neurologic deficits. The symptoms of a subarachnoid hemorrhage are occasionally confused with those of a migraine headache, but a CT scan of the brain usually reveals blood at the base of the brain. A lumbar puncture yields bloody cerebrospinal fluid (CSF) in hemorrhages of recent onset, and xanthochromic CSF in hemorrhages more than several days old. Neurosurgeons can occlude most ruptured aneurysms.[1]

There are also two different varieties of traumatic hemorrhages, in addition to the subarachnoid hemorrhages, that usually occur as intracerebral lesions and, in most cases, involve some type of brain impairment. An extradural hemorrhage occurs when the outer skull is fractured and a fragment ruptures a middle meningeal artery. Blood immediately flows into the epidural space. Patients may recover for brief periods after an injury of this sort, but they typically suffer relapse when the intracranial pressure rises. The pupil on the affected side becomes dilated and fixed, and there is contralateral hemiparesis.[16] This type of injury requires immediate neurosurgical intervention.

Subdural hematomas are equally serious hemorrhages that usually follow minor injuries to the brain. Subdural hematomas occur when one of the veins that suspends the brain from the sagittal sinus is ruptured. Blood gradually accumulates between the dura and the arachnoid layer, and symptoms may not develop until hours or days after the traumatic event. Chronic subdural hematomas are more likely to impair some form of consciousness and to affect movement, sensation, or vision, because most of their effect results from pressure rather than from specific nerve destruction. In the patient who presents with marked clouding of consciousness, or who is in coma without severe hemiparesis, a subdural hematoma is a far more likely possibility than an ischemic stroke.[24]

Hydrocephalus

A common consequence of a completed stroke is impaired circulation of the cerebrospinal fluid. This can pro-

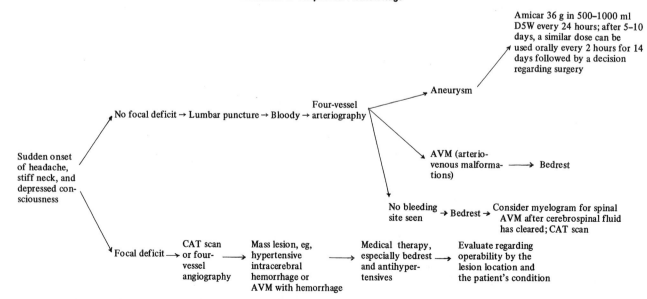

Figure 40–2. Clinical evaluation of a suspected intracranial hemorrhage. Abbreviations: AVM, arteriovenous malformation; CAT, computed (axial) tomography; D5W, 5% dextrose in water. (From Heilman KM, Watson RT, Greer M: Handbook for Differential Diagnosis of Neurologic Signs and Symptoms. New York, Appleton-Century-Crofts, 1977.)

duce normal-pressure hydrocephalus, which is largely characterized by three classic clinical symptoms: dementia, gait disturbance, and urinary incontinence. Treatment usually is a surgical procedure to shunt the cerebrospinal fluid from the lateral ventricles into the general circulation (ventriculoperitoneal shunt).[1, 4, 5]

CEREBROVASCULAR ACCIDENTS AND NEUROPSYCHIATRIC ABNORMALITIES

In contrast to the physical disabilities that often accompany the cerebrovascular disease process, a host of cognitive-emotional-behavioral disorders have been reported that can also be present as a prominent feature once a stroke has developed.[2–4, 12, 20, 22, 23, 26, 28, 29] Repeated vascular occlusions or small hemorrhages can produce a multi-infarct dementia in which the cognitive deficits become cumulative.

Multi-Infarct Dementia

Multi-infarct dementia accounts for 8% to 40% of all cases of dementia and in almost all cases is preceded by hypertensive cerebrovascular disease, which causes multiple small cerebral scars (lacunae).[1] With successive infarction, the neuropsychologic picture is characterized by rapid onset with a pattern of gradual deterioration, including intellectual decline and progressive physical impairments such as paresis, clumsiness, rigidity, and reflex abnormalities.[2, 26] There can be partial recovery after each successive attack, but the general clinical picture is one of gradual deterioration. The neurologic and behavioral signs are typically more dramatic than those seen in Alzheimer's disease, and memory function is more likely to be better preserved in the patient with multi-infarct dementia.[3, 20]

Locked-In Syndrome

In a relatively rare occurrence among cerebrovascular accidents, referred to as the *locked-in syndrome,* the patient is mute, quadriplegic, and unable to respond with conventional modalities. Careful neuropsychologic examination reveals that such a patient not only is mentally alert but can move the eyes and eyelids, and the mental capacity is usually preserved. This is important to note, because patients with the locked-in syndrome can be confused with those in coma, in a vegetative state, or with profound dementia.

Locked-in syndrome is the result of an infarction in the lower portion of the brain stem. The patient is mute because of bulbar palsy and quadriplegic because of an interruption along the corticospinal tract on both sides.[1, 23] The cerebral cortex and upper brain stem are usually well preserved and remain intact. The mute patient with a CVA who can blink the eyes meaningfully should be evaluated for the ability to see, hear, understand, and respond to yes/no questions using eye-blink responses. Further investigation may reveal that even though there is severe limitation to physical movement, the patient retains relatively intact cognitive processing.

Behavioral Disorders

Any cardiovascular disease process that interferes with the blood supply to the brain has the potential to produce neurologic or psychiatric symptoms, depending on the severity, localization, acuteness of onset, and reversibility of an organic assault.[2, 4, 20, 28, 29] For example, cardiovascular problems that produce global compromises of brain functioning are virtually indistinguishable from one another and from a wide variety of toxic or metabolic disorders. It is the focal CVAs that are of special interest to behavioral specialists because the study of localized functional deficits of blood supply can produce insights into the mental structure of the brain.

Patients with chronic, diffuse vascular disease present with a variety of vague complaints, including headaches, dizziness, decreased concentration, hypochondriasis, sleep disturbances, and mood swings. Eventually, symptoms of a typical organic brain syndrome begin to develop. Subtle personality changes can occur with diffuse vascular disease, which may manifest as a wide variety of neurotic symptoms.[20, 28, 30] The behavioral changes are often extensions or exaggerations of the patient's normal personality.

Other more common psychiatric presentations of vascular disease are the frontal lobe syndrome and various disturbances of consciousness. The patient demonstrates altered behavior, with a release of inhibitions and decline of social graces and moral restraints. Individuals can become inappropriate, and disruptive, and may manifest a wide variety of affective or emotional changes. There is a general loss of initiative, with apathy and indifference about the future. Associated symptoms include impairments in orientation, attention, learning new information, abstract thinking, memory, and perception, although overall intelligence on formal testing is not necessarily below normal.[27]

Global disruptions of consciousness, such as in states of delirium and coma, commonly occur with encephalopathies or with infectious, toxic, or metabolic conditions; however, focal lesions can produce the same symptomatology. Acute delirium has been reported with infarctions in the distribution of the anterior, middle, and posterior cerebral arteries. In addition, lesions involving the reticular activating system, subcortical structures like the thalamus, and the parietal, temporal, and occipital cortices are especially involved in disturbances of attention.[10, 26, 30]

Disorders of Affect and Mood

A large number of emotional disorders have been attributed to cerebrovascular disease over the years. Four of the most common are catastrophic reaction, indifference reaction, depressive disorder, and manic syndrome.[2] Signs and symptoms of catastrophic reaction are physical restlessness, hyperemotionality, sudden and uncontrollable lability, irritation, expressions of anger, cursing or swearing, displacement of anxiety on external events, and sharp refusal to continue with the interview or examination. Catastrophic reactions seem to occur more common among patients with left hemisphere lesions and aphasia than with other types of lesions.[2, 31]

The indifference reaction consists of apparent indifference toward future events, personal failures, tendency to joke in an unconcerned way, lack of awareness of cognitive or physical deficits, explicit denial of illness, and a tendency to attribute impairments to insignificant causes such as weariness or poor concentration. Indifference reactions seem to be commonly associated with right hemisphere lesions and left hemisphere neglect.[2]

The most common emotional disorders associated with cerebrovascular disease are major depressive disorders, which also include chronic low-level dysthymia (minor depression) and which occur in approximately 40% of patients after an acute stroke phenomenon.[2, 32] Clinical symptoms include depressed mood, anxiety, restlessness, loss of energy, increased worry, hopelessness, weight loss, early morning rising, irritability, and social withdrawal.

Mania following an acute stroke event usually involves a lateralized and focal lesion in the right hemisphere, particularly in the basal ganglia, thalamic, midbrain nuclei, or limbic portions of the frontal or temporal lobes.[20, 23] It typically consists of euphoric or irritable mood, hyperactivity, sleep disturbance, excessive or pressured speech, flight of ideas, grandiosity, and a lack of judgment, usually in the absence of gross cognitive impairment.[2]

Disorders of Communication and Thought

Acute cerebral infarctions may lead to sudden disruptions or disorganization of thought processes that are characteristic of delirium. Small, repetitive infarctions typically result in a gradual impoverishment of both the content and stream of thought processing. Over time, the patient becomes more literal and concrete, and the structure of sentences and vocabulary becomes less and less complicated. Speech becomes circumstantial, and ideas perseverative. Gradually, with obvious decline in intellectual capacity, evasiveness and defensiveness intrude into the patient's personality. With repeated strokes, dementia is the final outcome.[20]

Compromise of specific areas of either the dominant or nondominant cerebral cortex can produce varying discrete deficits of speech or language (aphasia). Most of these lesions result from infarction in the distribution of the middle cerebral artery.[20]

Pure word deafness results from the destruction of the primary auditory area of the temporal lobe or to the connections of this area with the posterior superior temporal region. This destruction produces a syndrome in which the patient has normal spoken language, writing, and reading comprehension but is unable to interpret speech.[27, 34, 35] Destruction of Wernicke's area itself results in more severe disturbances (sensory aphasia), in which not only comprehension but also expression is impaired (Wernicke's aphasia).[27]

Broca's aphasia (expressive or motor aphasia) is a nonfluent aphasia often accompanied by hemiplegia. The language of affected patients is characteristically telegraphic, impoverished, and agrammatical. Articles, prepositions, and normal punctuation may be omitted, and what little speech can be produced is made slowly and with great effort.[34, 35]

Conduction aphasia occurs when only the connections between Wernicke's and Broca's areas are damaged, but

the areas themselves are spared.[27, 34, 35] The lesion is usually deep in the parietal lobe just above the sylvian fissure. Although speech comprehension is intact, repetition, naming, and writing are poor. Reading comprehension and spontaneous speech are variably affected.[34, 35]

Global aphasia results in both receptive and expressive deficits and evolves from comparatively massive lesions that destroy both Wernicke's and Broca's areas.[27] The patient neither comprehends nor speaks and usually has severe hemiplegia.

Nominal aphasia develops with lesions in the angular gyrus or between the angular gyrus and the posterior part of the superior temporal gyrus of the dominant parietal lobe. In milder forms, the patient has difficulty naming familiar objects or shows evidence of circumlocution in the speech pattern.[11, 12, 28, 34, 35]

Amnesic aphasia is a rare occurrence that is also caused by lesions in the angular gyrus but sometimes can occur from a diffuse disease process such as arteriosclerosis. The patient develops poor speech impulse and limited vocabulary, and is unable to find the right words to express ideas.[12]

Agraphia, or the inability to write correctly, often accompanies aphasia; however, agraphia can also arise as an isolated phenomenon if the motor areas of either parietal lobe are infarcted. A specific constellation of symptoms known as Gurstmann's syndrome evolves from an infarction to the dominant parietal lobe.[5] It consists of agraphia, difficulty with calculations, confusion over right-left differences, and difficulty in naming the fingers.

Whereas the dominant parietal lobe is involved with language functioning, the nondominant parietal lobe appears to be significant for visual-spatial functions.[27] Patients with infarctions in the nondominant parietal lobe may show either deficits in depth perception or constructional dyspraxia (inability to assemble pieces into a whole or to construct a three-dimensional figure). Such patients may also have difficulty drawing maps or recognizing familiar people. Constructional apraxia is also seen with dominant parietal lobe lesions, but improvement in performing the various tasks can be achieved with repeated practice.[27]

Ideomotor apraxia, the most common type of apraxia, is usually seen with diffuse brain disease like arteriosclerosis. The patient is able to understand a request but unable to execute it. The patient may, however, be able to carry out the same task automatically.[3] For instance, a patient may not be able to tie shoelaces on command but may be observed doing so automatically. With ideational apraxia, the individual movements may be correct, but they cannot be assembled into a coherent plan of action in order to accomplish a particular task.[3] Dressing apraxia may be a mixture of constructional and ideational apraxia whereby the patient puts clothes on backward, upside down, inside out, or even on the wrong limbs.[2]

Aprosody has been described as an abnormality in the affective components of language, primarily involving prosody and emotional gesturing. Along with the use of facial, limbic, and body gestures, emotional speech is thought to be the dominant linguistic feature of the right cerebral hemisphere.

Similar to the aphasias, aprosody can be divided into motor, sensory, global, conduction, and transcortical aspects, depending on the location of the lesion. For instance, the patient with motor aprosody has marked difficulty in the spontaneous use of emotional inflection in language or in emotional gesturing, but retains intact comprehension of emotional inflection or gesturing. This disorder is associated with posterior inferior lesions of the right frontal lobe.[2, 36] Sensory aprosody is just the opposite, manifesting as spontaneous emotional inflection in language and gesturing in a patient whose comprehension of emotional inflection or gesturing is markedly impaired.[36] Sensory aprosody results from lesions in the right anterior parietal lobe. Both expression and comprehension of emotional inflection and gesturing are impaired in global aprosody. Repetition is impaired in conduction aprosody.[2, 27, 36]

Visual hallucinations commonly involve diffuse brain disease or states of delirium but can also occur with more focal lesions in the temporal, parietal, or occipital lobe. Visual hallucinations tend to arise from irritative rather than destructive lesions.[2, 3, 26, 28–30] Typically, patients report hallucinations in the context of their environment. For example, they see faces at the window or bugs crawling on the wall.[2]

In contrast, decreased blood flow in the vertebrobasilar arterial system and ischemia of the occipital lobe produce unformed visual hallucinations, such as white or black spots, irregular lines, or colored patches obscuring vision.[2, 20] Ischemia of the temporal lobe may produce more elaborate visual distortions in which movement and color are perceived much as in a psychedelic drug experience.[20]

Paranoid delusions or delusional thought processes can be observed with any form of cerebrovascular disease. In the acute phase, the delusions are more likely to be restricted to the immediate environment and generally lack the expansive, global, and universal qualities seen with the functional paranoid disorders.[20] Organically based paranoid delusions are unlikely to have the elaborate and internal consistency seen in the functional disorders. Maintaining a well-integrated and internally consistent delusional thought process requires attention, concentration, memory, and fairly intact intellectual capacity, all of which are often compromised in the patient with organically based paranoia.[20]

Disorders of Intellectual Function

Deficits involving recent memory and learning of new information with relative preservation of remote memory can be associated with almost any form of diffuse brain disease. They are commonly accompanied by other deficits in cognitive functioning, however, such as orientation, attention, concentration, mental calculations, thinking, reasoning, judgment, and problem-solving abilities. Isolated memory deficits are relatively rare but can develop through a focal disease process of vascular origin.

Perhaps the best known of the focal memory disorders is Korsakoff's syndrome, in which the patient is unable to retain any new memories.[12, 20, 26, 28–30] Information can be registered but is not processed further into memory, so the individual seems always to be living in the immediate present. Patients with Korsakoff's syndrome demonstrate disorientation, continuous anterograde amnesia, and confabulation (they try to fill in their memory gaps by recreat-

ing possible events that could have occurred but that have no basis in reality). Korsakoff's syndrome is usually associated with thiamine deficiency, seen in chronic or advanced stages of alcoholism, or infarction of the mammillary bodies.[20, 30]

Disturbances of higher-level, complex intellectual functioning, such as judgment, reasoning, and abstraction, are associated with frontal lobe lesions. Specific deficits such as acalculia (difficulty manipulating mathematical concepts) usually involve parietal lobe lesions.[12, 20, 26]

PROGNOSIS AND TREATMENT

Treatment of strokes usually involves hospitalization for medication, therapy, and, very possibly, surgery. Medication can help prevent new clots from forming or prevent existing clots from getting larger. Several studies have reported benefits from the use of intravenous tissue plasminogen activator (tPA) for nonhemorrhagic strokes if treatment is begun within 3 hours of symptom onset.[37] Surgery may be used to remove fatty deposits from clogged arteries that reduce blood flow to the brain and also increase the risk of clot formation.

At some point in the recovery process, rehabilitation aims to improve the patient's physical ability and to reduce dependence. The goal is to make the patient as productive as possible, with many programs focused on return to school or competitive employment, or improving the quality of life. Success depends on the extent of brain damage, the patient's attitude and level of motivation, the skill of the rehabilitation team, and the support of family and friends.

Case Study

A 20-year-old woman is brought to the emergency room by her family because she is suddenly unable to speak or to move her right side. She looks directly forward but does not follow any verbal commands. Inspection of her fundi shows that her eyes evert. She seems to respond to visual images in all fields. The right arm and leg are flaccid and immobile, although her face is symmetric. Deep tendon reflexes are symmetric, and no pathologic reflexes are elicited. She does not react to noxious stimuli on the right side of her face or body.

Questions

1. Where might the lesion be to cause these symptoms?
2. What pathologic features usually found with such a lesion are not present in the patient? What nonpathologic features are present?
3. What is the most likely etiology?
4. What readily available test would lend great support to this diagnosis?

Discussion

1. A patient who seems to have global aphasia and a right-sided hemiparesis would usually have a left hemispheric lesion.

2. This patient does not have the usual paresis of the lower (right) face, asymmetric deep tendon reflexes, Babinski's sign, or a right homonymous hemianopsia. Eversion of the eyes during examination is always a voluntary act. Inability to perceive noxious stimuli is rare in cerebral lesions, and a sharply demarcated sensory loss (splitting along the midline) is not neurologic. Hence, a psychogenic disturbance might be suspected.

3. Hysterical reaction, malingering, or another psychogenic disturbance is the most likely etiology.

4. A normal EEG or CT scan of the brain would support such a diagnosis.

References

1. Kaufman DM: Cerebrovascular disease. *In* Clinical Neurology for Psychiatrists, ed 2. Orlando, FL, Grune & Stratton, 1985.

2. Robinson RG, Forrester AW: Neuropsychiatric aspects of cerebrovascular disease. *In* Hales RE, Yudofsky SC (eds): The American Psychiatric Press Textbook of Neuropsychiatry. Washington, DC, The American Psychiatric Press, 1987.

3. Strub RL, Black FW: Cerebrovascular disease. *In* Organic Brain Syndromes: An Introduction to Neurobehavioral Disorders. Philadelphia, FA Davis, 1983.

4. Wells CE, Duncan GW: Cerebrovascular disease. *In* Neurology for Psychiatrists. Philadelphia, FA Davis, 1980.

5. Weisberg LA, Strub RL, Garcia CA: Stroke. *In* Essentials of Clinical Neurology. Baltimore, University Park Press, 1983.

6. Kannel W, Wolf P: Epidemiology of cerebrovascular disease. *In* Russell R (ed): Vascular Disease of the Central Nervous System. New York, Churchill Livingstone, 1983.

7. Marquardson J: The natural history of acute cerebrovascular disease. Acta Neurol Scand 38(suppl):11, 1969.

8. Oxbury J, Greenhall R, Grainger K: Predicting the outcome of stroke: Acute stage after cerebral infarction. Br Med J 3:125–127, 1975.

9. Walker A, Robins M, Weinfold F: Clinical findings in the National Survey of Stroke. Stroke 12(suppl 1):13–44, 1981.

10. Adams RD, Victor M: Cerebrovascular diseases. *In* Principles of Neurology, ed 2. New York, McGraw-Hill, 1981.

11. Berg R, Franzen M, Wedding D: Screening for Brain Impairment: A Manual for Mental Health Practice. New York, Springer-Verlag, 1987.

12. Brown GG, Baird SD, Shatz MW: The effects of vascular disease and its treatment on higher cortical functioning. *In* Grant I, Adams KM (eds): Neuropsychological Assessment of Neuropsychiatric Disorders. New York, Oxford University Press, 1986.

13. Wiederholt WC: Cerebrovascular disease. *In* Neurology for Non-neurologists. New York, Academic Press, 1982.

14. Garoutte B: Survey of Functional Neuroanatomy. Greenbrae, Calif, Jones Medical Publications, 1981.

15. Pansky B, Allen DJ: Review of Neuroscience. New York, Macmillan, 1980.

16. Parsons M: Color Atlas of Clinical Neurology. Chicago, Year Book Medical, 1983.

17. Wolf P, Kannel W: Controllable risk factors for stroke: Preventive implications of trends in stroke mortality. *In* Meyer J, Shaw T (eds): Diagnosis and Management of Stroke and TIAs. Reading, MA, Addison-Wesley, 1982.

18. Becan-McBride K: Cerebrovascular disease. *In* Bishop M, Duben-von Laufen J, Fody E (eds): Clinical Chemistry: Principles, Procedures, Correlations. Philadelphia, JB Lippincott, 1985.

19. Becan-McBride K: Cerebrovascular accidents. *In* Davis BG, Bishop ML, Mass D (eds): Clinical Laboratory Science: Strategies for Practice. Philadelphia, JB Lippincott, 1989.

20. Guynn RW: Psychiatric presentations of cardiovascular disease. *In* Psychiatric Presentations of Medical Illness. New York, Spectrum Publications, 1980.

21. Heilman KM, Watson RT, Greer M: Handbook for Differential Diagnosis of Neurologic Signs and Symptoms. New York, Appleton-Century-Crofts, 1977.

22. Ullman M, Gruen A: Behavioral changes in patients with strokes. Am J Psychiatry 117:1004–1009, 1960.

23. Kolb LC, Brodie HKH: Brain syndromes associated with cerebral arteriosclerosis and other cerebrovascular disturbances. *In* Modern Clinical Psychiatry. Philadelphia, WB Saunders, 1982.

24. Wolf JK: Practical Clinical Neurology. Garden City, NY, Medical Examination, 1980.

25. Kooi KA, Tucker RP, Marshall RE: Cerebral vascular and other circulatory disorders. *In* Fundamentals of Electroencephalography. Hagerstown, Md, Harper and Row, 1978.

26. Grant I, Adams KM: Neuropsychological Assessment of Neuropsychiatric Disorders. New York, Oxford University Press, 1986.

27. Lezak MD: Neuropsychological Assessment, ed 2. New York, Oxford University Press, 1983.

28. Benson DF, Blumer D (eds): Psychiatric Aspects of Neurological Disease, vol 2. New York, Grune & Stratton, 1982.

29. Fisher SH: Psychiatric considerations of cerebral vascular disease. Am J Cardiol 7:379–385, 1961.

30. Lishman WA: Organic Psychiatry: The Psychological Consequences of Cerebral Disorder. London, Blackwell Scientific, 1978.

31. Gainotti G: Emotional behavior and hemispheric side of lesion. Cortex 8:41–55, 1972.

32. Ross ED, Rush AJ: Diagnosis and neuroanatomical correlates of depression in brain damaged patients. Arch Gen Psychiatry 38:1344–1354, 1981.

33. Cummings JL, Mendez MF: Secondary mania with focal cerebrovascular lesions. Am J Psychiatry 141:1084–1087, 1984.

34. Benson DF: Psychiatric aspects of aphasia. Br J Psychiatry 123:555–566, 1976.

35. Benson DF: Aphasia, Alexia, Agraphia. New York, Churchill Livingstone, 1979.

36. Ross ED, Mesulam MM: Dominant language functions of the right hemisphere: Prosody and emotional gesturing. Arch Neurol 36:144–148, 1979.

37. The National Institute of Neurological Disorders and Stroke t-PA Stroke Study Group: Tissue plasminogen activator for acute ischemic stroke. N Engl J Med 333:1581–1587, 1995.

Seizure Disorders, Epilepsy, and Other Convulsive States

Alexander von Laufen

No single definition of epilepsy is either universally accepted or completely adequate to describe all the different types of seizure disorders and their various manifestations. Most neurologists today believe that epilepsy is not a disease process, but rather, a complex of symptoms characterized by periodic, transient episodes of altered states of consciousness, which may in turn be associated with convulsive movements or disturbances in thinking, feeling, or behavior, or disturbances involving all three components.[1]

From a strictly neurologic perspective, seizure activity can be considered a sudden and identifiable dysfunction in the central nervous system in which there is an abnormal occurrence of highly synchronized electrical activity in the brain. Abnormal electrical discharges are not always present on the electroencephalogram of an epileptic patient, however. More commonly, abnormal discharges are manifested on the physical examination in the absence of any observable behavioral disturbance.[2] Seizures and epilepsy are, therefore, not completely synonymous. Individuals with epilepsy continue to have recurring seizures throughout their lifetimes and, most likely, maintain or control the frequency of their seizures with antiseizure medication. An individual seizure, on the other hand, may occur as a result of almost any physiologic disease state, and does not necessarily indicate an epileptic disorder with repetitive seizure occurrence. The current perspective is to regard a seizure disorder as symptomatology of almost any medical or psychopathologic condition and not to classify it as a mental disorder.[3]

Reviews have suggested that approximately 1% of the American population has been identified with some form of epilepsy, defined as at least two or more seizure episodes in the absence of an obvious precipitating factor, at least one seizure having occurred within the past 5 years.[4] This estimate would place the prevalence somewhere between 4 and 6 cases per 1000 persons, or 1 in 200 individuals.[1] These figures are approximate at best, and the actual number of cases is probably even one-third greater.[4-6] The incidence of seizure activity in males is slightly greater than in females, probably because of the greater frequency of head trauma in males, both at birth and later in adult life. Moreover, between 5% and 10% of normal, healthy individuals exhibit abnormalities on EEG tracings very similar to those seen in epileptic patients.[1] Such individuals are probably predisposed to epilepsy, but the disturbance in cortical electrodynamics is not serious enough to result in overt seizure activity, unless the cerebral cortex suffers some pathologic alteration.[1]

ETIOLOGY AND PATHOPHYSIOLOGY

In 1929, Hans Berger of Jena discovered the technical methods of amplification that enable the recording of the electrical discharges accompanying cortical activity through the intact skull. This came to be known as the electroencephalogram or EEG, which began to demonstrate the continuous alterations in electrical (and therefore physiologic) activity within the brain.[1] When these currents are recorded onto an EEG tracing, they show a pattern of voltage and frequency (i.e., height and rate of the waves) that is more or less characteristic of the individual.

When neuronal activity becomes disorganized and nerve cells suddenly produce a burst of electrical activity that is greater than normal, a wave of electricity may be set up in the brain that causes an alteration in neurologic or psychologic function. This physiologic imbalance may cause problems associated with consciousness, thought processes, sensation, muscle strength, or coordination.[6] The EEG reveals the presence of dysrhythmic discharges but fails to reveal the underlying pathogenesis:[1]

- If the focal discharging electrical activity is in the parietal, occipital or frontal lobes, the resulting symptomatology is largely neurological.

• If the disorder is in one or both temporal lobes, the symptomatology is largely psychiatric or that of psychomotor epilepsy.[1]

During a seizure or epileptic episode, normal brain functioning is upset by focal or generalized disturbances in neuronal activity. The specific type of impairment that is actually manifested is largely determined by the location and severity of the nerve cell disturbances (Fig. 41–1). This accounts for the many different varieties of seizure disorders.[6, 7]

From a neurochemical perspective, acetylcholine (Ach) is a ubiquitous neurotransmitter that is found at nearly all levels in the brain. It is also the principal excitatory agent in the central nervous system (CNS), whereas γ-aminobutyric acid (GABA) is the principal inhibitory neurotransmitter. Pharmacologic evidence seems to support dysinhibition (i.e., a decrease in GABA) as the major neurochemical mechanism in the generation of seizure activity. Most antiseizure medication, used to treat epilepsy, facilitates this inhibitory system.[8]

The electrical activity of the brain results from these two different neuronal activities.[8] There is activity at the dendrite, where neurotransmitters polarize (GABA) or depolarize (Ach) the cell membrane through synaptic junctions. Polarizations are inhibitory; depolarizations are excitatory. When local excitatory potentials in the dendrite significantly override inhibitory potentials, a threshold may be reached, and an action potential may be generated. This action potential is actually an amplification of the electrical potential of the dendrite and is transmitted quickly down the axon of nerve terminals, with the consequent release of other inhibitory or excitatory neurotransmitters. These electrical action potentials can subsequently be recorded by surface electrodes on an EEG tracing.

The ability to monitor intracranial neuronal activity assists in the understanding of normal brain functioning. Electrical potentials recorded by surface electrodes reflect activities generated from a variety of brain regions. The alpha rhythm (α) is the basic resting rhythm of the brain and can be optimally recorded over the occipital region of the brain with the alert individual's eyes closed.

Beta activity (β) is usually a fast, low-amplitude activity seen predominantly in recordings over the central regions of the cortex. The entire cerebral cortex has the potential to generate this type of activity, but it is inconspicuous in the normal awake adult and is rarely a prominent rhythm.[8] The slowest electrical rhythms are theta (ϑ) and delta (δ). These slower rhythms, which are inconspicuous in the normal awake adult but become predominant during deeper stages of sleep, are typically of high amplitude.[8] Once brain wave patterns have been determined for normal intracranial activity, measured alterations and significant deviations in these patterns begin to take on a new meaning, especially when associated with the individual's neurobehavioral activity.

Symptomatic vs. Idiopathic Epilepsy

Epilepsy has traditionally been divided into two etiologic categories, symptomatic and idiopathic, on the basis of the presumed origin of the disorder.[2] *Symptomatic epilepsy* refers to those types of seizure disorders with which an identifiable cause is associated. For instance, certain

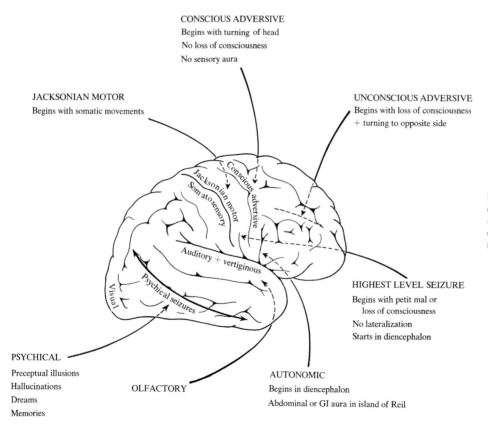

CONSCIOUS ADVERSIVE
Begins with turning of head
No loss of consciousness
No sensory aura

JACKSONIAN MOTOR
Begins with somatic movements

UNCONSCIOUS ADVERSIVE
Begins with loss of consciousness
+ turning to opposite side

Figure 41–1. Location and pattern of various nerve cell disturbances. (From Pansky B, Allen DJ: Review of Neuroscience. New York, Macmillan Publishing Company, 1980.)

HIGHEST LEVEL SEIZURE
Begins with petit mal or
    loss of consciousness
No lateralization
Starts in diencephalon

PSYCHICAL
Preceptual illusions
Hallucinations
Dreams
Memories

OLFACTORY

AUTONOMIC
Begins in diencephalon
Abdominal or GI aura in island of Reil

Box 41–1. Factors That May Precipitate Epileptic Seizures in Susceptible Individuals

Hyperventilation
Sleep (usually within the first 30 minutes or shortly
    before awakening)
Sleep deprivation
Sensory stimuli
    Flashing lights
    Reading-speaking, coughing
    Laughing, touch, pain
    Sounds (music, bells, etc.)
Trauma
Hormonal changes
    Menses, puberty, adrenal steroids
    Adrenocorticotropic hormone
Fever
Emotional stress
Drugs
    Phenothiazines, analeptics
    Tricyclic mood elevators, butyrophenones
    Antihistamines, alcohol
    Excessive anticonvulsants

types of cerebral trauma, brain tumors, encephalitis, and drug toxicity may be causal agents in the onset of epilepsy (Box 41–1). In these conditions, seizures are simply seen as symptoms of another disease state.

Idiopathic epilepsy is used to refer to those seizure disorders that do not have a prescribed cause or for which a cause has not yet been found. The idiopathic category applies to the vast majority of those individuals who are diagnosed as suffering from epilepsy which has the following characteristics: The seizure activity arises spontaneously. The seizure activity has a tendency to occur in the absence of other disorders of the nervous system.

The history of the disorder starts in childhood or adolescence. There might be a genetic predisposition for the convulsive state.

The age of the individual when the seizures first occur can be a very important clue in determining actual etiology (Fig. 41–2). For example, seizures that begin before the age of 6 months usually reflect some form of injury at

birth, a congenital defect of the nervous system, a metabolic error, or an infectious disease process. Seizures that begin between the ages of 2 and 20 years are usually regarded as having a strong genetic component and are most likely idiopathic. The onset of seizures between the ages of 20 and 35 years is relatively rare. If they do occur, they are most likely due to an external cause, such as head trauma, drug abuse, or infection. When seizures begin after the 35 years, vascular disease or brain tumors are common causes.[2] A thorough investigation into the family history of the patient is sometimes the only reliable source of information available to the clinician.

Neurogenic vs. Psychogenic Seizures

Perhaps even more important than the ability to attribute cause to a particular type of seizure is the need to determine differentially whether the presenting disorder is neurologic or psychologic in origin. Although the presenting symptomatology may be quite similar, the two groups of disorders not only have different causes but also respond in a different manner to various treatment modalities. In most instances, however, the clinician is not likely to be confronted with "pure" cases but encounters situations that display elements of both origins. Seizures have been classified generally as *partial* or *generalized;* and the International Classification of Epileptic Seizures can be seen in Box 41–2.[7]

CLINICAL MANIFESTATIONS

Partial Seizures

Partial seizures are classified into three groups, depending the symptomatology presented: (1) simple partial seizures, (2) complex partial seizures, and (3) simple or complex seizures that evolve into generalized seizures (see Box 41–2).

Partial seizures with elementary symptomatology have a localized area of focus that results in specific characteristics. There is generally no impairment of consciousness. If the seizure begins in the frontal, parietal, or occipital lobes of the brain, the initial signs or symptoms are focal ones of movement or sensation (see Fig. 41–3). This may involve jerking of an arm or leg.

If the seizure arises in the sensorimotor area adjacent to

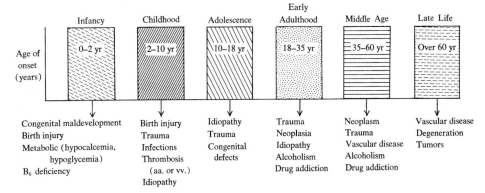

Figure 41–2. Etiology of seizures at different age levels. (From Pansky B, Allen DJ: Review of Neuroscience. New York, Macmillan Publishing Company, 1980.)

International Classification of Epileptic Seizures

I. Partial seizures (seizures beginning locally).
  A. Partial seizures with elementary symptoms (without impairment of consciousness).
    1. Motor symptoms (includes jacksonian seizures).
    2. Special sensory or somatosensory symptoms.
    3. Autonomic symptoms (rare).
    4. Compound forms (elementary and/or complex symptoms).
  B. Partial seizures with complex symptoms (with impairment of consciousness) (temporal lobe or psychomotor seizures).
    1. Impairment of consciousness only.
    2. Cognitive symptomatology.
    3. Affective symptomatology.
    4. "Psychosensory" symptomatology (hallucinations).
    5. "Psychomotor" symptomatology (automatisms).
    6. Compound forms.
  C. Partial seizures secondarily realized: tonic-clonic seizures developing from a partial seizure.
II. Generalized seizures (bilaterally symmetric and without local onset).
  A. Absences (petit mal).
  B. Bilateral massive epileptic myoclonus.
  C. Infantile spasms.
  D. Clonic seizures.
  E. Tonic seizures.
  F. Tonic-clonic seizures (grand mal).
  G. Atonic seizures (loss of tone).
  H. Akinetic seizures (loss of movement).
III. Unilateral seizures (predominantly): seizures with clinical features restricted to one side of the body.
IV. Unclassified epileptic seizures (due to lack of reliable information).

the central sulcus, symptoms of movement or sensation appear in one part of the body and generalize to larger areas. This type of seizure is called *jacksonian* (after the man who first described them), and the symptoms can actually be observed as they begin in the fingers and progressively move up to involve the entire arm.

Seizures that originate in the parietal area start with a sensation described as a breeze blowing on the skin or a light tingling or numbness. This sensation is referred to as an *aura* preceding the actual attack.

Seizures in the precentral region begin with a rhythmic twitching of the face, arm, or leg. Onset of seizures in the premotor area produces such contraversive movements as turning of the head and turning of the entire body. Seizures that originate in the occipital lobe begin with visual sensations, such as flashing colored lights (see Box 41–1).

Partial seizures with complex symptomatology have their origin in the temporal lobe and involve more mixed symptomatology related to more complicated thoughts and actions than the elementary movements and sensations of the focal seizures. The onset of a temporal lobe or psychomotor seizure can occur with or without impairment in consciousness, and the seizure can involve any or all of the features described for simple partial seizures.

In a more complicated fashion, temporal lobe seizures are usually characterized by changes in subjective experience (Fig. 41–3). These can be very idiosyncratic types of sensations, such as peculiar taste in the mouth, a visual hallucination of a person or scene, or an overwhelming feeling of familiarity with a place or an event (dejà vu). There may be the experience of strangeness, which involves the perception that objects are getting larger or smaller or are approaching the pattern or receding into the background. There may also be the experience of overwhelming anxiety or fear, or perhaps the inability to comprehend what is being said or to express oneself.[9, 10]

One of the more interesting aspects of temporal lobe seizure activity is the automatic behavior that can occur. Automatisms may be preceded by a brief loss of consciousness or simply by a subjective sensation. Repetitive and stereotyped movements, such as a continual scratching of the head or picking at the clothes, are common. Automatic types of behavior can vary from simple, uncoordinated movements all the way to complex activities. What is so unusual about this form of behavior, however, is that the individual is unaware of surroundings while performing the automatic behavior over and over again. Violent behavior during these episodes is very rare, but attempts at restraining the automatic behavior may be met with aggressive reaction.[4, 11]

Partial seizures secondarily generalized are seizures that begin in the simple phase and progress to generalized tonic-clonic seizures. They can also originate as complex seizures and evolve into a more generalized stage, or they can involve both processes.

Generalized Seizures

The second group of seizure disorders involves generalized seizures in which the electric overactivity in the brain is no longer focused but is more diffuse. Several different types of generalized seizures have been identified.

Absence seizures, or *petit mal epilepsy,* is a disorder characterized by a brief loss of awareness during which there is no motor activity other than a blinking or a rolling up of the eyes. An attack of this nature may be very brief, usually lasting less than 10 seconds, but may proceed for several minutes. Patients do not fall to the ground, and they rapidly return to full consciousness without retrograde amnesia or confusion, although they have no awareness of what took place during the attack. Petit mal epilepsy is typically found in children between the ages of 2 and 15 years, and is rarely seen in anyone older.[2, 4]

Myoclonic seizures are characterized by brief, repetitive jerking of the arms and trunk. Typically, the arms flex and the trunk jerks forward. The jerks are so quick that a lapse of consciousness is not evident; however, the jerks can become so rapid and repetitive that they begin to fuse into a generalized clonic seizure.[4] Myoclonic jerking sometimes occurs in nonepileptic individuals and may be experienced by anyone just before falling asleep when in a relaxed state.

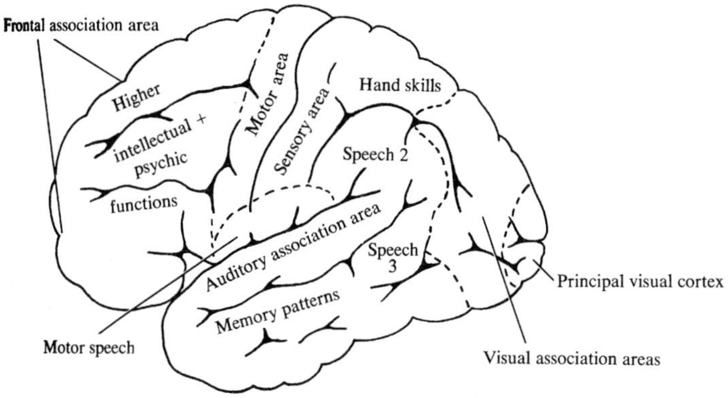

Figure 41–3. Functional regions of the left cortex. (From Pansky B, Allen DJ: Review of Neuroscience. New York, Macmillan Publishing Company, 1980.)

Tonic-clonic seizures, or *grand mal epilepsy,* is primarily generalized from the onset. There is a total loss of consciousness and stereotyped motor activity.[2] About 50% of patients with grand mal epilepsy have little or no warning that a tonic-clonic attack is imminent. In the initial tonic phase, the body suddenly becomes rigid, the extremities extend, and breathing stops. This is followed by a clonic phase, characterized by a rhythmic jerking of the extremities and trunk. Gradually, the jerking motions slow down, and they stop altogether after 2 to 10 minutes. The patient begins to regain consciousness, but may remain confused and drowsy for several minutes up to a day or two.

Akinetic seizures, which occur in children between the ages of 1 and 7 years, are characterized by a sudden loss of their antigravity muscles.[2] The child simply falls to the ground without any warning. This kind of attack is usually very brief, and after a few seconds, the child may get up without any postictal depression. Many authorities believe that seizures of this type are not actually akinetic but rather are myoclonic, because they result from a severe flexion of the neck and hips. Although the onset is quick and the actual duration of the attack lasts only a few seconds, most of these cases are associated with brain damage, and affected children usually do not develop normal intellectual functioning.

Infantile spasms, which always begin before the age of 2 years, are actually massive myoclonic spasms in which there is a sudden flexion or extension of the body. Seizures of this type often go unrecognized in infancy, because they are of such short duration and are frequently mistaken for a startle reaction. Infantile spasms generally resolve as the child grows older, or they may evolve into other clinical seizures. Because this type of epilepsy results in a profound disruption of the central nervous system and occurs at such a young age, it can be expected to be associated with fairly severe forms of mental retardation.

Diagnostic Evaluation

Although the epilepsies lend themselves to the preceding method of classification, and their behavioral manifestations can be described on the basis of symptomatology, only about one out of four patients diagnosed with an active form of epilepsy has no associated disabilities.[4] This fact suggests that the majority of patients seeking medical care for their seizures also have other disabilities, such as neurologic deficits, cognitive impairment, or behavioral and adjustment problems. Patient evaluation is, therefore, of the utmost importance, not only to differentiate between a true and a pseudo–seizure disorder, but also to determine the etiology and nature of the disorder as a basis for treatment.

LABORATORY ANALYSES AND DIAGNOSIS

The actual type of seizure itself commonly suggests the possible cause and, consequently, the most appropriate method of study. For instance, focal seizures are often caused by focal brain irritation.[12] Clinical studies are, therefore, more likely to include tests to identify those structural changes in the areas of the brain under consideration, for example, an electroencephalogram (EEG) or computed tomography (CT) scan of the brain. Because generalized seizures are more apt to be caused by problems affecting the entire brain, such as chemical abnormalities, infections, or poisons, patients with such seizures should undergo blood and chemical analyses as well as spinal fluid studies.[12] The evaluation procedure typically advances along the lines of a decision tree much like the one presented in Figure 41–4.

Preliminary evaluation of a seizure disorder usually comprises routine blood and urine tests and sometimes an analysis of the cerebrospinal fluid, all performed by the clinical laboratory scientist. A neurologic examination, electrophysiologic studies, a CT scan of the brain, and comprehensive neuropsychologic testing can also be beneficial (Box 41–3).

No clinical laboratory tests specifically indicate a diagnosis of seizure or epilepsy. Laboratory analysis is generally limited to the monitoring of anticonvulsant drugs in the blood of the patient. The laboratory scientist does, however, perform a number of other analyses that aid the physician in ruling out a diagnosis of epilepsy and in differentiating between seizures resulting from a particular disease or illness and seizures resulting from a primary neurologic disorder. Results of a complete blood count (CBC), blood chemistry tests, and urinalysis are all generally within the expected normal range, unless the seizures are associated with an underlying disease state. Analyses of the cerebrospinal fluid for glucose, total proteins, immunoglobulin G, and lactic acid all yield normal results in epilepsy.[13]

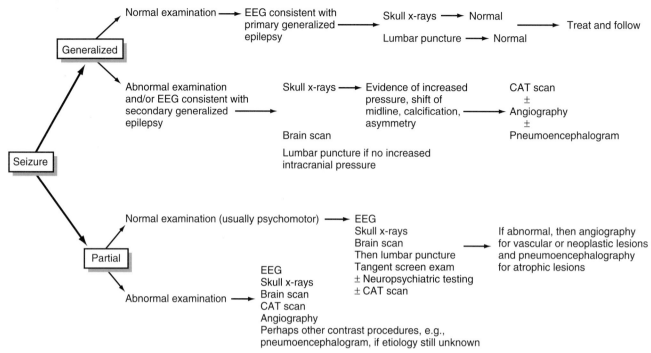

Figure 41–4. Diagnostic evaluation of seizures. Abbreviations: EEG, electroencephalogram; CAT, computed axial tomography.

TREATMENT OF ONGOING SEIZURE DISORDERS

Most of the many types of seizures can be managed effectively and treated successfully with anticonvulsant drugs. Alternative types of treatment, such as dietary manipulation, biofeedback, psychosurgery, and less conventional techniques, should be implemented only after a drug regimen is clearly proved nonbeneficial.[6] Anticonvulsant medication, however, should be kept as simple as possible. The goal is to reduce the frequency of occurrence and eventually to abolish the seizures themselves, with the least amount of the safest drugs possible.[14]

Generally, one anticonvulsant is begun at a time, and

Box 41–3. **Diagnostic Tests in the Evaluation of a Seizure Disorder**

Basic Diagnostic Tests

Hematologic studies	Complete blood count
Urine studies	Urinalysis
Biochemical studies	Serum calcium and phosphorus; fasting blood sugar
Serology	Studies to exclude tuberculosis, syphilis
Electrophysiologic studies	EEG
Radiologic studies	Skull x-ray, computed tomography scan of the brain
Psychologic studies	Psychologic, psychometric testing

Additional Studies in Select Cases

Biochemical studies	5-hour glucose tolerance test, amino acid screen
Genetic studies	Chromosomal analysis
CSF examination	Infections of the nervous system
Electrophysiologic studies	Special EEG activation procedures (sleep, telemetry, chemical)
Neuropsychologic studies	Psycholinguistic evaluation for learning problems

Special Studies

Electrophysiologic studies	24-hour video and EEG monitoring, brain surface and depth EEGs
Radiologic studies	Angiogram or air study

Table 41–1. Common Drugs Used in the Treatment and Management of Seizures

Generic Name	Trade Name	Total Daily Dose*	Type of Epilepsy Used for					
			Partial Elementary	Partial Complex	Major Motor	Petit Mal	Myoclonic	Infantile Spasms
Phenytoin	Dilantin	4–7	+	+	–			
Phenobarbital	Luminal	1–5	As added to DPH	+	–			
Primidone	Mysoline	10–25	+	+	–			
Carbamazepine	Tegretol	7–15	+	+	–			
Ethosuximide	Zarontin	20–30				+		
Trimethadione	Tridione	10–25				+		
Paramethadione	Paradione	10–25				+		
Mephenytoin	Mesantoin	7–12	+	+	–			
Ethotoin	Peganone	10–20	+	+	–			
Metharbital	Gemonil	2.5–10	+		–			
Mephobarbital	Mebaral	2.5–10	+		–			
Methsuximide	Celontin	10–20				+		
Phenacemide	Phenurone	25–45	+	+				
Acetazolamide	Diamox	5–15				+ and premenstrual		
ACTH		40–60 units total per day						+
Corticosteroids		5–60 mg total per day						+
Diazepam	Valium	0.15–2			Alcohol withdrawal	+ and status epilepticus		
Chlordiazepoxide	Librium	1–4			Alcohol withdrawal			
Paraldehyde		0.3–0.7 mL/kg		Tonic seizures				
Dextroamphetamine	Dexedrine	0.2–0.3		Tonic seizures				
Methylphenidate	Ritalin	0.2–0.3						
Clonazepam	Klonopin	0.1–0.2				+	+	

*Given as mg/kg body weight unless otherwise noted.

the dosage gradually increased, with serum blood levels periodically checked, before a second medication is added. The particular medication first instituted depends on several contributing factors. The age of the patient, the particular type and severity of the seizure disorder, past medical history, and the patient's prior experience with anticonvulsant drugs all influence the physician's decision about the medication to use. If the first drug fails, other drugs should be tried one at a time until all reasonable choices have been selectively exhausted.[6] If one drug cannot control the occurrence of a seizure, then perhaps two or more anticonvulsant drugs in combination can prove beneficial.

Clinical research over the last several years has established certain medications as the drugs of choice for each presenting seizure type (Table 41–1). The drug having the fewest adverse effects and the greatest efficacy is usually the one that is prescribed.[6] Most clinicians agree that phenytoin sodium (Dilantin) is still the most effective and safest drug available for treating generalized tonic-clonic seizures. Carbamazepine (Tegretol) is the first choice of many physicians for complex partial seizures. Primidone (Mysoline) can be a valuable, alternative if carbamazepine fails to control this type of seizure activity.[6] Generalized absence seizures are probably best managed with ethosuximide and sodium valproate. Focal motor and focal sensory seizures respond best to phenytoin.

An important advancement in the management of epilepsy was the introduction of certain techniques for measuring serum anticonvulsant levels. Evidence has now accumulated that the anticonvulsant properties and occurrence of potential neurotoxic side effects of specific drugs are better correlated with the concentration of the drug in the serum rather than with the dosage.[15] From research in this area, the concept of the *therapeutic drug range* has emerged—that is, the range of serum levels within which maximum seizure control can be expected with the minimum incidence of side effects.[15]

Serum concentrations of all drugs used as anticonvulsants can be measured periodically by commonly available blood tests (Table 41–2). The dosage required by a particular patient with seizures in order to maintain a therapeutic drug level in the serum can be measured precisely through periodic checking of the serum drug level. How often the serum drug level is checked depends on the rate at which the drug is metabolized in the body. The best time to check a serum drug level is usually at the end of the dose level,[6] that is, just before the patient takes another dose of the drug.

Case Study

A 27-year-old woman came to the attention of a referring psychiatrist, who diagnosed her symptoms as "free-floating" anxiety and prescribed Librium. Her background had been extremely traumatic, with mentally ill parents and institutionalization at an early age.

Psychodiagnostic assessment identified anxiety and depression, but also a marked perceptual confusion that required further differential diagnosis. The patient's past medical history was also significant, involving two head injuries at ages 5 and 11 years. Both injuries had resulted in a loss of consciousness. She developed severe headaches that were described as frequent and becoming worse. She also experienced blackout spells, dizziness, nausea, blurring of vision, tingling in her fingers, and altered state of consciousness, as well as a prescient feeling that something terrible was going to happen to her. On one occasion, she suddenly and inexplicably struck out and hit a companion.

The referring psychiatrist rejected the "psychologic" findings and decided to obtain a neurologic consultation. A second psychiatric opinion concluded that "the clinical picture is that of emotional instability that is probably secondary to her cerebral dysfunction and probably secondary to familial dysfunction."

Questions

1. Are the presenting symptoms "neurologic" or "psychologic" in nature? Is this diagnosis accurate, given the patient's medical and social history?

2. How might the psychiatrist treat the patient's various symptoms?

Discussion

1. Anxiety, depression, and emotional or behavioral disorders can commonly imitate (and often be mistaken for) an underlying neurologic process. The course in an individual largely depends on the preexisting personality of the patient, the functional area of the brain in which the physiologic imbalance occurs, and the speed at which the excitation spreads in the brain tissue. The actual diagnosis of this somewhat complicated case lies somewhere between a strictly neurologic and a psychologic explanation. Elements of both neurologic and psychologic reactions to that dysfunctioning come into play. It would be extremely difficult and nearly impossible to treat the "psychologic" symptoms if the underlying neurologic conditions were not first addressed. This "working" assumption is certainly a viable one, but it is also too obvious and, as a diagnosis, would also lend itself to very difficult treatment. An alternative diagnosis of post-traumatic seizures could explain some of the manifest symptomatology. However, the severity of the patient's developmental history should not be overlooked.

Table 41–2. Therapeutic Serum Levels of Common Anticonvulsant Drugs

Drug	Serum Levels (μg drug/ mL serum)	Starting Dose (mg)	Daily Dose
Phenytoin	10–20	900	300–400
Carbamazepine	6–10	100–200	600–1,200
Valproic acid	50–100	250	1,000–3,000
Ethosuximide	50–100	250	750–2,000
Primidone	6–12	50–125	750–1,500
Phenobarbital	15–35	30–60	100–150
Clonazepam	0.013–0.072	0.5	1–2

2. In this particular case, the patient was started on a therapeutic regimen of anticonvulsant medication (Dilantin) and quickly responded with improvement in nearly all her symptoms.

Not long afterwards, however, she returned to the clinic with continued complaints of increasing depression, irritability, restlessness, intellectual slowing, and relatively unstable mood swings. A blood sample was drawn as a routine procedure, and the serum level of Dilantin was subsequently checked. The anticonvulsant medication the patient was taking was found to be outside the therapeutic range of values and possibly causing toxic side effects. The dosage was reduced, and the patient's serum drug level was systematically monitored over the next several months. Her complaints gradually decreased, and her social worker reported greatly improved feelings with initial prospects for employment. The patient had to be kept on Dilantin therapy with occasional returns to the clinic in order to monitor the drug's effectiveness, but she returned to a normal and active life.

Although there is not conclusive proof that this patient's symptoms were directly related to seizure activity, her problems seemed to respond quickly to an appropriate level of anticonvulsant medication. The important thing to note here is that the drug of choice has to be monitored periodically (usually every 2 to 3 months), because it can easily cause negative side effects if not properly adjusted.

References

1. Kolb LC, Brodie HKH (eds): Brain Syndromes Associated with Convulsive Disorders (Epilepsy). *In* Modern Clinical Psychiatry, ed 10. Philadelphia, WB Saunders, 1982.
2. Pincus JH, Tucker GJ: Behavioral Neurology, ed 3. New York, Oxford University Press, 1985.
3. Diagnostic and Statistical Manual of Mental Disorders (DSM-IV), ed 4. Washington DC, American Psychiatric Association, 1994.
4. Masland RL: The Nature of Epilepsy. *In* Sands H (ed): Epilepsy: A Handbook for the Mental Health Professional. New York, Bruner/Mazel, 1982.
5. Strudler LA, Perlman LG (eds): Basic Statistics in the Epilepsies. Philadelphia, FA Davis, 1975.
6. Lechtenberg R: The Diagnosis and Treatment of Epilepsy. New York, Macmillan, 1985.
7. Gastaut H: Classification of the epilepsies: Proposal for an International Classification. Epilepsia 10(Suppl):2–19, 1969.
8. Stevenson JM, King JH: Neuropsychiatric aspects of epilepsy and epileptic seizures. *In* Vudofsky SC, Hales RE (eds): Textbook of Neuropsychiatry. Washington, DC, American Psychiatric Press, 1992.
9. Blumer D. Temporal Lobe epilepsy and its psychiatric significance. *In* Benson DF, Blumer D (eds): Psychiatric Aspects of Neurological Disease. New York, Grune & Stratton, 1975.
10. Blumer D, Benson DF: Psychiatric manifestations of epilepsy. *In* Benson DF, Blumer D (eds): Psychiatric Aspects of Neurological Disease, vol 2. New York, Grune & Stratton, 1982.
11. Berman SA, Rosenfield DB: Neurobehavior and temporal lobe epilepsy. *In* Fann WE (ed): Phenomenology and Treatment of Psychophysiological Disorders. New York, Spectrum Publications, 1982.
12. Svoboda WB: Learning About Epilepsy. Baltimore, University Park Press, 1979.
13. Berman JJ: Effects of Diseases on Laboratory Tests. Philadelphia, JB Lippincott, 1983.
14. Wells CE, Duncan GW: Neurology for Psychiatrists. Philadelphia, FA Davis, 1980.
15. Grant I, Adams KM: Neuropsychological Assessment of Neuropsychiatric Disorders. New York, Oxford University Press, 1986.

Bibliography

Bannister R: Brain's Clinical Neurology, ed 6. London, Oxford University Press, 1985.

Glaser GH: Epilepsy: Neuropsychological aspects. *In* Reiser MF (ed): American Handbook of Psychiatry: Organic Disorders and Psychosomatic Medicine, ed 2. New York, Basic Books, 1975.

Heilman KM, Watson RT, Greer M: Handbook for Differential Diagnosis of Neurological Signs and Symptoms. New York, Appleton-Century-Crofts, 1977.

Kaufman DM: Clinical Neurology for Psychiatrists, ed 2. New York, Grune & Stratton, 1985.

Kirkpatrick B, Hall RCW: Seizure disorders. *In* Hall RCW (ed): Psychiatric presentations of medical illnesses: Somatopsychic disorders. New York, Spectrum Publications, 1980.

Lechtenberg R: The Psychiatrist's Guide to Diseases of the Nervous System. New York, John Wiley & Sons, 1982.

Pansky B, Allen DJ: Review of Neuroscience. New York, Macmillan, 1980.

Soloman G, Plum F: Clinical Management of Seizures. Philadelphia, WB Saunders, 1976.

Strub RL, Black FW: Organic Brain Syndromes: An Introduction to Neurobehavioral Disorders. Philadelphia, FA Davis, 1981.

Wiederholt WC: Neurology for Non-Neurologists. New York, Academic Press, 1982.

Williams DT: The Treatment of Seizures. *In* Sands H (ed): Epilepsy: A Handbook for the Mental Health Professional. New York, Bruner/Mazel, 1982.

Hematologic Disorders

Chapter 42

The Anemias

Marian Schwabbauer

ETIOLOGY AND PATHOPHYSIOLOGY

All body cells need oxygen to function and survive. Erythrocytes, the major formed elements of the blood, carry oxygen to the cells via a carrier protein, hemoglobin. If there is not enough functional hemoglobin in the circulation to deliver the required oxygen levels, *anemia* is pres-

ent. Erythrocytes are produced in the bone marrow, circulate for approximately 120 days, and then are removed by the reticuloendothelial system (RES). Normally there is an equilibrium between the number of erythrocytes needed, produced, and removed from the circulation.

Anemia exists when the level of circulating hemoglobin is lower than that in healthy persons of the same sex and age group in the same environment as the patient.[1] Anemia can also be defined as a decrease in oxygen-carrying capacity of the blood caused by diminished hemoglobin function or availability. It is often, but not always, associated with decreased erythrocyte numbers (mass). Hemoglobin and erythrocyte reference ranges differ according to sex, age, geographic location, and ethnic origins. The physiologic needs of individuals also change with age, altitude, stress, and disease. Thus, the symptoms of anemia relate both to the level of physiologic need of the individual and to the extent of the reduced hemoglobin function or availability.

Anemia per se is usually not considered a primary diagnosis, but rather a manifestation of an underlying disease process.[2] Anemia is corrected by identifying and treating the underlying disease. To simply improve the diminished oxygen-carrying capacity by either increasing oxygen availability or replacing decreased erythrocyte numbers via transfusion does not resolve the underlying disease state and can mask important diagnostic clues. Except in extreme cases, the underlying disorder must be identified before treatment is begun.

In evaluation of anemia, the goal is to determine the etiology as efficiently as possible so that it can be treated quickly, appropriately, and cost-effectively. Along with the clinical symptoms, history and physical examination, pathophysiologic and morphologic classification systems based on laboratory data can be very helpful in determining

Table 42–1. Pathophysiologic Categorization of Anemias

Erythrocyte Kinetics	Examples	
	Shortened Erythrocyte Life Span	*Normal Erythrocyte Life Span*
Increased erythrocyte production	Compensated hemolytic anemias	Some deficiency anemias
Normal erythrocyte production	Uncompensated hemolytic anemia	Acute blood loss
Decreased erythrocyte production	Combinations of etiologies	Bone marrow failure

etiology. Six general etiologic categories are used in this discussion: deficiency anemias, hemolytic anemias, hemoglobinopathies, bone marrow failure, blood loss, and secondary anemias.

Because the etiologic possibilities are so varied, many factors must be assessed during the history and physical examination. The history should include age, sex, ethnic origin, diet, recent geographic habitation, toxic exposures including prescription and over-the-counter drugs, infection, neoplasm, bleeding tendencies, family history of diseases, and symptoms.[3] The physical examination should include observation of the skin for abnormal color changes, rashes, and ulceration; the tongue, nails, and hair for characteristic changes; and the lymph nodes, spleen, and liver. Secondary diagnostic tests may be needed to adequately determine the neurologic, endocrine, and nutritional status of the patient.

Classification of Anemias

The pathophysiologic classification of anemia is based on the mechanism of disease, for example, decreased bone marrow production of normally functioning erythrocytes or increased loss of erythrocytes by hemorrhage or hemolysis.[1] Anemias can be roughly divided into five general pathophysiologic categories using two criteria: the number of erythrocytes produced by the marrow and the rate of erythrocyte destruction, as shown in Table 42–1.

In the morphologic classification of anemias, physical characteristics of erythrocytes (shape, size, color, and presence or absence of inclusions) are used to make decisions about treatment as well as about further testing. Table 42–2 depicts this categorization scheme. Table 42–3 lists characteristics of the major anemic states discussed in this

Table 42–2. Morphologic Categorization of Anemias

Erythrocyte Morphology	Examples	
	Hypochromic	*Normochromic*
Microcytic	Iron deficiency	Chronic blood loss
Normocytic	Chronic blood loss	Acute blood loss
Macrocytic	Combination of etiologies	Megaloblastic anemia

chapter. The use of these or other schemes to classify anemias is often complicated by multiple etiologies that can give conflicting or confusing laboratory results.[4]

Deficiency Anemias

Deficiency anemias are anemias caused by the lack of one or more substances needed to produce functional erythrocytes or hemoglobin. This lack may be due to a diet deficient in these substances, to malabsorption, or to metabolic substitution or interference by drugs or toxins. Iron deficiency and megaloblastic anemias are the most common deficiency anemias.

Iron is required by all organs and systems in the body, and most of the iron in the body is found in hemoglobin. The normal diet provides 10 to 20 mg of iron per day, and only 5% to 10% of it is absorbed, although absorption is increased in iron deficiency. The four major causes of iron deficiency are blood loss, dietary deficiency, malabsorption, and increased requirements such as in pregnancy and growth spurts.

In megaloblastic anemias, the underlying problem is impaired DNA synthesis due to vitamin B_{12} or folate deficiency. Although all dividing cells in the body are affected, rapidly dividing cells, such as developing erythrocytes and leukocytes, are affected first. The cytoplasm develops relatively normally, but the nucleus does not, and there is no signal to divide. Macrocytosis develops owing to the smaller number of cell divisions. The nuclear material has a characteristic "open chromatin" pattern that is so abnormal that large numbers of developing cells are recognized as defective and are removed by the reticuloendothelial cells in the bone marrow before they reach the circulation. This "ineffective erythropoiesis" is a major contributing factor to the anemia.

Vitamin B_{12} is synthesized by microorganisms and is found in all animal tissues. It requires intrinsic factor for absorption and is then transported by transcobalamins I and II. The body's store, 2 to 5 mg, will last for several years after intake ceases. A deficiency of B_{12} may be due to inadequate intake of the vitamin, defective absorption, competition with the host for B_{12}, or pernicious anemia. Inadequate intake is seen only in strict vegetarians. Defective absorption of B_{12} is most often due to gastrointestinal disease, that is, malabsorption. Competition with the host for B_{12} is characteristic of infestation with *Diphyllobothrium latum*, a parasitic tapeworm, or certain intestinal bacteria. Pernicious anemia is thought to result from an autoimmunity to gastric parietal cells or intrinsic factor, with the subsequent loss of B_{12} absorptivity and resulting deficiency of this vitamin.

Folates, or folic acid, are widely present in foods, but the body's stores last only weeks if intake ceases. If there is a total dietary lack, serum folate level decreases within 3 weeks. At 11 weeks, hypersegmentation of neutrophils appears, and at 17 weeks, erythrocyte folate levels decrease. Megaloblastic anemias due to folate deficiency are similar to those due to B_{12} deficiency, except that leukopenia, thrombocytopenia, and central nervous system symptoms are less common. A folate deficiency can be due to nutritional inadequacy, pregnancy, intestinal disease, dialysis, or the administration of folic acid antagonists. Nutri-

Table 42–3. **Characteristics of Anemia**

Anemia	Defect	Effect	Usual Treatment
Aplastic	Often idiopathic, drugs, toxins, ↓ erythropoietin	Decreased red cells (relatively normal) produced, pancytopenia	Steroids Bone marrow transplant
Autoimmune hemolytic (AIHA)	Antibody present	Coated red cells removed prematurely from circulation by RES (spleen)	Steroids, etc, to reduce antibody production Remove antigenic stimulus

B$_{12}$ deficiency
  Pernicious anemia
  Malabsorption
	Lack of active intrinsic factor
	Lack of intestinal tract; bacterial overgrowth
		Unable to absorb B$_{12}$ needed for nucleic acid synthesis; macrocytic, normochromic cells, ↓RBCs, ↓WBCs, ↓platelets	B$_{12}$ by injection
			Treat malabsorption; replacement therapy

Chronic disease, inflammation	Multiple; iron not released from storage cells ↓ Erythropoietin activity	Slight hypochromia, microcytosis ↓life span of RBCs ↓ # of red cells produced	Treat underlying disease

Enzyme deficiencies
  G6PD
  Pyruvate kinase
	↓G6PD
	↓Pyruvate Kinase
		Cells susceptible to oxidation and Heinz body formation
		Impaired glycolysis; ↓RBC life span
			Remove oxidative agent
			Supportive therapy

Folate deficiency	Dietary Alcoholism (folate block) Chemotherapy	Unable to synthesize nucleic acids properly; macrocytic normochromic cells, ↓RBC, ↓WBC, ↓platelets	Folic acid Treat alcohol dependency Supportive therapy
Hereditary spherocytosis	Membrane protein defects	Rigid, spherical cells cannot move freely through microcirculation and are removed prematurely by RES (spleen)	Splenectomy to increase RBC life span
Hypersplenism	Increased splenic sequestration of RBCs	↓RBC life span	Splenectomy
Iron deficiency	Lack of iron (dietary or blood loss)	Unable to make enough hemoglobin to fill cells Microcytic hypochromic cells	Oral ferrous sulfate; correct blood loss
Lead poisoning	Decreased heme synthesis	Unable to make enough hemoglobin to fill cells Microcytic hypochromic cells	Chelation therapy
Microangiopathic hemolytic anemia	Vessel abnormalities, occlusion, DIC	Fragmentation of red cells, which are then removed early from the circulation	Treat underlying disease
Nutritional	Most often combined folate and iron deficiency	Unable to make enough hemoglobin to fill cells Microcytic hypochromic cells Unable to synthesize nucleic acids properly	Change nutritional status; nutritional supplements
Paroxysmal cold hemoglobinuria	Presence of biphasic antibody	Complement fixed in cold; cells lyse upon warming Hemoglobinuria	Avoid cold
Paroxysmal nocturnal hemoglobinuria	Increased susceptibility to complement	Intravascular hemolysis during night and/or periods of stress, resulting in hemoglobinuria	Avoid stress, infection
Pregnancy	Increased demand for iron and folate Increased plasma volume	Folate deficiency; iron deficiency Relative anemia, ↓Hct, RBC mass stays same	Supplemental folate, iron
Pyridoxine deficiency	Dietary, enzyme deficiency	Unable to fill cells with hemoglobin Hypochromic, microcytic RBCs; often 2 populations (dimorphic).	Vitamin B$_6$ (pyridoxine)
Sickle cell	Valine substituted for glutamic acid in 6th position	Crystallizing hemoglobin deforms cells, causing sludging and premature removal by RES (spleen)	Avoid ↓O$_2$ tension situations Molecular therapies being tried Supportive therapy

Sideroblastic
  Acquired
  Inherited
	Unable to incorporate iron to make heme	Unable to fill cells with hemoglobin
		Hypochromic, microcytic RBCs; often 2 populations (dimorphic)
		Basophilic stippling
			Vitamin B$_6$ (pyridoxine)
			Supportive therapy

Thalassemia	Decreased synthesis of one or more globin chains	Inability to fill cells with hemoglobin; microcytic hypochromic RBCs	Supportive therapy Genetic counseling
Unstable hemoglobin	Amino acid replacement or deletion	Hemoglobin denatures and precipitates as Heinz bodies	Supportive therapy

Abbreviations: G6PD, glucose-6-phosphate dehydrogenase; RES, reticuloendothelial system; RBC, red blood cell; WBC, white blood cell; DIC, disseminated intravascular coagulation; Hct, hematocrit.

Adapted from Schwabbauer MH: Understanding anemias. In-Service Reviews in Clinical Laboratory Science, Vol 6, No 8. Birmingham, AL, Educational Reviews, 1993.

tional inadequacy is commonly seen in underdeveloped nations and in alcoholics. In pregnancy, folate deficiency is due to the increased need to support the developing fetus. Intestinal disease often results in malabsorption of many substances, including folates. Folates can be lost during the dialysis process if not closely monitored and replaced. Folic acid antagonists, given to cancer patients in an effort to selectively decrease rapidly dividing malignant cells, also create a functional folate deficiency.

Bone Marrow Failure and Aplastic Anemia

Bone marrow failure can be due to marrow replacement with malignant cells or other nonfunctioning material, or it can be idiopathic (no apparent cause is known or can be determined). When bone marrow failure is idiopathic, it is usually termed aplastic anemia, even though there is a pancytopenia or decrease in all cell lines. Drugs and radiation can also damage bone marrow cells. In hemolytic anemia, infections, or hypersplenism, the demand for cells can be so overwhelming that the bone marrow is unable to keep up with the increased losses, and a relative bone marrow failure occurs. In these circumstances, a bone marrow evaluation is necessary to the diagnosis of marrow failure.

Hemolytic Anemias

Hemolytic anemia is an etiologic category comprising a wide variety of anemias due to a decreased erythrocyte life span and is, with few exceptions, inherited. Obtaining a family history of similar disorders is important. Hemolytic anemia due to extracellular influences is almost always an acquired disorder; reviewing a detailed history of recent illness or drug usage is imperative.

A chronic hemolytic process is ongoing and usually not life threatening, in contrast to an acute hemolytic process, which is sudden, devastating, and frequently life threatening. A chronic process may or may not be "compensated." The hemolytic process is considered "compensated" if the bone marrow is able to increase the production of erythrocytes each day to equal or surpass the number being destroyed and thus to maintain an adequate hemoglobin level. If the marrow is unable to do so, the hemolytic anemia is "uncompensated."

The increased hemolysis or cell destruction may take place primarily within or outside the vascular circulation or may be a combination of both. If cell destruction occurs within the circulation, it is termed *intravascular*. If the cell destruction occurs in reticuloendothelial organs such as the spleen, bone marrow, or liver, it is *extravascular*.

The usual approach to a hemolytic anemia consists of two steps. First, hemolysis is established, and then the specific etiology of the anemia is determined by means of appropriate laboratory tests. For effective utilization of the laboratory to delineate hemolytic anemias, the symptoms, defect, and effects of each hemolytic anemia must be understood (see Table 42–3).

The anemias due to increased destruction because of intracellular defects are characterized by greater hemolysis with a normal hemoglobin molecule. Some, such as heredi-

tary spherocytosis, are due to defects in the cell membrane. Others, such as glucose-6-phosphate dehydrogenase (G6PD) deficiency, are due to defects in the red cell enzyme system. The only commonly recognized hemolytic anemia due to an acquired membrane defect is paroxysmal nocturnal hemoglobinuria (PNH).

Always acquired rather than inherited, the immunohemolytic anemias can be categorized as autoimmune, alloimmune, or drug-induced. Autoimmune hemolytic anemias can be secondary to other diseases, such as viral or immune disorders, or they can be primary and of unknown origin. These anemias are unpredictable and vary widely in severity and duration. The cause of the increased cell destruction is an antibody directed against the patient's own erythrocytes. These antibodies can be of the warm antibody type, the cold antibody type, or the paroxysmal cold hemoglobinuria (PCH) type. Cold antibodies are most often either anti-I or anti-i. They are commonly secondary to leukemia, lymphoma, or infections, most often with *Mycoplasma pneumoniae* or the Epstein-Barr virus.

Drug-induced antibodies can be classified as drug adsorption (hapten) type, immune complex (innocent bystander) type, membrane modification (nonimmunologic protein adsorption) type, or induction of autoimmunity (unknown) type.

Alloimmune hemolysis is seen in transfusion reactions and in hemolytic disease of the newborn, which is discussed in detail in Chapter 67.

Non–antibody-related extracellular influences that can increase cell destruction are infections, exposure to toxic chemicals and drugs, physical agents such as heat, cold, and microangiopathic vessel disorders, and hypersplenism.

Hemoglobinopathies, Thalassemias, and Sideroblastic Anemias

The hemoglobinopathies are due to one or more qualitative defects or amino acid substitutions on one or more globin chains. The thalassemias, considered quantitative disorders, are caused by decreased synthesis of one or more globin chains. The sideroblastic anemias are a diverse group of disorders that have common clinical and laboratory features due to reduced porphyrin synthesis. Both the hemoglobinopathies and the thalassemias are considered to be due to intracellular defects and to be inherited rather than acquired. The sideroblastic anemias may be hereditary or acquired. The erythrocytes in most hemoglobinopathies and thalassemias have a shorter life span.

More than one amino acid substitution can occur in the same patient, and a quantitative defect, such as thalassemia, can occur along with a qualitative defect or hemoglobinopathy. For example, an anemia might be due to a combination of hemoglobin S (HbS) and β-thalassemia.

The most common abnormal hemoglobin is HbS, found in 8% to 10% of blacks, although fewer than 1% are homozygous for the defect. It is characterized by a substitution of valine for glutamic acid at the sixth position of the β-chain that is inherited as an autosomal codominant. This substitution allows the hemoglobin molecules to polymerize and crystallize under decreased oxygen tension. As the cell membrane conforms to the structure of the crystal, the cell assumes a characteristic sickle shape. The deformed cells have a tendency to sludge and block the microcirculation and are removed early from the circulation by the RES.

The next most common β-chain structural change, a lysine substitution for a glutamic acid, most often at the sixth position on the β-chain, is hemoglobin C (HbC) and its variants. Two percent to 3% of blacks have one or more β-chains with the substitution, which is also inherited as an autosomal codominant. The heterozygote is usually asymptomatic, with 30% to 40% HbC and a few target cells. In homozygotes, who usually have from 90% to 100% HbC, which tends to form a characteristic rhomboid crystal or tactoid, which deforms the erythrocyte.

Combinations of abnormal hemoglobins, such as SC, occur. The clinical and laboratory picture of SC is less severe than that of SS, with red cell morphologic characteristics of both S and C.

Another β-chain structural change is that of hemoglobin E, which occurs in as much as 30% of the population of certain areas in Southeast Asia.

Patients with methemoglobinemia do not have a low hemoglobin level but still may be hypoxic. The iron portion of the hemoglobin molecule can be oxidized owing to a NADH (nicotinamide adenine dinucleotide, reduced form) diaphorase deficiency, resulting in an abnormal hemoglobin molecule that resists reduction, or to an overwhelming exposure to toxic compounds, such as nitrates, aniline dyes, lidocaine, and sulfonamide drugs. Because methemoglobin does not transfer oxygen effectively, the hemoglobin level may be high in response to the resulting lack of tissue oxygen.

A number of other hemoglobins are considered unstable because of their inability to withstand mild thermal or mechanical trauma and their tendency to precipitate. An amino acid substitution decreases the binding of heme to globin chains, yielding the instability.

Thalassemias are caused by the decreased synthesis of one or more globin chains. The defect is approximately 10 times more common than amino acid substitutions and can occur simultaneously with an amino acid defect. Wide variations in clinical symptoms and laboratory values can occur in thalassemia, because each globin chain is under separate genetic control on a different chromosome pair, creating the possibility of many different combinations of quantitative defects. There is often a hemolytic component due to aggregation and precipitation of "excess" globin chain. The normally produced globin chains are in relative excess because not enough of the affected globin chains are produced to combine with the normal chains to form the hemoglobin tetramer. These aggregates can appear as Heinz bodies and lead to early removal of the affected erythrocytes by the spleen.

In β-thalassemia, production of β-chains is decreased. In the heterozygote, there is one gene for the normal production of β-chains and one for either reduced or absent β-chains. Affected patients commonly have compensatory elevations in hemoglobins F and A_2. Hemoglobin electrophoresis and determination of the A_2 level are usually included in the laboratory evauation, along with iron studies to rule out an iron deficiency; however, iron deficiency and thalassemia can coexist.

In the homozygote, both β-chains are affected. Infants with this disorder fail to thrive because they can make very little, if any, HbA, and few survive to adulthood. The diagnosis can be made before birth through chorionic villous sampling and DNA probes. Routine testing is difficult in the neonate, because the switch from γ-chain to β-chain production is not yet complete. Affected patients often require transfusion support and can become overloaded with iron after many transfusions, requiring treatment to remove excess iron.

α-Thalassemias are manifest at birth, because production of the α-chains needed to complete all hemoglobins is affected. The decrease in α-chains results in excess β-chains, which can form HbH, and excess γ-chains, which can form Bart's hemoglobin. There are many more variations of α-thalassemia than of β-thalassemia, because there are four genes for α-chain production, but only two genes for β-chain production. The characteristic gene defects are also dissimilar.

Continued production of HbF is often secondary to a hemoglobin disorder such as thalassemia but can also occur as a primary disorder. In hereditary persistence of hemoglobin F (HPHF), the production of γ-chains is not "turned off" as the infant matures, and elevated levels of HbF persist, although the hemoglobin is functional.

Sideroblastic anemias can be subdivided by etiology into acquired and hereditary. The acquired subgroup can be further divided into primary and secondary. The most common form of sideroblastic anemia is acquired primary sideroblastic anemia, also known as chronic refractory anemia with ringed sideroblasts (RARS). Although this form is considered idiopathic, there appears to be a clonal abnormality of the pluripotential stem cell. This results in impairment of the biosynthetic pathway of heme synthesis due to inadequate enzyme activity. Acquired secondary sideroblastic anemia is linked to the interference of drugs, toxins, or disease in the heme biosynthetic pathways.

Hereditary sideroblastic anemia comprises a heterogeneous group of rare disorders, some of which are X-linked. Among the inherited enzyme deficiencies that can cause a sideroblastic anemia are δ-aminolevulinic acid (ALA) synthetase, heme synthetase, and coproporphyrinogen oxidase. The course of these anemias may be complicated by iron overload.

Secondary Anemias

The secondary anemias are a large and varied group of anemias found in conjunction with other diseases or conditions. The anemia is usually not the primary concern, but it is an important symptom and may be due to several related causes. Some of the processes in which secondary anemias can be found are pregnancy, hypervolemia, chronic infections and inflammation, renal disease, alcoholism, nosocomial anemia, lead poisoning, and acute infections.

Anemia secondary to chronic diseases, such as infectious, inflammatory, and malignant processes, is considered by some to be the most common anemia in the United States. The anemia is usually due to a combination of a decreased erythrocyte life span, retention of iron in the reticuloendothelial cells so that it is unavailable to the maturing erythrocyte, and decreased erythrocyte production. Anemia may be a symptom in many other disorders. Some are systemic, such as the endocrine-related diseases and acquired immunodeficiency syndrome (AIDS), whereas others are related to hematologic dyscrasias, such as refractory anemia with excess blasts (RAEB).

CLINICAL MANIFESTATIONS

Anemia indicates decreased oxygen delivery capacity, resulting in reduced oxygenation of body tissues (hypoxia). Clinical symptoms range from minor fatigue to dyspnea, syncope, and angina. A reduction in circulating hemoglobin produces pallor and eventually hypotension. A compensatory increase in cardiac output leads to symptoms such as minor palpitations but may progress to actual heart failure if the hemoglobin capacity continues to decrease.[3]

Symptoms are also related to the etiology of the anemia and the rate at which it developed. For example, early nutritional anemias are often characterized by pallor and fatigue, whereas massive blood loss can result in hypoxia and heart failure. Most iron deficiencies are asymptomatic early in their course. As the patient becomes more iron deficient, symptoms such as easy fatigability, headache, rapid pulse, dyspnea, pallor, pica (the craving of unusual foods such as clay, starch, or ice), soreness and atrophy of the tongue, sore mouth, and abnormal, spoon-shaped nails, appear.

The clinical symptoms of chronic hemolytic anemia include those of decreased oxygen delivery, jaundice, splenomegaly and aplastic, hemolytic, or megaloblastic "crises." Symptoms of acute hemolysis are fever, pain, backache, muscle spasms, shock, acute renal failure, and disseminated intravascular coagulation (DIC). These symptoms are the result of attempts by the various organs and systems of the body to deal with the sudden increase in red cell breakdown products.

In sickle cell disease, the heterozygote is usually asymptomatic unless placed in a stressful or oxygen-poor environment. The homozygote typically suffers pain due to the blocked circulation and is anemic, primarily owing to decreased erythrocyte survival, but ineffective erythropoiesis and aplastic crises also occur.

LABORATORY ANALYSES AND DIAGNOSIS

Initial Studies

Timely, accurate, and precise laboratory data are very important to the diagnosis and treatment of anemia. A variety of laboratory tests are needed to establish the presence of anemia, evaluate its severity, and identify the etiology. Depending on the working diagnosis, it is usually more cost and time effective to perform certain groups of tests together rather than sequentially. For example, a hospitalized patient may be able to be discharged several days earlier if the physician orders the proper blood and other samples to complete the evaluation early, rather than waiting for the results of single tests before ordering follow-up tests. For this reason, many laboratories have instituted "profiles" for the diagnosis of anemia. Examples of some profiles for characterizing hemolytic anemias are shown in Box 42–1.

The initial screening profile or group of tests consists of

Box 42–1. Profiles for Evaluation of Hemolytic Diseases

The following are examples of batteries of laboratory studies organized to help diagnose hemolytic anemias. For example, the group of tests shown here are ordered as an initial screen to establish hemolysis and give direction for further testing.

Screening Profile

Reticulocyte count
Erythrocyte morphology
Bilirubin
Haptoglobin

If acute intravascular hemolysis is suspected, plasma and urinary hemoglobins, and a direct anti–human globulin test (DAT) may be ordered before moving on to the appropriate profile shown here:

Membrane Defect Profile

Osmotic fragility
Ham's test
Direct anti–human globulin (DAT)
Cold agglutinins
Protein electrophoresis
Donath-Landsteiner
Acetylcholinesterase

Enzyme Defect Profile

G6PD screen—assay if positive
Red cell glutathione assay and glutathione stability
Red cell pyruvate kinase
Heinz body test

Hemoglobin Defect Profile

A_2 quantitation
Sickle cell screen
Hemoglobin electrophoresis
Alkali denaturation for hemoglobin F
2,3-diphosphoglycerate
Heinz body test
Methemoglobin

Adapted from Schwabbauer MH: Understanding anemias. In-Service Reviews in Clinical Laboratory Science, Vol 6, No. 8. Birmingham, AL: Educational Reviews, 1993.

---

a complete blood count (CBC) and examination of erythrocyte and leukocyte morphology. These tests establish the presence of anemia and give direction to further testing to determine the etiology. Additional tests can then be selected on the basis of the history, erythrocyte indices, and erythrocyte morphology.

Once the presence of anemia has been established, the status of erythrocyte production or increased destruction must be determined. Erythrocyte morphology also provides important clues as to the etiology of the anemia and which additional laboratory tests would be the most helpful. Table 42–4 lists significant erythrocyte morphologic changes, the

Table 42–4. Erythrocyte Morphology and Inclusion Bodies

Type of Cell	Defect/Process	Clinical Disorder
Acanthocyte	Increased cholesterol/lecithin ratio	Abetalipoproteinemia, severe liver disease
Agglutination	Decreased zeta potential	Cold hemagglutinin disease (CHD)
Basophilic stippling	Ribosomal aggregation	Disordered hemoglobin synthesis
Bite or blister cells	Splenic pitting	Abnormal RBCs or RBC inclusions
Burr cell	Extracellular	Uremia, postsplenectomy
Dimorphic	Two distinct RBC populations	Sideroblastic, treated, alcoholic, transfused
Elliptocyte	Membrane defect	Hereditary elliptocytosis, megaloblastic
		Iron deficiency, thalassemia (thin RBCs)
Heinz bodies	Enzyme defect	G6PD deficiency
	Unstable hemoglobins	Hemoglobin H, thalassemia
Howell-Jolly bodies	Disturbed nuclear maturation	Megaloblastic cell production
	Decreased removal	Postsplenectomy
Hypochromia	Decreased hemoglobin synthesis:	
	Lack of iron	Iron deficiency anemia
	Defective globin synthesis	Thalassemia
	Defective porphyrin synthesis	Sideroblastic anemia
Pappenheimer bodies	Excess nonhemoglobin iron	Thalassemia, hemosiderosis
Polychromasia	Increased RNA; less mature RBCs	Normal response to increased need for RBC
Schistocyte (helmet, triangle, etc.)	Mechanical damage of RBCs	Microangiopathic hemolytic anemia; malignancy; physical agents
Sickle cell and oat cell	Aggregation of HbS	HbS disease
Spherocyte	Antigen/antibody complex	Immune hemolytic anemia
	Membrane defect	Hereditary spherocytosis
Stomatocyte	Defects in membrane; cation transport	Hereditary stomatocytosis; alcohol; malignancy
Target cell (codocyte)	Accumulation of cholesterol and phospholipid on RBCs	Liver disease, obstructive jaundice, postsplenectomy
	Uneven distribution of hemoglobin	Hb, C, S, thalassemia
Teardrop	Cell membrane stretched beyond ability to revert to normal shape	Myeloproliferative disorders, bone marrow failure

Abbreviations: RBC, red blood cell; G6PD, glucose-6-phosphate dehydrogenase; Hb, hemoglobin.
Adapted from Schwabbauer MH: Understanding anemias. In-Service Reviews in Clinical Laboratory Science, Vol 6, No. 8. Birmingham, AL, Educational Reviews, 1993.

underlying defect or process involved, and the clinical disorders in which the morphologic change can be seen. For example, spherocytes seen on the peripheral smear are an indication of either an underlying antigen-antibody complex, such as immune hemolytic anemia, or a membrane defect–related disorder, such as hereditary spherocytosis.

Figures 42–1 to 42–5 represent algorithms for laboratory testing in anemias.

Tests to Detect Erythrocyte Production

The two tests most commonly used to determine the number of erythrocytes being produced are the reticulocyte count and examination of the bone marrow for cellularity and myeloid-erythroid (M:E) ratio. If the bone marrow is not producing, as evidenced by decreased cellularity or a low reticulocyte count, the etiology is most likely bone

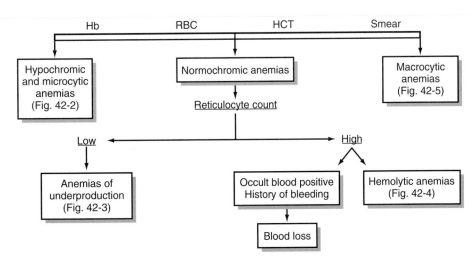

Figure 42–1. Laboratory characterization of anemias. Abbreviations: Hb, hemoglobin; RBC, red blood cell; HCT, hematocrit. (Adapted with permission from Schwabbauer MH: Understanding anemias. In-Service Reviews in Clinical Laboratory Science, Vol 6, Nos. 8 and 9. Birmingham, AL: Educational Reviews, 1993.)

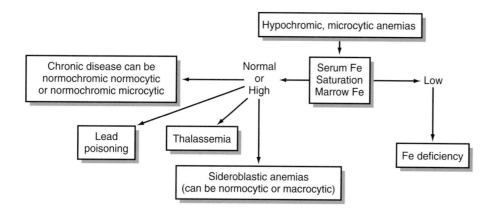

Figure 42–2. Hypochromic, microcytic anemias. Abbreviation: Fe, iron. (Adapted with permission from Schwabbauer MH: Understanding anemias. In-Service Reviews in Clinical Laboratory Science, Vol 6, Nos. 8 and 9. Birmingham, AL: Educational Reviews, 1993.)

marrow failure. Because the normal physiologic response to increased cell destruction or loss is to step up the production and release of young erythrocytes, a higher rate of erythrocyte production suggests those etiologic possibilities.

An increase in reticulocytes is the simplest and most reliable sign of accelerated erythrocyte production; however, the percentage of reticulocytes can be misleading when the red blood cell (RBC) count is low. In this event, the reticulocyte count should be either corrected for the hematocrit or reported in absolute numbers. In hemolytic anemia, the reticulocyte count commonly is 5% or higher after correction, although a normal reticulocyte count does not rule out hemolytic anemia. If the bone marrow is unable to respond to the need for replacement cells, the reticulocyte count would remain low or normal.

The M:E ratio compares the number of developing, immature myeloid cells with the number of developing, immature erythroid cells in the bone marrow. Normally, there are approximately three times as many myeloid precursors as erythroid precursors. In hemolytic anemia, or after treatment for a deficiency anemia, this number may even be reversed, with more erythroid than myeloid precursors present.

Tests to Detect Accelerated Erythrocyte Destruction

Bilirubin, a product of hemoglobin catabolism, is commonly used as an indicator of increased cell destruction but is neither a very sensitive nor specific index. As many as 45% of patients with hemolytic anemia have a normal bilirubin level. Even though large amounts of bilirubin are being produced, these patients are able to process the increase, and the circulating bilirubin levels are within the reference range. Because several hepatic disorders also produce elevated bilirubin levels, a high bilirubin value alone is not sufficient to establish a diagnosis of hemolytic anemia.

Free haptoglobin is a very sensitive index of hemolysis. Haptoglobin is a hemoglobin-carrying protein. Although free haptoglobin levels can be decreased in both intravascular and extravascular hemolysis because it can attach to any increased free hemoglobin to form hemoglobin-haptoglobin complexes, it is more decreased in intravascular hemolysis. As a rule of thumb, haptoglobin is absent whenever erythrocyte destruction exceeds twice the normal rate; however, haptoglobin levels increase with some infections, malignancies, and steroid therapy. Thus, a normal haptoglobin

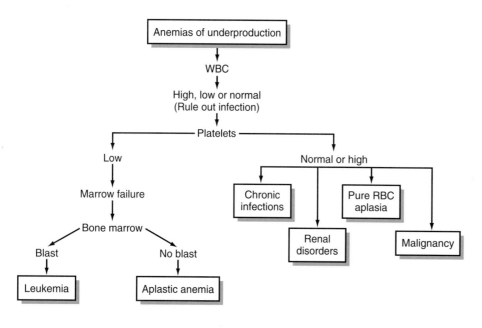

Figure 42–3. Anemias of underproduction. Abbreviations: WBC, white blood cell; RBC, red blood cell. (Adapted with permission from Schwabbauer MH: Understanding anemias. In-Service Reviews in Clinical Laboratory Science, Vol 6, Nos. 8 and 9. Birmingham, AL: Educational Reviews, Inc., 1993.)

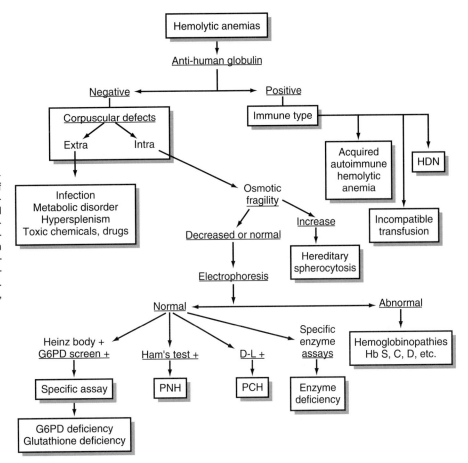

Figure 42–4. Hemolytic anemias. Abbreviations: HDN, hemolytic disease of the newborn; G6PD, glucose-6-phosphate dehydrogenase; PNH; paroxysmal nocturnal hemoglobinuria; PCH; paroxysmal cold hemoglobinuria; Hb, hemoglobin. (Adapted with permission from Schwabbauer MH: Understanding anemias. In-Service Reviews in Clinical Laboratory Science, Vol 6, Nos. 8 and 9. Birmingham, AL: Educational Reviews, Inc., 1993.)

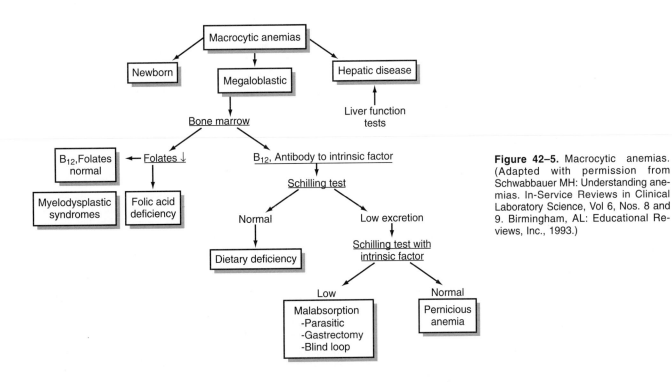

Figure 42–5. Macrocytic anemias. (Adapted with permission from Schwabbauer MH: Understanding anemias. In-Service Reviews in Clinical Laboratory Science, Vol 6, Nos. 8 and 9. Birmingham, AL: Educational Reviews, Inc., 1993.)

value in patients with such disorders may actually represent a significant decrease in haptoglobin due to hemolysis. Patients with liver disease may have a decreased haptoglobin due to reduced synthesis rather than to hemolysis.

Hemoglobinuria may cause the urine to appear faint pink to deep red or even cola-colored, owing to the presence of free hemoglobin and hemoglobin breakdown products. It is found only in severe intravascular hemolysis.

Hemosiderinuria refers to hemosiderin in the urine, which also is found only after episodes of intravascular hemolysis. It is more consistently present than hemoglobinuria in chronic intravascular hemolytic anemia. Hemosiderinuria occurs when free hemoglobin has been absorbed, converted, and stored as ferritin and hemosiderin by the proximal tubules in the kidney. The tubule cells then slough off and are excreted over a period of several days after the hemolytic episode.

Over time, patients with hemoglobinuria or hemosiderinuria can become iron deficient, because the iron is lost and not recycled. Patients with hemolytic anemia and only extravascular hemolysis do not become iron deficient as a result of their hemolytic disease.

Another sensitive but not specific test for hemolysis is the measurement of lactic dehydrogenase (LD) and its isoenzymes. LD, specifically fractions 1 and 2, is increased with erythrocyte breakdown. LD-1 and LD-2 are also markedly increased in megaloblastic erythrocyte production because of the destruction of enormous numbers of abnormally developing erythrocytes within the marrow. Plasma hemoglobin and fecal urobilinogen levels are infrequently used to detect hemolysis because of the technical difficulties of their analysis.

Nuclear medicine imaging studies can be used to document accelerated erythrocyte destruction. Not only can they give an indication of the average erythrocyte life span but they can also demonstrate sites of increased sequestration.

Deficiency Anemias

The laboratory features of iron deficiency anemia depend on the severity of the deficiency. In the first or iron depletion stage, there is only a lack of storage iron. If the decreased intake or increased loss of iron is not reversed, the next stage is iron deficiency without anemia. There is a decreased serum iron in addition to the lack of iron stores. The last stage is iron deficiency anemia with a microcytic, hypochromic anemia, decreased serum iron, and no storage iron.

In early iron deficiency, the erythrocytes are normochromic normocytic. They then become microcytic, because a cell does not get the signal to stop dividing even though there is no iron to incorporate into hemoglobin. Finally, the cells become hypochromic. In the later stages, poikilocytosis, target cells, elliptocytes, and other bizarre shapes may also be present. The bone marrow shows erythroid hyperplasia with no storage iron. The serum iron level is low, rarely normal. The serum ferritin value is decreased but may be normal if inflammation is also present. The free erythrocyte protoporphyrin level is increased.

Iron deficiency anemia must be differentiated from the hemoglobinopathies, especially the thalassemias and hemoglobin E; from the blockage of heme synthesis by chemicals; from lead poisoning; and from the anemia of chronic disease, all of which may also display microcytosis and hypochromia, as indicated in Figure 42–2. Anemias of underproduction are outlined in Figure 42–3.

In megaloblastic anemias, macrocytosis with oval macrocytes and hypersegmented neutrophils can be seen on the peripheral blood smear. Commonly, there is a pancytopenia. Megaloblastic erythropoiesis, giant bands, enlarged abnormal megakaryocytes, Howell-Jolly bodies, karyorrhexis, and basophilic stippling can be seen in the bone marrow and sometimes in the peripheral blood (see Fig. 42–5). To support a diagnosis of pernicious anemia, there should be some combination of the following findings: megaloblastic anemia; gastric achlorhydria; decreased B_{12} level; antibodies to parietal cells and/or intrinsic factor; elevated urine and serum methylmalonic acid; and elevated serum homocysteine level and a positive Schilling test.

Hemolytic Anemias

The hemolytic anemia screening profile consists of the reticulocyte count to detect accelerated erythrocyte production, a peripheral blood smear to check erythrocyte morphology, and bilirubin and haptoglobin measurements to detect accelerated erythrocyte destruction (see Fig. 43–4). If a membrane defect is suspected on the basis of the screening profile test results, membrane defect tests, such as the osmotic fragility, sucrose lysis, direct anti–human globulin, cold agglutinin or Donath-Landsteiner test, protein electrophoresis, or acetylcholinesterase measurement would be in order. If an enzyme defect is a possibility, selected enzyme defect profile procedures would be performed. If a hemoglobin defect is suspected, the appropriate tests listed in the hemoglobin defect profile would be performed (see Box 42–1).

Immunohemolytic anemias due to warm antibodies often yield a positive direct anti–human globulin test (DAT), and the peripheral blood smear may show spherocytes, anisocytosis, erythrophagocytosis, and polychromasia. Spherocytes are also common in hemolytic disease of the newborn due to ABO incompatibility. Cold antibody types usually yield a negative DAT result, and anemias due to drug-induced antibodies may yield either a positive or negative DAT result.

Hemoglobinopathies, Thalassemias, and Sideroblastic Anemia

The peripheral smear may show oat cells, target cells, polychromasia, basophilic stippling, Howell-Jolly bodies, and anisocytosis. Laboratory detection of sickle cell disorder often begins with a sickling or insoluble hemoglobin screening test. When an abnormal hemoglobin is detected, it must be further characterized by electrophoresis, immunologic tests, or isoelectric focusing. Sickling and solubility screening tests are rapidly being replaced by more definitive monoclonal antibody procedures, because HbS is not the only sickling or insoluble hemoglobin. Also, the traditional screening tests are unable to detect the presence of abnormal hemoglobins in newborns. Molecular pathology tests for differentiation and characterization of hemoglobinopathy such as DNA probes, Southern blots, and polymerase chain reaction (PCR), are being employed with increasing frequency in the clinical laboratory.

Target cells are characteristic in hemoglobin C. A prominent number are seen in the homozygote, but fewer are seen in the heterozygote. In other hemoglobinopathies, the peripheral blood smear may show poikilocytosis, anisocytosis, target cells, and basophilic stippling. Abnormal laboratory findings include Heinz bodies and decreases in heat and isopropanol stabilities. Hemoglobin electrophoresis is not generally useful when HbS exists in association with other abnormal hemoglobins or in the presence of hemoglobin variants with similar migration patterns, such as HbE, HbO$_{arab}$ and HbC. HbE disease can morphologically resemble anemia due to iron deficiency or thalassemias.

The characteristic red cell morphology observed in the thalassemias is microcytosis and hypochromia with target cells. RBC counts are often higher than 5.0×10^{12}/L. The heterozygote for α-thalassemia 1 and 2 exhibits mild hypochromasia and slight microcytosis. Bart's hemoglobin is present in the former condition.

Blood Loss

After an acute blood loss, the erythrocyte count, hemoglobin, and hematocrit decline once the system has had time to reestablish a volume equilibrium. A normochromic, normocytic anemia persists until the cells have been replaced by the bone marrow. Chronic blood loss results in significant loss of iron and the development of an iron deficiency anemia.

Secondary Anemias

In secondary anemias, the serum iron level is usually decreased but iron stores are increased. The erythrocyte morphology is most often microcytic and normochromic, although it may be microcytic and hypochromic. Occasionally, the red cells appear normal in size and color.

Chronic renal disease almost always has secondary anemia as a component. Erythrocyte survival is reduced along with erythropoietin activity and marrow output, and bleeding tendency is increased owing to decreased platelet function. The anemia secondary to alcoholism is usually macrocytic and normochromic with target cells but may also be hypochromic.

In hypervolemia, there is an increase in plasma volume, so the hematocrit may be low but the erythrocyte mass may be normal. Patients, especially newborns and infants, can suffer a nosocomial anemia from the sheer quantities of blood withdrawn to perform laboratory tests. In lead poisoning, there is an anemia, usually hypochromic microcytic with basophilic stippling, owing to blocked porphyrin synthesis, which in turn increases the excretion of δ-ALA and porphyrins.

TREATMENT

Unless an anemic state is due to marrow failure or acute blood loss, or there are cardiac manifestations, transfusion even of packed erythrocytes is seldom indicated and may even be dangerous if volume overload occurs. Treatment is directed toward the underlying cause of the anemia or, if it is incurable, to supportive therapy.[5]

Deficiency states generally respond well to replacement therapy.[6] In iron deficiency anemia, for example, iron replacement is simple and cost effective. Iron therapy is not appropriate, however, when there is no evidence of deficiency. Although absorption is regulated, iron overload can occur. Overload is a consideration in long-term therapy for the hemoglobinopathies, thalassemias, and sideroblastic anemias. The administration of vitamin B$_{12}$ or folic acid to deficient patients also results in dramatic improvement, with reticulocytosis observed 4 or 5 days after therapy is begun.

Hemolytic anemias due to membrane abnormalities, especially hereditary spherocytic anemia, respond to splenectomy. Immunohemolytic anemias often respond to corticosteroids, but when they do not, splenectomy may be considered. Patients with immunohemolytic disorders who need transfusions often present cross-match problems, and it may be difficult to provide suitable blood products.[7]

Anemias secondary to other disorders or to exposure to drugs or other toxins improve if the underlying condition is corrected or the drug discontinued. Primary disorders of the bone marrow, however, are often irreversible, with only supportive therapy available. Bone marrow transplants have become a more commonly chosen option in such cases.

Case Study 1

A 23-year-old female clinical laboratory scientist volunteered to have her blood used as a normal control for the laboratory. A CBC, including platelet and reticulocyte counts, was performed to confirm her "normal status." The results (with reference ranges) were as follows:

Hemoglobin (g/dL)	10.0	(11.6–14.8)
Hematocrit (%)	35	(34.2–43.7)
RBCs ($\times 10^{12}$/L)	5.50	(3.79–4.91)
Mean corpuscular volume (MCV) ($\times$ fL)	60	(83–94)
Mean corpuscular hemoglobin (MCH) (pg/cell)	18.2	(28.4–32.9)
Mean corpuscular hemoglobin concentration (MCHC) (%)	30.3	(32.5–33.5)
WBCs ($\times 10^9$/L)	7.5	(4.5–10.0)
Platelets (10^9/L)	285	(150–350)

The stained blood smear demonstrated the presence of oval macrocytic erythrocytes and hypersegmented neutrophils. The history and physical examination revealed an apparently healthy female with mild pallor of the conjunctiva and fatigue of several months' duration. An adequate diet was noted; there was no history of pregnancy, drug use, or excessive blood loss.

Questions

1. What is the most likely cause of anemia?
2. What laboratory tests will identify the primary etiology?
3. What other tests are needed to complete the diagnosis?
4. What other testing might follow?

Discussion

1. Megaloblastic anemia is most likely, given the presence of oval macrocytes.
2. Vitamin B_{12} and folate levels should indicate the primary etiology. Vitamin B_{12} deficiency is most likely in this case, considering the history and physical examination.
3. The Schilling test with and without intrinsic factor yielded a definitive diagnosis of pernicious anemia and ruled out malabsorption.
4. Thyroid testing is recommended, because the patient with pernicious anemia often has other autoimmune manifestations.

Case Study 2

A CBC was ordered for a 20-year-old black female during her first appointment at a prenatal clinic. The results (with reference ranges) were as follows:

Hemoglobin (g/dL)	9.9	(11.6–14.8)
Hematocrit (%)	28.5	(34.2–43.7)
RBCs ($\times 10^{12}$/L)	2.34	(3.79–4.91)
MCV ($\times$ fL)	123	(83–94)
MCH (pg/cell)	42.2	(28.4–32.9)
MCHC (%)	34.4	(32.5–33.5)
WBCs ($\times 10^9$/L)	4.8	(4.5–10.0)
Platelets (10^9/L)	98	(150–350)
Reticulocytes (%)	0.6	(0.5–2.0)
Corrected (%)	0.4	(0.5–2.0)

Microcytic, hypochromic red cells, some of which contained Pappenheimer's bodies, were noted on the stained blood smear. The history and physical examination revealed an apparently healthy, pregnant female. An adequate diet was noted; the patient reported that a brother and sister had been unable to give blood owing to a low hematocrit during a recent blood drive.

Questions

1. What is the most likely cause of anemia?
2. What laboratory tests will identify the primary etiology?
3. What other tests are needed to complete the diagnosis?
4. What other testing might follow?

Discussion

1. A hemoglobinopathy, thalassemia, or sideroblastic anemia is most likely, given the presence of Pappenheimer's bodies, presumably containing nonhemoglobin iron.
2. Iron studies and hemoglobin electrophoresis should indicate the primary etiology. Thalassemia is most likely in this case, considering the history and physical examination.
3. Normal iron studies with increased hemoglobins A_2 and F and the history indicated a diagnosis of thalassemia and ruled out iron deficiency.
4. The fetus could be tested in utero for an abnormal hemoglobin production gene, and genetic counseling could be provided.

References

1. Evatt BL: Anemia. Fundamental Diagnostic Hematology, ed 2. Atlanta, Centers for Disease Control, 1992.
2. Spaet TH: Anemia is a symptom [editorial]. Hosp Pract 15:17, 1980.
3. Wintrobe MM, Lukens JN, Lee GR: The approach to the patient with anemia. *In* Lee GR, Bithell TC, Forester J, et al: Wintrobe's Clinical Hematology, ed 9. Philadelphia: Lea & Febiger, 1993.
4. Schwabbauer MH: Understanding anemias. In-Service Reviews in Clinical Laboratory Science, Vol 6, Nos. 8 and 9. Birmingham, AL, Educational Reviews, 1993.
5. Swoyer J: The Anemias. *In* Davis BG, Bishop ML, Mass D: Clinical Laboratory Science Strategies for Practice. Philadelphia, JB Lippincott, 1989.
6. Bunn HF: Anemia. *In* Isselbacher KJ, Brunwald E, Wilson JD, et al (eds): Harrison's Principles of Internal Medicine. New York, McGraw-Hill, 1994.
7. Rosse LW, Bunn HF: Hemolytic Anemias. *In* Isselbacher KJ, Brunwald E, Wilson JD, et al (eds): Harrison's Principles of Internal Medicine. New York, McGraw-Hill, 1994.

Bibliography

Bessis MD: Blood Smears Reinterpreted. New York City, Springer International, 1977.
Bishop ML, Duben-Engelkirk JL, Fody EP: Clinical Chemistry: Principles, Procedures, Correlations, ed 2. Philadelphia, JB Lippincott, 1992.
Burtis CA, Ashwood ER: Tietz Fundamentals of Clinical Chemistry, ed 4. Philadelphia, WB Saunders, 1996.
Harmening DM: Clinical Hematology and Fundamentals of Hemostasis, ed 2. Philadelphia, FA Davis, 1992.
Henry JB: Clinical Diagnosis and Management by Laboratory Methods, ed 18. Philadelphia, WB Saunders, 1991.
Lotspeich-Steininger CA, Stiene-Martin EA, Koepke JA: Clinical Hematology: Principles, Procedures, Correlations. Philadelphia, JB Lippincott, 1992.
McClatchey KD (ed): Clinical Laboratory Medicine. Baltimore, Williams & Wilkins, 1994.
Rodak BF: Diagnostic Hematology. Philadelphia, WB Saunders, 1995.
Rudmann SV: Textbook of Blood Banking and Transfusion Medicine. Philadelphia, WB Saunders, 1995.
Tietz NW (ed): Clinical Guide to Laboratory Tests, ed 3. Philadelphia, WB Saunders, 1995.
Williams WJ, Beutler E, Erslev AJ: Hematology, ed 4. New York, McGraw-Hill, 1990.

Chapter 43

Leukocyte Abnormalities and Hematologic Malignancies

Karen Brown

Disorders of leukocytes may be broadly grouped into two categories, nonmalignant (benign) and malignant. Because leukocytes function as sentries to defend the body against invasion by foreign substances and organisms, they may respond physically in ways that can be detected or observed in the clinical laboratory. Such physical responses of leukocytes consist of either quantitative or qualitative (functional) variations. Quantitative changes reflect increases or decreases in the total number of circulating leukocytes. Qualitative variations affect the morphology and sometimes the functional capabilities of leukocytes. Malignant disorders can also cause physical variations in leukocytes, but these changes usually result from an inherently abnormal cell and do not reflect a normal response to a neoplasm.

Leukocytes can be classified on the basis of function as lymphocytes and nonlymphocytes, or myeloid cells. The formation and development of all leukocytes occurs in the bone marrow and are influenced by growth factors, inhibitors, and the microenvironment of the marrow; however, lymphocytes may also proliferate and differentiate in the thymus and, in response to an antigenic stimulus, in peripheral lymphoid tissues such as lymph nodes and spleen. Lymphocytes are further divided into T (thymus-dependent) lymphocytes and B (bone marrow–derived) lymphocytes. T and B lymphocytes each have numerous subclassifications based on cellular functions. Cytotoxic cells and helper cells are two subsets of T lymphocytes. B lymphocytes are classified according to specific immunoglobulins produced at various times in their maturation. Stimulated, end-stage B lymphocytes differentiate into immunoglobulin-producing plasma cells or plasmacytes (Fig. 43–1).

ETIOLOGY AND PATHOPHYSIOLOGY

Nonmalignant (Benign) Leukocyte Abnormalities

Quantitative and qualitative changes in leukocytes reflect normal responses to abnormal environmental factors; however, quantitative variations should be evaluated cautiously. The concentration of specific leukocytes, whether lymphocytes or nonlymphocytes, depends on the age and ethnic origin of individuals as well as numerous other genetic and environmental factors.[1] For example, children tend to have more circulating lymphocytes than adults, whereas adults have more myeloid cells.

Any evaluation of quantitative leukocyte variations should consider both increases and decreases in all numbers. Because neutrophils represent the greatest percentage of granulocytic leukocytes, neutropenia can be a serious condition resulting in greater susceptibility to infection. Neutropenia may be congenital or acquired and may result from one or more pathophysiologic processes. Decreased production of neutrophils by the bone marrow occurs in the rare, congenital neutropenias and has also been associated with chemicals, such as benzene, cytotoxic drugs used as chemotherapy, ionizing radiation, bone marrow replacement in malignancy, and nutritional deficiencies.

Neutropenia may also be acquired as a result of increased destruction or accelerated utilization in the periph-

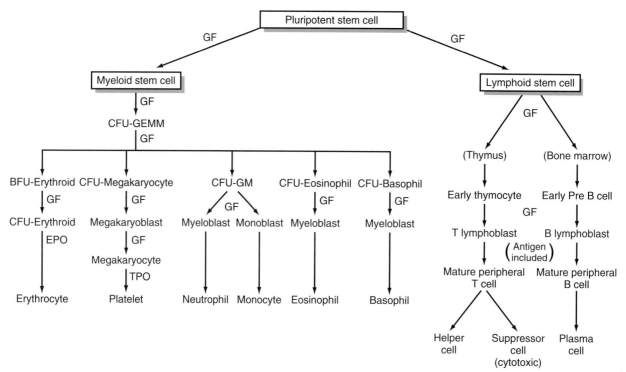

Figure 43–1. Development of leukocytes, indicating influence of growth factors (GF) and other cytokines. Abbreviations: CFU, colony-forming unit; GEMM, granulocyte/erythrocyte/monocyte/megakaryocyte; BFU, burst-forming unit; EPO, erythropoietin; TPO, thrombopoietin; GM, granulocyte/monocyte.

eral circulation. The mechanisms can involve immune reactions, infectious diseases, or drugs. Drug-induced neutropenia can arise as a dose-related phenomenon or as an immune process. Numerous drugs have been linked to this condition, including the phenothiazines, antithyroid medications, and chloramphenicol. An apparent neutropenia, or pseudoneutropenia, may occur because of a shift of neutrophils from circulating blood pools to marginated, tissue pools. This situation is temporary and has been associated with hypersensitivity reactions, bacterial infections that release endotoxins, and some viral infections. A false neutropenia may also result from the in vitro handling of blood specimens in the laboratory.

Neutrophilia is a common finding in malignant processes such as myeloproliferative disorders and myelogenous leukemia; however, several benign conditions can result in a neutrophilia as well, and it is important to recognize nonmalignant causes in the differential diagnosis of neutrophilia. In fact, a benign, extreme neutrophilia is referred to as a *leukemoid reaction,* because the elevation of the blood cell count is suggestive of a leukemic process; this underscores the importance of considering all possibilities in the diagnosis of neutrophilia.

The mechanisms that result in neutrophilia are a shift in the proportion of cells from marginated to circulating pools (pseudoneutrophilia); an accelerated release of cells from the bone marrow to the peripheral blood; an increase in bone marrow production of cells; and decreased utilization of cells. They may occur alone or in combination. Furthermore, these mechanisms may be stimulated by any number of physiologic factors (Box 43–1).

Qualitative disorders of neutrophils should also be considered in the evaluation of nonmalignant leukocyte abnor-

malities. Defects in neutrophils can be found in nearly every facet of normal functions, whether an impairment of phagocytosis or faulty biochemistry leading to impairment of cellular movement or organism killing.

Lymphocytes may also respond to environmental factors, as reflected in lymphocytopenia and lymphocytosis. Nonmalignant conditions associated with lymphocytopenia are stress, corticosteroid therapy, granulocytosis, acute inflammatory conditions, recent surgery, acute viral infection, platelet apheresis, zinc deficiency, and starvation. Likewise, a reactive lymphocytosis has many causes (Box 43–2). It is particularly important to define the etiology of a lymphocytosis, because several malignant conditions may be confused with nonmalignant processes (Box 43–3). In addition, several factors are useful in determining the nature of a leukocytosis, such as age of the patient, clinical

---

Box 43–1. Physiologic Factors Resulting in Neutrophilia

Exercise
Infections
Inflammation
Tissue necrosis
Drugs
Hormones
Toxins
Certain tumors
Metabolic and endocrinologic disease
Hematologic disorders
Congenital conditions

symptoms, polyclonality, viral antibody test results, and surface marker and gene rearrangement studies.

Several morphologic variations of leukocytes may be observed that do not impair the functional capabilities of the cells. They are important to recognize, however, as they reflect benign conditions and must be considered in differential diagnosis. In the Alder-Reilly anomaly, deposited mucopolysaccharides[2] or defects in cytoplasmic maturation[3] result in the appearance of large, purple granules in the cytoplasm of leukocytes. This intense granule deposition can be confused with toxic granulation, but the granules in this case are generally larger, are more intense in their staining, and are leukocyte alkaline phosphatase negative, unlike toxic granules.

The May-Hegglin anomaly is an uncommon inherited condition characterized by the presence of cytoplasmic inclusions that resemble Döhle bodies, thrombocytopenia, and enlarged platelets. Whereas the Döhle bodies seen in various infections represent a transient finding, the Döhle–like inclusions of May-Hegglin are always present. The thrombocytopenia and enlarged platelets are also consistently found and should not be confused with the atypical platelet morphology associated with myeloproliferative disorders and myelodysplastic syndromes.

In the Pelger-Huët anomaly, neutrophil nuclei fail to segment (hyposegmentation). This condition is important to recognize, from two perspectives. First of all, Pelger-Huët cells should not be confused with a neutrophilic left shift and the presence of increased numbers of band cells. Second, an acquired or pseudo–Pelger-Huët condition is associated with myeloproliferative disorders and myelodysplastic syndromes and must be distinguished from the benign, inherited Pelger-Huët anomaly.

Likewise, the variant, atypical lymphocytes seen in reac-

tive lymphocytosis should not be mistaken for malignant proliferations. Considerable variation in morphologic appearance can be associated with the lymphocytes of nonmalignant or reactive processes. Malignant lymphocytes, in contrast, display more homogeneity and monotony of appearance.

Malignant Conditions

The Leukemias

The *leukemias* are a group of hematologic malignancies characterized by the progressive, unregulated proliferation of one cell type in the bone marrow or peripheral blood. This cell type originates from a hematopoietic stem cell that has become disturbed. The disturbed stem cell is capable of self-renewal and differentiation, resulting in a malignant clone of cells. The dominant clone overruns the bone marrow and eventually replaces normal hematopoietic precursors. Malignant transformation of a stem cell may be caused by a mutation and the modified expression of specific genes called *oncogenes*[2]—normal genes that control the proliferation and differentiation of cells.

The actual stimuli or events that alter a normal oncogene and trigger a stem cell to undergo uncontrolled proliferation have not been firmly established. Several factors associated with the development of a leukemic process are (1) exposure to ionizing radiation, (2) exposure to chemicals and drugs, both occupational and therapy related, (3) genetic abnormalities, such as Down syndrome, (4) immunodeficiency states, (5) marrow dysfunction conditions such as myeloproliferative disorders, myelodysplastic syndromes, aplastic anemia, and paroxysmal nocturnal hemoglobinuria (PNH), and (6) some infectious agents, most notably viruses.[4]

Certain epidemiologic patterns are also associated with the leukemias. The overall incidence of leukemia in the United States is 8 to 10 new cases per 100,000 individuals each year. In general, males are more often affected than females, and adults develop leukemia at a higher frequency than children.

Leukemias may be classified on the basis of cell maturity and predominant cell type. In acute leukemias, the abnormal cells are primarily immature, undifferentiated blasts. Chronic leukemias are characterized by an accumulation of morphologically more mature and more differentiated cells. Leukemias may also be regarded as arising from lymphoid lineage or myeloid cell lines (nonlymphoid or nonlymphocytic); therefore, the four major types of leukemia are acute lymphocytic, acute nonlymphocytic (myelogenous), chronic lymphocytic, and chronic nonlymphocytic (myelogenous).

ACUTE LEUKEMIAS

In 1976, a group of French, American, and British hematologists devised a system to further standardize the classification and nomenclature of the acute leukemias.[5] This system has since been called the FAB classification. The original publication subdivides lymphocytic and nonlymphocytic leukemias into three groups and six groups, respectively. A seventh subgroup of acute nonlymphocytic leukemias, M7, was added in the mid 1980s.[6, 7] Acute nonlymphocytic leukemias are commonly referred to as acute myelogenous leukemia (AML), and acute lymphocytic leukemias are also termed acute lymphoblastic leukemia (ALL).

Acute Nonlymphocytic Leukemia. The FAB system is based on standard morphologic and cytochemical methods and specifies the following subgroups of AML:

- *AML-M0*[8] (acute myeloblastic leukemia, minimally differentiated): This relatively new classification represents 2% to 3% of all cases of AML[8] and is associated with a relatively poor prognosis.
- *AML-M1* (acute myeloblastic leukemia without maturation): More common in adults and rare in children, this leukemia represents nearly 20%[10] of all cases of AML and is generally associated with a poor prognosis.
- *AML-M2* (acute myeloblastic leukemia with maturation): The median age of onset for this subtype is 48 years, although about 40% of cases are seen in people 60 years or older.[2] This subset is also associated with a poor prognosis and accounts for 32% to 45% of AMLs.[9]
- *AML-M3* (acute promyelocytic leukemia): This disorder represents 10% to 16% of all acute leukemias.[9] The leukemic cells are abnormal promyelocytes that contain high concentrations of thromboplastic substances, which can precipitate disseminated intravascular coagulation (DIC) when released. A variant of AML-M3 is the microgranular or hypogranular form (M3m); the primary, promyelocytic granules are not easily visible on stained smears in this variant, although it is important to recognize because it is associated with a high incidence of DIC.
- *AML-M4* (acute myelomonocytic leukemia): This subtype is distinctive, in that both granulocytic and monocytic components are present. A relatively common condition, it constitutes 16% to 19% of the acute leukemias.[9] A small percentage of M4 cases (6%) are associated with higher number of eosinophils in the bone marrow; this variant is called M4e and is a significant finding. Cases of AML-M4e respond better to chemotherapy and have a higher remission rate than cases of typical myelomonocytic leukemia.[10]
- *AML-M5* (acute monocytic leukemia): Representing only 10% to 12% of AMLs,[9] this leukemia is divided into two subtypes, M5a and M5b. AML-M5a is a poorly differentiated condition in which monoblasts without significant maturation to promonocytes or monocytes are present; this subtype tends to affect younger adults and is associated with a poor prognosis. AML-M5b is a more differentiated subtype characterized by the presence of recognizable promonocytes and monocytes.
- *AML-M6* (acute erythroleukemia): A rare type of leukemia previously known as Di Guglielmo's leukemia, AML-M6 manifests as abnormal proliferation of erythroid precursors in the bone marrow and peripheral blood. Immature myeloid cells may also be seen.
- *AML-M7* (acute megakaryoblastic [megakaryocytic] leukemia): The least common type of AML, this type represents only 1% or fewer of all cases of AML.[9] Megakaryoblasts and atypical megakaryocytes predominate. This

type of leukemia is often associated with bone marrow fibrosis.

The FAB system is not adequate to classify all cases of acute nonlymphocytic leukemias (ANLL), especially when morphologic and cytochemical evaluations are inconclusive. Several additional types of ANLLs have been recognized:

- Acute basophilic or mast cell leukemia
- Acute mixed-lineage (myeloid and lymphoid components) leukemia
- Acute undifferentiated leukemia

Acute Lymphocytic Leukemia. Specific morphologic features define the FAB types of acute lymphoblastic leukemia. Cell size, nuclear chromatin, nuclear shape, nucleoli, amount of cytoplasm, basophilia of cytoplasm, and cytoplasmic vacuolation are features evaluated in order to classify ALL morphologically as: L1, L2, or L3 (Table 43–1). In addition, immunologic classification of ALLs through immunophenotyping of leukemic blasts using flow cytometry or immunocytochemistry has become important in distinguishing ALL from AML and also as a prognostic indicator.

Acute lymphoblastic leukemia is a common disorder in children, with nearly 70% of all cases occurring in those younger than 17 years.[9] The frequency of the different morphologic types varies according to the age group affected. Most pediatric cases of ALL are classified as L1, in contrast to adults, which usually are L2. ALL-L3 is associated with the lowest incidence in both groups as well as the poorest prognosis of any type of ALL.

CHRONIC LEUKEMIAS

Chronic Myelogenous Leukemia (CML). Approximately 20% of all leukemias are CML. The majority of cases are diagnosed in adults, although rare instances have involved infants and young children.

Chronic myelogenous leukemia is one of a group of conditions called the *myeloproliferative disorders* (MPDs). These malignancies are clonal, originating from an abnormality associated with a pluripotential hematopoietic stem cell. As a chronic leukemic process, CML manifests as some evidence of differentiation in the granulocytic series. Although immature myelocytic precursors may be evident, the predominance of blast cells seen in AML is absent in the initial phases of CML.

Chronic Lymphocytic Leukemia (CLL). Chronic lymphocytic leukemia, primarily a disease of the elderly, accounts for 30% of all leukemias in Western countries. It is a subtype of a larger group of conditions called the *lymphoproliferative disorders*. In CLL, mature-appearing lymphocytes overpopulate the bone marrow and peripheral blood. These lymphocytes, though morphologically normal, actually arise as malignant clones of immunologically incompetent cells. In contrast to other types of leukemia, development of CLL has not been linked to exposures to alkylating agents, radiation, or chemicals.[11] Generally, malignant lymphocytes of CLL are immunophenotypically

Table 43–1. Subgroups of Acute Lymphoblastic Leukemia (ALL)

Classification	Size	Nuclear Characteristics	Cytoplasmic Characteristics
L1	Small	Regular shape sometimes with clefting or indenting; generally inconspicuous nucleoli	Scant and moderately basophilic
L2	Large	Irregular shape often with clefting and indenting; one or more large nucleoli	Moderately abundant and basophilic
L3	Medium to large	Regular shape; one or more often prominent nucleoi	Moderately abundant with prominent vacuolation

classified as B cells incapable of responding to antigenic challenges.

Two morphologic transformations have been associated with CLL. Richter's syndrome represents a transition of CLL to a diffuse, large cell lymphoma and occurs in approximately 5% of patients with CLL. Another 15% of patients with CLL undergo a prolymphocytoid transformation. In addition to the typical mature-appearing lymphocytes, prolymphocytes are seen in the bone marrow and peripheral blood. Prolymphocytic leukemia (PLL) may also develop unrelated to CLL and is characterized by a predominance (more than 55%) of prolymphocytes. PLL manifests as a more aggressive disease with a poorer prognosis than either CLL or CLL with prolymphocytoid transformation.

Hairy Cell Leukemia (HCL). Hairy cell leukemia is a rare chronic disease primarily affecting males, with a peak incidence during the fifth decade of life. The malignant lymphocytes are B cell in origin, and the classic cells, with hairlike cytoplasmic projections, may be difficult to observe on stained peripheral blood or bone marrow smears. These cells often pack the marrow and spleen, leading to the characteristic pancytopenia and splenomegaly associated with this disease.

Other Lymphoid Leukemias. Several additional lymphoid leukemias have been characterized, including bone marrow and peripheral blood involvement by non-Hodgkin's lymphoma as well as Sézary's syndrome. Sézary's syndrome represents the peripheral blood involvement by mycosis fungoides, a primary T-cell lymphoma of the skin. Large granular lymphocyte leukemia (LGLL) and adult T-cell leukemia/lymphoma also represent T-cell proliferations that must be considered in the differential diagnosis of a lymphoproliferative condition.

Myeloproliferative Disorders

The myeloproliferative disorders (MPDs) are characterized by excessive proliferation of nonlymphoid cell lines. They are a group of closely related syndromes that share similar clinical and hematologic findings at some point during their progression. In addition, MPDs have a tendency to evolve into an acute leukemia.

The MPDs are clonal in origin. The development of the neoplastic clone occurs after commitment to myeloid, erythroid, or megakaryocytic lineage.[12] Besides CML, the MPDs comprise polycythemia vera, myelofibrosis with myeloid metaplasia, and essential thrombocythemia.

Polycythemia Vera. Sustained increases in red cell mass, hemoglobin level, and hematocrit value occur in polycythemia vera without any stimulation from erythropoietin or as a result of hypoxia. Some patients also demonstrate peripheral blood granulocytosis and thrombocytosis. Most patients who develop polycythemia vera are whites in their sixth decade of life.

A common transformation seen in approximately 15% of patients with polycythemia vera patients is the "spent" or postpolycythemic myeloid metaplasia (PPMM) phase. In this transitional stage, the bone marrow becomes progressively fibrotic, with resulting peripheral blood pancytopenia. Splenomegaly increases secondary to extramedullary hematopoiesis. Research indicates that a higher incidence of acute leukemia is associated with development of the spent phase.[13]

The type of therapy initiated for a patient with polycythemia vera also affects the level of risk for the onset of acute leukemia. Overall, 18% of individuals with polycythemia vera develop acute myelogenous leukemia.[12]

Myelofibrosis with Myeloid Metaplasia. Myelofibrosis with myeloid metaplasia is characterized by fibrosis in the bone marrow and by extramedullary hematopoiesis. Apparently, the bone marrow fibrosis is a secondary reaction to higher amounts of platelet-derived growth factor (PDGF). Abnormal megakaryocytes in myeloid metaplasia release PDGF, which in turn stimulates fibroblasts, causing the development of a fibrotic marrow. Extramedullary hematopoiesis is initiated when greater numbers of clonal stem cells are released into the peripheral circulation and eventually accumulate in the reticuloendothelial system and various other organs.[14]

This disorder is also primarily seen in older adults. The average length of survival is 5 years, but survival is extremely variable and depends on such factors as the severity of anemia and thrombocytopenia and the rate of production of fibrosis in the marrow. A small percentage of patients with myeloid metaplasia succumb to an AML.

Essential (Primary) Thrombocythemia. Uncontrolled and abnormal megakaryocytic proliferation defines essential thrombocythemia, a rare myeloproliferative condition. The extreme megakaryocytic production results in peripheral blood platelet counts commonly in excess of 600×10^9/L and often greater than 1000×10^9/L. Essential thrombocythemia generally occurs in a younger age group than other MPDs, although patients range in age from 25 to 70 years. It is estimated that 80% of patients with this disorder survive at least 5 years.[15]

Myelodysplastic Syndromes

The *myelodysplastic syndromes* (MDSs) are a heterogeneous group of hematopoietic stem cell disorders that result in ineffective and abnormal development in one or more cell lines. The MDSs were at one time called preleukemias because they had a common predilection to develop into an acute leukemia but lacked the obvious definitive characteristics of acute leukemia. The development of an acute leukemia from any MDS is very much related to the classification of the myelodysplasia. In general, 25% of patients with MDS progress to an acute leukemia, usually AML.[16] MDSs are rarely diagnosed in individuals younger than 50 years, and they affect males slightly more often than females.

Several pathophysiologic processes have been postulated to influence the progression of MDSs. Exposure to physical agents, such as alkylating chemotherapeutic drugs or radiation, may cause a somatic mutation of oncogenes that disturb normal hematopoiesis. Defects in the production or regulation of hematopoietic growth factors may upset the marrow microenvironment, so that usual hematopoietic processes are inhibited. Certain cytogenetic abnormalities may also contribute to myelodysplastic development.

The FAB cooperative group has proposed five categories of MDSs, and their classification system has been widely accepted. The classification is based on cytologic features, most notably the peripheral blood and bone marrow blast counts, but also utilizes other quantitative and morphologic criteria. Box 43–4 lists and defines the five major subtypes of myelodysplastic syndromes.

The subclasses RAEB (refractory anemia with excess blasts) and RAEB-t (refractory anemia with excess blasts in transformation) are associated with the highest rate of development to acute nonlymphocytic leukemia, with older patients having the greatest risk. Therapy-induced MDS and subsequent development of ANLL also occur. Survival rates for the myelodysplastic syndromes vary according to the particular subset and can range anywhere from several years to only several weeks or months.

Lymphoproliferative Disorders

In addition to acute and chronic lymphocytic leukemias, several other conditions can be classified as malignant lymphoproliferative disorders.

The Lymphomas

The lymphomas are a heterogeneous group of diseases that originate in lymphoid tissue. Unique to the lymphomas is disruption of normal histologic structure in affected lymph nodes as well as lymph node enlargement. Generally, peripheral blood involvement, with abnormal circulating cells, is not present in the lymphomas.

Two major categories of lymphomas have been defined, Hodgkin's disease and non-Hodgkin's lymphoma (NHL). Both groups are further subclassified on the basis of histologic features.

Hodgkin's disease is characterized by a bimodal age distribution pattern. One peak occurs in persons 15 to 45 years old, and a second peak is seen in those older than 50

Box 43–4. The Myelodysplastic Syndromes

Refractory anemia
  <100% blasts in peripheral blood
  <5% blasts in bone marrow
  Cytopenias
Refractory anemia with ringed sideroblasts (RARS)
  <1% blasts in peripheral blood
  <5% blasts in bone marrow
  Cytopenias
  >15% ringed sideroblasts
  Dimorphic RBC population
Refractory anemia with excess blasts (RAEB)
  <5% blasts in peripheral blood
  5%–20% blasts in bone marrow
  Cytopenias
  Dysgranulopoiesis, dyserythropoiesis, dysmega-
    karyopoiesis
Refractory anemia with excess blasts in transforma-
  tion (RAEB-t)
  5% or more blasts in peripheral blood
  20%–30% blasts in bone marrow
  Cytopenias
  Dysplastic hematopoiesis
  Auer's rods in blasts
Chronic myelomonocytic leukemia (CMML)
  <5% blasts in peripheral blood
  Absolute monocytosis (>1.0 × 10^9/L)
  WBC count may be increased

---

years. Approximately 8000 new cases of Hodgkin's disease are diagnosed in the United States each year.[17] As with many malignant conditions, the etiology of this disorder is unknown. Proposed factors include genetic conditions, infectious agents such as the Epstein-Barr virus, and environmental influences, although specific support for any factor is lacking. The origin of the neoplastic cells in Hodgkin's disease has not been identified. Immunohistologic techniques are inconclusive in establishing the cells as T or B lymphocytes or monocytes.

Non-Hodgkin's lymphomas (NHLs) are more common than Hodgkin's disease in the United States. Persons of all ages may be affected, but the incidence increases after about the age of 40 years. Like that of Hodgkin's disease, the etiology of NHL is unknown. Several predisposing conditions have been implicated, however, including both congenital and acquired immunodeficiency diseases, viruses, and such physical or chemical agents as ionizing radiation and chemotherapy. Malignant T or B cells may be produced in NHL, and it has been suggested that the abnormal clone of cells arises when lymphocyte transformation is inhibited.[18]

Plasma Cell Dyscrasias or Immunoproliferative Disorders

The plasma cell dyscrasias are a group of malignant disorders characterized by the overproduction of a monoclonal immunoglobulin. The abnormal cells responsible for this proliferation are usually either plasma cells or B lymphocytes. The classification includes multiple myeloma, Waldenström's macroglobulinemia, the heavy-chain diseases, and primary amyloidosis.

Multiple myeloma is the most common and significant immunoproliferative malignancy. It is rarely seen in individuals younger than 40 years, the mean age of onset being around 63 years. The incidence of multiple myeloma increases with age. Gender and race predispositions are also noteworthy, with males more often affected than females and blacks having a higher incidence than whites.

The etiology of multiple myeloma is unknown, but it is the result of a defect that appears very early in B cell development. Most patients with myeloma produce excessive amounts of immunoglobulin (Ig) G, although IgA proliferation also occurs. Production of IgD or IgE is rare, and IgM myeloma is most often separately classified as Waldenström's macroglobulinemia.

The clinical course and length of survival in patients with myeloma directly correlates to the progression of disease at the time of diagnosis. Patients in advanced stages have a survival rate of less than 2 years. The average length of survival is 3 years, although a small percentage of patients may live longer than 10 years after diagnosis.

CLINICAL MANIFESTATIONS OF MALIGNANT CONDITIONS

The major clinical manifestations of the acute leukemias result from decreased production of normal hematopoietic cells and organ infiltration by malignant populations of cells. The onset of symptoms tends to be more abrupt and nonspecific. Fatigue, malaise, pallor, and weakness reflect a developing anemia. Infection may indicate a secondary immunosuppression or neutropenia. Petechiae, ecchymoses, and bleeding are commonly associated with thrombocytopenia. Masses of malignant infiltrates may cause bone and joint pain as well as splenomegaly and lymphadenopathy. DIC and bleeding are especially seen in AML-M3 and AML-M5. The infusion of neoplastic cells into gums and other mucosal sites, such as the skin, are common features of the monocytic leukemias, AML-M4 and AML-M5.

In contrast to the acute leukemias, chronic leukemias generally have a more insidious onset. Symptoms of anemia are milder, and white blood cell (WBC) and platelet counts are usually higher than in acute leukemias.

The myeloproliferative disorders share similar clinical characteristics, although some variations exist depending on the primary abnormality. Patients may be asymptomatic at presentation or may demonstrate fatigue and bleeding. A consistent finding in the MPDs is splenomegaly.

Lymphoproliferative disorders are quite diverse in clinical manifestations. Bone pain, primarily in the chest and back, is a major complaint in multiple myeloma. Weakness, fatigue, pallor, weight loss, and infection may be additional initial findings. Although Waldenström's macroglobulinemia may also manifest as weakness and related symptoms of anemia, bone pain is absent. Lymphadenopathy, hepatosplenomegaly, and a hyperviscosity syndrome may persist, however.

Hodgkin's disease usually manifests as a painless swelling of one or more lymph nodes in the neck. The condition spreads to successive lymph node groups in a very predictable manner. Fever, night sweats, pruritis, and weight loss may be presenting symptoms. Hodgkin's disease is predominantly nodal. The non-Hodgkin's lymphomas also may first appear as a painless enlargement of lymph nodes; however, noncontiguous lymph node clusters are often involved, as are extranodal sites, especially in children and immunocompromised individuals.

Clinical manifestations in the myelodysplastic syndromes are nonspecific and reflect the extent of peripheral blood cytopenia that has developed. Early stages may be asymptomatic, but fatigue, weakness, and malaise are usual findings. Fever and bleeding are sometimes present.

LABORATORY ANALYSES AND DIAGNOSIS OF MALIGNANT CONDITIONS

Performing a complete blood cell count (CBC) and identifying specific cellular, nuclear, and cytoplasmic characteristics of cells in peripheral blood, bone marrow, and lymph nodes are essential to the diagnosis and classification of hematologic malignancies. Because the morphologic evaluation of cells has some shortcomings, several additional identification techniques have become useful. These methods are cytochemical stains, rare techniques using ultrastructural studies such as electron microscopy, cytogenetics, immunologic techniques like flow cytometry, and the utilization of DNA probes to help characterize lymphocytic leukemias and detect gene rearrangements. If clinically indicated, other routine laboratory procedures may be necessary, such as chemistry tests, coagulation studies, and serologic evaluations.

Acute Myelogenous Leukemia

One of the first considerations necessary in the evaluation of a suspected acute leukemia is to differentiate an acute nonlymphocytic (or myeloid) leukemia (AML) from an acute lymphocytic leukemia (ALL). The treatment protocols for these disorders vary significantly, so an accurate diagnosis is essential. In addition to clinical features such as patient age and type of onset, morphologic review and cytochemistry testing are important laboratory procedures that can aid in distinguishing these leukemias. Although blast cells are predominant in both AML and ALL, certain morphologic features characterize each type of leukemia. In addition, basic cytochemical reactions are helpful in the initial distinction of AML from ALL. Generally, the blasts in AML are myeloperoxidase (peroxidase) positive and Sudan black B (SBB) positive, and terminal deoxynucleotidyl transferase (TdT), and nonspecific esterase (NSE) negative. ALL blasts are usually peroxidase, SBB, and NSE negative; however, the FAB subclassifications of the acute leukemias are each associated with specific criteria that are used in defining the subtype.

AML-M0

Minimally differentiated AML must be classified by means of cytochemistry and monoclonal antibodies. The blast cells are large and lack granules. Morphologically, they most closely resemble the malignant cells associated with ALL-L2 or, rarely, the lymphoblasts in ALL-L1. Generally, peroxidase, NSE, and SBB staining are negative, although less than 3% of blasts may be positive. Myeloperoxidase activity may be detected by immunohistochemical methods or by flow cytometry. The cells are negative for T and B lymphocyte–associated antigens, with the exceptions of TdT, CD2, CD4, and CD7; these latter lymphoid antigens are relatively nonspecific and may be positive in some of these undifferentiated neoplasms. At least one myeloid antigen must be identified by monoclonal antibody, either CD13 or CD33. Myeloid markers such as CD14 or CD11b may also be positive.

AML-M1

In myeloblastic leukemia without differentiation, more than 30% of nucleated cells and more than 90% of nonerythroid cells in the bone marrow are myeloblasts. The remaining 10% of nonerythroid cells must be either granulocytic cells, varying from promyelocytes on through the various maturation stages, or monocytes.[19] The peroxidase and SBB reactions must be positive in at least 3% of blasts. NSE staining should be negative in more than 90% of blasts. This subtype may be easily confused morphologically with ALL-L2; however, the presence of Auer's rods in approximately 50% of cases is a useful distinguishing feature of AML-M1. The cytoplasm may also contain azurophilic granules. Immunophenotyping, in particular the antigen expression of CD13, CD33, and HLA-DR, is also valuable in differentiating AML from ALL, especially when the myeloperoxidase or SBB reactivity is minimal (<10%).

AML-M2

The FAB criteria for the classification of myeloblastic leukemia with maturation defines the leukemia by the presence of myeloblasts, composing greater than 30% of nucleated cells in the bone marrow. In this instance, however, blasts constitute less than 90% of the nonerythroid cells, and granulocytes constitute more than 10% of the remaining cells. Monocytes must represent less than 20% of nonerythroid cells. Myeloperoxidase or SBB staining is positive in more than 50% of blasts. The neutrophils and neutrophil precursors often display nuclear and cytoplasmic dysplastic changes, including pseudo–Pelger-Huët condition. Auer's rods may be present in approximately 70% of cases. About 25% of patients with AML-M2 have the chromosome translocation t(8;21)(q22;q11). This translocation has been associated with unique immunophenotypic characteristics that may prove useful in defining this subtype of acute leukemia, especially in pediatric cases.[20]

AML-M3

A high incidence of disseminated intravascular coagulation is common in patients with acute promyelocytic leukemia (APL) and is an important feature both to evaluate and manage. Abnormal coagulation studies reflect the DIC, including prolonged prothrombin time, activated partial thromboplastin time, and thrombin time tests. Fibrinogen levels are decreased, and positive fibrinogen degradation product (FDP) and D-dimer results are seen. Thrombocytopenia is generally more pronounced in AML-M3 than in other subtypes of AML.

Several morphologic characteristics are also unique to AML-M3. Abnormal promyelocytes are the predominant malignant cell type, with heavy, intense azurophilic granulation. In some cells, the granules may be larger than usual, completely obscuring the nucleus. Additionally, Auer's rods, many in bundles, may be seen in as many as 90% of cases of AML-M3. The nuclei in these hypergranulated cells are often bilobed or kidney-shaped. Both myeloperoxidase and Sudan black B reactions are strongly positive, and the NSE reaction is negative.

A variant of acute promyelocytic leukemia has also been identified. In this microgranular or hypogranular (M3m or M3v) form, the primary, azurophilic granules are small and sparsely distributed, and may not be easily visualized with Wright's stain. In addition, the prominent nuclear folding and convolutions within an abundant cytoplasm may make it difficult to distinguish these cells from the abnormal monocytes characteristic of AML-M4 or AML-M5; however, promyelocytic leukemias show strong peroxidase and Sudan black B staining, whereas AML-M4 or AML-M5 characteristically stains with NSE. In contrast to patients with typical AML-M3, patients with the microgranular variant usually have a higher total white blood cell (WBC) count.

Both types of acute promyelocytic leukemia have been associated with an abnormal chromosomal translocation, t(15;17)(q22; q12-21), which is present in most cases. The identification of this karyotype has significance with respect to response to newer treatment regimens, such as the use of tretinoin. This cytogenetic translocation specific to APL results in the rearrangement of the retinoic acid receptor–α (RAR-α), from chromosome 17 to the myl locus on chromosome 15. Consequently, a new fusion gene is produced. Research suggests that expression of this abnormal fusion gene is necessary for an effective response to tretinoin.[21]

Flow cytometry analysis may also be useful in defining APL. Most cases of AML-M3 have been associated with the absence of the human leukocyte antigen DR (1a) (HLA-DR1a), which is easily determined by flow cytometry.[10]

AML-M4

Acute myelomonocytic leukemia is characterized by the presence of both granulocytic and monocytic malignant cells. Adherence to the FAB diagnostic criteria[19] is especially important in defining AML-M4, in order to distinguish this subtype from either AML-M2 or AML-M5.

In bone marrow samples of AML-M4, blast cells (myeloblasts and monoblasts) constitute more than 30% of all the nonerythroid cells. The total percentage of myeloblasts, promyelocytes, myelocytes, and other granulocytes is greater than 30% but does not exceed 80% of the nonerythroid cells. Monoblasts, promonocytes, and monocytes account for 20% to 80% of bone marrow cells and 20% of peripheral blood cells. Cytochemistry is needed to confirm the monocytic origin of cells. For a diagnosis of AML-M4, 20% to 80% of bone marrow cells must be NSE positive.

Likewise, 20% to 80% of cells are peroxidase or SBB positive. Large amounts of lysozyme (muramidase) are released from monocytes and may also be detected; levels greater than 3 times normal in either serum or urine[11] suggest a diagnosis of AML-M4. If bone marrow and cytochemical staining do not provide enough information to distinguish this subtype from AML-M2, AML-M4 can still be established if the peripheral blood monocyte count exceeds 5×10^9 cells/L.

A variant of AML-M4 has also been identified. In AML-M4 with eosinophilia (M4e), 5% or more of nonerythroid cells in the bone marrow are eosinophils. The eosinophils are distinctly abnormal, having large basophilic granules in addition to the eosinophilic granules. The nuclei may also be monocytoid or unsegmented. These abnormal eosinophils stain positive with the chloroacetate esterase (specific esterase) and periodic acid–Schiff (PAS) reactions, unlike normal eosinophils. AML-M4e is also associated with a characteristic cytogenetic abnormality involving either a deletion or inversion of the long arm of chromosome 16.

AML-M5

Acute monocytic leukemia is divided into two subtypes: M5a, poorly differentiated, and M5b, well differentiated. Regardless of subtype, monoblasts, promonocytes, or monocytes account for at least 80% of all nonerythroid cells in the bone marrow. In M5a, 80% or more of the monocytic cells are monoblasts: whereas in M5b, monoblasts account for less than 80% or more of the monocytic cells, and promonocytes and monocytes predominate. The NSE stain is useful in characterizing both types of AML-M5. The leukemic monoblasts and promonocytes are NSE positive and generally myeloperoxidase negative.

As in AML-M4, lysozyme levels in serum or urine are often increased in AML-M5. Apparently, the amount of enzyme present is directly proportional to the extent of monocytic differentiation, with lysozyme levels more elevated in M5b than in M5a.[4]

Abnormalities in the long arm of chromosome 11 (11q) have also been associated with some cases of AML-M5.

AML-M6

In acute erythroleukemia, a predominance of primarily erythroid precursors is seen, although myeloid components may also be present. Erythroid cells constitute 50% or more of all nucleated cells in the bone marrow, whereas 30% or more of the remaining nonerythroid cells are myeloblasts. The erythroid cells often appear morphologically abnormal, commonly demonstrating megaloblastoid features as well as multinucleation, karyorrhexis, gigantism, and cytoplasmic vacuolation and budding. AML-M6 sometimes develops from a myelodysplastic syndrome or as a secondary complication in patients undergoing alkylating chemotherapy for different conditions. Likewise, some cases of diagnosed erythroleukemia may transform into acute processes indistinguishable from other acute myeloid leukemias, such as AML-M1, AML-M2, or AML-M4.

Cytochemistry and immunohistochemistry can be useful in diagnosing AML-M6. The PAS reaction is often positive in erythroid precursors. The NSE reaction with acetate as the substrate is commonly positive. Immunophenotyping with monoclonal antibodies directed to erythroid glycophorin A is also helpful in establishing the erythroid origin of the blast cells.

Because of the bizarre dyspoietic and megaloblastoid appearance of the erythroid cells, it is important to differentiate erythroleukemia from possible diagnoses of myelodysplastic syndromes, congenital dyserythropoietic anemias, and folic acid or vitamin B_{12} deficiency.

AML-M7

Acute megakaryoblastic leukemia is characterized by an abnormal proliferation of variably sized megakaryoblasts and atypical megakaryocytes. Blast cells must make up more than 30% of all cells in the bone marrow. Sometimes, the nuclear chromatin is dense and heavy, resembling the lymphoblasts seen in ALL-L1. Other times, the chromatin is loose and fine. Blasts in the bone marrow or peripheral blood may also display cytoplasmic projections or buds. Megakaryocytic fragments may be seen in the peripheral blood as well.

Cytochemistry, electron microscopy, and immunophenotyping are important procedures used to define acute megakaryoblastic leukemia. Megakaryoblasts do not stain with myeloperoxidase, Sudan black B, or NSE with butyrate as the substrate. The NSE reaction is positive when acetate is used as the substrate. PAS positivity can often be demonstrated in AML-M7. Electron microscopy may also reveal specific platelet peroxidase activity. Immunophenotyping is often the most acceptable method for classifying cases of AML-M7, and monoclonal antibodies directed against platelet glycoprotein receptors are particularly valuable. Two commonly used monoclonal antibodies are CD41, which recognizes the glycoprotein IIb/IIIa receptor (fibrinogen) on the surfaces of platelets, and CD61, the antibody to platelet glycoprotein IIIa. Antibodies against factor VIII–related antigen may also yield positive results in AML-M7. Box 43–5 summarizes the reactions that are useful in supporting an FAB diagnosis of AML.

Other AMLs

The FAB system does not classify all types of acute nonlymphocytic leukemias. In acute basophilic leukemia, basophilic granules can be recognized in differentiated cells using light microscopy. Some cases of poorly differentiated acute basophilic leukemia have also been demonstrated in which there are no or only a few basophilic granules visible on light microscopy. Likewise, myeloperoxidase activity is negative when evaluated using the light microscope, but positive with the electron microscope. The basophilic granules stain positively with toluidine blue.[8] Cases of undifferentiated leukemia are uncommonly encountered, because immunophenotyping and electron microscopy are usually capable of distinguishing acute leukemia when morphology and cytochemistry yield inconclusive results.

A true undifferentiated acute leukemia exists when the blast cells are morphologically unrecognizable, cytotechnical tests are negative, no cell antigens can be detected, electron microscopy does not provide any clues, and cytogenetic studies are unclear. In mixed-lineage acute non-

---

Box 43–5. Reactions Useful in Supporting a Diagnosis of Acute Nonlymphocytic Leukemia

To Support a Diagnosis of AML-M1, AML-M2, or AML-M3

Use Peroxidase, SBB, and NSE.

- AML-M1
- AML-M2 } Peroxidase positive; SBB positive; NSE negative
- AML-M3

To Differentiate AML-M4 from AML-M5

Use peroxidase, SBB, and NSE.

- AML-M4   Peroxidase positive; SBB positive; NSE positive
- AML-M5   Peroxidase negative; SBB negative; NSE positive

To Support a Diagnosis of AML-M6

Use NSE, PAS, and immunophenotyping.

- AML-M6   NSE positive with acetate but not with butyrate; PAS positive; immunophenotyping using monoclonal antibodies to erythroid glycophorin A

To Support a Diagnosis of AML-M7

Use NSE, PAS, PPO, and immunophenotyping.

- AML-M7   NSE positive with acetate but not with butyrate; PAS positive; PPO positive; immunophenotyping using anti-gp IIIa (antibody to platelet glycoprotein IIIa-CD61) or anti-gp IIb/IIIa (antibody to the platelet fibrinogen receptor-CD41)

Abbreviations: NSE, nonspecific esterase with acetate or butyrate substrates; PAS, periodic acid–Schiff staining; PPO, platelet peroxidase; SBB, Sudan black B.

---

lymphocytic leukemias, blast cells express myeloid and lymphoid characteristics as a mixed population, or myeloid and lymphoid features are demonstrated simultaneously in individual cells.

Acute Lymphoblastic Leukemia

The laboratory findings most characteristic of acute lymphoblastic leukemia (ALL) at presentation are leukocytosis, a normocytic, normochromic anemia, and thrombocytopenia. Circulating lymphoblasts are usually present. The bone marrow is almost always hypercellular with abundant lymphoblasts. Analysis of cerebrospinal fluid (CSF) may reveal lymphoblasts, because central nervous system involvement is a common manifestation of ALL. Once again, the first steps in identifying the abnormal population

should include a morphologic review and cytochemical evaluation of the leukemic cells.

The French-American-British cooperative group has devised a classification system for acute lymphoblastic leukemia based on cytologic characteristics of bone marrow lymphoblasts. The features evaluated are cell size, amount of cytoplasm, presence or absence of nucleoli, nuclear shape, nuclear chromatin structure, basophilia of cytoplasm, and the presence or absence of cytoplasmic vacuolation.

As previously described, the three subgroups of ALL are L1, L2, and L3 (see Table 43–1). ALL-L1 cells are generally small blasts with scanty cytoplasm and inconspicuous nucleoli. L2 blasts tend to be larger and heterogeneous with moderately abundant cytoplasm and prominent nucleoli. The most noteworthy characteristic associated with ALL-L3 is a deeply basophilic, moderately abundant cytoplasm with conspicuous vacuolation.

Myeloperoxidase staining, when positive, is important in distinguishing myeloblasts from lymphoblasts. PAS, NSE, and acid phosphatase reactions may be useful in defining specific FAB subgroups of ALL. ALL-L1 and ALL-L2 are usually PAS and acid phosphatase positive, whereas ALL-L3 cells show no reactivity with these stains. The NSE reaction is variably positive in ALL-L1 and ALL-L2 but generally negative in ALL-L3. Terminal deoxynucleotidyl transferase (TdT) is also a valuable lymphoid marker, in that more than 90% of lymphoblasts in ALL are TdT positive;[22] however, B-cell ALL with L3 morphology is TdT negative.

Acute lymphoblastic leukemia is actually a heterogeneous group of disorders. A morphologic and cytochemical classification of ALL is often inadequate to distinguish this disorder from AML or other lymphoproliferative conditions and provides little information as a prognostic indicator; therefore, the immunologic classification of ALL using monoclonal antibodies has become an important diagnostic and prognostic procedure. Table 43–2 relates ALL morphology to an immunologic classification of subgroups.

Gene rearrangement studies of the immunoglobulin and T-cell receptor genes are occasionally useful in determining cell lineage and clonality of certain cases of ALL.

Chronic Myelogenous Leukemia

Chronic myelogenous leukemia (CML) is characterized by very high leukocyte counts ($50–4000 \times 10^9$/L), normocytic, normochromic anemia, and normal or even elevated platelet counts. A striking feature of the peripheral blood smear is the variety of granulocytic precursors present. Myeloblasts and promyelocytes generally represent less than 10% of the circulating white blood cells, but myelocytes may often predominate, and metamyelocytes and more mature granulocytes are commonly seen. Eosinophilia and basophilia may also be observed. Morphologic findings are similar in a hypercellular bone marrow.

Cytochemical, cytogenetic, and molecular studies are important laboratory procedures used to diagnose CML. In uncomplicated cases of CML, the leukocyte alkaline phosphatase (LAP) score is usually near zero. The Philadelphia chromosome (Ph) can be demonstrated in almost all cases.

Table 43–2. Immunologic Classification of Subgroups of Acute Lymphoblastic Leukemia (ALL)

Subgroup	Morphology	CALLA	CD7	CD19	CIg	SIg	HLA-DR
Precursor B-cell ALL	L1/L2	−	−	+	−	−	+
Early pre–B-cell ALL	L1/L2	+	−	+	−	−	+
Pre–B-cell ALL	L1/L2	+	−	+	+	−	+
B-cell ALL	L3	−	−	+	−	+	+
T-cell ALL	L1/L2	−	+	−	−	−	−

Abbreviations: CALLA, common ALL antigen (CD10); CIg, cytoplasmic immunoglobulin; SIg, surface immunoglobulin; HLA, human leukocyte antigen.

The Ph chromosome can be further defined at the molecular level. The translocation of the long arm of chromosome 22 to chromosome 9, t (9;22), that results in the Ph creates a genetic relocation of the *c-abl* oncogene from chromosome 9 to the breakpoint cluster region (bcr) on chromosome 22. A rearrangement study to detect this bcr-*abl* hybrid is an important diagnostic procedure when a patient presents with peripheral blood and bone marrow findings consistent with CML but the LAP score is inconclusive and cytogenetics are negative for the Ph.

After the initial chronic phase, most CML patients progress through an accelerated phase, characterized by a continuing basophilia, an increase in peripheral blood myeloblasts, and promyelocytes, myelofibrosis, and thrombocytopenia.[23] This terminal phase of CML is termed *blast crisis*. The development of blast crisis in some cases of CML has been associated at the genetic level with alterations in the p53 cancer suppressor gene.[24] In this stage, blasts represent more than 30% of all leukocytes in the peripheral blood or bone marrow and may be myeloid or lymphoid in origin. Cytochemistry, especially the use of myeloperoxidase and TdT, is useful in classifying the blasts.

Chronic myelogenous leukemia must be differentiated from conditions with similar presenting hematologic features. Leukemoid reactions and other myeloproliferative disorders generally do not manifest as a low LAP or basophilia. Furthermore, the FAB cooperative group has suggested that subclassifications of CML may need to include Ph-negative, bcr-*abl*–negative cases as well as cases of atypical chronic myeloid leukemia and chronic myelomonocytic leukemia.[25]

Chronic Lymphocytic Leukemia

A persistent peripheral blood lymphocytosis is a common feature of chronic lymphocytic leukemia (CLL). Most of the lymphocytes appear small and morphologically mature, with condensed chromatin and scanty blue cytoplasm. Many smudge cells may be seen. Anemia is not always initially present but is usually normocytic and normochromic. An autoimmune hemolytic anemia develops in some cases, demonstrated by polychromatophilia and spherocytes on the peripheral blood smear and a positive direct antiglobulin test. The bone marrow is often hypercellular, and the malignant lymphocytes constitute more than 30% of all nucleated cells.

Chronic lymphocytic leukemia has been classified immunophenotypically as a B-cell disorder, and the cells classically express surface immunoglobulin with light-chain restriction, pan–B-cell antigens such as CD19, CD20 and CD24, and coexpress the traditional T-cell marker CD5.

Additional tests useful in defining CLL are serum immunoglobulin levels, which are generally decreased, and cytogenetic studies. Both numerical alterations, such as trisomy 12, and structural variations in chromosomes, such as 14q, 6q, and 11, have been identified.[26]

The transformation of CLL to Richter's syndrome is usually recognized from a biopsy of lymph nodes that reveal a large cell lymphoma. A prolymphocytic transformation is characterized by an increase in prolymphocytes in the peripheral blood. These cells are morphologically large with more abundant cytoplasm and distinct nucleoli in contrast to the small, mature-appearing lymphocytes of classic CLL.

Hairy Cell Leukemia

Hairy cell leukemia (HCL) is also a B-cell malignancy. The characteristic cells are larger than small lymphocytes and generally have round or oval nuclei. Nucleoli are usually indistinct in a finely stippled chromatin. Moderately abundant light blue cytoplasm surrounds the nucleus. The cytoplasm often has frayed projections.

Although this disorder is classified as a leukemia, it is not uncommon for patients with HCL to present with a pancytopenia. A bone marrow evaluation is essential in the diagnosis of HCL, but a dry tap often results. Hairy cells can usually be identified in biopsy specimens morphologically and by immunostaining with B-cell markers such as CD20. The tartrate-resistant acid phosphatase (TRAP) stain is useful in confirming HCL in bone marrow touch preparations or peripheral blood smears. Most hairy cells are TRAP positive.

Other Lymphoid Leukemias

The morphologic evaluation and immunophenotyping of peripheral blood and bone marrow specimens are the most useful techniques in identifying rare cases of lymphoid leukemia. The leukemic phase of non-Hodgkin's lymphoma, Sézary's syndrome, large granular lymphocyte leukemia, and adult T-cell leukemia/lymphoma are best recognized with these procedures.

Myeloproliferative Disorders

The myeloproliferative disorders (MPDs) share several laboratory findings, yet each has unique distinguishing features. Table 43–3 summarizes common laboratory findings in the MPDs.

Table 43–3. Laboratory Findings in the Myeloproliferative Disorders

Parameter	Chronic Myelogenous Leukemia	Polycythemia Vera	Myelofibrosis with Myeloid Metaplasia	Essential Thrombocythemia
WBC	Markedly ↑ (>50 × 10⁹/L)	Moderately ↑ (<30 × 10⁹/L)	Variable	Normal or ↑ (<30 × 10⁹/L)
Hemoglobin	Normal or ↓	Markedly ↑	↓	Variable
Platelet count	Variable	Normal or ↑	Variable	Markedly ↑
Peripheral blood morphologic changes				
WBCs	Immature granulocytes	None	Immature granulocytes	Occasional immature granulocyte
	Eosinophilia, basophilia	Occasional eosinophilia and basophilia	Occasional eosinophilia and basophilia	Mild eosinophilia and basophilia
RBCs	Normochromic normocyte	Normochromic normocytic	Anisocytosis, dacryocytes, nucleated RBCs	Normochromic normocytic
Platelets	Occasional giant	Megakaryocytic fragments	Megakaryocytic fragments and giant	Marked variation in size and shape
Leukocyte alkaline phosphatase (LAP)	Markedly ↓	↑	Normal or ↑	Normal or ↑
Philadelphia chromosome/bcr-*abl* gene rearrangement	Present	Absent	Absent	Absent
Marrow fibrosis	Progressively ↑	Progressively ↑	Markedly ↑	Progressively ↑

Lymphoproliferative Disorders

Hodgkin's disease is diagnosed when classic Reed-Sternberg cells, or any one of a number of variants, are observed on a lymph node biopsy specimen. Hematologic abnormalities are rarely seen in Hodgkin's lymphoma, although a mild to moderate normocytic, normochromic anemia may be evident. Some patients present with monocytosis, eosinophilia, and neutrophilia. Platelet counts are normal. Bone marrow involvement in Hodgkin's disease is also uncommon. Blood chemistry values, such as alkaline phosphatase and lactate dehydrogenase, are sometimes elevated. Immunophenotyping and gene rearrangement studies are additional techniques that may be useful in establishing a differential diagnosis of Hodgkin's disease.

The morphologic evaluation of tissue biopsy specimens, immunophenotyping, gene rearrangement studies, and cytogenetic analysis are also methods used to diagnose and classify the non-Hodgkin's lymphomas (NHLs). Peripheral blood and bone marrow involvement are more common in NHL than in Hodgkin's disease; however, the hematologic manifestations are variable, depending on the classification of the lymphoma. Blood cell counts are generally normal, but lymphoma cells may infiltrate the circulation in certain types of NHL. Routine serum chemistry tests are useful in evaluating liver and renal function, which may be impaired in NHL.

Several laboratory abnormalities characterize multiple myeloma. Most patients present with a normocytic, normochromic anemia with rouleaux prominent on the peripheral blood smear. A few plasma cells may be seen. The erythrocyte sedimentation rate (ESR) is markedly elevated as a result of increased serum immunoglobulins. More than 10% plasma cells must be noted in the bone marrow to establish a diagnosis of multiple myeloma. Monoclonal immunoglobulin is detected in both serum protein and urine electrophoresis or with various immunotechniques.

Increased amounts of monoclonal IgM distinguishes Waldenström's macroglobulinemia from multiple myeloma.

Serum viscosity is also elevated. Tests of platelet function and routine coagulation screening values may be abnormal because of the high levels of IgM.

Myelodysplastic Syndromes

The myelodysplastic syndromes (MDSs) are characterized by various degrees of erythroid, myeloid, and megakaryocytic abnormalities in both the peripheral blood and the bone marrow. The dyspoietic findings may be qualitative or quantitative. Dyserythropoiesis varies from mild to marked, depending on the classification of the MDS. Likewise, dysgranulopoiesis may be absent in some types of MDS but severe in others, and dysmegakaryopoiesis is a common feature of many of the myelodysplastic syndromes. In addition, the number of blasts in the bone marrow increases in the more severe classifications of MDS, although it never exceeds 30%. Table 43–4 summarizes the major hematologic manifestations of the myelodysplastic syndromes.

As the blast count increases in the more severe forms of MDS, the peripheral blood and bone marrow picture may more closely resemble that of AML. The FAB cooperative group has proposed a scheme for the differential diagnosis of MDS versus AML. Figure 43–2 illustrates the relationship between the MDSs and AML.[6]

TREATMENT

The Leukemias

Treatment protocols for the acute leukemias are designed to eliminate the malignant cells, to return the bone marrow to a normal disease-free functional state, and to support the patient as necessary. Responses to therapy vary considerably and are influenced by patient age, specific subtype of acute leukemia diagnosed, prior treatment regimens (for a previous MDS or other malignancy), and cytogenetic characteristics of the leukemia. In general,

Table 43–4. **Major Hematologic Manifestations of the Myelodysplastic Syndromes**

Syndrome	Peripheral Blood	Bone Marrow
Dyserythropoiesis	Anemia	Megaloblastoid erythropoiesis
	Oval macrocytes	Ringed sideroblasts
	Hypochromia	Binucleated or multinucleated red blood cells
	Dimorphism	Nuclear binding
	Howell-Jolly bodies	Uneven cytoplasmic staining
	Basophilic stippling	Erythroid hyperplasia
	Nucleated red blood cells	
	Poikilocytosis	
Dysgranulopoiesis	Neutropenia	Increased myeloblasts
	Hyposegmentation (pseudo–Pelger-Huët)	Reduced or giant granules
	Hypersegmentation	Myeloid hyperplasia
	Hypogranulation	Monocytosis
	Giant granules	Uneven cytoplasmic staining
	Immature granulocytes	
Dysmegakaryopoiesis	Thrombocytopenia	Variable number megakaryocytes
	Giant platelets	Micromegakaryocytes
	Micromegakaryocytes	Single, multiple, or odd-numbered nuclei
	Abnormal platelet granules	

treatment of the acute leukemias comprises combination chemotherapy, radiation therapy, and bone marrow transplantation in selected individuals. Newer compounds, especially for the treatment of acute myelogenous leukemias, have been developed. These agents function to stimulate maturation and differentiation in the leukemic cells that are frozen in an immature state. To date, the most significant of this new class of drugs is tretinoin, used in the treatment of acute promyelocytic leukemia.

A significant consequence of treatment in any of the leukemias is the development of pancytopenia which must be monitored carefully. The use of hematopoietic growth factors in elevating blood cell counts has proven to be an effective therapy.[27] Morphologic variations in cells may also be seen, and some cases of chemotherapy in acute lymphoblastic leukemia may be associated with the peripheral blood appearance of cytoplasmic fragments from disrupted lymphocytic cells.[28]

Treatment of chronic myelogenous leukemia (CML) fo-

cuses on reducing the excessively high WBC count and managing complications of hyperleukocytosis and rapid cell turnover, such as hyperuricemia and splenomegaly. Alkylating drugs and antimetabolites have been useful in suppressing the hyperleukocytosis, and allopurinol is an effective agent in reducing uric acid levels. Interferon-α is also associated with high rates of remission in patients with early-stage or chronic CML;[23] however, the only documented long-term disease-free survivals in CML are associated with allogeneic bone marrow transplants in suitable candidates. Chronic myelogenous leukemia invariably progresses from a chronic phase to a terminal, blast crisis. Effective treatments of blast crisis have not yet been established, although induction regimens for AML or ALL are minimally successful. Review of the peripheral blood smear of a treated CML patient still in the chronic stage shows some changes. The leukocyte count is generally decreased, though still often above 15.0×10^9/L, and the initially pronounced left shift is mild, with only few num-

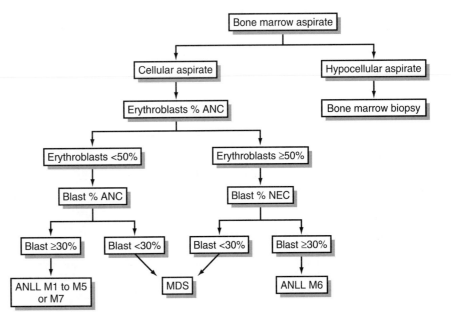

Figure 43–2. Relationship between the myelodysplastic syndrome (MDS) and acute nonlymphocytic leukemia (ANLL). Abbreviations: ANC, all nucleated cells; NEC, nonerythroid cells. (Adapted from Bennett JM, Catovsky D, Daniel MT, et al: Proposed revised criteria for the classification of acute myeloid leukemia. Ann Intern Med 103:626–629, 1985.)

bers of immature granulocytes. Basophilia may still be present.

Patients with chronic lymphocytic leukemia (CLL) who show no significant progression of the disease often do not receive treatment until it is clinically indicated. Therapy regimens usually include alkylating agents, which are used singly or combined with corticosteroids. Traditional drugs are chlorambucil, cyclophosphamide, and prednisone. Newer protocols include fludarabine, 2-chloro-2'-deoxy-adenosine (2-CdA), and 2-deoxycoformycin (pentostatin) as well as biotherapeutic substances like monoclonal antibodies, interferon-α, and interleukin-2.[26] In general, when the progression of CLL to variants such as prolymphocytic leukemia occurs, the response to customary treatment methods is poor. As with therapeutic measures in other types of leukemia, myelosuppression is always possible in the treatment of CLL. Granulocytopenia, thrombocytopenia, and anemia are commonly observed in treated CLL patients.

Advances in treatment of HCL are beginning to replace splenectomy as the method of choice in controlling progression of the leukemic cells. Interferon-α, 2-CdA, and pentostatin are effective against HCL.[29]

Myeloproliferative Disorders

The myeloproliferative disorders, polycythemia vera, agnogenic myeloid metaplasia, and essential thrombocythemia, each have specific treatment regimens; however, myelosuppressive agents, such as hydroxyurea, are eventually employed to reduce the mass of abnormally proliferating cells. Polycythemia vera is initially treated with phlebotomy. Numerous antifibrosing drugs are undergoing evaluation as possible therapy for myelofibrosis with myeloid metaplasia.[30] Plateletpheresis is used in cases of essential thrombocythemia. Anagrelide, a megakaryocyte inhibitor, and interferon-α have now been added to the treatment protocol.[30] Patients with polycythemia who have undergone long-term phlebotomy may develop an iron deficiency. The use of some types of cytotoxic drugs has been associated with the development of an acute leukemia in all types of myeloproliferative disorders.

Lymphoproliferative Disorders

Treatment for Hodgkin's disease depends on clinical stage. Radiation therapy, combination chemotherapy, and combined radiation therapy and chemotherapy are the standard choices. Likewise, treatment for non-Hodgkin's lymphomas (NHLs) is formulated around the clinical stage of the disease as well as the histologic classification. Chemotherapy and radiation therapy are often used, but surgery, biotherapeutic agents, and bone marrow transplantation have also been effective in managing certain types of lymphomas.

Immunoproliferative Disorders

Patients with symptomatic multiple myeloma are usually treated with chemotherapy and corticosteroids. Several clinical trials suggest that combination chemotherapeutic regimens may yield higher response rates than single-drug

protocols.[31] Interferon-α has also been effective in controlling the disease. In addition, bone marrow transplantation has been successful in the treatment of multiple myeloma. As with other lymphoproliferative and myeloproliferative conditions, supportive therapy is always critical in managing a patient with multiple myeloma. The laboratory results that indicate effective treatment of multiple myeloma are decreases in erythrocyte sedimentation rate and serum proteins, and an elevation of peripheral blood cell counts. Plasmapheresis is used in treating patients with Waldenström's macroglobulinemia who develop symptoms of hyperviscosity. Chemotherapeutic drugs, either as single agents or in combination with other alkylating drugs or corticosteroids, are utilized in controlling cell proliferation in this disorder. Waldenström's macroglobulinemia may also be successfully managed through the use of recombinant human interferon.

Myelodysplastic Syndromes

Several treatment methods have been used in patients with any one of the myelodysplastic syndromes (MDSs). Most individuals require at least some type of supportive therapy, generally including transfusion of blood components. More aggressive protocols depend on the age of the patient and the clinical severity of the MDS. In advanced disease in older patients, aggressive chemotherapeutic drugs have been used. Patients in younger age groups (less than 50 years old) may respond to bone marrow transplantation. Hematopoietic growth factors, such as granulocyte colony–stimulating factor, granulocyte-macrophage colony–stimulating factor, interleukin-3, and recombinant human erythropoietin, have been minimally effective in managing the MDSs. Drugs that promote differentiation of precursor cells, like some derivatives of vitamin D, retinoic acids, and interferons, are other possible treatment agents.[32]

Case Study 1

A 60-year-old man in remission from a previously diagnosed acute lymphoblastic leukemia was admitted to the hospital. The results of laboratory testing (with reference ranges) completed to evaluate his leukemic relapse were as follows:

WBCs ($\times 10^9$/L)	45.0	(3.6–9.0)
RBCs ($\times 10^{12}$/L)	13.5	(4.71–5.77)
Hemoglobin (g/dL)	10.0	(14.9–17.1)
Hematocrit (%)	29.0	(44.9–51.1)
Mean corpuscular volume (fL)	76.0	(86.0–96.0)
Mean corpuscular hemoglobin (pg)	27.2	(29.1–32.7)
Mean corpuscular hemoglobin concentration (g/dL)	36.1	(32.0–36.0)
Platelets ($\times 10^9$/L)	19	(140–440)

Differential blood cell count (%)		
Lymphocytes	4	(16–47)
Monocytes	1	(0–9)
Blasts	95	(0)

Cytochemical staining showed the cells to be peroxidase negative and TdT positive. Immunophenotyping revealed that more than 90% of the lymphoid cells in the peripheral blood expressed CD10, HLA-DR, and CD19, a weak CD20 expression was present, but not surface immunoglobulin.

Questions

1. On the basis of the laboratory results provided, does this patient still have ALL?
2. How do the cytochemistry and immunophenotyping results help in classifying this leukemic relapse?
3. What types of therapy may be beneficial to this patient?

Discussion

1. Yes, this patient still has acute lymphoblastic leukemia, as indicated by the high blast count, cytochemical results, and cell marker studies.
2. Abnormal lymphoid cells in lymphoblastic leukemia are usually peroxidase negative and TdT positive. In addition, the lymphoblasts can be immunologically classified as B cells.
3. In older adults, only a small percentage of leukemias are curable. This patient may still show response to cytotoxic chemotherapeutic agents; however, supportive therapy for the anemia and thrombocytopenia and to control possible infections are important in managing this patient's disease.

Case Study 2

A previously healthy 20-year-old female initially presented to the emergency room after a sledding accident in which she suffered abdominal trauma. Surgery repaired a lacerated right ovary, but the patient received significant amounts of blood during surgery and packed red blood cells postoperatively. Three days postoperatively, she developed wound bleeding, epistaxis, and vaginal bleeding, with the following laboratory results (with reference ranges):

	Values	Reference Range
WBCs ($\times 10^9$/L)	10.1	(3.6–9.0)
RBCs ($\times 10^{12}$/L)	2.7	(4.71–5.77)
Hemoglobin (g/dL)	8.1	(14.9–17.1)
Hematocrit (%)	24.2	(44.9–51.5)
Platelets ($\times 10^9$/L)	21.0	(140–440)

Prothrombin time (sec)	19.1	(10–13)
Fibrinogen (mg/dL)	75	(200–400)
FDP (mg/dL)	>1.0	(<0.5)

Differential blood cell count (%)		
Segmented neutrophils	27	(45–79)
Band neutrophils	8	(0–5)
Lymphocytes	10	(16–47)
Promyelocytes	48	(0)
Myelocytes	5	(0)
Metamyelocytes	2	(0)

Questions

1. What is the most likely diagnosis of this patient's condition, on the basis of clinical features and hematologic test results?
2. What additional tests are needed to confirm a diagnosis?
3. What coagulopathy has developed in this patient?

Discussion

1. This patient has acute promyelocytic leukemia (AML-M3).
2. Cytochemistry, including myeloperoxidase staining and a TdT, should be performed. In addition, cytogenetics may be performed. Patients with AML-M3 who have the characteristic t(15;17)(q22;q12-21) chromosomal translocation generally respond better to newer treatment protocols.
3. Disseminated intravascular coagulation (DIC) has developed. The release of large numbers of promyelocytic granules with procoagulant activity can initiate this complication in AML-M3.

References

1. Dale CD: Neutrophil disorders: Benign, quantitative abnormalities of neutrophils. *In* Williams WJ (ed): Hematology, ed 4. New York, McGraw-Hill, 1990.
2. Turgeon ML: Clinical Hematology: Theory and Procedures, ed 2. Boston, Little, Brown, 1993.
3. Beck WS: Hematology, ed 4. Cambridge, Mass, MIT Press, 1985.
4. Perkins ML: Introduction to leukemia and the acute leukemias. *In* Harmening DM (ed): Clinical Hematology and Fundamentals of Hemostasis, ed 2. Philadelphia, FA Davis, 1992.
5. Bennett JM, Catovsky D, Daniel M-T, et al: Proposals for the classification of the acute leukaemias. Br J Haematol 33:451–458, 1976.
6. Bennett JM, Catovsky D, Daniel M-T, et al: Criteria for the diagnosis of acute leukemia of megakaryocyte lineage (M7). Ann Intern Med 103:460–462, 1985.
7. Bennett JM, Catovsky D, Daniel M-T, et al: Proposal for the recognition of minimally differentiated acute myeloid leukaemia (AML-M0). Br J Haematol 78:325–329, 1991.
8. McKenna R: Acute myeloid leukemia. *In* Kjeldsberg CR (ed): Practical Diagnosis of Hematologic Disorders, ed 2. Chicago, ASCP Press, 1995.
9. Goasguen J, Bennett JM: The acute myeloid leukemias: Morphology and cytochemistry. *In* Bick RL (ed): Hematology: Clinical and Laboratory Practice, vol 2. St Louis, CV Mosby, 1993.
10. Moriarty AT: Acute and chronic leukemias. *In* Rodak BF (ed): Diagnostic Hematology. Philadelphia, WB Saunders, 1995.

11. Foon KA, Rai KR, Gale RP: Chronic lymphocytic leukemia. *In* Bick RL (ed): Hematology: Clinical and Laboratory Practice, vol 1. St Louis, CV Mosby, 1993.

12. Bick RL, Laughlin WR: Myeloproliferative syndromes. Lab Med 24:770–776, 1993.

13. Wolf BC, Neiman RS: The morphology of the myeloproliferative disorders. *In* Bick RL (ed): Hematology: Clinical and Laboratory Practice, vol 2. St Louis, CV Mosby, 1993.

14. Griep J: Myeloproliferative disorders. *In* Rodak BF (ed): Diagnostic Hematology. Philadelphia, WB Saunders, 1995.

15. Silverstein MN: The myeloproliferative diseases. *In* Bick RL (ed): Hematology: Clinical and Laboratory Practice, vol 2. St Louis, CV Mosby, 1993.

16. Ward PCJ: The myelodysplastic syndromes. *In* Bick RL (ed): Hematology: Clinical and Laboratory Practice, vol 2. St Louis, CV Mosby, 1993.

17. Kjeldsberg CR: Hodgkin's disease. *In* Kjeldsberg CR (ed): Practical Diagnosis of Hematologic Disorders, ed 2. Chicago, ASCP Press, 1995.

18. Kjeldsberg CR: Non-Hodgkin's lymphoma. *In* Kjeldsberg CR (ed): Practical Diagnosis of Hematologic Disorders, ed 2. Chicago, ASCP Press, 1995.

19. Bennett JM, Catovsky D, Daniel M-T, et al: Proposed revised criteria for the classification of acute myeloid leukemia. Ann Intern Med 103:626–629, 1985.

20. Hurwitz CA, Raimondi SC, Head D, et al: Distinctive immunophenotypic features of t(8;21)(q22;q22) acute myeloblastic leukemia in children. Blood 80:3182–3188, 1992.

21. Berman E: New drugs in acute myelogenous leukemia: A review. J Clin Pharmacol 32:296–309, 1992.

22. McKenna R: Acute lymphoblastic leukemia. *In* Kjeldsberg CR (ed): Practical Diagnosis of Hematologic Disorders, ed 2. Chicago, ASCP Press, 1995.

23. Kantarjian HM, Deisseroth A, Kurzrock R, et al: Chronic myelogenous leukemia: A concise update. Blood 82:691–703, 1993.

24. Foti A, Ahuja HG, Allen SL, et al: Correlation between molecular and clinical events in the evolution of chronic myelocytic leukemia to blast crisis. Blood 77:2441–2444, 1991.

25. Bennett JM, Catovsky D, Daniel M-T, et al: The chronic myeloid leukaemias: Guidelines for distinguishing chronic granulocytic, atypical chronic myeloid, and chronic myelomonocytic leukemia. Br J Haematol 87:746–754, 1994.

26. Peterson LC: Chronic lymphocytic leukemia and other lymphoid leukemias. *In* Kjeldsberg CR (ed): Practical Diagnosis of Hematologic Disorders, ed 2. Chicago, ASCP Press, 1995.

27. Williams L: Clinical applications of hematopoietic growth factors. Clin Lab Sci 6:283–290, 1993.

28. Hobson AS: Acute lymphoblastic leukemias. *In* Lotspeich-Steininger CA, Steine-Martin EA, Koepke JA, et al (eds): Clinical Hematology: Principles, Procedures, Correlations. Philadelphia, JB Lippincott, 1992.

29. Starr C, Ramsey MK, Roberts GH: Hairy cell leukemia: A case history. Clin Lab Sci 8:292–297, 1995.

30. Bick RL, Laughlin WR: Myeloproliferative syndromes. Lab Med 24:770–776, 1993.

31. Aller RD: Laboratory diagnosis of polycythemia. *In* Bick RL (ed): Hematology: Clinical and Laboratory Practice, vol 1. St Louis, CV Mosby, 1993.

32. Bick RL, Laughlin WR: Myelodysplastic syndromes. Lab Med 24:712–716, 1993.

Chapter 44

Hemostatic Disorders

Rebecca Jensen and Gordon E. Ens

PLASMA COAGULATION SYSTEM

In most cases, the clotting proteins circulate as inactive precursors and become active enzymes (serine proteases) after proteolytic cleavage or conformational change. The clotting system traditionally has been divided into two pathways, the intrinsic and the extrinsic, whose actions and reactions result in the production of activated factor X (factor Xa).[1] Factor Xa then participates in the common pathway, ultimately leading to fibrin formation.

Although the division of clot formation into extrinsic and intrinsic pathways may be useful for in vitro interpretation of hemostatic abnormalities, it appears doubtful that this simplified model represents in vivo coagulation. More likely, the intrinsic pathway, influenced by the tissue factor/factor VIIa complex, serves to amplify and sustain coagulation following initiation by the extrinsic pathway.[2] The intrinsic pathway is initiated by the surface-mediated reactions intrinsic to the vessel, whereas the extrinsic pathway requires tissue factor activation. This classic waterfall-cascade mechanism of blood coagulation is being revised, in part owing to the relatively new discovery of tissue factor pathway inhibitor (TFPI)[3] (Fig. 44–1).

The newer model of coagulation includes the formation of a tissue factor/factor VIIa complex that activates both factor X and factor IX. TFPI is capable of inactivating tissue factor/factor VIIa complex and factor Xa. Further formation of factor Xa occurs only via the action of factors IXa and VIIIa on factor X. This mechanism explains the need for both an extrinsic and an intrinsic component for adequate hemostasis and provides some rationale regarding the lack of bleeding in patients with contact factor deficiencies.[4]

The intrinsic pathway begins with the activation of factor XII. The extrinsic pathway begins with the release of tissue factor from an injured vessel. Tissue factor then acts as a cofactor with calcium ion (Ca^{2+}) and factor VII to activate factor X. After factor X is activated to Xa, the extrinsic pathway is identical to the intrinsic pathway activation of prothrombin and fibrinogen.

PLATELETS

When platelets are activated, a membrane phospholipid (platelet factor 3) is exposed. The phospholipid is involved in several steps in the coagulation pathway, including the activation of factors II, X, and XI, as well as the activation of factor XII by kallikrein. Once the coagulation mechanism is activated and thrombin is formed, platelets are reinforced with a fibrin mesh.

Platelets undergo many changes as they are activated, in shape, secretion, adhesion, internal contraction, and aggregation. Platelets also appear to undergo two types of adhesion. With minor breaks in the endothelium, platelets adhere to the endothelial cells and seal over the injury; no aggregation appears to take place with this type of injury. With more extensive injury, platelets adhere within seconds to the subendothelium and exposed collagen.

Adhesion requires platelet surface glycoprotein Ib (GPIb), factor VIII/von Willebrand factor (vWF) as a cofactor, and exposed connective tissue elements of the subendothelium following vascular injury. The platelet membrane GPIb appears to act as the surface receptor of vWF; therefore, absence of either GPIb or vWF results in defective platelet adhesion.

With more extensive injury, when the subendothelial tissue is exposed, it is rapidly covered by a layer of adhering platelets. This is usually rapidly followed by the formation of platelet aggregates on top of the adhering platelets. Platelet aggregometry by adenosine diphosphate (ADP) requires platelet membrane GPIIb, GPIIIa, Ca^{2+}, and fibrinogen, and platelets will not aggregate if any of these

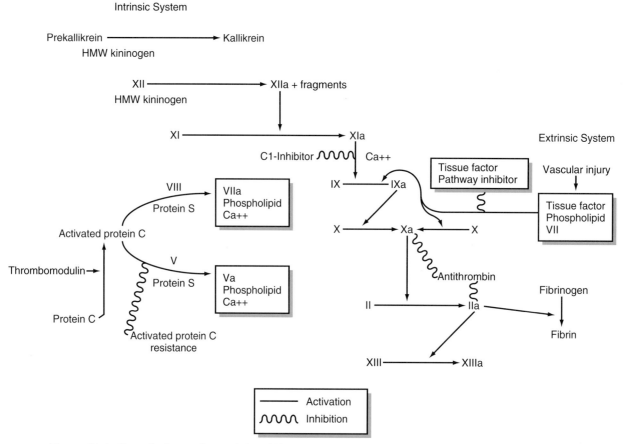

Figure 44–1. Cascade theory of coagulation. Abbreviations: HMW, high-molecular-weight; XII, Hageman factor (contact factor); XI, plasma thromboplastin antecedent; IX, plasma thromboplastin component (Christmas factor); VIII, antihemophilic factor; X, Stuart-Prower factor; VII, stable factor; V, labile factor (proaccelerin); II, prothrombin; IIa, thrombin; XIII, fibrin-stabilizing factor; a, activated.

components are missing. Platelet aggregation occurs in two stages, primary and secondary. The shape change and primary aggregation are reversible reactions. Higher concentrations of agonists cause secondary aggregation, which tends to be irreversible.

During the aggregation process, the platelets degranulate. Platelets contain both α-granules and dense bodies. The α-granules contain platelet factor 4, β-thromboglobulin, factor VIII/vWF, factor V, fibrinogen, fibrinonectin, mitogenic factor, and thrombospondin. The dense bodies contain ADP, serotonin, and Ca^{2+}. During secondary aggregation, ADP and other substances are released from the platelet granules and secreted into the surrounding plasma. In the plasma, ADP may increase by as much as 7 times. Secondary aggregation and secretion are mediated primarily by released ADP and thromboxane A_2 and are mostly irreversible.

The aggregated platelets are loosely bound until a fibrin mesh, mediated through the clotting system and thrombin, stabilizes the clot. The platelets eventually retract into a dense thrombus. It is useful to think about platelet abnormalities in relation to the four steps described: adhesion, aggregation, release, and interaction of the clotting system.

PROSTAGLANDINS

Thromboxane A_2 is generated by the action of cyclooxygenase on arachidonic acid and found in membrane phos-

pholipid. The prostaglandins formed are then acted upon by two different enzymes. If thromboxane synthetase acts on prostaglandin, the result is the production of thromboxane A_2, a powerful platelet aggregant and vasoconstrictor. If prostacyclin synthetase is the enzyme, prostacyclin, a powerful inhibitor of platelet aggregation and a vasodilator, is produced. Anything that increases the synthesis of thromboxane A_2 or decreases the production of prostacyclin increases platelet aggregation. Aspirin affects the secondary aggregation of platelets by irreversibly inhibiting cyclooxygenase, blocking the production of prostaglandins from arachidonic acid.

SYNTHESIS OF VITAMIN K–DEPENDENT FACTORS

The vitamin K–dependent factors (factors II, VII, IX, and X, proteins C and S) are produced by the liver, but they require vitamin K to carboxylate the glutamic portions of their molecules. Without carboxylation, the protein cannot bind calcium ions, although the protein has the same antigenic determinants as a functional factor. The binding of calcium ions is important, because the calcium forms bridges to phospholipid surfaces and allows the trace plasma proteins to be concentrated enough for activation and interaction with cofactors and substrates. Without vitamin K, there is no calcium ion binding, and the factors circulate with markedly impaired clotting activity. Factors made in the absence of vitamin K are called *proteins induced in vitamin K absence* (PIVKAs).

FIBRINOLYSIS

The fibrinolytic mechanism is primarily an enzymatic process that removes fibrin deposits and reestablishes flow in vessels. This mechanism is directed by the activation of plasminogen. Plasminogen activation occurs through the intrinsic coagulation system, by extrinsic activators, and by exogenous activators. Activation of the intrinsic components—factor XII, prekallikrein, and high-molecular-weight kininogen (HMWK)—gives rise to plasmin; however, the exact mechanism of contact activation of fibrinolysis is not well understood.

Extrinsic activators are thought to be the most important physiologic activators of plasminogen. Extrinsic activators are those from tissue, called tissue-type plasminogen activators (t-PAs), and those from secretions, urokinase-like plasminogen activators (u-PAs).[5]

Initial cleavage of the fibrinogen molecule by thrombin releases fibrinopeptides A and B. The degradation of fibrinogen and non–cross-linked fibrin by plasmin results in X and Y fragments that further break down to the end product fragments D and E. The initial degradation of fibrinogen also results in the release of B beta 1–42. Thrombin catalyzes the conversion of factor XIII to factor XIIIa, which stabilizes the fibrin clot by cross-linking fibrin strands. When cross-linked fibrin is degraded by plasmin, soluble cross-linked derivatives such as D-dimer are observed.

INHIBITORS

The body must have ways of controlling clot formation if coagulation is initiated in vivo. Regulation usually occurs from the presence of naturally occurring inhibitors, many of which are serine protease inhibitors. The major inhibitors are antithrombin, protein C, and protein S. Antithrombin primarily neutralizes thrombin (IIa); however, it can also neutralize factors Xa, IXa, and XIIa, and kallikrein. Protein C, after activation by the thrombin/thrombomodulin complex, and in the presence of cofactor protein S, inactivates activated factors V and VIII, decreasing the activity of the plasma coagulation system. Other naturally occurring inhibitors are α_2-macroglobulin, α_1-antitrypsin, C1 esterase inhibitor, and α_2-antiplasmin. A powerful inactivator of plasmin, α-2-antiplasmin helps control the lysis of clots. Deficiency of antithrombin III, protein C, or protein S can lead to a thrombotic tendency, whereas deficiency of α-2-antiplasmin can lead to a bleeding tendency.

The discovery of a familial thrombophilia characterized by a poor anticoagulant response to activated protein C has contributed to the elucidation of genetic defects that predispose for thrombosis primarily due to a mutation in the factor V gene. This is called *activated protein C resistance* (APCR) and is the most commonly inherited cause of thrombosis. In patients with thrombosis, the prevalence of APCR is between 40% and 60%.[6]

ETIOLOGY AND PATHOPHYSIOLOGY

Hemorrhagic Disorders

Bleeding disorders constitute a major risk for patients deficient in one or more of the blood coagulation proteins. Although uncommon, the clinical significance of both qualitative and quantitative deficiencies suggests the importance of evaluating patients presenting with histories of easy bruising or excessive blood loss.

Both congenital and acquired disorders have been observed. Early childhood bleeding histories generally reflect congenital defects, whereas adult-onset bleeding indicates an acquired factor deficiency.

Hereditary Hemorrhagic Disorders

Von Willebrand's disease (factor VIII/vWF deficiency) is the most common hereditary abnormality, followed by hemophilia A (factor VIII deficiency) and hemophilia B (factor IX deficiency).[7] The other factor deficiencies are rare.

Acquired Hemorrhagic Disorders

Physical examination and thorough evaluation of patient history are essential in diagnosing patients with bleeding disorders. The use of drugs that affect platelet function, especially aspirin and ibuprofen, may confuse the clinical picture in an otherwise healthy subject. Additionally, infection and chemical exposure can alter hemostatic function. It is incumbent upon the physician to access the presence of petechiae, purpura, ecchymoses, hemarthroses, and other indications of abnormal bleeding. Additionally, a positive family bleeding history or any previous bleeding episode requiring transfusion should be investigated.[8]

Thrombotic Disorders

Although much is known about bleeding in patients, thromboembolic disease is less clearly understood. Several physiologic variables can influence the formation of a thrombus, or blood clot, in a vessel or heart chamber. They are the flow rate of the vessel, alteration of the vessel wall, entry of large quantities of activators of coagulation into the blood stream, defects in the natural inhibitors of coagulation, and a decrease in the ability of the fibrinolytic system to lyse a clot.

The flow rate of an artery usually is undisturbed and rapid; thus, the clot is often a *white thrombus,* consisting mostly of platelets and fibrin deposits. Because the flow rate of a vein may be disturbed and slower, activated coagulation factors become more important, and a *red thrombus,* consisting of trapped red blood cells and fibrin, is more likely. The thrombus that forms may adhere to the side of the vessel, allowing blood to flow, or it may be occlusive and block the vessel. If a white thrombus is occlusive, red thrombi may form behind it, because the flow of blood is decreased behind the blockage.

Alterations in the vessel wall are important, because exposure of the subendothelium uncovers collagen, which can activate platelets and the plasma coagulation system. The activated platelets not only adhere to the surface and aggregate together but also provide a phospholipid surface on which the coagulation system can act. The end point of the coagulation system, thrombin, converts factor XIII to factor XIIIa, which stabilizes the clot.

Some situations do not require endothelial damage for thrombus formation. One example is the release of large quantities of activators of coagulation into the blood stream. During surgery, large quantities of tissue factor or thromboplastin may be released and activate the coagulation system, leading to thrombi in the circulation. Other conditions associated with activation of coagulation in vivo are malignancies, injection of snake venom, and bacteremia; these may lead to thrombosis or disseminated intravascular coagulation (DIC), depending on the rates of production and consumption of the hemostatic factors.

Defects in the fibrinolytic system can also lead to thrombosis because the body has less ability to lyse clots once they form. Some examples are excess of α2-antiplasmin, dysfunctional plasminogen, and plasminogen activator inhibitor–1. Patients with suspected plasminogen deficiency should undergo tests for both immunologic and functional plasminogen, because genetically abnormal plasminogen has been reported. The mechanism for thrombosis in some dysfibrinogenemias may be a fibrinogen resistant to lysis. It is important to remember that stasis is a critical element, whatever the cause of thrombosis. The more venous stasis is present, the greater the risk of thrombosis.

Hereditary Thrombotic Disorders

The discovery of inherited risk factors of thrombosis has improved the ability to diagnose thrombotic disorders as well as to identify individuals at greater risk for thrombosis. The primary factors responsible for thrombosis are quantitative and qualitative deficiencies of protein C, protein S, antithrombin, resistance to activated protein C (APCR), antithrombin, and antiphospholipid antibody (Table 44–1).

ACTIVATED PROTEIN C RESISTANCE

The newest reported cause of familial thrombosis, APCR, is found in 3% to 5% of the general population and is responsible for 20% to 40% of thrombosis cases. Individuals heterozygous for this gene trait are at 5 to 10

times greater risk of thrombosis, whereas those who are homozygous are at 50 to 100 times greater risk.

PROTEIN C

Heterozygous protein C deficiency occurs with a prevalence of 1 in 200 to 300; however, associated thrombosis probably occurs in less than 1 in 10,000 individuals. Homozygous protein C deficiency, causing life-threatening thrombosis unless treated, typically manifests as purpura fulminans neonatalis immediately following birth.

ANTITHROMBIN

In patients who present with thrombosis, antithrombin (AT) deficiency is found less commonly than some other inherited deficiencies. The prevalence of AT deficiency is estimated at 1 in 2,000 to 5,000 individuals. A positive family history of recurrent thrombosis typically begins in youth and is associated with trauma or surgery.

PROTEIN S

Protein S circulates in the blood approximately 60% bound to C4b binding protein (C4bBP) and 40% able to function as an anticoagulant. Clinical conditions resulting in elevated levels of C4b binding protein may cause a deficiency of functional protein S.[9]

Acquired Thrombotic Disorders

Both protein S and protein C are decreased in patients receiving oral anticoagulant therapy. Acquired protein S deficiency commonly occurs during pregnancy, oral contraceptive use, and nephrotic syndrome. Acquired AT deficiency may develop in patients following 3 or more days of intravenous heparin administration and is associated with liver disease, DIC, nephrotic syndrome, and asparaginase therapy. Oral contraceptive use can result in a 10% to 20% reduction in AT concentration.[9]

Antiphospholipid antibodies are autoantibodies directed against phospholipid cellular components that result in clinically evident arterial and venous thrombosis.[10] The two most common antiphospholipid antibodies are anticardiolipin antibodies (ACAs) and lupus anticoagulant (LA). The continuing associations of LA with venous and arterial thrombosis, and with recurrent fetal loss, have supported advances in the diagnosis of this phenomenon.

Acquired protein C deficiency occurs in liver disease, DIC, the postoperative state, and adult respiratory distress syndrome, and in association with L-asparaginase therapy.

Acquired Coagulation Disorders

Liver Disease

A combination of coagulation abnormalities is common in liver disease, owing to the liver's involvement in many facets of hemostasis, including the synthesis of many clotting factors, the clearance of activated clotting factors from the circulation, and fibrinolysis. Approximately 85% of patients with liver disease have at least one hemostatic abnormality, and 15% have clinical bleeding. A low platelet

---

Table 44–1. Estimated Incidence of Hereditary Defects in Patients with Venous Thrombosis

Defect	Incidence (%)
Activated protein C resistance	20–40
Protein S deficiency	5–8
Protein C deficiency	2–5
Antithrombin III	2–4
Antiphospholipid syndrome	2–3
Plasminogen deficiency	1–2
Fibrinogen deficiencies	1
Heparin co-factor II deficiency	1
Fibrinolytic abnormalities (not well defined)	10–15

count often is seen; it may be due to folate deficiency, increased splenic pooling, or decreased bone marrow production from ethanol abuse. Higher-than-normal levels of fibrin(ogen) degradation products in the plasma, perhaps due to decreased clearance, may lead to platelet function abnormalities or prolonged bleeding time. DIC may accompany liver disease.

Vitamin K Deficiency

The usual sources of vitamin K in humans are dietary intake (green plants) and synthesis by gastrointestinal flora. As previously described, vitamin K is required in the synthesis of functional factors II, VII, IX, and X. An acquired defect may occur in patients with malabsorption syndrome in which fat-soluble vitamins A, D, E, and K are low. Antibiotics that destroy vitamin K–producing gastrointestinal flora may also result in low levels of these factors, although there are enough stores of vitamin K in the human body to last approximately 2 weeks; thus, dietary deficiency alone is rarely seen. Neonates have low levels of coagulation proteins owing to the immaturity of the liver.[7] Hemorrhagic disease of the newborn is due partly to a lack of vitamin K in the diet (breast milk is a poor source of vitamin K) and a sterile gut. Bleeding usually occurs on the second or third day after birth. Although many neonates do not bleed, vitamin K is now administered to most newborns at birth.

Platelet Defects

Qualitative Disorders

Acquired qualitative platelet defects are fairly common and accompany a wide range of diseases and drugs.[10] Drug effect, through a variety of mechanisms, causes the largest number of platelet dysfunctions. Aspirin is probably the most common drug causing platelet dysfunction. Aspirin ingestion is characterized by a defective secondary wave of aggregation and, often, a mild increase in the bleeding time. Although aspirin affects the function of the platelet for the life of the platelet, or about 8 days, many other drugs affect the function of the platelet only as long as the drug is in the circulation. Platelet function returns to normal when the drug is metabolized.

Uremia also produces platelet dysfunction, which seems to intensify as the amounts of metabolic products increase in the blood; however, dialysis removes the metabolic products.

Increased fibrin(ogen) degradation products (FDPs) can cause mild platelet dysfunction. This condition can be difficult to evaluate, because higher levels of FDPs often are accompanied by many other hemostatic abnormalities.

Dysproteinemias or hyperfibrinogenemia (as seen in hemophiliac patients receiving large quantities of cryoprecipitate) can cause platelet dysfunction. The mechanism for this effect is not known, but it may be due to interference by the protein at the reaction site on the platelet membrane surface.

Patients with myeloproliferative disorders (polycythemia vera, chronic myelogenous leukemia, agnogenic myeloid metaplasia, essential thrombocytosis) may exhibit platelet dysfunction. The abnormality demonstrated varies from patient to patient. Abnormal platelet aggregation, especially with epinephrine, is common.

Quantitative Disorders

Platelet counts and peripheral smears can be used to detect thrombocytopenia. Although thrombocytopenia generally is defined as a platelet count of less than $150 \times 10^9/L$, spontaneous bleeding rarely occurs when the platelet count is greater than $50 \times 10^9/L$. Functional platelet abnormalities, a probable cause of hemorrhage, are reflected in laboratory tests by prolonged bleeding times, abnormal platelet aggregation, and decreased platelet factor–3 (PF3) availability.

Metabolic platelet abnormalities, including interference in the binding of vWF to glycoprotein Ib, platelet serotonin, storage pool defects, and abnormal prostaglandin synthesis, may contribute to platelet dysfunction.

When the thrombocytopenia is present with hemorrhage, a complete blood count should be performed to determine whether other cell lines are decreased. Pancytopenia is suggestive of acute leukemia, aplastic anemia, or myelodysplastic syndrome.

Thrombotic thrombocytopenia purpura, when untreated, is associated with a mortality as high as 95%; therefore, the finding of microangiopathic hemolytic anemia warrants investigation. When the peripheral smear is normal except for thrombocytopenia, drug-induced thrombocytopenia should be considered. Heparin is one of the drugs most commonly associated with thrombocytopenia, which occurs in 1% to 10% of treated patients, depending on the source of heparin.

The majority of cases of bleeding and thrombocytopenia in the presence of a normal complete blood count are a result of idiopathic thrombocytopenia. A bone marrow aspirate and biopsy can rule out primary bone marrow disorders.[11]

Disseminated Intravascular Coagulation

DIC is a syndrome that has been given various names, such as defibrination syndrome, consumption coagulopathy, and intravascular coagulation-fibrinolysis syndrome. It describes a condition in which platelets and fibrinogen are consumed. DIC is always a secondary phenomenon, the process being triggered by some underlying condition in the patient. Several mechanisms initiate DIC. One of these is extensive endothelial damage, with exposure of collagen. Collagen may activate the intrinsic pathway of coagulation or provide a surface for platelets to adhere and thus form a plug. Another means of initiating DIC is the release of thromboplastic substances into the blood stream, with the subsequent activation of the extrinsic pathway of coagulation. A third means of triggering DIC is exposure to specific proteases, such as snake venoms, trypsin, or some commercial factor IX concentrates. Thus, DIC can be initiated by activation of the intrinsic pathway, the extrinsic pathway, platelets, or any combination of these.

Many clinical conditions are associated with DIC, the most common being infection, obstetric disorders, malignancy, surgery, and shock. It is important to remember that whenever the coagulation system is activated, the fibrinolytic system is also activated, leading to the degradation of fibrin(ogen) and factors V and VIII.

DIC may be associated with thrombosis, bleeding, or no abnormality, depending on the rates of production and consumption of the various components. When only a small amount of thrombin is generated, levels of fibrinogen and platelets actually may increase, leading to thrombosis; this is observed in some cancers in which the slow destruction of cells releases a small amount of thromboplastin. The thromboplastin, in turn, causes small amounts of thrombin to be generated, raising the risk of thrombosis.

Normal hemostasis is observed in patients who are able to manufacture enough hemostatic components to compensate for the increased destruction. Greater utilization in these patients can be demonstrated only with research tests such as survival studies of radiolabeled components such as ^{51}Cr-platelets and ^{125}I-fibrinogen.

Bleeding occurs because the components of coagulation are being consumed faster than they are being produced. In patients with DIC, bleeding occurs through three main mechanisms, either alone or in combination. One mechanism is the reduction in levels of coagulation factors, including fibrinogen. In a second mechanism, if enough platelets are consumed, thrombocytopenia occurs. Finally, the increased lysis of fibrin(ogen) leads to degradation that may interfere with normal platelet function.

Massive Transfusion

Blood that is stored in the blood bank retains normal levels of most of the coagulation factors, except factors V and VIII. If a patient is transfused with large quantities (10–20 units) of stored bank blood, cryoprecipitate also may be required to increase the concentration of factor VIII and fibrinogen. Thrombocytopenia is common in massively transfused patients; therefore, platelet concentrates may be needed. A platelet count near $100 \times 10^9/L$ is desirable.

Inhibitors

Some inhibitors of clotting can be found in normal plasma, including antithrombin, α_1-antitrypsin, α_2-antiplasmin, C1 esterase inhibitor, and α_2-macroglobulin. Circulating inhibitors also may be acquired after a blood component transfusion, following therapeutic drug administration, or accompanying certain diseases, and some arise spontaneously, especially in the elderly. Inhibitors may or may not be associated with a bleeding tendency.

The most common specific factor inhibitor is directed against factor VIII. Approximately 10% to 15% of hemophiliacs develop antibodies directed against factor VIII. Antibodies against factor VIII also may develop in postpartum women and spontaneously in the elderly. The clinical picture of such a patient may resemble that of the hemophiliac patient, because the antibodies have destroyed the patient's factor VIII. The resulting bleeding diathesis may be mild to life threatening.

CLINICAL MANIFESTATIONS

Clinical manifestations of inherited abnormalities are variable, ranging from severe bleeding to normal clotting.

The milder forms of the diseases occur with more frequency than the severe forms. The diagnosis of severe forms usually is made clinically and is confirmed by laboratory tests. Mild forms may be recognized only when a patient is challenged hemostatically, and laboratory evaluation may be difficult.

Unlike the clinically indistinguishable defects in naturally occuring anticoagulants predisposing to thrombotic events, bleeding disorders commonly manifest unique features that can aid in diagnosis.[11]

A useful way to approach clinical findings is to determine whether the hemostatic abnormality involves the primary or the secondary mechanism. Bleeding involving the primary or platelet system often is characterized by immediate bleeding that stops when direct pressure is applied. Hemorrhages into the skin and mucous membrane are common, as are petechiae and frequent bruises after minor trauma. Patients with an abnormal primary hemostasis mechanism often have epistaxis, menorrhagia, and genitourinary and gastrointestinal hemorrhages.

The congenital deficiencies of antithrombin, protein C, and protein S, so-called inherited thrombophilia, lead to the alteration of the hemostatic balance in favor of thrombosis. The initial presentation of a thrombotic event occurs before 40 years in approximately 80% of patients with congenital deficiencies. No triggering event is evident in approximately one-half of patients who present with thrombosis. Hereditary protein S deficiency typically manifests as deep vein thrombosis of the legs. The median age of onset is in the late 20s, with men presenting at an earlier age than women. The family history commonly is positive for thrombosis.

For patients with acquired deficiencies of antithrombin, protein C, or protein S, the thrombotic event generally accompanies the clinical condition responsible for the deficiency. The most common presentations are thrombophlebitis and deep vein thrombosis of the lower extremities, and pulmonary embolism.

Antiphospholipid antibody syndrome should be considered in patients with a cerebrovascular event prior to age 50 years, in women with a history of two miscarriages in the first trimester or one fetal death after the first trimester, and in patients with thrombosis who have a history of therapy with such agents as chlorpromazine and phenothiazine.[9]

LABORATORY ANALYSES AND DIAGNOSIS

Clinical manifestations and thorough evaluation of patient history represent the first steps in identification of a bleeding diathesis in the patient with a known or suspected hemostatic disorder. The clinical history can provide important clues as to which component in the hemostatic mechanism is responsible for the aberration, can help determine the severity of the derangement, and can help establish whether the disorder is congenital or an acquired alteration of hemostasis. Such information can be elicited with questions about neonatal bleeding during childhood, hemorrhage after delivery, or postoperative hemorrhage (Box 44–1).

The laboratory evaluation of patients with a thrombotic

- Is there a family or personal history of bleeding related to circumcision or the umbilical cord following birth?
- Is there a family or personal history of nosebleeds, easy bruising, or joint bleeding in childhood?
- Is there a family or personal history of excessive bleeding following tooth extractions or spontaneous gum bleeding?
- Is there a family or personal history of excessive menstrual bleeding or hemorrhage following childbirth?
- Is there a family or personal history of easy bruising or hematomas without known trauma?
- Is there a family or personal history of blood in the urine or stool?
- Is there a family or personal history of transfusion, especially platelets?
- Are you taking or have you taken within the last 7 days, aspirin or aspirin-containing medication such as Alka-Seltzer, Coricidin, Dristan, Florinal, Percodan, or Triaminicin?

event should be directed by the clinical picture, personal history, and family history after other clinical conditions associated with thrombosis, such as malignancy, pregnancy, infection, myeloproliferative disease, hyperlipidemia, postoperative state, and nephrotic syndrome, have been ruled out. Location of the thrombi, onset, and duration are important to note during the physical examination.[12] Hereditary or acquired disorders of antithrombin, protein C, protein S, and activated protein C resistance cannot be differentiated from the clinical presentation. Patients in whom these disorders are suspected initially should be tested with functional assays, when the patient is not anticoagulated, and after allowing sufficient time after the clinical event for protein C, protein S, and antithrombin levels to return to baseline, because they may have been consumed during the thrombotic process.[13]

Laboratory Approach to Bleeding Disorders

When the information from the history and physical examination is combined with data from the screening tests such as the platelet count, peripheral smear examination, bleeding time, prothrombin time, activated partial thromboplastin time, thrombin time, and fibrinogen level, a decision usually can be made about whether the hemostatic problem is in the primary or secondary system. A schematic of the laboratory approach to a defect in the primary mechanism is shown in Figure 44–2. The first consideration is whether the platelet count is normal or low. A low platelet count—thrombocytopenia—can be caused by decreased platelet production, increased platelet destruction, or changes in distribution. Because approximately one-third of the body's platelets are stored in the spleen, any condition that increases the size of the spleen will decrease the platelet count in the peripheral circulation. A bone marrow

examination may help determine the cause of the thrombocytopenia as well as the presence or absence of underlying marrow diseases. If the megakaryocyte number appears normal or increased in the bone marrow, the cause of the thrombocytopenia probably is accelerated destruction or a change in distribution. If the megakaryocyte count is reduced, the cause probably is decreased production. Disorders associated with thrombocytopenia are displayed in Figure 44–2. If a patient is thrombocytopenic, other laboratory tests that may be indicated are an antiglobulin test for autoantibodies, antinuclear antibody testing, and, on occasion, an ultrastructural examination or platelet antibody studies.

If the platelet count is normal in a patient with a history of bleeding, the next test performed usually is the bleeding time. If the bleeding time is also normal, a blood vessel disease should be suspected. If the platelet count is normal and the bleeding time is prolonged, a qualitative platelet disorder should be suspected. These platelet abnormalities may be inherited or acquired, and most are associated with a mild bleeding tendency unless the hemostatic challenge is severe. The hereditary platelet abnormalities listed in Box 44–2 are rare. The laboratory tests usually used to distinguish these conditions are platelet count with peripheral smear, bleeding time, and platelet aggregation studies. Storage pool deficiencies can be of either α-granules or dense granules. The gray platelet syndrome is defined as a nearly complete absence of α-granules in the platelet, whereas the patient with Hermansky-Pudlak syndrome platelet lacks dense granules and, thus, ADP. The type of abnormalities seen in the laboratory tests vary with the missing granule.

Figure 44–2 also contains a schematic for laboratory evaluation of the secondary or plasma coagulation system. The prothrombin time (PT) is used to test for levels of factors VII, X, V, II, and I, whereas the activated partial thromboplastin time (APTT) tests for levels of factors XII, and XI, HMWK, prekallikrein (Fletcher's factor), and factors IX, VIII, X, V, II, and I. If the PT is long and the APTT is normal in a patient with a single factor deficiency, the patient probably has factor VII deficiency. If the APTT is long and the PT is normal, the patient probably has factor XII or XI, HMWK, prekallikrein, or factor IX or VIII deficiency; because factor VIII and IX deficiencies occur with higher frequency, it is probably one of these. If both the PT and APTT are prolonged, the patient probably has factor X, V, II, or I deficiency. Thrombin times are then measured to ensure that enough fibrinogen is present to produce a clot or that the fibrinogen is normal (dysfibrinogen [qualitative defect]), and also to check for the pressure of heparin.

The preceding scheme is useful for single factor deficiencies but is not sufficient if multiple deficiencies are present. Many disease states, such as liver disease, DIC, and vitamin K deficiency, as well as warfarin treatment produce multiple deficiencies and prolonged PT and APTT. It is important to note that the screening tests do not detect deficiency of factor XIII or α2-antiplasmin. These disorders must be detected by history and subsequent special testing. An inhibitor may be suspected when a prolonged PT or APTT is not corrected by a 1:1 mixture of the patient's plasma and normal plasma.

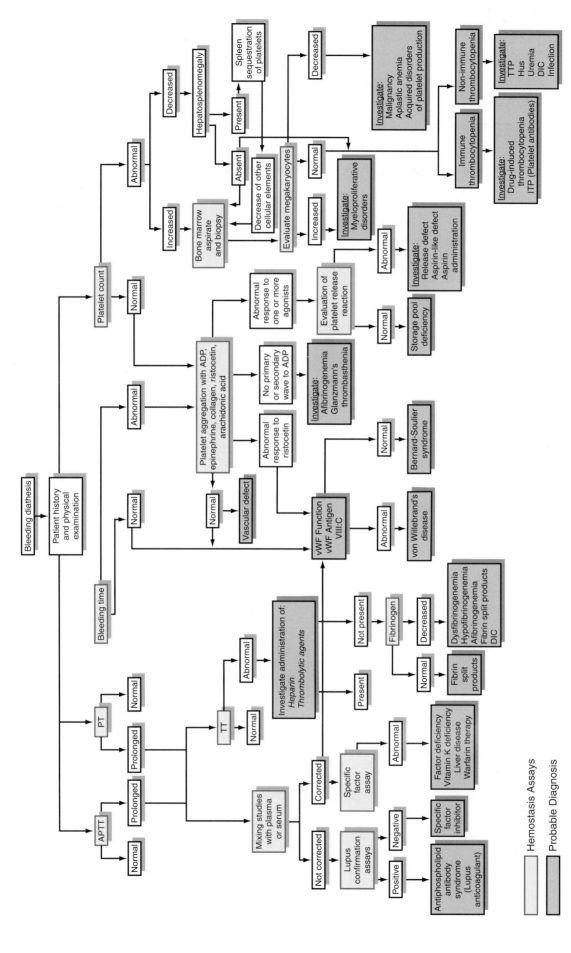

Figure 44-2. Diagnostic approach to bleeding diathesis. Abbreviations: APPT, activated partial thromboplastin time; PT, prothrombin time; TT, thrombin time; ADP, adenosine diphosphate; vWF, von Willebrand's factor; DIC, disseminated intravascular coagulation; ITP, immune thrombocytopenia; TTP, thrombotic thrombocytopenic purpura. (Redrawn from Jensen R, Ens GE: Cost-effective diagnosis of hemorrhagic disorders. Clin Hemost Rev 9:1, 1995; with permission of Clinical Hemostasis Review.)

<table>
<tr><td colspan="2">

Box 44–2. Hereditary Platelet Disorders

Glanzmann's thromboasthenia
Storage pool deficiency
Hermansky-Pudlak syndrome
Wiskott-Aldrich syndrome
Gray platelet syndrome
Bernard-Soulier syndrome

</td></tr>
</table>

Once the PT and APTT are performed and the factor deficiency has been narrowed to one area of the plasma coagulation scheme, specific factor assays should be performed to arrive at a definitive diagnosis for patients with a single factor deficiency. Identifying the specific factor deficiency in the patient determines treatment with replacement products. If inherited multiple factor deficiencies are suspected, specific factor assays should be performed to identify them.

Hemophilia A and von Willebrand's Disease

The laboratory diagnosis of hemophilia A is usually made with a specific factor VIII assay. These patients typically demonstrate a normal PT, prolonged APTT, normal bleeding time, and normal platelet count. It is important to remember that several physiologic conditions, such as stress, exercise, and pregnancy, can increase the level of factor VIII, possibly masking slightly low factor VIII activity in mild hemophiliacs.

The diagnosis of von Willebrand's disease (vWD) typically is more difficult. Tests commonly performed to aid in the diagnosis and classification of vWD are the platelet count, APTT, bleeding time, factor VIII clotting activity, von Willebrand's factor (vWF) antigen, vWF function, ristocetin-induced platelet aggregation (RIPA), and multimeric analysis of the vWF molecule. There are four general types of von Willebrand's disease: 1, 2A, 2B, and 3.[14] Table 44–2 compares the laboratory findings in

hemophilia A and vWD. Several problems can arise in the evaluation of von Willebrand's disease. Physiologic conditions such as stress and exercise can result in the release of vWF from storage sites in endothelial cells, causing a transient elevation in vWF levels and masking mild von Willebrand's disease. Another problem is the variability in laboratory results in an individual over time. Patients with a history suggestive of von Willebrand's disease that is not confirmed by laboratory testing should undergo repeat studies.

Other Factor Deficiencies

Factor IX deficiency is clinically indistinguishable from factor VIII deficiency. Definitive diagnosis must be made with specific factor assays. Diagnosis is important, because treatments for these two diseases are different.

The diagnosis of afibrinogenemia, hypofibrinogenemia, or dysfibrinogenemia should be made by means of a coagulation assay and an immunologic assay for fibrinogen.

Other factor deficiencies should be diagnosed with specific factor assays to confirm the factor absence.

It is important to remember that factor XIII deficiency is not detected in any coagulation screening test. If factor XIII deficiency is suspected from the history, a clot stability test using 5 M urea should be performed as a screening test. Specific assay of factor XIII will then confirm the diagnosis.

Vitamin K Deficiency

In vitamin K deficiency, PT is prolonged and APTT may be normal or abnormal, depending on the severity of the deficiency. Typically, the PT becomes prolonged before the APTT, because factor VII has the shortest in vivo half-life and depletes most rapidly. The thrombin time (TT) should be normal. When the PT and APTT are both moderately prolonged, the differentiation of vitamin K deficiency from DIC may be difficult. A factor V evaluation may be helpful, because factor V is not vitamin K dependent; therefore, factor V activity should be normal in vitamin K deficiency, but decreased in DIC as a result of consumption.

Table 44–2. Comparison of Laboratory Findings in Hemophilia and von Willebrand's Disease

| Parameter | Hemophilia A | von Willebrand's Disease ||||
		Type 1	*Type 2A*	*Type 2B*	*Type 3*
COAGULATION ASSAY					
Bleeding time	Normal	Prolonged	Prolonged	Prolonged	Prolonged
F VIII: C	Decreased	Decreased	Normal or decreased	Normal or decreased	Very decreased
vWF: Ag	Normal or increased	Decreased	Normal or decreased	Normal or decreased	Very decreased
vWF: RCo	Normal or increased	Decreased	Decreased	Normal or decreased	Very decreased
RIPA	Normal	Normal or decreased	Decreased	Normal or increased*	Variable
Multimers	Normal	Normal	Abnormal	Abnormal	Variable

*Increased = hyperresponse to low levels of ristocetin
Abbreviations: F VIII: C, procoagulant factor VIII; vWF: Ag, von Willebrand factor antigen; RCo, ristocetin cofactor; multimers, multimeric structure components of vWF plasma.

Liver Disease

The PT and APTT often are prolonged in liver disease, owing to decreases either in production of coagulation factors or in carboxylation of the vitamin K–dependent factors, leading to reduced function. The TT may be prolonged if the fibrin(ogen) degradation products are greatly increased. DIC may accompany liver disease and confuse the diagnosis and treatment.

DIC

The diagnosis of DIC is based on the clinical condition of the patient and on laboratory tests. If the patient has a disease often associated with DIC and is bleeding or has signs of thrombosis, screening tests should be performed. The screening tests should consist of platelet count, PT, APTT, TT, and fibrinogen level, fibrin(ogen) degradation products, and D-dimer levels. A diagnosis of DIC is indicated if the platelet count and fibrinogen levels are very low or are falling in a successive series of tests. The examination of a blood smear for fragmented red blood cells sometimes is suggested as a screening test for DIC, but it seldom proves useful. Fibrin(ogen) degradation products are usually increased in DIC but are not diagnostic of DIC. A factor V assay may be helpful in differentiating DIC from vitamin K deficiency, as described previously. In vitamin K deficiency, the platelet count and fibrinogen also are often normal. The differential diagnosis of DIC from liver disease can be difficult. A factor VIII level may be helpful, because factor VIII is often elevated in mild liver disease. If the liver disease is more advanced, the factor VIII level may be low in both conditions.

Massive Transfusion

Most coagulation screening tests are affected in massively transfused patients who have been given stored bank blood. The PT, APTT, TT, and bleeding time may all be prolonged. The fibrinogen and platelet counts may be low. Because the screening tests are similar in massively transfused patients and in patients with DIC or liver disease, massive transfusion should always be considered in the differential diagnosis.

Inhibitors

Deficiency in inhibitors of fibrinolysis can cause a bleeding tendency. Some patients deficient in α_2-antiplasmin have been reported to bleed excessively. Screening tests for this condition are whole blood clot lysis or euglobulin clot lysis. Specific α_2-antiplasmin assays may be run to confirm the diagnosis.

Laboratory Approach to Thrombosis

Laboratory tests are most commonly used to identify patients with increased thrombotic risk and to evaluate components of the naturally occurring anticoagulant systems (Box 44–3) and the fibrinolytic system.[15]

Antithrombin

The assay most commonly performed and most useful for measuring antithrombin (AT) is the AT-III heparin

---

> **Box 44–3.** **Laboratory Tests to Evaluate Thrombotic Risk**
>
> Activated protein C resistance
> Antithrombin
> Homocysteine
> Protein C
> Protein S
> Plasminogen
> Tissue plasminogen activator
> Plasminogen activator inhibitor–1

---

cofactor assay utilizing a chromogenic substrate. This method detects abnormalities at the activated serine protease–binding site and at the heparin-binding site. Immunologic assays by rocket immunoelectrophoresis or radial immunodiffusion techniques can be performed to determine whether a deficiency is a type I or type II.

Protein C

The protein C level is determined quantitatively by enzyme-linked immunosorbent assay (ELISA) or rocket immunoelectrophoresis and functionally by synthetic substrate or clot-based assays. The clot-based assay is more sensitive to all defects but is affected by heparin and warfarin in the sample, unlike the synthetic substrate method.

Protein S

Protein S circulates in plasma partially complexed to C4bBP, and the remaining portion is biologically active. Total Protein S is determined quantitatively by ELISA or rocket immunoelectrophoresis. Functional protein S is determined by a clot-based assay or by removing the complexed protein S from the plasma through absorption with polyethylene glycol and then measuring the remaining (free) protein S with ELISA or rocket immunoelectrophoresis.

Activated Protein C Resistance

Resistance to activated protein C (APC) is the most common hemostatic defect associated with venous thrombosis. The disorder can be detected by determining the ratio of a routine (baseline) APTT to a second APTT after the addition of a known concentration of APC, as shown in the following equation:

$$\text{APCR Ratio} = \frac{\text{APTT with APC}}{\text{APTT without APC}}$$

Test results are invalid if the baseline APTT is abnormal. If the patient is receiving heparin or oral anticoagulant therapy, the test must be modified to obtain accurate results. Individuals testing positive should be tested for genetic confirmation of the factor V gene mutation to determine whether they are heterozygous or homozygous for the gene trait.

Fibrinolytic System

When the fibrinolytic system fails to appropriately break down fibrin, the risk of thrombosis rises. A number of components regulating the fibrinolytic system can be measured.

Euglobulin Clot Lysis

The euglobulin clot lysis time (ECLT) commonly is used to screen for abnormalities of plasminogen, tissue plasminogen activator (t-PA), and tissue plasminogen activator inhibitor–1 (PAT-1). A prolonged ECLT is suggestive of an abnormality. Fibrinogen levels lower than 100 mg/dL may cause abnormal results.

The euglobulin precipitate, prepared by diluting and acidifying plasma, contains substantially all of the plasminogen and t-PA present in the plasma and a portion of PAI-1. The supernatant contains most of the inhibitors of fibrinolysis, including α_2-antiplasmin and α_2-macroglobulin; however, PAI-1 is only partially removed.

ECLTs are determined by dissolving the euglobulin precipitate in buffer, clotting with thrombin, and observing for clot lysis at 37 °C.

Plasminogen

Plasminogen functional activity typically is assayed by activating plasminogen with streptokinase, subsequently generating plasmin, which is measured with a chromogenic substrate.

Tissue Plasminogen Activator

Activity levels of t-PA are determined indirectly by activating plasminogen in the presence of a fibrin-related stimulator and measuring the plasmin generated. Quantitative levels of t-PA are determined by enzyme immunoassay.

α_2-Antiplasmin

Activity of α_2-antiplasmin is determined by adding plasmin in excess to patient plasma and measuring residual plasmin activity utilizing a chromogenic substrate.

Plasminogen Activator Inhibitor–1

PAI-1 activity is evaluated indirectly by adding an excess of t-PA and measuring the residual t-PA. Because plasma contains additional t-PA inhibitors, the assay may not be very specific.

Considerations in Specific Laboratory Analyses

Platelet Count

Platelet counts usually are performed utilizing electronic cell counters, although very low counts should be manually determined using phase microscopy. It is important to review the peripheral smear before reporting a platelet count result, because some clinical situations can cause false results: a clotting specimen, EDTA-associated platelet satellitism, cold agglutinins, and administration of chemotherapy (which may fragment white cells that may then be counted as platelets).

Examination of the Peripheral Smear

The examination of the peripheral smear should consist of an estimate of the number of platelets, size of the platelets, variation in the size and granularity of the platelets, granule distribution, and whether there are any pseudopods on the platelet. The peripheral smear may also suggest other diseases that affect hemostatic status.

Bleeding Time

The Ivy template bleeding time is the recommended method for performing bleeding time tests. Commercially made bleeding time apparatus is available. It is important to remember that the bleeding time is inversely related to the circulating platelet count when it falls below 100×10^9/L. It is a good practice to obtain the platelet count before beginning the bleeding time test, so that the test may be avoided in patients with low platelet counts.

A patient with a long bleeding time but a platelet count greater than 100×10^9/L is said to have platelet dysfunction. More specific tests of platelet function, such as platelet aggregation, usually are needed to establish a specific diagnosis.

Prothrombin Time

The prothrombin time test measures the extrinsic pathway of coagulation (factors I, II, V, X, and VII). When the test is performed, thromboplastin is added as a source of tissue extract and phospholipid. Thromboplastin is combined with calcium ions and platelet-poor plasma, and the formation of a fibrin clot is observed. The final result depends on the concentration and source of thromboplastin, calcium concentration, and the method used to detect clot formation. Therefore, results may vary a great deal from laboratory to laboratory.

International Normalized Ratio

The International Normalized Ratio (INR) was established as a means of standardizing the PT for oral anticoagulant monitoring. Thromboplastins are calibrated against an international standard and assigned an international sensitivity index (ISI). The lower the ISI, the more sensitive the reagent. The INR is calculated as follows:

$$INR = \frac{(PT\ [sec]\ Patient)^{ISI}}{(Mean\ [sec]\ of\ Normal\ Range)}$$

ISI values have been shown to vary among instruments, creating a potential source of error in INR reporting.

Activated Partial Thromboplastin Time (APTT)

The APTT test measures the intrinsic pathway of coagulation (factors I, II, V, X, VIII, IX, XI, and XII, prekallikrein, HMWK). The term *activated* refers to the fact that an inert substance (such as kaolin, celite, elegiac acid, or micronized silica) is added to the test to maximally activate the contact factors. The other reagents in the test are a source of phospholipid and calcium ions. The end point is the formation of a fibrin clot, which depends on the concentration and source of activator, the phospholipid and calcium concentrations, as well as the method used for fibrin detection.

Factors I, II, V, and X are measured by both the prothrombin time and partial thromboplastin time. Deficiencies in any of these factors may result in the prolongation of both tests, depending on the severity of the defect. In most laboratories, the APTT is more sensitive to factor deficiencies than the PT.

Thrombin Time

The thrombin time (TT) measures the time it takes for fibrinogen to be converted to a fibrin clot. It does not measure any other coagulation factors. The reagent used in the test is a dilute thrombin. Because calcium is added, the formation of the fibrin clot depends on the thrombin-fibrinogen reaction. Conditions resulting in prolongation of the TT include heparin therapy, dysfibrinogenemia, severe hypofibrinogenemia, and increased fibrin(ogen) degradation products.

Fibrinogen

Many methods are available for the measurement of fibrinogen, including the modified thrombin time test, various clottable protein methods, and immunologic methods. Fibrinogen levels also may be derived from the prothrombin time when it is performed on certain instruments. High levels of fibrin(ogen) degradation products or heparin may influence modified thrombin time methods. Fibrinogen is an important consideration in all clotting assays, because the conversion of fibrinogen to fibrin is the end point for these tests. In general, a fibrinogen level below 100 mg/dL influences the PT, APTT, and TT.

Other Hemostatic Studies

To establish a definite diagnosis, coagulation studies other than screening tests may be indicated. Many of these tests are difficult to perform and are best done in a reference laboratory that performs them on a regular basis and so maintains proficiency.

Specific Factor Assays

Specific factor assays for clotting activity can be performed on dilutions of the patient plasma using either the PT or APTT plus a substrate deficient in a specific factor. The clotting results for the patient are compared with a standard reference curve for the specific factor, and the answer is expressed as a percentage of normal. Commercial chromogenic assays also are becoming available for many of the specific factors. Factor XIII is analyzed by a clot stability test using 5 M urea. Immunologic tests can also be performed for most coagulation factors, indicating only that the protein is present, not whether it is functional.

Fibrin(ogen) Degradation Products

Split products represent the result of plasmin digestion of both cross-linked and non–cross-linked fibrin or fibrinogen and thus provide an early indication of fibrinolysis. The FDP assay measures all fragments but does not differentiate between those derived from fibrinogen and those from fibrin.

Tests for fibrin(ogen) degradation products are usually semiquantitative methods performed by slide agglutination. Any substance that causes fibrinogen or fibrin to be digested increases the FDP value.

D-Dimer

When fibrin cross-linking occurs, two D regions and one E region fuse. Degradation by plasmin then releases D-dimer fragments measurable by assays that utilize monoclonal antibodies raised against these fragments. Cross-reactivity with FDPs does not occur, and the assay is specific for fibrin degradation, indicating the presence of thrombin and plasmin.

Platelet Aggregation

The ability of platelets to aggregate is usually tested using a platelet aggregometer. A platelet agonist is added to stirred platelet-rich plasma. As the platelets aggregate, the increase in light transmission is recorded. The four main characteristics that can be detected on the tracing are changes in platelet shape, primary aggregation due to the addition of the agonist, secondary aggregation due to the release of the platelets' own internal constituents, and disaggregation. The platelet shape change and primary aggregation are reversible, whereas secondary aggregation is usually irreversible. Agonists often used are ADP, epinephrine, collagen, thrombin, arachidonic acid, and ristocetin. With a special aggregometer that measures luminescence, the release of ATP by platelets can be detected. The instrument allows measurement of the time relationship between platelet aggregation and secretion of adenosine triphosphate (ATP).

Inhibitors

Some patients develop circulating anticoagulants that may be directed against a specific coagulation factor or, as in the case of lupus anticoagulant, may be less specific. These can be assayed in two ways. One is to make serial dilutions of patient plasma in a normal plasma and test the dilutions, using either PT or APTT, at 0 time and after 2 hours incubation at 37 °C; some antibodies are time dependent and require the incubation time to react. The other way is to run specific factor assays to observe the effect of the inhibitor on the coagulation factor; an example of this type of assay is the Bethesda assay, done for factor VIII inhibitors.

Other anticoagulants, such as the lupus anticoagulant, typically act immediately. Assays utilizing increased or decreased amounts of phospholipid in the reagent are available to assist in identifying a lupus anticoagulant. The most commonly performed assays are the dilute Russell viper venom test and the platelet neutralization procedure. Additionally, anticardiolipin antibody testing to IgG and IgM is available to help diagnose the antiphospholipid antibody syndrome.

TREATMENT

Heparin

Heparin is a widely prescribed anticoagulant for both prophylactic and therapeutic purposes and is commonly the first agent administered in patients with thrombotic disease. Heparin's anticoagulant effect is primarily attributable to its high affinity for antithrombin.

The anticoagulant response of an individual can be influenced by the availability of antithrombin, other concomitant drug therapies, and the patient's weight. Because the individual response to heparin varies widely, instituting a standard protocol for heparin administration often results in inadequate protection against thromboembolic disease.

The most common complication of heparin administration is bleeding. Serious and life-threatening hemorrhage is estimated to occur in 1% to 7% of patients. An additional complication of heparin therapy is heparin-induced thrombocytopenia (HIT), which occurs in approximately 1% to 5% of patients receiving standard heparin regardless of route of administration. HIT is less often associated with administration of low-molecular-weight heparin.

Vitamin K Antagonists

Vitamin K antagonists such as sodium warfarin, a derivative of 4-hydroxycoumarin, are widely used for prophylaxis and treatment of venous and arterial thrombosis, primarily because they can be given orally with a highly predictable and well-characterized onset of action and duration of effective therapy. Achieving appropriate dosage requires monitoring, most commonly with the PT.

Replacement of Coagulation Factors

Products used for replacement therapy in factor-deficient individuals include fresh-frozen plasma, cryoprecipitate, human factor concentrates, and factor concentrates produced by recombinant technology. The use of products for replacement therapy requires knowledge of various products, their efficacy and potency, and the biochemical characteristics of the factor itself.

Fresh-frozen plasma is processed from single blood donors by separating the plasma from the cells and storing the plasma at −50 °. Patients should be given ABO and Rh blood group–specific fresh-frozen plasma except in emergency cases, when group AB plasma may be given to other blood groups.

Cryoprecipitate is collected from single donors and, following a multiple centrifugation and freezing process, yields 5 to 10 mL of precipitate. Cryoprecipitate is utilized in the treatment of fibrinogen, factor II, factor VIII, and von Willebrand factor deficiencies. The factor activity level in each bag varies and depends on the donor levels. Each bag is generally thought to contain 100 to 120 units of factor VIII and von Willebrand factor, and approximately 200 mg of fibrinogen. Cryoprecipitate is rather easily produced by the blood bank, available, and low in cost.

When massive quantities of a factor are required for treatment, factor concentrates provide the best support. Concentrates can bring factor levels to 100%, control severe bleeding events, or provide adequate hemostasis for surgery. Factor concentrates are prepared from large pools of carefully screened donors. Viral inactivation processes are utilized to remove transmissible agents, and the concentrate is then analyzed for factor concentration using national coagulation factor standards. Factor concentrates currently are available for factors II, VII, VIII, IX, and X, fibrinogen, and vWF. Inactivated as well as activated prothrombin complex concentrates are available for the treatment of patients with hemophilia A.

With the discovery of the factor VIII and factor IX gene in the 1980s, the development of monoclonal products for transfusion became possible. Recombinant factor replacement products are now commercially available. These products have shown in vivo recovery and efficacy comparable with those of plasma-derived products.[16]

Plasma half-lives of the various factors must be considered when replacement therapy is necessary. The bioavailability of the transfused product and the pharmacokinetics of the clotting factor are important in determining the need for further transfusions. Clotting factor replacement therapy can be represented by a biphasic exponential disappearance curve. The first phase is a rapid disappearance curve, thought to reflect the equilibration of the concentration in the intravascular and extravascular space and the biologic degradation of the factor molecule. The second phase represents the metabolic rate of the molecule and is characterized by a gradual disappearance. Investigators have reported that for factor VIII concentrates, the first and second phase half-disappearance times ($T_{1/2}$) are 7 and 12 hours, respectively. For factor IX concentrates, $T_{1/2}$ has been reported at 2 to 4 hours for the first phase and 24 hours for the second phase. Booster transfusions can be given subsequently to saturate the extravascular compartment and maintain the necessary level.

Factor X has a half-life of 40 hours, whereas factor II has a half-life of 60 to 80 hours. Factor VII has a $T_{1/2}$ of 3 to 4 hours, necessitating booster transfusion every 4 hours. Factors V and XI have long half-lives, approximately 36 hours. Factor XIII deficiency can be treated with plasma or cryoprecipitate. It has an extremely long half-life of 7 to 14 days. Fibrinogen has a half-life of 3 to 5 days, necessitating booster injections only every third to fifth day.[16]

Appropriate therapy for vWD is based on the accurate diagnosis of the disorder in an individual, determination of the vWD type, and the response to therapy as established from prior management or from laboratory assays.[17]

DDAVP

The administration of DDAVP (1-deamino-8-D-arginine-vasopressin) is widely used for mild cases of vWD to regain hemostasis in bleeding episodes and provide adequate levels of vWF for dental extractions and minor invasive procedures. DDAVP can be given intravenously, subcutaneously, or intranasally. The response to DDAVP is usually consistent in an individual from one administration to another. This agent has been observed to induce thrombocytopenia. No triggering event is evident in type 2 vWD, and therefore DDAVP is contraindicated in this population. Because patients with type 3 vWD have essentially no stores of vWF, there is no response to administration of DDAVP.[17]

Case Study

A 37-year-old white woman presented to the emergency room with a sudden onset of left lower extremity and left groin pain that had progressively worsened. The lower extremity was markedly swollen and turned bluish. She was admitted with a diagnosis of cerulea dolens.

Her personal and family history were negative for thrombotic events. She revealed that she was taking oral contraceptives at the time. A venogram showed an iliofemoral venous thrombosis. The patient was taken to the operating room for an iliac venolysis and thrombectomy on the iliac vein as well as creation of an arteriovenous fistula. The patient was then anticoagulated with heparin and coumarin with a target INR with coumarin of 3.0.

Although she reached the target INR by day 5 postoperatively, she complained of persistent left groin and flank pain. A CT scan revealed a large left retroperitoneal hematoma. The patient received 3 units of packed red blood cells as well as 3 units of fresh-frozen plasma, and coumarin was discontinued. The hematoma subsequently was removed surgically, and the postoperative course was uncomplicated. The patient was discharged on postoperative day 9 and restarted on coumarin, tolerating a regular diet, ambulating, and with no signs of further bleeding or hematoma.

She remained on oral anticoagulant therapy for 6 months, maintaining an INR of approximately 2.0. One month after stopping oral anticoagulants, she was evaluated for the commonly associated inherited thrombotic risk factors—activated protein C resistance, antithrombin, protein C, and protein S—all of which were normal. The patient was then referred to a laboratory for a more comprehensive evaluation of thrombotic risk factors, including lipoprotein (a) measurement, which was markedly elevated.

Question

What factor or factors contribute to the thrombotic events experienced by this patient?

Discussion

Thrombosis originates as a result of the impairment of blood flow, pathologic activation of platelets, or im-

balance of the procoagulant and anticoagulant factors of the plasma. Although the exact cause of this patient's thrombosis is uncertain, she appears to have experienced a "multiple hit," with three factors possibly contributing to the thrombosis. Clearly, the anatomic narrowing of the vein and the subsequent scarring contributed to slow blood flow through the area, possibly causing stasis. Oral contraceptives, which she was taking at the time of the events, have been shown to increase fibrinogen and factor VIII levels, decrease antithrombin and protein S levels, and enhance platelet aggregation, contributing to a thrombotic risk state. Elevated lipoprotein (a) levels, as found in this patient, are thought to accelerate the atherosclerotic disease process.

References

1. Hathaway WE, Goodnight SH: Physiology of hemostasis and thrombosis. *In* Disorders of Hemostasis and Thrombosis. New York, McGraw-Hill, 1993.
2. Jensen R, Ens GE: Intrinsic factor deficiencies. Clin Hemost Rev 8:1, 1994.
3. Broze GJ: The tissue factor pathway of coagulation. *In* Loscalzo J, Schafer Al (eds): Thrombosis and Hemorrhage. Boston, Blackwell Scientific, 1994.
4. Jensen R, Ens GE: Tissue factor pathway inhibitor. Clin Hemost Rev 6:1, 1992.
5. Jensen R, Ens GE: The fibrinolytic pathway. Clin Hemost Rev 8:1, 1994.
6. Jensen R, Ens GE: Activated protein C resistance. Clin Hemost Rev 9:1, 1995.
7. Hill, RJ, Ens GE: Factor deficiencies. Clin Hemost Rev 1:1, 1987.
8. Weiss AE: The hemophilias. *In* Corriveau DM, Fritsma GA (eds): Hemostasis and Thrombosis in the Clinical Laboratory. Philadelphia, JB Lippincott, 1988.
9. Jensen R, Ens GE: Cost-effective diagnosis of thrombotic disorders. Clin Hemost Rev 9:1, 1995.
10. Goodnight SH: Antiphospholipid antibodies and thrombosis. *In* Adamson JW (ed): Current Review of Hematology 1995. Philadelphia, Current Science Ltd, 1995.
11. Rao AK, Carvalho ACA: Acquired qualitative platelet defects. *In* Colman RW, Hirsh J, Marder VJ, Salzman EW (eds): Hemostasis and Thrombosis: Basic Principles and Clinical Practice, ed 3. Philadelphia, JB Lippincott, 1994.
12. Jensen R, Ens GE: Diagnostic approach to easy bruising. Clin Hemost Rev 4:1, 1990.
13. Jensen R, Ens GE: Cost-effective diagnosis of hemorrhagic disorders. Clin Hemost Rev 9:1, 1995.
14. Ware J, Zaverio RM: The molecular bases of von Willebrand disease. *In* High KA, Roberts HR (eds): Molecular Basis of Thrombosis and Hemostasis. New York, Marcel Dekker, 1995.
15. Ens GE: Disorders leading to thrombosis. *In* Lotspeich-Steininger CA, Stiene-Martin EA (eds): Clinical Hematology: Principles Procedures Correlations. Philadelphia, JB Lippincott, 1992.
16. Jensen R, Ens GE: Management of coagulant factor deficiencies. Clin Hemost Rev 9:1, 1995.
17. Jensen R, Ens GE: Diagnosis and management of von Willebrand disease. Clin Hemost Rev 9:1, 1995.

Chapter 45

Acquired Immunodeficiency Syndrome (AIDS)

Karen James

ETIOLOGY AND PATHOPHYSIOLOGY
Origin of the Acquired Immunodeficiency Syndrome

Reports of young, white, homosexual males suffering from a rare skin cancer, Kaposi's sarcoma, which was previously only seen in severely immunocompromised individuals, began to appear in the late 1970s. Simultaneously, other young men were being diagnosed with a rare pneumonia caused by *Pneumocystis carinii*. Other homosexual men were manifesting enlarged lymph nodes and non-Hodgkin's lymphoma. The common observations among these various reports were an impaired immune system, depletion of T cells, and male homosexuality. It was soon determined that these same symptoms were appearing in intravenous (IV) drug abusers, hemophiliacs, others who had received blood transfusions, and female partners of male IV drug abusers. Because people were dying of this "new" disease, there was great fear about an epidemic of a previously unknown virus. The disease was first called acquired immunodeficiency syndrome (AIDS) in 1981, described as causing susceptibility to opportunistic infections and associated with Kaposi's sarcoma.

433

Human retroviruses, "viruses that work backward," had been discovered in the early 1970s following reports of the isolation from viruses of an unprecedented enzyme, *reverse transcriptase* (RT). This enzyme used viral RNA as a template to manufacture a complementary negative strand of DNA that could insert itself into the host DNA. The retrovirus found in infected cells of certain adult T-cell leukemias was designated human T-cell lymphotropic virus (HTLV). A few years later, the retrovirus that causes AIDS, human immunodeficiency virus (HIV), was discovered. Some investigators believe that HIV originated as a simian immunodeficiency virus (SIV) transmitted from monkeys to humans.[2]

Isolation of Human Immunodeficiency Virus

The virus associated with AIDS was first isolated in France in 1983[3] and called the lymphadenopathy-associated virus (LAV). In 1984, two American groups identified similar viruses, termed HTLV-II[4] and AIDS associated retrovirus.[5] All three viruses have been shown to be the same; in 1985, by consensus, the virus was named the human immunodeficiency virus (HIV). It has subsequently been shown that HIV has two variants, HIV-1 and HIV-2. HIV-1 is the predominant HIV type found worldwide, and HIV-2 is found almost exclusively in West Africa.

Several related viruses have also been isolated, including human T-cell lymphotropic virus (HTLV) I and II, SIV, feline immunodeficiency virus, bovine immunodeficiency virus and equine infectious anemia virus. These viruses constitute the family of retroviruses in the taxonomic group of lentiviruses. In contrast to other retroviruses, lentiviruses are non-oncogenic, have a complex genome organization, and are responsible for a slow disease course.

HIV is an enveloped, single-stranded RNA retrovirus (Fig. 45–1). It contains three structural genes:[2]

1. The group-specific *gag* gene directs the synthesis of a protein precursor (p55) that consists of (a) p24, the major capsid protein; (b) p7/p9, nucleocapsid protein; and (c) p17, matrix protein.
2. The polymerase *(pol)* gene encodes for RT, which copies the viral RNA into DNA, circularizes the DNA, and inserts it into the cellular genome of CD4+ T cells.
3. The envelope *(env)* gene encodes a precursor glycoprotein (gp160), which is cleaved to yield gp41 and gp120.

HIV-1 and HIV-2 share 60% nucleotide homology in the conserved *gag* and *pol* genes, but less in the *env* region.

HIV can be isolated from CD4+ cells, but not from CD8+ lymphocytes. The cellular receptor for HIV-1, HIV-2, and SIV is the CD4 molecule,[6] the cell surface antigen that distinguishes T-helper cells. CD4 molecules are also found on monocytes/macrophages, and HIV can infect those phagocytic cells. Viral replication is much slower in monocytes than in lymphocytes, and monocytes do not appear to be killed by the virus. Other monocyte-derived cells, such as microglia of the brain, may be infected with HIV, resulting in neurologic complications. Virus amplification occurs in the major trafficking area for lymphocytes, the lymph node, which is rich in follicular denditric cells (FDCs).[7] FDCs are rich in CD4 molecules and Fc receptors,

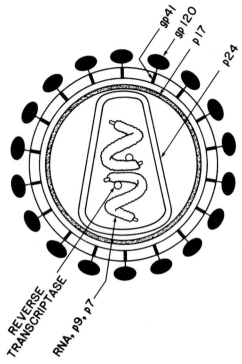

Figure 45–1. Schematic representation of the morphologic structure of HIV-1, which include *env* gene products, gp120 and gp41; *gag* gene products, p7, p9, p17, and p24; and *pol* gene product reverse transcriptase. (*From* Borkowsky W, Wilfert CM: Acquired immunodeficiency syndrome. *In* Krugman S, Katz SL, Gershon AA, et al (eds): Infectious Diseases of Children. St Louis, Mosby–Year Book, 1992.)

both of which serve to accumulate high concentrations of HIV virions. After the virus binds to the CD4 molecule on cells, the viral envelope and the cell membrane fuse, resulting in the formation of multinucleated giant cells (syncytia). Syncytia of lymphoid origin can be found in lymph nodes; those of monocyte origin can be found in the brain and lungs of patients with HIV infections. The HIV-infected cells become activated during infection, resulting in apoptosis, cell death, and depletion of the CD4 population.[8]

Genetic Diversity of HIV

There is significant sequence variability of HIV isolates between and within patients.[2] The distribution of individual viral variants changes during the course of the infection, with the ability to infect cells increasing as the disease progresses. Viral mutants develop resistance to antiviral drugs and escape neutralizing antibodies and cytotoxic T cells.[9] At least eight subtypes/genotypes (A through H) have been classified on the basis of *env* sequences. These subtypes constitute the major group of HIV-1, group M.[10] Divergent strains outside group M are categorized as HIV-1, group O. The geographic distribution of the various subtypes is just beginning to be elucidated. Initial studies in the United States indicate that approximately 50% of patients are infected with HIV-1, group M, subtype B. The more divergent HIV-1 strains, particularly group O, may not be well detected by HIV screening tests commonly used in the United States, especially those that use recombinant antigens or synthetic peptides.[10]

Two viral biologic or functional groupings have been identified, rapid/high syncytium-inducing (SI) and slow/low non–syncytium-inducing (NSI) isolates, which differ in tropism for cells of different lineages.[9] Chemokine receptors that serve as cofactors to the primary CD4 receptor have also been described.[11] The polymorphism of these chemokine receptors plays a major role in determining susceptibility or resistance of certain cell types to infection by HIV and resistance or susceptibility of virally infected cells to antiretroviral therapy. Much remains to be done in HIV surveillance to correlate the subtypes with functional groupings and chemokine receptors to categorize HIV-1 infections. In the future, HIV phenotyping may provide additional information to physicians and patients about whether a particular HIV infection will remain asymptomatic for prolonged periods or will progress rapidly. Phenotyping may also accurately predict which forms of therapy specific infections will respond to.

Mechanisms of HIV Transmission

The *env* gene product of HIV, a glycosylated protein (gp 160), is proteolytically cleaved, resulting in gp41 and gp120. The carboxy-terminal end of gp120 is the critical domain for fusion with the CD4 receptor site on T-helper cells that results in HIV viral infection.[7] This CD4-binding domain of gp120 is conserved between HIV-1, HIV-2, and SIV. An immunodominant region on gp41, also highly conserved, is responsible for antibody production in HIV infections.

Understanding of the viral life cycle has changed dramatically since the development of methods to measure viral load, and the introduction of anti-retroviral therapy. It is now known that although the infection might be clinically latent, HIV is replicating at high rates ($\sim10^9$ virions/day) and CD4+ cells are being destroyed soon after transmission.[2, 12]

After the HIV virus enters the cell through fusion with the CD4 receptor, viral RNA is inserted in the cytoplasm of the cell. RT then translates or copies the viral RNA into proviral DNA, which can be integrated into the nuclear DNA of the cell (Fig. 45–2). The pathogenic potential of HIV viruses varies in the host cells they infect and the tropism for specific cells. Perinatally infected infants generally develop the disease in 6 months, transplant patients in 2 years, transfusion patients of all ages within 6 years, otherwise immunologically normal homosexual men in 10 years, young patients with severe hemophilia in 14 years, and those with mild hemophilia in 20 years.[13]

There is evidence that the lymph node follicular dendritic cells further virus amplification after the primary infection. As previously described, FDCs have CD4 molecules and Fc receptors on their surfaces as well as crablike interstices that serve to trap infectious agents and lymphocytes traveling through the lymph nodes.[7] The CD4 molecules on FDC cells trap HIV, accumulating high concentrations of HIV virions. The physical architecture of the lymph node with FDC serves to trap lymphocytes, exposing them to infection and resulting in generalized lymphadenopathy.

When a stimulus provokes productive replication, viral RNA and viral proteins are transcribed from mRNA that is

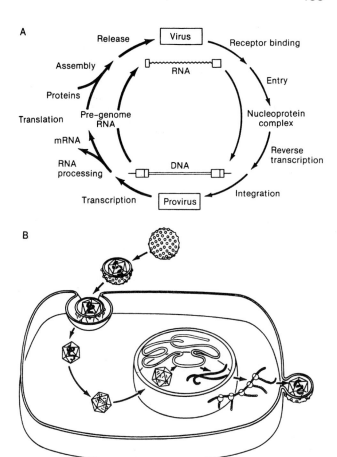

Figure 45–2. Different representations of viral replication. On entry into the infected cell, the reverse transcriptase enzyme makes a DNA copy (proviral DNA) of the RNA genome. Infected cells can contain both unintegrated and integrated proviral DNA. The latter allows for latent nonproductive viral infection. During productive replication, RNA transcripts are made from proviral DNA and complete virions are assembled and released from infected cells. (From Varmus H, Brown P: Retroviruses. *In* Berg DE, Howe MM (eds): Mobile DNA. Washington, D.C., American Society for Microbiology, 1989.)

transcribed from proviral DNA. Viral RNA and viral proteins are then reassembled into complete HIV virions that can be released from cells (see Fig. 45–2). Viral replication in CD4+ lymphocytes results in loss of expression of CD4, formation of syncytia, and shortened survival of CD4+ cells.

The natural history of HIV infection is also influenced by nonviral factors. The immunologic and psychosocial mechanisms that precipitate the progression of HIV are still being characterized. Alcoholism[14, 15] and drugs of abuse[16] are proposed mechanisms. Previous or concurrent infections with other infectious agents involved in sexually transmitted diseases have also been proposed as supplemental factors—for example, *Trichomonas* infections,[17] other parasitic infections, particularly in African AIDS,[18] and cytomegalovirus.[19]

Mechanisms of Immune Destruction by HIV

One immunologic marker of AIDS is a marked depletion of CD4+ lymphocytes, both phenotypically and functionally. The absolute number of CD4+ lymphocytes in the peripheral circulation is inversely correlated with the duration of HIV infection and subsequent progression to AIDS. To illustrate the effect this virus has on the immune system, it is important to understand the significant central role that the CD4+ lymphocyte plays in the development and maintenance of the body's response to foreign invaders (Fig. 45–3). Macrophages present antigen to CD4+ helper lymphocytes in association with MHC (major histocompatibility complex) class II antigens and cytokines, to activate this class of T cells. Activated CD4+ lymphocytes then stimulate the differentiation and maturation of CD8+ lymphocytes, which differentiate into cytotoxic T cells and T-suppressor cells. Activated CD4+ lymphocytes provide "help" for antigen-specific differentiation of B cells into antibody-producing cells. Activated CD4+ lymphocytes and the cytokines produced by activated T cells also serve to activate natural killer (NK) cells and macrophages.

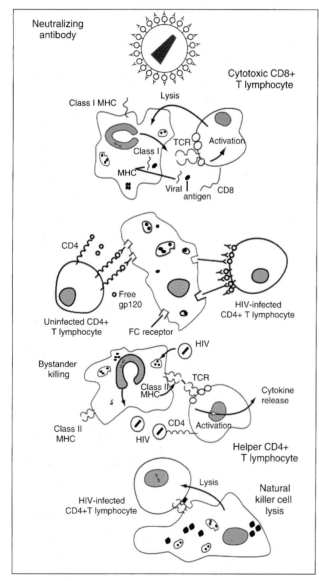

Figure 45–3. The central role of the CD4+ lymphocyte in the development of response to antigen. (From Fauci A, Braunwald E, Isselbacher K, et al (eds): Harrison's Principles of Internal Medicine. New York, McGraw-Hill, p 1814.)

CD8+ cytolytic T lymphocytes (CTLs) expand during primary infection, apparently eliminating virus-infected cells during this expansion, but then disappear from circulation. Other clones of CD8+ lymphocytes that recognize the same viral epitope may partially control viral replication in the peripheral blood but not in lymphoid tissue, the main site of viral replication. In this way, HIV establishes chronic infection by forming a large pool of infected cells that cannot be eliminated by virus-specific CTLs.

The HIV virus, trophic for CD4+ lymphocytes, is cytopathic to or disturbs the function of these cells. Mechanisms of CD4+ lymphocyte reduction could directly or indirectly involve HIV infection of CD4+ cells. Figure 45–4 illustrates the absolute numbers of CD4+ and CD8+ lymphocytes and the extent of viremia over the duration of an HIV infection. During the period of asymptomatic infection, CD4+ cell numbers can remain relatively constant for extended periods, but once CD4+ cells begin to decrease, the onset of full-blown AIDS is precipitous. It is likely that mechanisms other than killing of CD4 cells are also involved in depleting CD4 cells during HIV infection. Indirect mechanisms for which there is experimental support include apoptosis, anergy, superantigen-induced cell proliferation and depletion, defective signaling, molecular mimicry, and autoimmunity.[20] More than one mechanism of CD4 depletion might be involved during different phases of the HIV infection.

Another marker for HIV replication and disease progression is measurement of HIV-1 plasma viral RNA. Monitoring patients by means of viral load quantitation has become an important tool in the management of HIV-infected patients and is discussed later.

Spectrum of Immune Dysfunction in AIDS

Derangement of CD4+ function would produce most of the abnormalities associated with AIDS, including lymphopenia, diminished proliferative response to antigens, decreased cytotoxic responses of both NK cells and cytotoxic T cells, impaired monocyte function, ablated primary antibody response, and increased levels of circulating immune complexes. Although AIDS patients mount a poor primary antibody response to foreign antigens (such as vaccines), their existing clones of B cells are in a constant state of polyclonal stimulation, resulting in mild hypergammaglobulinemia early in the disease process. The absolute number of B cells in AIDS patients is normal, but those B cells are highly activated in vivo, perhaps owing to the loss of immunoregulatory T-cell control. The defect in primary antibody response is at the level of antigen presentation or T-cell help, because matrix-bound antigen can induce an antibody response whereas soluble antigen does not.

HIV-specific, MHC-restricted cytotoxic T lymphocytes are present in the peripheral blood, providing a vigorous lymphocyte response during HIV infection. Viral antigens recognized by primary CTLs include *env* (envelope), *gag* (core), and *pol* (reverse transcriptase) gene products.[21] The antiviral CTL response depends on the route of antigen presentation of viral proteins but does not result in destruc-

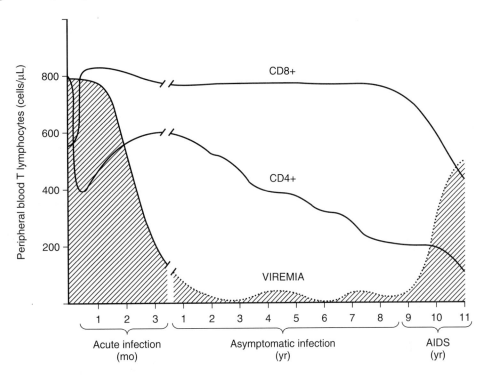

Figure 45–4. A schematic illustration of the natural history of HIV infection. The concentrations of peripheral blood (and lymph node) CD4+ and CD8+ lymphocytes are plotted over duration of the infection. Viremia, indicated by the shaded area under the dotted-line curve, is based on the relative frequency of detection of HIV in peripheral blood during infection. (From McChesney MB, Oldstone MBA: Virus-induced immunosuppression. Adv Immunol 45:335–380, 1989.)

tion of autologous HIV-infected cells, suggesting antigen-specific anergy.

Monocyte chemotaxis is decreased during HIV infection, but microbicidal activity, lipopolysaccharide (LPS)–induced interleukin-1 (IL-1) secretion, and accessory functions for mitogen and antigen stimulation of T cells are normal. Response to soluble antigens injected intradermally (purified protein derivative [PPD], tetanus toxoid, *Candida*) are all decreased in vivo; however, if corrected for the number of CD4+ cells in vitro, HIV-infected patients' lymphocytes can still mount a proliferative response to those antigens. Early in the course of the disease, NK cell numbers and responsiveness are normal. As the disease progresses, many of these monocyte, T-cell, and NK cell functions become depressed or severely depleted.

Infection with HIV results in a strong humoral immune response, a primary, transient immunoglobulin (Ig) M response, and a sustained IgG response. Antibodies are principally directed to *env* (gp41) and *gag* (p24) gene products. Immune complexes of HIV antigen and antibody are detectable during asymptomatic as well as early and late symptomatic stages of the infection. In small numbers of patients, the presence of immune complexes in antigen excess can result in failure to detect HIV antibodies in serum; this is particularly true in HIV-infected infants. One assay system dissociates the immune complexes prior to detection of the antibody or the antigen.[22] Decline in antibody titer or loss of antibody to p24 core antigen is strongly associated with progression to AIDS.

Serum complement does not inactivate the virus, and antibody plus complement does not lyse virus-infected cells. Neutralizing antibody may be present in low titers during HIV infection but does not appear to alter the course of the disease. Antibodies to circulating red cells, platelets, and granulocytes may represent polyclonal B-cell activation, because their presence does not correlate with development of blood cytopenias.[23]

Although HIV infection was initially considered to evolve slowly, it is now known to be a dynamic process. Even when the infection is clinically latent, up to 10^9 virions can be produced daily, the virion pool can turn over every 48 hours, and the plasma virus half-life is 6 hours.[24, 25] HIV particles are actively replicating in the germinal follicles of lymphoid tissues, where they are stored until their release into circulation.[26]

CLINICAL MANIFESTATIONS

AIDS Risk Factors

In North America and Europe, the primary risk group for AIDS has been homosexual or bisexual men, who in 1996 constituted 54% of reported cases of AIDS. Overall, reported cases have decreased for the first time since AIDS reporting began in 1984.[27] Intravenous drug abusers are the fastest-growing risk group (31%), followed by female sexual partners of males at risk for or known to have HIV (10%). The incidence of HIV in hemophiliacs and recipients of transfusions continues to decrease as screening and testing of blood donors have improved. The rate of neonatal AIDS is growing because of the increasing numbers of infected females giving birth to infected infants. The age, race, and sex distributions of AIDS patients correspond to the nature of the risk groups. Behavioral factors within each risk group increase the chances of infection, for example, high promiscuity, sharing of needles, number of exposures. The disproportionate increase in HIV among racial minorities (blacks and Hispanics) is considered to be attributable to behavioral factors rather than race or ethnicity.[27]

By late 1982, the mechanisms of transmission of HIV were understood. Virtually all HIV transmissions have resulted from (1) sexual contact, (2) IV inoculation of body fluids by intentional (i.e., IV drug use, blood transfusion, or receipt of coagulation factor concentrates) or unintentional (e.g., needlesticks) means, or (3) mother-to-child transmission. Sexual practices that traumatize the rectal or vaginal mucosa are more dangerous to the receptive partner. Female-to-male coital transmission is less efficient, on the basis of studies from heterosexual partners of patients who obtained HIV from a blood transfusion, unless the females have genital ulcers that harbor large quantities of the virus or the male is uncircumcised.[7] Sharing of needles and syringes has been a deadly practice for IV drug abusers, the population in which the incidence of AIDS continues to increase.

Nonsexual, non-IV transmission of the disease is very rare. Since the advent of testing blood donors for HIV antibodies and requesting high-risk donors to refrain from donation, the risk of transmission of HIV per blood component exposure has decreased to 1 in 420,000 donor units.[28, 29] Needlesticks have resulted in occupational transmission of HIV to health care workers at an efficiency rate of 0.3 percent.[30] A very small number of occupational HIV transmissions have occurred in health care workers whose damaged skin was exposed to contaminated blood or body fluids. Risk factors for seroconversion include deep injury, injury with a device visibly contaminated with patient's blood involving a needle placed in an artery or vein, and exposure to an AIDS patient within 2 months of the patient's death.[30] Post-exposure prophylaxis with AZT (zidovudine) appears to protect individuals who have experienced occupational HIV transmission, but a protease inhibitor should be added for those with the highest risk.[31]

In most of the Third World countries, where AIDS is overwhelmingly a heterosexually transmitted disease, the numbers of cases in females equal or exceed those in males. In the United States, women accounted for 14% of AIDS cases in 1992, 17.5% in 1995, and 19% in 1996. The proportion is growing rapidly, especially among women in their teens and early 20s.[27] Of the 3000 women a day who become infected with HIV, 70% are between the ages of 15 and 25. The factors that put young women at much greater risk include behavior (low rate of condom use), high rate of anal intercourse with older men, anatomy (vaginal mucosa very thin in early adolescence), and physiology (transition zone of cells outside the cervical opening vulnerable to infection).

Individuals infected with other microorganisms that produce a cellular immune response tend to be more susceptible to HIV infections and to progress to AIDS faster than those not otherwise infected. People who live in countries where parasitic infections such as schistosomiasis are prevalent appear to be less resistant to AIDS.[18] Greater susceptibility to HIV infections also appears to be associated with prior exposure to other infectious sexually transmitted diseases, such as syphilis, *Chlamydia*, herpes simplex lesions, and gonorrhea.[7]

Congenital and Neonatal AIDS

The rate of congenital transmission of the HIV virus is rapidly increasing. As women of childbearing age are contracting the disease, they are passing the virus on to their fetuses transplacentally. The AIDS Clinical Trials Group (ACTG)[32] showed that transmission of HIV from pregnant mothers to their infants occurred in 25.5% of

untreated women, compared with 8.3% of women who received AZT.[32] For women with high viral loads, the transmission rate was as high as 40%.[33] AZT was effective at reducing transmission of HIV regardless of the viral load or CD4 count, and it is now recommended for all HIV-infected pregnant women. Studies in progress by some ACTG subgroups show that "viral load in children can be variable due to compliance (failure to receive the drugs prescribed), age (younger children have higher viral loads), infections and immunizations (temporarily increase viral load), drug effects (different drug combinations differ in their ability to reduce viral load), and resistance (HIV viruses can develop resistance to drugs)."[34]

AIDS Indicator Diseases

Because there are no mandated screening programs except in the blood donor population, HIV infections are commonly suggested by the clinical presence of an indicator disease, in the absence of another cause for immunodeficiency, with or without the detection of HIV antibodies (Box 45–1). Some of the HIV-1 strains are not reliably

---

Box 45–1. Indicator Diseases Suggesting HIV Infection*

Candidiasis—of bronchi, trachea, or lungs; esophageal
Cervical cancer—invasive†
Coccidioidomycosis, disseminated or extrapulmonary
Cryptococcosis—extrapulmonary
Cryptosporidiosis—chronic diarrhea persisting > 1 month
Cytomegalovirus disease—other than liver, spleen or nodes
Cytomegalovirus retinitis (with loss of vision)
Encephalopathy, HIV-related
Herpes simplex: chronic ulcers (> 1 month duration); or bronchitis, pneumonia, or esophagitis
Histoplasmosis, disseminated or extrapulmonary
Isosporiasis, chronic intestinal (> 1 month duration)
Kaposi's sarcoma
Lymphoma, Burkitt's (or equivalent term)
Lymphoma, primary, of brain
Mycobacterium avium complex or *M. kansasii*—disseminated or extrapulmonary
Mycobacterium tuberculosis, any site (pulmonary) or extrapulmonary†
Mycobacterium, other species or unidentified species, disseminated or extrapulmonary
Pneumocystis carinii pneumonia
Pneumonia, recurrent†
Progressive multifocal leukoencephalopathy
Salmonella septicemia, recurrent
Toxoplasmosis of the brain
Wasting syndrome of HIV

*Conditions listed in the AIDS surveillance case definition (AIDS-Indicator Conditions). Data from MMWR Morb Mortal Wkly Rep 41 (RR-17):1–19, 1992.
†Added in 1993.

detected by all antibody screen tests currently being used.[35, 36] Regardless, the more esoteric tests (i.e., p24 antigen, HIV RNA, and HIV cultures) should be reserved for individuals who present with AIDS indicator diseases but do not have detectable HIV antibodies.

The majority of patients exposed to a significant HIV inoculum become infected. A chronic HIV infection can span a few months to 20 years. Many such patients are well and asymptomatic, with the only evidence of HIV infection being a positive serologic result that is most often discovered serendipitously. On physical examination, approximately a third of these asymptomatic patients have a persistent generalized lymphadenopathy with nodes that are symmetric, mobile, and nontender.

If constitutional symptoms arise (fatigue, debilitating diarrhea, night sweats, fever) or if the lymphadenopathy becomes asymmetric or the nodes are tender or enlarging, opportunistic infections must be excluded. A lymph node biopsy is recommended to exclude mycobacterial infections, lymphoma, and lymph node involvement by Kaposi's sarcoma. The features of chronic HIV infection associated with opportunistic infections are commonly found on the skin (viral, fungal, or bacterial infections), in the oropharynx (candidiasis, herpes simplex, hairy leukoplakia, or dental disease), and in the nervous system.

Neurologic Complications of AIDS

HIV infection can manifest as an acute viral infection with glandular-like fever and, less commonly, acute neurologic syndromes. The neurologic complications include the effects of the viral infection on the central nervous system (AIDS-related dementia, cytomegalovirus encephalitis, HIV-related meningitis), effects of intracranial mass lesions on the central nervous system (cerebral toxoplasmosis, lymphoma), effects on the peripheral nervous system (neuropathies, myeloradiculitis), or opportunistic infections, such as cryptococcal meningitis or neurosyphilis. The most common neurologic complication, AIDS-related dementia

(30% of patients with neurologic complications), manifests as a history of cognitive or behavioral changes, such as memory loss, apathy, and impaired concentration. The neurologic findings in these patients include hyperreflexia, hypertonia, myelopathy (paresthesia, leg weakness, ataxia, incontinence), and polyneuropathy (inflammatory demyelinating disease, e.g., Guillain-Barré syndrome).

LABORATORY ANALYSES AND DIAGNOSIS

The mean time from initial infection to symptoms that lead to the diagnosis of AIDS is more than 8 years, but most persons (>95%) develop enzyme immunoassay (EIA)–detectable antibody within 4 to 12 weeks of acquiring the infection. The serologic profile of HIV infection is shown in Figure 45–5. Repeatable EIA reactivity for HIV antibody remains the first step in diagnosing AIDS. Although current tests have specificities of 99.9%, the potential impact of a false-positive test mandates confirmation by a test with even greater specificity, the Western blot to detect antibodies to specific HIV proteins (gp41, p24, p55, or gp110 bands indicate a positive result for AIDS) in order to confirm HIV antibody specificity. The two most common causes of false-positive EIA results for HIV are HLA-DR antibodies in multiparous women and polyclonal hypergammaglobulinemia.

Most EIA methods for HIV-1 and HIV-2 antibody were designed for high-volume analysis of blood donor sera. A rapid EIA assay for HIV antibody in a single-use device,[37] disposable test system makes it feasible for small laboratories or clinics to perform HIV-1 antibody testing on individuals in a timely manner. An oral mucosal transudate (OMT) sampling device, which concentrates IgG antibodies to a level 4-fold greater than in saliva, has been approved by the U.S. Food and Drug Administration (FDA), and testing of OMT has been found to be equivalent to testing to serum.[38] An experimental EIA for screening for HIV antibody in urine has been reported.[39]

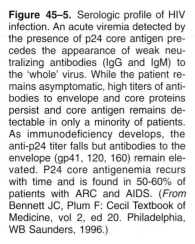

Figure 45–5. Serologic profile of HIV infection. An acute viremia detected by the presence of p24 core antigen precedes the appearance of weak neutralizing antibodies (IgG and IgM) to the 'whole' virus. While the patient remains asymptomatic, high titers of antibodies to envelope and core proteins persist and core antigen remains detectable in only a minority of patients. As immunodeficiency develops, the anti-p24 titer falls but antibodies to the envelope (gp41, 120, 160) remain elevated. P24 core antigenemia recurs with time and is found in 50-60% of patients with ARC and AIDS. (*From* Bennett JC, Plum F: Cecil Textbook of Medicine, vol 2, ed 20. Philadelphia, WB Saunders, 1996.)

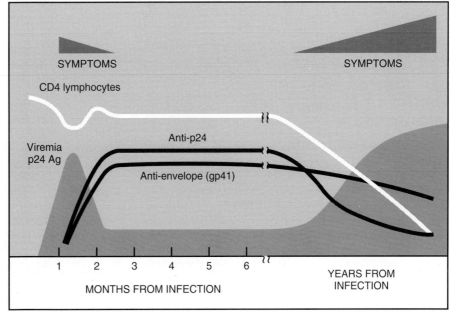

HIV antigen can be detected by a capture EIA for p24 antigen. This test may be useful for that very small group of patients who present with AIDS indicator diseases but do not demonstrate HIV antibody. Although initial large clinical trials found no situation in which p24 antigen was detected without a positive EIA for HIV antibodies,[40, 41] three transfusions with p24 antigen–positive, anti-HIV–negative blood resulted in transfusion-associated HIV infections in recipients.[28] Since 1996, the FDA has recommended that all blood and plasma donations be screened with tests for HIV-1 p24 antigen.[28] Although p24 antigen testing reliably detects HIV infection approximately one week before antibodies appear and reduces the "window period" from 22 days to 16 days, it does so at a significant cost (~$5/unit).[29] As HIV RNA testing methods evolve to the point where they can be used for mass screening, it may prove efficacious to test all blood donors to reduce the "window" to 11 days to ensure an even safer blood supply, but at an even greater cost.

The immune complex–dissociated HIV (ICD-HIV) assay is useful to detect p24 core protein in neonates that may be masked by maternal antibody.[22] This assay and the p24 antigen assay by itself are important tools to detect HIV infections in infants and children. Another proposed application for the ICD-HIV assay or p24 antigen assay was to increase the sensitivity of detection of disease progression, but the quantitation of HIV RNA has been shown to be more sensitive for this purpose.[42] HIV RNA detection is available and has been used in rare cases for diagnosis when HIV infection is suspected but the antibody and p24 antigen tests are both negative.

Viral culture is feasible, but not practical. HIV culture requires separation of peripheral blood mononuclear cells (PBMCs) from other blood components by density gradient centrifugation, incubation of the PBMCs with PBMCs from an HIV-seronegative donor for 4 weeks in the presence of IL-2, phytohemagglutinin (PHA), and fresh PBMCs every 4 days. Detection of a positive HIV culture requires assaying culture supernatant for the presence of p24 antigen as an indicator of viral replication. HIV culture is not warranted in the routine diagnosis and management of HIV infection but may be useful in establishing the diagnosis in neonates and infants, in adults with acute primary infection prior to seroconversion, and in high-risk adults with indeterminate Western blot results.

LABORATORY ANALYSES TO MONITOR TREATMENT OR PROGRESSION

Progressive depletion of CD4+ T cells in HIV-positive patients is associated with increasing clinical complications. The absolute number of CD4+ T cells is a prognostic indicator in patients with HIV. These data are used to determine when antiviral therapy should be initiated and when prophylaxis for *Pneumocystis carinii* pneumonia should be started, and to monitor the efficacy of treatment. Because of the importance of accuracy in quantifying CD4+ T cells, the Centers for Disease Control and Prevention (CDC) have published guidelines for the flow cytometry performance of immunophenotyping for CD4:CD8 ratio and quantitation of the absolute number of CD4+ T cells.[43]

Measuring viral load by quantifying virion-associated RNA in plasma has become the marker of choice for therapeutic monitoring. Viral load can currently be quantitated by three different methods[44]:

- Reverse transcriptase polymerase chain reaction (RT-PCR), which amplifies the target RNA molecules in plasma to detectable levels
- Nucleic acid–based sequence amplification (NASBA), an in vitro version of the natural replication of retroviral RNA
- Branched DNA (bDNA) assay, which amplifies the signal (the DNA probe that binds to the viral RNA) as the means of detection

Each of these assays has different calibration methods and gives somewhat different results, and their results trend but do not necessarily match, so only one test should be used to monitor an HIV-infected patient. Studies show that viral load is correlated with disease stage and effectiveness of therapy.[44] When the virus becomes resistant to therapy, the viral load increases (Fig. 45–6). High levels of HIV RNA measured within a year of seroconversion predict long-term progression to AIDS.[42] Viral RNA measurements are more direct, more accurate, and more meaningful markers of HIV infection than the surrogate marker (the CD4 cell count) and p24 antigen detection.

TREATMENT

By the end of 1997, 11 antiretroviral agents (ARVs) had been approved by the FDA,[45] and more were in the approval process. The ARVs fall into three classes: (1) protease inhibitors (PIs), (2) nucleoside analog reverse transcriptase inhibitors (NRTIs), and (3) nonnucleoside reverse transcriptase inhibitors (NNRTIs).[46] The initial triple-drug regimen usually consists of two NRTIs and one PI; the alternative therapy is 2 NRTIs and 1 NNRTI.

The major issue to consider is when to begin therapy. ARV treatment is potent, expensive, and complex and has numerous potentially toxic side effects. The virus can become resistant to many of these drugs, so HIV-infected patients who are clinically well might choose to delay initiating therapy. The International AIDS Society–USA Panel recommends that asymptomatic patients begin ARV treatment when the CD4+ count falls below 500 cells/μL or the HIV RNA level exceeds 10,000 copies/mL.[46]

Because of the differences between the viral load measurement assays, individual patients should always be monitored with the same assay system.[44] Patients must be totally committed to following the drug regimen once it has begun, because nonadherence may result in virus breakthrough and appearance of drug-resistant strains.

The cost of the triple-drug regimen is approximately $1,000/month.[45] Side effects range from headache, nausea, and fatigue to peripheral neuropathy, diarrhea, and kidney stones. It is not known whether eradication of the virus might be possible with early treatment by ARVs. It is also not known at this time whether ARV therapy can be discontinued after a prolonged period; clinical trials are ongoing.

Pneumococcal vaccine and *Haemophilus influenzae* vaccine should be given to HIV-infected patients as early in

HIV levels during antiviral therapy

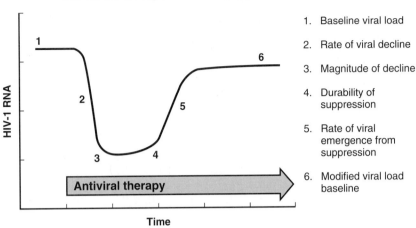

Figure 45–6. HIV levels during antiviral therapy. HIV RNA as detected by RT-PCR or by bDNA assay during course of antiviral therapy. (*From* Effect of antiviral therapy on HIV levels. CAP Today 19:20, 1995.)

1. Baseline viral load
2. Rate of viral decline
3. Magnitude of decline
4. Durability of suppression
5. Rate of viral emergence from suppression
6. Modified viral load baseline

the course of the disease as possible. Patients with a history of a positive PPD should receive isoniazid (INH) prophylaxis.

AZT prophylaxis continues to be recommended for women to prevent perinatal transmission of HIV. If a woman who is already taking an ARV regimen becomes pregnant, she is advised to continue the course of therapy and become part of a study group to determine whether ARV might be as effective as AZT in decreasing the likelihood of vertical transmission of HIV.[46] A soluble form of recombinant CD4 (sCD4) was developed as a potential therapeutic agent intended to bind to the virus and prevent the virus from binding to CD4 on lymphocytes. Unfortunately, it demonstrated no efficacy in vivo despite achievement of acceptable drug levels in serum.[47]

VACCINE DEVELOPMENT

Effective vaccines against HIV have proved elusive, although many investigators have worked toward this goal for the past decade. Mutations in the HIV genome occur at a very high frequency, resulting in rapidly changing variations in HIV proteins, with the surface envelope glycoprotein gp120 being the most variable. Antibody-based vaccines have been unsuccessful at binding to primary viruses isolated from patients. It is possible that a vaccine effective against a dominant strain in one community may not be effective against other strains now or in the future.

To provide insight into HIV vaccine development, investigators have reviewed the natural course of HIV infection in many patients. Most HIV-infected persons develop AIDS. In the typical natural history of HIV infection, as shown in Figure 45–4, patients are asymptomatic for a number of years; however, about 10% of HIV-infected patients have an accelerated course and develop full-blown AIDS within the first 2 to 3 years of infection (rapid progressors). At the other end of the spectrum, 10% to 15% of individuals remain disease free for as much as 10 years (nonprogressors).[48] Rapid progressors have lower concentrations of HIV antibodies, especially neutralizing antibodies, lower levels of CD8 anti-HIV cytotoxic T-lymphocyte (HIV suppressor) reactivity, and higher levels of HIV RNA than do nonprogressors. Researchers developing vaccines conclude that the HIV immunogen may

need to: (1) generate neutralizing antibody to HIV primary isolates, (2) be population or cohort HLA-based to optimize reactivity, (3) be designed for specific geographic locations and/or for specific ethnic groups, and (4) be accepted as being less than 100% effective.[48]

Vaccines available for several viral diseases do not prevent infection but do prevent the pathologic consequences of the infection. For example, feline leukemia virus (FeLV) does not prevent cats from being infected, but does prevent viremia and limits dissemination of FeLV to distant lymphoid tissues.[49] Identifying immunologic factors associated with nonprogressors, in combination with accepting vaccines that prevent the pathologic consequences of infection, may be the method of choice for HIV vaccine development.

Vaccines for viral diseases have traditionally been live, attenuated or killed viruses, but because of the implications of possible infectivity, such vaccines are not considered safe for HIV. Many candidate HIV vaccines have been or are being studied in clinical trials worldwide using various vectors and methods of delivery. Vaccines under development fall into four categories: (1) synthetic peptide, (2) recombinant subunit, (3) live recombinant vector, and (4) combination of live recombinant vector and recombinant subunit.[49] All of the vaccine candidates have been well tolerated, have stimulated the production of HIV antibodies that have blocked HIV infectivity of lymphocytes in culture, and have induced HIV-specific immunologic memory cells in phase I and phase II trials. However, because most of the vaccines have not stimulated HIV-neutralizing antibodies for viral isolates obtained directly from infected individuals, none has progressed to the phase III (large-scale human efficacy) trials. Some investigators believe that an effective HIV vaccine must elicit a cell-mediated immune response rather than an antibody response.[50]

Case Study

SP, a 23-year-old male homosexual, was admitted to the hospital after a grand mal seizure. He had no prior history of seizures, and his HIV status was unknown. He had four to five sexual partners over the last 5 years, but had been with his current partner for 6 months. He did not use condoms. He had two episodes of disorientation in the past 6 weeks for which he had been seen at an Urgent Care center, where the differential diagnosis included infectious mononucleosis, otitis media, brain tumor, cerebral abscess, and arteriovenous malformation. Upon his admission to the hospital, computed tomography and magnetic resonance imaging of his brain showed lesions suggestive of *Toxoplasma*.

CBC, blood chemistry profile, and UA were within normal limits. Acute hepatitis viral assessment was negative, and rapid plasma reagin test was nonreactive. The urine drug screen showed only salicylates. HIV Ab by EIA was positive, confirmed by Western blot. Toxoplasma antibodies were as follows: IgG 1:80, IgM <10.

T cell studies yielded the following results:

	Absolute No. (μ/L)	Reference Range	Percentage (%)	Reference Range
Lymphocyte	2,208	(1500–3000)		
CD5	1,724	(500–2500)	85	(70–90)
CD4	284	(350–1500)	14	(35–55)
CD8	1,460	(200–1000)	72	(19–37)
CD4:CD8 ratio	0.2	(0.9–3.5)		

Questions

1. What diagnosis has been confirmed by the clinical picture, imaging, and laboratory test results?

2. What is the most likely cause of the seizure and other neurologic symptoms?

3. What tests should be used to monitor the treatment and prognosis of this disease?

Discussion

1. The patient has an indicator disease and a positive HIV antibody test. According to CDC criteria, this patient has AIDS.

2. The most likely cause of the seizure and neurologic symptoms is toxoplasmosis of the brain, although other neurologic complications of AIDS have not been ruled out.

3. The patient should be monitored with CD4 counts and HIV-RNA viral load testing and should be treated with antiretroviral therapy that is adjusted according to viral load quantitation.

References

1. Radetsky P: The Invisible Invaders: The Story of the Emerging Age of Viruses. Boston, Little, Brown, 1991.
2. Barré-Sinoussi F: HIV as the cause of AIDS. Lancet 348:31–35, 1996.
3. Barré-Sinoussi F, Chermann JC, Rey F, et al: Isolation of a T-lymphotrophic retrovirus from a patient at risk for acquired immuno-deficiency syndrome (AIDS). Science 220:868–871, 1983.
4. Gallo RC, Saluhuddin SZ, Popovic M, et al: Frequent detection and isolation of cytopathic retroviruses (HTLV-3) from patients with AIDS and at high risk for AIDS. Science 224:500–503, 1984.
5. Levy JA, Hoffman AD, Kramer SM, et al: Retroviruses from San Francisco patients with AIDS. Science 225:840–842, 1984.
6. Levy JA: The transmission of HIV and factors influencing progression to AIDS. Am J Med 95:86–100, 1993.
7. Kaplan MH: Pathogenesis of HIV. Infect Dis Clin North Am 8:279–289, 1994.
8. Gougeon ML, Montagnier L: Apoptosis in AIDS. Science 260:1269–1270, 1993.
9. Mellado MJ, Cilleruelo MJ, Ortiz M, et al: Viral phenotype, antiretroviral resistance and clinical evolution in human immunodeficiency virus-infected children. Pediatr Infect Dis J 16:1032–1037, 1997.
10. Hu DJ, Donderoo TJ, Rayfield MA, et al: The emerging genetic diversity of HIV: The importance of global surveillance for diagnostics, research, and prevention. JAMA 275:210–216, 1996.
11. Bjorndal A, Deng H, Jansson M, et al: Coreceptor usage of primary human immunodeficiency virus type 1 isolates varies according to biological phenotype. J Virol 71:7478–7487, 1997.
12. Gostin LO, Ward JW, Baker AC: National HIV case reporting for the United States. N Engl J Med 337:1162–1167, 1997.
13. Root-Bernstein RS: Five myths about AIDS that have misdirected research and treatment. Genetica 95:111–132, 1995.
14. Balla AK, Lischner HW, Pomerantz RJ, et al: Human studies on alcohol and susceptibility to HIV infection. Alcohol 11:99–103, 1994.
15. Wang Y, Watson RR: Is alcohol consumption a cofactor in the development of acquired immunodeficiency syndrome? Alcohol 12:105–109, 1995.
16. Pillai R, Nair BS, Watson RR: AIDS, drugs of abuse and the immune system: A complex immunotoxicological network. Arch Toxicol 65:609–617, 1991.
17. Krvavac S: Pre-existing chronic intraepithelial *Trichomonas* invasion with consecutive immunodepression enables progression of human immunodeficiency virus: A new concept of acquired immunodeficiency syndrome pathogenesis. Med Hypotheses 39:225–228, 1992.
18. Duesberg PH: AIDS acquired by drug consumption and other noncontagious risk factors. Pharmacol Ther 55:201–277, 1992.
19. Fiala M, Mosca JD, Barry P, et al: Multi-step pathogenesis of AIDS—role of cytomegalovirus. Res Immunol 142:87–95, 1991.
20. Gougeon ML, Colizzi V, Dalgleish A, et al: New concepts in AIDS pathogenesis. AIDS Res Hum Retroviruses 9:287–289, 1993.
21. Walker BD, Flexner C, Paradis TJ, et al: HIV-1 reverse transcriptase is a target for cytotoxic T lymphocytes in infected individuals. Science 240:64–66, 1988.
22. Miles SA, Balden E, Magpantay L, et al: Rapid serologic testing with immune complex dissociated HIV p24 antigen for early detection of HIV infection in neonates. N Engl J Med 328:297–302, 1993.
23. Aboulafia DM, Mitsuyasu RT: Hematologic abnormalities in AIDS. Hematol Oncol Clin North Am 5:195–214, 1991.
24. Ho DD, Neumann AU, Perelson AS, et al: Rapid turnover of plasma virons and CD4 lymphocytes in HIV-1 infection. Nature 373:123–126, 1995.
25. Wei X, Ghosh SK, Taylor ME, et al: Viral dynamics in human immunodeficiency virus type 1 infections. Nature 373:117–122, 1995.
26. Haase AT, Henry K, Zupancic M, et al: Quantitative image analysis of HIV-1 infection in lymphoid tissue. Science 274:985–989, 1996.
27. Centers for Disease Control and Prevention: Update: Trends in AIDS incidence—United States, 1996. MMWR 46:861–867, 1997.
28. Centers for Disease Control and Prevention: U.S. Public Health Service guidelines for testing and counseling blood and plasma donors for human immunodeficiency virus type 1 antigen. MMWR 45:1–9, 1996.
29. AuBuchon JP, Birkmeyer JD, Busch MP: Cost-effectiveness of expanded human immunodeficiency virus-testing protocols for donated blood. Transfusion 37:45–51, 1997.
30. Cardo DM, Culver DH, Ciesielski CA, et al: A case-control study of HIV seroconversion in health care workers after percutaneous exposure. N Engl J Med 337:1485–1490, 1997.
31. Centers for Disease Control and Prevention: Update: Provisional public health service recommendations for chemoprophylaxis after occupational exposure to HIV. MMWR 45:468–472, 1996.
32. Conner EM, Sperling RS, Gelber R, et al: Reduction of maternal-infant transmission of human immunodeficiency virus type 1 with zidovudine treatment. Pediatric AIDS Clinical Trials Group Protocol 076 Study Group. N Engl J Med 331:1173–1180, 1994.
33. Sperling RS, Shapiro DE, Coombs RW, et al: Maternal viral load, zidovudine treatment, and the risk of transmission of human immunodeficiency virus type 1 from mother to infant. Pediatric AIDS Clinical Trials Group Protocol 076 Study Group. N Engl J Med 335:1621–1629, 1996.

34. Sever JL: HIV viral load measurements for evaluating and monitoring infected patients. AMLInteractions 2:1–2, 1997.

35. Loussert-Ajaka I, Ly TD, Chaix ML, et al: HIV-1/HIV-2 seronegativity in HIV-1 subtype O infected patients. Lancet 343:1393–1394, 1994.

36. Schable C, Zekeng L, Pau CP, et al: Sensitivity of United States HIV antibody tests for detection of HIV-1 group O infections. Lancet 344:1333–1334, 1994.

37. Carter S, Carter JB, James K: Rapid HIV-1 antibody screening using the Murex single use disposable system (SUDS). Lab Med: 26:339–342, 1995.

38. Gallo D, George JR, Fitchen JH, et al: Evaluation of a system using oral mucosal transudate for HIV-1 antibody screening and confirmatory testing. JAMA 277:254–258, 1997.

39. Berrios DC, Avins AL, Haynes-Sanstad K, et al: Screening for human immunodeficiency virus antibody in urine. Arch Pathol Lab Med 119:139–141, 1995.

40. Lackritz EM, Satten GA, Aberle-Grassee J, et al: Estimated risk of HIV transmission by screened blood in the United States. N Engl J Med 333:1721–1725, 1995.

41. Schreiber GB, Busch MP, Kleinman SH, et al: The risk of transfusion-transmittal viral infections. N Engl J Med 334:1885–1890, 1995.

42. Mellars JW, Kingsley LA, Rinaldo CR, et al: Quantitation of HIV-1 RNA in plasma predicts outcome after seroconversion. Ann Intern Med 122:573–579, 1995.

43. Centers for Disease Control: Guidelines for the performance of CD4+ T cell determinations in persons with human immunodeficiency virus infection. MMWR 41:1–17, 1992.

44. Revets H, Marissens D, DeWit S, et al: Comparative evaluation of NASBA HIV-1 QT, Amplicor-HIV Monitor, and Quantiplex HIV RNA assay: Three methods for quantification of human immunodeficiency virus type 1 RNA in plasma. J Clin Microbiol 34:1058–1064, 1996.

45. Henry K, Stiffman M, Feldman J: Antiretroviral therapy for HIV infection. Postgrad Med 102:100–119, 1997.

46. Carpenter CCJ, Fischi MA, Hammer SM, et al: Antiretroviral therapy for HIV infection in 1997. JAMA 277:1962–1969, 1997

47. Daars ES, Ho DD: Relative resistance of primary HIV-1 isolates to neutralization by soluble CD4. Am J Med 90:22S–26S, 1991.

48. Haynes BF: HIV vaccines: where we are and where we are going. Lancet 348:933–937, 1996.

49. Lee TH: Acquired immunodeficiency disease vaccines: Design and development. *In* Curran J, Essex M, Fauci AS (eds): AIDS: Etiology, Diagnosis, Treatment, and Prevention. Philadelphia, Lippincott-Raven, 1997.

50. Stricker RB: The Maginot line and AIDS vaccine. Med Hypotheses 48:527–529, 1997.

Bibliography

Borkowsky W, Wilfert CM: Acquired immunodeficiency syndrome. *In* Krugman S, Katz SL, Gershon AA, et al (eds): Infectious Diseases of Children. St Louis, Mosby–Year Book, 1992.

Shaw GM: Biology of human immunodeficiency viruses. *In* Bennett JC, Plum F (eds): Cecil Textbook of Medicine, ed 20. Philadelphia, WB Saunders, 1996.

Fauci AS, Lane HC: Human immunodeficiency virus (HIV) disease: AIDS and related disorders. *In* Fauci AS, Braunwald E, Isselbacher K, et al (eds): Harrison's Principles of Internal Medicine, ed 14. New York, McGraw-Hill, 1998.

McChesney MB, Oldstone MBA: Virus-induced immunosuppression. Adv Immunol 45:335–380, 1989.

Chapter 46

Primary Immunodeficiencies

Hal S. Larsen

During the 1990s, knowledge of the immune system has expanded at an exponential rate. The crucial role of cell-mediated immunity (CMI) in host defense, the role of the mononuclear phagocyte in the generation of an immune response, and the role of the major histocompatibility complex (MHC) in health and disease are but a few examples of the great variety of immunologic information that has direct impact on the clinical laboratory.[1-3]

The most primitive cellular response is phagocytosis, mediated by granulocytes and monocyte-derived cells. Humoral and cellular immunity are provided by the lymphoid cells. The activity of these cellular systems is augmented by the biologic amplification systems, primarily complement, and the acute-phase proteins.

Within the marrow, lymphoid stem cells are stimulated to differentiate by chemical influences termed the *lymphopoietic inductive microenvironment*. The resulting prelymphocytes migrate into the peripheral blood and then to the primary lymphoid organs.

The primary lymphoid organs, the thymus and the bone marrow, are responsible for immunologic programming. Prelymphocytes within the thymus are referred to as *thymocytes*. These cells are programmed under the influence of thymopoietins and interactions with MHC antigens on thymic stromal cells, resulting in the deletion of autoreactive clones. The mature cell is released into the peripheral blood as a thymus-derived cell (T cell). The lymphocytes mediating humoral immunity are presumably processed in a similar fashion in the bone marrow, hence the term B cells.

Following differentiation and programming, immunocompetent T and B cells migrate into the peripheral lymphoid organs. The major secondary lymphoid organs are the spleen, lymph nodes, tonsils, and gut-associated lymphoid tissue (GALT), which provide a systemic network of antigen-responsive cells. Within secondary lymphoid tissue, T and B cells occur in relatively discrete regions with macrophages dispersed throughout. This sequence of maturation is depicted in Figure 46–1.

The primary stimulus for the generation of an immune response is the interaction of immunogen and the mononuclear phagocyte system (MPS). The MPS is a body-wide collection of specialized fixed macrophages. Immunogens are phagocytized by these cells and partially degraded. The processed antigen is then displayed on the cell membrane. These antigen-presenting cells (APCs) interact with lymphocytes through MHC membrane proteins. Simultaneously, APCs begin secreting the immunoregulatory monokine interleukin-1 (IL-1), a lymphocyte-activating factor that triggers the clonal expansion of both T and B cells.

The interaction of the APC with the T cell triggers dedifferentiation into a T lymphoblast, followed by intense proliferation of the stimulated clone. This clonal expansion

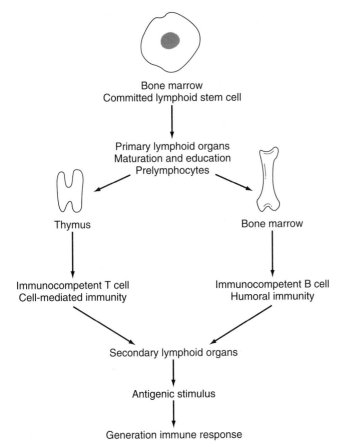

Figure 46–1. Maturation of the immune system.

heterogeneous group of glycoproteins classed as lymphokines (Table 46–1).

A humoral immune response is produced by the interaction of APCs and T and B cells, which stimulate the production of long-lived memory cells and short-lived antibody-secreting plasma cells. Primary immune responses produce predominantly immunoglobulin M (IgM); however, prolonged exposure or reexposure to immunogen will produce an immunoglobulin class switch, promoted by the helper T cell. The plasma cells will now secrete predominantly immunoglobulin G (IgG) or A (IgA). Antibody production is regulated by the suppressor T cell, which acts by inhibiting the helper T cell or the B cell itself (Fig. 46–3). Table 46–2 lists the five major Ig classes and their biologic activities.

ETIOLOGY AND PATHOPHYSIOLOGY

All immunodeficiencies (IDs) can be classed as either primary (congenital) or secondary (acquired). Within these broad groups the abnormality may be the result of an embryologic abnormality, a defective or absent enzyme, or an idiopathic cause. The presenting symptoms and clinical course of each deficiency state are a reflection of the particular defense mechanism affected.

B-Cell Deficiency States

The B-cell deficiency states range from a virtual absence of all Ig classes to selective defects in one class. The clinical symptoms and therapy depend on the immunoglobulin class affected and the totality of that defect. Because of the relative ease of detecting a hypogammaglobulinemic condition, patients are usually diagnosed promptly, permitting rapid therapeutic intervention.

BRUTON'S AGAMMAGLOBULINEMIA

Bruton's agammaglobulinemia, an immunodeficiency state also termed *X-linked infantile hypogammaglobulinemia*, was described by Bruton in a male child in 1952, which is considered the first description of a primary ID.

results in a number of T-cell subpopulations (Fig. 46–2), which are classed as effector, memory, or regulatory. Effector T cells promote cell-mediated cytotoxicity (CMC) and delayed-type hypersensitivity (DTH). Memory T cells are responsible for anamnesis. The regulatory T cells are the helper/inducer and suppressor cells. The relative proportion of these two populations of cells regulates the strength and duration of both cellular and humoral immune responses, often directly mediated by the elaboration of a

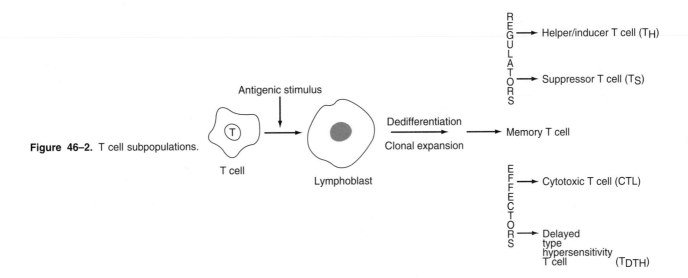

Figure 46–2. T cell subpopulations.

Table 46–1. Lymphokines Secreted by Antigen-Stimulated T Lymphocytes

Lymphokine	Other Names	Biologic Activities
Interleukin-2	IL-2 T cell growth factor	Stimulates division of T cells to enhance immune response
γ-Interferon	Macrophage-activating factor (MAF)	Stimulates macrophage phagocytosis and NK cell killing; antineoplastic; regulates antibody production
B cell growth factor	—	Stimulates B cell growth and plasma cell differentiation
Lymphotoxin	—	Cytotoxic
Chemotactic factor	—	Attracts macrophages to site of antigen
Migration inhibition factor	—	Enhances macrophage adherence at site of antigen

It has been estimated that 1:100,000 males may be affected. Although there is an absence of mature B cells in the peripheral blood, recent investigations have detected pre-B cell populations in the bone marrow. These cells fail to mature and do not secrete immunoglobulin, probably as a result of an as-yet-undetermined maturation block or an absence of helper T cell interactions.[4–6]

TRANSIENT NEONATAL HYPOGAMMAGLOBULINEMIA

Transient neonatal hypogammaglobulinemia mimics Bruton's agammaglobulinemia in some ways. At present, the etiology is unknown. In isolated cases, maternal antibodies to IgG allotypic markers have been found that could produce a transient suppression of IgG-secreting cells. Alternatively, a selective defect in helper T cells has been proposed.[5–8]

ACQUIRED HYPOGAMMAGLOBULINEMIA

Although the etiology of acquired hypogammaglobulinemia, also called *variable unclassifiable immunodeficiency*, is not known, these patients do have normal levels of circulating B cells. This has led to a hypothesis that implicates either an increase in suppressor T cells or a decrease in helper T cells.[5–8]

SELECTIVE IgA DEFICIENCY

A selective lack of IgA is the most common ID state to be identified, with reported incidence ranging from 1:600 to 1:800. It appears that IgA deficiency, like other ID states, predisposes the affected individual to a number of other diseases. As in most ID states, the pathogenesis of selective IgA deficiency is not definitively known. Studies have demonstrated normal levels of circulating IgA-bearing

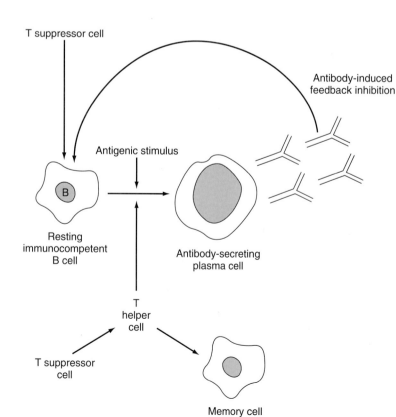

Figure 46–3. Regulation of the antibody response.

Table 46-2. Immunoglobulin Class and Biologic Activities

Class	Subclass	M.W.	Biologic Activity
IgG	IgG1–IgG4	150,000	Antiviral Antibacterial Antifungal Opsonizing
IgM	IgM1 and IgM2	900,000	Antiviral Antibacterial Antifungal
IgA	IgA1 and IgA2	160,000 or 400,000	Mucosal immunity
IgE	—	190,000	Allergy Antiparasitic
IgD	—	180,000	B-lymphocyte differentiation

B cells. A subpopulation of patients have suppressor T cells that inhibit IgA production from B cells of normal individuals. Drug-induced IgA deficiencies have been described in cases in which the deficiency often resolved upon removal of the drug.[5]

Cell-Mediated Immunodeficiencies

Because of the interactions between T and B cells, a pure T-cell ID state is rare. Generally speaking, any defect in T-cell number or function will result in some aberration in immunoglobulin synthesis. Patients with CMI deficiencies are prone to develop acute or chronic infections with numerous viral, fungal, or protozoal pathogens.

DiGeorge's Syndrome

Also known as *congenital thymic aplasia*, DiGeorge's syndrome is a result of an embryologic malformation producing physical abnormalities and ID. Between the sixth and eighth weeks of gestation, an unknown embryologic insult perturbs the normal development of the thymus and parotid glands. They are either totally absent or partially developed in an abnormal anatomic location. It has also been suggested that some cases may be the result of failure of thymopoietin production and faulty T-cell maturation.[5–9]

Combined Humoral and Cell-Mediated Immunodeficiency

Several different etiologies have been proposed for the different classifications of severe combined immunodeficiency disease (SCID), ranging from partially depressed immunity to a complete lack of responsiveness. Genetically, SCID may be inherited as an X-linked recessive (X-linked lymphopenic agammaglobulinemia) or as an autosomal recessive (Swiss-type lymphopenic agammaglobulinemia) trait. Because many of the affected children die before a diagnosis can be made, the exact incidence of SCID is unknown. There are two theories about the origin of SCID and its variants. The first assumes a failure of the lymphoid stem cells to differentiate into mature lymphocytes. The second theory is that normal stem cells exist, but the primary lymphoid organs are nonfunctional. *Nezelof's*

syndrome is a loose grouping of variable immunologic deficiencies with no known etiology, characterized by marked cell-mediated defects and variable humoral abnormalities. *Ataxia-telangiectasia* involves not only the immune system, but also the nervous, endocrine, and vascular systems. *Wiskott-Aldrich syndrome* is an X-linked ID characterized by hypercatabolism of immunoglobulins. No satisfactory etiology has been advanced for ataxia-telangiectasia or Wiskott-Aldrich syndromes.[5–8, 10] A summary of disorders involving lymphocytes may be found in Table 46–3.

Adenosine Deaminase/Nucleoside Phosphorylase Deficiency

Adenosine deaminase (ADA) and nucleoside phosphorylase (NP) are both involved in the normal catabolism of purines (Fig. 46–4). Deficiencies in either of these enzymes results in a gradual buildup of biochemically toxic intermediates.[5–8, 11]

Phagocytic Cell Deficiencies

The primary deficiencies of phagocytic function (Box 46–1) are usually related to an inability to complete the bactericidal pathway, often due to an enzyme deficiency.[2–6, 12] Generally, little difficulty is encountered when responding to viral infection.

Chronic Granulomatous Disease

There are numerous biochemical defects described that produce chronic granulomatous disease (CGD), but the most common is defective or absent nicotinamide adenine dinucleotide/nicotinamide adenine dinucleotide phosphate (NADH/NADPH). This results in decreased oxygen metabolism and, consequently, ineffective bactericidal activity. It is inherited predominantly as an X-linked disorder, although a female variant has been described.[13]

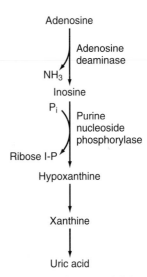

Figure 46–4. Enzyme-induced immunodeficiencies. Abbreviation: P_i, inorganic phosphate.

Immunodeficiency Disorders Affecting Phagocytic Cells

Defective Bactericidal Enzyme Systems

NADH/NADPH oxidase, NADH reductase (CGD)
Lysosomal proteases (Chédiak-Higashi syndrome)
Glucose-6-phosphate dehydrogenase
Myeloperoxidase
Alkaline phosphatase

Defective Chemotactic Responses

Tuftsin deficiency
Lazy leukocyte syndrome
Hyper-IgE syndrome
Glycogen storage diseases

CHÉDIAK-HIGASHI SYNDROME

Chédiak-Higashi syndrome is an autosomal recessive multisystem disorder. The bactericidal defect is seen as an increased killing time, likely due to abnormal lysosomal enzymes. Natural killer (NK) cell activity is also reduced.[5–8, 11]

Complement Deficiencies

Activated components of the complement cascade are necessary for optimal bactericidal activity, neutrophil chemotaxis, and immune adherence. The etiology of complement component deficiency is most often a result of either decreased synthesis or increased catabolism.[1, 2, 14, 15]

Secondary Immunodeficiency States

Secondary ID states (Table 46–4) are the result of some exogenous influence. These may be disease related (as with tumors or infectious agents), drug induced, or even dietary. Depending on the etiology, secondary IDs may be transient or permanent.[1–3]

CLINICAL MANIFESTATIONS

Very often the presenting symptoms provide the first indication as to which part of the immune system is abnormal. For example, abnormalities in humoral immunity of-

Table 46–3. Features of Some Human Primary Immunodeficiency Disorders Involving Lymphocytes

Disorder	Functional Deficiencies	Presumed Cellular Level of Defect	Molecular Level of Defect
X-linked agammaglobulinemia	Antibody	Pre-B cell	Xq22; B-cell-specific tyrosine kinase (BTK)
Immunodeficiency with elevated IgM	IgG and IgA antibodies	IgG, IgA B lymphocytes; "switch" T cells	Xq26–27 (qp39, ligand for CD40) in X-linked type
Common variable immunodeficiency (acquired hypogamma-globulinemia)	Antibody	B lymphocyte	?6p21.3
Selective IgA deficiency	IgA antibody	IgA B lymphocyte	?6p21.3
IgG subclass deficiencies; κ-chain deficiency	Antibody	B lymphocyte; immunoglobulin heavy- or light-chain gene deletions	2p11; 14q32.3
X-linked lymphoproliferative disease	IgG subclasses; anti–Epstein-Barr early antigen antibody	B cell; ?also T cell	Xq25–26
DiGeorge's syndrome	T cellular; some antibody	Dysmorphogenesis of third and fourth branchial pouches	22q11 submicroscopic deletions
Severe combined immunodeficiency syndromes (autosomal recessive; ADA deficiency; X-linked recessive; reticular dysgenesis)	Antibody and T cellular; phagocytic in reticular dysgenesis	Unknown; metabolic defect(s); T, B, and NK cells; ?stem cell; ?recombinase deficiency	Xq13.1–21.1 (γ chain of IL-2R in X-linked); 20qter (ADA deficiency)
Nezelof's syndrome (including with purine nucleoside phosphorylase [PNP] deficiency)	T cellular, some antibody	Unknown; ?thymus; ?T cell; metabolic defects	14q3.1 (PNP deficiency)
Cartilage-hair hypoplasia	T cellular	G1 cycle of many cells	Unknown
Wiskott-Aldrich syndrome	Antibody, T cellular	Unknown	Xp11–11.3
Ataxia-telangiectasia	Antibody, T cellular	B lymphocyte; helper T lymphocyte	11q22.3
MHC antigen deficiencies	Humoral and cellular	Defective synthesis of class I or II antigens	Unknown
Leukocyte adhesion deficiencies (LAD 1 and LAD 2)	Cytotoxic lymphocytes, phagocytic cells	All leukocytes	21q22.3; 95-kD β chain (CD18) of CD11a (LFA-1), CD11b (CR3), and CD11c (p150, 95); Sialyl-Lewis X ligand of E selectin
Hyperimmunoglobulinemia E	Specific immune responses; excessive IgE	Unknown	Unknown

From Paul WE: Fundamental Immunology. ed 3. New York, Raven Press, 1993. Used with permission.

Table 46–4. Secondary Immunodeficiency Disorders

Etiologic Agent	Affected Immune Parameters
Pathogens	
Rubella	Decreased T-cell function
	Decreased antibody response
	Immunoglobulin deficiency
Leprosy/tuberculosis	Decreased delayed-type hypersensitivity (DTH) response
	Hyper-Ig in leprosy
Coccidioidomycosis	Decreased T-cell function
Cytomegalovirus (CMV)	CMI anergy to CMV
	Hyper-IgM and -IgA
Human immunodeficiency virus	T cell lysis; depressed interleukin-2 (IL-2)
Malignant/Autoimmune Disease	
Leukemias/lymphomas	Variable T- or B-cell defects
Myelomas	Abnormal antibody response
Nonhematopoietic tumors	Increasing T- and B-cell anergy with tumor burden
Connective tissue disease	Decreased T-cell levels
	Abnormal T-cell function
	Hypergammaglobulinemia
	Variable complement defects
Chronic hepatitis	Decreased T-cell numbers
	Decreased T-cell function
	Hypergammaglobulinemia
Miscellaneous Clinical Conditions With Variable Deficiencies	
Diabetes	
Alcoholism	
Malnutrition	
Burns	
Sarcoidosis	
Splenectomy	
Sickle cell disease	
Uremia	
Down syndrome	
Immunosuppressive Regimens	
Steroids	Short-term decrease in T- and B-cell numbers
	Reduced Ig synthesis
	Reduced phagocytosis
Antimetabolites	Generalized suppression
Alkylating agents	
Radiation	
Antithymocyte globulin	Variable effects on T-cell numbers and function, some T-dependent antibodies depressed
Cyclosporine	Depressed synthesis of Il-2

ten result in chronic or recurrent infections with pyogenic bacteria. Patients with defects in CMI are subject to disseminated viral and fungal infections (Box 46–2). Recurrent gram-negative infections may signal a phagocytic function deficiency. Patients generally exhibit pallor, malaise, and appear chronically ill.

B Cell Immunodeficiencies

BRUTON'S AGAMMAGLOBULINEMIA

The majority of individuals affected by Bruton's agammaglobulinemia do not encounter any clinical problems for the first 4 to 6 months of life because of the protective effect of maternal IgG. Beyond this age, however, the affected child will begin to suffer from chronic, recurrent bacterial infections. Diagnosis may be delayed at this point because of a good response to antibiotic therapy. The most common presenting symptoms are otitis media, bronchitis, pneumonia, meningitis, dermatitis, and, rarely, arthritis and malabsorption. Generally, the infections are of a pyogenic nature, with *Streptococcus pneumoniae* and *Haemophilus influenzae* implicated most often. Gram-negative infections are also common. One indication that hypogammaglobulinemia may be present is an incomplete response to antimicrobials, or failure to clear infections completely.

Chronic low-grade infections often result in progressive tissue damage, especially respiratory or neurologic. There also appears to be an increased risk of developing leukemia or lymphoma. For the most part, patients with defective antibody synthesis have an intact cell-mediated response and are not usually at risk for viral or fungal infections.[1, 3, 5, 9, 16, 17]

TRANSIENT NEONATAL HYPOGAMMAGLOBULINEMIA

Transient, or physiologic, hypogammaglobulinemia mimics Bruton's agammaglobulinemia in many of the clinical manifestations, and a differential diagnosis must be made with care.[9]

ACQUIRED HYPOGAMMAGLOBULINEMIA

Patients with variable unclassifiable ID will present with the classic symptoms of X-linked immunoglobulin deficiency. Recurrent upper respiratory tract infections with pyogenic bacteria are common. A small percentage will progress to a protein-losing malabsorption syndrome. The two major differences are that the acquired condition does not appear until later in life, typically 15 to 30 years, and that both sexes are affected. This group of immunodeficient patients may also present with cell-mediated abnormalities, and seems to be more prone to a variety of autoimmune diseases and tumors.[1, 3, 5, 9]

SELECTIVE IgA DEFICIENCY

As might be expected, the most common presenting symptom in patients with selective IgA deficiency is recur-

---

Box 46–2. Presenting Symptoms in Immunodeficiency Disorders

Often Found

- Chronic or recurrent infections
- Opportunistic or unusual pathogens
- Incomplete response to therapy
- Failure to thrive

Occasionally Found

- Rash/eczema
- Chronic diarrhea/malabsorption
- Hepatosplenomegaly
- Growth retardation
- Abscesses
- Autoimmune disease

rent infections, chiefly viral or bacterial sinopulmonary events. A strong linkage exists between selective IgA deficiency and atopy. Of clinical importance is the subgroup of IgA-deficient individuals who produce high titers of IgG anti-IgA, which place them at risk for anaphylactic reactions to plasma proteins.

Because of the role of IgA in mucosal immunity, it is not surprising that these patients suffer from a variety of gastrointestinal disorders. Celiac disease, ulcerative colitis, and regional enteritis are all associated with IgA deficiency. IgA-deficient individuals are also at increased risk for pernicious anemia, with autoantibodies to both intrinsic factor and gastric parietal cells. IgA deficiency also predisposes the individual to other autoimmune disorders, particularly systemic lupus erythematosus and rheumatoid arthritis. Other autoimmune disease associations described are thyroiditis, Coombs'-positive hemolytic anemia, and chronic hepatitis.[5, 6, 9]

Cell-Mediated Immunodeficiencies

DiGeorge's Syndrome

The congenital physical abnormalities of DiGeorge's syndrome are usually the means of early diagnosis. The embryologic trauma results in a newborn with structural defects in the eyes, ears, and mouth; hypoparathyroidism; and congenital heart disease. The most common symptoms in a patient with DiGeorge's syndrome is early-onset refractory hypocalcemia. Should the newborn survive the gross anatomic abnormalities, the immunologic defects will become manifest. Chronic infections with numerous pathogens may produce pneumonia, diarrhea, mucosal candidiasis, and failure to thrive.[1, 3, 5, 9]

Combined Humoral and Cell-Mediated Immunodeficiencies

Severe Combined Immunodeficiency Disease

SCID patients are prone to infection with any potential pathogen. In fact, they rarely survive longer than 1 year after birth. Maternal IgG offers only limited protection. Presenting symptoms of individuals with SCID include pneumonia, sepsis, oral candidiasis, otitis media, and a generalized failure to thrive. These patients are particularly susceptible to the opportunistic pathogens, notably *Candida*, cytomegalovirus, and *Pneumocystis carinii*.[3, 5, 18, 19]

Symptoms of the SCID variants is similar, with some exceptions. Nezelof's syndrome often presents with lymphadenopathy and hepatosplenomegaly.

Ataxia-telangiectasia can be identified by neurologic and endocrine disorders. Selective IgA deficiency and consistently elevated levels of α-fetoprotein are common findings.

Patients with Wiskott-Aldrich syndrome develop recurrent bacterial infections beginning at the age of about 6 months. Viral infections occur as the patient ages. Nonimmunologic manifestations include thrombocytopenia present from birth, with bleeding tendencies during infectious episodes. Eczema is found at about the age of 1 year.[3, 5, 20, 21]

Phagocytic Deficiencies

Chronic Granulomatous Disease

Patients with CGD often present in early childhood with recurrent infections caused by a variety of nonpathogenic or opportunistic organisms. Draining nodes, lymphadenopathy, and hepatosplenomegaly are also seen.[5]

Chédiak-Higashi Syndrome

The major symptomatology in Chédiak-Higashi syndrome includes recurrent bacterial infections, hepatosplenomegaly, central nervous system defects, natural killer (NK) cell dysfunction, and increased risk of lymphoreticular neoplasms.[5, 16, 19]

Complement Deficiencies

Depending on which specific component of complement is defective or absent, there may be a range of clinical effects as follows:

C1 deficiency has been described in individuals with other IDs and some autoimmune disorders. The degree of increased risk of bacterial infection will vary sharply.

C2 deficiency has been strongly linked to systemic lupus-like disorders with renal disease and positive antinuclear antibodies.[22] These patients are at risk for bacterial infections.

C3 deficiency has been described in several patients, with increased risk of infection and nephritis.

C4 abnormalities have been found in a range of patients, from those who are asymptomatic to those with lupus-like syndromes. Human leukocyte antigen (HLA) associations have been noted in some cases. These patients exhibit decreased chemotactic responses and diminished immune adherence.

C5, C6, C7, and C8 deficiencies have been seen in numerous cases, predisposing the affected individual to repeated meningococcal or gonococcal infections. C7 deficiency is strongly linked to connective tissue disease.

Secondary Immunodeficiencies

In general, the clinical manifestations of secondary IDs are extremely variable and are largely dependent on the agent producing the deficiency. Any or all combinations of humoral, cellular, phagocytic, or complement defects have been described.

LABORATORY ANALYSES AND DIAGNOSIS

A summary of laboratory tests for the evaluation of ID states is shown in Box 46–3.

B Cell Deficiency States

Bruton's Agammaglobulinemia

Diagnosis of a hypogammaglobulinemic state can be made easily, based on serum electrophoresis and serum immunoglobulin class quantitation. In most cases, total

Box 46–3. Laboratory Tests in the Evaluation of Immunodeficiency Disorders

Cell-Mediated Immunity

Absolute lymphocyte count
Monoclonal analysis of T-cell subpopulations
Mitogen- and antigen-induced proliferation (blastogenesis)
Delayed-type hypersensitivity skin testing

Humoral Immunity

Absolute lymphocyte count
Monoclonal analysis of total B cells, surface immunoglobulin (SIg) subpopulations
Quantitation of immunoglobulin levels
In vitro antibody production to mitogen or antigen challenge

Phagocytic Function

Phagocytosis, with and without antibody-coated particles
Chemotaxis
NBT reduction and chemiluminescence
Myeloperoxidase levels

Complement

Total hemolytic complement
Quantitation of individual components
Chemotactic activity of serum

---

serum Ig levels are in the range of 200 to 250 mg/dL, with IgG constituting about 80% of the total immunoglubin. Levels of the other four classes of antibody a loss of B cells, depending on the severity of the immunoglobulin deficiency. Tests for CMI, such as DTH skin testing or mitogenic stimulation, most often prove normal in individuals more than 1 year of age.[5, 9, 16, 17]

Transient Neonatal Hypogammaglobulinemia

Laboratory evaluation is essential in a differential diagnosis of transient neonatal hypogammaglobulinemia and Bruton's agammaglobulinemia. This is done by determining the levels of individual Ig classes. Although the levels of IgM and IgA are abnormal in Bruton's agammaglobulinemia, patients with transient hypogammaglobulinemia have normal age-matched levels of these two immunoglobulin classes.[23] Serial Ig level determinations indicate increasing levels of IgM and IgA, which further supports the diagnosis of a temporary physiologic aberration in immunoglobulin production.[5, 9]

Acquired Hypogammaglobulinemia

Patients with acquired hypogammaglobulinemia do have normal levels of circulating B cells, but lymph node biopsy specimens reveal an absence of plasma cells. Immunoglobulin levels are usually in the region of 300 mg/dL, and IgG is usually less than 250 mg/dL. Both IgA and IgM levels vary. Cell-mediated immune abnormalities include absence of DTH response in patient when tested, depressed mitogen stimulation, and low levels of circulating T cells.[5, 9]

Selective IgA Deficiency

By convention, IgA deficiency occurs when an individual presents with an IgA serum level of less than 5 mg/dL, with normal or increased levels of the other immunoglobulin classes. The number of circulating peripheral B cells is in the normal range. Generally, all tests of CMI are normal. Patients who have cell-mediated defects must be carefully monitored for the possible development of ataxia-telangiectasia.[9]

Cell-Mediated Immunodeficiencies

DiGeorge's Syndrome

Because of the immaturity of the cell-mediated immune response in a normal neonate, the functional immunologic testing required to determine a T-cell defect must be interpreted with caution. Nevertheless, the total T-cell count is usually depressed ($<1200/\mu L$), and determination of T-cell numbers with monoclonal antibodies reveals a striking decrease in T-cell populations. Functional studies of the immune system, such as DTH or lymphocyte mitogen stimulation, usually result in negative responses.

Another nonimmunologic laboratory test that helps to establish a diagnosis of DiGeorge's syndrome are radiographs, which can determine the absence of a thymic shadow. When coupled with the demonstration of elevated serum phosphorus, low serum calcium, and absent parathyroid hormone levels, these findings are strongly supportive of DiGeorge's syndrome.[1, 3, 5, 9]

Combined Humoral and Cell-Mediated Immunodeficiencies

Severe Combined Immunodeficiency Disease

Humoral immune responses in suspected SCID patients should be evaluated by serial determinations of IgM and IgA levels, which normally increase with time. Serum IgG is more difficult to assess because of the presence of maternal IgG. However, a continually declining IgG level combined with a failure of IgM and IgA to increase is an important finding, especially in infants with repeated infections. Most SCID patients have severely depressed or totally absent peripheral B-cell levels.

Likewise, tests for CMI are abnormal, and peripheral T-cell levels are significantly depressed. Functional studies such as mitogen stimulation or mixed lymphocyte culture generally show no response. DTH testing does not provide meaningful data. Because of the possibility of SCID resulting from a deficiency in enzymes of the purine metabolic pathway, differential diagnosis must include a determination of ADA and NP levels, both of which should be in the normal range.[17]

NEZELOF'S SYNDROME

All laboratory tests of immune function are variable in patients with Nezelof's syndrome. Although the levels of circulating B cells are usually within normal limits, the levels of each immunoglobulin class will vary. There is no specific antibody response following immunization. A differential diagnosis based on these findings can be difficult. It is often necessary to do further nonimmunologic testing to rule out ataxia-telangiectasia or Wiskott-Aldrich syndrome.

ATAXIA-TELANGIECTASIA

The immunologic defects seen in ataxia-telangiectasia are similar to those seen in Nezelof's syndrome in that most cell-mediated and humoral immune parameters are affected to a variable degree in each patient. Selective IgA deficiency is a common finding. The presence of neurologic and endocrine disorders is important in establishing a differential diagnosis. Consistently elevated levels of α-fetoprotein are a common finding.[9]

WISKOTT-ALDRICH SYNDROME

Early in the Wiskott-Aldrich syndrome, CMI is within normal limits, but it may decline progressively with age. Normal levels of circulating B cells are present, but serum immunoglobulin analysis reveals levels of decreased IgM and increased IgA and immunoglobulin E (IgE). This pattern may not appear until 1 year of age. Paraproteinemia may also be present.[9, 18, 19, 21]

Phagocytic Deficiency States

CHRONIC GRANULOMATOUS DISEASE

The peripheral white blood cell count is often elevated in CGD, even when no active infection is present. Immunoglobulin and complement levels may be elevated, with normal function. CMI is normal. The best diagnostic test indication for CGD is the failure to reduce nitroblue tetrazolium (NBT), which would indicate a lack of effective bactericidal capacity. Chemotactic assays are normal, and a correlation presents between CGD and McLeod's phenotype on red blood cells.[9]

CHÉDIAK-HIGASHI SYNDROME

On routine peripheral blood smears, giant cytoplasmic granular inclusion bodies can be found in both white blood cells and platelets in cases of Chédiak-Higashi syndrome. The bactericidal defect of the phagocytic cells is seen as an increased killing time due to abnormal lysosomal enzymes.[5, 16, 19]

Complement Deficiencies

Very often an abnormal hemolytic complement level is the first indication of a complement deficiency. Quantitative analyses of the individual components will be necessary to establish a firm diagnosis.

Secondary Immunodeficiencies

Because of the diverse etiologies of secondary IDs, diagnosis can be difficult. A close examination of the medical history can often give a clue. A screening panel of immunoglobulin and complement levels, absolute lymphocyte count, and evolution of phagocytosis should provide further information.

TREATMENT

B Cell Immunodeficiencies

BRUTON'S AGAMMAGLOBULINEMIA

The treatment of choice for hypogammaglobulinemic patients is intramuscular preparations of γ-globulins supported by broad-spectrum antibiotics. The dose and timing of the γ-globulin should be tailored to the patient's clinical course. Antibiotics should be continued even when no infection is evident, as this appears to decrease the incidence of irreversible tissue damage. It has been suggested that fresh plasma infusions be given occasionally to replace the IgA that is virtually absent in commercial γ-globulin preparations. The major adverse reaction seen in these patients is anaphylaxis, most likely a result of intravenous delivery of aggregated IgG.

Serial determinations of IgG and IgM levels should be performed after each dose of γ-globulin to monitor effective serum levels and to determine when additional doses are required.[9]

TRANSIENT NEONATAL HYPOGAMMAGLOBULINEMIA

If therapy for transient, physiologic neonatal hypogammaglobulinemia is required, it is identical to that for the X-linked condition. In some cases transient hypogammaglobulinemia has lasted for 18 to 24 months before spontaneously normalizing.[5, 9]

SELECTIVE IgA DEFICIENCY

At the present time, no effective immunologic replacement therapy for selective IgA deficiency is available. Patients should not be transfused with plasma or immunoglobulin fractions because of the increased risk of immunization against IgA and subsequent anaphylactic reactions. Broad-spectrum antibiotic therapy is the treatment of choice for this ID state.

Although some patients with selective IgA deficiency have had normal life spans, the majority of affected individuals present with clinical problems within the first 10 years of life. Careful monitoring and aggressive antibiotic intervention are necessary.[9]

Cell-Mediated Immunodeficiencies

DIGEORGE'S SYNDROME

Once a diagnosis of congenital thymic aplasia has been made, a fetal thymic transplant should be performed as soon as feasible. To avoid potential graft-vs.-host reactions, the thymus should be obtained from a fetus of less than 14 weeks of gestation. Alternatively, treatment with thymosin or other thymic hormones has been attempted with mixed success. The prognosis for the individual with DiGeorge's syndrome is guarded at best. Although there are some reports of good short-term survival, the numbers of patients who have received thymic grafts is insufficient to draw any firm conclusions. Those with successful grafts have displayed a variable reconstitution of their immune functions. An added problem is that patients who have been successfully engrafted may still suffer morbidity and mortality from their other congenital anomalies.[5, 9]

Combined Humoral and Cell-Mediated Immunodeficiencies

SEVERE COMBINED IMMUNODEFICIENCY DISEASE

Unless heroic measures are taken, the overwhelming majority of SCID individuals do not survive the first year. The major goal is to prevent systemic infections and the ensuing complications. Supportive therapy consists of aggressive antibiotic treatment and γ-globulin infusions as often as required. The only definitive therapy for SCID is bone marrow transplantation. A successful transplant results in the appearance of some immune functions.[5, 9, 24]

NEZELOF'S SYNDROME

Therapy consists of aggressive antibiotic support and γ-globulin infusions. Experimental therapies have included bone marrow and thymic transplants, but neither has proven beneficial. Patients rarely survive beyond the age of 18 years.[5, 9]

ATAXIA-TELANGIECTASIA

Prophylactic antibiotics and γ-globulin lessen the severity of the recurrent infections, but no curative therapy is available. Although some patients have survived into their fifth decade, the majority will succumb earlier to infection or neoplasm.[5, 9]

WISKOTT-ALDRICH SYNDROME

Intravenous γ-globulin and antibiotic therapy are used, although bone marrow transplantation has been performed. Therapy is complicated by the concurrent thrombocytopenia. Although the prognosis has improved somewhat, patients who survive infectious complications often develop lymphoreticular or hematopoietic neoplasms.[5, 9, 16, 21]

ADA/NP DEFICIENCY

ADA-deficient individuals have been treated with red blood cells as a temporary source of the enzyme, but the definitive treatment for either enzyme deficiency remains bone marrow transplantation. Successful engraftment will result in normalization of enzyme levels. ADA deficiency has been successfully treated with gene therapy. Bone marrow cells are removed and normal copies of the defective gene are inserted by means of a virus vector. The treated

cells are returned to the host's circulation. Successful gene transfer into long-lasting progenitor cells, producing a functional multilineage progeny, has been accomplished.[25–27]

Phagocytic Deficiency States

CHRONIC GRANULOMATOUS DISEASE

In the absence of a definitive cure, aggressive broad-spectrum antibiotic therapy is the treatment of choice to prevent or reduce the severity of the inevitable bacterial infection. Bone marrow transplantation is an effective therapy when long-term antibiotic and interferon therapy are used concurrently. Although improved diagnosis and therapy have produced survival into the second decade, chronic infection and organ dysfunction remain the major causes of morbidity and mortality.[5, 9, 17]

CHÉDIAK-HIGASHI SYNDROME

Treatment with antibiotics alone is ineffective. Bone marrow transplantation is the treatment of choice.[16, 17, 28]

Complement Deficiencies

No specific therapy other than antibiotics has been accepted for C1 deficiency.[5, 9] For C2 deficiency, complement replacement therapy is unwise due to the increased risk of immune complex–mediated tissue damage. The basic therapy involves treating the autoimmune disease and giving antibiotics when infection occurs.[5, 9] Therapy for C5 through C8 deficiencies are limited to specific antibiotics during infectious episodes, although there have been some reports of successful reconstitutive therapy.[5, 9]

Secondary Immunodeficiencies

Because of the diversity of exogenous agents that can produce ID states, the best therapy remains identification and removal (if possible) or replacement of the causative agent. Laboratory testing is helpful in identifying the specific immunologic defect and determining when these parameters have normalized. If the defect is found to be permanent, then selective support or replacement therapy is indicated.

Case Study

A 17-week-old male infant, weighing 9 lb, 2 oz, was seen for chronic diarrhea and sinus infection. *Staphylococcus aureus* was isolated and antibiotics were prescribed. The response was rapid and complete. At 6, 10, and 14 months the child was seen for respiratory tract infections, which partially responded to antibiotics. At 23 months, the child was hospitalized for *H. influenzae* pneumonia. Both height and weight were significantly below normal. Laboratory analyses at this time revealed normal levels of lymphocytes in the peripheral blood. Further analysis by flow cytometry detected normal levels of T cells but less than 1% B cells (normal 5% to 15%). Serum immunoglobulin levels were quantitated, and IgG, IgM, and IgA were all found to be significantly depressed (normal <10%). No other family members were found to have problems.

Questions

1. During the first year of life, what two IDs must be considered, given this patient's history?
2. Given the patient's history over the first 2 years of life and the laboratory findings at the time of hospitalization, what is the most likely diagnosis?
3. What therapy is appropriate with this diagnosis and what is the role of the laboratory in monitoring its effectiveness?

Discussion

1. Bruton's agammaglobulinemia and transitory neonatal hypogammaglobulinemia should be considered.
2. Bruton's agammaglobulinemia is the most likely diagnosis. Recurrent infections in a male infant with only partial response to antibiotics is typical of Bruton's agammaglobulinemia. In addition, the decreased number of B cells, normal level of T cells, and a decrease in immunoglobulins of all classes are consistent with this diagnosis. Only γ-globulin would be decreased in transient neonatal hypogammaglobulinemia.
3. Intramuscular injection of immunoglobulin on a periodic basis is the appropriate treatment in this case, with laboratory monitoring of the immunoglobulin levels.

References

1. Paul WE (ed): Fundamental Immunology, ed 3. New York, Raven Press, 1993.
2. Roitt IM: Essential Immunology. ed 8. Oxford, Blackwell Scientific Publications, 1994.
3. Frank MM, Austen KF, et al (eds): Samter's Immunologic Diseases, ed 5. Boston, Little, Brown & Co, 1995.
4. De la Concha EG, Garcia-Rodriquez MC, Zabay JM, et al: Functional assessment of T and B lymphocytes in patients with selective IgM deficiency. Clin Exp Immunol 49:670, 1982.
5. Waldmann TA, Nelson DL: Inherited immunodeficiencies. *In* Frank MM, Austen KF, et al (eds): Samter's Immunologic Diseases, ed 5. Boston, Little, Brown & Co, 1995.
6. Buckley RH: Primary Immunodeficiency Diseases. *In* Paul WE (ed): Fundamental Immunology, ed 3. New York, Raven Press, 1993.
7. Tiller TL, Buckley RH: Transient hypogammaglobulinemia of infancy: Review of the literature, clinical and immunologic features of 11 new cases, and long-term followup. J Pediatr 92:347, 1978.
8. Siegel RL, Isseekutz T, Schwaber J, et al: Deficiency of T helper cells in transient hypogammaglobulinemia of infancy. N Engl J Med 305:1307, 1981.
9. Knutsen AP, Fischer TJ: Primary Immunodeficiency Diseases. *In* Lawlor GJ, Fischer TJ, Adelman DC (eds): Manual of Allergy and Immunology, ed 3. Boston, Little, Brown & Co, 1995.
10. Pahwa SG, Pahwa RN, Good RA: Heterogeneity of B lymphocyte differentiation in patients with recurrent pyogenic infections. J Clin Invest 66:543, 1980.
11. Hirshorn R, Martin DW: Enzyme defects in immunodeficiency diseases. Semin Immunopathol 1:299, 1978.
12. Quie PG, Root RK, Metcalf JA: Phagocytic defects. Springer Semin Immunopathol 1:323, 1978.
13. Johnston RB, Baehner RL: Chronic granulomatous disease: Correlation between pathogenesis and clinical findings. Pediatrics 48:730, 1971.
14. Agnello V: Complement deficiency states. Medicine 57:1, 1978.
15. Muller-Eberhand HJ: Complement abnormalities in human disease. Hosp Pract 13:65, 1978.
16. Paller AS: Immunodeficiency syndromes. Dermatol Clinics 13:65, 1995.
17. Arbiser JL: Genetic immunodeficiencies: Cutaneous manifestations and recent progress. J Am Acad Dermatol 33:82, 1995.
18. Hitzig WH, Martin DW: Severe combined immunodeficiency diseases. Springer Semin Immunopathol 1:238, 1978.
19. Hague RA, Rassam S, Morgan G, Cant AJ: Early diagnosis of severe combined immunodeficiency syndrome. Arch Dis Child 70:260, 1994.
20. Ochs HD, Slichter SJ, Harker LA: The Wiskott-Aldrich syndrome: Studies of lymphocytes, granulocytes, and platelets. Blood 55:243, 1980.
21. Peacocke M, Siminovitch KA: Wiskott-Aldrich syndrome: New molecular and biochemical insights. J Am Acad Dermatol 27:507, 1992.
22. Day NK: C2 deficiency: Development of lupus erythematosus. J Clin Invest 52:1601, 1973.
23. Schur PH, Rosen F, Norman ME: Immunoglobulin subclasses in normal children. Pediatr Res 63:301, 1979.
24. Filipovich AH: Unrelated donor bone marrow transplantation for correction of lethal congenital immunodeficiencies. Tranfus Sci 12:135, 1991.
25. Bordignon C, Notarangelo LD, Nobili N, et al: Gene therapy in peripheral blood lymphocytes and bone marrow for ADA-immunodeficient patients. Science 270:470, 1995.
26. Blaese RM, Culver KW, Miller AD, et al: T lymphocyte-directed gene therapy for ADA-SCID: Initial trial results after 4 years. Science 270:475, 1995.
27. Dubé ID, Cournoyer D: Gene therapy: Here to stay. Can Med Assoc J 152:1605, 1995.
28. Haddad E, Le Deist F, Blanche S, et al: Treatment of Chediak-Higashi syndrome by allogenic bone marrow transplantation: Report of 10 cases. Blood 85:3328, 1995.

Chapter 47

Allergies

Hal S. Larsen

ETIOLOGY AND PATHOPHYSIOLOGY

The immune system is an essential part of our defenses against pathogenic microorganisms and environmental exposures. In the majority of cases, this response is beneficial, although in certain situations, hypersensitivity results in immune-mediated disease.

Types of Hypersensitivity

The various types of allergies result from immunologic hypersensitivities, which have been classified into four general categories. These categories are based on kinetics of the response and the mechanisms of tissue injury. The four types of hypersensitivity reactions (types I, II, III, and IV), as first classified by Gell and Coombs, are summarized in Table 47–1.[1] Although this classification is useful, it is important to keep in mind that, except for anaphylactic reactions, human disease processes involving hypersensitivity usually include mechanisms from more than one type.

Type I (Immediate) Hypersensitivity

Type I, or "immediate," hypersensitivity is characterized by an immune response within 15 minutes following contact with the antigen. The allergic response can be either generalized, as in anaphylactic shock, or localized, as in allergic rhinitis and asthma. This type of hypersensitivity depends on specific triggering of immunoglobulin (Ig) E–sensitized mast cells by the antigen, followed by release of powerful pharmacologic mediators and cytokines (Fig. 47–1A). Cross-linking of the IgE molecules serves as the most important event in the release of mast cell substances. These released substances cause greater vascular permeability as well as a number of other inflammation-related effects.[1, 2]

The mast cell and basophil are important sources of substances that mediate the clinical effects of immediate hypersensitivity. Mast cells are widely distributed in the connective tissues and are especially prevalent along small blood vessels. Their cytoplasm is filled with granules that are the source of the mediators of inflammation. Basophils are found in very low numbers in the circulation and are rarely seen in the tissue of normal individuals. They resemble mast cells, in that they contain deep violet-blue granules when stained with Wright's stain that contain pharmacologic mediators, and they bind IgE. The two types of cells metabolize arachidonic acid in similar ways; however, they differ in a number of other characteristics, and it is believed that the origins of mast cells and basophils are different.[3, 4]

An increase in eosinophils may also be seen in individuals with type I hypersensitivity. These cells appear at the site of the hypersensitivity reactions and produce substances that inhibit the release or action of some of the mast cell mediators.[2, 4]

Type II (Cytotoxic) Hypersensitivity

Type II, or cytotoxic, reactions (Fig. 47–1B) are mediated by binding of cell-bound antigen with either IgG or IgM antibody. The binding activates the complement cascade and causes destruction of the cell that was binding the antigen. Examples of diseases that result from type II hypersensitivity are immune hemolytic anemia and hemo-

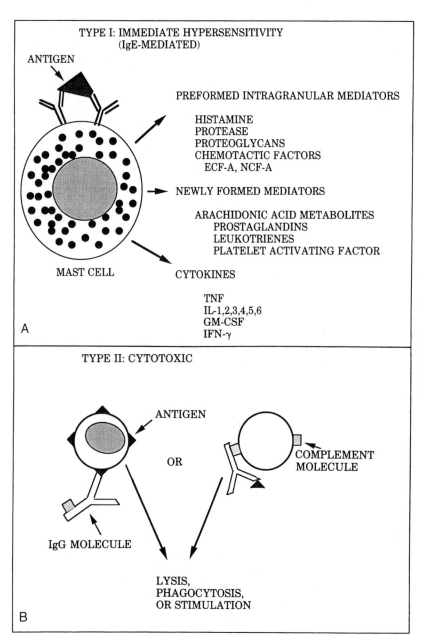

Figure 47–1. Four classifications *(A–D)* of allergic reactions: *(A)* Immediate Hypersensitivity, *(B)* Cytotoxic, *(C)* Immune complex mediated reactions, and *(D)* Cell-mediated delayed hypersensitivity. Abbreviations: TNF, tumor necrosis factor; IL, interleukin; GM-CSF, granulocyte/monocyte–macrophage colony-stimulating factor; IFN-8, interferon-8; ECE-A, eosinophil chemotactic factor of anaphylaxis; NCF, neutrophil chemotactic factor. (From Lawlor GJ, Fischer TH, Adelman DC: Manual of Allergy and Immunology, ed 3. Boston, Little, Brown & Co, 1995.)

Table 47–1. **Pathways of Inflammation**

Type	Name	Antigen	Immune Response	Time After Antigen Exposure	Mediators	Pathology
I*	Immediate hypersensitivity	Soluble	IgE antibody	15 min	Histamine, LTC4	Mast cell degranulation
II	Cytotoxic	Cell bound	IgG or IgM antibody	—	Complement-dependent cytotoxicity or antibody-dependent cell-mediated cytoxicity	Antibody deposition; tissue damage
III	Immune complex	Soluble	IgG antibody	4–6 hr	Complement (C5a); neutrophil proteases	Neutrophil accumulation
IVA	Delayed hypersensitivity	Soluble	Lymphokine-producing T cells	>24 hr	Lymphokines (e.g., IFN); macrophage proteases	Macrophage infiltrate
IVB	—	Cell bound	CTL	—	CTL-mediated cytotoxicity	CTL infiltrate; tissue damage

*LPR (late-phase response) with inflammatory infiltrate of eosinophils and other cells are characteristic of IgE-dependent reactions but do not occur immediately; see text.

From Paul WE: Fundamental Immunology, ed 3. New York, Raven Press, 1993.

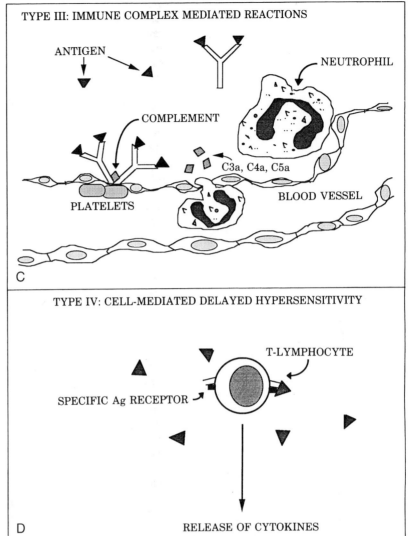

Figure 47–1 *Continued*

lytic disease of the newborn. Myasthenia gravis and autoimmune hyperthyroidism are the results of immune cytotoxic reactions.[2, 4, 5]

Type III (Immune Complex) Hypersensitivity

Type III reactions are also referred to as immune complex reactions (Figure 47–1*C*). The antigen-antibody complexes are deposited in tissues or blood vessel walls and produce an acute inflammatory reaction. The reaction occurs 4 to 6 hours after antigen-antibody binding. The neutrophil plays a major role in this reaction. Complement components such as C3a, C4a, and C5a activate neutrophils to release proteases, which induce tissue injury. Examples of type III reactions are serum sickness and immune complex glomerulonephritis.[2, 4, 5]

Type IV (Delayed) Hypersensitivity

Delayed or type IV hypersensitivity reactions occur 24 hours or longer after antigen-sensitized lymphocyte interaction (Fig. 47–1*D*). Unlike the first three types of hypersensitivity, type IV is a result of sensitized lymphocytes that secrete cytokines following antigen contact. A mononuclear cell infiltrate forms at the site in response to the immune mediators. A diagram of the cellular responses involved in this type of hypersensitivity is shown in Figure 47–2. Examples of type IV reactions are the tuberculin skin test, contact dermatitis, and the chronic granuloma seen in some infectious processes.[2, 4, 5]

CLINICAL MANIFESTATIONS

Type I Immediate Hypersensitivity Disorders

The common allergic respiratory diseases affect millions of persons. The clinical manifestations of allergic disease are summarized in Table 47–2. Nearly 10% of the population suffer to some extent with allergies to extrinsic allergens.[5] Inhalant allergens are most commonly involved and are usually derived from natural organic sources, such as house dust, mold spores, insect products, pollens, and animal epithelial products.

Seasonal allergic disease is usually due to pollens such as ragweed, molds, and insects. Inhalant allergens are most

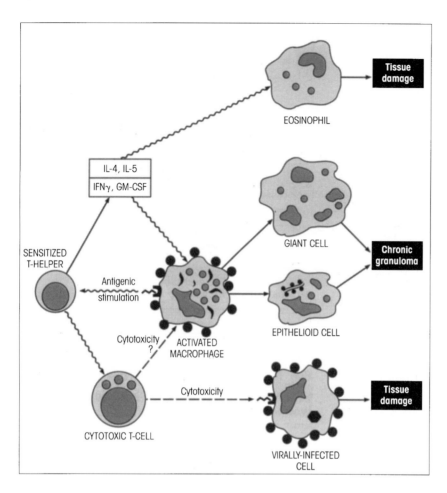

Figure 47–2. The cellular basis of type IV hypersensitivity. (From Roit IM: Essential Immunology, ed 8. Oxford, Blackwell Scientific Publications, 1994. Reprinted by permission of Blackwell Science, Inc.)

often responsible for rhinitis, conjunctivitis, and asthma, and they occasionally cause urticaria or systemic anaphylaxis. Year-round allergies are due to exposure to nonseasonal allergens, such as dust, animal danders, some plant products, and molds. In addition, occupational exposure to certain chemicals has been shown to be a growing cause of allergic rhinitis, asthma, or both.

The dose of exposure, the route of exposure, and the genetic background of the host all interact to determine the magnitude of the IgE response to allergens.[1] The allergen makes contact with IgE-bound mast cells found in the

bronchial tree, nasal mucosa, and conjunctival tissues. The localized release of the mast cell substances gives the symptoms of asthma, allergic rhinitis, and hay fever, respectively.

Allergic Asthma

Allergic asthma is an IgE-mediated problem in which patients have a specific sensitivity to common inhaled substances, such as house dust, mold spores, and other "indoor" allergens. Cytokine and mediator pathways lead to many of the symptoms of asthma (Fig. 47–3). Other aspects of the disease, however, have yet to be attributed to known mechanisms.[6]

Asthma, the most common chronic lung disorder, is seen in persons of all ages. Onset is usually before 5 years of age, but symptoms may begin at any age. The course of disease, diagnosis, and treatment can be complex. Asthma involves the large and small bronchi and is characterized by wheezing and breathlessness, often with cough and sputum production. There is reduction in the airway diameter owing to constriction of smooth muscle, edema of the mucous membranes and bronchial wall tissues, accumulation of thick tenacious secretions, and inflammatory changes in the bronchial mucosa. This obstruction of the air flow can be reversed with medication or with time. Infection, atelectasis, and cardiovascular complications may occur secondary to an acute or chronic asthmatic

Table 47–2. Clinical Manifestations of Allergic Disease

Site of Antigen Exposure	Diseases
Respiratory	Allergic rhinitis
	Asthma
	Hypersensitivity pneumonitis
Cutaneous	Atopic dermatitis
	Urticaria
	Angioedema (anaphylaxis)
Digestive	Food allergy
	(Urticaria)
	(Angioedema)
	(Anaphylaxis)
Anaphylaxis	Anaphylaxis due to allergenic extracts, drugs, insect stings, food

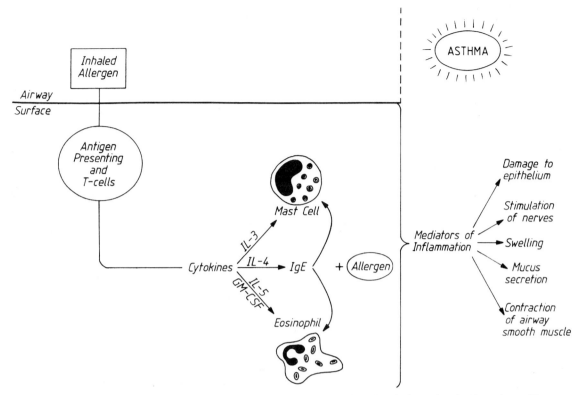

Figure 47–3. Relation of allergen exposure, cytokine release, and disordered airway function in asthma. (From Bradding P, Freezer NJ, Sheffer AL, et al: Asthma. *In* Frank MM, Austen KF, Claman HN, et al (eds): Samter's Immunologic Diseases, ed 5. Boston, Little, Brown & Co, 1995.)

attack. Asthma is classified as extrinsic, intrinsic, mixed, or occupational.

Extrinsic asthma results from exposure to environmental allergens. Onset is usually before 20 years of age. This type is associated with atopy or a type I (allergic) reaction.

Symptoms of *intrinsic asthma* are unrelated to allergen exposure (nonallergic). Infection, exercise, psychologic stimuli, and climatic changes trigger a reaction. This type is more common in patients older than 30 years. Some patients with intrinsic asthma have a clinical intolerance to aspirin that manifests as rhinitis, nasal polyps, or exacerbations of asthma. The mechanism of aspirin-induced asthma is associated with manipulation of arachidonic acid metabolism. The formation of leukotrienes and other substances result in bronchospasm, increased mucus production, and airway edema.[6]

In *mixed asthma,* symptoms are caused by both allergic and nonallergic factors. This is the type most common in childhood.

Occupational asthma is as a result of workplace exposure to specific proteins or low-molecular-weight chemicals. Materials such as chemicals, wood dusts, metals, dyes, animal and plant products, and vegetable gums (latex) have been shown to cause occupational asthma.[1, 2, 5, 7]

Allergic Rhinitis

Symptoms of allergic rhinitis can occur when the sensitized individual inhales allergen. The IgE-mediated reaction initiates a rapid release of various mediators from mast cells (see Fig. 47–1*A*). These mediators cause vasodilation

and edema (nasal congestion), increased mucus secretion and cellular recruitment (rhinorrhea), and increased capillary and mucosal permeability. The mediators probably also disturb the balanced nervous control of nasal function, leading to direct and reflex vascular dilation and hypersecretion and also lowering the sneezing threshold. Symptoms are usually seasonal but may be perennial if the allergen is constantly present. Complications such as sinusitis, ear infections, or nasal polyps can occur.

A variety of types of rhinitis and other nasal conditions must be considered in the differential diagnosis of allergic rhinitis. They include eosinophilic nonallergic rhinitis, vasomotor rhinitis of pregnancy, vasomotor rhinitis, rhinitis medicamentosa, and disturbance of nasal function associated with a number of clinical conditions (tumors, ciliary dyskinesia, hypothroidism, aspirin intolerance, and others). A significant percentage of cases of chronic rhinitis are assigned to one of these poorly understood categories.

Allergic rhinitis is associated with symptoms of nasal discharge or obstruction, sneezing, itching of the nose, eyes, palate, pharynx, and conjunctivae, and mucous discharge. Patients may show irritability, fatigue, depression, and anorexia. Maxillofrontal headache, postnasal discharge, and persistent nasal stuffiness may indicate complicating inflammatory sinusitis. Symptoms related to accompanying serous otitis and eustachian tube dysfunction may also be present, particularly in children.[8, 9]

Hypersensitivity Pneumonitis

Hypersensitivity pneumonitis is a general term that identifies a variety of clinical conditions, all with more fanciful descriptions. "Pituitary snufftaker's lung," "doghouse disease," "farmer's lung," "wheat weevil disease," and "bird fancier's lung" are a few of the clinical descriptions. All of these illnesses have in common the inhalation of organic material that leads to airway and lung parenchymal hypersensitivity reactions in susceptible persons.[6] The reaction that occurs in patients susceptible to hypersensitivity pneumonitis is different from that seen in asthma, in that the allergic reaction does not occur immediately following inhalation of the allergen. The onset of signs and symptoms is 4 to 6 hours after exposure, commonly with cough, fever, and dyspnea.[9]

Food Allergies

Food allergies result from ingesting allergen-containing foods, which induce an IgE antibody response.[10] This response may induce vomiting and diarrhea. In addition, the allergen may enter the body when this local inflammation causes a change in gut permeability resulting in skin or lung reactions. This latter process explains how eating certain foods may result in hives or asthma in sensitized individuals.[5] Foods primarily accounting for an allergic response are milk, egg, peanut, nut, wheat, soy, fish, and shellfish. Food allergy in infants often disappears after age 2 years.

Allergic reactions to drugs are quite common. Because many of the drugs are of low molecular weight, they are immunogenic only if they bind to endogenous proteins and serve as a hapten. Penicillin is a classic example.

Hypersensitivity to Latex Rubber

A problem that has become more pronounced over the last several years is immediate hypersensitivity to latex rubber. The allergens appear to be the proteins in the latex, which are contaminants from the rubber plants or are added during latex processing. Severe reactions may occur in medical personnel who wear latex gloves.[1]

Allergic Skin Diseases

Allergic skin diseases are common problems that occur in all age groups. They include atopic dermatitis, urticaria, and angioedema. The exact role of IgE sensitization in these conditions is unclear.

Atopic dermatitis is a difficult disease to characterize and define. The cause(s) are not completely known. It is a common dermatitis characterized by severe pruritus, common onset in infancy, a strong familial propensity, and a tendency to chronicity.

The dermatitis usually begins on cheeks in the first few months after birth. The face, scalp, neck, diaper area, and extensor surface of the extremities are the areas most commonly affected in an infant. The patches are erythematous and edematous and may have weeping or crusted surfaces. During childhood, the face is involved less often, whereas the sides of the neck show lesions. The teenager or adult tends to have localized plaques of dry, thickened skin with varying degrees of redness and scaling.

Patients with atopic dermatitis often have higher levels of serum IgE, have family histories of allergic disease, and develop of allergic rhinitis or asthma.[2, 11]

Urticaria-angioedema is a common problem that has its highest incidence in young adults. It affects 10% to 20% of individuals at some time during their lives. Each lesion may persist for up to 24 hours. *Urticaria,* or hives, appears as pruritic, circumscribed, and elevated erythematous areas of cutaneous edema that involve the superficial portions of the dermis. When the edema extends deeper into the skin or mucous membranes, it is referred to as *angioedema.* A number of conditions may result in urticaria; they include increase in body temperature, friction, sunlight, cold, and exercise.[12]

A common response to aspirin ingestion is development of urticaria-angioedema. Aspirin and related compounds inhibit the biosynthesis of prostaglandin E_2 from arachidonic acid, favoring the synthesis of both prostaglandin F_2, which is a bronchoconstrictor, and leukotrienes.[2]

Anaphylaxis

Symptoms of anaphylaxis may begin within seconds or may take up to an hour to develop. Onset is usually within 5 to 10 minutes. The cardiovascular system, respiratory tract, gastrointestinal tract, and skin are the major organs affected. The most common manifestations of anaphylaxis are urticaria, flushing, and angioedema, although symptoms involving multiple organ systems may be seen. Reactions involving the cardiovascular and respiratory systems are the most serious, and deaths have occurred as the result of laryngeal edema and shock.[13]

Type II (Cytotoxic) Hypersensitivity Disorders

The direct binding of an antibody to an antigen on the surface of a cell produces damage to that cell. The mechanisms of damage may involve either activation of the complete complement sequence, with lysis of the cell, or opsonic effects mediated by receptors for Fc or C3b, which result in phagocytosis and destruction of the cell by phagocytes. Examples of the clinical disorders associated with Type II hypersensitivity are listed in Box 47–1.

Transfusion Reactions

The transfusion of ABO-incompatible blood can have serious consequences. The anti-A and anti-B antibodies found in the circulation of people with type O blood readily react with the A and B blood group substances. Those with type A blood have anti-B antibodies, and those with type

---

Box 47–1. **Type II Hypersensitivity Reactions**

- Transfusion reactions
- Rh incompatibility reaction
- Autoimmune hemolytic anemia
- Drug-induced reactions
- Anti-receptor antibody disease
  Myasthenia gravis
  Graves' disease

B blood have anti-A antibodies, which also react strongly with the corresponding blood group substances. The reacting IgM antibodies are very efficient at binding to the red cells and activating complement. The result is destruction of the red cells. Affected patients may suffer kidney damage from blockage by large amounts of the red cell membrane as well as possible toxic effects from the release of the heme complex.

Rh Incompatibility Reaction

An Rh-negative mother who has been immunized with Rh-positive cells during birth may form anti-Rh antibodies. Subsequent Rh-positive children will be at risk for an Rh incompatibility reaction as a result of IgG antibodies, which cross the placental barrier and reach the fetal circulation. These antibodies bind to the Rh antigen on the red cells of the fetus. The red cells do not agglutinate, because the low density of antigenic sites does not allow for antibody bridges to be formed unless albumin or an anti-immunoglobulin serum (Coombs') is added. The antibody-coated cells are destroyed by the opsonic effect of the Fc portions of the IgG, which bind with the receptors on phagocytic cells. This results in destruction of the fetal or newborn red cells a decreased ability for oxygen transport as well as jaundice from the breakdown products of hemoglobin.

Autoimmune Hemolytic Anemia

Autoantibodies against a patient's own red cells may result in anemia. The autoantibody binds to the red cells and shortens their life span. These cells are cleared by phagocytes when they pass through the liver, spleen, and other tissues of the reticuloendothelial system. The destruction occurs over time, so the anemia is progressive. If the antibody produced binds to the red cells only at lower temperatures, it is called a cold agglutinin. In this case, lowering of the body temperature, such as may occur at the extremities, leads to antibody binding and destruction of the red cells.

Drug-Induced Reactions

Drugs may act as haptens and, when coupled to body components, induce antibody formation. The antibody combines with cells coated with the drug and causes cytotoxic damage. The type of injury depends on the cell type that binds the drug. Binding to platelets results in thrombocytopenia and can give rise to bleeding. Some drugs bind to white blood cells, and others to red blood cells; this binding results in agranulocytosis and hemolytic anemia, respectively.

Antireceptor Antibody Disease

Antibodies against cell receptor molecules on cells can lead to a number of clinical disorders. In myasthenia gravis, for example, antibody to the acetylcholine receptors on motor end plates of muscles leads to muscle weakness of striated muscle groups. Graves' disease results from antibodies to the thyroid-stimulating hormone receptor of thyroid cells and gives rise to hyperthyoidism.

Type III (Immune Complex) Hypersensitivity Disorders

Exposure to an excess of antigen over time (persistent infection, autoimmunity, environmental antigens) may lead to the formation of insoluble antigen-antibody complexes within body sites. This results in acute inflammatory reactions with all of the accompanying problems, such as the Arthus reaction, serum sickness, immune complex disease, and hypersensitivity pneumonitis.

Arthus Reaction

When antigen diffuses toward blood vessels that contain the circulating antibody, the antigen and antibody may form an insoluble complex that accumulates in or near vessel walls. Complement may be bound, and activation of the complement cascade occurs. This increases local permeability of blood vessels, with resulting edema. Neutrophils and platelets are attracted to the site, which may cause stasis of blood flow and blockage of the blood vessels. The vessel wall may hemorrhage, and necrosis of local tissue may occur.[14] The Arthus reaction is uncommonly seen.

Serum Sickness

Serum sickness is seen after therapeutic injection of foreign material that is potentially antigenic as well as therapeutic. Historically, it was caused by repeated injection of horse serum containing the antibodies to bacterial toxins. Affected individuals showed a pruritic rash, fever, arthralgia, swollen joints, and lympadenopathy. Cases of serum sickness are rarely seen today.

Immune Complex Disease

Some individuals produce antibody that cross-reacts with their own normal tissue. This process may result from an infection (e.g., rheumatic fever following streptococcal pharyngitis) or for unknown reasons. Antibody that binds to the basement membrane in the lung and kidney fixes complement and causes membrane damage. The resulting clinical condition is Goodpasture's syndrome, which leads to pulmonary hemorrhage and glomerulonephritis. Rheumatic fever may follow a group A streptococcal infection. The cross-reactive antibodies induced as a result of the infection react with normal cardiac and glomerular antigens. Rheumatoid arthritis occurs from an IgM autoantibody that binds to the Fc portion of normal IgG. The immune complexes deposit in the joints and cause inflammation. Occupational antigens (e.g., moldy hay, dust from pigeon droppings, sugar cane fiber.) may cause a hypersensitivity pneumonitis. This leads to a reaction in the lungs that is similar to the Arthus reaction.

Type IV (Delayed) Hypersensitivity Disorders

Type IV, or delayed hypersensitivity (DH), reaction is characterized by a reaction consisting mainly of erythema and induration. The cellular interactions and mediators involved in DH are very complex. Unlike other forms of hypersensitivity, type IV depends on sensitized T lymphocytes rather than antibodies. Also, the reaction that occurs following intradermal injection of antigen into a sensitized individual peaks within 24 to 48 hours.

Allergic Contact Dermatitis

A common dermatologic problem is allergic contact dermatitis, characterized by a 48-hour delayed eczematous response to the antigen. The most common contact-sensitizing antigens encountered in clinical practice are plants (poison ivy, oak, or sumac), paraphenylenediamine, nickel compounds, rubber compounds, and the dichromates. The diagnosis is based on the distribution of the lesions, medical history, and examination for environmental exposures. The diagnosis can be confirmed by patch testing, which consists of applying the suspected antigen to the patient's skin and covering it with a dressing for 48 hours. An eczematous reaction at the site of the patch test constitutes a positive response. The patch test is important, because an eczematous reaction is not otherwise pathognomonic of allergic contact dermatitis.

Tuberculin-Type Hypersensitivity

Tuberculin-type hypersensitivity is characterized by local induration and swelling, with or without a fever. There is an intense infiltration by mononuclear cells, of which about 50% are lymphocytes, and the remainder monocytes. As the lesion develops, it may become a granulomatous reaction. This type of reaction is often associated with the presence of an infectious agent, such as *Mycobacterium tuberculosis*. Nonmicrobial antigens may also induce this type of reaction, and it may be seen in individuals treated with bacille Calmette-Guérin vaccine.

Allograft Rejection

The rejection of transplants is, to a large extent mediated by sensitized T cells. An inflammatory reaction ensues, causing destruction of the vessels that have vascularized the transplanted tissue. The result is necrosis and death (rejection) of the graft.

LABORATORY ANALYSES AND DIAGNOSIS

Laboratory findings are of little value in anaphylaxis, because the diagnosis must be made and treatment begun in a very short time. On the other hand, diagnosis of the less acute allergic diseases can be aided by the proper in vitro and in vivo studies.

Establishing the diagnosis of chronic allergic rhinitis is difficult, because there is not objective test whose result is pathognomonic. Consequently, diagnosis must be made on the basis of medical history and interview, examination, and laboratory data, including a nasal smear and skin tests. Seasonal allergic rhinitis due to pollens seldom presents a problem in diagnosis, except in efforts to differentiate it from the common cold.[2]

Complete Blood Count

A complete blood count (CBC) should be performed for all patients suspected of having allergic disease. Eosinophilia is a not uncommon finding that, when consistent with the patient's allergic signs and symptoms, often requires no further investigation. Unexplained numbers of eosinophils, particularly in the absence of allergic disease, may indicate parasitic infestation, collagen vascular diseases, malignancy, or drug reactions. In general, allergic diseases are associated with eosinophilia, although it is not a consistent finding. Diagnosis, in most cases, is made on the basis of physical findings and history, with the CBC playing a minor role. Patients with food allergy, however, may demonstrate anemia due to occult gastrointestinal bleeding. In this case, a CBC, whether or not it reveals eosinophilia, is of diagnostic importance.

Although relative eosinophilia is usually determined by the use of the peripheral blood differential counts, absolute eosinophil counts may be more useful in some cases.

Nasal Smear

Nasal smears for eosinophils can be used to evaluate patients with chronic rhinitis. When correlated with historical data and physical findings, these results aid in the determination of the type of rhinitis present. Nasal cytologic examination can be performed on expelled mucus, but a more satisfactory specimen is obtained by scraping the nasal turbinates and mucosal surfaces with a flexible nasal probe. Nasal smears are usually limited to cases with questionable diagnosis and to determinations of chronic allergic rhinitis.

Total Serum IgE

Total serum IgE levels are elevated in many, but not all, patients with allergic (IgE-mediated) disease. Some nonallergic diseases are also associated with an increase in serum IgE, including parasitic, infectious, immunologic, and cutaneous diseases.[2] The total serum IgE level, therefore, does not precisely correlate with the presence or absence of allergy in a patient.

Specific IgE

Measurement of specific IgE can be accomplished by epicutaneous skin tests. In vitro testing for allergen-specific IgE is reserved for situations involving extraordinary sensitivity to allergen, abnormal skin conditions, or required medication that interferes with skin test results. The standard in vitro test uses specific allergen attached to a solid-phase support (allergosorbent) as the test substrate. Serum is added to the allergosorbent to allow any specific antibody to bind; unbound antibody is washed away, labeled anti-IgE is added, and the amount of bound labeled IgE is measured as a reflection of the allergen-specific IgE concentration. This test is called a radioallergosorbent test (RAST) when the anti-IgE antibody is labeled with a radionuclide. It is also possible to use enzyme-labeled anti-IgE in this test, as in an enzyme-linked immunosorbent assay (ELISA).[15]

Leukocyte Histamine Release

Basophils release histamine when challenged by the antigen to which they have been sensitized. An in vitro test (leukocyte histamine release) is available for measurement of this release. The test is expensive, time-consuming, and difficult to perform and so is not practical as a routine diagnostic procedure.

Arterial Blood Gases

The determination of arterial blood gases is an important method of laboratory evaluation of the asthmatic patient, especially in an acute episode. Arterial blood gas determinations are indicated if the patient is steroid dependent, fails to respond to therapy rapidly, or has a history of frequent hospitalizations for asthma. Blood should be obtained when the patient is breathing room air and not receiving supplemental oxygen. The abnormalities are usually revealed are respiratory alkalosis and hypocarbia followed by hypoxia.

Skin Testing

Direct skin tests are the most commonly used of all tests in clinical allergy. Testing may be performed by intradermal or prick-puncture methods, with the latter being preferred in most cases. Testing sites (back or forearm) are cleansed, and a drop of antigen solution is placed on the skin. A needle or prick-puncture device is inserted into the skin through the antigen. Only superficial penetration is made, and no bleeding should occur. The antigen is removed by blotting 1 minute after puncture, and the site is observed for a wheal-and-flare reaction 15 minutes later. Skin testing is inexpensive, rapid, precise, and sensitive. In addition, a multitude of antigens are available.

Considerations in skin testing include the potential for anaphylaxis, skin disease, the potential for sensitizing the patient, and the age of the patient (infants and elderly individuals can be difficult). In general, skin testing is a reproducible, accurate (particularly with food antigens), sensitive, and patient-accepted method of allergy testing that has been found to be very helpful in a number of allergic conditions.

TREATMENT

Table 47–3 summarizes the various components or steps in the treatment of allergic disease, including what therapeutic interventions are currently used and what might be possible in the near future.

Type I (Immediate) Hypersensitivity Disorders

The treatment of an allergic disease may be as "simple" as removing the offending antigen from the patient's environment or as complex as individualized asthma treatment protocols.

Table 47–3. Therapeutic Intervention in Allergic Disease

Steps in Allergic Disease	Therapeutic Intervention	Theoretical Intervention
Genetically susceptible individual		Gene therapy to change susceptibility genes
Allergen exposure	Reduce allergen exposure, especially in infancy	
IgE antibody production	"Immunotherapy with allergens"	Immunotherapy with peptides (tolerance induction?); oral immunotherapy (tolerance induction?); peptides that block antigen presentation; agents that inhibit IL-4 or other cytokines; agents that inhibit functions of IgE-bearing B cells; agents that interfere with memory IgE responses
IgE binding to mast cell and basophil FcεRI		Receptor blockade/interference, by receptor-derived peptides, IgE-derived peptides, or high levels of "nonspecific" IgE
Allergen reexposure	Reduce allergen exposure	
Signal transduction in mast cells and basophils, resulting in mediator secretion	Inhibit signal transduction; use β-adrenergic agents (including epinephrine)	Anti–tyrosine kinase(s)?, anti-PKC (?), anti-PLC (?), blockade of histamine versus LTC versus cytokine secretion (?)
Mediator effects on blood vessels and smooth muscle	Block mediator effects: use antihistamines (histamine₁ receptor antagonists)	Anti-LTC (?), anti-PAF (?), anticytokine (?)
Mediator effects on blood vessels and smooth muscle	Counteract mediator effects: use β-adrenergic agents (including epinephrine) and glucocorticoids (?)	
Induction of inflammation	Inhibit induction of inflammation; use glucocorticoids	Other anti-inflammatory agents (?), anticytokine
Action of inflammatory mediators on tissues		Anti-eosinophil products (?), others (?)

Abbreviations: FcεRI, surface receptor on basophil; IL-4, interleukin-4; LTC, leukotriene C; PAF, platelet activating factor; PKC, protein kinase C; PLC, phospholipase C.

From Paul WE: Fundamental Immunology, ed 3. New York, Raven Press, 1993.

For some conditions, such as seasonal allergic rhinitis, the use of an antihistamine may be adequate for relief. A number of new antihistamines—terfenadine (Seldane), astemizole (Hismanal), and loratadine (Claritin)—are available that have fewer of the classic side effects of the first-generation antihistamines (drowsiness, dizziness, nervousness). Some patients require more aggressive immunotherapy such as antigen desensitization.

Immunotherapy employs subcutaneous injections of gradually increasing doses of allergens for the purpose of altering the immune response. The effects probably result from the production of IgG-blocking antibody, lowering of specific IgE antibodies, a decrease in sensitivity of the basophil and the mast cell to histamine release, and modulation of T-cell responses. Most patients achieve some allergy relief within 12 to 24 months. The average patient receives 3 to 5 years of immunotherapy. Allergic rhinitis responds well to immunotherapy, but urticaria, angioedema, food allergy, and atopic dermatitis do not.[2]

The primary goal of treatment for asthma is to keep the patient as symptom-free as possible with a minimum of medication. The therapeutic modalities are many and include psychologic, physical, and supportive therapies as well as a considerable number of drugs that can be used when symptoms are manifested. These drugs include adrenergic stimulants (e.g., isoproterenol), methylxanthines (e.g., theophylline), and glucocorticoids. The last are known to have deleterious side effects when administered orally; however, inhaled forms are effective without the severity of side effects seen with the oral forms.[16] Among other medications that have become available for the treatment of asthma are leukotriene inhibitors. In addition, secondary problems that may develop over the course of the disease further complicate treatment. Patient education probably plays the most important role in most cases.

Hypersensitivity pneumonitis is not affected by immunotherapy. The best treatment, if possible, is avoidance of the offending antigen. When symptoms continue, corticosteroid therapy (prednisone) is used.

Food allergies are best treated by eliminating the offending food. Patient education is very important. Patients are taught to carefully read ingredients labels and to be aware of cross-reacting foods. Antihistamines are sometimes helpful in preventing urticaria and angioedema but are not effective in preventing anaphylactic reactions. In the case of severe reactions, epinephrine is indicated.

A problem faced by a significant number of health care workers is latex allergy. The only effective treatment at this time is avoidance of latex products (gloves, catheters, tourniquets, etc.).

The treatment of atopic dermatitis is tailored to the individual. The three major approaches to treatment are (1) reduce itching and scratching, (2) keep skin moisturized, and (3) prevent inflammation. Antihistamines are used to control pruritus, and moisturizers, and corticosteroids may be used to ameliorate the other symptoms.

The treatment of urticaria and angioedema is very similar to that of other conditions, in that, whenever possible, elimination and avoidance of the offending allergens or conditions is the best course of action. The most commonly used drugs are the antihistamines. Epinephrine is used in emergencies when an anaphylactic or rapidly progressing acute urticaria is seen.

A patient in anaphylaxis is in a potentially very grave situation. Depending on the severity of the reaction, death may result; therefore, immediate treatment is essential. Epinephrine is administered subcutaneously, although this has considerable risk for elderly patients and patients with cardiovascular or cerebrovascular disease. A detailed discussion of the treatment of anaphylaxis is beyond the scope of this chapter; however, a thorough medical history to determine significant allergies, proper monitoring of patients after injections of drugs, identification of allergies by the wearing of wrist bracelets or necklaces, and having epinephrine and other drugs available for emergency injection will prevent most cases of anaphylaxis.

Type II (Cytotoxic) Hypersensitivity Disorders

If signs and symptoms of a transfusion reaction develop, the transfusion should be stopped immediately. Treatment for shock, acute intravascular hemolysis, and urticaria is initiated, if necessary. The laboratory plays an important role in investigating the reaction, including demonstrating the presence of bacterial contamination, identifying antibodies that may be present, and performing blood chemistry analyses to monitor renal function.

Treatment of Rh incompatibility can be started during the last trimester of pregnancy if the fetus is in distress. Compatible blood is injected into the abdominal cavity of the fetus and is absorbed into the circulation. Intrauterine transfusions are possible. Following delivery, exchange transfusions of the newborn may be needed.

Treatment of autoimmune hemolytic anemia is directed at correcting the underlying disease process, which may require corticosteroids, splenectomy, or transfusion.

Drug-induced reactions may be managed by removal of the drug. If symptoms continue or have intensified, treatment is directed at the results of the reactions (e.g., platelet transfusions if thrombocytopenia is present).

The most effective treatment of myasthenia gravis involves the use of anticholinesterase drugs. The removal of antiacetylcholine receptor antibodies by plasmapheresis is also of value. Definitive therapy for Graves' disease involves the removal of the thyroid gland.

Type III (Immune Complex) Hypersensitivity Disorders

Treatment for type III hypersensitivity reactions is often symptomatic. Aspirin and antihistamines are used with corticosteroids if symptoms are severe. Treatment of Goodpasture's syndrome, glomerulonephritis, and rheumatic fever may eventually result in transplantation of the affected organ.

Type IV (Delayed) Hypersensitivity Disorders

Treatment of contact dermatitis involves avoidance of the offending antigen or application of corticosteroid cream if dermatitis is present. Treatment and elimination of infectious agents are the primary therapy for tuberculin-type hypersensitivity. The use of corticosteroids and other agents that interfere with T-cell activation, lymphokine release, and cell-to-cell communication are used to prevent graft rejection.

Case Study 1

A 7-year-old girl demonstrated conjunctivitis and rhinitis during August and September. She had sunken, dark-appearing infraorbital areas and constantly rubbed the tip of her nose upward with the palm of her hand. On examination, the tympanic membranes were well visualized and were normal in appearance and in mobility. Hearing was normal. The nasal mucosa was boggy, glistening, and bluish gray, with swelling over the inferior turbinates.

Laboratory findings for this patient were as follows:

Hematocrit	38%
Hemoglobin	13.5 g/dL
WBC	8.5×10^9/L
Neutrophils	56%
Lymphocytes	29%
Monocytes	4%
Eosinophils	11%

Serum immunoglobulin measurements showed IgA, IgG, and IgM levels to be within normal range, and IgE to be markedly elevated. Examination of a nasal smear revealed many eosinophils. Urinalysis results were normal.

Questions

1. A presentation such as this could have an infectious etiology. Which tests distinguish between infectious and allergic processes?
2. Are any other tests indicated?

Discussion

1. This case demonstrates the laboratory findings seen in allergic rhinitis: eosinophilia, positive nasal smear, and elevated serum IgE value.
2. Nasal cultures could be done. However, on the basis of cost, treatment for an allergic condition should be attempted first.

Case Study 2

A 26-year-old man with an 8-year history of asthma was admitted to the hospital for acute shortness of breath. Laboratory results showed the CBC to be normal except for 7% eosinophils, and urinalysis to be normal. No eosinophils were seen in nasal and sputum smears. Arterial blood gas valves were as follows:

pH	7.50
$Paco_2$	37 mm Hg
Pao_2	70 mm Hg
Bicarbonate	25 mEq/L

Questions

1. Does lack of nasal or sputum eosinophils cast doubt on the allergic basis for the patient's condition?
2. Evaluate the arterial blood gas results. How can they be explained in this patient?

Discussion

1. Although peripheral blood eosinophilia is demonstrated, no eosinophils were seen in the sputum or nasal smear. The presence of eosinophils is not essential for the diagnosis, although both specimens often contain eosinophils.
2. The arterial blood gas levels are compatible with a diagnosis of respiratory alkalosis with hypoxemia. There is often an early decrease in arterial Pao_2, with a greater decrease as severity of the condition increases. Early in an asthma attack, hyperventilation often causes a decrease in $Paco_2$ and respiratory alkalosis. If the attack is not responsive to treatment, however, the $Paco_2$ rises with time resulting in respiratory acidosis.

Case Study 3

A 53-year-old woman who was hospitalized for congestive heart failure developed eosinophilia (9%) after a normal peripheral blood (PB) differential count on admission. Two days later, a severe pruritic rash appeared all over her body, and the eosinophil count rose to 24%. Therapy was initiated with antihistamines, and in 10 days, the rash had cleared. The PB differential showed 1% eosinophils at that time.

Question

Are any other laboratory tests indicated?

Discussion

Because treatment with antihistamines was successful, no further tests are necessary. If further problems occur, however, a more complete evaluation would be indicated.

References

1. Paul WE: Fundamental Immunology, ed 3. New York, Raven Press, 1993.
2. Lawlor GJ, Fischer TJ, Adelman DC: Manual of Allergy and Immunology, ed 3. Boston, Little, Brown, 1995.
3. Gurish MF, Austen KF: Different mast cell mediators produced by different mast cell phenotypes. *In* Chadwick D (ed): IgE, Mast Cells and the Allergic Response. (Ciba Foundation Symposium 147.) New York, John Wiley & Sons, 1989.
4. DeJarnatt AC, Grant JA: Basic mechanisms of anaphylaxis and anaphylactoid reactions. Immunol Allergy Clin North Am 12:501, 1992.

5. Roitt IM: Essential Immunology, ed 8. Oxford, Blackwell Scientific, 1994.
6. Bradding P, Freezer NJ, Sheffer AL, et al: Asthma. *In* Frank MM, Austen KF, Claman HN, et al (eds): Samter's Immunologic Diseases, ed 5. Boston, Little, Brown, 1995.
7. Mathews DP: Respiratory atopic disease. JAMA 248:2587, 1982.
8. Kaplan AP (ed): Allergy. New York, Churchill Livingstone, 1985.
9. Middleton E, Reed CE, Ellis EF (eds): Allergy: Principles and Practice, ed 4. St Louis, CV Mosby, 1993.
10. Sampson HA, Metcalfe DD: Food allergies. JAMA 268:2840, 1992.
11. Buckley RH, Mathews KP: Common "allergic" skin diseases. JAMA 248:2611, 1982.
12. Berzofsky JA: Immunogenicity and antigenicity. *In* Frank MM, Austen KF, Claman HN, et al (eds.): Samter's Immunologic Diseases, ed 5. Boston, Little, Brown, 1995.
13. Patterson R, Valentine M: Anaphylaxis and related allergic emergencies including reactions due to insect stings. JAMA 248:2632, 1982.
14. Terr AI: Immune-complex allergic disease. *In* Stites DP, Terr AI (eds): Basic and Clinical Immunology, ed 7. Norwalk, CT, Appleton & Lange, 1991.
15. Fleisher TA: Immunologic methods. *In* Frank MM, Austen KF, Claman HN, et al (eds): Samter's Immunologic Diseases, ed 5. Boston, Little, Brown, 1995.
16. McFadden ER Jr: Asthma. *In* Isselbacker KJ, Braunwald E, Wilson JD, et al (eds): Harrison's Principles of Internal Medicine. New York, McGraw-Hill, 1994.

Autoimmune Diseases

David L. Smalley

Autoimmune diseases are disorders of immunoregulation with increased autoantibody production or inappropriate cellular proliferation that result in immune complex formation, cell death, tissue damage, or altered function. On the humoral side of the immune system, autoantibody specificity may be directed toward a ubiquitous self-antigen, a neoantigen, a cross-reactive antigen, or a chemical or viral antigen. The subsequent antibody production or overproduction may be due to genetic predisposition, polyclonal activation of B lymphocytes, alteration of the ratio of T-suppressor to T-helper cells, alteration of idiotypic–anti-idiotypic network (antibodies produced by one individual), or impaired C4 activation–macrophage phagocytosis. The immune injuries that may result include the following:

- *Vasculitis, arthralgias, neurologic syndromes, glomerulonephritis, myalgias,* and other disorders caused by circulating immune complexes
- *Innocent bystander syndrome,* due to cross-reactivity of tissue antigen and organisms such as bacteria and viruses
- *Cell death,* due to an autoantibody to a specific tissue antigen
- *Tissue damage,* due to cellular and humoral immune response to altered self-proteins

- *Altered function* of a specific tissue, due to the autoantibody to a receptor or specific antigen

Drug-induced disorders may result from impaired clearance of immune complexes, because the drug impairs C4 activation and, consequently, macrophage phagocytosis. Chemically or environmentally induced autoimmune syndromes have been a major target of investigation in autoimmune disorders. In all of these general disorders, clinical manifestations and laboratory findings are related to the specificity of the autoantibody or directed T cells and the resultant immune injury mechanism.

The term *autoimmune disease* specifically refers to an immunopathologic condition caused by autoimmunization to "self" components. Although nonpathologic autoimmune responses to self components occur naturally, the immune response seems to exhibit either a controlled or a noncontrolled loss of tolerance to self in autosensitization. The effects are variable, and autoimmune disorders may be organ/tissue-specific or non–organ/tissue-specific in scope. The autoimmune response may destroy, mimic, or enhance the target. The disorder can range in severity from only an irritation to death.

Autoimmune diseases have a major impact on medical care in this country. For example, there are nearly 6.5 million cases of rheumatoid arthritis in the United States, and type I diabetes mellitus, an insulin-dependent autoimmune disease, is the leading cause of end-stage renal disease.[1] Aside from the immunopathology associated with the development of autoimmune response or autoimmune disease, it is important to understand the etiologic factors that permit autoimmunization to self components.

ETIOLOGY AND PATHOPHYSIOLOGY

A normal, immunocompetent individual has an intact autorecognition system that distinguishes self from nonself. The causes of the phenotypic change in autorecognition are not clearly understood; however, etiologic factors have been implicated that serve as nonself or foreign recognition factors. Some of these factors are viral and chemical modifications of self, defective immune regulation, hyperimmunization, and immunogenetic alterations. In the assessment of the implications of each of these broad-based etiologic factors, certain etiologies are more attributable to specific autoimmune disease than others.[2]

Viral or Chemical Modifications

Autoimmune diseases with suspected chemical or viral etiologies may be organ/tissue-specific disorders, whereas others initiate a general or non–organ/tissue disorder. Among the organ/tissue-specific disorders, type I diabetes has been reported to be a result of a previous infection with coxsackievirus, and the autoantibodies that develop cross-react with the islet cells of the pancreas. The resultant autoantibody disrupts normal production of insulin, thereby causing an insulin-dependent diabetes mellitus (IDDM). Chemical modifications of lung basement membrane by gasoline fumes have been implicated in the development of Goodpasture's syndrome. In viral stimulation, it is believed that the immune response (antibody and/or lymphokine) cross-reacts to a self-antigen or exposes a hidden antigen that is new, rather than self.[2–4]

General or non–organ/tissue-specific disorders have been reported to be caused by a variety of environmental agents. For example, crystalline silica and amorphous silica have been recognized for many years as immunogenic agents in the organ-specific disease of the lungs commonly referred to as silicosis or pneumoconiosis; however, it is very common for these agents also to cause non–organ-specific disorders such as arthralgias, myalgias, and other rheumatic-type symptoms related to silicosis. Another well-studied chemical agent shown to be immunogenic is beryllium. Lung disease was common in the original exposures to beryllium, but as with silicosis, general autoimmune disorders have also been reported in affected individuals. In addition, other so-called light metals have been implicated as causative agents in autoimmune syndromes. These include nickel, cadmium, chromium, zinc, and gold. These agents appear to stimulate T cells as a monocyte-dependent, or major histocompatibility gene complex (MHC) class II response, which most likely occurs as a hapten linked with normal body proteins. The same phenomena have been seen with certain drugs, such as penicillin.

Another agent that has received significant publicity in recent years is silicone used in manufacturing silicone breast implants. Silicone, a manufactured substance, is derived from silica and appears to biodegrade in the environment as well as in the human body.[5–7] Although there is great controversy currently, a body of literature implicates silicone or its metabolites as being immunogenic. The resulting autoimmune syndrome mimics various disorders such as systemic lupus erythematosus (SLE), scleroderma, and rheumatoid arthritis.

Defective Immune Regulation

Defective immune regulation is a potential cause of autoimmune disease, both organ/tissue-specific and non–organ/tissue-specific. Mouse models for SLE demonstrate both hyperactivity of B lymphocytes to T-helper cell–produced lymphokines and hyperactivity of T-helper cells in lymphokine production.

Hyporeactivity of the immune system has been implicated in a number of investigations into loss of T-suppressor cell function or decrease in these cells. At specific times during the course of autoimmune disease, the number of circulating T-suppressor cells is diminished, but this state does not seem to be consistent throughout the course of the disease. A relationship between these diseases and the CD4+ (T-helper) to CD8+ (T-suppressor) cell ratio has been suggested, as have differences in disease occurrence between males and females; however, these relationships have not yet been confirmed. T-suppressor cell levels can be depressed and can influence disease severity but in themselves are not the etiologic factors for autosensitization.[8] An example of T-suppressor cell shift is seen in multiple sclerosis. Prior to an active episode of the disease, levels of both CD8+ cells and 2H4+ suppressor-inducer cells are typically decreased.[9] In this situation, the shifts in immune regulation reflect a antigenic stimulation that controls the immune cell delivery but does not reflect the source of the etiologic stimulation.

Another aspect of immune regulation that has been widely investigated in autoimmune disease is the role of the idiotypic–anti-idiotypic antibodies in the remission-relapse cycles of certain diseases. Idiotypic–anti-idiotypic networks can be both suppressive and stimulatory to the immune system. Investigations suggest that cross-reactive monoclonal idiotypes found in lymphoproliferative disorders are specific for DNA antibodies found in SLE. The implication is that the cells that produce the autoantibodies are more subject to neoplastic transformation.[8] This finding has also been suggested in immune stimulation in animal models, in which, ultimately, monoclonal gammopathy or plasmacytomas develop after exposure to certain substances.[10, 11]

Another view of autoidiotypes suggests that the ability to produce certain autoantibodies is endogenous, although this ability in itself does not constitute the immunopathology. The shift from nonpathologic to pathologic autoantibody production occurs when a "minor" idiotypic antibody (Ab1) expands into a major antianti-idiotypic antibody as a result of genetic alteration. These alterations occur because the antianti-idiotypic antibody (Ab3) does not really "see" the originating antigen (immunogen), but instead responds to conformational idiotypes that are self-antigens. Because of sharing in the idiotype of the originating antibody, the Ab1 and Ab3 become part of a regulatory idiotype. This suggests that autoimmune diseases may be a multi-step, multi-gene process in which specific etiologic factors or specific genetic factors trigger autosensitization by a "minor" idiotypic response resulting in immunopathologic tissue destruction. An example would be a bacterial antigen that stimulates production of an antibody sharing a common idiotype with a DNA antibody. The original Ab1 binds only the bacterial antigen, not DNA; however, the resultant antianti-idiotypic antibody (Ab3) binds DNA but not the original bacterial antigen. The anti-DNA is not necessarily immunopathologic, unless there is a shift in production of antibody-producing cells that changes them from a minor subpopulation to a major population.[8]

Another concept being explored is genetic modification of the variable regions of the CD3+ antigen receptors, which might enhance autoimmunization or at least modulate the response. The autoepitopes (autoantigens) seen by the immune response mechanism are unique substances. Their structure has to be easily accessible to the immune response, whether the antigen is a virus, a chemical modification, or a shared idiotype.[2, 4] There is clearly a role for genetic factors in certain autoimmune diseases thought to be associated with human leukocyte antigens (HLAs). Many autoimmune disorders have been associated with certain HLA-DR phenotypes. For example, rheumatoid arthritis has been associated with HLA-DR4, multiple sclerosis with HLA-DR2, and SLE with HLA-DR3.

The autoepitopes found in the SLE and SLE-related groups are of interest. Suggested autoepitopes include the spectrum of histones—H1, H2A, H2B, H3, H4; histidyl-t-RNA synthetase (Jo-1); cyclin, snRNP, and the like. Some of these are autoepitopes of DNA bases, nucleic acid–binding proteins, or the Fc region of IgG. Because SLE is a multisystem disorder, multiple autoantibodies occur not only to nuclear-associated epitopes but also to red blood cell antigens and to leukocyte antigens, either HLA-specific or granulocyte-specific.[8]

It has been suggested that autoantibodies are naturally occurring mechanisms that function in the elimination of degraded antigens. The subsequent loss of immunoregulation could occur from defects in enzyme systems or immunoregulation, or any combination.[8]

Pathologic Effects

The autoantibody that occurs in some of these autoimmune disorders may not be pathologic per se, but the resulting immune complexes may be, as in SLE. In other instances, the autoantibody may be cytotoxic to cell-bound antigens that then become pathologic to the body, as in autoimmune hemolytic anemia or Goodpasture's syndrome. In other instances, the autoantibody can impair function of a cell, as in myasthenia gravis, in which the autoantibody inhibits the binding of the acetylcholine to its receptor in the neuronal synapse. Autoantibodies can be stimulatory, as in thyroid immunoglobulin (TIg). In this instance, the autoantibody binds to the thyroid-stimulating hormone (TSH) receptor and functions as TSH to stimulate thyroxin (T_4) production by the thyroid. Autoimmune diseases are not all autoantibody mediated but may be cell mediated, with destruction of target cells. Hashimoto's thyroiditis is an example of cellular proliferation and destruction of the target organ.[2–4] Another example is the immune granulomatous disease demonstrated by beryllium- or silica-induced disease.[12, 13]

The common thread in autoimmune disease is the autoimmunization to self components with eventual immunologically mediated injury. The mechanism of injury is as varied as are the target organs, tissues, and symptoms. The immunopathologic injury may be an antibody-mediated cytotoxic (type II) reaction, immune complex deposition (type III) reaction, or cell-mediated (type IV) reaction. The cell-mediated disorders usually involve cellular toxicity and release of lymphokines that can enhance the cellular proliferative response.[2–4] The targets of autoimmune disorders include cell receptors, specific cellular antigens and components, products of cells, catabolized fragments of cells, and organelles.

Autoimmune disorders can be categorized as organ/tissue-specific or non–organ/tissue-specific. Non–organ/tissue-specific disease are the systemic rheumatoid disorders, such as SLE, rheumatoid arthritis, ankylosing spondylitis, necrotizing angiitis (vasculitis), polymyositis, dermatomyo-

sitis, scleroderma, mixed connective tissue disease (MCTD), and Sjögren's syndrome. Many of these disorders have specific tissue or organ involvement as well as generalized systemic effects.

Non–Organ/Tissue-Specific Diseases

Systemic Lupus Erythematosus

SLE, one of the most studied autoimmune disorders, affects females 6 to 9 times more commonly than males. The disease often manifests in women 20 to 30 years of age, although it is sometimes known to strike younger females in their teens. SLE has an estimated prevalence of 15 to 50 cases per 100,000 persons in the United States.

The etiology of classic SLE is still unknown, although tissue damage is thought to be due to autoantibodies that react to normal tissue during an inflammatory response. The disease often has an insidious onset, but it can prove to be fatal at a very early age. Immune complex deposition in SLE can produce serious lesions in the kidney, blood vessels, and heart. Central nervous system (CNS) involvement occurs in 50% of patients with SLE, and fatalities are usually attributable to renal failure or cerebral hemorrhage.[2–4] A family history of SLE occurs in a limited number of cases. In identical twins, concordance of disease occurs in about 25% of the cases, whereas dizygotic twins have concordance of disease in only about 2% of the cases.[14] The limited occurrence of disease in both monozygotic twins reflects the possibility that other factors may influence the development of the disease, such as occupational, environmental, or infectious agent exposure.

Revised criteria for diagnosis of systemic lupus erythematosus were established by the American Rheumatism Association in 1982.[15] In one study of pediatric cases of SLE, the female-to-male ratio was 5.5:1. In this study, the clinical features in pediatric-onset SLE were basically the same as for adult-onset SLE. Cardiopulomonary disease was more common in the adults than in children, but the pediatric patients had greater likelihood of renal disorders and significantly higher rates of hematologic disease than adults.[16]

Drug-induced lupus accounts for about 10% of all cases of SLE. Some of the more common agents associated with this disorder are hydralazine, procainamide, and methyldopa. Drug-induced lupus varies with the drug, but the overall response is inappropriate stimulation of the immune cells or T cells.[17] Generally, when drug-induced lupus is encountered, elimination of the drug abates the disease process over time. Yung and associates[18] found that normal antigen-specific T cells can become autoreactive through a relatively simple drug treatment, suggesting that similar changes could occur within the body. As the cells become autoreactive, they could potentially cause an autoimmune disease. Certain chemicals and foods and other environmental agents have been implicated as causative agents in the induction of lupus.[19–21]

Rheumatoid Arthritis

Rheumatoid arthritis (RA) is commonly grouped with the SLE and SLE-like disorders because of the shared symptomatology of arthralgias. Unlike other disorders in the group, RA usually results in bilateral or symmetric joint involvement. Rheumatoid arthritis occurs four times more commonly in females than in males, and its estimated incidence in the United States is 1000 cases per 100,000 persons. RA is an autoimmune inflammatory disease that affects the joints, resulting in pain, tenderness, and joint swelling. Arthritis of the adult type is rare in children, and although the disease favors women, it has not been associated with any specific race. As seen in other autoimmune disorders, rheumatoid arthritis is more common in persons with HLA-DR4+ haplotypes. Histopathologic examinations commonly reveal lymphocytic infiltrates within the synovium, and immunophenotyping shows the lymphocytes to be T cells.[22] The American Rheumatism Association has also established criteria for the classification of rheumatoid arthritis.[23]

Ankylosing Spondylitis

Ankylosing spondylitis (arthritis of the spine) is the opposite of most other autoimmune diseases, in that the male-to-female ratio is 9:1. The estimated incidence of ankylosing spondylitis in the United States is 0.5 to 1.0 cases per 100,000 people. This disorder has no known etiology, and it primarily affects joints and tissue of the axial skeleton. Sacroiliac joint involvement is the hallmark of the disease, followed by bony ankylosing.[24] Other forms of similar diseases exist, including Reiter's syndrome, psoriatic arthritis, and enteropathic arthritis. Patients with ankylosing spondylitis often have radiologically abnormal sacroiliitis and may have spondylitis, but a common feature is asymmetric peripheral arthritis. Criteria for diagnosis of ankylosing spondylitis have been established and revised since 1961.[24, 25] Ankylosing spondylitis typically occurs before the age of 40 years (15 to 40 years). Anterior uveitis occurs in about 25% of patients with active disease.[24]

There is a strong association between the presence of HLA-B27 and ankylosing spondylitis, which should be considered along with family history. For example, 1% to 10% of the white population with HLA-B27 develop ankylosing spondylitis, as do more than 20% of first-degree relatives with HLA-B27.[26] More than 90% of the ankylosing spondylitis patients have HLA-B27. Most patients with this disease have episodic periods of active disease that may last from a few weeks to a year or longer. The most common episodes last for about 3 months.[27]

HLA-B27 also occurs in about 85% of patients with Reiter's syndrome. This disorder manifests as a triad of symptoms, consisting of non-specific urethritis, acute polyarthritis, and conjunctivitis.

The laboratory findings in ankylosing spondylitis are not particularly helpful. Affected patients are typically negative for ANA and rheumatoid factor, but as many as 75% have elevated erythrocyte sedimentation rates during active episodes and may have increases in haptoglobin and C-reactive proteins.[28] T cells from synovial fluid and tissue have expressed HLA-DR and IL-2 receptors, indicating that activation of T cells has occurred.[29] Diminished mitogenic response to phytohemagglutinin and pokeweed mitogens have been reported, with correction following short-term corticosteroid therapy.[30]

Polymyositis/Dermatomyositis

Polymyositis and dermatomyositis can manifest as acute or chronic inflammatory diseases of the muscle and skin. These diseases affect females twice as often as males. The estimated incidence of disease in the United States is 0.5 to 1.0 cases per 100,000 people.

These disorders are characterized by symmetric muscle weakness, dysphagia, abnormal electromyographic studies, elevation of muscle-associated enzymes such as creatine kinase, degeneration of muscle fibers on biopsy, and skin changes. Polymyositis occurs commonly around the age of 50 years, whereas dermatomyositis generally occurs between the ages of 50 and 60 years. Approximately 50% of affected patients develop an antimyosin antibody, and 40% also have a positive ANA.[31] Another autoantibody found in these disorders is called the PM-1.[32] A number of studies have indicated that activated T cells are common and that the myositis is specifically associated with activation of the cell-mediated immune system.[33, 34]

Scleroderma (Systemic Sclerosis)

Scleroderma is characterized by increased connective tissue deposition resulting in hardening of the skin. It is not uncommon to find fibrotic changes in muscle and joints in affected patients. Scleroderma has been subdivided into two subsets, diffuse cutaneous and limited cutaneous, both of which are characterized by skin involvement. Raynaud's phenomenon, esophageal dysmotility, sclerodactyly, and other disorders have been associated with the latter form, and visceral disease is more likely in the former.[3]

The relative rarity of scleroderma has limited appropriate epidemiologic studies.[35] The American Rheumatism Association has established criteria for the diagnosis of systemic sclerosis,[36] which are guidelines for differential diagnosis. The median age of onset is typically between 50 and 60 years; occurrence in children is rare.[37] Environmental hazards have also been reported in some patients with systemic sclerosis, including vinyl chloride, trichlorethylene, solvents, silica, silicone, and bleomycin.[38]

As with other autoimmune diseases, T cells appear to play a major role in the pathogenesis of scleroderma. The majority of the lymphocytes present in skin lesions are T cells,[39] and studies have confirmed that activation of the cell-mediated immune system leads to cytokine release, which plays a role in connective tissue metabolism. It is likely that the development of fibrosis is a direct result of the chronic inflammatory response.

Multiple Sclerosis

Multiple sclerosis is a relapsing disease with active phases of exacerbation followed by periods of remission. A demyelinating disorder, multiple sclerosis affects males and females equally, and onset usually occurs between the ages of 20 and 40 years. Epidemiologic studies reveal certain high-risk areas in the world, suggesting a possibility of a transmissible agent; however, occupational exposure to zinc has been implicated by epidemiologic studies and in studies of the immune response of T cells to zinc compounds.[40, 41] The estimated incidence of multiple sclerosis in the United States is 100 cases per 100,000 people.

Sjögren's Syndrome

Sjögren's syndrome, also called sicca syndrome, is a chronic inflammatory disease that can afflict multiple organs, although the primary target tissue appears to be secretory glands such as the lacrimal and salivary glands. It is also common for females with this disorder to complain of vaginal dryness. Sjögren's syndrome has 9 times greater incidence in females than in males, and the estimated incidence in the United States is 0.5 to 1.0 cases per 100,000 persons.

Organ/Tissue-Specific Diseases

The organ- or tissue-specific disorders commonly have specific autoantibodies, rather than the multiplicity of antibodies seen in SLE and SLE-like diseases. In some of the endocrine disorders, multiple autoantibodies are commonly present. The antibody-mediated disorders involve cytotoxic injury with or without complement activation, and inhibitory or stimulatory responses of specific tissue. Cell-mediated injury is also commonly present.[8]

Cytotoxic Reactions

Cytotoxic reactions may be exhibited by some patients. For example, autoimmune hemolytic anemia with either a warm or cold antibody demonstrates cytotoxic reactions with or without complement activation. If the autoantibody is non–complement-fixing and nonlytic, the destruction of red blood cells is due to splenic sequestration. The clinical results are anemia and spherocytosis. Other examples with similar mechanisms are seen with autoantibodies to platelets, granulocytes, lymphocytes, and other cellular components.

Other cytotoxic reactions may be directed at basement membrane to kidneys or lungs, as in Goodpasture's syndrome, heart tissue, as in the case of rheumatic fever, or desmosomes, as in pemphigus vulgaris. The autoantibody involved is specifically targeted to the tissue. Cytotoxic reactions also occur in demyelinating disorders, with demonstrable antibodies to myelin; in thyroid disease, with autoantibodies to thyroglobulin and/or microsomes; in gastric atrophy or pernicious anemia, with antibodies to intrinsic factor and/or parietal cells; and in biliary cirrhosis, with mitochondrial antibodies.

Modifications of the cytotoxic type of immunologic injury are the enhancement autoantibody and inhibitory autoantibody. Both are demonstrable in tissue-specific disorders. In myasthenia gravis, the autoantibody is against the acetylcholine receptor. It inhibits the binding of acetylcholine to its natural receptor in the neuronal synapses, compromising normal nerve impulse conduction. Occasional instances of myasthenia gravis have been shown to have an anti-idiotypic antibody that can mimic acetylcholine binding and facilitate continuation of low-level nerve impulse. As the disease progresses, the anti-idiotypic response is negated by increasing idiotypic antibody, and total impairment of nerve impulse occurs. Most of the idiotypic–anti-idiotypic antibodies described have been cross-reactive idiotypes, suggesting that they are not individual-specific but autoantibody-specific—that is, the anti-idiotypic antibody inhibits the binding of idiotypic antibodies from several different individuals to the choline receptor in an in vivo test.[8]

Enhancement or Inhibitory Reactions

An enhancement reaction occurs when the autoantibody mimics a natural hormone or peptide, or binds to a receptor, stimulating a specific response. Thyroid immunoglobulin, also known as LATS (long-acting thyroid stimulator), binds to the TSH receptor and mimics TSH stimulation of the thyroid. TIg as an autoantibody is present in a significant but small percentage of patients with hyperthyroidism. TIg is the specific autoantibody, but its mechanism is stimulatory to that of its receptor antigen rather than inhibitory or cytotoxic.[2, 4]

Cell-Mediated Reactions

One mechanism seen in organ-specific disorders is cell mediated (lymphokine mediated) rather than antibody mediated. The proliferative or cytotoxic T lymphocytes with their lymphokine products are the causative factors in organ destruction. Hashimoto's thyroiditis is due in part to a mononuclear cell infiltrate that disrupts the organ structure and function. In this disorder, the thyroid becomes enlarged, tender, and inflamed owing to T-proliferative cells, their lymphokines, and the infiltrating macrophages. Allergic encephalomyelitis is similar, except that it is infiltration by T-proliferative cells into the central nervous system, specifically the meninges, with subsequent inflammation that causes the symptoms. The autoantigen in both of these disorders is a particulate cell-bound antigen that is more stimulatory to the cell-mediated system than to the antibody-mediated immune response. Even though the principal pathologic response is lymphokine mediated, antibody-mediated response occurs as well and accounts for some of the injury.[2]

CLINICAL MANIFESTATIONS

Clinical symptoms of the non–organ/tissue-specific disorders are very similar. They comprise joint pain, complaints associated with vasculitis, and skin lesions. The organ/tissue-specific disorders involve blood components, endocrine glands, kidney, the gastrointestinal (GI) tract, central nervous system, skin, liver, lungs, muscle, and eye. The organ/tissue-specific disorders are more easily defined because they have a specific target. Examples are red blood cells in autoimmune hemolytic anemia, platelets in idiopathic thrombocytopenia purpura, and kidney and lung in Goodpasture's syndrome.[2-4]

Non–Organ/Tissue-Specific Diseases

The first symptoms of SLE may occur during puberty, with a common complaint of joint pain or sun sensitivity. A red rash across the upper cheeks and bridge of the nose that has a characteristic "butterfly" shape may be present. This rash is the origin of the name—*lupus* (wolf) and *erythematosus* (red). Light sensitivity among SLE patients is common. It is thought that ultraviolet light induces keratinocytes to release interleukin-1, which stimulates the immune response and subsequent release of the other cytokines.[42]

Clinically, SLE symptoms may vary from case to case; however, the most common symptoms (and their relative frequencies) are as follows: fatigue (90%); arthralgia (90%); low-grade fever (80%); alopecia (70%); lymphadenopathy (70%); anorexia (60%); facial butterfly rash (60%); photosensitivity (40%); and myalgia (30%). Arthritis in SLE is most commonly seen in the hands, wrists, and knees. Morning stiffness is another common complaint among patients with SLE. Diffuse alopecia or hair loss is common, and Raynaud's phenomenon occurs spontaneously, commonly after cold exposure. Peripheral neuropathies are seen to a lesser degree, usually without central nervous system disease.[43] Spontaneous abortion occurs frequently in women with SLE and is most commonly attributed to the presence of an autoantibody referred to as an antiphospholipid antibody.

Patients with rheumatoid arthritis or Sjögren's syndrome commonly present with arthralgias, and those with Sjögren's present with a possible sicca syndrome (dry eyes and/or mouth). Mixed connective tissue disease (MCTD) frequently causes arthralgias and esophageal dysphagia but no renal complications. Patients with dermatomyositis have both skin and muscle complaints. Polymyositis causes joint and muscle pain.[2-4, 8]

Sarcoidosis is another autoimmune disorder with no known etiology. A common clinical presentation is respiratory tract involvement that on biopsy shows granulomatous lesions; however, lesions of this type may develop in almost any organ. There is no particular sex preference in this disorder but females are somewhat more commonly afflicted, and their symptoms generally appear between the ages of 20 and 40 years. In the United States, blacks are affected more often than whites. As with other autoimmune diseases, T cells are significantly increased in lesions of affected patients.

Organ/Tissue-Specific Disease

In organ-specific disorders, whether cell directed, membrane directed, or receptor directed, the clinical presentation is usually specific. For example, it may be muscle weakness as in myasthenia gravis, hyperthyroidism as in Graves's disease, or insulin-dependent diabetes mellitus as in the case of an islet cell antibody.[2]

Antibody-mediated kidney disease is not uncommon in SLE. In this situation, antibody-antigen complexes create an inflammatory response in the glomeruli, leading to deposition of antibody and irreversible kidney disease. Other organs may demonstrate the same or similar pathology. One of the characteristic lesions found in SLE is vasculitis, particularly around small blood vessels. Chronic inflammatory reactions are characterized by the presence of lymphocytes and, in some cases, plasma cells.

LABORATORY ANALYSES AND DIAGNOSIS

Most of the antibody-mediated autoimmune disorders demonstrate a polyclonal gammopathy, usually of the immunoglobulin G (IgG) type; chronic inflammatory re-

sponse; possible classic complement activation with circulating immune complexes; and alteration in function or numbers of autoantibody targets. Other components that may be affected are the immune regulatory system, such as decreased CD8+ (T-suppressor) cells; the function of kidneys, lungs, blood flow, and neuromuscular system; and multiple autoantibody activities. Specific substrate and disease associations are shown in Table 48–1.

Systemic Lupus Erythematosus

Laboratory findings in SLE comprise a glomerular permeability type of proteinuria, a polyclonal increase in IgG, complement activation via the classical pathway with decreases in components C3 and C4, a positive rheumatoid factor test, possible positive cryoglobulin tests, circulating immune complexes, possible anemia and/or leukopenia, and a positive antinuclear antibody (ANA) test.

The presence of ANAs may be due to a number of autoantibodies to specific nuclear components, such as ds-DNA, DNP, SS-A, Smith (Sm), and Ma. The most definitive ANA specificity are ds-DNA and the Sm autoantibody, complement-fixing antibodies that are particularly damaging. Sm antibody occurs in approximately 40% of all patients with SLE. The ANA is not specific for SLE, because approximately 3% to 7% of the normal population, 40% of the elderly population, and patients with other disorders such as rheumatoid arthritis can have positive reactions. High titers of ANA, especially those with solid or rim reaction patterns, are suggestive of SLE. The diagnosis can be established with more confidence if the ANA specificity can be attributed to ds-DNA and also to Sm. Cross-reactivity or false-positive serologic reactions do occur in SLE, and false-positive tests for syphilis have been reported in as many as 15% of SLE patients.

Antiphospholipid antibodies have been found to be associated with thrombosis, thrombocytopenia, and spontaneous abortion in SLE.[44, 45] One of the most commonly used laboratory tests to detect these problems in SLE patients is the anticardiolipin antibody test. Because of the predictive value of this test, Hughes and colleagues[46] have proposed a new subset classification for SLE called the anticardiolipin syndrome. Serial studies of patients with positive cardiolipin antibodies suggest that two further subsets exist. The first is a group who have antibodies to cardiolipin that persist over time and pose a higher risk for thromboses and spontaneous abortion during pregnancy. The second group shows positive antibodies to cardiolipin only during active phases of SLE.[47]

Discoid lupus, a variant of SLE, may not exhibit proteinuria. Quite often, patients with this variant are not ds-DNA positive, although they commonly have SS-A antibodies. The finding of SS-A antibody in pregnant women has been associated with congenital heart disease in newborns and with high-risk infants. The infant of such a woman may or may not be positive for SS-A antibody. In addition, spontaneous abortions have been associated with antibodies to cardiolipin and to SS-A. SS-A antibodies usually result in a speckled ANA pattern when HEp-2 (human laryngeal tumor) cells are used as the substrate.[48, 49]

ANA-negative SLE was originally reported to be associated with antibodies to single-stranded DNA (ss-DNA).

Table 48–1. Autoantibody Detection by Immunofluorescence

Autoantibody	Substrate	Reaction Site	Disease Correlation
Nuclear (ANA)	Rat kidney HEp 2 cells	Nucleus	Collagen vascular disease, SLE, SLE-related disease, drug-induced
Mitochondrial (AMA)	Rat kidney	Mitochondria	Primary biliary cirrhosis
Smooth muscle (ASMA)	Rat stomach	Actin	Acute and chronic hepatitis, lupoid hepatitis, acute infectious mononucleosis
Parietal cell (APCA)	Rat stomach	Parietal cell	Pernicious anemia, microsomes, atrophic gastritis
Reticulin	Rat kidney	Reticulin	Malabsorption syndrome, sprue, celiac disease
Glomerular	Rat kidney	Basement membrane	Chronic active hepatitis, Goodpasture's syndrome
Striated muscle	Rat striated muscle	Myoid cell striations	Myasthenia gravis
Skin	Human skin	Epithelial basement membrane	Bullous, pemphigoid
Myelin	Rat sciatic	Myelin sheath	Demyelinating disease
Islet cell	Human pancreas (blood group O)	Islet cell cytoplasm	Diabetes
Salivary	Human salivary	Salivary duct cytoplasm	Sjögren's syndrome
dsDNA	Crithidea	Kinetoplast	SLE
Histone	Acid-treated rat kidney	Nucleus—no reaction indicates presence of histone antibodies (if DNA and reconstituted histone are positive)	Drug-induced lupus

About 5% of patients with SLE are ANA negative, but nearly half of these individuals ultimately develop systemic disease. Many of the ANA-negative mouse kidney reactions may demonstrate weakly positive speckled ANA patterns on HEp-2 cells. Single-stranded DNA antibodies are commonly present in SLE, but usually in association with other nuclear-specific antibodies. The variation between substrates for ANA can often be correlated with differences in titer and, to some extent, with the pattern observed. For example, some autoantibodies are demonstrable on mouse kidney but not on HEp-2 cells, and vice versa. In addition, most autoantibodies that are associated with disease are usually IgG, but IgM and IgA classes of antibodies have been reported.[48, 49]

SLE-Like Disorders

The SLE-like disorders have physical and clinical symptoms similar to those seen in SLE, but with specific physical-clinical variations and differences in autoantibody specificities. Another distinction is that complement activation is not as striking in the SLE-related disorders as it is in SLE. In MCTD, the ANA is a high-titered speckled reaction with ribonucleoprotein (RNP) specificity.

The autoantibodies of Sjögren's syndrome are demonstrated as a speckled ANA in which the specificity is SS-B or SS-A, and SS-B is an autoantibody to salivary duct.

In polymyositis, the positive speckled ANA occurs in approximately 50% of patients, with the specificity being PM-1 or JO-1.

The ANA in dermatomyositis is commonly a nucleolar pattern with RNA specificity. Scleroderma also is characterized by an ANA nucleolar reaction but may show a speckled or a centromere pattern. The ANA reaction in the CREST (calcinosis cutis, Raynaud's phenomenon, esophageal dysfunction, sclerodactyly, and telangiectasia) syndrome of scleroderma is characterized by a large speckled pattern that is actually the centromere antibody seen in dividing or mitotic cells. In addition, a spindle pattern has

also been detected. One antibody specificity associated with scleroderma is the SCL-70.[48, 49]

The entire group of SLE-related diseases commonly exhibit speckled ANA patterns with specificities directed to what was originally called *extractable nuclear antigens* (ENAs) because they were present in the saline wash of calf thymus extraction for DNA. Since their discovery, characterization of these substances with respect to their true specificity has been continuing. RNP and Sm both appear to be endonucleases; PM-1 appears to be related to a polymerase, and SCL-70 is a 70-kDa ribsomal protein.[48] The type of autoantibody specificity and the manifestation of the disease process are currently of great interest to researchers. Some have suggested that Z-DNA may be more "immunogenic" than B-DNA. There are also occasional reports of anti-idiotypic antibodies, both cross-reactive and individual, that have been demonstrated in patients with SLE and SLE-like diseases. This finding has led to speculation that these anti-idiotypes may be responsible for some of the cyclic patterns observed in patients with remission-relapse sequences.

Patients with rheumatoid arthritis have high titers of rheumatoid factor, a polyclonal gamma increase, and little or no complement consumption or circulating immune complexes. The serum protein pattern may reflect a chronic inflammatory response with increased α_1- and α_2-globulins. Not all patients with RA have classic rheumatoid factor (anti-IgM with IgG specificity); some may have an IgG or IgA class of rheumatoid factor (seronegative). Complement levels in the synovial fluid are reduced, compared with a normal value one-third the serum value.

The triggering event for rheumatoid arthritis may be Epstein-Barr virus (EBV). Whether it is EBV or some other event, the synovium becomes activated, with mononuclear infiltrate, plasmacytosis, and antibody production. The antibody produced has been shown to have the capability of reacting as an EBV nuclear antigen, and it reacts with an antigen called RANA (rheumatoid-associated nuclear antigen). RANA is demonstrable in a cell extract of Wil-2 cell line along with SS-A. RANA exhibits a speckled pattern when Wil-2 cells are used as the substrate for ANA. Other laboratory findings are leukocytosis, decreased hyaluronidase, and increased protein in the synovial fluid.[8, 48]

In other studies of lymphocytes from RA patients, decreased mitogenic response was seen in severe disease;[50] however, synovial lymphocytes did respond effectively to specific antigens.[51] Cytokine release has also been noted among RA patients, particularly, interleukin-2, which is produced by activated T cells.[52] Besides RF, antibodies to collagen have been reported by several laboratories.[53, 54]

Organ/Tissue-Specific Disease

In autoimmune hemolytic anemia, the antibody may be complement fixing or hemolytic. In either case, the circulating red blood cells are lysed, resulting in intravascular hemolysis with decreased haptoglobin and hemopexin. The autoantibody may or may not be detectable, depending on its specificity. Nonspecific autoantibodies can create significant clinical management problems in certain patients, because compatible blood is not available. Specific red blood cell autoantibodies, such as those of the Ii system, can be detected, and compatible blood can be found.[2, 8]

In Goodpasture's syndrome, the autoantibody is usually of insufficient concentration or cross-reactivity to be detected in the patient's serum by the usual indirect fluorescent immunomicroscopy. A biopsy of the affected tissue for direct fluorescent immunomicroscopy or specific immunoassays using target tissue are the methods of choice for demonstrating the presence of the autoantibodies. In biopsy studies, the autoantibody is usually of the IgG class, and there is no evidence of complement fixation.[2, 8]

Often, several disorders manifest similar clinical-pathophysiologic pictures. Autoantibody tests become useful, therefore, not only as positive diagnostic indicators but as tools to rule out disorders. In evaluating ANA reactions, it is well to remember that endocrine disorders may exhibit multiple antibodies, so that a positive parietal cell antibody test does not always mean gastric atrophy or pernicious anemia. Moreover, certain autoantibodies require primate tissue for demonstration, for example, basement membrane in pemphigoid. If human tissue is used as the substrate, it should be from O-negative individuals; otherwise, reactions may be blood-group related rather than a "true antibody."[8, 48]

Chronic Autoimmune Hepatitis

Tissue-specific autoimmune disorders are becoming more commonly recognized. For example, chronic active autoimmune hepatitis is a progressive liver disease with an increased prevalence in women.[55] Onset of illness usually occurs between the ages of 30 and 40 years, but children have also been found with this disorder.[56] Nearly half of these patients ultimately develop secondary manifestations, such as arthritis, thyroiditis, or hemolytic anemia. Chronic autoimmune hepatitis has been subdivided into two basic types. Type I is considered a lupoid or lupus-like illness; affected patients typically have positive ANA and smooth-muscle antibody titers. Type II chronic autoimmune hepati-

tis is characterized by a positive antibody to liver-kidney microsomal proteins.[57] Type I chronic autoimmune hepatitis has been shown to have an HLA association with increased prevalence among HLA-DR6 haplotypes.[58]

Primary Biliary Cirrhosis

Primary biliary cirrhosis is another form of chronic autoimmune hepatitis. Characterized by spontaneous destruction of bile ducts leading to liver failure, the disease commonly affects middle-aged women. Laboratory tests used for detection of primary biliary cirrhosis include antimitochondrial antibody tests and M2 immunoblots. There are at least nine mitochondrial antigens, referred to as M1 through M9.[59] M2 appears to be specific for primary biliary cirrhosis. The M2 peptides have been shown to be components of the 2-oxo-acid dehydrogenase enzyme system.[59] Antimitochondrial antibodies can be detected by immunofluorescence or by enzyme immunoassays. The M2 antibodies are typically detected by Western blot analysis for identification of antibodies to the mitochondrial polypeptides with molecular weights of 74, 58, and 47 kD.

Primary Sclerosing Cholangitis

An inflammatory disease affecting the common bile duct, known as primary sclerosing cholangitis (PSC), manifests as large-duct sclerosis. A common laboratory finding is the presence of antineutrophil cytoplasmic antibodies, which are also seen in Wegener's granulomatosis and systemic vasculitis.

Another aberrant of small-duct PSC with either negative or atypical antimitochondrial antibodies has been described as autoimmune cholangitis.[60] Affected patients typically are ANA positive and anti–mitochondrial antibody negative, and some have anti–smooth muscle antibody.

TREATMENT

Autoimmune disorders are complex and sometimes frustrating for both the clinician and the patient. A variety of possibilities, many of which are still not understood, must be kept in mind for treatment. Most of the autoimmune disorders are currently treated with steroids to reduce antibody production, and possibly with therapeutic plasmapheresis to remove immune complexes or autoantibodies. If steroids do not prove useful, an immunosuppressive drug such as cytoxan may be used. In organ-specific disease, supportive therapy only may be used initially, until cellular destruction or malfunction can be slowed.[2, 8]

Studies of the clinical effects of cyclosporin on autoimmune diseases are still at an early stage. The preventive effects of cyclosporin in experimental models are comparable to those seen in transplantation. These data clearly show that cyclosporin may be suppressing the autoimmune disorder but does not cure the disease process. As with other drugs, the implications of long-term therapy and side effects must be addressed when cyclosporin is being considered.[61] Extensive investigation of hormonal therapy to control the pathogenic effects seen in autoimmune disorders has been conducted, and hormones are considered modulating agents of the immune system.[62]

Systemic Lupus Erythematosus

Avoidance of ultraviolet light is highly recommended for patients with SLE. Moderation of exercise is also recommended. Drug treatment varies, depending on organ involvement and severity of disease. One of the most common therapeutic agents used in SLE is an antimalarial known as hydroxychloroquine. It has been used in treatment of skin involvement but also has been used successfully for joint pain and other symptoms.[63] In addition, nonsteroidal anti-inflammatory drugs, such as aspirin, ibuprofen, ketoprofen, and naproxen, have been used for joint pain and other manifestations.

In patients with organ involvement, the use of short bursts of corticosteroids is common. Corticosteroids are widely used in renal involvement, but much controversy has evolved over the toxicity associated with their long-term use. Other agents used in this disease are azathioprine, chlorambucil, and cyclophosphamide, which appears to be one of the most beneficial.[64]

In drug-induced lupus, which mimics SLE in symptomatology, the patient is often being treated for cardiac arrhythmias with procainamide or tocainide. After the drugs are discontinued, the ANA titer gradually disappears in relation to the half-life of IgG, and the symptoms abate. In a small number of affected patients, the ANA titer does not revert to normal, however, and they exhibit symptoms and findings of SLE indefinitely.

Rheumatoid Arthritis

Nonsteroidal anti-inflammatory drugs are the agents most commonly used for treatment of RA. Aspirin, indomethacin, ibuprofen, and naproxen are among a few that are widely used. Other agents are antimalarials such as hydroxy chloroquines, penicillamine, and gold, as well as immunosuppressive agents such as azathioprine and cyclosphosphamide. The action of gold is thought to interfere with the macrophage function and lessen the activation of T cells.[65] The basic problem with long-term gold injections is the induction of immune recognition of the gold salts by recipient T cells, and treatment failure due to an immunologic response to the gold.[66]

Penicillamine, also thought to suppress the T cell function, is one of the treatments used in patients in whom gold treatment has failed. Steroids are typically used in the more severe stages of RA, and short-term treatments are preferred for remission of symptoms. Methotrexate, also used in treatment of RA, is thought to interfere with DNA synthesis as a folic acid antagonist, with a subsequent anti-inflammatory effect.[67]

Other SLE-like Disorders

Colchicine has been used widely for patients with scleroderma; however, toxic effects have now limited its utility. Corticosteroids have also been widely used in treatment of serious or organ-specific conditions. Nonsteroidal anti-inflammatory drugs are the typical treatment used.

Artificial tears or wetting solutions are commonly recommended for the sicca syndrome or dry-eye effect in Sjögren's syndrome. Corticosteroids are also used in Sjögren's syndrome, especially in more severe cases.

Case Study 1

A 30-year-old woman presented to her physician complaining of low-grade fever, anorexia, joint pain, fatigue, and unusual rashes on her face and chest. The onset of symptoms had been gradual, occurring over the past year.

The patient's laboratory findings were as follows:

FANA	Positive (titer of 1:320 with a homogeneous pattern)
Anti–ds-DNA	Positive
Anti-RNP	Negative
Anti–SS-B	Negative
Anti-Sm	Negative
Anti–SS-A	Negative

Questions

1. What is the most likely condition the physician should consider?
2. Do the laboratory findings support this diagnosis?

Discussion

1. In a woman of this age group with symptoms as described, SLE would be highly probable.
2. Laboratory data clearly support the diagnosis. The presence of a high-titer ANA is common to SLE, but the presence of antibodies to ds-DNA is highly suggestive of SLE. The anti-Sm Titer is negative, but only about 30% of patients with SLE demonstrate a positive test for Smith antibody.

Case Study 2

A 40-year-old woman presented with Raynaud's phenomenon, a rash on her chest, joint pain with swelling, muscle aches, respiratory distress, and short-term memory loss. She had been a factory worker for the past 20 years and had no previous medical problems. She had no family history of autoimmune diseases or arthritis, and no implantable devices. Upon careful history, the physician noted that she worked around toxic chemicals, including beryllium, silica, and silver salts.

The laboratory findings were as follows:

FANA	Positive (titer of 1:80; speckled pattern)
Rheumatoid factor	Negative
Anti–ds-DNA	Negative
Anti-Sm	Negative
Anti-RNP	Negative
Anti–SS-A	Negative
Anti–SS-B	Negative
Erythrocyte sedimentation rate	8 mm/hr

T cell response to beryllium	Strong proliferative response
Concanavalin A response	Normal response
T cell response to silica	Nonresponsive

Questions

1. Considering the occupational exposure and clinical presentation, what condition is suggested?
2. Do the laboratory findings support such a diagnosis?

Discussion

1. On the basis of the long-term exposure to several chemicals that have known immunogenic effects, the physician should consider an occupationally induced autoimmune syndrome that may mimic SLE or scleroderma. An important point that should be considered is the duration of exposure. Many environmentally or occupationally induced disorders have a significantly long latency, of 10 or more years.

2. This patient demonstrates a positive ANA, but it is low titer. The other markers used for classic autoimmune or rheumatic diseases are negative. Special testing for a cell-mediated immune response shows a proliferation of cells responsive to beryllium but not to silica. The concanavalin A response represents a normal T cell mitogen response. Proliferation of T cells responsive to beryllium is an important clinical marker and identifies the chemical responsible for the atypical autoimmune disorder seen in this patient. Nonexposed patients do not show proliferative T cells upon exposure, and such a test can be extremely useful in determining the specific agent involved. Tests for specific antibodies to beryllium have not been useful.

References

1. Retig RA, Levinsky NG: Kidney Failure and the Federal Government. Washington, DC, National Academy Press, 1991.
2. Stites D, Stobo J, Fudenberg H, et al: Basic and Clinical Immunology, ed 5. Los Altos, Calif, Lange Medical, 1984.
3. Bryant NJ: Laboratory Immunology and Serology, ed 2. Philadelphia, WB Saunders, 1986.
4. Roitt I: Essential Immunology, ed 5. Boston, Blackwell Scientific, 1984.
5. Garrido L, Pfleiderer B, Papisov M, et al: In vivo degradation of silicones. Magn Res Med 29:839–843, 1993.
6. Shanklin DR: Late tissue reactions to silicone and silica: The natural history of silicone-associated diseases with special reference to infections and immunological markers in tissue. In Stratmeyer ME (ed): Silicone in Medical Devices. Baltimore, USHHS/FDA 92–4249, 1991.
7. Pfleiderer B, Ackerman JL, Garrido L: Migration and biodegradation of free silicone from silicone gel-filled implants after long-term implantation. Magn Res Med 30:534–543, 1993.
8. Schwartz R, Rose N: Autoimmunity: Experimental and clinical aspects. Ann N Y Acad Sci 475:146–156, 1986.
9. O'Gorman M, Oger J: Cell-mediated immune functions in multiple sclerosis. Pathol Immunopathol Res 6:241–272, 1987.
10. Potter M, Morrison S, Wiener F, et al: Induction of plasmacytomas with silicone gel in genetically susceptible strains of mice. J Natl Cancer Inst 86:1058–1065, 1994.
11. Potter M, Boyce C: Induction of plasma neoplasms in strain BALB/c mice with mineral oil and mineral oil adjuvants. Nature 193:1086–1087, 1962.
12. Hanifen JM, Epstein WL, Cline MJ: In vitro studies of granulomatous hypersensitivity to beryllium. J Invest Dermatol 55:284–288, 1970.
13. Haustein UF, Ziegler V, Herrmann K, et al: Silica-induced scleroderma. J Am Acad Dermatol 22:444–448, 1990.
14. Deapen D, Escalante A, Weinrib L, et al: A revised estimate of twin concordance in systemic lupus erythematosus. Arthritis Rheum 35:311–318, 1992.
15. Tan EM, Cohen AS, Fries JF, et al: The 1982 revised criteria for the classification of systemic lupus erythematosus. Arthritis Rheum 25:1271–1277, 1982.
16. Tucker LB, Menon S, Schaller JG, et al: Adult- and childhood-onset systemic lupus erythematosus: A comparison of onset, clinical features, serology, and outcome. B J Rheumatol 34:866–872, 1995.
17. Litwin A, Adams LE, Hess EV, et al: Hydralazine urinary metabolites in systemic lupus erythematosus. Arthritis Rheum 16:217, 1973.
18. Yung RL, Johnson KJ, Richardson BC: Biology of disease: New concepts in the pathogenesis of drug-induced lupus. Lab Invest 73:746–759, 1995.
19. Wilson GB, Dixon FJ: Antiglomerular basement membrane antibody induced glomerulonephritis. Kidney Int 3:74, 1973.
20. Bohme J, Haskins K, Stecha P, et al: Transgenic mice with I.A. on islet cells are normoglycemic but immunologically intolerant. Science 244:1179–1183, 1989.
21. Love LA: New environmental agents associated with lupus-like disorders. Lupus 3:467–471, 1994.
22. Meijer CJLM, Graaff-Reitsma CB, Lafeber GJM, et al: In situ localization of lymphocyte subsets in synovial membranes of patients with rheumatoid arthritis with monoclonal antibodies. J Rheumatol 9:359–365, 1982.
23. Arnett FC, Edworthy SM, Bloch DA, et al: The American Rheumatism Association 1987 revised criteria for the classification of rheumatoid arthritis. Arthritis Rheum 38:315–324, 1988.
24. Khan MA: Ankylosing spondylitis. In Calin A (ed): Spondyloarthropathies. Orlando, Fla, Grune & Stratton, 1984.
25. Bennet PH, Burch IA: Population studies of rheumatic diseases. Amsterdam, Excerpta Medica, 1968.
26. Van der Linden S, Khan MA: Spondylitis in HLA-B27 individuals: A reappraisal [editorial]. J Rheumtol 11:727, 1984.
27. Keat AC: Reiter's syndrome and reactive arthritis in perspective. N Engl J Med 309:1606, 1983.
28. Kendall MJ, Lawrence DS, Shuttleworth GR, et al: Hematology and biochemistry of ankylosing spondylitis. B Med J 2:235, 1973.
29. Burmester GR, John B, Gramatzki M, et al: Activated T cells in vivo and in vitro: Divergence in expression of Tac and Ia antigens in the nonblastoid small T cells of inflammation and normal T cells activated in vitro. J Immunol 133:1230, 1984.
30. Richter MB, Woo P, Panayi GS, et al: The effects of intravenous pulse methylprednisolone (MTP) on immunologic and inflammatory processes in ankylosing spondylitis. Clin Exp Immunol 43:51, 1983.
31. Steigerwald JC: Polymyositis-dermatomyositis—the inflammatory myopathies. In Samter M, Talmadge DW, Frank MM, et al (eds): Immunological Diseases, ed 4. Boston, Little, Brown, 1988.
32. Wolfe JF, Adelstein E, Sharp GC: Antinuclear antibody with distinct specificity for polymyositis. J Clin Invest 59:176, 1977.
33. Rowe DJ, Isenberg DA, McDougall J, et al: Characterization of polymyositis infiltrates using monoclonal antibodies to human leucocyte antigens. Clin Exp Immunol 45:290, 1981.
34. Watson AJS, Dalbow MH, Stachura I, et al: Immunologic studies in cimetidine-induced nephropathy and polymyositis. N Engl J Med 308:142, 1983.
35. Medsgar TA, Masi AT: Epidemiology of progressive systemic sclerosis. Clin Rheum Dis 5:15, 1979.
36. Subcommittee for Scleroderma Criteria of the American Rheumatism Association, Diagnostic and Therapeutic Criteria Committee: Preliminary criteria for the classification of systemic sclerosis (scleroderma). Arthritis Rheum 23:581–590, 1980.
37. Kornreich HK, King KK, Bernstein BH, et al: Scleroderma in childhood. Arthritis Rheum 20:343–350, 1977.
38. Haustein UF, Ziegler V: Environmentally induced systemic sclerosis-like disorders. Int J Dermatol 24:147–151, 1985.

39. Kondo H, Rabin BS, Rodnan GP: Cutaneous antigen-stimulating lymphokine production by lymphocytes of patients with progressive systemic sclerosis (scleroderma). J Clin Invest 58:1388, 1976.

40. Stein EC, Schiffer RB, Hall J, Young N: Multiple sclerosis and the workplace: Report of an industry-based cluster. Neurology 37:1672–1677, 1987.

41. Ruhl H, Kirchner H: Monocyte-dependent stimulation of human T cells by zinc. Clin Exp Immunol 32:484–488, 1978.

42. Linker-Israeli M, Bakke AC, Kitridou RC, et al: Defective production of interleukin 1 and interleukin 2 in patients with systemic lupus erythematosus (SLE). J Immunol 130:2651–2655, 1983.

43. Sedwick LA, Burde RM: Isolated sixth nerve palsy as initial manifestation of systemic lupus erythematosus: A case report. J Clin Neurol Ophthamol 3:109, 1983.

44. Harris EN, Gharavi AE, Boey ML, et al: Anticardiolipin antibodies: Detection by radioimmunoassay and association with thrombosis in systemic lupus erythematosus. Lancet 2:1211–1214, 1983.

45. Lockshin MD, Druzin ML, Goei S, et al: Antibody to cardiolipin as a predictor of fetal distress or death in pregnant patients with systemic lupus erythematosus. N Engl J Med 313:152–156, 1985.

46. Hughes GR, Harris NN, Gharavi AE: The anticardiolipin syndrome. J Rheumtol 13:486–489, 1986.

47. Ishii Y, Nagasawa K, Mayumi T, et al: Clinical importance of persistence of anticardiolipin antibodies in systemic lupus erythematosus. Ann Rheum Dis 49:387–390, 1990.

48. Nakamura R, Peebles C, Rubin R, et al: Autoantibodies to Nuclear Antigens (ANA), ed 2. Chicago, American Society of Clinical Pathologists, 1985.

49. Rose N, Friedman H, Fahey J: Manual of clinical laboratory immunology, ed 3. Washington, DC, American Society for Microbiology, 1986.

50. Lance EM, Knight SC: Immunologic reactivity in rheumatoid arthritis response to mitogens. Arthritis Rheum 17:513–520, 1974.

51. Peterson J, Andersen V, Bendixen G, et al: Functional characteristics of synovial fluid and blood mononuclear cells in rheumatoid arthritis and traumatic synovitis. Scand J Rheumatol 11:75–80, 1982.

52. Wilkins JA, Warrington RJ, Sigurdson SL, et al: The demonstration of an interleukin-2 activity in the synovial fluids of rheumatoid arthritis patients. J Rheumatol 10:109–113, 1983.

53. Andriopoulos NA, Mestecky J, Wright GP, et al: Characterization of antibodies to the native human collagens and to their component alpha-chains in the sera and the joint fluids of patients with rheumatoid arthritis. Immunochemistry 13:709–712, 1976.

54. Menzel J, Steffen C, Kolarz G, et al: Demonstration of anticollagen antibodies in rheumatoid arthritis synovial fluids by c-radioimmunoassay. Arthritis Rheum 21:243–248, 1978.

55. Czaja AJ: Natural history, clinical features and treatment of autoimmune hepatitis. Semin Liver Dis 4:1–12, 1984.

56. Mistilis SP, Blackburn CRB: Active chronic hepatitis. Am J Med 48:484–495, 1970.

57. Hornberg JC, Abuaf N, Bernard N, et al: Chronic active hepatitis associated with antiliver/kidney microsome antibody type 1: A second type of "autoimmune" hepatitis. Hepatology 7:1333, 1987.

58. Fainboim L, Marcus Y, Pando M, et al: Chronic active autoimmune hepatitis in children: Strong association with a particular HLA-DR6 (DRB1*1301) haplotype. Human Immunol 41:146–150, 1994.

59. Berg PA, Klein R: Heterogeneity of antimitochondrial antibodies. Semin Liver Dis 9:103–116, 1989.

60. Taylor SL, Dean PJ, Riely CA: Primary autoimmune cholangitis: An alternative to antimitochondrial antibody-negative primary biliary cirrhosis. Am J Surg Pathol 18:91–99, 1994.

61. Borel JF, Gunn HC: Cyclosporin as a new approach to therapy of autoimmune diseases. Ann New York Acad Sci 475:307–319, 1986.

62. Ansar Ahmed S, Penhale WJ, Talal N: Sex hormones, immune responses, and autoimmune diseases: Mechanisms of sex hormone action. Am J Pathol 121:531–551, 1985.

63. Rudnick RD, Gresham GE, Rothfield NF: The efficacy of antimalarials in systemic lupus erythematosus. J Rheumatol 2:323, 1975.

64. Stenberg AD: The treatment of lupus nephritis. Kidney Int 30:769, 1986.

65. Ugai K, Ziff M, Lipsky PE: Gold-induced changes in the morphology and functional capacities of human monocytes. Arthritis Rheum 22:1352, 1979.

66. Romagnoli GA, Spinas GA, Sinigaglia F: Gold-specific T cells in rheumatoid arthritis patients treated with gold. J Clin Invest 89:254–258, 1992.

67. Samter M, Talmadge DW, Frank MM, et al: Immunological Diseases, ed 4. Boston, Little, Brown, 1988.

Chapter 49

Transplantation Immunology

David L. Smalley

Since the late 1970s, transplantation of tissues and whole organs has become a reality because of the gradually emerging understanding of the immune response system and the ability to suppress it to avoid tissue rejection. This progress is almost totally attributable to the proliferation of knowledge in the science of immunology, although the contributions of genetics, biochemistry, and pharmacology, as well as the development of new surgical techniques, have also been major factors in the success of transplantation. To appreciate the development of transplantation sciences, the basic role of the immune system in recognizing foreign tissue, the cellular and humoral immune responses, and the novel approaches in controlling the immune reaction to avoid rejection of the transplanted tissue must also be examined.

CONDITIONS LEADING TO TRANSPLANT

Transplantation replaces damaged tissues or organs with those that are functional. The most commonly transplanted organ is the kidney. Kidney transplantation has been accomplished successfully since 1958. The most frequent cause of end-stage renal disease requiring subsequent transplantation is diabetes; renal disease secondary to systemic lupus erythematosus (SLE) is second most frequent. As the kidney fails, urea and ammonia build in the body, and multiorgan failure can result. In the United States approximately 10,000 renal transplants are performed annually, about 80% of which use cadaver kidneys.[1] The success rate of a single kidney transplant is approximately 87%, and the success rate increases to almost 95% with a sibling kidney transplant. Transplanted kidneys may last for years, and the average renal transplant lasts for more than 5 years. Niepp and colleagues[2] report that the survival rate of 52 renal transplant recipients younger than 6 years was 90% for more than 5 years.

The second most commonly transplanted organ is the heart. The first heart transplant was performed in 1960, and the recipient lived approximately 98 days. The first successful human heart transplant was performed in 1967 by Dr. Christiaan Barnard in South Africa, and the recipient lived for 18 days afterward. The primary indication for heart transplantation is chronic coronary muscle deterioration or cardiomyopathy. The average life expectancy after surgery for a heart transplant recipient is 1 year in about 80% of cases.[3] Cardiac transplantation has not been considered appropriate for all patients dying of heart disease. Contraindications include active infection, recent pulmonary infarction, renal or hepatic dysfunction, diabetes mellitus, malignancy, and peptic ulcer disease.[4] In many instances heart transplants are combined with lung transplants; the first heart-lung transplant was performed in 1981 at Stanford University.[5] Because it is not uncommon for cardiomyopathic disease to also diminish pulmonary function, the simultaneous transplant of the two organs improves the likelihood of successful transplantation and the subsequent health of the patient.

Lung transplants have been performed without the heart but with less success. The primary indication for lung transplantation is end-stage pulmonary disease. The frequency of this procedure is restricted by the short time frame allowed to remove the lungs from the donor to implant into the recipient. Lung transplant recipients often have major complications with acute rejection and major infections of the implanted lungs.

Another frequently transplanted organ in the United States is the liver. The most common indications for liver transplant are primary malignancy of the liver, cryptogenic cirrhosis, posthepatitis as a consequence of hepatitis, and other less common disease states.[6] Much of the early liver transplantation work was done by Starzl and colleagues,[7] who performed the first successful human liver transplant in 1963.[8] In an analysis of 5180 liver transplants from 1982 to 1991, Kilpe and colleagues[9] reported a 79% survival rate after 1 year and a 60% survival rate at 5 years. Improved survival was noted for cirrhosis, primary biliary cirrhosis, alcoholic cirrhosis, primary sclerosing cholangitis, and Wilson's disease. Poor survival was reported in patients with hemochromatosis. Five-year survival was 67% for children younger than 13 years. As the age of the patient increases, survival rates decline until adults older than 55 years experience a five-year survival rate of less than 65%.

Keeffe and Esquivel[10] report that liver transplants for alcoholic cirrhosis have become less controversial because the great majority of recipients do not resume drinking postoperatively. Hepatitis B continues to be problematic in transplant patients, with 80% to 90% reinfection of the allografts. Liver cancer patients have only a 20% to 30% long-term survival rate, although typically they are cured of the malignancy. Liver atresia is the most common indication for transplant in children. Starzl and colleagues reported that children are almost always suitable candidates for grafting and have been some of the longest survivors.[8] Partial liver wedges have been transplanted successfully from mother to child; however, the removal of liver tissue from a living donor is too dangerous to be routinely recommended.

In 1913 the first pancreas segment was grafted into a dog by Duffy and Calne with a resulting drop in blood glucose.[11] In 1966 Kelly and colleagues[12] performed pancreas transplants on 14 diabetic patients, only one of whom survived more than 1 year. Failures were thought to be due to the limitations of immunosuppressive therapy available at the time. Cyclosporine has recently been shown to be effective in immunosuppressive therapy in pancreatic transplantation.[13] In 1983 Najarian and Sutherland[14] suggested that diabetics with end-stage renal disease were poor candidates for transplant, whereas diabetics with microangiopathy and no renal disease were suitable candidates. More than 6000 pancreas transplants have been performed worldwide, with recipients primarily consisting of diabetic persons. Because of the associated nephropathy in diabetic patients, in 1995 Sutherland and Gruessner[15] reported that combined pancreas-kidney transplants are becoming more frequent. The survival rate of more than 5 years for this combined procedure varies from 74% to 100%.

TISSUE COMPATIBILITY VS. REJECTION

Immunologic Reactions and Tissue Rejection

Almost all nucleated human cells carry specific antigens known as *human leukocyte antigens* (HLA). These antigens are coded by the genes of the major histocompatibility complex (MHC) system and consist of three antigen classes, two of which are important in tissue matching for transplantation. The loci of human HLA antigens are found on the short arm of chromosome 6. Class I antigens have three loci: HLA-A, HLA-B, and HLA-C. Class II antigens were originally defined as HLA-D but are now recognized as DR- and D-related antigens and include HLA-DR, HLA-

DQ, and HLA-DP. The loci for class I and II antigens on each chromosome are inherited together as a *haplotype*. Therefore, each individual has two haplotypes, one from each parent. The numerous alleles for each locus generally result in great variation of HLA haplotypes, and except for identical twins, who share identical haplotypes, each non-twin individual has a unique HLA genotype. Thus, the immune system of one individual recognizes nucleated cells from another individual as foreign, and any tissue or organ transplanted has the potential for rejection by the recipient's immune system. One way to prevent this is to minimize the foreignness by what is commonly called *tissue matching*. This permits transplantation of donor tissue most similar in HLA type to that of the recipient.

Tissue rejection is a process by which the recipient's immune system recognizes the transplanted tissue as foreign and attempts to destroy or eliminate it. The rejection process follows the usual physiologic process by which the macrophage (antigen-presenting cell) identifies the tissue as being foreign or "nonself" and undertakes degradation or processing of the tissue for presentation to the T lymphocytes. This occurs by identification of two structural points: the foreign antigen and the MHC class II protein, which facilitates the recognition of the foreign antigen by the T cells. As this identification is accomplished, the macrophage releases interleukin-1 (IL-1). This cytokine activates and recruits more helper T cells in a manner analogous to the mobilization of forces for battle. As the T cells receive the antigen presented and become activated, they also release interleukin-2 (IL-2), which further recruits T and B cells to the site.

The activation of the additional lymphocytes initiates the second phase of foreign tissue destruction—an attack by cytotoxic T cells. These cells release lymphotoxins, which destroy the tissue cells and make the transplanted cells more susceptible to other immune attacks. As the process of rejection and destruction of the tissue continues, B cells are activated, which, upon transformation to plasma cells, produce antibodies directed at the foreign HLA antigens that are present on the donor tissue surface. These antibodies attach, initiate the complement cascade, and increase the pace of tissue injury, particularly in the endothelium of the donor organ. As the cells lose their integrity, they undergo lysis and die. The longer the tissue is attacked by the recipient's immune system, the more likely that the tissue will ultimately be rejected or become nonfunctional. Thus the control of the immune system response by suppressing immune activation has become an essential component of successful transplantation.

In tissue transplant recipients the immune-regulated rejection of the grafted tissue is primarily T-cell based, although both cellular and humoral elements of the immune response system are involved. The speed of rejection depends on the particular components involved and has been characterized as *hyperacute, accelerated, acute,* and *chronic.* Hyperacute reactions are due to preformed HLA and ABO antibodies in the recipient, and rejection of the donor tissue begins to occur almost immediately. Acute rejection takes place within days to weeks and is the most frequently occurring type of rejection. It is a result of cell-mediated immunity[16] in which the foreign antigen initiates the interaction, primarily with CD4 + or helper/inducer T cells. Activated T cells then respond by releasing IL-2, which activates CD8+ or cytotoxic T cells, and also by releasing other lymphokines that recruit and activate macrophages and other effector cells. This results in direct cytolysis and damage to the donor tissue in addition to the recipient cells.[17] The expression of MHC antigens in grafted or donor tissue initiates the recognition of reacting T cells. Rejection is typically accompanied by an increased expression of MHC class I and II proteins on the cells. Muller-Ruchholtz reported that in rat kidney grafts the induction of class I antigens occurs in about 24 hours, whereas in rat heart grafts the class I antigens are induced in about 72 hours. Class II antigens occur in both types of transplants after 3 to 4 days, but the MHC expression can increase as much as 30- to 40-fold within 5 days.[17]

Two major groups of humoral factors are reported to occur in transplantation immune response and are designated as *nonspecific* and *specific*, respectively. The nonspecific factors include interleukins and growth and differentiation factors for B and T cells. The specific factors are the antibodies that are directed against the MHC antigens. The role of antibodies in acute rejection of a first-time recipient depends on the tissue but is typically limited. Accelerated rejection takes place upon second exposure to tissue antigens, resulting in both T and B cell response.[16] Circulating antibodies seem to play a more significant role in chronic rejection, which can occur months or years following transplantation. In chronic rejection syndromes, the target tissue is most often vascular endothelium and results in complement activation, which can cause direct cell damage.

In a review of the pathology of kidney rejection, Thiru found that the stages of transplanted tissue rejection were described as early as 1943.[18, 19] The rejection of allografts with destruction of tissue was described as being due to specific immune responses provoked by antigens from the foreign tissue. Kidney transplantation survival has improved because of improved preservation of donor tissue, better facilities, improved understanding of tissue typing and matching, and development of immunosuppressive agents.[18] In 1944 Medawar described the presence of mononuclear cell infiltration, which started within a few hours after transplantation, as a prominent feature of all first-set allografts in animals.[20] It is now known that the cells described were, in fact, T cells, which when sensitized initiate the first-set rejection by two mechanisms. In the first mechanism, cytotoxic T cells mount a direct attack on the graft cells. In the second mechanism, T cells initiate a delayed hypersensitivity reaction, which recruits more immune cells. The resulting vascular damage compromises the graft.[21]

Another well-recognized response of importance in transplantation is the immune recognition of foreign HLA proteins of the recipient by the graft cells. Immune recognition uses the same mechanism as described earlier, but in this case, the process, called *graft vs. host response*, can initiate tissue damage to the recipient. Muller-Ruchholtz suggested that four major factors affect the incidence of graft vs. host response. The first factor is the degree of antigenic disparity between the donor and recipient. As described above, immune-induced response does not occur either in the host or the graft in bone marrow grafts between identical twins. The risk of graft response to the

host, however, increases as the number of HLA incompatibilities increases. The second factor of graft vs. host response depends on the number of lymphocytes transferred in the grafted tissue. For example, the response is more likely to occur in solid organ transplantation when a large portion of lymphoid tissue is present in the grafted tissue. The third factor is the presence of microbial flora and infection. Some viral infections appear to amplify the graft vs. host response. The fourth factor appears to be the age of the recipient. The older the recipient the more likely that such a response occurs, a poorly understood phenomenon.[17] Of all the common transplants, bone marrow is the tissue in which graft vs. host response is of greatest importance.

Protected Tissue

Several tissues seem to be protected from the immune response of transplantation, and the most frequently transplanted tissue with limited immune recognition is the cornea. More than 40,000 corneal transplants were performed by 1991.[22] It is thought that these tissues probably do not include MHC surface proteins and that the cornea has limited vascularity, which limits transport of the immune-activating cells to the site of implantation. The most common rejection of this type of protected tissue occurs as a result of postoperative infections. Primary corneal grafts have a greater than 90% success rate with a 2-year survival.[23] Increased rejection syndromes occur with two types of corneal transplant recipients: those with vascularized corneas and those with previous history of rejection syndromes.[24, 25] Opinions vary about the need for HLA matching. In a 3-year study of 419 transplant patients, Hahn reported that the development of antibodies to class I HLA antigens was associated with immune-mediated graft rejection and that the development of such antibodies was an indicator of impending graft rejection.[24, 25, 26, 27]

CLINICAL MANIFESTATIONS OF REJECTION

Kidney

Fever, swelling, oliguria, and pain above the area of the allograft are early signs of rejection, although these inflammatory signs may be diminished by cyclosporine. If renal function was good prior to transplantation, an increase in serum creatinine level and a decrease in creatinine clearance may be the only signs of possible rejection.[28]

Heart and Heart-Lung

Early signs of rejection of the transplanted heart can be minimal, and necrosis may occur before there is any overt warning. Although monitoring of activated T lymphocytes in the peripheral blood can provide some indication of ensuing rejection, biopsies are often required to ascertain the status of the transplanted tissue. Heart-lung transplants are somewhat more complicated because rejection of the lungs can occur separately from the heart. Endobronchoscopic biopsies are necessary if rejection is suspected. Unrecognized rejection may lead to obliterative bronchiolitis, limiting long-term survival.[29]

Lung

Rejection of the transplanted lung is characterized by fever, cough, dyspnea, deterioration of pulmonary function, and infiltrates detected radiographically. Because these signs are also observed in infection, differentiation between rejection and infection is important. Biopsy is more useful to establish the onset of rejection than bronchoalveolar lavage, which is limited to the diagnosis of infection.[30]

Liver

Fever, right upper quadrant pain, and reduced production of bile pigment (bilirubin) and volume are clinical signs of rejection. Biopsy is necessary to establish the correct diagnosis because these symptoms may also occur in a number of other complications associated with liver transplant.[31]

Bone Marrow

In rejection of the marrow graft by the recipient, peripheral blood counts suddenly drop, biopsy results reveal a lack of cellular elements, and myeloid tissue disappears. In acute graft vs. host disease the first sign may be a rash. Diarrhea may occur with abdominal pain.[32]

LABORATORY ANALYSES

ABO Grouping

ABO grouping is performed to ensure a donor-recipient match because of the presence of ABO antigens on many cell types and the need to avoid incompatibility with the high-titered, complement-binding antibodies of this system.[16]

HLA Typing

HLA matching of donor and recipient has demonstrated benefit for kidney transplant patients. Yoon and colleagues found a 26% difference in graft survival after 5 years when the graft recipient received tissue with zero vs. two HLA-DR mismatches. With grafts of tissue from living donors the 5-year graft survival rate went from 84% with zero HLA-DR mismatches to 39% with two mismatches.[33] Although the role of HLA antigen matching in pancreas grafting has not been as clearly defined, the likelihood of immune-based rejection remains high. Islet cells of the pancreas are not considered to be highly immunogenic, but "passenger leukocytes" play a major role in immune recognition and subsequent attack on the graft by the recipient's immune system.[11]

One of the oldest techniques used in tissue typing is the *lymphocytotoxicity test*, using lymphocytes from the patient, antibody to specific HLA antigens, and rabbit complement. If the specific antibodies recognize and attach to the counterpart antigen, the lymphocytes are killed and can be visualized microscopically using a vital stain such as trypan blue or eosin dye. Live cells, undamaged by the antigen-antibody-complement–mediated attack because of their intact cell membranes, remain unstained by the dye.

Milford has provided an excellent review of the proce-

dure for HLA typing, discussing in detail cell preparation and recovery of lymphocytes from blood, lymph nodes, and spleen tissue. Detecting class I antigens by reagent sera uses T cells from the recipient; class II antigen screens require B cells.[1] Commercial panels of cells are also available for screening the recipient's serum for HLA antibodies. Another technique used is the National Institutes of Health Amos technique, which is a crossmatch or crosschecking for preformed donor antibodies to antigens present in the recipient, and vice versa.[1] Several modifications of this technique have been reported, including the use of an antiglobulin crossmatch and B-cell crossmatches.

Mixed Lymphocyte Reaction Testing

Mixed lymphocyte reaction (MLR) tests the match between donor and recipient by assessing the degree of stimulation of the recipient's T lymphocytes by donor cells. Because the procedure requires approximately 1 week to complete, performing this test is useful when sufficient time before transplantation is available.[16] In the future, polymerase chain reaction (PCR) testing for DNA sequence coding for class II antigen alleles may prove useful.

Flow Crossmatching

In flow cytometric crossmatching, non–complement-binding antibodies can be detected in the serum of the recipient. Lymphocytes are recovered from the blood or tissue, and the patient's serum is added. After a short incubation, the cells are washed, and anti-human antibody is added, which has been tagged with a fluorescent compound such as fluorescein isothiocyanate. After incubation, the cells undergo flow cytometric analysis.[1] Each laboratory must establish its own criteria for a positive response. A two-color crossmatch can also be performed in which a second fluorescent dye, such as phycoerythrin, which emits red florescence, is used. This allows two antibodies to be used simultaneously to identify specific T or B cells and the presence of antibody.[1]

IMMUNOMODULATION AND TREATMENT

Although total body irradiation was once applied to recipients of kidney grafts, classic drug immunosuppressive agents, such as corticosteroids, have been used successfully since the 1950s. These agents prevent IL-1 release and antigen-induced activation of T cells. Cyclosporine, discovered in 1972, is now known to play a major immunosuppressive role by blocking IL-2 release from activated T cells. This prevents the cytokine cascade of interleukins and interferons from activating further immunologic reaction.[17] Certain antibodies may reduce the graft vs. host reaction. In one of the oldest modes of treatment, antilymphocyte antibodies can eliminate T cells because antibodies are directed specifically at CD3+ or mature T cells. This technique has recently been replaced with one that uses antibodies specific for T cells (OKT3). New immunosuppressive drugs include FK-506, a macrolide derived from *Streptomyces*. The mechanism of action appears to be similar to that of cyclosporine, blocking the release of IL-2.[17]

Orloff and colleagues[34] reported that chronic rejection is the major cause of graft failure in solid tissue transplantation after the first year. In their studies, tolerance induction was considered as a possible immunomodulating effect that would prevent chronic rejection. Tolerance induction by autologous bone marrow transplants and intrathymic inoculations were both found to be effective.

In the early 1980s Stoin reported that immunosuppression was the major means to control moderate to severe rejection of transplanted tissue.[35] Mild rejection was treated with short bursts of increased steroids, with a repeat biopsy performed in a week to detect changes. The agents used successfully were antithymocyte globulin and azathioprine or steroids and the more commonly used agent today, cyclosporine. Bieber and colleagues reported that the antithymocyte globulin typically reduced the patient's circulating T-cell populations from about 70% to 80% of the lymphocytes to about 5%.[35] However, cyclosporine simply reduced the activation of T cells by blocking the release of IL-2. A newer agent, FK-506, also blocks IL-2 release. Among a group of 204 adults who received kidney transplants and FK-506, an effective graft survival rate of 94% 1 year after transplant was achieved.[37] In this study the addition of azathioprine to FK-506 was not more effective than the FK-506 alone.

Recently, antilymphocyte-specific serum and monoclonal antibodies directed at CD3 + cells (OKT3) have been used in lung, heart, and pancreas transplants during acute rejection phases. The basic problem with this treatment is the stimulation of the recipient's immune system to develop an antibody to the murine proteins in some cases, thus inactivating the monoclonal antibodies.

mismatching would be predictive of potential rejection in the future as the recipient responded to the foreign HLA antigens.

References

1. Milford EL: Immunologic testing for renal transplantation. *In* Rose NR, De Macario BC, Fahey JL, et al (eds): Manual of Clinical Laboratory Immunology, ed 4. Washington, DC, American Society for Microbiology, 1992.
2. Neipp M, Oldhafer KJ, Offner G, et al: Renal transplantation in children under six years of age. Transplant Proc 27:3439, 1995.
3. Duquesnoy RJ, Zeevi A: Immunological monitoring of heart and lung transplant patients. *In* Rose NR, De Macario BC, Fahey JL, et al (eds): Manual of Clinical Laboratory Immunology, ed 4. Washington, DC, American Society for Microbiology, 1992.
4. Wallwork J: Heart and heart-lung transplantation. *In* Calne RY (ed): Transplantation Immunology: Clinical and Experimental. Oxford, Oxford University Press, 1984.
5. Reitz BA: Heart-lung transplantation: A review. Heart Transpl 4:291–297, 1982.
6. Rolles K, Calne RY: Liver transplantation. *In* Calne RY (ed): Transplantation Immunology: Clinical and Experimental. Oxford, Oxford University Press, 1984.
7. Starzl TE, Kaupp HA, Brock DR, et al: Studies of rejection of the transplanted homologous dog liver. Surg Gynecol Obstet 112:135–144, 1961.
8. Starzl TE, Marchiori TL, Von Kualla KN, et al: Homotransplantation of the liver in humans. Surg Gynecol Obstet 117:659–676, 1963.
9. Kilpe VE, Krakauer H, Wren RE: An analysis of liver transplant experience from 37 transplant centers as reported to Medicare. Transplant 56:554–561, 1993.
10. Keeffe EB, Esquivel CO: Controversies in patient selection for liver transplantation. West J Med 159:586–593, 1993.
11. Duffy TJ, Calne RY: Pancreas and islet cell transplantation. *In* Calne RY (ed): Transplantation Immunology: Clinical and Experimental. Oxford, Oxford University Press, 1984.
12. Kelly WD, Lillehei RC, Merkel FK, et al: Allotransplantation of the pancreas and duodenum along with the kidney in diabetic nephropathy. Surgery 61:827–837, 1967.
13. Calne RY, Rolles K, White DJG, et al: Cyclosporin A in clinical organ grafting. Transplant Proc 13:349–357, 1981.
14. Najarian JS, Sutherland DER: In workshop on transplantation of the pancreas. Transplant Proc 15:1509, 1983.
15. Sutherland DER, Gruessner A: Long-term function (> 5 years) of pancreas grafts from the International Pancreas Transplant Registry database. Transplant Proc 27:2977–2980, 1995.
16. LaChapelle R, Huot AE: Transplantation and tumor immunology. *In* Stevens CD: Clinical Immunology and Serology. Philadelphia, FA Davis, 1996.
17. Muller-Ruchholtz W: The immunopathology of transplantation. *In* Sale GE (ed): The Pathology of Organ Transplantation. Boston, Butterworths, 1990.
18. Thiru S: Pathology of rejection—kidney. *In* Calne RY (ed): Transplantation Immunology: Clinical and Experimental. Oxford, Oxford University Press, 1984.
19. Gibson T, Medawar PB: The fate of skin homografts in man. J Anat 77:299–316, 1943.
20. Medawar PB: The behaviour and fate of skin autografts and skin homografts in rabbits. J Anat 78:176–199, 1944.
21. McCluskey RT, Benacerraf B, McCluskey JW: Studies of the specificity of the cellular infiltrate in delayed hypersensitivity reactions. J Immunol 90:466–477, 1963.
22. Eye Bank of America: Activity Report. Washington, DC, Eye Bank Association of America, 1992.
23. Khoudadoust AA: The allograft rejection reaction: The leading cause of late failure of clinical corneal grafts. *In* Corneal Graft Failure, Ciba Foundation Symposium. Amsterdam, Elsevier Science Publishers, 1973, p 151.
24. Hahn AB, Foulks GN, Enger C, et al: The association of lymphocytotoxic antibodies with corneal allograft rejection in high risk patients. Transplant 59:21–27, 1995.

Case Study

A 35-year-old male presented to his physician with end-stage renal disease secondary to long-term, uncontrolled diabetes. The transplant team elected to place him on the renal and pancreas transplant list for a potential donor.

Laboratory Findings

Recipient HLA type	A1B5Cw3/A2B8Cw3
Donor HLA type	A1B3Cw3/A1B8Cw3

Questions

1. Does the HLA type show any mismatching?
2. If the crossmatch for the patient is compatible, does this mean that there is no chance of rejection syndrome?

Discussion

1. There is one mismatch for the HLA-A and one mismatch for the HLA-B.
2. The crossmatch measures whether the recipient has preformed antibodies and does not measure incompatibilities of the HLA matching. In this case, the

25. Batchelor JR, Casey TA, Gibbs DC, et al: HLA matching and corneal grafting. Lancet 1:551, 1976.
26. Wilson ST, Kaufman HE: Graft failure after penetrating keratoplasty. Ophthalmol 98:1177, 1991.
27. Ehlers N, Kissmeyer-Nielsen F: Corneal transplantation and histocompatibility. Acta Ophthalmol 49:513, 1971.
28. Carpenter CB, Lazarus JM: Dialysis and transplantation in the treatment of renal failure. *In* Isselbacher KJ, Braunwald E, Wilson JD, et al (eds): Harrison's Principles of Internal Medicine, ed 13. New York, McGraw-Hill, 1994.
29. Schroeder JS: Cardiac transplantation. *In* Isselbacher KJ, Braunwald E, Wilson JD, et al (eds): Harrison's Principles of Internal Medicine, ed 13. New York, McGraw-Hill, 1994.
30. Trulock EP, Cooper JD: Lung transplantation. *In* Isselbacher KJ, Braunwald E, Wilson JD, et al (eds): Harrison's Principles of Internal Medicine, ed 13. New York, McGraw-Hill, 1994.
31. Dienstag J: Liver transplantation. *In* Isselbacher KJ, Braunwald E, Wilson JD, et al (eds): Harrison's Principles of Internal Medicine, ed 13. New York, McGraw-Hill, 1994.
32. Thomas ED: Bone marrow transplantation. *In* Isselbacher KJ, Braunwald E, Wilson JD, et al (eds): Harrison's Principles of Internal Medicine, ed 13. New York, McGraw-Hill, 1994.
33. Yoon YS, Jin DC, Yang CW, et al: The effect of HLA mismatching on graft survival in living-donor kidney transplants: Catholic Medical Center, 1984–1993. Clin Transplant 18:275–283, 1993.
34. Orloff MS, DeMara EM, Coppage ML, et al: Prevention of chronic rejection and graft arteriosclerosis by tolerance induction. Transplant 59:282–288, 1995.
35. Stoin PGI: The morphology of myocardial rejection and transplantation pathology. *In* Calne RY (ed): Transplantation Immunology: Clinical and Experimental. Oxford, Oxford University Press, 1984.
36. Bieber CP, Griepp RB, Oyer PE, et al: Relationship of rabbit ATG serum clearance rate to circulating T-cell level, rejection onset, and survival in cardiac transplantation. Transplant Proc 9:1031–1036, 1977.
37. Shapiro R, Jordan ML, Scantlebury VP, et al: A prospective randomized trial of FK-506–based immunosuppression after renal transplantation. Transplant 59:485–490, 1995.

Chapter 50

Tumor Immunology and Tumor Markers

Karen James

Etiology and Pathophysiology

ETIOLOGY AND PATHOPHYSIOLOGY

Development of Tumors

Physicians, scientists, and patients often use terms such as *cancer, neoplasm, tumor,* and *malignancy* as if synony-

mous. *Cancer* is a layman's term, however, used to indicate a process of malignant neoplasia. *Neoplasia* means new growth, and *tumor* actually refers to swelling or to a defined mass of tissue that is different from normal physiologic growth.[1, 2] *Malignancy* is a tendency to progress in virulence, and defining a tumor or neoplasm as *malignant* denotes its ability to become progressively worse, resulting in death. *Metastasis* is the transfer of disease from one organ or part of the body to another not directly connected with it and distant from the primary site.

Benign plasias or growths (hyperplasia, metaplasia) may cause clinical disease by affecting the functions of normal tissues or by producing hormones with functional activity. Anaplasia or dysplasia refers to alterations in the size, arrangement, and organization of cells in a specific tissue.[2] A neoplasm is a relatively autonomous growth of tissue, essentially a parasite that establishes a relationship with a host. This relationship is referred to as a *tumor-host interaction.* Neoplasias cause symptoms of disease when they attack normal tissue, grow quickly, and deplete the nutrient resources of normal tissues. The behavioral characteristics of benign and malignant neoplasms are listed in Table 50–1.[3] Malignant tumors are characterized by infiltrating, erosive growth that penetrates the surrounding tissues, making their surgical removal exceedingly difficult. Compared with normal cells, some of the unusual characteristics that cancer cells display are (1) decreased cohesiveness that facilitates shedding of cancer cells into natural channels (e.g., bladder cancer cells found in urine, cervical cancer cells found in vaginal secretions), (2) loss of contact inhibition, whereby cancer cells continue to grow when contacting other cells, unlike normal cells, which would

Table 50–1. Behavioral Characteristics of Benign and Malignant Neoplasms

Benign	Malignant
Encapsulated	Non-encapsulated
Noninvasive	Invasive
Highly differentiated	Poorly differentiated
Rare mitoses	Mitoses relatively common
Slow growth	Rapid growth
Little or no anaplasia	Anaplastic to varying degrees
No metastases	Metastases

Reprinted from Pitot HC: Fundamentals of Oncology. New York, Marcel Dekker, 1978, by courtesy of Marcel Dekker, Inc.

cease to proliferate, and (3) elaboration of enzymes or other products that facilitate invasiveness, such as the induction of osteoblastic activity by metastasizing cancers of the breast and prostate.

Neoplasms are grouped according to the types of tissue from which they have arisen. Tumors arising from embryonic ectoderm or endoderm are termed *carcinoma,* whereas malignant neoplasms arising from the epithelium of the stomach, the pancreas, or the breast are termed *adenocarcinoma.* A malignant neoplasm arising from the mesodermal (mesenchymal) embryonic germ layer is termed *sarcoma.* The suffix *-blastoma* denotes certain types of neoplasms that have primitive appearances resembling embryologic structures (e.g., neuroblastoma). Malignant neoplasms of multiple-tissue origin are known as *teratomas.*

A *carcinogen* is an agent whose administration leads to a greater incidence of malignant neoplasms in animals, including humans. A large number of materials have been implicated as carcinogenic, including many naturally occurring chemicals as well as synthetic chemicals that have been associated with specific types of neoplasms.[3]

Hormones have been shown to have teratogenic (if not carcinogenic) properties. For example, the estrogenic compound diethylstilbestrol (DES) causes adenocarcinoma of the vagina or cervix in females who were exposed to this compound in utero.[3] Other synthetic steroids have been associated with carcinoma of the liver. Endocrine-related neoplasms (breast, prostate) are primarily affected by the growth-stimulating effects of the hormones.

Long-term exposure to radiation is carcinogenic and leukemogenic.[3] The incidence of leukemia in radiologists in the first half of the 20th century was 3 to 4 times that in the general population. Survivors of the atom bomb blasts in Japan have an incidence of leukemia twice that of the general population. Treatment of goiter and other lesions of the thyroid with radioactive iodine in young individuals in the 1950s has resulted in higher incidence of thyroid carcinoma later in these patients' lives. Many individuals exposed to radium while painting the dials of watches developed osteogenic sarcomas 15 to 25 years after exposure.

Viruses are also known to cause cancer. Human papillomavirus (HPV) is the best characterized oncogenic DNA virus, implicated as a causative agent in squamous cell carcinoma of the cervix.[4] Other DNA viruses that have been statistically linked with human tumors are Epstein-Barr virus (EBV) with Burkitt's lymphoma and nasopha-ryngeal carcinoma, and hepatitis B virus (HBV) infections with primary liver cancer.[5] RNA viruses, such as retroviruses, have within their virions the reverse transcriptase enzyme that enables them to transcribe a DNA copy of the viral genome, which is then integrated into the genome of the host cell. Integration of the viral genome into the host genome results in the constant production of virus by the transformed cell (illustrated in Fig. 45–2, Chapter 45). Examples of oncogenic RNA viruses in humans are human T-cell leukemia virus (HTLV I and II) which are associated with certain T-cell leukemias. Others attack various species of animals.

Many types of cancer have some genetic predisposition in combination with a variety of environmental factors. Familial polyposis of the colon is an autosomal dominant disease that predisposes individuals to colon cancer. Bilateral retinoblastoma is inherited as a mendelian dominant characteristic. Although only a fraction of total neoplasias can be categorized as genetic, there is much evidence of a genetic predisposition to developing cancer in many more individuals. The incidence of breast cancer in relatives of patients with premenopausal breast cancer is three times greater than in relatives of patients with postmenopausal breast cancer.

Tumor Immunology

The study of tumor immunology began in the 1950s, when tumors induced by carcinogens (methylcholanthrene) were used to immunize inbred mice. These immunized mice could reject a graft of the same tumor, a phenomenon that provided them protection from the same tumors, but no protection against other tumors.[6] Antigens on the chemically induced tumors were unique for the individual tumor and could be passed in vivo or in vitro without being lost. Immunity to carcinogen-induced tumors could be passed on to other mice through lymphocytes, suggesting that T cells were involved in the immune responsiveness to tumors. By using tumor-associated antigens as immunogens in the effort to control tumor growth, tumor immunologists continue to explore potential therapeutic mechanisms.[7]

For many years, scientists have hypothesized that the immune system plays a key role in tumor immunity, basing their assumptions on the observation that mononuclear cell infiltrates are present when solid tumors are removed from humans during surgery, which implies an immune response to the cancer. The theory that the immune system detects and destroys tumor cells that are constantly arising during the life of all individuals has been termed "immune surveillance."

Immune Responsiveness to Tumors

Tumor Antigens

Antigens on the surfaces of tumor cells were thought at first to be unique immunogens, identified by the immune system as being different from molecules on the surfaces of normal cells. Chemically induced tumors were extensively studied to understand the nature of these antigens; however, nearly every tumor had unique antigens, even when induced by the same carcinogen using the same strain of animals, a fact that confounded scientists. After many years of study, four classes of tumor-associated antigens have been characterized.[7]

- Tumor-specific peptides that require major histocompatibility gene complex (MHC) interaction to elicit an immune response
- Virus-induced tumor antigens that must be associated with MHC antigens on the surface of tumor cells to generate an immune response
- Genome-encoded tumor antigens with point mutations of oncogenes that induce unbridled cellular proliferation
- Expression of normally dormant differentiation antigens

TUMOR-SPECIFIC PEPTIDES

Tumor-specific peptides are derived from fragmented proteins presented by MHC products on the cell surface during antigen processing.[8] Antigen processing and presentation for T-cell recognition follows two primary pathways, the exogenous pathway and the endogenous pathway.[7]

Exogenous protein presentation involves several processes: (1) endocytosis of the foreign protein by antigen-presenting cells called APCs (macrophages and B cells), (2) degradation of the protein into short peptides of eight to nine amino acids within the APCs, and (3) binding of these peptides to class II MHC molecules within the APCs. When the MHC-peptide complexes reach the cell surface, they are recognized by T cells expressing the CD4 molecule (CD4+ T cells).

Endogenous protein presentation involves insertion of the peptides into class I MHC molecules within the endoplasmic reticulum of the cell. When these MHC-peptide complexes reach the cell surface, they are recognized by T cells expressing the CD8 molecule (CD8+ T cells).

The existence of two mechanisms of MHC-peptide interaction makes it clear that intracellular proteins (not only surface antigens) can be displayed on the surfaces of tumor cells; that is, these proteins are integral to the mechanism for dysregulation in tumor cells that become visible to the immune system.[9]

VIRUS-INDUCED TUMOR ANTIGENS

Virus-induced tumor antigens on murine neoplasms were the first antigenic structures detectable on tumor cells as targets for T-cell immunity.[10] Virus-related specific antigens have analogous or cross-reactive specificities, even if induced in different species of animals. Cancer-causing viruses in animals include the polyomavirus, Moloney virus, Gross virus, and simian virus (SV40). Oncogenic viruses that affect humans, as already mentioned, include Epstein-Barr virus, associated with Burkitt's lymphoma; human papillomaviruses, which cause epithelial proliferative diseases (cervical cancer); human T-cell leukemia virus (HTLV-I), the causative agent of adult T-cell leukemia; and hepatitis B virus, associated with primary hepatoma. Peptides originating from EBV nuclear antigens (EBNA-3, EBNA-4, EBNA-6) and associated with certain HLA antigens have been shown to elicit specific cytotoxic T-cell (CTL) responses.[11]

GENOME-ENCODED TUMOR ANTIGENS

Single-point mutations in oncogenes and tumor suppressor genes (TSGs) lead to single amino acid substitutions in the protein products of those genes and become genome-encoded tumor antigens that may elicit specific immunity against cancer cells.[7] Malignant cells have altered genes; multiple oncogenes or TSGs must be affected for normal tissue to become malignant.[12] More than 10 TSGs and nearly 100 oncogenes have been identified. One TSG and three of the more common oncogenes are addressed briefly here.

Mutated p53 Proteins. The most common oncogenetic mutation seen in humans involves spontaneous alterations in the p53 TSG cell cycle inhibitor.[7] Approximately 70% of colon cancers, 30% to 50% of breast cancers, 50% of lung cancers, nearly 100% of small cell carcinomas of the lung, and several "hereditary cancers" have been shown to include p53 mutations.[13] Observed point mutations on p53 have been shown to generate 63 peptides that induce CD8+ cytotoxic T-lymphocyte (CTL) clones.

***bcr/abl* Oncogenes.** The translocation of the *abl* oncogene on chromosome 9 to the *BCR* (breakpoint cluster region) on chromosome 22 produces the Philadelphia chromosome, which leads to the creation of the fusion gene *bcr/abl*. The *bcr/abl* gene is found in more than 95% of patients with chronic myelogenous leukemia (CML). A smaller proportion of patients with acute lymphoblastic leukemia (10% of children and 25% of adults with a poorer prognosis) have a related, but different oncogene abnormality, one that translocates the *abl* gene to a different region of the *bcr* gene on the 22nd chromosome.[14] Synthetic peptides that correspond to the *bcr/abl* joining region, when used to immunize mice, have elicited peptide-specific CD4+ CTL clones.

***ras* Oncogenes.** Mutations in *ras* oncogenes (K-*ras,* N-*ras,* or H-*ras*) are commonly found in human malignancies. Nearly 90% of pancreatic carcinomas, 50% of colorectal carcinomas, and 25% of acute myelogenous leukemias (AMLs), but less than 5% of breast tumors, show *ras* mutations.[7] Single amino acid substitutions activate *ras* oncogenes in three specific codons, genetic alterations that are well characterized. Murine CD8+ CTL clones have been established using *ras* oncogenes. Human CTL clones, reactive to multiple *ras* oncogenes, have been identified by combining lymphocytes from healthy donors with mutated peptides derived from *ras* oncogenes.[15]

***myc* Oncogenes.** c-*myc* is strongly linked to lymphocyte activation and the proliferative capacity of cell populations. Deregulation of *myc* expression prohibits cells from leaving the activation cycle, a limitation that results in a state of continuous replication. *myc* is one of several oncogenes translocated in lymphomas and lymphocytic leukemias.

EXPRESSION OF NORMALLY DORMANT DIFFERENTIATION ANTIGENS

Oncofetal antigens are normally silent differentiation antigens that are expressed only during malignant transformation. Two examples of these antigens are α-fetoprotein (AFP), produced by human hepatomas, and carcinoembryonic antigen (CEA), expressed by colorectal carcinomas. These oncofetal antigens were the first human tumor-associated antigens to be identified and were originally thought to be tumor specific.

Natural Immunity to Tumors

Natural immunity spontaneously occurs in normal individuals, mirroring the innate immunity of the acute-phase response to inflammation. Natural immunity is independent of previous exposure to tumor cells. Its activity can increase very rapidly (within hours or a few days) and may be the first line of defense against malignancies. The cells involved in natural immunity are macrophages, natural killer (NK) cells, killer (K) cells, lymphokine-activated killer (LAK) cells, and tumor-infiltrating lymphocytes (TILs).

Macrophage-mediated cytotoxicity is the tumoricidal function of activated macrophages.[16] Macrophages from normal individuals (inactive) show only minimal levels of tumor cytotoxicity and have characteristic surface markers. Activated macrophages, however, can distinguish between tumor cells and normal cells and can selectively kill tumor cells, leaving normal cells untouched. Unlike CTLs, macrophage tumoricidal activity is independent of the recognition of MHC molecules or other constituents of self. Macrophage-mediated tumor cytotoxicity occurs regardless of genetic factors, including species barriers.

A host of events can activate macrophages, including infections with intracellular organisms such as *Mycobacterium, Listeria,* and *Toxoplasma.*[17] Endotoxins (lipopolysaccharides), soluble products of bacteria, and the cytokine T-cell interferon (IFN-γ), can stimulate macrophages as well.[18] Immune complexes (antigen-antibody) and complexes containing C-reactive protein have also been shown to activate macrophage-mediated cytotoxicity in vitro.[16]

Killing of tumor cells by macrophages requires close physical contact between the macrophage and the tumor cell (Fig. 50–1).[19] In vitro studies using labeled lysosomes show that the cytotoxic macrophage directly transfers its lysosomal contents to the tumor cell while the two cell membranes are fused.[17] Stimulated macrophages contain higher numbers of lysosomes and secrete large amounts of the cytokine tumor necrosis factor (TNF-α).

One of the primary causes of death from malignancies is metastases. The metastasized cells have the same surface antigens and other characteristics as the primary tumor and are found in another, formerly normal area of the body. The lymph nodes, lung, and liver are most susceptible to metastasis. Activated macrophages have proved to be quite effective at decreasing the incidence of metastasis in several animal tumor models.[16]

NK cells can identify and lyse a number of tumor cells and other cell lines in vitro. There is a broad specificity for the NK effector function that may include target cells from the following sources[20]: syngeneic (e.g., identical twins), allogeneic (same animal species, different genetic background), and xenogeneic (different species with different genetic background). NK cells are also named LGLs (large granular lymphocytes) because of the azurophilic granules in their cytoplasm and their high cytoplasm-to-nucleus ratio. NK cells have low-affinity FcγIII receptors and CD16 and NKH-1/Leu 19 surface markers. Mice that are congenitally athymic or have been thymectomized as neonates and have no distinguishable T cells do have detectable and functional NK cells.

The lytic action of NK cells involves a complex series of events leading to the destruction of target cells. This lysis can be divided into at least four distinct stages,[21] as follows:

1. Target cell binding when physical contact is made between effector cells and target cells.
2. Programming for lysis, during which the effector cell cytoskeletal components and Golgi apparatus move within the cytoplasm to the area of the effector cell that has physical contact with the target cell.
3. Secretion of factors such as NK cytotoxic factor (NKCF), granule cytolysin, and interleukin-1 (IL-1) by the LGL effector cell.
4. The cell-independent phase of the lytic event, in which the NK cells are no longer needed because soluble factors complete the killing process.

Just as macrophages can be activated, NK cells can also be stimulated by the cytokines IFN-γ and interleukin-2 (IL-2). In contrast to T cells and B cells, activation of NK cells does not evoke immunologic memory. No primary response is detectable for NK cells, only a proliferative response that is apparently triggered by IL-1 during the acute inflammatory process. NK cells are suppressed by certain factors known to be produced by tumor cells as well as by macrophages (e.g., prostaglandin E$_2$). NK activity is age-dependent, beginning with low levels in neonates, peaking at puberty, and steadily declining with advancing age. NK effector function apparently plays no role in immunity to established solid tumors. The antitumor effects of NK cells are likely to be the first line of defense against growing tumors and metastasis.

The sensitivity of tumor cells to NK cells in vitro is inversely proportional to the level of MHC class I antigens expressed on the surface of the tumor cells. This relationship suggests that MHC class I expression can lead to escape from NK cells in vivo.[7] The "missing self" hypothesis[22] states that NK cells regularly survey their environment for MHC class I expression. Cells that have lost MHC surface antigens are identified as targets and killed.

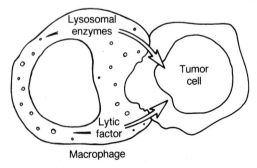

Figure 50–1. Macrophage-mediated tumor cytotoxicity. (*From* James K: Tumor immunology. *In* Sheehan C (ed): Clinical Immunology: Principles and Laboratory Diagnosis. Philadelphia, JB Lippincott, 1990.)

One theory proposes that MHC molecules inhibit the lytic action of NK cells that have bound to target cells.

LAK cells, which specifically respond to IL-2, appear to have many of the same cell surface antigens as NK cells and could be latent NK cells.[23] Like NK cells, LAK cells are LGLs that do not express the T-cell CD3 receptor. LAK activity mirrors the potency of IL-2 both to stimulate cytotoxic activity and to increase the population(s) of natural effector cells.

Nonimmunologic Tumor Development

Tumor development and spread take place in a sequence of nine phases, beginning with transformation from normal/benign to malignant cells and their unrestricted growth progressing to invasion of the surrounding tissues by the tumor cells and their intravasation/release of individual tumor cells into the blood stream and ending with metastases to other sites and tumor growth there.[24] Throughout each phase, nonimmunologic mechanisms as well as immunologic mechanisms can affect the progression of the malignancy. Many of the intercellular interactions depend on integrins, a class of molecules that causes cells to adhere to one another.[25] Proteolysis of tissue barriers is an essential mechanism of tumor cell invasion and metastasis. Enzymes, such as metalloproteinases produced by tumor cells,[26] degrade collagens and proteoglycans, thereby allowing tumor invasion.

T Cell–Mediated Immunity to Tumors

T cell–mediated immunity to tumor antigens is similar to the body's response to other T cell–dependent antigens, such as transplantation antigens. In vitro experiments have shown that tumor antigens provoke the proliferation of T cells of all subpopulations (helper, suppressor, and cytotoxic). The amplification of effector functions (Fig. 50–2) of these cells necessitates the production of antigen nonspecific, low-molecular-weight mediator molecules, or cytokines, which are released from nucleated cells.[19] Specific cytokines are secreted by stimulated T cells (lymphokines) and macrophages (monokines).

Cytokines involved in tumor immunity are listed in Table 50–2. Interleukin-1 (IL-1) and TNF-α are discrete cytokines that originate from antigen-presenting cells. IL-1, which promotes the reproduction and activation of T cells, B cells, and natural killer (NK) cells, is the endogenous pyrogen that evokes the fever response to inflammation.[27] TNF-α is similar in its action to IL-1 but also functions as a cytotoxin to cause necrosis of the tumor cells.[28] IL-2 is secreted by activated CD4+ T cells and NK cells and stimulates the proliferation and further activation of T cells and NK cells, thus augmenting the cytotoxic abilities of both cell types. IFN-γ, generated by activated CD4+ T cells and NK cells, serves to activate macrophages and enhance the cytocidal effects of natural killer cells. Secreted by activated CD4+ T cells and APCs, IL-6 acts in concert with IL-1 and TNF to stimulate T cells. IL-6 stimulates the acute-phase response of the liver.[18]

Cytokines secreted by tumor cells that have immunosuppressive activity include transforming growth factor (TGF-β) and IL 10. TGF β inhibits other cytokines, including IL-2, IL-4, IFN-γ, and TNF-α. TGF-β also blocks NK cytolysis, downregulates IL-2 receptor and MHC expression, and hinders the manufacture of T cells, B cells, LAK cells, and CTLs.[29] IL-10 blocks the proliferation of NK cells and inhibits cytokine synthesis by macrophages. IL-10 has been found in the supernatant of several human cancer cell lines, as well as in the peritoneal fluid and serum of patients with ovarian cancer and other intraperitoneal cancers.

Cytotoxic T lymphocytes can directly lyse tumor cells that carry antigens to which these immune T cells have been previously exposed (also referred to as "primed"). The CTL response begins with the cell surface interactions identifying the tumor antigens. The primary pathway of interactions between CTLs and tumor cells includes the recognition of the class II MHC antigens, identifying those tumor antigens or peptides as self through an interaction with the CD3 T cell receptor.

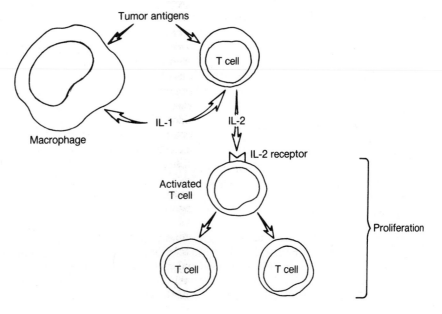

Figure 50–2. Amplification of effector functions of T cells. (*From* James K: Tumor immunology. *In* Sheehan C (ed): Clinical Immunology: Principles and Laboratory Diagnosis. Philadelphia, JB Lippincott, 1990.)

Table 50–2. Cytokines in Tumor Immunity

Cytokine	Produced by	Action
IL-1	APCs	Activates T, B, and NK cells
TNF-α	APCs	Activates T, B, and NK cells
		Involved in tumor cell necrosis
IL-2	CD4+ T cells, NK cells	Activates T and NK cells to proliferate and become cytotoxic
IFN-γ	CD4+ T cells, NK cells	Activates macrophages and NK cells
IL-6	CD4+ T cells, APCs	Stimulates T cells, stimulates the acute-phase response (APR)
TGF-β	Tumor cells	Inhibits IL-2, IL-4, IFN-γ, TNF-α
		Blocks NK cytolysis, downregulates IL-2 receptor and MHC expression
IL-10	Tumor cells	Blocks NK proliferation, inhibits macrophage cytokine synthesis

The second step in the T cell–mediated response to tumors is specific proliferation of the activated (primed) CTLs. Cytokines are produced in tandem with this clonal proliferation. At the same time, the CTLs seek out the tumor cells that express the tumor-specific antigen/peptide and MHC, lysing the tumor cells.

Mechanisms of Escape From Immune Surveillance

Although the theory of immune surveillance has not been substantiated with experimental data, there is much evidence that natural immunity and antigen-specific responses do appear to provide a surveillance function to prevent the development of selected tumors. The failure of the immune system to detect and prevent tumor growth has led to investigations into why the immune response is ineffective. Mechanisms used by tumor cells to circumvent a potentially effective immune response include (1) selection of less immunogenic or antigen-negative variants of tumor cells, (2) antigenic modulation to minimize the expression of tumor-specific antigens, (3) noncytolytic antibody that serves to block or suppress effector functions, (4) cytokines secreted by tumor cells that suppress immunologic responsiveness, and (5) development of specific suppressor cells that suppress T cell–mediated tumor cytotoxicity.[28]

CLINICAL MANIFESTATIONS OF CANCER

Persistent changes in normal physiologic functions are the typical ways that patients present clinically with cancer; in other words, the seven warning signals of cancer as defined by the American Cancer Society:

- Change in bowel or bladder habits
- A sore that does not heal
- Unusual bleeding or discharge
- Thickening of a lump in the breast or elsewhere
- Indigestion or difficulty in swallowing
- Obvious change in wart or mole
- Nagging cough or hoarseness

Recurrent pain, recurrent unexplained fever, steady weight loss, and appearance of bleeding from orifices are typical presentations that must be examined and explained. Patients older than 40 years should be screened for localized lesions in the skin, uterus, mouth, breast, lungs, rec-

tum, prostate, and thyroid in order to find cancers at a stage for which therapy can be successful.[5] It is essential to detect the cancer while it is still localized, and specific, periodic examinations are recommended for early detection of cancer in asymptomatic persons (e.g., Papanicolaou smear, mammography).[30]

LABORATORY ANALYSES OF TUMOR MARKERS

"The perfect tumor marker would be one that was produced solely by a tumor and secreted in measurable amounts into body fluids, it should be present only in the presence of cancer, it should identify cancer before it has spread beyond a localized site, its quantitative amount in body fluids should reflect the bulk of the tumor, and the level of the marker should reflect responses to treatment and disease progression."[31] The perfect tumor marker does not exist. If perfect tumor markers existed, they could be used to screen asymptomatic individuals for the presence of occult cancer. Most tumor markers are found in low concentrations in normal individuals and in higher quantities in individuals with inflammatory and other conditions that are not malignant. Prostate-specific antigen (PSA) is the first tumor marker to be approved by the U.S. Food and Drug Administration (FDA) for screening of cancer patients when used in conjunction with the digital rectal examination.[32, 33] Other tumor markers may be appropriately used for screening "at risk" populations.

Chemical Classes of Tumor Markers

Tumor markers are seldom useful in detecting or diagnosing cancer because most tumor markers have also been found in benign conditions; however, many tumor markers have a definite role in confirming diagnoses, detecting recurrence of the cancer, monitoring responses to therapy, and estimating prognosis.[34] Useful tumor markers are divided into five categories: (1) glycoproteins, (2) mucinous glycoproteins, (3) enzymes, (4) hormones, and (5) molecules of the immune system.

Glycoproteins

Glycoprotein tumor markers are derived from fetal or placental tissue and are found in small amounts in normal adult tissue; therefore, these markers are not tumor specific. Most glycoprotein tumor markers contain less than 20%

carbohydrate (CEA is the exception, with 60% carbohydrate), have *N*-linked glycosyl residues without repeating units, and express their antigenic determinants on polypeptide chains. Examples of glycoprotein tumor markers are CEA, AFP, human chorionic gonadotropin (β-HCG), tissue-polypeptide antigen (TPA), squamous cell carcinoma antigen (SCC-A), and PSA.

CEA was first identified in 1965 in extracts from human colon carcinoma and fetal colon cells. CEA exists in low levels on normal colon mucosa, lung, and breast tissue, and is found in serum associated with several malignancies. Purified CEA is quite heterogeneous, owing to varying amounts of sialic acid. CEA molecules are involved in cell recognition and intercellular adhesion and may play a role in tumor metastasis.[34]

CEA is used in the monitoring of gastrointestinal tumors, particularly colon cancer. It is normally synthesized and secreted by cells lining the gastrointestinal (GI) tract, and in normal situations, the marker is eliminated through the bowel. In disorders of the GI tract, CEA can be found circulating through the blood stream when the mucosal surface of the tract has been damaged. Such GI disturbances include inflammatory bowel disease, ulcerative colitis, Crohn's disease, multiple polyps, and tumors of the GI tract. Certain types of tumors have been shown to secrete CEA, including adenocarcinoma of the colon, pancreas, liver, and lung, particularly when there is metastasis to the liver. In fact, the highest CEA levels are found in metastatic disease. Forty percent to 70% of patients with colon cancer have elevations of CEA. When present, CEA correlates with tumor histology and pathologic stage. Very high preoperative levels are prognostic for high recurrence rates and decreased survival rates. If the tumor secretes CEA, the glycoprotein can be used to monitor the effectiveness of surgical removal of the tumor as well as to monitor for recurrence of disease.[35]

Preoperative CEA measurements are useless, however, in other cancers where CEA can be found, that is, breast, lung, and gastric cancers. Elevated postoperative CEA values in other cancers, however, indicate recurrent or metastatic disease. CEA measurement is useful in monitoring for bone metastasis in patients with breast cancer. This measurement is not recommended for use as a screening test for cancer, however, because of the incidence of CEA elevation in other inflammatory diseases.

AFP is a major plasma glycoprotein of the early human fetus. It is synthesized by the fetal liver, and its levels peak during gestation at 14 weeks, then fall to adult normal levels by 6 to 10 months after birth. AFP is highly elevated in fetal serum, maternal serum, and serum of adults with hepatomas and testicular teratoblastomas.[31] Not all hepatomas or teratoblastomas produce AFP, but those that do synthesize it in copious amounts. It should be noted that elevations of AFP are not always associated with malignancy, and that AFP levels can be raised in inflammatory diseases of the liver, such as viral hepatitis, chronic hepatitis, and cirrhosis. High levels of AFP can also be present in inflammatory diseases of the bowel, such as Crohn's disease and ulcerative colitis, that also produce elevations of CEA. AFP determination is useful as a screening test for liver cancer only in patient populations at risk for developing hepatoma (Alaskan Eskimos, Chinese, and Japanese); it is useless for most patients because of the significant elevations of this glycoprotein in benign conditions.

AFP measurements are useful in obstetrics. High levels of AFP are found in amniotic fluid associated with neural tube defects of the fetus. The serum of patients who are at risk for having a baby with certain types of nephrosis or with neural tube defects such as spina bifida can be screened for high levels of AFP.

β-HCG is secreted by placental syncytiotrophoblasts. The α-chain of this molecule shares sequence homology with luteinizing hormone (LH), but the β-chain is unique. β-HCG is normally present in serum and urine only during pregnancy. It is also found, however, in 10% of patients with benign inflammatory bowel disease, duodenal ulcers, and cirrhosis. In addition, β-HCG is found in nearly 100% of patients with trophoblastic tumors and in 10% to 40% of non–germ cell tumors, such as carcinoma of the lung, breast, GI tract, and ovary. In patients with trophoblastic (germ cell) tumors (seminoma, teratoma, choriocarcinoma), β-HCG is very useful in diagnosing, monitoring therapy, forecasting metastasis, and predicting treatment failure or relapse. When measured in combination with AFP, this glycoprotein is particularly useful in detecting seminomatous tumors. Increased β-HCG indicates probable nonseminomatous elements or metastatic disease, whereas increased AFP signals the presence of yolk sac elements. The observation of AFP and/or β-HCG correlates with the stage of nonseminomatous tumors.

Tissue polypeptide antigen is found in the serum of patients with squamous cell carcinoma of the head and neck, lung, and bladder, but is also found in benign conditions, such as wound healing, pregnancy, and inflammatory diseases. In addition, TPA is found in 20% of benign breast disease, making it too nonspecific to be useful in either diagnosing or monitoring cancer.[31]

Squamous cell carcinoma antigen, subfraction of tumor antigen 4 (TA-4), is elevated in squamous cell carcinoma of the uterus, endometrium, and other genital tract carcinomas. TA-4 and SCC-A are also present in high levels in squamous cell tumors of the head and neck, lung, and cervix. SCC-A is useful for monitoring therapy in those tumors, but not for diagnosis.[31]

Prostate specific antigen is a glycoprotein with proteolytic enzyme activity that dissolves seminal gel formed after ejaculation. PSA is found in normal, benign, and malignant prostatic tissue and seminal plasma and is produced in the cytoplasm of prostatic acinal cells and ductal epithelium.[36] Other tissues of cloacal origin contain immunochemically detectable PSA.[37] In serum, PSA is bound to α1-antichymotrypsin (ACT), a phenomenon that may affect the measurement of PSA in serum because different vendors' PSA assays contain widely varying proportions of PSA-ACT.[38–40] The differences are great enough to potentially affect patient results if assay methods are changed indiscriminately.

PSA levels are elevated in prostate cancer, the most common cancer in men older than 75 years. High PSA levels are also found in benign prostatic hypertrophy and acute or chronic prostatitis. PSA levels correspond directly with prostate volume, with the stage of prostate cancer, and with response to therapy.[31] Healthy men or women usually have no detectable PSA in their serum. Prostate carcinoma is the only form of cancer in men in which PSA is detectable in the serum. PSA is recommended, in combination with the digital rectal examination, for use in the detection of prostate cancer.[41] PSA is superior to prostatic acid phosphate (PAP) as a tumor marker in prostate cancer and has replaced it for screening, diagnosis, and monitoring.

Mucinous Glycoproteins

Mucinous glycoproteins are high-molecular-weight cell surface antigens with a polypeptide backbone attached to oligosaccharides by O-glycoside linkages. They are 60% to 80% carbohydrate and bear structural resemblance to the Lewis blood group antigens A and B[42] (Fig. 50–3). Mucinous glycoprotein epitopes expressed on epithelial surfaces unmasked by modified glycosyl transferases include CA 15-3, MCA, CA 19-9, and CA 125. These epitopes are recognized by bimonoclonal immunoassays, in which one monoclonal antibody "captures" the antigen, and a second monoclonal antibody (MAb) is used to identify the bound antigen by binding to the molecule at a different site from the capturing monoclonal antibody. The antibodies currently defined are proprietary, that is, they have been licensed by one vendor. Other vendors are developing analogous MAbs and obtaining FDA approval for assays that use other MAbs to detect similar epitopes on mucinous glycoproteins.

CA 15-3 is expressed during mammary differentiation and is detected on lactating mammary cells, lung epithelium, and carcinoma of the breast, ovary, pancreas, stomach, and liver. Low levels of CA 15-3 can be found in nonmalignant conditions such as chronic hepatitis, cirrhosis, sarcoidosis, tuberculosis, and systemic lupus erythematosus. Elevated levels of CA 15-3 are detected in epithelial malignancies such as ovarian, lung, and liver carcinoma. CA 15-3 levels are diagnostically indiscriminate and pro-

vide questionable prognostic ability. If bone or liver metastases are present, CA 15-3 levels are highest; the levels decrease with response to chemotherapy. Serial measurements of CA 15-3 has predicted relapses of breast cancer before clinical examination indicated recurrence.[43]

Mucinous-like cancer antigen (MCA) is found on most breast cancer cells regardless of histologic grade. Levels are highest in metastatic breast carcinoma and correspond closely with CA 15-3 levels.

CA 19-9 is a muciglycoprotein identical in structure to sialated Lewis A antigen, and whose expression depends on Lewis antigen expression, except in pancreatic cancer.[44] CA 19-9 is detected in acute and chronic pancreatitis and benign liver disease as well as pancreatic cancer. Levels of this muciglycoprotein in excess of 70 U/mL are the best serologic means of confirming pancreatic carcinoma. CA 19-9 decreases after curative resection and predicts recurrence 3 to 9 months before clinical symptoms appear.

CA 125 is a large muciglycoprotein with a low carbohydrate content that is expressed on embryonal coelomic epithelium and found in several benign diseases. High levels of CA 125 indicate ovarian carcinoma in postmenopausal women but do not indicate a malignancy in premenopausal women.[45] Monitoring levels of CA 125 is, however, very useful during treatment of ovarian cancer for women of all ages.

Enzymes

Neuron-Specific Enolase (NSE) in the gamma form is elevated in sera from patients with neuroblastoma, small cell lung carcinoma, melanoma, pancreatic islet cell carcinoma, and hypernephroma. In neuroblastoma, NSE correlates with prognosis but is not helpful in monitoring for recurrence. The primary use of NSE is in small cell lung carcinoma. Seventy percent of patients have high NSE levels with this disorder, and NSE can be used to monitor effects of therapy and to detect release before there is clinical evidence.[31]

Elevations of *lactate dehydrogenase (LD)* have been noted in almost every malignancy, values in neoplasia overlapping with values in nonmalignant diseases. Although LD has no value as a screening tumor marker, it is somewhat useful in monitoring therapy in hematologic malignancies. Extremely high LD levels are found in cases of pediatric leukemia and non-Hodgkin's lymphoma for which treatment has failed.[31]

Hormones

Calcitonin, a peptide hormone produced by C cells of the thyroid, plays a role in calcium regulation. Calcitonin is present in high concentrations in pregnancy and in several nonmalignant diseases, such as hyperthyroidism, Paget's disease, and pernicious anemia. In addition, calcitonin is elevated in specific malignancies (breast cancer, hepatoma, hypernephroma, and lung cancer) but is notably elevated in medullary carcinoma of the thyroid (MCT).[31] As a tumor marker for MCT, calcitonin level correlates with the severity of the disease, is helpful for monitoring therapy, and is used as a screening assay for families with autosomal dominant transmission of MCT.

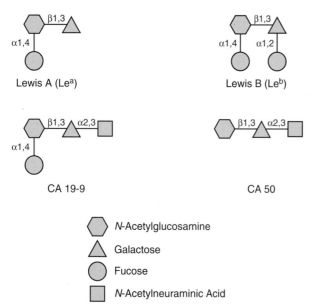

Figure 50–3. Relationship of Lewis antigen structure to mucinglycoprotein epitopes. (*From* Jacobs EL, Haskell CM: Clinical use of tumor markers in oncology. Curr Probl Cancer Nov/Dec: 301, 1991.)

Thyroglobulin, a glycoprotein created by thyroid follicular cells, is required for proteolysis and release of thyroxine (T_4) and triodothyronine (T_3) into circulation. High levels of thyroglobulin are present in nearly all thyroid disorders; therefore, it is useless for determining benign or malignant disease. Thyroglobulin is a useful tumor marker, however, after total thyroidectomy or radioiodine ablative therapy, when thyroglobulin levels can predict metastasis.[31]

Catecholamine metabolites vanillylmandelic acid (VMA) and homovanillic acid (HVA) are found in the urine in pheochromocytoma and neuroblastoma. Pretreatment levels correspond with stage of disease, and serial determinations are useful in monitoring therapy.

Molecules of the Immune System

Monoclonal immunoglobulins (M proteins) were the first-known tumor markers. They are recognized by serum or urine protein electrophoresis and characterized by serum or urine immunofixation as immunoglobulin (Ig) G (IgG), IgA, IgM, IgD, IgE, or κ or λ free light chains. M proteins are present in nearly 1% of adults, but 25% of those proteins are of undetermined significance.[46] Half of the M proteins identified indicate multiple myeloma. Approximately 4% of patients with monoclonal immunoglobulins have Waldenström's macroglobulinemia, a malignancy of primed B lymphocytes that secrete large quantities of IgM. Nearly 15% of patients with M proteins have a B-cell lymphoproliferative malignancy, such as chronic lymphocytic leukemia or lymphoma.

β_2-*Microglobulin* (β_2-M) is located on the membrane surface of nearly all nucleated cells and is released into circulation during membrane turnover. β_2-M aids in predicting treatment failures and poor survival in lymphoma patients.

Oncogenes and Gene Products as Tumor Markers

The next generation of tumor marker detection will comprise detection of mutations in oncogenes, quantitation of proteins coded for by oncogenes, or perhaps autoantibodies that are produced to oncoproteins. Detection of single-point mutations in oncogenes has been shown to be useful for diagnosis as well as for monitoring for recurrence after treatment. Chromosomal translocations, some of which can be detected by cytogenetic techniques, can also be detected by gene rearrangement studies using Southern hybridization with radioactive probes, including *bcr/abl* in chronic myelogenous leukemia, *bcl-2* in follicular lymphomas, and *myc* in lymphomas and certain other leukemias.[47]

Tumor suppressor genes (TSGs) regulate cell growth by stopping cell proliferation. Mutations in TSGs known to be involved with neoplasia include inactivation of the *Rb* gene found in familial retinoblastoma; the *APC* gene in familial colonic polyposis; *WT-1* in Wilms' tumor; and p53 found in a wide variety of tumors (epithelial, leukemia, lymphoma, sarcoma, and neurogenic).[48] An immunofluorometric assay for quantitating p53 protein accumulation in ovarian cancer and breast cancer has been described.[49]

Oncogenes encode for oncoproteins, which resemble normal proteins, but without regulation. Oncoprotein production in transformed cells does not depend on growth factors or other external signals. Some growth factors become oncoproteins in neoplastic disease, for example, platelet-derived growth factor (PDGF) in astrocytoma and osteosarcoma. Overexpression of the epidermal growth factor receptor (EGF-R) *erb-B2* is found in certain forms of breast cancer, ovarian cancer, lung cancer, and other epithelial neoplasias. Immunohistochemical detection of *erb-B2* is routinely performed as a prognostic indicator in breast cancer. Point mutations in proteins of the *ras* gene, involved in signal transduction (e.g., guanine triphosphate [GTP]), are the most common abnormality of the dominant oncogenes in human neoplasias, including those of lung, colon, and pancreas, and many leukemias.[48] The oncoprotein fragment HER-2 *neu* can be found in the serum of breast cancer patients and is detectable with a commercially available solid-phase enzyme immunoassay.[50]

Autoantibodies to oncoproteins have also been described.[51] In one study, approximately 25% of sera from cancer patients had anti-p53, whereas none of the control sera did. Twenty-two percent of patients with negative tumor marker assays were anti-p53 positive, suggesting that assaying for anti-p53 might be a relevant tool to use in combination with current tumor marker assays.

LABORATORY ANALYSES TO MONITOR TREATMENT OR PROGRESSION

Appropriate Uses of Tumor Markers

There is no "perfect" tumor marker, and most tumor marker assays should not be used to screen for the presence of cancer. Table 50–3 summarizes the currently available tumor markers that have clinical applicability. PSA is the only marker currently approved by the FDA, in combination with a digital rectal examination, for screening males for prostate cancer. AFP is appropriately used as a screening test in selected "at risk" populations (Chinese, Japanese, and Alaskan Eskimos). Calcitonin can be used as a screening test for cancer in families of patients with MCT that has an autosomal dominant transmission.

Several tests are effective in the differential diagnosis

Table 50–3. **Summary of Applications for Tumor Markers**		
Tumor Marker	**Screening**	**Monitoring**
CEA	No	Yes
AFP	Hepatoma (at risk)	Yes
β-HCG	No	Yes
CA-125	No	Yes
CA 15-3	No	Breast cancer
CA 19-9	No	Yes
PSA	Prostate	Yes
LDH	No	Lymphomas
NSE	No	Small cell lung cancer
Calcitonin	MCT	Yes
Catecholamines	No	Yes
M proteins	No	Yes
β_2-microglobulin	No	Lymphoma

of specific tumors. AFP and β-HCG are useful in establishing a differential diagnosis of nonseminomatous germ cell tumors in the appropriate clinical setting.[31] CA 125 is used in the diagnostic evaluation of ovarian masses, but with reservation.[52] Although CA 125 has been shown to be elevated prior to the clinical detection of ovarian cancer, less than half of the patients with early-stage disease have elevated CA 125 levels. Conversely, in premenopausal women, several benign conditions are associated with mild elevations of CA 125. A combination of assays using CA 125, CA 15-3, and TAG72 (monoclonal antibody specific for urinary gonadotropin fragment) has demonstrated a specificity of 99.9% in detecting ovarian cancer in early stages,[53] but the numbers of patients were insufficient to extrapolate to the general population.[52]

Detecting M proteins with serum protein electrophoresis (SPE) is not useful for screening for myeloma, because only 50% of the patients found to have monoclonal protein have multiple myeloma. Diagnosis, prognosis, and the monitoring of therapy depend not only on the detection of a monoclonal protein but also on characterization of the Ig type, which must be performed using immunofixation. Patients with IgA myeloma have significantly reduced survival rates, shorter durations, and more severe complications of their disease than patients with IgG myeloma or light-chain disease. Once the M protein is characterized for immunoglobulin type, the level of monoclonal protein is best monitored by SPE, integrating the M-spike to determine concentration.[54] Immunoglobulins can be quantitated by nephelometry; however, the antisera used in that procedure were prepared against polyclonal immunoglobulins and have limited specificity toward each immunoglobulin subgroup (e.g., IgG_1, IgG_2, IgG_3, IgG_4). This feature may result in underestimation or overestimation of a monoclonal protein.

All of the tumor markers listed in Table 50–3 have applicability in monitoring for progression of disease or effectiveness of therapy. The frequency of monitoring is not standardized, but an appropriate sequence of monitoring would be testing monthly postoperatively, for the first 6 months, then every other month for the next 6 months, then quarterly for the next year, and twice yearly thereafter. Table 50–4 shows the appropriate tumor markers to be used

for specific neoplasms, characterized as either established markers or investigational markers.

Role and Responsibilities of the Laboratory in Tumor Marker Testing

Most tumor markers are detected by enzyme immunoassay (EIA) using monoclonal antibodies. The methodology is streamlined considerably from the multi-step CEA assay of the 1970s that required extraction and dialysis prior to assay.[35] Many manufacturers use different monoclonal antibodies with different antibody specificities and different binding characteristics, depending on the nature of the antigen found in serum, and differences between manufacturers' assays can be significant. Additionally, because most tumor markers are glycoproteins, the percentage of carbohydrate in the molecules can vary as well as the tumor marker's binding characteristics to other serum proteins. With all laboratories moving toward cost containment, and with the continual introduction of new immunoassay analyzers, it is highly likely that a given laboratory will frequently change assay methods for tumor markers. For those reasons, it is recommended that each laboratory involved in tumor marker testing maintain a database on all patients tested for tumor markers. Levels "within reference range" are still relevant and should be retained, because the patients may be monitored after surgical removal of their tumors. A subsequent test might show an elevation, and it would be important to know whether the previous level was at the low end or the high end of the reference range.

Database entries should be discarded only when the patient has not been retested after 18 months. The 18-month time frame is necessary because some physicians monitor patients annually, but patients may not schedule appointments precisely a year apart.

It is recommended that statistically significant elevations[55] of tumor markers since the last laboratory evaluation be phoned or verbally reported to physicians as "critical values." Statistically significant elevations that should be brought to physician attention do *not* include already high levels (e.g., CEA >100 ng/mL). Rather, a statistically significant level for CEA would be a change from 2.0 ng/mL to 4.0 ng/mL, because at this range, if there is a recurring tumor, it is likely to still be resectable. The physician should be advised that such a change is a statistically significant elevation (not attributable to laboratory standard deviation; Fig. 50–4). The physician can elect to perform another tumor marker assay sooner than would normally be scheduled or to perform any additional testing that might be indicated to confirm or refute a change in the patient's tumor status.

The reason to personally notify physicians of statistically significant changes in CEA levels is to ensure that the laboratory report comes to the physician's attention in a timely way, before the patient's next "routine" appointment. If the patient's next appointment were to be 3, 6, or 12 months in the future, the tumor growth might have progressed to the stage of being nonresectable.

Patients being monitored for effects of treatment or recurrence of cancer with tumor marker assays must be tested using both the old and new assay method whenever assay systems or kits are changed. The differences between

Table 50–4. **Role of Tumor Markers in Specific Malignancies**		
Neoplasm	**Established Marker**	**Investigational**
Breast	CEA	CA 15-3
Ovarian	CA 125	CA 15-3, TAG72
Prostate	PSA	
Colon	CEA	
Pancreas		CA 19-9
Small cell lung cancer		NSE
Hepatoma	AFP	
Trophoblastic	β-HCG	
Testicular	β-HCG and AFP	
MCT	Calcitonin	
Multiple myeloma	M protein	$β_2$-microglobulin
Neuroblastoma	VMA/HVA	NSE
Thyroid	Thyroglobulin	

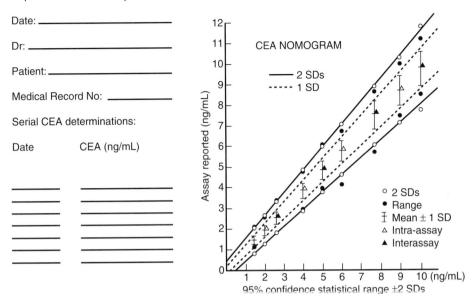

Figure 50–4. The nomogram illustrated was developed for carcinoembryonic antigen (CEA) by calculating interassay and intra-assay variability, plotting one and two standard deviations (SD) from the mean. The nomogram is used by locating the two reported assay values on the vertical axis and drawing lines that correspond to those values parallel to the horizontal axis. Where the parallel lines intersect the nomogram, draw lines parallel to the vertical axis. If the upper and lower limits of assay variability for the two assay values overlap, the results are not statistically significantly different from each other.

St. Elsewhere's Medical Center, 1234 Main Street, Anytown USA
Department of Laboratory Medicine

Date: _____

Dr: _____

Patient: _____

Medical Record No: _____

Serial CEA determinations:

Date   CEA (ng/mL)

The above patient demonstrates a statistically significant elevation of CEA since the last evaluation. The following conditions have been associated with elevations in CEA: (1) Recurrent cancer, (2) Liver malfunction (hepatitis, cirrhosis), and (3) Inflammatory conditions.

Suggest re-evaluation of the CEA level to ascertain whether this evaluation is transient or persistent.

_____ M.D.
Medical Director

PSA kits already described illustrate the need to establish a trend for each patient when a new assay system is adopted. A minimum of two simultaneous assays is recommended to establish trends between assays, and both sets of values should be reported.[56] A recommended decision algorithm for monitoring patients being tested for tumor markers is shown in Figure 50–5.

TREATMENT

There are basically four approaches to treating cancer: surgery, radiotherapy, chemotherapy, and immunotherapy. Often a combination of therapies is necessary to relieve or limit the tumor burden.

Surgical Excision of the Tumor

Surgical responsibilities in clinical oncology include biopsy for tissue diagnosis, staging, surgical resection of the tumor, and patient follow-up.[57] Surgery is the first method of treatment to decrease the solid tumor burden in early stages of breast cancer, colon cancer, lung cancer, and prostate cancer—the four major cancers in humans, representing more than 50% of solid tumors.[58] In these and other types of cancers, the tumor may grow parasitically, advancing unnoticed until it restricts a necessary function of the host's body and signals its presence. Once recognized, it may be necessary to excise the tumor to prevent loss of function of the body part.

Radiation Therapy

Radiotherapy can be either a primary therapy or an adjuvant (supplementary) therapy. Primary radiotherapy is recommended for cancer of the head and neck and in Hodgkin's disease, in which the radiotherapy is targeted to affected lymph nodes in different regions of the body. Radiotherapy is less disfiguring and more effective in treating tumors of the soft tissue in areas adjacent to the jaw and nasal passages. For other solid tumors, radiotherapy of draining lymph nodes after surgical removal of the primary tumor has been found to increase the 5-year survival rate.[59] Radiation therapy is often used as palliation to relieve distressing symptoms, avert impending symptoms, or prolong useful or comfortable survival.[60] The most extreme use of radiotherapy is whole-body radiation. This procedure is used prior to bone marrow transplantation in patients with certain types of acute leukemia that are refractory to chemotherapy, as well as for other solid tumors (e.g., breast cancer) that have recurred after several years of remission.

Chemotherapy Regimens

Chemotherapy is treatment with drugs that interfere with nucleic acid or protein synthesis or antimetabolites and thereby will kill proliferating tumor cells.[61] The drugs, either singly or in combination, are administered to the highest levels the patient can tolerate. Chemotherapy is given in "courses," allowing the normal body cells to

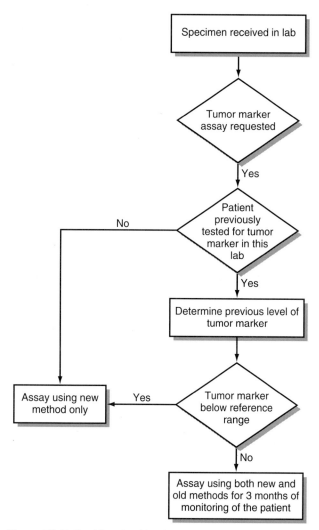

Figure 50–5. Decision algorithm flow diagram for specimen testing for tumor markers when method is changed.

recover before the patient is given a subsequent dose. Leukemias are most effectively treated with chemotherapy. Acute childhood leukemias are very responsive to appropriate regimens of chemotherapy that are administered in accordance with the cellular classification of the leukemia. Solid tumors also respond to chemotherapy when used in conjunction with surgery or radiotherapy. Most therapeutic regimens have been formulated as a result of experimentation with combinations of drugs or other therapies.[62]

Immunomodulatory Therapy

Immunoprophylaxis with vaccines to certain viruses has successfully prevented disease in animals,[63] but there is currently no vaccine available to protect against any human tumors.

Immunotherapy of cancer is the attempt to destroy tumor cells by manipulating the immune system to overcome the poor immune responses provoked by tumors. Several types of immunotherapy have been used to augment the MHC expression on tumor cells including chemical coupling, enzyme treatment, infection of tumor cells with vaccinia virus, and introduction of IFN-γ and other cyto-

kine genes into tumor cells to upregulate the expression of self MHC molecules.[7] It is now generally accepted that in murine tumor models, defects in immune regulation, not the absence of tumor antigens, result in failure to elicit an antitumor immune response. Investigators are now working to modify the local tumor cell immunologic environment either to enhance the presentation of tumor-specific antigens or to activate tumor-specific lymphocytes.[7]

Monoclonal antibodies to particular tumor antigens enhance radioimmunodetection (RAID) of occult tumors and facilitate their destruction by directed chemotherapy or radiotherapy.[64] RAID can help determine whether a lesion is a malignancy or a scar from previous surgery or radiotherapy and can indicate the extent of disease (staging) for patients being evaluated for different therapy options. Radioimmunoguided surgery (RIGS) uses a γ-detecting probe during surgery to locate recurrent disease during second-look laparotomy.[65] Radiolabeled MAbs can also be used to target micrometastases in patients with cancer[66] and to increase delivery of drug molecules or therapeutic toxins to a tumor.[64] It is hoped that immunoconjugates of drugs or toxins would be significantly less toxic than unconjugated drugs. MAbs are generally made in mice and consequently are a foreign protein to humans. They are potentially immunogenic, resulting in serum sickness, urticaria, fever, and anaphylaxis.[64] Laboratory tumor marker assays can show false elevation or be misinterpreted when immunotherapeutic MAbs compete with assay reagent MAbs.

In vitro stimulation of the patient's lymphocytes, NK cells, or macrophages is an alternative approach to chemotherapy. Rosenberg and colleagues[67] have had some success with systemic administration of autologous LAK cells plus recombinant IL-2 in achieving tumor regression in certain patients with cancer. The toxic effects of this type of immunotherapy, however, prohibit its use in all but the most resistant forms of cancer that are unresponsive to conventional therapies.

Molecular biologic approaches to cancer are the future of tumor immunology. Cancer therapy is changing because of the discovery of oncogenes. Oncogenic proteins seem to act on normal cells at different stages of differentiation, "freezing" their development to one particular stage. The protein products of oncogenes can help identify the stage at which the interference occurred. Therapy can then be tailored to known susceptibilities of cells at that single stage of differentiation. As other protein products of oncogenes are identified and characterized, more rational approaches to cancer therapy can be developed.

Case Study

ML was diagnosed with breast cancer initially detected by mammography at age 36. The tumor was surgically removed in a "lumpectomy," and the patient was diagnosed as having stage T_1 (lesion <2 cm), N_0 (no detectable lymph node involvement), M_0 (no detectable metastases) cancer. Estrogen and progesterone receptor assays were negative, indicating a probable lack of response to adjuvant hormonal therapy.

ML was monitored at 6-month intervals with serum

alkaline phosphatase and liver enzyme determinations (inexpensive screening tests for bone or liver metastasis) and CEA measurements. Three years later, when CA 15-3 testing became available, that test was added to her monitoring schedule. All monitoring tests were within normal limits for 4 years. She used the same laboratory for postoperative monitoring. Mammography and breast examinations were negative.

The 5-year check-up for ML showed complete blood count, live enzyme levels, and urinalysis values to be within normal limits. Other laboratory findings (with reference ranges) were as follows:

Alkaline phosphatase (IU/L)	130	40–125
CEA (ng/mL)	4.1	<2.5 for non-smokers
CA 15-3 (U/mL)	32	<35

Questions

1. What additional information should the laboratory provide to assist the physician in interpreting these laboratory results?
2. What additional tests should be performed?
3. What is the most probable explanation for these results?
4. What are the patient's treatment options?

Discussion

1. The laboratory should provide the serial monitoring results for CEA and CA 15-3 even though the physician should have that information in the patient's record (Fig. 50–6).
2. CEA and CA 15-3 testing should be repeated to confirm that the levels are increasing and that the values seen on this evaluation are not spurious.
3. CEA is useful in predicting bone metastases in breast cancer. Review of alkaline phosphatase results over the 3-year span showed persistent increases (although still within the reference range), which also might suggest bone metastases. Increased alkaline phosphatase would be consistent with bone metastasis. The bone scan was positive.

This case study provides the opportunity to discuss the concept of "reference ranges." Reference ranges for tumor markers (and many other serum proteins) are obtained by testing large groups of purportedly healthy individuals, using either 2 standard deviations from the mean or an arbitrary cut-off level that would put 95% of the normal population into the "reference range." In monitoring tumor markers over time, however, the reference range is irrelevant. Sequential values establish the individual patient's baseline level. (ML's baseline value for CA 15-3 is probably <30 U/mL, whereas the reference range is <35 U/mL.) It is necessary to establish and report reference ranges, but laboratorians should be aware that when monitoring patients for other serum proteins in addition to tumor markers (e.g., C3 and C4 in systemic lupus erythematosus), physicians should be encouraged to make therapeutic decisions on the basis of patient-established baselines rather than on reference ranges.

4. The treatment options explained to the patient were radiation therapy, chemotherapy, and bone marrow transplant. Although bone marrow transplant would incur the most risk, it also offered the best chance for long-term survival, if successful. The patient chose bone marrow transplant and is currently disease free.

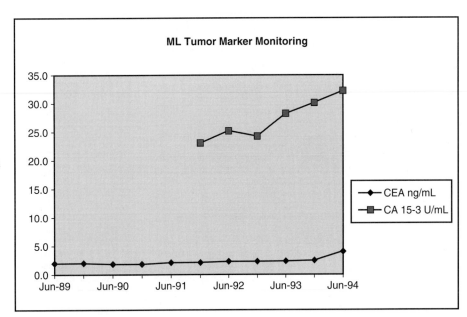

Figure 50–6. Malignant lymphoma (ML) tumor marker monitoring.

References

1. Willis RA: The Spread of Tumors in the Human Body. London, Butterworth, 1952.

2. Robbins SL: Pathologic Basis of Disease. Philadelphia, WB Saunders, 1974.

3. Pitot HC: Fundamentals of Oncology. New York, Marcel Dekker, 1978.

4. Caussy D, Marrett L, Worth A, et al: Human papillomavirus and cervical intraepithelial neoplasia in women who subsequently had invasive cancer. J Can Med Assoc 142:311–317, 1990.

5. Rubin P, Cooper RA: Statement of the clinical oncological problem. *In* Rubin P, McDonald S, Qazi R (eds): Clinical Oncology: A Multidisciplinary Approach for Physicians and Students. Philadelphia, WB Saunders, 1993.

6. Prehn RT, Main JM: Immunity of methylcholanthrene induced sarcomas. J Natl Cancer Inst 18:69, 1957.

7. Roth C, Rochlitz C, Kourilsky P: Immune response against tumors. Adv Immunol 57:281, 1994.

8. Babbit BP, Allen PM, Matsueda G, et al: Binding of immunogenic peptides to Ia histocompatibility molecules. Nature (London) 317:359, 1985.

9. Kourilsky P, Jaulin C, Ley V: The structure and function of MHC molecules: Possible implication for the control of tumor growth by MHC-restricted T cells. Cancer Biol 2:275, 1991.

10. Klein G: Immunovirology of transforming viruses. Curr Opin Immunol 3:665, 1991.

11. Gavioli R, Kurilla MG, DeCampos-Lima PO, et al: Multiple HLA-A11 restricted CTL epitopes of different immunogenicity in the Epstein-Barr virus (EBV) encoded nuclear antigen-4 (EBNA4). J Virol 67:1572, 1993.

12. Fearon ER, Vogelstein B: A genetic model for colorectal tumorigenesis. Cell 61:767, 1990.

13. Hollstein M, Sidransky D, Vogelstein B, et al: p53 mutations in human cancer. Science 253:49, 1991.

14. Maurer J, Jannsen JW, Thiel E, et al: Detection of chimeric bcr-abl genes in acute lymphoblastic leukemia by the polymerase chain reaction. Lancet 337:1055, 1991.

15. Jung S, Schluesener HJ: Human T lymphocytes recognize a peptide of single point-mutated oncogenic ras proteins. J Exp Med 173:273, 1991.

16. Deodhar SD, Barna BP: Macrophage activation: Potential for cancer therapy. Clev Clin Quart 53:223, 1986.

17. Adams DO, Nathan CF: Molecular mechanisms in tumor cell killing by activated macrophages. Immunol Today 4:166, 1983.

18. Taramelli D, Holden HT, Varesio L: Endotoxin requirement for macrophage activation by lymphokines in a rapid microcytotoxicity assay. J Immunol Methods 37:225, 1980.

19. James K: Tumor Immunology. *In* Sheehan C (ed): Clinical Immunology: Principles and Laboratory Diagnosis. Philadelphia, JB Lippincott, 1990.

20. Whiteside TL, Herberman RB: The role of natural killer cells in immune surveillance of cancer. Curr Opin Immunol 7:704–710, 1995.

21. Wright S, Bonavida B: Studies on the mechanisms of natural killer cell cytotoxicity. III: Activation of NK cells by interferon augments the lytic activity of released natural killer cytotoxic factors (NKCF). J Immunol 130:2960, 1984.

22. Ljunggren N, Karre K: In search of the "missing self": MHC molecules and NK recognition. Immunol Today 11:237, 1990.

23. Herberman RB, Balch C, Golub S, et al: Lymphokine-activated killer cell activity: Characteristics of effector cells and their progenitors in blood and spleen. Immunol Today 8:178, 1987.

24. Hart IR, Saini A: Biology of tumor metastasis. Lancet 339:1453, 1992.

25. Hynes RO: Integrins: Versatility, modulation, and signaling in cell adhesion. Cell 69:11, 1992.

26. Liotta LA, Steeg PS, Stetler-Stevenson WG: Cancer metastasis and angiogenesis: An imbalance of positive and negative regulation. Cell 64:327, 1991.

27. Oppenheim JJ, Kovacs EJ, Matsushima K, et al: There is more than one interleukin 1. Immunol Today 7:45, 1986.

28. Oppenheim JJ, Ruscetti FW, Faltynek CV: Cytokines. *In* Stites DP, Terr AI, Parslow TG (eds): Basic & Clinical Immunology. Los Altos, Cal, Lange Medical, 1994.

29. Sulitzeanu D: Immunosuppressive factors in human cancer. Adv Cancer Res 60:247, 1993.

30. Williams PA: A productive history and physical examination in prevention and early detection of cancer. Cancer 47:1146–1150, 1981.

31. Jacobs EL, Haskell CM: Clinical use of tumor markers in oncology. Curr Probl Cancer 15:299–360, 1991.

32. Hybritech Inc: Premarket approval of Tandem-R, E, and ERA PSA assays. Federal Register. October 14, 1994; 59:52169.

33. Catalona WJ, Richie JP, Ahmann FR, et al: Comparison of digital rectal examination and serum prostate-specific antigen in the early detection of prostate cancer: Results of a multicenter clinical trial of 6630 men. J Urol 151:1283–1290, 1994.

34. Seleznick MJ: Tumor markers. Primary Care 19:715, 1992.

35. Martin EW, James KK, Minton JP: The use of CEA as an early indicator for gastrointestinal tumor recurrence and second-look procedures. Cancer 29:440, 1977.

36. Wang MC, Papsidero LD, Kuriyama M, et al: Prostatic antigen: A new potential marker for prostatic cancer. Prostate 2:89, 1981.

37. Frazier HA, Humphrey PA, Burchette JL, et al: Immunoreactive prostatic specific antigen in male periurethral glands. J Urol 147:246, 1992.

38. Graves HCB: Standardization of immunoassays for prostate-specific antigen. Cancer 72:3141, 1993.

39. Zucchelli GC, Pilo A, Chiesa MR, et al: Poor standardization of PSA immunoassays emerging from data of an international EQA program. Clin Chem 41:S219, 1995.

40. Strobel S, Esgate J, Norton K, et al: Discordance between commercial prostate specific antigen (PSA) assays: How PSA forms affect assay results. Clin Chem 41:S225, 1995.

41. Gerber GS, Goldberg R, Chodak GW: Local staging of prostate cancer by tumor volume, prostate-specific antigen, and transrectal ultrasound. Urology 40:311, 1992.

42. Virji MA, Mercer DW, Herberman R: New immunologic markers for monitoring of cancer. Ann Chir Gynaecol 78:13, 1989.

43. Colomer R, Ruibal A, Genolla J, et al: Circulating CA 15-3 levels in postsurgical follow-up of breast cancer patients and in non-malignant diseases. Breast Cancer Res Treat 13:123, 1989.

44. Masson P, Palsson B, Andre-Sandberg A: Cancer-associated tumor markers CA 19-9 and CA-50 in patients with pancreatic cancer with special reference to the Lewis blood cell status. Br Cancer 62:118, 1990.

45. Malkasian GD, Knapp RC, Lavin PT, et al: Preoperative evaluation of serum CA 125 levels in premenopausal and postmenopausal patients with pelvic masses: Discrimination of benign from malignant disease. Am J Obstet Gynecol 159:341, 1988.

46. Ameis A, Ko HS, Pruzanski W: M components: A review of 1242 cases. Can Med Assoc J 114:889, 1976.

47. Mattson JC, Crisan D, Wilner F, et al: Clinical problem solving using bcl-2 and bcr gene rearrangement analysis. Lab Med 25:648–653, 1994.

48. Weinberg RA: Oncogenes and tumor suppressor genes. CA Cancer J Clin 44:160–170, 1994.

49. Levesque MA, Diamandis EP, Yu H, et al: Immunofluorometrically quantified p53 protein as a prognostic indicator in ovarian carcinoma. Clin Chem 41:S224, 1995.

50. Mercer DW, Klein K, Yann V: HER-2 *neu* oncoprotein monitoring in sera of patients with breast cancer: Comparison with CA 15-3. Clin Chem 41:S226, 1995.

51. Volkmann M, Müller M, Meyer M, et al.: Anti-p53 autoantibodies as serological marker in different tumor entities. Clin Chem 41:S221, 1995.

52. Teneriello MG, Park RC: Early detection of ovarian cancer. CA Cancer J Clin 45:71–87, 1995.

53. Jacobs IJ, Oram DH, Bast RC Jr: Strategies for improving the specificity of screening for ovarian cancer with tumor-associated antigens CA 125, CA 15-3, and TAG 72.3. Obstet Gynecol 80:396–399, 1992.

54. James K: Quantitation of monoclonal proteins by SPE. ASCP News Jan/Feb, 1988.

55. James K: Immunoserology. (Listen, Look and Learn Series for the Clinical Laboratory Sciences.) Chicago, Health & Education Resources, 1990.

56. James K, Carter S, Carter JB: An automated method for prostate-specific antigen: A clinical evaluation of the Tosoh AIA-Pack PSA immunoassay. Lab Med 26:746–750, 1995.

57. Langmuir VK, Schwartz SI: Principles of surgical oncology. *In* Rubin

P, McDonald S, Qazi R (eds): Clinical Oncology: A Multidisciplinary Approach for Physicians and Students. Philadelphia, WB Saunders, 1993.

58. Wingo PA, Tong T, Bolden S: Cancer statistics, 1995. CA Cancer J Clin 45:8–30, 1995.

59. Harris JR, Hellman S, Kinne DW: Limited surgery and radiotherapy for breast cancer. CA Cancer J Clin 36:120, 1986.

60. Rubin P, Siemann DW: Principles of radiation oncology and cancer radiotherapy. *In* Rubin P, McDonald S, Qazi R (eds): Clinical Oncology: A Multidisciplinary Approach for Physicians and Students. Philadelphia, WB Saunders, 1993.

61. Bakemeier RF, Qazi R: Basic concepts of cancer chemotherapy and principles of medical oncology. *In* Rubin P, McDonald S, Qazi R (eds): Clinical Oncology: A Multidisciplinary Approach for Physicians and Students. Philadelphia, WB Saunders, 1993.

62. Bennett JM: Basic concepts in investigational therapeutics. *In* Rubin

P, McDonald S, Qazi R (eds): Clinical Oncology: A Multidisciplinary Approach for Physicians and Students. Philadelphia, WB Saunders, 1993.

63. Jarrett W, Mackey L, Jarrett O, et al: Antibody response and virus survival in cats vaccinated against malignant lymphoma. Nature 253:71, 1975.

64. Goldenberg DM: New developments in monoclonal antibodies for cancer detection and therapy. CA Cancer J Clin 44:43–64, 1994.

65. LaValle GJ, Chevinsky A, Martin EW: Impact of radioimmunoguided surgery. Semin Surg Oncol 7:167, 1991.

66. Goldenberg DM, Deland F, Kim E, et al: Use of radiolabeled antibodies to carcinoembryonic antigen for the detection and localization of diverse cancers by external photoscanning. N Engl J Med 198:1384, 1978.

67. Rosenberg SA, Lotze MT, Muul LM, et al: Special report: Observations on the systemic administration of autologous lymphokine-activated killer cells and recombinant interleukin-2 to patients with metastatic cancer. N Engl J Med 313:1485, 1985.

Infectious Diseases

Chapter 51

Sexually Transmitted Diseases

Lauren Roberts

Sexually transmitted diseases are infections transmitted through sexual activity involving contact between the genitalia of one partner and the genitalia or other mucosal surface of the other partner.[1] Sexually transmitted diseases (STDs) have long been a major health problem; however, the emergence of acquired immunodeficiency syndrome (AIDS) in the 1980s has brought greater awareness of these infections. In the past two decades, there have been significant changes in the epidemiology and the understanding of clinical manifestations of STDs. Although these infections are considered as a group, they encompass a broad variety of specific illnesses caused by biologically dissimilar microbial agents. The spectrum of STDs has expanded from the five traditional venereal diseases— gonorrhea, syphilis, chancroid, lymphogranuloma venereum, and granuloma inguinale—and now includes clinical syndromes caused by more than 25 pathogenic organisms and viruses[2, 3] (Box 51–1). AIDS is discussed in Chapter 45.

The changing emphasis in the field of STDs is due to several factors, including the emergence of new pathogens, such as human immunodeficiency virus (HIV), as well as the long-term effects of infections with *Chlamydia trachomatis*, herpes simplex virus (HSV), and human papilloma virus (HPV). Unlike the traditional venereal diseases that respond well to antimicrobial therapy, the newer pathogens cause incurable or fatal diseases. Improvements in laboratory testing have improved the ability to accurately diagnose these infections and assess their prevalence, thereby aiding epidemiologic investigations. In addition, there has been an increase in infections with pathogens that are not usually spread by sexual transmission, such as hepatitis B virus (HBV), cytomegalovirus (CMV), and certain enteric pathogens. Lastly, the impact of STDs on maternal and neonatal health has become an important women's health issue.

EPIDEMIOLOGIC CONSIDERATIONS

Even though the diagnosis and treatment of STDs have been greatly improved, these infections remain epidemic in all societies. The Centers for Disease Control and Prevention (CDC) estimates that approximately 12 million residents in the United States acquire an STD each year.[4] These diseases provide a classic example of the influence that behavioral and demographic factors have on an infec-

Box 51–1. Sexually Transmitted Pathogens

Bacteria

Neisseria gonorrhoeae
Chlamydia trachomatis
Ureaplasma urealyticum
Treponema pallidum
Haemophilus ducreyi
Calymmatobacterium granulomatis
Shigella species
Campylobacter species

Fungi

Candida species
Other yeasts

Ectoparasites

Phthirus pubis
Sarcoptes scabiei

Viruses

Human immunodeficiency virus (HIV)
Herpes simplex virus (HSV)
Human papillomavirus (HPV)
Cytomegalovirus (CMV)
Hepatitis B virus (HBV)
Molluscum contagiosum virus (MCV)

Protozoan Parasites

Trichomonas vaginalis
Giardia lamblia
Entamoeba histolytica

tious disease. The rate of spread of an STD pathogen within a population is influenced by three factors: the rate of partner change in the population, the length of time the pathogen is infectious, and the efficiency of transmission to a susceptible host. Prevention and control efforts attempt to shorten the duration of infectiousness through early diagnosis and treatment, and to decrease the efficiency of transmission and the rate of partner change through educational efforts about barrier protection and sexual behavior consequences.[4]

Most persons with active symptoms of STD cease sexual activity and seek medical attention. Infected individuals who transmit STDs to their partners are likely to be asymptomatic or to have mild symptoms whose implications they do not understand. Asymptomatic individuals continue sexual activity, providing a reservoir for disease transmission. It is important, therefore, to screen patients in a high-risk category. Another critical issue in the management of the current STD epidemic is partner notification. Examination and treatment of the partner are of paramount importance to eliminate re-infection and spread.

Anyone who is sexually active is at some risk of acquiring STD infections. The principal risk factor for exposure to STDs is sexual behavior, which consists of number of partners and rate of partner change, contact with casual sex partners, sexual preference, and specific sexual practices.[2, 5] The AIDS epidemic has forced an awareness of sexual behavior, because avoiding exposure through behavioral intervention is the most important factor in the control of this disease.

Additional risk factors for acquisition of STDs are co-infection with other STDs, lack of circumcision, drug abuse, prostitution, and methods of contraception. Infection with one STD predisposes an individual to further STDs. This is most evident in the transmission of HIV, in which it has been determined that individuals with genital ulcers have a greater susceptibility to HIV. The exchange of sex for drugs, especially crack cocaine, has resulted in a resurgence of gonorrhea, syphilis, and chancroid.[5]

Rates of traditional STDs have fallen in most industrialized countries, except in the United States, where they have risen because of the widespread use of cocaine. In developing nations, however, STDs continue to spread with no evidence of declining rates. The populations of developing nations and the poor populations of inner city and rural areas in the United States have similar social profiles that influence the spread of STDs. These two groups—in developing nations and U.S. inner city/rural areas—have the following social conditions in common:

- High proportion of sexually active adolescents and young adults
- High population growth rate
- High levels of transience
- Unstable economic and political factors that contribute to social disintegration

Prostitution and drug abuse arise as a result of all these social conditions and contribute to the transmission of STDs.[6]

Although many clinical syndromes are associated with STDs, six major illnesses account for the vast majority of cases: gonorrhea, *Chlamydia* infection, genital herpes, syphilis, viral hepatitis, and AIDS. Data on the frequency and distribution of STDs are limited, because there is a serious problem of underreporting, and not all diseases are reportable[7] (Table 51–1). Although 448,984 cases of *Chlamydia* infection were reported in 1994, the estimated incidence of this disease is more than 4 million. Genital herpes is not a reportable disease, and it is estimated that as many as 30 million individuals in the United States

Table 51–1. Reported Sexually Transmitted Diseases in the United States, 1994

Disease	No. Reported Cases
AIDS	78,279
Chancroid	773
Chlamydia	448,984*
Gonorrhea	418,068
Granuloma inguinale	3
Hepatitis B	12,517
Lymphogranuloma venereum	235
Syphilis	81,696

*Reported from 47 states.

may have genital HSV. The true incidence of STDs is not known.

ETIOLOGY AND PATHOPHYSIOLOGY
Host-Parasite Interactions

The transmission of microorganisms from the urogenital tract is usually a result of mucosal contact between an infected individual and a susceptible host. Some of the most successful sexually transmitted pathogens induce a discharge that allows the organisms to be shed as they are carried over epithelial surfaces. Other pathogens are effectively transmitted from mucosal sores or ulcers and gain entrance to a new host through minor breaks in the skin surface.[8]

The urogenital tract possesses various defense mechanisms against invasion by sexually transmitted pathogens. A natural mechanism to eliminate pathogens is the flushing effect of urine over the urethra. The normal flora and mucosal secretions of the vagina serve as the primary defense against infectious agents in females. The pH of the vagina also inhibits colonization of most organisms except lactobacilli, certain other streptococci, and diphtheroids. In order for organisms to colonize and invade, they must have specific mechanisms to breach the host defenses, or they must take advantage of impaired host defenses.

Successful sexually transmitted pathogens have developed specialized mechanisms that allow them to gain entrance and replicate. Gonococci, for example, possess abundant pili that mediate attachment on the surface of human genital cells and prevent the organisms from being washed away by the flow of urine or the normal vaginal discharge.[9] Other organisms, like the chlamydiae, induce host epithelial cells to phagocytize them. Once they gain entrance into these "nonprofessional phagocytes," the chlamydiae begin their replication process.[10] The mucous membranes of the genital tract provide an appropriately moist surface for the transmission of vital agents that will not survive on environmental surfaces.

Common Syndromes in Men

Urethritis, the response of the urethra to inflammation of any etiology, is the most common clinical STD syndrome in males. The primary etiologic agents associated with urethritis are *Neisseria gonorrhoeae* and *C. trachomatis* (Table 51–2). Urethritis is generally classified as gonococcal (GU) or nongonococcal (NGU), depending on the presence or absence of gonococci in the urethral discharge.[11] Although the overall incidence of NGU is greater than that of GU, there is a variation in the infection rates among different populations. In STD clinics, the frequencies are about the same, but on college campuses, more than 85% of urethritis is NGU.[6]

The etiology of NGU is varied. *C. trachomatis* is responsible for 30% to 40% of cases, and *Ureaplasma urealyticum* has been implicated as a probable cause in many *Chlamydia*-negative patients. The significance of *U. urealyticum* remains controversial, however, because this organism has been found to colonize the urethra of men without urethritis.[6] Other etiologic agents of NGU are herpes simplex virus, *Trichomonas vaginalis*, *Bacteroides ureolyticus*,

Table 51–2. Common STD Syndromes in Men

Syndrome	Causative Agents
Urethritis	*N. gonorrhoeae*
	C. trachomatis
	U. urealyticum
Epididymitis	*C. trachomatis*
	N. gonorrhoeae
Hepatitis	Hepatitis A, B, C(?), D(?) viruses
Intestinal syndromes	
Proctitis	*N. gonorrhoeae*
	C. trachomatis
	Herpes simplex virus
	T. pallidum
Proctocolitis	*E. histolytica*
	Campylobacter species
	Shigella species
	C. trachomatis (LGV serotypes)
Enteritis	*G. lamblia*

Mycoplasma genitalium, and *Haemophilus* species. Coliform bacteria are rare causes of urethritis, most often seen in homosexual men.

Some individuals may be infected with more than one organism, and dual infections with gonorrhea and chlamydiae are common. *Postgonococcal urethritis* is a condition that occurs in men who have been treated for urethral gonorrhea and either develop symptoms following therapy or remain symptomatic. *C. trachomatis* is responsible for the majority of these cases. This condition demonstrates the longer incubation period of chlamydiae and is found in men with concurrent chlamydial infections who have been treated with antimicrobials that are effective only against *N. gonorrhoeae*.

Epididymitis is another common syndrome found in males. Inflammation of the epididymis can result from trauma or chemical irritation, but most cases of acute epididymitis are infectious. This condition is usually, but not always, associated with urethritis. *C. trachomatis* and *N. gonorrhoeae* are the agents most commonly found in heterosexual men younger than 35 years. In men older than 35 years, and in homosexual men, urinary tract pathogens such as *Escherichia coli* and *Pseudomonas aeruginosa* are usually responsible.[12]

Sexually transmitted intestinal infections are primarily seen in homosexual or bisexual men. These infections have a complex clinical and etiologic spectrum that has been greatly altered by the AIDS epidemic. The number of sexually transmitted infections has decreased in this group, probably owing to the implementation of safe sex practices, but the number of opportunistic intestinal infections has risen because of the immunosuppression of HIV. In patients without AIDS, sexually transmitted intestinal infections can be separated into three clinical syndromes: proctitis, proctocolitis, and enteritis.[6, 13]

Proctitis refers to inflammation confined to the rectal mucosa and results from direct rectal inoculation of typical STD pathogens. It is found most often in men who practice unprotected passive rectal intercourse, and the most common etiologic agents are *N. gonorrhoeae*, *C. trachomatis*, herpes simplex virus, and *Treponema pallidum*. *Proctocolitis* involves inflammation that extends from the rectum to the colon, and *enteritis* involves only the small intestine;

these infections are usually acquired by ingestion of typical intestinal pathogens through oral-anal contact. Proctocolitis is most often due to *Campylobacter* species, *Shigella* species, *Entamoeba histolytica*, and lymphogranuloma venereum (LGV) strains of *C. trachomatis*. Enteritis is primarily associated with *Giardia lamblia*. These infections are complicated not only by the normal bacterial flora of the intestinal tract but also by the fact that the patients commonly have multiple pathogens.

Common Syndromes in Women

In general, STDs are associated with more long-term complications in women than in men. Some infections are more readily transmitted from male to female than the reverse, owing to the prolonged exposure of the mucous membranes in the vaginal canal. In addition, women are more likely to have asymptomatic infection, allowing the infection to become more severe. STDs in women may lead to higher risk of genital cancer, a loss of reproductive capability, and transmission of a serious infection to the fetus and newborn.

As with men, *C. trachomatis* and *N. gonorrhoeae* are the leading causes of urethritis in women. Cervicitis may also be present. These pathogens may also result in the urethral syndrome, in which dysuria and frequency occur in the absence of bacteriuria.[14] Herpes simplex virus may also produce urethritis, especially during a primary infection (Table 51–3).

Vulvovaginitis—inflammation of the vulva and the vagina—is one of the most common reasons why women in their childbearing years visit physicians. Most cases of vulvovaginitis can be assigned to one of three categories: bacterial vaginosis (BV), which accounts for 40% to 50% of cases; vulvovaginal candidiasis, which accounts for 20% to 25% of cases; and trichomoniasis, which accounts for 15% to 20% of cases.[15] These conditions have long been recognized as a nuisance to the patient, but it has now been realized that they may have more serious implications for the patient. Bacterial vaginosis and trichomoniasis during pregnancy can lead to obstetric complications, and trichomoniasis may increase susceptibility to HIV infection.[4, 6]

Unlike vulvovaginal candidiasis and trichomoniasis, BV

is not associated with a single etiologic agent and is not a true inflammatory process. This condition represents a disturbance of the vaginal microflora in which the normal lactobacilli decrease, and anaerobes, genital mycoplasmas, and *Gardnerella vaginalis* begin to predominate. No host factor is recognized that increases susceptibility to this condition, and it is not established that BV is sexually transmitted.[16]

Candida albicans is responsible for the majority of vulvovaginal yeast infections, with *Torulopsis glabrata* and other species of *Candida* causing the remaining cases. *Candida* species are found in the genital tract of approximately 20% of asymptomatic, healthy women of childbearing age. Predisposing factors, such as pregnancy, use of oral contraceptives, diabetes, and antibiotic therapy, lead to increased growth of the colonizing yeast, and infection results.

The protozoan flagellate *Trichomonas vaginalis* is primarily transmitted through sexual intercourse. The prevalence of this infection is related to the level of sexual activity in the population studied. Epidemiologic studies indicate a decrease in this infection in industrialized nations, where women have access to medical care. In the United States, the incidence of this infection is greatest in women seen at STD clinics, where it is noted that trichomoniasis is often an indication of gonorrhea or other STDs.[15]

Cervicitis is often referred to as the "silent partner" of urethritis in men, because it is equally common but is more difficult to detect.[4] Infections of the cervix serve as a reservoir for sexual transmission, but they can also lead to further sequelae by ascending. For example, cervicitis during pregnancy may lead to obstetric complications, and *endocervicitis* (mucopurulent cervicitis)—inflammation of the columnar mucus-secreting cells of the cervical canal—may develop. *C. trachomatis* and *N. gonorrhoeae* are the most common causes of endocervicitis; rarely, herpes simplex virus is involved. *Ectocervicitis*, which involves infection of the squamous epithelium cells that project into the vagina, is associated with infections by herpes simplex virus, *T. vaginalis*, and *C. albicans*. In some cases, however, the exact etiologic agent is not identified. Anaerobic organisms and genital mycoplasmas may also be potential causes of cervicitis, because mucopurulent cervicitis often accompanies bacterial vaginosis.[17]

Pelvic inflammatory disease (PID) is the most important complication of sexually transmitted pathogens, as well as the major medical and economic consequence of these infections. It is caused by ascending spread of organisms to the endometrium, fallopian tubes, or adjacent structures. Thus, PID can result in endometritis, parametritis, salpingitis, peritonitis, and abscess formation.[3] There are several predisposing factors for the development of PID: sexual activity with multiple partners, previous episode of PID, use of an intrauterine device, and adolescence.

The organisms most commonly responsible for PID are *C. trachomatis* and *N. gonorrhoeae*. Cases of gonorrheal PID have decreased in most industrialized countries, whereas cases of chlamydial PID are increasing. Other pathogens involved in this syndrome are the organisms associated with BV, various anaerobes, and *M. hominis*.

Syndrome	Causative Agents
Urethral syndrome	*C. trachomatis*
	N. gonorrhoeae
	Herpes simplex virus
Vulvovaginitis	*C. albicans*
	Other yeasts
	Trichomonas vaginalis
Bacterial vaginosis	*G. vaginalis*, genital mycoplasmas, and several anaerobes
Cervicitis	*N. gonorrhoeae*
	C. trachomatis
	Herpes simplex virus
Pelvic inflammatory disease	*C. trachomatis*
	N. gonorrhoeae
	Mixed bacteria

Table 51–3. Common STD Syndromes in Women

Many cases of PID are caused by more than one organism, and, commonly, the etiology is not established.[6]

Salpingitis, the most serious complication of female genital tract infections, is the major cause of ectopic pregnancies and infertility. Among women who have had salpingitis, about 17% become infertile from tubal occlusion, and 6% have an ectopic pregnancy.[17] The probability of becoming infertile increases with each episode of PID.

Sexually transmitted intestinal infections are not common in women, but they do occur. Women can acquire these infections through anal intercourse, but most cases of anorectal infections are probably the result of contiguous spread from the genitalia.

Genital Skin Lesions

Skin lesions of the genitalia are categorized as ulcerative or nonulcerative (Table 51–4). The nonulcerative sexually transmitted infections are genital warts, *Candida* balanitis or vulvitis, genital molluscum contagiosum, and infestation with scabies or crab lice. Of these, genital warts have the greatest clinical significance.

Genital warts are epidermal tumors caused by infection of the epidermis by specific types of human papillomaviruses. More than 20 different genital types of HPV have been recognized, some of which are associated with dysplasia and carcinoma.[18] There has been a marked increase in genital warts over the last several years, and they are considered the most common viral STD. Because many cases are subclinical, the extent of this infection is unknown.

Ulcerative lesions of the genitalia are complex STDs with a diverse clinical presentation and etiology. These infections are currently of great importance, because they have been recognized as major risk factors in the transmission of HIV. The incidence and etiology of genital ulcers vary in different parts of the world, and they are usually more common in developing nations. In North America and Europe, genital herpes is the most common infection, although syphilis has also been increasing in these nations. Other ulcerative diseases, such as chancroid, LGV, and granuloma inguinale (GI), are more common in Africa, Asia, Latin America, and tropical countries. Trauma resulting from sexual activity may produce abrasions and ulcer lesions that may become infected with staphylococci or streptococci.

Table 51–4. Genital Lesions

Lesions	Causative Agents
Genital herpes	Herpes simplex virus
Syphilis	*T. pallidum*
Chancroid	*H. ducreyi*
Lymphogranuloma venereum	*C. trachomatis*, serotypes L1, L2, L3
Granuloma inguinale	*C. granulomatis*
Genital warts	Human papillomavirus
Candida balanitis	*C. albicans*
Molluscum contagiosum	Molluscum contagiosum virus
Scabies	*S. scabiei*
Pubic (crab) lice	*P. pubis*
Trauma	

Systemic or Disseminated STDs

Some STDs begin as a localized infection in the genitalia and may extend beyond the local site to other areas, as in epididymitis and salpingitis. Other STDs quickly enter the blood stream and spread to other organs. Syphilis and AIDS represent two classic diseases in which the most common means of acquisition is sexual, yet the clinical complications occur in infection at other sites.

N. gonorrhoeae usually invades the transitional and columnar epithelial surfaces of the genitourinary tract; however, infection can be acquired through other mucosal sites, such as the conjunctiva, pharynx, and anal canal. In addition, hematogenous dissemination can occur. Disseminated gonococcal infection, also called arthritis-dermatitis syndrome, is manifested in two stages, bacteremic and arthritic. The prevalence of disseminated infection among total gonorrhea cases is less than 1%. It is more common in women, and the risk is greatest during menstruation and pregnancy. Meningitis and endocarditis are also complications that can occur with untreated or inadequately treated gonococcal infections; however, they develop infrequently.[19]

Syphilis is a chronic systemic STD caused by the spirochete bacterium *T. pallidum*. The organism gains entrance through inapparent breaks in the skin, replication takes place in the local tissues, and dissemination occurs via the lymphatics. Primary chancres usually occur at the point of entry of the spirochetes into the body. Because the primary lesions are self-limiting and generally painless, patients may not seek medical care, and the disease progresses to further stages.[20] The most destructive forms of the disease affect the cardiovascular system and the central nervous system.

Lymphogranuloma venereum, caused by *C. trachomatis* serotypes L1, L2, and L3, is another form of a systemic STD. Upon entry, the chlamydiae invade and multiply within local macrophages. They are then carried from the site of infection through the lymphatics to the regional lymph nodes, resulting in inflammatory processes. These organisms are also capable of spreading through the blood stream to the central nervous system.[21]

Other viral agents that are transmitted sexually, but are not considered primary sexual pathogens, are cytomegalovirus and hepatitis viruses.[6] CMV and HBV are carried in the blood and shed in genital secretions; thus, they can be transmitted through sexual and perinatal exposure. Hepatitis A virus (HAV) is shed by the fecal-oral route and can be acquired through anal-oral sex. Vaccines are available for HAV and HBV, providing a mechanism of prevention for STDs caused by these agents.

Reiter's syndrome is a reactive arthritic condition associated with various forms of inflammation. It usually occurs following an infection of the genital tract or intestinal tract. The STDs associated with Reiter's syndrome are chlamydia and gonorrhea.[6]

Maternal–Neonatal Transmission

The consequences of STDs are an important health-care issue for women and their offspring. Women who have or acquire an STD during pregnancy are likely to transmit the infection to the fetus. Table 51–5 lists the various STDs that are transmitted from a mother to her newborn.

Infection in the newborn can occur in several ways. Some microorganisms that are present in the maternal blood may reach the fetus through hematogenous spread. *T. pallidum*, CMV, and HSV are three etiologic agents that can spread to the fetus in utero with devastating results. Other organisms infect the fetus either by progressively ascending from the endocervix, or at delivery, when the newborn passes through the birth canal. *C. trachomatis* and *N. gonorrhoeae* represent common STD pathogens transmitted in this fashion. Other STD syndromes, such as BV and trichomoniasis, may not cause significant infection in the newborn but may lead to obstetric complications that pose a risk to the infant. Routine prenatal screening is an important component in the prevention of these infections; however, many of the women who give birth to children with these infections have not received adequate prenatal care.

CLINICAL MANIFESTATIONS

STDs produce a variety of clinical manifestations, including genital discharge, itching, lesions or ulcers, dysuria, and pain.

Urethritis and Epididymitis

The clinical manifestations of urethritis include dysuria, a urethral discharge, or itching at the end of the urethra. Although there are some differences in symptoms between GU and NGU, it is not usually possible to distinguish between them on the basis of clinical criteria. Gonorrhea has an incubation period of 2 to 6 days and an abrupt onset, and produces a more purulent discharge.[11, 19] Nongonococcal urethritis, particularly *Chlamydia* infections, have a longer incubation period (1 to 5 weeks) and produce a milder urethritis with a less purulent discharge.[11, 14]

Symptoms of urethritis in females may be associated with acute urethral infection or a urinary tract infection. The acute urethral syndrome is associated with signs of a urinary tract infection, including dysuria and frequency. Culture of the urine in these patients is negative, or fewer than 100 colony-forming units (CFUs) per mL are recovered.[14] This syndrome is recognized in women with gonorrhea or chlamydial infections.

Table 51–5. Neonatal Infections With Sexually Transmitted Organisms

Disease in the Neonate	Causative Agents
Conjunctivitis	*C. trachomatis*
	N. gonorrhoeae
Pneumonia	*C. trachomatis*
Hepatosplenomegaly/jaundice	Hepatitis B virus
	Cytomegalovirus
	Herpes simplex virus
	T. pallidum
Meningoencephalitis	Cytomegalovirus
	Herpes simplex virus
	T. pallidum
	Group B streptococci

Epididymitis associated with a sexually transmitted organism can be a complication of urethritis. Inflammation of the epididymis results in scrotal pain and swelling. The onset is usually acute, and the pain is unilateral. A urethral discharge may or may not be present.[12]

Vaginitis and Cervicitis

Vulvovaginal infections produce one or more of the following symptoms: increased volume of vaginal discharge, bad odor, vulvar pruritus or burning, external dysuria, and painful intercourse. The predominant symptom in patients with yeast vulvovaginitis is vulvar pruritus. Vaginal discharge is not significantly increased, but the consistency is often cottage cheese–like or homogeneously thick. Trichomoniasis typically produces an increase in the quantity of vaginal discharge, which is described as yellow and purulent. The chief complaint in patients with BV is a fishy vaginal odor that is noted to increase in the presence of semen. An abnormal gray to white discharge with a milky consistency is also noted.[16]

Patients with mucopurulent cervicitis may note an increase in a purulent vaginal discharge. Other indications of this syndrome are dysuria and intermenstrual bleeding. Salpingitis and other forms of PID manifest as a dull lower abdominal pain. The patient often has fever and may complain of increased vaginal discharge. These symptoms are nonspecific and can be associated with a variety of other clinical conditions, including urinary tract infection, appendicitis, tubal pregnancy, and proctocolitis.

Genital Lesions

Ulcerative lesions of the genitalia are clinically evaluated according to the number of lesions present, the size and morphology, and whether or nor they are painful and associated with lymphadenopathy.

The primary stage of syphilis begins when a painless papular lesion develops at the site of entry.[20] The chancre heals spontaneously, but if no treatment is provided, symptoms of secondary syphilis occur several weeks later. Secondary syphilis is a systemic infection, in which the patient experiences malaise, fever, headache, lymphadenopathy, and rash. Untreated, the patient develops latent syphilis, which is usually asymptomatic. The most progressive form of the disease, tertiary syphilis, occurs years later. This stage manifests as large granulomatous lesions or gummas along with neurologic and cardiovascular damage.

Although most primary herpes infections are asymptomatic, lesions that do occur are vesicular. Painful multiple lesions develop and continue to appear for a week or longer. The lesions progress to a pustule and eventually crust and heal as reepithelialization occurs.[22] General constitutional symptoms, including headache, fever, and malaise, are often present during the first few days. Patients may experience dysuria, vaginal or urethral discharge, and tenderness of the inguinal lymph nodes. Recurrent genital herpes is usually milder, and the duration is shorter.

The less common ulcerative STDs are chancroid, lymphogranuloma venereum, and granuloma inguinale. In chancroid, soft papular lesions develop after infection with *Haemophilus ducreyi*. The lesions are quite painful, become pustular, and rapidly ulcerate. Inguinal adenopathy follows, and buboes may appear 7 to 10 days after the lesion. If untreated, the buboes rupture and form draining abscesses.[23]

The primary lesion in LGV is a painless ulcer that is often asymptomatic or inconspicuous. As the chlamydiae are carried to the regional nodes, general constitutional symptoms may develop. Untreated, regional lymphadenopathy leads to suppurative buboes.[24] In homosexual men and in some women, LGV may manifest as a hemorrhagic proctitis.

The lesions in GI, also known as donovanosis, are painless papules that enlarge slowly over months to years. Lymphadenitis is uncommon, but as the enlarging lesion ulcerates, it often extends onto the inguinal area, forming pseudobuboes.[24]

The clinical manifestations of genital HPV infection range from no evidence of epithelial abnormalities to warts that are visible to the naked eye. Occasionally, patients complain of pruritus and burning. Warts may be flat, or they may appear as condyloma acuminata, which are soft, fleshy, cauliflower-like lesions.[25]

Infestation with scabies or lice can also result in genital lesions. Scabies represent one of the rare STDs that is commonly transmitted in households through nonsexual contact. Pubic lice, on the other hand, are considered to be transmitted primarily through sexual contact. The main symptom in these infestations is severe pruritus, which is caused by an immune response against the ectoparasite. The continued scratching leads to erythema, irritation, and inflammation.[26]

LABORATORY ANALYSES AND DIAGNOSIS

Specimen Collection

Appropriate collection and handling of the specimens for detection of STD pathogens are essential to obtain reliable results. The recommended specimen for collection depends on the STD syndrome involved and the suspected etiologic agent. Table 51–6 is an overview of recommended specimen sites and laboratory examinations.

Genital discharge material can be collected to detect *N. gonorrhoeae, C. trachomatis, U. urealyticum, T. vaginalis,* and yeast, as well as the agents involved in BV.[27] Discharge material is appropriate for most of these organisms; however, chlamydiae reside intracellularly, and it is necessary to remove urethral or endocervical cells if this agent is suspected. Dacron- or rayon-tipped swabs are recommended, because cotton and other materials are toxic for some pathogens. In males with a purulent discharge, the discharge can be collected directly onto the swab. If no discharge is evident, a thin urethrogenital swab is inserted 2 to 4 cm into the urethra, gently rotated, and left in place for 1 or 2 seconds before being withdrawn. Vaginal secretions are collected from the mucosa high in the vaginal canal. Exudate from the endocervix is collected after removal of vaginal secretions and mucus.

In ascending infections of the female pelvis and male genital organs, aspirated material represents the best specimen. Intrauterine contents, aspirates from the fallopian

Table 51–6. Recommendations for Genital Tract Evaluation

Syndrome	Specimen	Etiologic Agent/ Laboratory Tests
Urethritis	Urethral discharge	Gram stain Culture for *N. gonorrhoeae*
	Endourethral swab	Tests for *C. trachomatis*
Vaginitis	Vaginal secretions	Wet mount exam to detect: *T. vaginalis* Yeast Clue cells (BV) Gram stain for BV
Cervicitis	Endocervical mucus	Gram stain Culture for *N. gonorrhoeae*
	Endocervical cells	Tests for *C. trachomatis*
Genital lesions	Exudate material	Tests for HSV (culture, direct antigen) Dark-field exam for *T. pallidum* Gram stain for *H. ducreyi*
Lymphadenopathy/ buboes	Aspiration	Tests for *C. trachomatis* (serotypes L1–L3) Gram stain

tubes, and endometrial specimens are collected at surgery or during laparoscopy. Specimens from males may be collected by aspirating material from the epididymis or following prostatic massage.

Genital lesions are examined to detect the presence of *T. pallidum,* HSV, *H. ducreyi,* LGV strains of *C. trachomatis,* and *Calymmatobacterium granulomatis.*[27] If a lesion has a crust, the crust is removed, and the lesion scraped to express fluid and cells. Lesions that do not have crusts can be aspirated.

Once the specimens have been collected, the material needs to be submitted to the laboratory as soon as possible for examination. Because of the fastidious nature of certain microorganisms, it is often necessary to place the swab or aspirated material in a transport device. Swabs collected for *N. gonorrhoeae* can be transported in a protective medium, or the specimens can be inoculated directly onto selective enriched media. Several transport media for *N. gonorrhoeae* specimens are commercially available, which provide the appropriate medium for the organism as well as an increased carbon dioxide atmosphere. Specific transport media are also available for recovering chlamydiae and viruses.

Direct Microscopic Examination

Microscopic examination of the patient specimen allows direct visualization of pathogens and provides rapid results. Several microscopic examinations are useful in the evaluation of STDs, including wet mount preparations and stained preparations.

The Gram stain is an excellent tool for the detection of *N. gonorrhoeae* in urethral exudates. The presence of gram-negative intracellular diplococci in a symptomatic male is presumptive evidence of gonorrhea.[19] The presence of white blood cells with no organisms characteristic of *N. gonorrhoeae* is an indication of NGU. In specimens from females, normal cervical and vaginal flora may resemble gonococci, and the Gram stain cannot be relied on to diagnose gonorrhea; however, the Gram stain is very helpful in female specimens to detect the presence of BV. A grading system has been developed that establishes a diagnosis of BV according to the lack of normal vaginal bacteria and the presence of BV associated organisms.[28, 29] Lastly, the Gram stain should be used to evaluate genital lesions, particularly when chancroid is suspected. The presence of *H. ducreyi* is observed in the lesion material as small, pleomorphic, gram-negative bacilli arranged in chains and groups.[27]

The causative agent of vulvovaginal infections can often be determined by a microscopic examination of the vaginal discharge. A wet mount of a vaginal or urethral discharge or prostatic secretion should be prepared and examined promptly to detect the motility of *T. vaginalis*. Candidiasis can also be visualized in the wet mount preparation. The addition of 10% potassium hydroxide (KOH) to the preparation dissolves host cell protein and enhances the visibility of fungal elements. Addition of KOH to the specimen may also result in a fishy, amine-like odor that is often noted in the vaginal secretions of patients with BV. The presence of "clue cells," which are indicative of BV, is also noted in the wet mount examination. Clue cells are epithelial cells that are so heavily covered with coccobacillary bacteria that the borders of the cells are obscured.

The diagnosis of bacterial vaginosis is made when three of the following four clinical criteria are met[29]:

- Vaginal pH of greater than 4.5
- Milky homogeneous vaginal discharge
- Presence of clue cells in the vaginal fluid
- Elaboration of an amine odor after the addition of 10% KOH to the vaginal fluid.

Table 51–7 provides a summary of the current differential diagnosis of vaginal infections. If a patient has more than one of these vaginal syndromes, the results may be difficult to interpret.

Fluorescein-conjugated monoclonal antibody systems are also available for the direct detection of certain STD pathogens, including *C. trachomatis*, HSV, and *T. vaginalis*. Genital ulcers that are suggestive of syphilis are examined by dark-field microscopy to detect the presence of spiro-

chetes. The success of this method depends on the quality of the specimen that is collected and the ability to visualize and distinguish the motility of the treponemes. Dark-field microscopy should not be performed on lesions from the oral cavity because of the presence of other treponemes.

Culture Methods

Even though developing technology in clinical microbiology focuses on rapid nonculture methods for detecting infectious agents, the isolation and identification of a viable organism still provides the most definitive diagnosis of infectious diseases. Culture methods are not available for every STD pathogen, but a variety of organisms can be isolated, including bacteria, yeast, viruses, and parasites.

The isolation of *N. gonorrhoeae* is the diagnostic standard for gonorrhea.[6] The Gram stain may provide a presumptive diagnosis in symptomatic males, but culture is necessary to conclusively identify the organism and to perform antimicrobial studies. The primary specimens for culture are from the urethra and the endocervix. In certain situations, it is appropriate to culture specimens from the conjunctiva, pharynx, and anal canal.

Cultures of the vaginal canal are performed to detect the presence of group B streptococci (GBS). Although these organisms are not true STD pathogens, colonization of the vaginal canal in pregnant women can lead to life-threatening infections in the neonate. Neonatal disease can be prevented by screening pregnant women for GBS and treating those who are colonized.[3, 30] The greatest yield of GBS is obtained when the specimen is inoculated into an enrichment broth.

The isolation of *U. urealyticum* in males with NGU is difficult to achieve. These organisms are extremely susceptible to adverse environmental conditions, making it difficult to maintain their viability during specimen transport. Selective media are commercially available to isolate genital mycoplasmas, but few laboratories provide this service.

Culture is not usually necessary for the diagnosis of the majority of commonly encountered vaginal infections. Yeast vulvovaginitis can usually be diagnosed through microscopic examination of the vaginal secretions. A culture for yeast is indicated in symptomatic patients only when the microscopic preparation is negative.[6] Bacterial vaginosis is best diagnosed utilizing the Gram stain and the clinical criteria previously described. In the past, the isolation of *G. vaginalis* was used as an indicator of this syndrome, but this organism can be found in normal vaginal secretions, so culture is not now recommended.[29] Culture is the most sensitive method to detect *T. vaginalis*, although it is not the most practical approach.[6] A plastic envelope method is commercially available that improves the ability to culture this parasite.[27]

Isolation of HSV in tissue culture provides a sensitive and specific method for the diagnosis of genital herpes. The earlier in the disease process the specimen is processed, the greater the likelihood of a successful culture.[22] Lesions that are crusted should not be cultured. Herpes simplex virus grows rapidly in tissue culture, and the cytopathic effect may be visible within 24 hours.

The most sensitive and specific test for the detection of chlamydial infections is isolation in tissue culture.[14, 31] This

Table 51–7. Differential Diagnosis of Vaginitis/Vaginosis

Characteristic	Bacterial Vaginosis	Yeast	Trichomoniasis
pH	>4.5	<4.5	>4.5
Amine-like odor	Yes	No	No
Appearance	Homogeneous and milklike	Flocculent and thick	Homogeneous and frothy
Color	White to gray	White	White, yellow to green
Microscopic exam	Clue cells	Yeast	Motile trichomonads

technique is technically complex, and the specimen quality greatly affects the outcome; therefore, culture for chlamydiae is not readily available.

Nonculture Methods

Although culture remains the diagnostic standard in the detection of infectious diseases, certain situations limit its use. Some organisms, like *T. pallidum*, cannot be cultured on artificial media. Cultivation of other organisms requires technically complex methods that are not practical for routine laboratories to perform. Finally, some pathogens may be extremely sensitive to transport conditions or may require prolonged incubation for growth to occur. These limitations restrict the ability of the clinician to make early patient care decisions. Nonculture methods can be used to provide rapid results as a supplement to culture, and in certain situations, they may serve as the mainstay of diagnosis. These methods are antigen detection, demonstration of antibody, and nucleic acid hybridization.

The diagnosis of syphilis often depends on the detection of antibodies.[20] Two types of antibody tests are performed: nontreponemal tests, including the RPR (rapid plasma reagin) and the VDRL (Venereal Disease Research Laboratory); and treponemal tests, including the FTA-ABS (fluorescent treponemal antibody absorption) and the MHA-TP (microhemagglutination assay for *T. pallidum*). Nontreponemal tests are nonspecific, because they measure an antibody directed against cardiolipin, a normal component of many tissues. These antibodies are found in most patients with *T. pallidum* infection, but they may be seen in patients with other illnesses as well. Nontreponemal tests have two important applications. First, they are rapid and inexpensive to perform, making them useful for screening large populations. Second, these tests revert to negative when a patient with syphilis has been effectively treated; therefore, they can be used to monitor therapy. To determine whether a positive nontreponemal test is the result of syphilis, a treponemal test is subsequently performed that measures antibodies directed against *T. pallidum*. The development of enzymatic assays, antibody-capture assays, and polymerase chain reaction (PCR) to detect DNA in the patient sample should offer improved detection methods for this infection, but these are complex, expensive tests at present.

The etiology of viral hepatitis is also determined by detection of antigens and antibodies. See Chapter 26 for a discussion of hepatitis.

Nonculture methods are an aid in the diagnosis of gonorrhea and chlamydial infections. *N. gonorrhoeae* can be detected directly in clinical samples using an enzyme immunoassay (EIA). This method is equivalent to the Gram stain for the detection of this infection in male urethral specimens. In endocervical specimens, however, EIA results are considered only presumptive and must be confirmed with culture. Direct nucleic acid detection and amplification methods are available, and if economically justified, they are highly sensitive alternatives to detect gonorrhea.

Direct fluorescent antibody testing and enzyme immunoassay have been very useful in the diagnosis of chlamydial infections. The greatest limitation in the detection of this organism has been inadequate collection of specimens. Newer methods being introduced are DNA probes, PCR, and ligase chain reaction. In addition, some of these methods are performed on urine samples. The fact that a test requires a less invasive specimen allows it to be used as a screening test. This advantage will improve the detection methods for chlamydial disease and prevent the long-term sequelae associated with it. In the future, rapid methods such as these will be available for all STDs, so that rapid diagnosis and treatment will minimize the spread of these diseases. The cost of these tests will have to be balanced with their social, economic, and health benefits.

The diagnosis of genital warts is often based on the characteristics noted during the physical examination. Human papillomavirus cannot be grown in tissue culture; therefore, suspicious warts can be examined for the presence of HPV by biopsy. DNA hybridization methods are useful for detecting the type of HPV present.[18, 25] Infestation with scabies or lice is also diagnosed during physical examination.[26] The clinician can detect the presence of mites by scraping the burrow and examining the contents with a microscope. Pubic lice can be observed by examining the patient and observing lice or nits.

TREATMENT AND CONTROL

The prevention and control of STDs are based on four major concepts:

1. Education of those individuals at risk.
2. Detection of disease in asymptomatic individuals.
3. Effective diagnosis and treatment of infected individuals.
4. Evaluation, treatment, and counseling of sexual partners of individuals with STDs.[32]

Empiric therapy for STDs is often selected according to the syndrome present. Therapy is instituted to cover the most likely agents while laboratory results are pending. Rapid tests may be used to narrow the selection of therapy. An important factor in the selection of therapy is the possibility that the patient is infected with multiple STD pathogens. Many patients infected with *N. gonorrhoeae*, for example, are also infected with *C. trachomatis*. It is important to perform a thorough evaluation, using appropriate laboratory tests, to establish the etiologic agent or agents.

The prevention and control of STDs has become more complex over the years as viral agents have increased. Whereas the control of bacterial STDs depends on early diagnosis and therapy, the viral STDs are incurable and lifelong diseases; therefore, control depends on avoiding exposure. This situation requires public health education to discourage high-risk behaviors in the general public as well as individualized counseling of infected carriers.

A comprehensive guide to the treatment of STDs is published periodically by the CDC. Table 51–8 provides an overview of the CDC guidelines published in 1993.[32]

Table 51–8. **STD Treatment Guidelines**

Disease	Recommended Treatment	Follow-Up and Comments
Chlamydial infections and nongonococcal urethritis	Doxycycline or azithromycin	Test-of-cure not necessary after treatment with doxycycline or azithromycin, unless symptoms persist or re-infection is suspected
Gonococcal infections	Ceftriaxone *or* cefixime *or* ciprofloxacin *or* ofloxacin *plus* treatment effective against co-infection with *C. trachomatis*	Patients treated for gonorrhea should be serologically tested for syphilis
		Test-of-cure not necessary if uncomplicated gonorrhea is treated with regimen indicated
Genital herpes	Acyclovir or famciclovir	To reduce signs and symptoms only
Syphilis	Benzathine penicillin G *or* doxycycline if patient is penicillin allergic	Serologic follow-up at 3 and 6 months
Trichomoniasis	Metronidazole	Resistance is rare
		Treatment of sex partners is indicated
Bacterial vaginosis	Metronidazole	Routine treatment of sex partners is not recommended
Vulvovaginal candidiasis	Butoconazole *or* clotrimazole *or* miconazole *or* tioconazole *or* terconazole	Self-medication with over-the-counter preparations advised only for women who have been diagnosed previously
Chancroid	Azithromycin or ceftriaxone or erythromycin	Ulcers clinically improved after 7 days
		Clinical resolution of lymph nodes is slower
		Patients should be tested for HIV infection
Lymphogranuloma venereum	Doxycycline	Patients should be followed clinically until signs and symptoms resolve
Genital warts		
External	Cryotherapy *or* podofilox *or* podophyllin	Women with cervical warts should be evaluated for dysplasia before treatment
Internal (cervical/vaginal)	Cryotherapy *or* TCA *or* podophyllin	Retreatment may be indicated after 7 days
Pediculosis pubis	Lindane *or* permethrin *or* pyrethrins with piperonyl butoxide	Clothing and bedding should be decontaminated
Scabies	Perethrin *or* lindane	Pruritus may persist for several weeks
		Additional treatment may be necessary
		Clothing and bedding should be decontaminated

Data from Centers for Disease Control and Prevention: 1993 Sexually transmitted diseases: Treatment guidelines. MMWR 42 (No. RR-14), 1993.

Case Study

A 27-year-old woman presented to her gynecologist with complaints of a malodorous vaginal discharge. Although the quantity of discharge was only slightly increased, she described the fishy odor as more problematic. In addition, the odor became more obvious following sexual intercourse. She did not complain of abdominal pain, itching, or burning upon urination.

Upon examination, the physician noted a white, nonfloccular, homogeneous discharge adhering to the vaginal walls. The vaginal fluid pH was measured and found to be greater than 4.5. The "whiff test" was performed, and the release of an amine-like odor was noted when a drop of 10% KOH was added to the vaginal fluid on a microscope slide. A wet mount preparation of the vaginal fluid demonstrated the presence of clue cells.

Questions

1. What is the probable diagnosis?
2. What other conditions must be differentiated?
3. What is the recommended treatment? Is treatment of the patient's sexual partner indicated?
4. Are any other laboratory tests necessary to diagnose this condition?
5. What complications may arise from this condition?

Discussion

1. The most likely diagnosis in this patient is bacterial vaginosis (BV).

2. BV must be differentiated from other vaginal infections, including yeast vaginitis and trichomoniasis.

3. This patient was treated with 500 mg of metronidazole orally for 7 days. Treatment of male sex partners of women with BV is not indicated, because it has not been shown to alter the clinical course of BV in women, or the rate of relapse.

4. The clinical criteria noted during the examination were sufficient to diagnose this condition.

5. BV is now considered an important vaginal syndrome, because it may predispose women to develop pelvic inflammatory disease. It is also a significant condition in pregnant women, as it can lead to obstetric complications.

References

1. Drew WL: Sexually transmitted diseases. *In* Ryan KJ (ed): Sherris Medical Microbiology, ed 3. Norwalk, Conn., Appleton & Lange, 1994.
2. Handsfield HH: Sexually transmitted diseases. *In* Gorbach SL, Bartlett JG, Blacklow NR (eds): Infectious Diseases. Philadelphia, WB Saunders, 1992.
3. Sweet RL, Gibbs RS: Infectious Diseases of the Female Genital Tract, ed 2. Baltimore, Williams & Wilkins, 1990.
4. Holmes KK, Handsfield HH: Sexually transmitted diseases. *In* Isselbacher KJ, Braunwald E, Wilson JD, et al (eds): Harrison's Principles of Internal Medicine, ed 13. New York, McGraw-Hill, 1994.
5. Aral SO, Holmes KK: Epidemiology of sexual behavior and sexually transmitted diseases. *In* Holmes KK, Mardh PA, Sparling PF, et al (eds): Sexually Transmitted Diseases, ed 2. New York, McGraw-Hill, 1990.
6. Adimora AA, Hamilton H, Holmes KK, Sparling PF: Sexually Trans-

mitted Diseases Companion Handbook, ed 2. New York, McGraw-Hill, 1993.

7. Centers for Disease Control: Summary of notifiable diseases, US 1994. MMWR 43(53), 1995.

8. Mims CA, Playfair JHL, Roitt IM, et al: Medical Microbiology. St Louis, CV Mosby, 1993.

9. Robinson EN, McGee Z: The Neisseriae: Gonococcus and meningococcus. *In* Schaechter M, Medoff G, Schlessinger D (eds): Mechanisms of Microbial Disease. Baltimore, Williams & Wilkins, 1989.

10. Robinson EN, McGee Z: Chlamydiae and a common sexually transmitted disease. *In* Schaechter M, Medoff G, Schlessinger D (eds): Mechanisms of Microbial Disease. Baltimore, Williams & Wilkins, 1989.

11. Bowie WR: Urethritis in males. *In* Holmes KK, Mardh PA, Sparling PF, et al (eds): Sexually Transmitted Diseases, ed 2. New York, McGraw-Hill, 1990.

12. Berger RE: Acute epididymitis. *In* Holmes KK, Mardh PA, Sparling PF, et al (eds): Sexually Transmitted Diseases, ed 2. New York, McGraw-Hill, 1990.

13. Quinn TC, Stamm WE: Proctitis, proctocolitis, enteritis, and esophagitis in homosexual men. *In* Holmes KK, Mardh PA, Sparling PF, et al (eds): Sexually Transmitted Diseases, ed 2. New York, McGraw-Hill, 1990.

14. Martin DH: Chlamydial infections. Med Clin North Am 24:1367, 1990.

15. Sobel JD: Vulvovaginitis. *In* Hoeprich PD, Jordan MC, Ronald AR (eds): Infectious Diseases, ed 5. Philadelphia, JB Lippincott, 1994.

16. Mead PB: Epidemiology of bacterial vaginosis. Am J Obstet Gynecol 169:446, 1993.

17. Brunham RC, Embree JE: Cervicitis, endometritis, and salpingo-oophoritis. *In* Hoeprich PD, Jordan MC, Ronald AR (eds): Infectious Diseases, ed 5. Philadelphia, JB Lippincott, 1994.

18. Eron LJ: Human papillomaviruses and anogenital disease. *In* Gorbach SL, Bartlett JG, Blacklow NR (eds): Infectious Diseases. Philadelphia, WB Saunders, 1992.

19. Morse SA, Holmes KK: Gonococcal infections. *In* Hoeprich PD, Jordan MC, Ronald AR (eds): Infectious Diseases, ed 5. Philadelphia, JB Lippincott, 1994.

20. Musher DM: Syphilis. *In* Gorbach SL, Bartlett JG, Blacklow NR (eds): Infectious Diseases. Philadelphia, WB Saunders, 1992.

21. Perine PL: Lymphogranuloma venereum. *In* Hoeprich PD, Jordan MC, Ronald AR (eds): Infectious Diseases, ed 5. Philadelphia, JB Lippincott, 1994.

22. Goodman JL: Infections caused by herpes simplex viruses. *In* Hoeprich PD, Jordan MC, Ronald AR (eds): Infectious Diseases, ed 5. Philadelphia, JB Lippincott, 1994.

23. Ronald AR: Chancroid. *In* Hoeprich PD, Jordan MC, Ronald AR (eds): Infectious Diseases, ed 5. Philadelphia, JB Lippincott, 1994.

24. Ronald AR, Alfa MJ: Chancroid, lymphogranuloma venereum, and granuloma inguinale. *In* Gorbach SL, Bartlett JG, Blacklow NR (eds): Infectious Diseases. Philadelphia, WB Saunders, 1992.

25. Fife KH: Papillomaviruses and human warts. *In* Hoeprich PD, Jordan MC, Ronald AR (eds): Infectious Diseases, ed 5. Philadelphia, JB Lippincott, 1994.

26. Billstein SA, Mattaliano VJ: The "nuisance" sexually transmitted diseases: Molluscum contagiosum, scabies, and crab lice. Med Clin North Am 74:1487, 1990.

27. Baron EJ, Peterson LR, Finegold SM (eds): Bailey & Scott's Diagnostic Microbiology, ed 9. St Louis, CV Mosby, 1994.

28. Nugent RP, Krohn MA, Hillier SL: Reliability of diagnosing bacterial vaginosis is improved by a standardized method of Gram stain interpretation. J Clin Microbiol 29:297, 1991.

29. Hillier SL: Diagnostic microbiology of bacterial vaginosis. Am J Obstet Gynecol 169:455, 1993.

30. Centers for Disease Control and Prevention: Prevention of perinatal group B streptococcal disease: A public health perspective. MMWR 45(No. RR-7), 1996.

31. Arno JN, Jones RB: Venereal chlamydial infections. *In* Hoeprich PD, Jordan MC, Ronald AR (eds): Infectious Diseases, ed 5. Philadelphia, JB Lippincott, 1994.

32. Centers for Disease Control and Prevention: 1993 Sexually transmitted diseases: Treatment guidelines. MMWR 42(No. RR-14), 1993.

Chapter 52

Skin and Soft Tissue Infections

Connie R. Mahon

Etiology and Pathophysiology
Clinical Manifestations
Laboratory Analyses and Diagnosis
Treatment
Case Studies

Skin infections are among the most commonly encountered infectious diseases in the community as well as in the hospital environment. Infections can result from the invasion of a wide variety of bacterial, fungal, parasitic, or viral agents. Skin infections can occur either as primary manifestations, without preexisting conditions, or as secondary to previous injury, trauma, or systemic spread of the invading organism.[1]

The healthy intact skin is the body's first line of defense and is an effective physical barrier to infection. Very few organisms can initiate an infection through intact skin; most require breaks in the skin surface to cause infection. The skin is made up of several layers. Figure 52–1 shows the structure of normal skin.

The epidermis, the outermost layer, is composed of stratified squamous epithelial cells. Stratum corneum, the outermost layer of the epidermis, is made up of flat, dead cells containing a protein called keratin. These cells are continously shed and replaced, reducing the amount of bacteria on skin surfaces. This epidermal layer serves as an effective barrier against physical, chemical, and bacterial invaders.[2] In addition, Langerhans' cells of the epidermis have the ability to process and present antigens to lymphocytes.[3]

The second layer of the skin, the dermis, is made up of a thick layer of connective tissues and elastic fibers. It contains a dense network of capillaries and lymphatic vessels that make immunoglobulins and other humoral defense factors available. Numerous glands, such as sebaceous and eccrine sweat glands, and hair follicles are embedded in the dermis. Sebaceous and eccrine glands secrete substances such as lysozymes, lipids, and fatty acids that are inhibitory to most organisms.[2, 3]

The skin also contains normal bacterial flora that serve as a protective mechanism against potential microbial colonizers. The composition of the normal skin flora depends on the ability of the organisms to survive the high salt concentrations and the antimicrobial effects of lipids and fatty acids present on the skin. The skin flora consist of resident or permanent colonizers as well as transient colonizers. Gram-positive cocci, such as streptococci and coagulase-negative staphylococci, are common permanent

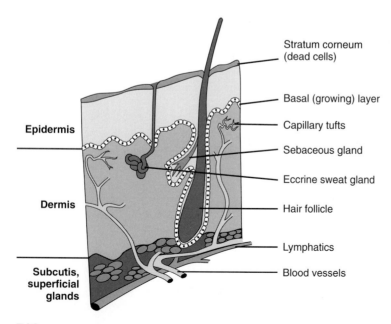

Labels:
- Stratum corneum (dead cells)
- Basal (growing) layer
- Capillary tufts
- Sebaceous gland
- Eccrine sweat gland
- Hair follicle
- Lymphatics
- Blood vessels
- Epidermis
- Dermis
- Subcutis, superficial glands

Figure 52–1. Structure of the skin.

colonizers of the skin. Diphtheroids, *Propionibacterium acnes*, *Micrococcus* species, and yeasts are others.[4, 5] Transient organisms may include coagulase-positive *Staphylococcus aureus.* Members of the resident flora do not usually cause disease, but rather, prevent potential pathogens from establishing infection. Resident flora help maintain a low pH, compete for nutrients, and produce bactericidal substances. The amount of skin bacteria may be reduced as much as 90% by washing, but the numbers return to normal shortly thereafter. Nevertheless, washing eliminates transient organisms such as *S. aureus,* which is a potential pathogen. Table 52–1 lists the common microbial flora on the skin.[6]

ETIOLOGY AND PATHOPHYSIOLOGY

Infectious diseases of the skin may be grouped according to etiologic agents (e.g., bacterial, fungal, parasitic, or viral). They may also be classified either as primary, when there is no obvious underlying skin disease present, or as secondary to trauma, injury, or systemic spread, as previously mentioned. This section discusses the most commonly encountered and clinically relevant infections of the skin and soft tissues and their etiologic agents.[7]

The most common primary pyodermas are folliculitis, impetigo, erysipelas, furuncle, carbuncle, and forms of cellulitis. Table 52–2 lists common primary pyodermas and their associated etiologic agents. *Folliculitis,* usually caused by *S. aureus,* is an infection and inflammation of the hair follicles. It is usually seen in areas of heavy friction and enormous sweat gland activity, such as the neck, face, axillae, and buttocks. Blockage of ducts by accumulated sebum produced by the sebaceous glands is a contributing factor in establishing the infection. This type of infection appears as small papules that may form pustules. The pustules subside when the associated factors no longer exist. *Pseudomonas aeruginosa* has also been associated with this infection. Outbreaks occur in facilities where hot tubs and whirlpools are not adequately and properly maintained.[1, 7]

Impetigo is a common pyodermal infection. Usually caused by *Streptococcus pyogenes* (group A streptococci), impetigo may become secondarily infected by *S. aureus.* The lesion of impetigo begins as a small vesicle that appears at the initial site of colonization.[8] The vesicle later pustulates and ruptures, releasing a thick, yellow fluid that becomes crusted when it dries. Bullous impetigo, caused by phage II strains of *S. aureus,* is an infection characterized by large blisters (bullae) filled with serous fluid. When

Table 52–1. Normal Microbial Skin Flora

Common	Less Common
Candida species	*Streptococcus* species
Micrococcus species	*Acinetobacter calcoaceticus*
Staphylococcus species	*Bacteroides* species
Clostridium species	Gram-negative rods (fermenters
Lactobacillus	and nonfermenters)
Diphtheroids	*Moraxella* species

Adapted from Larsen HS: Host parasite interaction. *In* Mahon CR, Manuselis G (eds): Textbook of Diagnostic Microbiology. Philadelphia, WB Saunders, 1995.

Table 52–2. Most Common Primary Pyodermas

Infection	Organism(s)	Comments
Impetigo	*Streptococcus pyogenes,* occasionally; *Staphylococcus aureus,* if bullous	Children affected most; communicable; no fever
Erysipelas	*S. pyogenes,* occasionally; other β-hemolytic streptococci or *S. aureus*	Distinct raised borders; fever common
Cellulitis	*S. pyogenes, S. aureus; Haemophilus influenzae* in children	Erythema, tenderness, pain, edema, warmth; fever common
Folliculitis	*S. aureus*; gram-negative bacilli or *Candida* if predisposing conditions	Papules around hair follicles; areas exposed to whirlpool bath (*Pseudomonas aeruginosa*)
Furuncle	*S. aureus*	Fluctuant, painful nodules, often in intertriginous areas
Carbuncle	*S. aureus*	Multiple abscesses
Paronychia	*S. aureus,* gram-negative bacilli, *Candida*	Peringual swelling

From Castiglia M, Smego RA: Skin and soft tissue infections. *In* Mahon CR, Manuselis G (eds): Textbook of Diagnostic Microbiology. Philadelphia, WB Saunders, 1995.

the blister ruptures, it dries into a crust. A highly contagious infection that primarily occurs in children, bullous impetigo can be easily transmitted by direct contact or fomites.[9] Large, bullous gangrenous lesions can also be caused by *Pseudomonas, Clostridium,* and gram-negative bacilli.[10, 11]

Erysipelas, also caused by *S. pyogenes,* is described as a painful form of cellulitis that involves not only the superficial epidermal layer but also the deeper layers of the dermis and lymphatics. The infection is associated with edema, erythema, and systemic symptoms such as fever and lymphadenopathy. Bacteremia may occur, making erysipelas a serious, possibly life-threatening infection.[12]

A *furuncle,* sometimes referred to as a boil, is a small purulent abscess that usually develops in the area of the hair follicle. Furuncles caused by *S. aureus* may eventually involve the dermis and subcutaneous tissues, resulting in a more critical and extensive infection. Multiple abscesses, a *carbuncle,* may arise in the area. Fever, chills, and malaise are systemic manifestations that may occur with carbuncles.[4, 9]

Cellulitis, fasciitis, myonecrosis, and tissue-necrotizing infections are types of soft tissue infections. The organisms isolated from these types of wound infections include both strict anaerobes, such as *Bacteroides fragilis, Clostridium perfringens,* and anaerobic cocci, and facultative anaerobes, such as *S. aureus, S. pyogenes,* and enteric gram-negative bacilli.[1, 10, 11] The incidence of necrotizing fasciitis caused by *S. pyogenes* has been rising and is particularly troubling. Transient bacteremia is the likely source of the organisms, although many patients do not report an antecedent infection.[13] Facial cellulitis in children is most often caused by *Haemophilus influenzae* type b. Gangrenous cellulitis in compromised hosts can be caused by *P. aeruginosa,* various species of phycomycetes, and *Aspergillus* species.[10]

Table 52-3. Infections Secondary to Preexisting Lesions

Infection	Major Pathogen(s)
Surgical wound infection	
Clean	*Staphylococcus aureus*, gram-negative bacilli
Contaminated, such as colon	Plus anaerobes, streptococci
Intravenous infusion sites	*S. aureus*, coagulase-negative staphylococci
Trauma	
Soil contamination	*Pseudomonas aeruginosa*, clostridia
Freshwater contamination	*Aeromonas, Plesiomonas*
Saltwater contamination	*Vibrio vulnificus*
Bites	
Human	Oral aerobes and anaerobes, *S. aureus*
Dog, cat	*Pasteurella multocida, S. aureus*, anaerobes
Rat	*Streptobacillus moniliformis, Spirillum minus* (minor)
Decubitus ulcer	Streptococci, *S. aureus*, coliforms, *Pseudomonas*, anaerobes including *Bacteroides fragilis*
Foot ulcer in diabetic patients	*S. aureus*, streptococci, coliforms, *P. aeruginosa*, anaerobes
Hidradenitis suppurativa	*S. aureus*, streptococci, coliforms, *Pseudomonas*, anaerobes
Burns	*S. aureus, Candida, P. aeruginosa*

From Castiglia M, Smego RA: Skin and soft tissue infections. *In* Mahon CR, Manuselis G (eds): Textbook of Diagnostic Microbiology. Philadelphia, WB Saunders, 1995.

Secondary skin infections and infections of the soft tissue can result when organisms are introduced following external trauma or internal damage such as that caused by atherosclerosis or allergic vasculitis. Necrotizing infections are of particular concern in surgical wounds. Secondary infections can be caused by a wide variety of bacteria, such as *S. aureus,* group A streptococci, *Proteus, Pseudomonas,* and *Escherichia coli,* as well as fungi and viruses.[12] Table 52–3 lists infections that occur secondary to trauma or injury.

Healthy living tissue has a high concentration of oxygen, and hence, a high oxidation-reduction potential (eH). When injuries that interfere with local blood flow occur, decreased oxygen, decreased eH, tissue necrosis, and decreased leukocyte activity follow. This type of environment becomes favorable for the growth of strictly anaerobic and facultatively anaerobic organisms that produce gas and enzymes, leading to further necrosis and spread of infection.[1, 10, 11]

Tissue infections that result from penetrating injury or burns are often polymicrobic. *P. aeruginosa* and *S. aureus* are commonly isolated from burn wounds. Isolates may also reflect the aerobic and anaerobic flora present on the particular body site, surrounding skin, and mucous membranes of the host. Postoperative infections, for example, that develop in the abdominal area may yield organisms that make up the colon flora. Fungal infections, such as sporotrichosis, chromomycosis, and mycetomas, are subcutaneous infections that occur after abrasions or penetrating injury. *Sporothrix schenckii* infection progresses along the lymphatics. Chromomycosis, caused primarily by de-

matiaceous soil saprobes, is a host-induced granulomatous response. Mycetomas, deep lesions that can progress to the bone, are caused by a wide variety of fungal and bacterial species. Actinomycotic mycetoma is caused by aerobic actinomycetes such as *Nocardia* species, whereas eumycotic mycetoma is commonly caused by the fungal agent *Pseudallescheria boydii*.[14]

Fungal infections of the stratum corneum, also known as ringworm or tinea, are caused by dermatophytes of the genera *Microsporum, Epidermophyton,* and *Trichophyton.* These fungi can hydrolyze the keratin on skin, hair, and nails and are well suited to these sites. These organisms rarely invade deeper tissues, because they fail to grow at 37 °C, but they may persist in the stratum corneum for years. *Candida albicans* and other normal flora yeasts can cause cutaneous infections in moist or lacerated areas of the skin, especially in the immunocompromised host, or they can colonize pre-existing skin conditions.[14, 15]

Skin and tissues can also become infected as a result of generalized systemic infection or by extension from other foci. Box 52–1 shows conditions that may lead to systemic spread of a bacterial infection.

Vibrio vulnificus and *Aeromonas hydrophila* are organisms found to cause severe cellulitis and tissue necrosis following a bacteremic spread. Primary septicemia due to *V. vulnificus* has been associated with the ingestion of raw oysters or other types of shellfish. Infections due to other halophilic vibrios and *Aeromonas* species are acquired when wounds are contaminated by fresh or marine water.[16] Disseminated *Neisseria gonorrhoeae* and bacteremic episodes of *N. meningitidis* produce erythematous macules, petechiae, and purpura that later progress to gray, hemorrhagic, necrotic lesions.[7]

Staphylococcal scalded skin syndrome (SSSS), a serious disease of young children, especially neonates, is caused by strains that produce an exfoliative toxin. This toxin splits layers of epidermis, which later exfoliate, so that affected patients look very similar to burn patients. The foci of staphylococcal infection are usually remote from the site of exfoliation.[17]

Group A streptococcus has been associated with toxic shock similar to that produced by *S. aureus.* Exotoxin-producing strains of group A streptococcus produce an invasive infection of the skin and mucous membranes, characterized as toxic-shock–like syndrome.[18] Such infections often begin as a severe necrotizing fasciitis and pro-

---

Box 52–1. Cutaneous Involvement in Systemic Bacterial Infections

Infective endocarditis
Bacteremia and sepsis
Scarlet fever
Toxic shock syndrome
Staphylococcal scalded skin syndrome
Enteric fever

From Castiglia M, Smego RA: Skin and soft tissue infections. *In* Mahon CR, Manuselis G (eds): Textbook of Diagnostic Microbiology. Philadelphia, WB Saunders, 1995.

gress to a necrotizing myositis. The disease progresses rapidly, and without intervention, mortality is high.

S. aureus is a normal colonizer of the anterior nares and perineum of healthy individuals. These sites become the sources of infections for the carrier and other susceptible individuals. Virulence factors associated with *S. aureus* include hemolysins, leukocidin, epidermolytic toxins, coagulase, fibrinolysin, nucleases, lipases, hyaluronidase, and protein A, a cell-wall component that binds to the Fc portion of immunoglobulin (Ig) G.[9] Similarly, *S. pyogenes* and *C. perfringens* produce hemolysins, spreading factors, and other extracellular enzymes that contribute to their pathogenicity.[11]

Microorganisms or their products elicit an inflammatory response in the skin. Staphylococci, streptococci, enteric gram-negative bacilli, and pseudomonads frequently cause an acute inflammatory reaction, with polymorphonuclear leukocytes (PMNs) predominating. In some infections, such as those caused by mycobacteria, actinomycetes, and fungi, a chronic inflammatory response follows the acute phase, owing to the persistence of antigen in the area. Monocytes, macrophages, and lymphocytes replace PMNs as predominant cells, and a granuloma is formed. The ready presence of immunoglobulins and lymphocytes also makes the skin a prime location for manifestations of immediate and delayed sensitivity.[19]

Skin and tissue infections can also be caused by a wide variety of viruses, rickettsiae, mycobacteria, fungi, and other bacteria. Although the more common conditions are usually diagnosed from their clinical presentations, laboratory tests are often needed to establish the etiology of the infection.

CLINICAL MANIFESTATIONS

Pyogenic infections such as those caused by *S. aureus* trigger acute inflammatory reactions. Pus-filled abscesses tend to become swollen, red, warm, and painful, and PMNs accumulate in the area. Necrotic tissues may surround the area. Bullous impetigo presents as a localized blister-like lesion containing seropurulent material. Scalded skin syndrome, an exfoliative dermatitis, begins as a localized lesion similar to a bullous impetigo, then progresses to a generalized condition. A cutaneous erythema is followed by extensive sloughing off of the epidermal layer of the skin. Streptococcal impetigo lesions begin as pustular vesicles that develop into superficial or deep ulcers with a honey-colored crust. Cellulitis appears as tender, red, edematous areas, and invasion of bacteria, especially with group A streptococcus, causes red streaking as the infection progresses into the lymphatics.[19] The necrotizing fasciitis caused by group A streptococci is usually of acute onset and is accompanied by severe pain at the involved site, fever, and chills. The rapid spread of the infection leads to dusky erythema and edema and often to shock, multiorgan failure, and death.[13]

The host response to soluble fungal antigens diffuses into the epidermis and dermis. The response varies from no reaction to diffuse scaly patches, to defined rings of inflammation, to inflammatory exudative lesions. *C. albicans* lesions, usually found in skin folds, appear as red, weeping areas with scalloped edges, surrounded by satellite

eruptions. Yeast can also cause a pustular folliculitis. Sporotrichosis is characterized by nodular ulcerations that progress along the lymphatics, whereas chromomycosis is described as localized warty, cauliflower-like lesions. Mycetomas appear as swollen, deformed areas of abscess with draining sinuses. Granules containing the etiologic agent are collected from these draining sinuses. Mycetomas are usually found on the hands or feet.[20]

Indicators of soft tissue infection, especially anaerobic infection, are gas in the tissues, foul smell, black discoloration, and exudates with granules. The classic signs of inflammation may occasionally be absent. In the case of any bacterial skin infection, fever may indicate septicemia and systemic spread of the organism.[10]

Systemic viral and rickettsial diseases can produce rashes, vesicles, or other types of skin lesions. Herpes simplex virus causes primary vesicular or bullous lesions. The virus establishes in the ganglia and becomes latent. It later reactivates, after various types of stress to the host occur. Mycobacterial skin infections usually manifest as granulomatous ulcers. Table 52–4 describes some of the typical lesions of skin infections.[21]

LABORATORY ANALYSES AND DIAGNOSIS

Although diagnosis of common skin infections is usually based on the clinical appearance of the lesions, culture and antimicrobial susceptibility tests may be needed to confirm the diagnosis and guide therapy. Skin scrapings or other material from lesions should be collected after the lesion and surrounding area have been carefully disinfected to eliminate irrelevant organisms. Any crusts and surface debris should also be removed. Specimens from draining sinus tracts of mycetomas should be examined for granules that will contain the organism.

Because swabs contain trapped oxygen and cotton is toxic to some anaerobes, special anaerobic swabs and transport tubes should be used if anaerobic organisms are suspected. In most cases, material from the center of the lesion should be obtained, although material from the periphery of lesions is necessary for isolation of dermatophytes. When fungi are suspected, a sterile scalpel can be used to carefully obtain skin scrapings. Swabs should not be used, because their fibers may be misleading when direct preparations are examined under the microscope.

Pus or fluid from closed lesions should be obtained with a needle and syringe. Material collected in the syringe is suitable for aerobic and anaerobic culture and for viral culture. Specimens for viral culture or analysis should be collected and transported in special viral transport media and stored at $-70\,^{\circ}C$ if they cannot be processed within 24 hours. Chronic localized infections, burns, necrotizing infections, and wounds may require biopsy. Histologic evaluation of granulomatous lesions helps to differentiate infection from neoplasm. For example, observation of brown sclerotic bodies in tissue is diagnostic of fungal chromomycosis rather than carcinoma.[22]

Several rapid direct methods can aid in the diagnosis of skin infections. Direct smear examination of clinical material submitted to the laboratory is a very important tool. Gram-stained smears can lead to presumptive identification

Table 52–4. Clinical Manifestations of Skin Infections

Etiologic Agent/ Disease	Lesion
Staphylococcus aureus	
Folliculitis	Pustules
Boils or furuncles	Circumscribed abscesses that become filled with pus
Carbuncles	Aggregates of boils
Impetigo	Bullous lesions with subsequent varnish-like crusts
Scalded skin syndrome	Large, flaccid bullae; epidermis separating into sheets with red, moist surface beneath
Streptococcus pyogenes (group A streptococci)	
Impetigo	Pustular vesicles developing into ulcers with honey-colored crusts
Erysipelas	Red thickening of the skin
Cellulitis	Flat, reddened areas of the skin
Lymphangitis	Red streaks following the lymphatic channels
Pseudomonas aeruginosa	
Burn infection	Greenish discoloration
Ecthyma gangrenosum	Brown or black, spreading, bullous lesions
Folliculitis	Pustules
Anaerobic or mixed bacterial tissue infections	
Anaerobic cellulitis	Spreading necrosis of tissue, usually with gas formation (crepitation)
Gas gangrene	Severe form of spreading anaerobic cellulitis with dusky discoloration, surface bullae formation
Dermatophyte fungi	
Ringworm (tinea)	Scaly patches; ring inflammation with healing center; persistent papules, pustules, abscesses
Candida albicans	
Intertriginous infection	Reddened areas with scalloped edges and pustules
Folliculitis and diaper rash	Pustules
Sporothrix schenckii	
Sporotrichosis	Ulcerating nodules progressing along lymphatic channels
Saprobic fungi	
Chromomycosis	Raised, warty lesions resembling cauliflower heads
Saprobic fungi, actinomycetes, bacteria	
Mycetoma	Massive swollen area with draining sinus tracts that discharge granules
Herpes simplex virus	Vesicles on a reddened base filled with clear fluid
Mycobacterium species	Granulomatous ulcers, nodules

and can help guide culture methods, test selection, and even initial treatment. This is of critical importance in rapidly progressing situations, such as necrotizing fasciitis, because treatment must begin immediately. Acid-fast stains should be performed on granules or granulomatous specimens that may contain actinomycetes or mycobacteria. Potassium hydroxide (KOH) preparations are necessary when fungi are suspected. Calcofluor white, a fluorescent compound, can be mixed with KOH to give a good fungal contrast, to visualize fungal elements with the use of a fluorescence microscope.[22]

Culture of abscesses should include methods to recover the variety of bacteria and fungi previously described. Quantitative culture of biopsy material may be requested, because knowledge of the number and type of organisms present helps the surgeon determine the best time for wound closure or for skin grafts on burns. Culture may also help to establish the etiology of invasive infections by establishing the identity of the predominant organism.

Culture of the affected site usually reveals the infecting organism. Routine culture of primary infections should include nonselective media, such as blood and chocolate agars, and selective media, such as MacConkey agar. Phenylethyl alcohol (PEA) and Columbia colistin–nalidixic acid (CNA) agars are additional selective media that may be used when a mixture of gram-positive and gram-negative bacteria is suspected. Similarly, because most anaerobic infections are polymicrobic, anaerobic culture media must include those that are selective for gram-positive and gram-negative bacteria. Identification of bacterial isolates is performed using various conventional or automated methods, sometimes a combination of both.

Blood cultures may or may not yield etiologic agents of skin infections that manifest as secondary to systemic spread. In cases in which the manifestation is a result of toxin, such as in scalded skin syndrome, the organism is rarely recovered from the blood or from the sloughed-off epidermal layer. The organisms are usually present at a distant focus of infection.[9, 17]

Except for group A streptococcus, which has remained consistently susceptible to penicillin G, antibiotic susceptibility tests are necessary for most isolates, such as enteric bacilli, pseudomonads, and staphylococci, owing to their unpredictable susceptibility patterns as well as emerging resistance to most prescribed antimicrobials.

Because viruses reproduce only within living cells, it is necessary to use tissue cultures to recover viral agents. Viruses produce inclusions or distinctive cytopathic effects (CPEs) on different types of tissue cell lines, which aid in their identification. Inclusions and viral antigens may be detected with fluorescent antibody stains. Various immunodiagnostic tests are available to detect humoral antibody response to most viral and rickettsial antigens.[21]

TREATMENT

Treatment of skin infections may consist of draining of pus-filled abscesses, debridement of necrotic tissue, topical agents, and systemic antibiotics. Table 52–5 indicates recommended treatment for various agents causing infection.[23–28]

Staphylococcal abscesses may heal following drainage, but in severe infections, systemic antibiotics are required. Penicillin G is the antibiotic of choice for susceptible organisms, because it is 10 to 100 times more active than the β-lactamase–resistant penicillins. Penicillin and methicillin resistance, however, has been a problem during the past several years. Topical therapy supresses but does not eliminate the carrier state and must be continued for prolonged periods to be effective. Nasal cultures may be performed to determine whether the carrier state has been eliminated.

In soft tissue infections, abscesses should be drained

Table 52–5. **Treatment for Skin and Tissue Infections**

Organism	Therapy
Staphylococcus aureus	Penicillin G, if *S. aureus* is susceptible
	Penicillin with clavulanic acid* or ceftriaxone alone if *S. aureus* is a β-lactamase producer
	Clindamycin or erythromycin for penicillin-allergic patients
	Vancomycin for severe hospital infection
	Rifampin or topical neomycin for nasal carriers
Group A streptococci	Penicillin G
	Clindamycin or erythromycin for penicillin-allergic patients
Anaerobes, mixed infection	Penicillin with clavulanic acid
	Metronidazole with gentamicin
Dermatophytes	Topical miconazole alone or with anti-inflammatory agent
	Topical triclosan
	Griseofulvin for severe infection
Candida	Topical miconazole
	Ketoconazole
Sporothrix	Topical and oral potassium iodide
Agents of chromocycosis	5-Flucytosine
	Thiabendazole
Pseudallescheria boydii	Miconazole
Nocardia, Actinomyces	Sulfamethoxazole-trimethroprim with streptomycin
Herpes simplex	Acyclovir

*Clavulanic acid is a β-lactamase inhibitor.

and foreign material and necrotic tissue removed. Early and aggressive surgical intervention is essential in cases of necrotizing fasciitis, myositis, and gangrene.[13] Because many of the bacteria present in mixed infections have different susceptibilities, mode of treatment must be based on tests for susceptibility and resistance of the individual organisms.[1]

Burn wounds are rarely sterile. Therefore, their bacterial population should be monitored by culture throughout healing, because septicemia is a serious consequence of uncontrolled bacterial populations in burns.

In fungal infections, topical treatments of antifungal agents combined with anti-inflammatory agents are often used. Systemic agents such as amphotericin B may be needed for severe systemic infections. Mycotic mycetomas are very difficult to treat, because drugs do not penetrate into fibrotic areas of the granulomatous lesions. Actinomycotic mycetomas may respond better to treatment with antibacterial agents.[20] In serious herpes simplex infections, initial lesions respond well to acyclovir.[21]

Case Study 1

A 45-year-old diabetic man was seen by his family physician because of multiple boils and abscesses on his thighs. He also reported flu-like symptoms and inability to eat for the preceding 12 hours. Except for a temperature of 101 °F, the physical examination was normal. A glucose test performed immediately in the office showed that the patient's blood glucose level was 185 mg/dL. The patient controlled his diabetes with insulin injections in his thighs, and the abscesses appeared to be located at the injection sites. The abscesses were drained, and a pus specimen was sent to the local hospital laboratory for culture and sensitivity, along with a nasal swab to be cultured for *Staphylococcus aureus.*

A course of oral dicloxacillin was given during the first 24 hours. The next day, the patient's temperature was normal, and his fasting blood glucose level was 130 mg/dL. Antibiotic therapy was changed to penicillin G when the laboratory reported that *S. aureus* had been isolated from the pus specimen and was sensitive to dicloxacillin. The nasal culture was also positive for *S. aureus,* and the physician added cloxacillin to the penicillin G therapy.

One month after treatment, the patient's nasal culture was negative, his fasting blood glucose level was 120 mg/dL, and the abscesses had healed.

Questions

1. What is the likely explanation for the development of *S. aureus* skin lesions in this patient?

2. What further complication might be suspected from the physical findings?

3. Why was cloxacillin added to the therapeutic regimen?

Discussion

1. Diabetics whose treatment needs adjustment often develop boils of the sort described in this case. Moreover, people who use needles regularly, such as diabetics receiving insulin injections, have higher nasal carrier rates for *S. aureus.* The organisms are thus readily available for invasion of the injection sites.

2. Temperature of 101 °F and the symptoms reported by the patient suggested bacteremia. The course of dicloxacillin resulted in a normal temperature within 24 hours.

3. Cloxacillin is effective in eliminating the nasal carrier state, which otherwise could be a source of recurrent episodes of staphylococcal infection for this patient.

Case Study 2

A 55-year-old Hispanic man presented to the emergency department with fever, scleral icterus, and swelling of the lower right leg with developing exudate. Examination revealed the patient to have a slightly enlarged liver, right pleural effusion, diarrhea, and symptoms of nephrotic syndrome. Heart tachycardia was also noted.

The patient, a non–insulin-dependent diabetic, revealed a history of alcohol abuse. He also had a history of hepatitis in childhood. Four weeks prior to admission, the patient had eaten raw oysters and experienced episodes of diarrhea that lasted for 2 to 3 weeks. His condition was diagnosed as systemic toxicity.

Cultures of urine showed no growth. A smear made from the exudate showed many gram-negative bacilli, and the culture grew what was identified as *Vibrio vulnificus*. The same organism was isolated from the blood cultures. It was found susceptible to ampicillin, cephalothin, cefoxitin, chloramphenicol, gentamicin, and clindamycin.

The patient was started on antimicrobial therapy with ampicillin, gentamicin, and clindamycin. Despite the broad-spectrum antimicrobial therapy, the cellulitis worsened. It was decided to amputate the lower right leg just above the knee to resolve the necrotizing cellulitis. The patient recovered successfully from surgery and was released from the hospital in stable condition.

Questions

1. What is the most likely source of the infection?
2. What risk factors predisposed this patient to this type of infection?

Discussion

1. *Vibrio vulnificus*, a halophilic vibrio commonly found in coastal waters, has been known to cause severe necrotic cellulitis and primary sepsis. Infections are usually acquired when wounds are exposed to marine water or by direct contact with shellfish. Ingestion of raw oysters has been associated with primary septicemia due to *V. vulnificus*.

2. Patients with chronic liver disease as well as diabetics, renal patients, and patients immunocompromised for other reasons are highly susceptible to primary septicemia due to *V. vulnificus*. Susceptibility of patients with alcoholic cirrhosis is also greatly increased.

References

1. Magnussen CR: Skin and soft tissue infections. *In* Reese RE, Douglas RG (eds): A Practical Approach to Infectious Diseases, ed 2. Boston, Little Brown, 1991.
2. Tortora GJ, Anagnostakos NP: Principles of Anatomy and Physiology, ed 3. New York, Harper & Row, 1981.
3. Roitt I, Brostoff J, Male D: Immunology. St. Louis, Mosby–Year Book, 1989.
4. Leyden JJ: Pathophysiology of certain bacterial diseases. *In* Soter NA, Baden HP (eds): Pathophysiology of Dermatologic Diseases. New York, McGraw-Hill, 1991.
5. Gonzalez E: Pathophysiology of certain fungal diseases. *In* Soter NA, Baden HP (eds): Pathophysiology of Dermatologic Diseases. New York, McGraw-Hill, 1991.
6. Larsen HS: Host parasite interaction. *In* Mahon CR, Manuselis G (eds): Textbook of Diagnostic Microbiology. Philadelphia, WB Saunders, 1995.
7. Castiglia M, Smego RA: Skin and soft tissue infections. *In* Mahon CR, Manuselis G (eds): Textbook of Diagnostic Microbiology. Philadelphia, WB Saunders, 1995.
8. Shulman ST: Bacterial infections of the upper respiratory tract. *In* Shulman ST, Phair JP, Sommers HM (eds): The Biologic and Clinical Basis of Infectious Disease. Philadelphia, WB Saunders, 1992.
9. Sheagren JN: *Staphylococcus aureus:* The persistent pathogen. [Medical Progress.] N Engl J Med 310:1368–1373, 1984.
10. Mader JT, Wallace W: Bone and necrotizing soft tissue infections. *In* Baron S (ed): Medical Microbiology, ed 3. New York, Churchill Livingstone, 1991.
11. Lewis RT: Necrotizing soft issue infections. Infect Dis Clin North Am 3:693, 1992.
12. Swartz MN: Cellulitis and superficial infections. *In* Mandell GL, Douglas RG Jr, Bennett JE (eds): Principles and Practice of Infectious Diseases. New York, Churchill Livingstone, 1990.
13. Stevens DL: Infections of the skin, muscle and soft tissues. *In* Isselbacher KJ, Braunwald E, Wilson JD et al (eds): Harrison's Principles of Internal Medicine. New York, McGraw-Hill, 1994.
14. Swartz MN: Subcutaneous tissue infections and abscesses. *In* Mandell GL, Douglas RG Jr, Bennett JE (eds): Principles and Practice of Infectious Diseases. New York, Churchill Livingstone, 1990.
15. Aly R: Microbiology of skin and nails. *In* Baron S (ed): Medical Microbiology, ed 2. Menlo Park, Calif, Addison-Wesley, 1986.
16. Warnock EW, MacMath TL: Primary *Vibrio vulnificus* septicemia. Emerg Med 11:153–156, 1993.
17. Elias PM, Fritsch P, Epstein E: Staphylococcal scalded skin syndrome. Arch Dermatol 113:201, 1977.
18. Stevens DL, Tanner MH, et al: Severe group A streptococcal infections associated with a toxic shock–like syndrome and scarlet fever toxin A. N Engl J Med 321:1–7, 1989.
19. Madri JA: Inflammation and healing. *In* Kissane JM (ed): Anderson's Pathology, ed 9, vol 1. St. Louis, Mosby–Year Book, 1990.
20. Rippon JW: Medical Mycology: The Pathogenic Fungi and Pathogenic Actinomycetes, ed 3. Philadelphia, WB Saunders, 1988.
21. Davison VE, Aldersen GL: Clinical virology. *In* Mahon CR, Manuselis G (eds): Textbook of Diagnostic Microbiology. Philadelphia, WB Saunders, 1995.
22. Isenberg HD, Washington JA II, Doern G, et al: Specimen collection and handling. *In* Balows A, Hausler WJ Jr, Hermann KL, et al (eds): Manual of Clinical Microbiology, ed 5. Washington, DC, American Society for Microbiology, 1991.
23. Leyden JJ, Kligman AM: Topical antibiotic in the prophylaxis of experimental *S. aureus* and *S. pyogenes* infections in humans. *In* Maibach H, Aly R (eds): Skin Microbiology: Relevance to Clinical Infection. New York, Springer-Verlag, 1981.
24. Finegold DS, Taplin D: Infections and infestations of the skin. J Am Acad Dermatol 11:971–974, 1984.
25. Blumer JL, O'Brien CA, Lemon E, et al: Skin and soft tissue infections: Pharmacologic approaches. Pediatr Infect Dis 4:336–341, 1985.
26. Davis JM, Dineen P: Antibacterial drugs. *In* Modell W (ed): Drugs of Choice 1984/1985. St Louis, CV Mosby, 1984.
27. Rosenblatt JE: Antimicrobial susceptibility testing of anaerobic bacteria. *In* Lorian V (ed): Antibiotics in Laboratory Medicine, ed 2. Baltimore, Williams & Wilkins, 1991.
28. Grabill JR, Drutz DJ: Ketoconazole for management of mucocutaneous candidiasis syndrome. *In* Maibach H, Aly R (eds): Skin Microbiology: Relevance to Clinical Infection. New York, Springer-Verlag, 1981.

Parasitic Infections

Lynne S. Garcia

During the past few years, the field of diagnostic medical parasitology has seen some dramatic changes, including the discovery of new parasitic organisms and diseases, the development of new molecular methods, and an increased awareness of parasitic infections. It is important that the laboratory and clinician maintain close communication, particularly regarding the clinical relevance of diagnostic procedures. Therapy often depends on laboratory results, and the clinician must be aware of the limitations of each test method and the results obtained. Medical parasitology has also risen in significance because of an increase in world travel and thus, an increased risk of exposure to organisms not ordinarily encountered by individuals and their physicians. The main emphasis for the physician is to include the possibility of parasitic disease in the differential diagnosis, particularly if the patient has a relevant travel history and/or a history of having lived in other parts of the world. In some cases, the history may be relevant over a 20 to 30 year time frame, rather than just a few weeks. Table 53–1 contains a list of possible parasites recovered from various sites of the body.

ETIOLOGY AND PATHOPHYSIOLOGY
Gastrointestinal Tract

Diarrheal diseases are one of the leading causes of morbidity and mortality worldwide and are second only to cardiovascular diseases as a cause of death. Diarrhea is the leading cause of childhood death and, in developing areas of the world, is responsible for more deaths than all other causes combined. Although often caused by bacteria and viruses, parasites, primarily protozoa and helminths, must be considered as potential etiologic agents of diarrheal disease. A range of symptoms—from those patients who are asymptomatic to those with severe, acute disease—is seen. Risk factors and relevant events include travel, drug-associated diarrhea, male homosexuality, acquired immunodeficiency syndrome (AIDS), and diarrhea in family members or other group contacts.

The pathophysiology seen in gastrointestinal parasitic diseases varies, often depending on the organism involved, numbers of organisms present, and the patient's age and immune status. A number of intestinal protozoa cause diarrheal disease, some of which can be life-threatening.

Entamoeba histolytica infects the colon and can produce ulcers through adhesion, cytolysis, and proteolysis. Through hematogenous spread it may also cause extraintestinal infections, although only 10% of *E. histolytica* infections progress to extraintestinal amebiasis. Pathogenic *E. histolytica* is considered to be the etiologic agent of amebic colitis and extraintestinal abscesses. Nonpathogenic *E. dispa,* although very similar morphologically, produces no intestinal symptoms, and is not invasive in humans. Differentiation of these two amebae on the basis of morphology is almost impossible, and monoclonal-based reagents are not yet widely available. The therapeutic approach to the patient continues to be based on all clinical findings, even though the laboratory report indicates *"Entamoeba histolytica"* (based on morphology only).

Blastocystis hominis is another possible cause of diarrheal illness. It may be the most common protozoan found within the population of the United States (4% to 30% or more), but it is not routinely reported by all laboratories because there is debate about its pathogenicity. To help correlate diagnostic findings with patient symptoms, this organism should be quantitated on the laboratory report (e.g., rare, few, moderate, many, packed).

Giardia lamblia, a flagellate, is found in the proximal small bowel. Pathogenic mechanisms include disruption of the brush border, mucosal invasion (rare), and stimulation of an inflammatory infiltration leading to villous flattening. Attachment to the mucosa via the sucking disk is also thought to cause irritation and prevent the parasites from being cleared by peristalsis. Malnutrition, hypogammaglob-

Table 53–1. Body Sites and Possible Parasites Recovered*

Site	Parasites†	Site	Parasites†
Blood		**Intestinal tract**	*Hymenolepis diminuta*
Red cells	*Plasmodium* spp.	*(Continued)*	*Taenia saginata*
	Babesia spp.		*Taenia solium*
White cells	*Leishmania donovani*		*Diphyllobothrium latum*
	Toxoplasma gondii		*Clonorchis sinensis (Opisthorchis)*
Whole blood/plasma	*Trypanosoma* spp.		*Paragonimus westermani*
	Microfilariae		*Schistosoma* spp.
Bone marrow	*Leishmania donovani*		*Fasciolopsis buski*
Central nervous system	*Taenia solium* (cysticerci)		*Fasciola hepatica*
	Echinococcus spp.		*Metagonimus yokogawai*
	Naegleria fowleri		*Heterophyes heterophyes*
	Acanthamoeba/Hartmanella spp.	**Liver, Spleen**	*Echinococcus* spp.
	Toxoplasma gondii		*Entamoeba histolytica*
	Microsporida		*Leishmania donovani*
	Trypanosoma spp.		Microsporida
Cutaneous ulcers	*Leishmania* spp.	Lung	*Pneumocystis carinii*‡
Intestinal tract	*Entamoeba histolytica*		*Cryptosporidium* spp.‡
	Entamoeba coli		*Echinococcus* spp.
	Entamoeba hartmanni		*Paragonimus* spp.
	Endolimax nana		Microsporida
	Iodamoeba bütschlii	Muscle	*Taenia solium* (cysticerci)
	Blastocystis hominis		*Trichinella spiralis*
	Giardia lamblia		*Onchocerca volvulus* (nodules)
	Chilomastix mesnili		*Trypanosoma cruzi*
	Dientamoeba fragilis		Microsporida
	Trichomonas hominis	Skin	*Leishmania* spp.
	Balantidium coli		*Onchocerca volvulus*
	Cryptosporidium parvum		Microfilariae
	Isospora belli	Urogenital system	*Trichomonas vaginalis*
	Microsporida		*Schistosoma* spp.
	Ascaris lumbricoides		Microsporida
	Enterobius vermicularis	Eye	*Acanthamoeba* spp.
	Hookworm		*Toxoplasma gondii*
	Strongyloides stercoralis		*Pneumocystis carinii*
	Trichuris trichiura		*Loa loa*
	Hymenolepis nana		Microsporida

*Note: This table does not include every possible parasite that could be found in a particular body site. However, the most likely organisms have been listed.
†Includes trophozoites, cysts, oocysts, spores, adults, larvae, eggs, amastigotes, and trypomastigotes.
‡Disseminated in severely immunosuppressed individuals.

ulinemia, achlorhydria, reduced levels of immunoglobulin A (IgA) and other immunodeficiencies are associated with increased susceptibility and difficulty in eradicating the infection. *Dientamoeba fragilis* is also a flagellate, but, morphologically, it looks more like an ameba.

Coccidia (protozoa) cause diarrheal illnesses that include *Cryptosporidium parvum, Cyclospora cayetanensis,* and *Isospora belli.* Although these coccidia can cause severe diarrhea, the infections tend to be self-limiting in the immunocompetent individual but life-threatening in the compromised host. *Cryptosporidium* has been implicated in nosocomial infections, day care center outbreaks, multiple waterborne outbreaks in many areas of the world, and severe watery diarrhea in AIDS patients. *Cyclospora* cases are sporadic and exhibit a self-limiting diarrhea in both immunocompetent and immunosuppressed patients. *Isospora* infections are rare and are often associated with AIDS.

Several genera within Microsporida (protozoa) cause severe diarrheal illness in humans, primarily those afflicted with AIDS. The two most common organisms, *Enterocytozoon bieneusi* and *Encephalitozoon intestinalis* are found in the intestinal tract and can disseminate to other body sites. The majority of these patients tend to be severely immunosuppressed with CD4 cells usually at or below 200 and often below 100 cells per μ/L.

A number of helminths can cause diarrheal illness, with symptoms depending on the type of worm, the worm burden, the host's immune status, and the presence or absence of other intestinal parasites. Both anatomic and physiologic damage can occur with helminth infections. Specific information on intestinal protozoa and helminths can be found in Table 53–2.

Liver and Billary Tract

It is always important to distinguish between an infection in a patient with liver disease and an infection in the liver itself. Many parasites within protozoa and helminths can infect the hepatobiliary system (Table 53–3).

E. histolytica has been discussed as a potential cause of liver abscess, particularly if left untreated. The trophozoites can penetrate *the* intestinal mucosa and can be carried via the blood stream to other body sites, primarily the right upper lobe of the liver. Some of these organisms may survive and begin to multiply, leading to a liver abscess.

It is now well documented that members of the order Microsporida can also infect the liver, particularly in disseminated infections. As indicated before, these infections are seen in AIDS patients with low CD4 counts.

Helminths that are involved with hepatobiliary disease include various nematodes (roundworms), such as *Toxocara canis* or *T. cati* (cause of visceral or ocular larva migrans); cestodes (tapeworms), such as *Echinococcus* spe-

Table 53–2. Parasitic Infections in the Gastrointestinal Tract

Clinical Manifestations

Diarrhea with or without blood and/or mucus
Abdominal pain
Flatulence
Anorexia
Fatigue (chronic)
Steatorrhea
Malabsorption
Obstruction
Worm migration

Parasites

Entamoeba histolytica
Dientamoeba fragilis
Giardia lamblia
Cryptosporidium parvum
Cyclospora cayetanensis
Isospora belli
Microsporida
  Enterocytozoon bieneusi
  Encephalitozoon intestinalis
Ascaris lumbricoides
Strongyloides stercoralis

Diagnostic Tests

MICROBIOLOGY
O&P
  Concentrate, permanent stained smear
  Duodenal aspirate
  Entero-Test
  Special stains
OTHER TESTS
Sigmoidoscopy
Biopsy
Radiography
Serology

Comments

E. histolytica: Serology recommended for extraintestinal amebiasis
D. fragilis: Permanent stained smear mandatory for identification, trophozoite form only
G. lamblia: O&P and duodenal specimens recommended; waterborne, day care, nosocomial infections; can use ELISA, or FA
C. parvum: Immunocompetent = self-cure; AIDS = chronic watery diarrhea; waterborne, day care, nosocomial infections; use modified acid-fast stains, EIA, or FA; oocysts 4–6 μm
C. cayetanensis: Sporadic cases, looks like *C. parvum*, but oocysts are twice size (8–10 μm); modified acid-fast stains, autofluorescence
I. belli: Rare, but may be seen in AIDS patients; modified acid-fast positive
Microsporida: Modified trichrome stains, calcofluor, experimental FA; spores very difficult to identify (1–2 μm)
Helminths: May see abnormal migrations with adult *Ascaris* (fever, anesthesia, therapy); symptoms with *S. stercoralis* related to disseminated strongyloidiasis (hyperinfection syndrome) seen in immunocompromised patients

Abbreviations: O&P, ova and parasites; ELISA, enzyme-linked immunosorbent assay; FA, fluorescent antibody; AIDS, acquired immunodeficiency syndrome.

Table 53–3. Parasitic Infections in the Liver and Biliary Tract

Clinical Manifestations

Hepatitis (with or without jaundice), fever, diarrhea
Hepatomegaly (with or without tenderness)
Referred pain, often to right scapula
Abscesses (may be elevation and fixation of right diaphragm)
Cirrhosis with ascites, splenomegaly and portal hypertension
Space-occupying lesions in liver
Biliary obstruction with cholecystitis
Eosinophilia (20–70 + %)

Parasites

Entamoeba histolytica
Microsporida
Toxocara canis or *T. cati*
Echinococcus spp.
Clonorchis sinensis
Fasciola hepatica
Schistosoma mansoni
Leishmania donovani

Diagnostic Tests

MICROBIOLOGY
O&P
  Concentrate, permanent stained smear
Special stains
  Modified trichrome
  Giemsa
Hatching test
SEROLOGY
Available for:
  Amebiasis
  Toxocariasis
  Hydatid disease
  Schistosomiasis
  Leishmaniasis
Check with local or state public health laboratory or CDC—local or reference laboratories may offer amebiasis
OTHER TESTS
Scans, MRI, biopsy
CBC
Liver function

Comments

E. histolytica: Serology recommended for extraintestinal amebiasis; GI tract findings may be negative
Microsporida: Modified trichrome stains, calcofluor, experimental FA; spores very difficult to identify (1–2 μm); PAS, tissue Gram stains, silver, Giemsa stains on tissue may be helpful
Toxocariasis: Serology recommended; cause of visceral or ocular larva migrans (eye infections very serious); retinitis, chorioretinitis; elevated eosinophilia
Echinococcus spp. (Hydatid Disease): Cyst fluid examined by laboratory; serology helpful; cyst rupture/leakage may cause anaphylaxis; cyst tissue can regenerate as secondary cysts if released into body during surgery; unilocular or multilocular cysts
Clonorchis, Fasciola: Generally find eggs in stool; *C. sinensis* eggs may be found in duodenal specimens
S. mansoni: Any suspected patient with schistosomiasis, collect both stool and urine without preservatives; laboratory report should mention egg viability rather than just egg identification
Leishmaniasis: Hepatosplenomegaly seen with *L. donovani* (visceral), cause of Kala Azar (all parts of the reticuloendothelial system—spleen, liver, bone marrow, etc.); all immunoglobulins increased

Note: Malaria can also cause hepatosplenomegaly.
Note: Spurious infections with certain helminths may occur from ingesting infected (egg-containing livers)—rare; eggs passed in stool do not represent true human infection.
Abbreviations: O&P, ova and parasites; GI, gastrointestinal; FA, fluorescent antibody; PAS, periodic acid-Schiff; CDC, Centers for Disease Control and Prevention; MRI, magnetic resonance imaging; CBC, complete blood cell count.

cies; and trematodes (flukes), such as *Schistosoma mansoni, Clonorchis sinensis,* and *Fasciola hepatica.*

Toxocariasis is caused by ingestion of infective dog or cat ascarid eggs from the soil. The human becomes the accidental host with extensive tissue migration of larvae through the liver and other parts of the body, including the eye. The most outstanding feature of the disease is a high peripheral eosinophilia, which may reach 90%. The larvae may become encapsulated in the liver and/or lungs; those that continue to migrate may cause inflammation and granuloma formation. These larvae are unable to complete their life cycle in the human host.

Echinococcus species are cestodes that are associated with infections in which the human becomes the accidental intermediate host after the ingestion of tapeworm eggs from the carnivore (dogs, wolves) intestine. After hatching, the larvae travel via the blood stream to the liver, where a hydatid cyst (*E. granulosus*) is formed. Unless the cyst grows to a large size, the patient may remain completely asymptomatic. If *E. multilocularis* is involved, then the cyst grows throughout the tissue like a metastatic cancer rather than being confined in a single limiting membrane.

Respiratory Tract

Although *Pneumocystis carinii* has now been reclassified with the fungi, it is often discussed with parasitic infections. Considering the increased number of immunocompromised patients, *P. carinii* is probably the most common "parasitic" infection in the respiratory tract, particularly in patients with AIDS. Reports of this infection in immunocompetent adults are rare. Extrapulmonary *P. carinii* infection is now being recognized more frequently; organisms have been found in lymph nodes, spleen, liver, bone marrow, adrenal glands, gastrointestinal tract, kidneys, thyroid gland, heart, pancreas, pleural space, temporal bone, brain, eyes, and ears.

E. histolytica can infect the lungs if a liver abscess is located close to the diaphragm. The abscess may rupture through or erode the diaphragm, leading to invasion of the lung and possible recovery of trophozoites in sputum or other respiratory specimens. This clinical situation is relatively rare.

Some Microsporida can also be recovered from the lung. The mode of transmission is speculated to be inhalation. AIDS patients with low CD4 counts are more at risk for such an infection.

Another organism that is associated with the lung is the trematode *Paragonimus westermani* or *P. mexicanus.* This infection is acquired by humans via the ingestion of metacercariae from freshwater crabs. The worms mature in the lung and release their eggs into bronchi or bronchioles. Eggs escape from the encapsulated tissue (location of the adult worm) and are coughed up and voided in the sputum or are swallowed and passed out in the stool.

S. stercoralis is a nematode that is found in the intestine; however, the life cycle includes a larval migratory phase through the lungs, like that seen with *Ascaris* and hookworms. In a case of disseminated strongyloidiasis, larvae may be found in any tissue of the body, including the lung and in sputum (Table 53–4).

Table 53–4. Parasitic Infections in the Respiratory Tract

Clinical Manifestations

Cough (with or without blood-flecked sputum)
Shortness of breath
Chronic bronchitis
Inflammatory reaction in lung
Pleurisy, with or without pleural effusion
Pneumonia, right lower lobe

Parasites

Pneumocystis carinii (fungi)
Entamoeba histolytica
Microsporida
Paragonimus spp.
Strongyloides stercoralis

Diagnostic Tests

MICROBIOLOGY
Respiratory specimen examinations (induced sputum, BAL, etc.—not expectorated sputum)
O&P
   Concentrate, permanent stained smear
Duodenal aspirate
Sputum examination
Special stains
   Modified trichrome
   Silver
FA
SEROLOGY
Available for:
   Amebiasis
   Paragonimiasis
Check with local or state public health laboratory or CDC—local or reference laboratory may offer amebiasis
OTHER TESTS
Scans, MRI, biopsy
CBC
Liver function

Comments

P. carinii: Now classified with the fungi; causes pneumonia in the compromised patient, particularly those with AIDS; also seen in other compromised patients (chemotherapy, transplants)
E. histolytica: Serology recommended for extraintestinal amebiasis; rupture of liver abscess through diaphragm into lung has been reported (rare); GI tract findings may be negative
Microsporida: Modified trichrome stains, calcofluor, experimental FA; spores very difficult to identify (1–2 μm); PAS, tissue Gram stains, silver, Giemsa stains on tissue may be helpful; spores easier to see in nonstool specimens
Paragonimus spp: Examination of both sputum and stool
S. stercoralis: Larvae may be seen in respiratory specimens (larval migration through lung); symptoms based on worm burden and possibility of hyperinfection in compromised patient; occult infection (30 yrs+ after patient has left endemic area); compromised patients (respiratory symptoms, intestinal pain, repeated episodes of meningitis and/or sepsis with Gram negative, intestinal flora).

Abbreviations: BAL, bronchoalveolar lavage; AIDS, acquired immunodeficiency syndrome; O&P, ova and parasites; GI, gastrointestinal; FA, fluorescent antibody; PAS, periodic acid-Schiff; CDC, Centers for Disease Control and Prevention; MRI, magnetic resonance imaging; CBC, complete blood cell count.

Nervous System

Although primary amebic meningoencephalitis (PAM) caused by *Naegleria* is rare, it is an acute, suppurative infection of the brain and meninges. With very rare exceptions, the disease in humans is fatal. PAM may mimic acute purulent bacterial meningitis and may be difficult to differentiate. Most cases are associated with exposure to contaminated water. An incubation period of 2 to 15 days occurs prior to the onset of clinical symptoms, and mental confusion and coma usually occur 3 to 5 days before death. Usually hemorrhagic necrosis is concentrated in the area of the olfactory bulbs and the base of the brain.

Granulomatous amebic meningoencephalitis, also caused by free-living amebae (*Acanthamoeba* and Leptomyxida amebae), may present as a subacute or chronic disease with focal granulomatous lesions in the brain. The incubation period is unknown but may take several weeks to months. Central Nervous System (CNS) invasion is thought to be hematogenous, with the primary site being skin or lung; and acute onset has also been reported. Most, although not all, infections have been associated with the compromised host.

Although most infections with *Toxoplasma gondii* are benign, severe symptoms can be seen in patients with congenital infections or in patients who are immunocompromised. Infection can occur through ingestion of rare or raw meats, accidental ingestion of oocysts from feces of animals in the cat family, and transfusion. The organism can be found in two forms in the human, very slow-growing stages called *bradyzoites* and actively proliferating intracellular forms called *tachyzoites*. Congenital infections may be particularly severe if the mother acquires the infection during the first or second trimester of pregnancy. *Immunosuppression* in a host can lead to severe CNS complications such as diffuse encephalopathy, meningoencephalitis, or cerebral mass lesions. More than 50% of immunocompetent patients show altered mental state, motor impairment, seizures, abnormal reflexes, and other neurologic sequelae. Statistics indicate that approximately 2.5% of AIDS patients will be diagnosed with cerebral toxoplasmosis.

Worldwide, cysticerci of *Taenia solium* (pork tapeworm) in the brain represents the most frequent parasitic infection of the human nervous system. Symptoms are directly related to space-occupying lesions in the brain. Computed tomography (CT) or magnetic resonance imaging (MRI) scans may reveal the lesions in the brain, and calcified larvae can be seen on x-ray examination. Although not a common infection, the number of cases within the United States is increasing due to immigration from Latin America.

Trypanosoma brucei, T. brucei gambiense, and *T. brucei rhodesiense* are hemoflagellates that cause African sleeping sickness and are transmitted to the human via the bite of the tsetse fly. The trypomastigote can be found at the bite site, in the lymph nodes, and, later in the course of the infection, in the spinal fluid. This parasite has the capability of expressing variable antigen types, thus stimulating a sustained immunoglobulin in (IgM) level. In an immunocompetent host, the absence of an elevated serum IgM rules out African trypanosomiasis. On invasion of the CNS, symptoms progress to coma and death, usually from secondary infection.

T. cruzi, the cause of South American trypanosomiasis or Chagas' disease, can also cause CNS disorders in children, usually in those younger than five years.

In a case of disseminated strongyloidiasis, larvae can invade the CNS, as in other tissues. This most often occurs in an immunosuppressed individual and is the result of hyperinfection (Table 53–5).

Heart

A primary cause of cardiac disease is *T. cruzi,* (Chagas' disease, South American trypanosomiasis). The infective organism is transmitted to the human via the feces of the reduviid or "kissing bug." The insect usually takes a blood meal from sleeping humans, then defecates immediately after feeding, and the human scratches the infective forms into the bite site. There may be a lesion at the bite site. The infective forms are spread to the lymph nodes via the blood stream (Table 53–6).

Vascular System

Malaria infects more than 250 million people throughout the world; more than 1 million die each year, most of whom are children. Of the four species that infect humans, *Plasmodium vivax* and *P. falciparum* account for approximately 95% of infections, with speculation that *P. vivax* may account for about 80%. *P. ovale* and *P. malariae* account for many fewer infections. After injection of the sporozoite by the female anopheline mosquito, the pre-erythrocytic stages develop within the liver parenchymal cells. Once these merozoites leave the liver, they invade the red blood cells (RBCs) and initiate the erythrocytic cycle. In *P. vivax* and *P. ovale,* a "true relapse" can be initiated at a later time from quiescent stages that remain in the liver; this does not occur in *P. malariae* or *P. falciparum.* Once the RBC cycle is synchronized, the patient may experience the classic paroxysm, which included a cold phase, fever, and sweats. Patients who present to the emergency department may have no periodic fevers, and their symptoms may mimic those of many other infections. It *is critical to remember that these parasites can be missed using automated blood differential instruments.* Also, it is important to remember that one set of negative blood films may not "rule out" malaria. The key objective in malaria diagnosis is to rule out the possibility of *P. falciparum* infection, the most pathogenic species of the four, possibly leading to severe or fatal complications such as cerebral malaria. Malaria can also be acquired through shared needles, transfusion, or congenital transmission.

Babesiosis is a tick-borne infection that is becoming more widely observed on the West Coast and not just in southern New England; transfusion-induced infections have also been reported. The organism morphology mimics *P. falciparum* ring forms, and the most severe illness occurs in splenectomized patients. Diagnosis is determined by blood smear examination.

Although not endemic within the United States, certain filarial infections have a large geographic range, particularly in the tropics. *Wuchereria bancrofti, Brugia malayi,* and *B. timori* microfilariae can be seen in the peripheral blood. The adult worms inhabit the lymphatic system. Depending on the particular parasite involved, clinical symptoms range from none to elephantiasis, lymphangitis, filarial abscess, and hydrocele.

Diphyllobothrium latum is a freshwater fish tapeworm that infects humans; although most patients are asympto-

Table 53–5. **Parasitic Infections in the Nervous System**

Clinical Manifestations

Headache, fever
Drowsiness
Meningoencephalitis
Retinochoroiditis
Hydrocephalus
Seizures
Disorientation and/or dementia
Swollen lymph nodes (Winterbottom's sign)

Parasites

Naegleria fowleri
Acanthamoeba spp.
Toxoplasma gondii
Taenia solium
Trypanosoma brucei gambiense
Trypanosoma brucei rhodesiense
Trypanosoma cruzi
Strongyloides stercoralis

Diagnostic Tests

MICROBIOLOGY
CSF wet and stained smears; calcofluor white; culture most sensitive
Tissue culture isolation from CSF
Giemsa-stained blood; CSF smears; special concentration
Xenodiagnosis
O&P
Concentrate, permanent stained smear
SEROLOGY
Available for:
　Naegleria
　Acanthamoeba
　Toxoplasma
　Trypanosoma spp.
Check with local or state public health laboratory or CDC—local or reference laboratories may offer serologic tests
OTHER TESTS
Scans, MRI, biopsy
CSF analysis
Immunoglobulin levels—particularly IgM

Comments

N. fowleri (PAM) Free-living amebae (soil, water); acute infection in brain; will mimic bacterial meningitis; history of swimming; usually fatal; culture recommended
Acanthamoeba spp. (Granulomatous Amebic Encephalitis): Free-living amebae (soil, water); chronic infection in AIDS; can mimic bacterial meningitis; history of swimming; may be fatal; culture recommended
T. gondii: CNS manifestations in AIDS; serious congenital infections (mental retardation); eye lesions may also occur; Giemsa, silver, monoclonal-based reagents; tissue culture isolation helpful (CSF, recommended specimen for CNS symptoms)
T. solium (cysticercosis): Space-occupying lesions, primarily in brain, but can be in other tissues; epileptic-like symptoms common; calcified cysts can be seen on scan
T. brucei spp: Gambian form chronic (progress to sleeping sickness), Rhodesian form more acute; examination of CSF, lymph node aspirates, blood; IgM must be elevated for disease confirmation
T. cruzi: Chagas' disease; involves striated muscle (GI tract, heart); xenodiagnosis using "clean" lab-raised bugs (feed on suspect patient, forms develop in hindgut of bug—confirmation of infection)
S. stercoralis: Larvae may be seen in CNS specimens in compromised patients (respiratory symptoms, intestinal pain, repeated episodes of meningitis and/or sepsis with Gram negative, intestinal flora) with disseminated strongyloidiasis—may be fatal even with immediate treatment

Note: Cerebral involvement can also occur with other organisms such as *Plasmodium falciparum.*

Abbreviations: O&P, ova and parasites; CSF, cerebrospinal fluid; PAM, primary amebic meningoencephalitis; AIDS, acquired immunodeficiency syndrome; CNS, central nervous system; CDC, Centers for Disease Control and Prevention; IgM, immunoglobulin M; MRI, magnetic resonance imaging; GI, gastrointestinal.

---

matic, some exhibit a vitamin B_{12} deficiency that resembles pernicious anemia.

Trypanosomiasis and the recovery of trypomastigotes in the blood stream has been discussed earlier (Table 53–7).

Skin and Mucous Membranes

Leishmania tropica complex (Old World cutaneous leishmaniasis), *L. mexicana* complex (New World cutaneous leishmaniasis), and *L. braziliensis* (mucocutaneous leishmaniasis) are transmitted to humans via the bite of the sandfly. Amastigotes are found in the macrophages of the skin and mucous membranes. Organisms that cause New World cutaneous leishmaniasis have been reported from southern Texas.

Onchocerca volvulus (cause of "river blindness"), is transmitted to humans via the bite of the blackfly, and the adult worms become encapsulated in fibrous tissue capsules in the dermis and subcutaneous tissues. Pathology in this infection is generally caused by ocular lesions, which are a result of the host's immune response to microfilariae.

Cutaneous larva migrans (CLM) is caused by migrating larvae of the dog or cat hookworm larvae, *Ancylostoma braziliense,* that accidentally infect the human. Infection is acquired by skin penetration of the larvae from the soil; linear tracts in the skin (elevated and vesicular) are then produced. Intense scratching may lead to secondary infec-

Table 53–6. **Parasitic Infections in the Heart**

Clinical Manifestations

Myocarditis
Tachycardia
Fever
Romaña's sign (unilateral orbital edema)
Abnormal ECG
Megaesophagus and/or megacolon

Parasites

Trypanosoma cruzi (South American trypanosomiasis, Chagas' disease)

Diagnostic Tests

MICROBIOLOGY
Giemsa-stained blood smears
SEROLOGY
Available for:
　Chagas' disease
Check with local or state public health laboratory or CDC—local or reference laboratories may offer some serologic tests
OTHER TESTS
ECG
Biopsy of lymph nodes

Comments

T. cruzi: May cause acute infection in children, particularly those <5 yrs old; in adults mortality not high, morbidity very high; chronic disease, often leading to cardiac failure; in the acute phase, death may occur due to myocardial insufficiency or cardiac arrest; symptoms in chronic disease are related to damage sustained during acute phase; chronic disease may develop years or decades after the initial infection or diagnosis of acute disease; most frequent sign is cardiomyopathy (cardiomegaly and conduction changes)

Note: Current discussions underway regarding potential testing of blood supply; tests being performed in endemic areas of the world; no decisions yet on areas within the United States

Abbreviations: ECG, electrocardiogram; CDC, Centers for Disease Control and Prevention.

Table 53-7. Parasitic Infections in the Vascular System

Clinical Manifestations

Paroxysm, with or without periodicity
Hepatosplenomegaly
Anemia
Lymphadenitis and/or lymphangitis
Hematuria
Vitamin B_{12} deficiency
Disseminated intravascular coagulation (DIC)

Parasites

Plasmodium vivax
P. ovale
P. malariae
P. falciparum
Babesia spp.
Wuchereria bancrofti
Brugia malayi
B. timori
Trypanosoma spp.

Diagnostic Tests

MICROBIOLOGY
Giemsa-stained blood smears, special concentrations (malaria,
    Babesia, filariasis, trypanosomiasis)
O&P
    Concentrate, permanent stained smear (*Diphyllobothrium
    latum*—changes in differential)
SEROLOGY
Available for:
    Malaria
    Babesia
    Filariasis
    Trypanosomiasis
Check with local or state public health laboratory or CDC—local or
    reference laboratories may offer some serologic tests
OTHER TESTS
Radiography (filariasis)
CBC
IgM (African trypanosomiasis)

Comments

Plasmodium spp: *P. falciparum* is always considered a medical
    emergency and all laboratory testing should be ordered stat; severe
    disease can be seen in patients with a low parasitemia
    (demonstrated death with only 8% infected RBCs); typical
    parasitemias seen in the United States are often ≤2%; multiple
    blood specimens must be sent—one negative specimen does not
    "rule out" malaria
Babesia spp: Can cause serious disease and death in
    immunocompromised patients, particularly those who have been
    splenectomized; transmitted by ticks; parasitemia often low; ring
    forms only seen in blood smears
Filariasis: Confirmation of the infection by demonstrating
    microfilariae in the blood can be difficult, particularly if the
    infection is long term and chronic; special concentrations also
    available
T. brucei spp: Gambian form chronic (progress to sleeping sickness),
    Rhodesian form more acute; examination of CSF, lymph node
    aspirates, blood; IgM must be elevated for disease confirmation
T. cruzi: Chagas' disease; involves striated muscle (GI tract, heart);
    xenodiagnosis using "clean" laboratory-raised bugs (feed on
    suspect patient, forms develop in hindgut of bug—confirmation of
    infection); demonstration of trypomastigotes in blood can be
    difficult

Note: These parasites can be transmitted via blood transfusions; confirmation
and identification of the parasites will not be accomplished using automated hematology instruments designed for routine blood profile analysis; routine thick and
thin blood smears should be prepared and sent for manual examination (300 fields
using oil immersion objective—total magnification of 1000×)
    Abbreviations: O&P, ova and parasites; RBCs, red blood cells; CDC, Centers
for Disease Control and Prevention; CSF, cerebrospinal fluid; IgM, immunoglobulin M; CBC, complete blood cell count; GI, gastrointestinal.

tion; deeper tissue migration to the lungs with pneumonitis may also occur. Eosinophilia may be present in the peripheral blood, in addition to the presence of eosinophils and Charcot-Leyden crystals in the sputum (Table 53–8).

Urinary Tract

Schistosoma haematobium adult worms reside in the vesicle and pelvic plexuses of the venous circulation. Eggs are most concentrated in the tissues of the bladder and lower ureter. As eggs become trapped in the tissues, granulomas lead to fibrosis and ulceration. Obstruction of the ureters and periportal fibrosis with hepatomegaly and splenomegaly have also been noted. Carcinoma of the bladder has also been linked with this infection.

P. falciparum (described earlier) may cause *blackwater fever,* a sudden, intravascular hemolysis that results in hematuria; it has been postulated that this is somehow linked to quinine sensitivity.

Microsporidial infections involving the kidneys are now well documented. *Encephalitozoon intestinalis* (formerly called *Septata intestinalis*) disseminates from the gastroin-

Table 53-8. Parasitic Infections in the Skin and Mucous Membranes

Clinical Manifestations

Lesions (dry or wet, on face or limbs)
Nodules on limbs, truck, or head
Serpiginous tunnels
Lymphadenitis or "hanging groin"

Parasites

Leishmania tropica
L. braziliensis
L. mexicana
Onchocerca volvulus
Ancylostoma braziliense (cutaneous larva migrans—CLM)

Diagnostic Tests

MICROBIOLOGY
Giemsa-stained touch preps, culture (leishmaniasis)
Skin snips (onchocerciasis)
SEROLOGY
Available for:
    Leishmaniasis
    Onchocerciasis
    CLM
Check with local or state public health laboratory or CDC—local or
    reference laboratories may offer some serologic tests
OTHER TESTS
Biopsy
CBC
Urine examination for microfilariae (rarely positive for *Onchocerca*)

Comments

Leishmaniasis: Specimens must be collected aseptically, bacterial
    contaminants will overgrow cultures; punch biopsies for histology
    and separate specimens for microbiology recommended (taken at
    the margin of the lesion—not the center); organisms found only at
    site of lesion
Onchocerciasis: Cause of eye disease (river blindness—caused by
    microfilariae)
CLM: Human is accidental host when dog or cat hookworm larvae
    penetrate skin of the host—life cycle can not be completed;
    serpiginous tunnels in skin cause severe itching; high eosinophilia

Abbreviations: CDC, Centers for Disease Control and Prevention; CBC, complete blood cell count.

testinal (GI) tract; spores can be found in the urine sediment. Occasionally, other Microsporida have been reported from this body site.

In some cases of filariasis, obstruction of the retroperitoneal lymphatics may cause the renal lymphatics to rupture into the urinary tract, leading to chyluria. In some studies, half of the patients had renal abnormalities with proteinuria and hematuria (Table 53–9).

Genital Tract

The most common parasitic infection in this site is *Trichomonas vaginalis* and should be considered in any case with vaginal or vulval pruritus and discharge. Infection in the male may be latent with no symptoms or self-limited, persistent, or recurring urethritis (Table 53–10). *T. vaginalis* is considered to be a sexually transmitted organism.

Enterobius vermicularis may occasionally cause vaginitis and salpingitis in young females, primarily as a result

---

Table 53–9. Parasitic Infections in the Urinary Tract

Clinical Manifestations

Hematuria
Proteinuria
Nephrotic syndrome
Renal failure

Parasites

Schistosoma haematobium
Plasmodium falciparum
P. malariae
Microsporida

Diagnostic Tests

MICROBIOLOGY
Urine sedimentation (schistosomiasis, Microsporida)
Giemsa-stained thick and thin blood smears, QBC tube, monoclonal-based reagents (malaria)
SEROLOGY
Available for:
  Schistosomiasis
  Malaria
Check with local or state public health laboratory or CDC—local or reference laboratories may offer some serologic tests
OTHER TESTS
Hatching test (schistosome egg viability test)
Biopsy

Comments

S. haematobium: Any suspected patient with schistosomiasis, collect both stool and urine without preservatives; laboratory report should mention egg viability rather than just egg identification
Malaria: P. falciparum can cause multiple organ failure (including kidneys); hemolysis of RBCs can produce "blackwater fever"—release of hemoglobin into the urine; *P. malariae* can form antigen/antibody complexes in the glomeruli of the kidneys (nephrotic syndrome)
Microsporida: Modified trichrome stains, calcofluor, experimental FA; spores very difficult to identify (1–2 μm); spores easier to see in urine than stool—will represent disseminated infection from GI tract (*Encephalitozoon intestinalis*)—AIDS patients with low CD4 count

Abbreviations: QBC, qualitative buffy coat; CDC, Centers for Disease Control and Prevention; RBCs, red blood cells; GI, gastrointestinal; AIDS, acquired immunodeficiency syndrome.

Table 53–10. Parasitic Infections in the Genital Tract

Clinical Manifestations

Vaginitis, with or without discharge
Dysuria
Salpingitis

Parasites

Trichomonas vaginalis
Enterobius vermicularis
Wuchereria bancrofti

Diagnostic Tests

MICROBIOLOGY
Direct wet smear, culture (trichomoniasis)
Scotch tape or paddle (enterobiasis)
Giemsa stain of thick blood films, special concentrates (filariasis)
SEROLOGY
Available for:
  Filariasis
Check with local or state public health laboratory or Centers for Disease Control and Prevention—local or reference laboratories may offer some serologic tests
OTHER TESTS
Hatching test (schistosome egg viability test)
Biopsy

Comments

T. vaginalis: This flagellate is the most common cause of genital tract problems; male may be asymptomatic; culture "pouch" system excellent for transport and growth; considered sexually transmitted disease
E. vermicularis (pinworm: Probably most common parasite throughout world; many asymptomatic; may cause rare problems in genital tract (female children); 6 consecutive negative tapes required to "rule out" infection; symptomatic individuals are often treated without confirmation of pinworm infection
Filariasis: Obstructed genital lymphatics may lead to hydrocele or scrotal lymphedema; renal lymphatics may rupture into urinary tract

---

of the female worms migrating from the perianal skin to other sites.

Some filarial infections can cause elephantiasis of the scrotum, the result of lymphadenitis and fibrosis of the lymphatics.

CLINICAL MANIFESTATIONS

The majority of the clinical manifestations seen in parasitic infections are consistent with many other possible etiologic agents (see Tables 53–2 through 53–11). However, because many of the drugs used to treat parasitic infections have serious side effects, therapy is normally not initiated without confirmation of the suspect parasite.

Patients with parasitic infections of the GI tract may be asymptomatic or may present with one or more of the following symptoms: diarrhea, with or without blood or mucus; abdominal pain, with or without cramping; nausea; flatulence; anorexia; chronic fatigue; steatorrhea; malabsorption; obstruction; or passage of adult worms or parts of worms in the stool (e.g., *Ascaris,* tapeworms).

Involvement of the liver or biliary tract with parasites can produce the following symptoms: hepatitis, with or without jaundice; fever; diarrhea; hepatomegaly, with or without tenderness; referred pain, often to the right scapula; abscesses with potential elevation and fixation of the right diaphragm; cirrhosis with ascites, splenomegaly and portal hypertension; space-occupying lesions of the liver; biliary obstruction with cholecystitis; and hepatosplenomegaly.

Respiratory tract parasitic infection symptoms include cough, nonproductive or with blood-flecked sputum; pneumonia; shortness of breath; chronic bronchitis; and pleurisy, with or without pleural effusion.

In AIDS patients, a nonproductive cough is typical and may progress to diminished respiratory capacity. Although respiratory distress may be significant, the clinical findings may not be that abnormal. The patient may be afebrile, the white blood cell count is normal or slightly elevated, and eosinophilia may be present. Infants younger than 3 months old experience cough, tachypnea, and episodes of apnea.

Patients with AIDS may have a longer incubation time, lasting up to 1 year with weight loss, malaise, diarrhea, nonproductive cough, progressive dyspnea, and low-grade fever. Chest x-ray findings may be normal (28%) and physical signs in the chest may be minimal or absent. Cotton-wool spots in the fundus of the eye should also alert the physician to the possibility of infection, particularly if diabetes or hypertension is not present.

Symptoms in the patient with paragonimus infection of the lung depend on the initial worm burden and may be mild in chronic cases. As the cough develops, there may be chest pain, dyspnea, and chronic bronchitis. The most serious complication is cerebral involvement, which include the following symptoms: fever, headache, nausea, vomiting, visual disturbances, motor weakness, localized or generalized paralysis, and possibly death.

Patients with parasitic infections involving the nervous system exhibit symptoms such as headache and fever, drowsiness, meningoencephalitis, retinochoroiditis, hydrocephalus, seizures, disorientation and/or dementia, coma, and swelling of posterior cervical lymph nodes (Winterbottom's sign, primarily seen in West African sleeping sickness).

At birth, or soon thereafter, symptoms in infants with congenital toxoplasmosis may include retinochoroiditis, cerebral calcification, and occasionally hydrocephalus or microcephaly.

Clinical manifestations of parasitic infections of the heart include: myocarditis; tachycardia; fever; unilateral edema of the eye (Romaña's sign); abnormal (ECG); and mega-esophagus and/or megacolon.

Acute symptoms of trypanosomiesis may occur, particularly in children, around week 2 or 3 and include high fevers, hepatosplenomegaly, myalgia, rash, and acute myocarditis. Amastigotes multiply within the cardiac muscle cells, causing conduction defects and loss of cardiac contractility. The most frequent clinical sign of chronic Chagas' disease is cardiomyopathy (cardiomegaly and conduction changes). The clinical course may vary from heart failure to a slow but continuous loss of cardiac function. Although less common, some patients are more likely to have dilation of the digestive tract, with or without cardiomyopathy. Dysphagia, heartburn, malnutrition, constipation, abdominal pain, and inability to discharge feces are symptoms seen in the esophagus and colon.

Clinical findings related to parasitic infections of the vascular system include typical paroxysms caused by malaria (sudden onset of shaking chills followed by a period of high fever and sweating, with or without periodicity), hepatosplenomegaly, anemia, disseminated intravascular coagulation, lymphadenitis and/or lymphangitis, and vitamin B_{12} deficiency.

Parasitic infections of the skin and mucous membranes appear as lesions, either dry or wet; nodules on the trunk, limbs, or head; serpiginous tunnels formed by migrating larvae (CLM); or "hanging groin" due to lymphadenitis. Often cutaneous or mucocutaneous lesions become secondarily infected with bacteria or fungi; specimens must be collected aseptically so subsequent cultures do not become contaminated and overgrown.

Leishmaniasis can be manifest as papules, nodules, or ulcers, often with spontaneous healing. In mucocutaneous disease, spread to the nasal or oral mucosa may occur immediately or many years after the primary lesion. Ulceration may lead to loss of the lips, soft parts of the nose, and soft palate.

Urinary tract infections with parasites can lead to hematuria and proteinuria. Damage to the kidney can occur with *P. falciparum,* and the nephrotic syndrome occurs with *P. malariae,* in which long-term infections lead to antigen/antibody complex formation in the glomeruli of the kidneys. Occasionally, microfilariae may also be recovered in urine. Probably the most common parasite found in urine is *T. vaginalis;* organism motility is detected when the urine sediment is examined during a routine urinalysis. Vaginitis, with or without discharge, often accompanies infection with *T. vaginalis.* Dysuria may also occur. Vaginitis and salpingitis may be associated with *E. vermicularis* infection when it rarely invades the genital tract.

Parasitic infections in individuals with a normal immune system are not uncommon and can even be fatal, and clinical manifestations seen in the immunocompetent host may also be seen in the compromised host. Individuals with immune defects, however, have an abnormally high susceptibility to infections with nonvirulent and minimally pathogenic organisms. Many of these individuals contract parasitic infections in addition to numerous infectious episodes with bacterial, viral, and fungal organisms.

Although any parasitic infection may be more severe in the immunosuppressed host, certain organisms tend to produce greater pathologic sequelae in these patients, whereas other organisms occur with a higher frequency in individuals with certain other immune deficiencies. Organisms include *E. histolytica, G. lamblia, T. gondii, P. carinii, C. parvum, I. belli,* the Microsporida, and *S. stercoralis.* A summary of clinical findings in normal and compromised hosts can be seen in Table 53–11.

LABORATORY ANALYSES AND DIAGNOSIS

The importance of having personnel adequately trained in the recovery and identification of parasites cannot be overemphasized, especially because many therapeutic decisions are directly based on the specific gross or microscopic identification of a particular parasite. Often specialized techniques must be used, some of which are not routinely performed by many laboratories. This will necessitate the use of a reference laboratory with personnel proficient in these types of diagnostic procedures.

Table 53–11. Parasitic Infections: Clinical Findings in Normal and Compromised Hosts

Organism	Normal Host	Compromised Host
Entamoeba histolytica	Asymptomatic to chronic–acute colitis; extraintestinal disease may also occur (primary site: right upper lobe of liver)	Diminished immune capacity may lead to extraintestinal disease
Giardia lamblia	Asymptomatic to malabsorption syndrome	Certain immunodeficiencies tend to predispose an individual to infection
Toxoplasma gondii	Approximately 30–50% of individuals have antibody and organisms in tissue, but are asymptomatic	Disease in compromised host tends to involve the central nervous system (CNS) with various neurologic symptoms
Pneumocystis carinii	Most individuals are probably carriers/asymptomatic	Disease state develops as pneumonia; disseminated disease well documented (now classified with the fungi)
Cryptosporidium parvum	Self-limiting infection with diarrhea and abdominal pain	Due to autoinfective nature of life cycle, will not be self-limiting, may produce fluid loss of over 10 L/day and there may be multisystem, disseminated involvement; no known totally effective therapy
Isospora belli	Self-limiting infection with mild diarrhea or no symptoms	May lead to severe diarrhea, abdominal pain, and possible death (rare case reports); repeated therapy often required in acquired immunodeficiency syndrome (AIDS) patients

Microsporida
  Nosema
  Encephalitozoon
  Enterocytozoon
  Pleistophora
	Very little known about these infections in the normal host	Can infect various parts of the body; diagnosis usually depends on histologic examination of tissues; can probably cause death; patients are typically those with AIDS and a CD4 count <200 μ/L

Strongyloides stercoralis	Asymptomatic to mild abdominal complaints; can remain latent for many years due to low level infection maintained by internal autoinfective life cycle	Can result in disseminated disease (hyperinfection syndrome due to autoinfective nature of life cycle); abdominal pain, pneumonitis, sepsis-meningitis with Gram negative bacilli, eosinophilia may or may not be significant

Nonserologic Procedures

The basic approach to diagnostic parasitology should be no different than that used in other areas of microbiology. There are published guidelines that contain recommended procedures for this field which qualified laboratories follow.[1-10] The clinician must be advised of the recommended number and types of specimens to be collected (Table 53–12), limitations of each test method (Table 53–13), and results obtained.

The main emphasis should be on the importance of recognizing what potential parasitic infections may occur, which procedures may provide confirmation of the diagnosis, and what are the implications and limitations of information provided to the physician. If there is an incomplete understanding of requirements for quality diagnostic testing, then incomplete information is transmitted to the clinician. It is the responsibility of both the laboratory and the clinician to develop a greater awareness of the importance of these requirements.

Serologic Procedures

Parasitic organisms infecting humans either multiply within the host (protozoans) or never multiply but mature within the host (schistosomes, *Ascaris*). Host immunity is usually not protective, and any immunity that does develop is usually species-specific and even strain- or stage-specific. Protozoan pathogens that multiply within the host produce continuous antigenic stimulation of the host's immune system as the infection progresses. In these instances, a posi-

tive correlation is usually present between clinical symptoms and serologic test results.

Some helminths migrate through the body and pass through a number of developmental stages before becoming mature adults. These infections are usually difficult to confirm serologically. Most antigens used in serologic procedures are heterogeneous mixtures that are not well-defined, resulting in cross-reactions or inadequate sensitivity.

Few serology tests for parasitic infections can be used to confirm an infection or predict disease outcome. Test result interpretation may also present problems, particularly because some titers may reflect exposure rather than actual disease.

Although serologic procedures have been available for many years, they are not routinely offered by most clinical laboratories due to sensitivity, specificity, and interpretation. Standard techniques that have been used include complement fixation (CF), indirect hemagglutination (IHA), indirect fluorescent antibody (IFA), soluble antigen fluorescent antibody (SAFA), bentonite flocculation (BF), latex agglutination (LA), double diffusion (DD), counterelectrophoresis (CEP), immunoelectrophoresis (IE), radioimmunoassay (RIA), and intradermal tests.

Two newer serologic tests are the Falcon assay screening test enzyme-linked immunosorbent assay (FAST-ELISA), and the enzyme-linked immunoelectrotransfer blot (EITB). The FAST-ELISA is a quantitative assay in which patient serum samples tested as a single dilution are referred to a standard curve to determine the levels of reactivity. FAST-ELISA is very sensitive and can be used with

Text continued on page 533

Table 53–12. **Body Sites and Specimen Collection**

Site	Specimen Options	Collection Method
Blood	Smears of whole blood	Thick and thin films Fresh (first choice)

	Anticoagulated blood	Anticoagulant (second choice)
		  EDTA (first choice)
		  Heparin (second choice)

Bone marrow	Aspirate	Sterile
Central nervous system	Spinal fluid	Sterile
Cutaneous ulcers	Aspirates from below surface	Sterile plus air-dried smears
	Biopsy	Sterile, non-sterile to histopathology (formalin acceptable)
Eye	Biopsy	Sterile (in saline), nonsterile to histopathology
	Scrapings	Sterile (in saline)
	Contact lenses	Sterile (in saline)
	Lens solution	Sterile, unopened commercial solutions not acceptable
Intestinal tract	Fresh stool	1/2 pint waxed container
	Preserved stool	5% or 10% formalin, MIF, SAF, Schaudinn's, PVA
	Duodenal contents	Fresh, PVA or Schaudinn's smears
	Anal impression smear	Entero-Test or aspirates
	Adult worm/worm segments	Cellulose tape (pinworm examination) Saline, 70% alcohol
Liver, spleen	Aspirates	Sterile, collected in 4 separate aliquots (liver)
	Biopsy	Sterile, nonsterile to histopathology
Lung	Sputum	True sputum (not saliva)
	Induced sputum	No preservative (10% formalin if time delay)
	Bronchoalveolar lavage (BAL)	Sterile Air-dried smears
	Transbronchial aspirate	Same as above
	Tracheobronchial aspirate	Same as above
	Brush biopsy	Same as above
	Open lung biopsy Aspirate	Sterile
Muscle	Biopsy	Fresh, squash preparation, nonsterile to histopathology Nonsterile to histopathology (formalin acceptable)
Skin	Scrapings	Aseptic, smear or vial
	Skin snip	No preservative
	Biopsy	Sterile (in saline) Nonsterile to histopathology
Urogenital system	Vaginal discharge	Saline swab, transport swab, (no charcoal), culture medium, plastic envelope culture Air-dried smear for FA
	Urethral discharge	Same as above
	Prostatic secretions	Same as above
	Urine	Single unpreserved specimen, 24 hr unpreserved specimen, early morning

Abbreviations: MIF, merthiolate-iodine-formalin; SAF, sodium acetate-acetic acid-formalin; PVA, polyvinyl alcohol; FA, fluorescent antibody; EDTA, ethylenediamine-tetraacetic acid.

Table 53–13. Body Site, Specimen, Diagnostic Procedure(s)

Body Site	Specimen	Recommended Diagnostic Procedure	Comments

GASTROINTESTINAL TRACT	Stool
	Sigmoidoscopy material
	Duodenal contents
	Entero-Test capsule
		O&P
		  Concentrate, permanent stained smear
		  Trichrome or iron hematoxylin
		    Intestinal protozoa
		  Modified trichrome
		    Microsporida
		Monoclonal reagents (EIA, FA)
		  Entamoeba histolytica, Giardia lamblia,
		  Cryptosporidium parvum (modified acid-fast
		  stain), Microsporida
			Although trichrome or iron hematoxylin stains can be used on almost all specimens from the intestinal tract, actual worm segments (tapeworm proglottids) can be stained with special stains or injected with India ink. Fluorescent detection kits are also available for the identification of *G. lamblia* and *C. parvum.* Modified Trichrome stains, Calcofluor White, or experimental FA reagents can be used for microsporida; confirmation may require EM studies. Sigmoidoscopy smears should be stained with Trichrome or iron hematoxylin stains. Duodenal contents should be centrifuged at 500 Xg for 10 min and examined as wet or permanent stained preparation.

	Anal impression smear Adult worm or worm segments	No stain, scotch tape prep India ink injection; carmine stains (rarely used)	It takes 6 negative tapes to rule out an infection. Patient diagnosed with *Taenia* infection should use good personal hygiene prior to therapy to prevent accidental ingestion of mature *T. solium* eggs, leading to cysticercosis.

	Biopsy	Hematoxylin and eosin (routine histology)
		  Amebae
		  G. lamblia
		  Coccidia
		  Microsporida
			Tissue Gram stains, silver stains, PAS, or Giemsa stains may be used for the diagnosis of microsporidiosis.

LIVER, BILIARY TRACT, SPLEEN	Aspirates Biopsy	Giemsa, culture Leishmaniae Routine histology, culture	Aspirates and/or touch preparations from biopsy material can be routinely stained with Giemsa stain; specimens should also be cultured using NNN and/or Schneidere's medium. There are definite risks associated with spleen aspirates and/or biopsy. Other parasites, such as larval cestodes, trematodes, or amebae could be seen and identified from routine histologic staining. The hatching test for schistosome egg viability could also be performed.

RESPIRATORY TRACT	Sputum
	Induced sputum
	Bronchoalveolar lavage
	Transbronchial aspirate
	Tracheobronchial aspirate
	Brush biopsy
	Open lung biopsy
		Silver methenamine stain
		Calcofluor (cysts only)
		  Pneumocystis carinii
		Giemsa (trophozoites only)
		  P. carinii
		Modified acid fast stains
		  C. parvum
		Hematoxylin and eosin (routine histology)
		  S. stercoralis
		  Paragonimus spp.
		  Amebae
		Silver methenamine, PAS, acid-fast, modified
		  trichrome stains, EM
		  Microsporida
			P. carinii is the most common parasite recovered and identified from the lung using silver or Giemsa stains or monoclonal reagents (FA). There are also monoclonal reagents (FA) available for the diagnosis of pulmonary cryptosporidiosis. Routine histology procedures would allow the identification of any of the helminths or helminth eggs present in the lung.

NERVOUS SYSTEM	Spinal fluid
	Brain biopsy
		Giemsa
		  Trypanosomes, *Toxoplasma gondii*
		Giemsa, modified trichrome, or calcofluor
		  Amebae (*Naegleria; Acanthamoeba*)
		Giemsa, acid-fast, PAS, modified trichrome, silver
		  methenamine
		  Microsporida
		Routine histology
		  Larval cestodes
			If CSF is received (with no suspect organism suggested), Giemsa would be the best choice; however, Calcofluor is also recommended as a second stain; a wet exam of CSF on a slide (not in counting chamber) is recommended for suspect cases of primary amebic meningoencephalitis (PAM). If brain biopsy material is received (particularly from an immunocompromised patient), routine histology should be sufficient to allow the identification of the microsporida.

EYE	Biopsy
	Scrapings
	Contact lens
	Lens solution
		Calcofluor (cysts only)
		  Amebae (*Acanthamoeba*), Giemsa (trophozoites, cysts)
		  Amebae
		Hematoxylin and eosin (routine histology)
		  Cysticerci
		  Loa loa
		  T. gondii
		Silver methenamine stain, PAS, acid-fast, EM
		  Microsporida
			Some free-living amebae (most commonly *Acanthamoeba*) have been implicated as a cause of keratitis. Although Calcofluor will stain the cyst walls, it will not stain the trophozoites. Therefore, in suspect cases of amebic keratitis, both stains should be used. Hematoxylin and eosin (routine histology) can be used to detect and confirm cysticercosis. The adult worm of *Loa loa*, when removed from the eye, can be stained with a hematoxylin-based stain (Delafield's) or can be stained and examined via routine histology. *Toxoplasma* infection could be diagnosed using routine histology and/or serology results. Microsporida confirmation is usually possible using routine histology.

Table continued on following page

Table 53–13. **Body Site, Specimen, Diagnostic Procedure(s)** *Continued*

Body Site	Specimen	Recommended Diagnostic Procedure	Comments

BLOOD	Whole or anticoagulated blood	Giemsa
		  All blood parasites
		Hematoxylin-based stain
		  Microfilariae (sheathed)
		NOTE: The QBC tube (capillary blood) has also been recommended as a screening method for blood parasites (hematocrit tube contains acridine orange) and has been used for malaria, *Babesia*, trypanosomes, leishmania, and microfilariae.
			Most drawings and organism descriptions of blood parasites were originally based on Giemsa-stained blood films. Although Wright's stain (or Wright-Giemsa combination stain) will work, stippling in malaria will normally not be visible and the organism colors will not match the descriptions. However, using other stains (those listed above, in addition to some of the "quick" blood stains), the organisms should be visible on the blood film.

BONE MARROW	Aspirate	Giemsa All blood parasites	See comments listed above for BLOOD

CUTANEOUS ULCERS	Aspirate
	Biopsy
		Giemsa
		  Leishmaniae
		Hematoxylin and eosin (routine histology)
		  Acanthamoeba spp.
		  E. histolytica
			Most likely causative agent would be leishmaniae, all of which would stain with Giemsa
			Hematoxylin and eosin (routine histology) could also be used to identify these organisms.

SKIN	Aspirates
	Skin snip
	Scrapings
	Biopsy
		See CUTANEOUS ULCERS above
		Hematoxylin and eosin (routine histology)
		  Onchocerca volvulus
		  Dipetalonema streptocerca
			Any of the potential parasites present could be identified using routine histology procedures and stains.

MUSCLE	Biopsy	Hematoxylin and eosin (routine histology)
		  Trichinella spiralis
		  Cysticercerci
		Silver methenamine, PAS, acid-fast stains, EM studies for Microsporida
			If *Trypanosoma cruzi* were present in the striated muscle, the organisms could be identified from routine histology preparations. Microsporida confirmation may require EM studies.

UROGENITAL SYSTEM	Vaginal discharge
	Urethral discharge
	Prostatic secretions
	Urine
	
	Biopsy
		Giemsa
		Monoclonal reagents (FA)
		  Trichomonas vaginalis
		Delafield's hematoxylin
		  Microfilariae
		Hematoxylin and eosin (routine histology)
		  Schistosoma haematobium
		  Microfilariae
			Although *T. vaginalis* is probably the most common parasite identified, there are others to consider, the most recently implicated organisms being in the microsporida group. Microfilariae could also be recovered and stained.

Abbreviations: O&P, ova and parasites; EIA, enzyme immunoassay; FA, fluorescent antibody; EM, electron microscopy; PAS, periodic acid-Schiff; NNN, Novy, MacNeal, Nicolle; CSF, cerebrospinal fluid; QBC, quantitative buffy coat.

Table 53–14. Serologic Tests Performed in the Parasitology Division (CDC) for the Diagnosis of Parasitic Diseases

Disease	Test	Diagnostic Titers
Amebiasis	IHA	≥1: 256
Babesiosis	IIF	≥1: 64
Chagas' disease	IIF, CF	≥1: 32, ≥1: 8
Cysticercosis	IB	Bands
Echinococcosis	IHA, IB	≥1: 256, bands
Leishmaniasis	IIF, CF	≥1: 16, ≥1: 8
Malaria	IIF	≥1: 64
Paragonimiasis	IB	Bands
Schistosomiasis	FAST-ELISA, IB	10 OD units, bands
Strongyloidiasis	EIA	≥1: 64
Toxocariasis	ELISA	OLM ≥1: 8, VLM ≥1: 32
Toxoplasmosis	ELISA, IFA-IgG, IFA-IgM	≥1: 16, ≥1: 256, ≥1: 16
Trichinosis	BFT	≥1: 15

Abbreviations: BFT, bentonite flocculation; CF, complement fixation; ELISA, enzyme-linked immunoassay; IB, Immunoblot; IHA, indirect hemagglutination; IIF, indirect immunofluorescence; FAST-ELISA, Falcon assay screening test–enzyme-linked immunoassay; EIA, enzyme immunoassay; IFA-IgG, indirect fluorescent antibody-immunoglobulin G; IFA-IgM, indirect fluorescent antibody-immunoglobulin M; OD, optical density; OLM, ocular larva migrans; VLM, visceral larva migrans.

crude, synthetic, and recombinant antigens. EITB has been used in the diagnosis of cysticercosis, paragonimiasis, and echinococcosis, using crude or semipurified extracts of adult or larval stages. The EITB is 98% sensitive and 100% specific for cysticercosis. The test can detect a single parietal cyst and also subcutaneous infections without neurologic involvement.

Recombinant protein techniques which develop better defined antigens and DNA probes also offer unique opportunities for direct detection of infection and may become more widely used in the future.

The detection of parasite-specific IgM has been useful in the diagnosis of toxoplasmosis. However, detection of IgM or IgA antibodies for the diagnosis of other parasitic infections is generally not recommended because of the inability to interpret results and the lack of test sensitivity.

The Centers for Disease Control and Prevention (CDC) in Atlanta, Georgia, offer a number of serologic procedures for diagnostic purposes, some of which are not available elsewhere. Because regulations regarding submission of specimens may vary from state to state, each laboratory should check with its own county or state department of public health for the appropriate instructions. Additional information on procedures, availability of skin test antigens, and interpretations of test results may be obtained directly from the CDC.

Criteria used by the CDC for the interpretation of serologic test results have been published and serve as guidelines. Changing titers, paired specimens, and multiple test procedure results are recommended and help in determining clinical relevance. Additional information on available serologic tests can be seen in Table 53–14.

TREATMENT

Many of the drugs used to treat parasitic infections have serious side effects; therefore, before initiating therapy, physicians must consider the following factors: the accuracy of the original diagnosis, the potential drug toxicity, and the need for follow-up examinations to monitor therapy. Specific information can be obtained from the CDC Parasitic Drug Service. One can also obtain drugs from the CDC that are not commercially available in the United States.

Drug failure may be very difficult to assess, particularly if there is some question as to the patient's compliance with the drug regimen. It is often recommended that the drug of choice be used for a second course of therapy rather than using alternative therapy that may be more toxic. Information on available drugs can be found in Table 53–15.

Table 53–15. Drugs for Treatment of Parasitic Infections

Infection	Drug	Possible Follow-up Measures
Acanthamoeba	Amphotericin B and sulfadiazine or sulfisoxazole	Follow clinical course
Ancylostoma duodenale	Mebendazole or pyrantel pamoate	Fecal examinations 2–4 wk after therapy; if eggs are rare in fecal concentrations, no need to repeat therapy
Angiostrongylus cantonensis	Mebendazole	Follow clinical course
Angiostrongylus costaricensis	Thiabendazole	Follow clinical course
Anisakis	Surgical or endoscopic removal	Follow clinical course
Ascaris lumbricoides	Mebendazole or pyrantel pamoate	Fecal examinations 2–4 wk after therapy
Babesia	Clindamycin plus quinine	Follow clinical course, repeat blood smears if symptoms persist
Balantidium coli	Tetracycline	At least 3 negative fecal examinations 1 mo after therapy
Blastocystis hominis	Metronidazole or iodoquinol (clinical significance is controversial)	Fecal examinations 2 wk to 1 mo after therapy (must include permanent stain)
Brugia malayi	Diethylcarbamazine or ivermectin	Blood smears, Knott concentration, and membrane filtration of blood for microfilariae 2–4 wk after treatment
Capillaria philippinensis	Mebendazole	Multiple fecal examinations for eggs several months after completion of therapy

Table continued on following page

Table 53–15. Drugs for Treatment of Parasitic Infections *Continued*

Infection	Drug	Possible Follow-up Measures
Clonorchis (Opisthorchis) sinensis	Praziquantel	Fecal examinations for eggs 1 and 3 mo after therapy
Cryptosporidium	No effective treatment	Clinical response and stool examinations during and after experimental therapy (acid-fast stain or direct fluorescent antibody [DFA] test)
Cyclospora	Trimethoprim-sulfamethoxazole	Follow clinical course and stool examination using acid-fast stain
Cutaneous larva migrans (*Ancylostoma duodenale*)	Thiabendazole	Clinical response to therapy
Dientamoeba fragilis	Iodoquinol or paromomycin or tetracycline	Fecal examinations 2–4 wk after therapy (must include permanent stained smear)
Diphyllobothrium latum	Praziquantel or niclosamide	Fecal examinations for eggs and proglottids 1 and 3 mo after therapy
Dipylidium caninum	Praziquantel or niclosamide	Fecal examinations for eggs and proglottids 1 and 3 mo after therapy
Echinococcus granulosus (Hydatid cyst)	Surgery and/or albendazole	Clinical response to therapy; follow-up with computed tomography (CT), ultrasonography, and radionucleotide scans
Entamoeba histolytica Asymptomatic cyst passer	Paromomycin or iodoquinol	Fecal examinations 2 wk to 1 mo after therapy (must include permanent stained smear)
Non-dysentery, intestinal	Metronidazole followed by iodoquinol	As above
Dysentery, intestinal	Metronidazole followed by iodoquinol	As above; careful clinical follow-up to rule out extraintestinal disease
Extraintestinal disease	Metronidazole followed by iodoquinol	Clinical response to therapy; follow with CT, ultrasonography, and scans
Entamoeba polecki	Metronidazole	Fecal examinations 2 wk to 1 mo after therapy (must include permanent stained smear)
Enterobius vermicularis	Pyrantel pamoate or mebendazole	Clinical response; follow-up scotch tape check of perianal area if symptoms persist (may take 4–6 consecutive negative tapes to rule out infection)
Fasciola hepatica	Bithionol	Fecal examinations for eggs 1 mo after therapy
Fasciolopsis buski	Praziquantel	Fecal examinations for eggs 1 mo after therapy
Giardia lamblia	Quinacrine HCl or metronidazole	Fecal examinations 2 wks to 1 mo after therapy (must include permanent stained smear); Entero-Test if stools are negative and patient is symptomatic
Gnathostoma spinigerum	Surgical removal or mebendazole	Check for additional migratory swellings
Heterophyes heterophyes	Praziquantel	Fecal examinations for eggs 1 mo after therapy
Hymenolepis nana	Praziquantel	Fecal examinations for eggs and proglottids 2 wk and 3 mo after therapy
Isospora belli	Trimethoprim-sulfamethoxazole	Fecal examinations 1–2 wk after therapy
Leishmania spp.	Stibogluconate sodium or meglumine antimoniate	For *L. donovani,* follow clinical response to therapy; other *Leishmania,* smear and culture of lesions 1–2 wk after therapy
Loa loa	Diethylcarbamazine or ivermectin	Blood smears, Knott concentration, and membrane filtration of blood for microfilariae 2–4 wk after therapy
Metagonimus yokogawai	Praziquantel	Fecal examinations for eggs 2–4 wk after therapy
Mansonella ozzardi	Ivermectin	
Mansonella perstans	Mebendazole	
Mansonella streptocerca	Diethylcarbamazine	
Microsporida *Enterocytozoon Encephalitozoon Microsporidium Nosema Pleistophora*	Albendazole for some genera	
Naegleria fowleri	Amphotericin B	Follow clinical response and organisms in cerebrospinal fluid (CSF), direct wet mounts of CSF and cultures
Necator americanus	Mebendazole or pyrantel pamoate	Fecal examinations 2–4 wk posttherapy; if eggs are rare in fecal concentrations, no need to repeat therapy
Onchocerca volvulus	Ivermectin	Skin snips for microfilariae 3–6 mo after therapy or sooner if symptoms reoccur
Paragonimus westermani	Praziquantel	Sputum examination for eggs 2–4 wk after therapy; fecal examinations for eggs 1–2 mo after therapy
Pediculus humanis (body lice)	Lindane	Examine clothing and bedding for nits and lice
Pediculus humanis (head lice)	Lindane	Examine hair 1 wk after treatment for nits and lice
Phthirus pubis	Permethrin	Examine clothing, bedding, and hair for nits and lice
Plasmodium Chemoprophylaxis Chloroquine-sensitive areas	Chloroquine phosphate	Follow clinical course

Table 53–15. **Drugs for Treatment of Parasitic Infections** *Continued*

Infection	Drug	Possible Follow-up Measures
Plasmodium (Continued)		
Chloroquine-resistant areas	Mefloquine	Thick and thin blood smears
Treatment of all *Plasmodium* except chloroquine-resistant *P. falciparum*	Oral chloroquine phosphate or parenteral quinidine gluconate	
Chloroquine-resistant *P. falciparum*	Oral quinine sulfate plus pyrimethamine-sulfadoxine or parenteral quinidine gluconate	Thick and thin blood smears with quantitation of the parasitemia
Radical cure	Primaquine phosphate	
Pneumocystis carinii	Trimethoprim-sulfamethoxazole or pentamidine	Follow clinical course; repeat bronchial washings and/or biopsy after therapy
Sarcoptes scabei	Lindane	Follow clinical course; may need mild steroid cream in sensitive individuals
Schistosoma haematobium	Praziquantel	Urine examinations for eggs 1 mo after therapy; bladder or rectal biopsy
Schistosoma intercalatum	Praziquantel	Fecal examinations for eggs 1 mo after therapy; rectal biopsy
Schistosoma japonicum	Praziquantel	Fecal examinations for eggs 1 mo after therapy; rectal biopsy
Schistosoma mansoni	Praziquantel	Fecal examinations for eggs 1 mo after therapy; rectal biopsy
Schistosoma mekongi	Praziquantel	Fecal examinations for eggs 1 mo after therapy; rectal biopsy
Strongyloides stercoralis	Thiabendazole	Fecal examinations and/or culture 1 mo after therapy
Taenia saginata	Praziquantel or niclosamide	Fecal examinations for eggs or proglottids 1 mo after therapy
Taenia solium	Praziquantel or niclosamide	Same as *T. saginata*
Cysticercosis	Praziquantel or albendazole	Follow clinical course and computer-assisted tomography (CAT) scans
Toxocara canis, T. cati	Diethylcarbamazine	Follow clinical course
Toxoplasma gondii	Pyrimethamine plus sulfadiazine	Follow clinical course and serology
Trichinella spiralis	Mebendazole plus corticosteroids	Follow clinical course; muscle biopsy in severe cases
Trichomonas vaginalis	Metronidazole	Pelvic examination 1 mo after therapy
Trichostrongylus	Pyrantel pamoate or albendazole	Fecal examinations 2–4 wk after therapy
Trichuris trichiura	Mebendazole or albendazole	Fecal examinations 2–4 wk after therapy
Trypanosoma brucei gambiense or *rhodesiense*		
Early stages (hemolymphatic)	Suramin	Thick and thin blood smears 1–2 mo after therapy
Late stage with CNS disease	Melarsoprol	Cerebrospinal fluid analysis during and after therapy
Trypanosoma cruzi	Nifurtimox	Thick and thin blood smears or xenodiagnosis 1–2 mo after therapy; follow serology and electrocardiograms (EKGs)
Wuchereria bancrofti	Diethylcarbamazine or ivermectin	Thick blood smears, Knott concentration, and membrane filtration of blood 2–4 wk

Case Study 1

A 28-year-old woman was seen in the emergency department with complaints of general malaise, headache, low grade fever (101 °F), aches, and diarrhea. The patient had been feeling ill for several days and indicated she had the "flu" or flu-like symptoms. She has just returned from a work-related trip abroad with several stops in different parts of Southeast Asia and reported taking malaria prophylaxis during the time she was abroad, although it was somewhat sporadic. No laboratory data were available.

Questions

1. Considering the travel history and patient symptoms what are the possible diagnoses?
2. What laboratory tests should be ordered?
3. What potential diagnostic problems does this case represent?

Discussion

1. The possible diagnoses could include intestinal parasites, malaria, and a number of other bacterial or viral infections.
2. Blood films for malaria should be examined on a "stat" (immediate) basis and stools should be submitted for culture and ova and parasites (O&P) examinations. The blood should be submitted for "presumptive diagnosis: malaria"—manual microscopic review is required (submission of purple top ethylenediaminetetraacetic acid (EDTA) anticoagulant recommended).
3. This patient will probably have a very low parasitemia with *P. falciparum* (less than 2% parasitized RBCs). If the blood is examined using automated differential instrumentation, the infection will almost certainly be missed. If the patient has taken any chloroquine during the past 48 hours (prophylaxis or

"just a pill to make me feel better"), the number of infected RBCs on the blood smears may be somewhat reduced and the laboratory should be given this information. However, if the *P. falciparum* is chloroquine resistant, then the numbers of infected RBCs will begin to increase. Many of the patients who present with malaria to the emergency department tend to have low parasitemia; an elevated, but not periodic, fever; and general flu-like symptoms. The life cycle of the malaria parasites will not yet be synchronized, thus the patient's presentation will not resemble any malaria case as presented in most textbooks.1

Laboratory and Therapeutic Follow-up

The Giemsa-stained thick and thin blood films revealed ring forms only with some RBCs containing two rings per cell (parasitemia of 1.8%). No crescent-shaped gametocytes were seen; the infection was too early for gametocytes to have formed. Based on the ring morphology, a diagnosis of *P. falciparum* malaria was made. Treatment was begun immediately with chloroquine and the patient was monitored with repeat blood specimens each day (parasitemia was determined and reported as a percentage of infected RBCs).

Case Study 2

A 22-year-old man, known to be seropositive for HIV-1, complained of chronic diarrhea and weight loss for approximately 4 to 5 weeks. The diarrhea was nonbloody and seemed to get worse and more watery after eating. The diarrhea did not respond to the usual treatment with Imodium A-D or Pepto-Bismol. The patient appeared to be somewhat dehydrated. Previous stool cultures were negative for bacterial enteric pathogens, and the stool was also negative for *Clostridium difficile* toxin.

Questions

1. Considering the patient's history and symptoms, what are the possible diagnoses?
2. What additional laboratory tests should be ordered?
3. What potential diagnostic problems does this case represent?

Discussion

1. Other possible causes for the diarrhea include intestinal parasites, such as *C. parvum, I. belli, C. cayetanensis,* or Microsporida (*E. bieneusi, E. intestinalis*).
2. Stools should be submitted for intestinal coccidia and Microsporida.
3. The routine O & P examination will not reveal these organisms. Special stains and/or the use of monoclonal-based diagnostic kits are required for identification. The one exception would be *I. belli,* which

should be identified on the wet concentration sediment examination. If the patient has a low CD4 count, then the chances of the diarrhea being caused by Microsporida increase. Also, approximately one third of AIDS patients who have cryptosporidiosis, also have infections with Microsporida.

Laboratory and Therapeutic Followup

Modified acid-fast stains revealed the presence of oocysts measuring approximately 4 to 6μm, characteristic of *C. parvum.* Because there is no specific therapy for cryptosporidiosis, the patient was followed and treated for symptomatic relief. During the next 6 months, the diarrhea would diminish somewhat and then increase with an increased fluid loss of approximately 6 L/day. Special trichrome stains and optical brightening agents (Calcofluor white) for Microsporida were negative.

References

1. College of American Pathologists: Commission on Laboratory Accreditation. Chicago, College of American Pathologists, 1992.
2. Committee on Education American Society of Parasitologists: Procedures suggested for use in examination of clinical specimens for parasitic infection. J Parasitol 63:959–960, 1977.
3. Isenberg, HD:Clinical Microbiology Procedures Handbook: Parasitology section Washington, DC, American Society for Microbiology, 1992.
4. National Committee for Clinical Laboratory Standards: Protection of Laboratory Workers from Infectious Disease Transmitted by Blood and Tissue: Proposed Guideline, M29-P1. Villanova, Pa, National Committee for Clinical Laboratory Standards, 1987.
5. National Committee for Clinical Laboratory Standards: Clinical Laboratory Waste Management: Tentative Guideline, GP5-T. Villanova, Pa, National Committee for Clinical Laboratory Standards, 1991.
6. National Committee for Clinical Laboratory Standards: Protection of laboratory workers from infectious disease transmitted by blood, body fluids, and tissue: Tentative guideline, M29-T2. Villanova, Pa, National Committee for Clinical Laboratory Standards, 1991.
7. National Committee for Clinical Laboratory Standards: Approved guideline, GP2-2A. *In* Clinical Laboratory Procedure Manuals, ed 2. Villanova, Pa, National Committee for Clinical Laboratory Standards, 1992.
8. National Committee for Clinical Laboratory Standards: 1992, Use of blood film examination for parasites. Tentative Guideline M15-T, National Committee for Clinical Laboratory Standards, Villanova, PA,
9. National Committee for Clinical Laboratory Standards: Procedures for the recovery and identification of parasites from the intestinal tract: Proposed Guideline M28-P, National Committee for Clinical Laboratory Standards, Villanova, Pa.
10. Parasitology Subcommittee Microbiology Section of Scientific Assembly American Society of Medical Technology: Recommended procedures for the examination of clinical specimens submitted for the diagnosis of parasitic infections. Am J Med Technol. 44:1101–1106, 1978.

Bibliography

Garcia LS, Bruckner DA: Diagnostic Medical Parasitology, ed 2. Washington, DC, American Society for Microbiology, 1993.
Gorbach SL, Bartlett JG, Blacklow NR (eds): Infectious Diseases, Philadelphia, WB Saunders. 1992.
Mandell GL, Bennett JE, (eds): Principles and Practice of Infectious Diseases, ed 4. New York, Churchill Livingstone, 1995.
Markell EK, Voge M, John DT: Medical Parasitology, ed. 6, Philadelphia, WB Saunders, 1986.

Septic Shock

Vickie S. Baselski and Linda L. Ross

Septic shock constitutes a dramatic culmination of a host response to injury in which additional tissue injury occurs. Recent estimates suggest that in the United States more than 500,000 cases of septic shock occur annually with approximately 100,000 deaths and accrued health care costs of $5 to $10 billion. This statistic represents an increase of 139% from 1979 to 1987 alone.[1] Sepsis is a confusing and complex disorder marked by multiple etiologies, multiple management strategies, and many apparently conflicting signs and symptoms, and many different laboratory tests are required for a proper diagnosis. Consequently, a vocabulary has recently emerged that seeks to stage the events of septic shock.[2] The interrelationships are shown schematically in Figure 54–1, with definitions established by a consensus conference of the American College of Chest Physicians and Society of Critical Care Medicine.

Injury to many types of tissues leads to inflammation

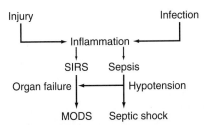

Figure 54–1. Interrelationships of terminology used in defining the continuum of events leading to septic shock. Abbreviations: SIRS, systemic inflammatory response syndrome; MODS, multiple organ dysfunction syndrome.

that may become generalized as the systemic inflammatory response syndrome (SIRS). SIRS is manifested by two or more of the following criteria: (1) temperature greater than 38 °C (hyperthermia) or less than 36 °C (hypothermia), (2) heart rate greater than 90 beats/minute (tachycardia), (3) respiratory rate greater than 20 breaths/minute (tachypnea) or arterial partial pressure of carbon dioxide ($Paco_2$) less than 32 mm Hg, and (4) white blood cell count greater than 12.0×10^9/L, less than 4.0×10^9/L, or greater than 10% immature band forms. When the injury is an infection this response is termed *sepsis.*

Sepsis is considered severe when associated with organ dysfunction, hypoperfusion, or hypotension. Inadequate organ perfusion may be demonstrated by hypoxemia, lactic acidosis, oliguria, or an acute alteration in mental status. *Sepsis-induced hypotension* is defined as a condition in which the systolic blood pressure is less than 90 mm Hg, or a reduction of 40 mm Hg or more from baseline occurs in the absence of other causes of hypotension. The term *septic shock* is used in extreme circumstances of severe sepsis with hypotension despite adequate fluid resuscitation. Sepsis and SIRS may lead to altered critical organ function termed *multiple organ dysfunction syndrome* (MODS). When severe, the term *multiple systems organ failure* (MSOF) has also been applied.

ETIOLOGY AND PATHOPHYSIOLOGY

The causes of SIRS and sepsis can be divided into two primary defining categories: noninfectious and infectious. Noninfectious injuries are many and include hepatic failure, pancreatitis, ischemia, inflammatory bowel disease, multiple trauma (blunt or penetrating), burns, wounds (including surgical), hemorrhagic shock, immune-mediated organ injury, and unintentional exogenous administration of infectious organism components (e.g., endotoxin) or immune mediators (as in transfusion).[2–4] The remainder of this chapter focuses primarily on sepsis.

Infection may occur at any number of anatomic locations, may result from many varied etiologic agents, and may or may not be accompanied by the presence of the organism in the circulating blood stream. Blood stream infections are termed according to the organism type (e.g., bacteremia, fungemia, viremia, parasitemia). Of the many potential etiologic agents, gram-negative bacteria are of particular note because the presence of *endotoxin,* a lipopolysaccharide (LPS) in the cell walls, which is a particularly potent and provocative substance in sepsis.[4–6]

Many situations may predispose a person to infection and subsequent development of sepsis. Risk factors include treatment with broad-spectrum antibiotics, use of immunosuppressive agents, frequent use of invasive devices (particularly catheters), advanced age, and increased survival of individuals with progressive syndromes (e.g., malignancy, diabetes, human immunodeficiency virus [HIV] infection).[3, 7]

The pathophysiology of SIRS and sepsis are as complex as the terminology used to define the process. A schematic diagram of the events postulated to occur is shown in Figure 54–2. The initial injury to the host provokes an expected inflammatory response that results in the sequential or simultaneous release of soluble immunomodulatory host factors (cytokines). In the unique situation of exposure to endotoxin, additional stimulation occurs through binding of LPS to lipopolysaccharide binding protein (LBP), and subsequent activation of macrophage mediator release through a CD14 receptor interaction. Endotoxin also triggers additional inflammation by direct activation of the alternate complement pathway.[4, 5]

Abnormal mediator excess develops in SIRS or sepsis, although the reasons for this situation are unclear but probably relate both to type and extent of initial injury as well as host-defined susceptibility. Followed by systemic dissemination of the mediators, widespread and profound effects occur on multiple organs and tissues.[3, 8] It has also been proposed that endothelial cell damage plays a central role in the destruction and dysfunction that occur. This is also a likely contributing factor in development of hypotension and disseminated intravascular coagulation (DIC), both of which are sepsis-defining events.[3] Even before current knowledge of cytokines evolved, the concept of *too much of a good thing* was described by Lewis Thomas as follows: ". . . all of these effects represent perfectly normal responses, things done every day in the course of

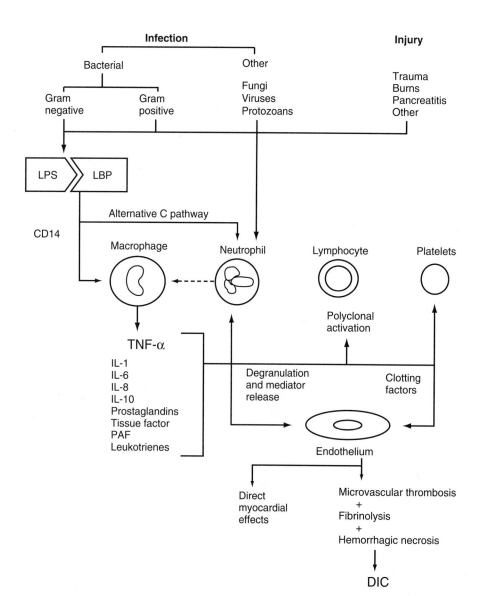

Figure 54–2. Schematic pathophysiologic events in the sepsis/SIRS cascade. Abbreviations: LPS, lipopolysaccharide; LBP, lipopolysaccharide binding protein; TNF, tumor necrosis factor; IL, interleukin; PAF, platelet activating factor; DIC, disseminated intravascular coagulation.

normal living. What makes it a disaster is that they are turned on all at once by the host, as though in response to an alarm signal, and the outcome is widespread tissue destruction . . ."[9]

Evidence that cytokines play a central role in sepsis can be consolidated into three key observations: (1) Certain plasma and body fluid cytokine concentrations are increased in clinical disease, (2) Experimental exogenous administration of key cytokines results in a clinically similar syndrome, and (3) specific blockers of cytokine activity can ameliorate or abort the clinical and physiologic findings associated with sepsis.[10] Although many mediators are known and may contribute to the disease process,[3] at present four key cytokines, which are released sequentially in experimental models, have been identified and serve as targets for novel therapeutic approaches. Tumor necrosis factor-α (TNF-α) and interleukin-1β (IL-1β) are considered early key mediators.[11] Both serve as endogenous pyrogens, increase catabolism, induce hepatic synthesis of acute-phase proteins, and result in hypotension and tachycardia. In experiments exogenous administration mimicked sepsis. TNF-α is released principally from macrophages and has multiple effects on other inflammatory cells, endothelial cells, and other cell types.[11] Although apparently central to development of sepsis, its multiple effects and phasic appearance have confounded attempts to use antibodies to it therapeutically.[12] IL-1β is also released predominantly from mononuclear cells and has similar ill-defined multiple effects. Not surprisingly, preliminary results from trials using agents to block its effects are also inconclusive. Interleukins 6 and 8 (IL-6, IL-8) appear predictably later in the progression of sepsis.[8] They appear to be important secondary mediators, but their specific roles are unclear. IL-6 is a pyrogen and lymphocyte activator, and its concentration has shown a strong correlation with severity of disease. IL-8 is a potent promoter of neutrophilic inflammation, but unlike IL-6, its concentration decreases regardless of disease severity.

In addition to specific mediators, the role of specific endogenous antagonists has recently been evaluated. Measurable levels of the cytokine antagonists termed *soluble TNF receptors* (sTNF-r) and *interleukin-1 receptor antagonists* (IL-1ra) have both been demonstrated.[12] Both serve to block and probably regulate cytokine function through slightly different mechanisms. Both substances have been suggested as potential therapies on the basis of their role in inhibiting cell activation and mediator release. However, because of their normal presence in a sepsis response, their usefulness in therapy may be confounded.

Additional secondary mediators or factors important in the evolution of sepsis include those that are vasoactive and those that influence the coagulation process. The former include prostaglandins, leukotrienes, and thromboxane A.[4] The latter includes platelet-activating factor (PAF) and factors that disrupt balance in procoagulant and fibrinolytic mechanisms through effects on clotting factors.[13]

Thus, although it is well accepted that the pathophysiology of sepsis is a result of excessive activation of endogenous mediators, our knowledge of exact mechanisms, sequences, and many complex interactions is still incomplete, as is our knowledge of similar processes in a normal response. This, at present, compromises our ability to use such information for diagnostic, prognostic, or therapeutic purposes.

CLINICAL MANIFESTATIONS

The diagnosis of sepsis is made when a combination of clinical and laboratory findings support a generalized state of "metabolic anarchy."[14] A summary of commonly used parameters for monitoring specific organ systems is given in Table 54–1. Significant biochemical derangements that mark this state often suggest organ dysfunction or failure, coagulative disorders, myocardial depression, generalized inflammation, and a hypermetabolic stress response. The changes all result from the combined effects of the mediators previously discussed. The normal nonspecific response to injury results in well-described cardiovascular changes including increases in heart rate, contractility, and cardiac output. Metabolic responses include oxygen consumption and accelerated protein catabolism. Additional neuroendocrine release of catecholamines, cortisol, antidiuretic hormone, growth hormone, glucagon, and insulin promote further metabolic derangements manifested by tachycardia, tachypnea, and a general hypermetabolic state. The latter is demonstrated by electrolyte and acid-base imbalances, hyperglycemia, and elevated lactate. The generalized inflammatory response resulting in mediator release promotes a sustained hypermetabolic state in addition to other signs

Table 54–1. Key Parameters Commonly Used in Defining System Dysfunction in Sepsis

System Category	Key Parameters*	
	Clinical	*Laboratory*
General hypermetabolism	Heart rate Respiratory rate	Electrolytes Blood pH Blood glucose Serum lactate*
General inflammation	Temperature	CRP ESR WBC count and differential*
Respiratory	Requirement for oxygen or mechanical ventilation	Blood gases PaO₂/FIO₂*
Renal	Urine output	Serum creatinine*
Hepatic	Jaundice	Serum bilirubin* Hepatic enzymes Serum albumin
Coagulation	Bleeding	Platelets* D-dimer PT/APTT FDP
Central nervous	Glasgow coma scale*	None
Cardiovascular	Blood pressure*	None
Gastrointestinal	Tolerance to enteral feeding*	None

*Indicates parameters considered to be most useful.[15]

Abbreviations: CRP, C-reactive protein; ESR, erythrocyte sedimentation rate; PaO₂, arterial partial pressure of oxygen; FIO₂, fractional concentration of inspired oxygen; PT, prothrombin time; APTT, activated partial thromboplastin time; FDP, fibrin degradation products; WBC, white blood cell.

Data from Beal A, Cevra F: Multiple organ failure syndrome in the 1990's: Systemic inflammatory response and organ function. JAMA 271:226, 1994.

of inflammation including fever, hematologic abnormalities (e.g., leukocytosis, leukopenia, or shift to the left), and presence of acute phase reactants (e.g., C-reactive protein [CRP], erythrocyte sedimentation rate [ESR]).[15, 16]

Hypotension is a key event in the progression of sepsis; however, the mechanisms by which it occurs are not completely understood. It may result from the nonspecific effects of endogenous mediators on the heart, or it may represent effects of a mediator specific for myocardial tissue. TNF has been recognized as a probable candidate for both mechanisms. In either case, the resultant cardiopathy, when combined with severe vascular paralysis, causes an inability to regulate blood flow to peripheral circulation, and blood pressure decreases.[3, 4] As vasomotor tone falls, capillary leakage also occurs, resulting in significant blood volume loss. A requirement for adequate fluid resuscitation ensues, frequently in conjunction with a requirement for vasopressor agents to correct blood pressure.

More recently, nitric oxide has also been implicated in sepsis-induced hypotension. This compound is an endogenous vasodilator that also functions as an immune modulator and may be directly cytotoxic. Thus, a role in pathogenesis of sepsis has been proposed, and inhibition of the enzyme leading to its production has been evaluated as an experimental strategy. At the present time, however, neither a role for nitric oxides in sepsis nor its inhibition in therapy has been firmly established.[17]

One of the most striking clinical manifestations is that of DIC. DIC is the extreme result of coagulopathy that is characterized by a dynamic process of microvascular thrombosis with consumption of platelets and coagulation proteins accompanied by stimulation of the fibrinolytic system. Hemorrhage and necrosis develop, which in a severe form may be marked by peripheral gangrene. Widespread microembolization is also likely a major contributor to multiple organ dysfunction and failure.[13, 18, 19]

Transition from a hypermetabolic, hypotensive, and thrombohemorrhagic state to one of overt organ failure probably depends on the extent and duration of the generalized response. MODS is the most common, with the respiratory, renal, hepatic, central nervous, cardiovascular, and gastrointestinal systems involved. The diagnosis of MODS usually involves measurement of both clinicophysiologic and laboratory parameters, although measures of the progression from organ dysfunction to irreversible organ failure have not been well-defined.[15, 20]

The clinical assessment of disease severity is an important component of monitoring sepsis patients. Many elaborate systems have evolved that score or grade clinical, physiologic, and laboratory abnormalities.[3, 10, 20] One of the most common is the Acute Physiology and Chronic Health Evaluation (APACHE) score. Use of such systems is important in monitoring disease progression, evaluating therapeutic efficacy, and controlling effective resource utilization.[21]

LABORATORY ANALYSES AND DIAGNOSIS

The central events in the pathophysiologic process and in diagnostic strategies for sepsis are similar, but the ordering of the events varies, as does the relative importance of clinical vs. laboratory findings. Current laboratory testing is two-fold in purpose. First, a variety of tests identify altered metabolic, inflammatory, and organ-function states. These tests are used both diagnostically and prognostically. Second, the use of cultures and other techniques to document an infectious etiology, and in particular to note its presence or absence in the blood stream, is key in optimal patient management. Documented or presumed infections, especially when in the blood stream, denote increased severity and poorer outcome.[1, 6] Additionally, specific identification and, if appropriate, antimicrobial susceptibility testing are essential to optimize the therapeutic strategy. For both purposes the laboratory plays an essential role in recognizing sepsis syndrome. The major laboratory analyses used in establishing and determining progression of sepsis are summarized in Table 54–1.

Hypermetabolic Changes

Lactic acid increases to greater than 130 mg/dL (normal, 4.5 to 19.8 mg/dL) in arterial blood samples due to a primary abnormality in glycolysis. Normal liver function ordinarily clears most lactic acid and other toxic by-products, so progressive liver dysfunction can exaggerate this effect. Plasma glucose levels also increase as a result of lactic acid (anaerobic) metabolism. Monitoring arterial blood gases early in the development of sepsis is also important for recognizing possible respiratory failure. Hypoxemia and respiratory and metabolic acidosis are indicated by a decrease in $Paco_2$ and a decrease in blood pH to less than 7.35 (normal, 7.35–7.45). Fever, altered metabolism, and reduced systemic vascular resistance may result in fluid losses; consequently, serum electrolyte imbalances must also be monitored.[5, 15]

Generalized Inflammation

A generalized state of inflammation may be manifest by a number of abnormal laboratory values. Early white blood cell (WBC) counts are elevated to greater than $12.0 \times 10^9/L$ (normal, 5.0 to $10.0 \times 10^9/L$) but may later decrease to less than $4.0 \times 10^9/L$ as tissue disposition occurs.[3] Either case may be accompanied by a significant left shift with greater than 10% immature band forms present. Mediator effect on hepatic function may also increase concentration of many acute phase reactants, most notably CRP. Early increases in fibrinogen or γ-globulins may also increase the ESR.[15]

Coagulopathic Changes

Sepsis is frequently associated with DIC, which can be induced by the endotoxin of gram-negative bacteria, the superantigen exotoxins of gram-positive organisms, and the cytokines endotoxins and exotoxins induce.[18] The laboratory tests employed demonstrate evidence of procoagulant activation, fibrinolytic activation, or inhibitor consumption. Laboratory findings in severe DIC include thrombocytopenia, prolonged prothrombin time (PT), activated partial thromboplastin time (APTT), decreased fibrinogen, and increased fibrin degradation products. To maximize cost-effective laboratory utilization, "DIC panels" have been

Table 54–2. Suggested Screening Tests for Disseminated Intravascular Coagulation

Test	Laboratory Finding
Platelet count	↓ ↓
Prothrombin time	Normal or ↑
Activated partial thromboplastin time	Normal or ↑
Fibrinogen	↓
Fibrin degradation products	↑
D-Dimer assay	Positive
Anti-thrombin III level	↓

developed to aid in efficient diagnosis and monitoring of DIC (Table 54–2). Although numerous laboratory tests can be employed, the test that best supports the diagnosis of DIC is establishing the presence of fibrin degradation products (FDP) using either a conventional FDP assay or a D-dimer test, a simple latex agglutination procedure.[18, 19] The test that best monitors progressive dysfunction, however, is the platelet count.[20]

Organ Dysfunction

The laboratory plays a key role in recognizing organ dysfunction and monitoring its progression (to outright failure for certain key organ systems). Early monitoring of arterial blood gases in septic shock is essential to detecting respiratory dysfunction and possibly preventing adult respiratory distress syndrome (ARDS). Hypoxemia results from both consumption demands and acute lung endothelial injury compromising alveolar function.[3, 14] Adequate oxygen delivery generally depends on supplemental oxygen, frequently by mechanical ventilation. The best monitor for respiratory failure appears to be a reduction in the *hypoxemia score*.[20] The hypoxemia score is defined as the ratio of arterial oxygen tension divided by the inspired oxygen concentration (PaO_2/FiO_2) and reflects both disease severity and oxygenation difficulty.

Common renal manifestations of sepsis include oliguria, azotemia, and active urinary sediment. Urinalysis may reveal a low specific gravity and proteinuria. In patients with sepsis, urinary sediment contains red blood cells and casts. In serum, blood urea nitrogen (BUN) rises above the normal range of 20 mg/dL and creatinine may increase to levels greater than 1.4 mg/dL. The BUN/creatinine ratio may be abnormal, and electrolyte levels of potassium, sodium, and chloride should be monitored to maintain normal balance.[5, 14]

Hepatic function is best monitored by measurement of total serum bilirubin;[20] however, elevations in other hepatic enzymes are typically noted. Ischemia may also cause pancreatic dysfunction and lipase elevation. Amylase may show similar elevation but this is not specific to pancreatic damage.[14] Adrenal insufficiency resulting from hemorrhagic necrosis may also be demonstrated by metabolic imbalances and reduced plasma adrenocorticotropic hormone (ACTH) levels.

For other organ systems, the laboratory plays a minor role in diagnosis and monitoring of dysfunction, with clinical assessment being of primary importance. For the systems previously discussed, however, many institutions have selected groups of tests, such as a "renal profile panel" or "hepatic profile panel," to assess these organ systems without the expense of additional and often unnecessary or irrelevant tests. Panels such as these and single order tests are cost-effective means of monitoring potential progression of single organ system dysfunction to MODS or MSOF.

Microbiologic Testing

Isolation and identification of the etiologic agents of sepsis are a key aspect of patient management.[16] Infections that promote development of sepsis may be found at many anatomic locations; as a result, a systematic approach that enables recognition of actual infection sites is important.[22] Table 54–3 identifies the most common anatomic sites and the clinical and microbiologic findings associated with making a diagnosis. For establishing a clinical differential diagnosis, it is especially important to identify aspects of the patient's history and physical findings that may suggest etiologic agents. In microbiologic testing, it is especially important for the laboratory to be aware of suspected etiologic agents to use methods for their optimal detection.

For infections at all sites, documentation of the presence of organisms in the blood is of particular importance because it is associated with increased severity, mortality, and MODS.[16] Positive results from blood culture specimens should always be immediately reported as alert values. Laboratory tests for bacteria and fungi, the most frequent organisms found in the blood of patients with sepsis, have a number of critical technical features that are known to influence the reliability of results.

Whenever possible, collection of blood cultures before initiation of antibiotic treatment is advised. A minimum collection of two separate blood cultures for each febrile episode and an inoculation of at least 20 mL of blood from adult patients into each set (aerobic and anaerobic bottles) of blood culture bottles is recommended and is usually sufficient for detection of bacteria and fungi.[23] For practical reasons, collection of between 1 to 5 mL of blood and

Table 54–3. Clinical and Laboratory Aspects of Common Infections Potentially Leading to Sepsis

Clinical Situation	Laboratory Diagnosis
Bacteremia, Fungemia, Viremia, Parasitemia	Blood culture
Catheter-related infection (intravascular)	Quantitative blood culture
Gastroenteritis	Stool culture
Meningitis	Cerebrospinal fluid culture Antigen detection tests
Peritonitis	Peritoneal fluid culture
Pneumonia	Lower respiratory tract culture Quantitative bronchoscopic specimen culture
Sinusitis	Sinus aspirate culture
Wound infection	Wound culture
Urinary tract infection	Quantitative urine culture

inoculation into a single bottle is appropriate for pediatric or venous-access compromised patients.

Timing between collection of blood cultures is an area of continued controversy; however, data suggest that randomly spaced, multiple cultures may improve detection compared to cultures obtained sequentially. Aseptic skin preparation using 2% tincture of iodine at the venipuncture site followed by alcohol or double alcohol skin preparation is critical to avoid contamination by skin flora.[23]

Processing blood cultures in the laboratory is method-dependent, with many laboratories using more than a single technique (e.g., broth-based manual, semi-automated, or automated methods and lysis/centrifugation) for isolation of bacteria, fungi, and mycobacteria. In fact, detection sensitivity of many different etiologic agents varies considerably with the method used. Instrumentation is currently available for continuous monitoring of blood culture bottles for rapid detection of positive results; however, cost, availability of trained personnel, and patient demographics are factors to be considered when selecting the most acceptable blood culture system appropriate for use in a particular laboratory setting.[23] As mentioned previously, collection of blood cultures before initiation of antimicrobial therapy is recommended; however, blood culture bottles are commercially available that contain antimicrobial removal devices such as resins, charcoal particles, or physical separation methods that remove most of the commonly used antibiotics. Their use has remained controversial. Once the etiologic agent has been isolated and identified, susceptibility testing can be performed whenever appropriate by conventional agar disk diffusion, broth dilution, or automated rapid susceptibility systems (see Chapter 58).

Alternative Test Methods

Due to delayed time for bacterial growth detection in culture and frequency of culture-negative sepsis in patients in whom an infectious agent is suspected but cannot be isolated, several non–culture-dependent methods have been evaluated. The *Limulus* amebocyte lysate (LAL) assay for endotoxin of gram-negative organisms has been used to attempt rapid diagnosis of gram-negative bacteremia, but low sensitivity related to organism concentration and presence of inhibitors in blood have compromised its utility.[4, 6] Antigen detection tests primarily using latex agglutination have been useful adjuncts to culture in select community-acquired meningitis cases, when culture is compromised by antecedent antibiotic therapy. Most promising, perhaps, is the application of nucleic acid amplification techniques, including polymerase chain reaction (PCR), which have the potential to detect a single microbe in a patient blood sample. Use of reagents designed to broadly amplify all members of a given group (e.g., gram-positive or gram-negative bacteria, fungi) may form the basis of future "rapid sepsis screens" for selection of appropriate therapeutic strategies.[24]

TREATMENT

Therapeutic strategies for sepsis can be divided into three basic categories, all of which may be dependent on supporting laboratory data for optimization.[25] Essential therapies are those that seek to either remove or correct the inciting event, or stabilize the physiologic derangements. These therapies are generally well accepted in the management of the septic patient. When an infection is documented, surgical drainage or debridement may accomplish the former, but of equal importance is the use of appropriate antimicrobial agents based on identification and, if indicated, susceptibility testing of the organism. Physiologic stabilization requires meeting increased oxygen need, supporting increased metabolic activity, restoring fluid and electrolyte balance, and using appropriate cardiotropic agents to manage hemodynamic complications. Management of DIC requires agents to inhibit thrombosis, replenish essential coagulation factors, and possibly inhibit fibrinolysis.[18] The use of anti-endotoxin antibodies is not recommended because these agents have had conflicting performance data.[26] This is presumably due to inability to stratify patients into groups likely to benefit (i.e., those with endotoxin-induced sepsis). For all essential therapies, laboratory data are necessary to support a desired return to homeostasis.

Many therapeutic agents considered controversial have been used in attempts to subvert the cascading events in sepsis. These agents are not universally accepted in management of patients, largely because the mechanisms of action are ill-defined, and the literature frequently fails to establish significant improvement in outcome.[11] Of particular note are the use of steroids (which appear to act by blocking mediator translation),[27] naloxone (opiate antagonists with hemodynamic effects), pentoxifylline or amrinone (which disrupt intracellular signaling and presumably mediator transcription), and cyclooxygenase inhibitors (e.g., ibuprofen, which reduces concentrations of thromboxane and prostacyclin metabolites with consequent hemodynamic stabilization).[5] Also in this category are inhibitors of nitric oxide synthesis.[17] Agents used prophylactically or as early therapy to enhance immune response in infection are also controversial. Examples include granulocyte transfusions and use of G-CSF (granulocyte colony-stimulating factor). Despite the controversy surrounding their use, laboratory data would again be necessary to monitor return to homeostasis.[25]

A third category of potential immunomodulatory agents has recently emerged. These agents may act by one of several possible mechanisms: (1) the specific inhibition of cytokine synthesis through effects on transcription or translation, (2) the use of antibody reagents to block activity of specific cytokines, and (3) the use of soluble agents, which block cytokine-receptor cell surface interactions, thus inhibiting cytokine mediated responses.

Conflicting and confusing research data on the use of novel, potential immunomodulatory agents has prevented their general use and has contributed to the inadequacies of current understanding of the processes.[25, 28] The complexities of the sepsis cascade may actually require concomitant or sequential use of several therapeutic agents, and their prophylactic use in at-risk patients may also be indicated.[29] The development of new and probably rapid laboratory assays (e.g., quantitative cytokine assays) will be required to facilitate the identification of patients likely to benefit because these new agents will undoubtedly be expensive.

Case Study

An 80-year-old male nursing home patient with advanced Alzheimer's disease was noted to be increasingly lethargic and unresponsive to external stimuli. Nursing records indicated a reduced urine output in his catheter drainage bag for the preceding 24 hours. Urinalysis showed the presence of protein, hemoglobin, leukocyte esterase, and nitrite. On microscopic examination of urinary sediment many WBCs, RBCs, and bacilli were observed. His blood pressure (BP) was 120/84 mm Hg; temperature, 97 °F; heart rate, 120 beats/minute; and respiratory rate, 30 breaths/minute; these findings suggested development of urosepsis, and he was transferred to the hospital.

At admission, additional abnormal laboratory findings included the following:

WBCs	3.8 × 10⁹/L (85% PMN, 10% bands, 5% lymphs)
Platelets	80 × 10⁹/L
Lactate (mg/dL)	27
Glucose (mg/dL)	200
Bilirubin (mg/dL)	2.0
Creatinine (mg/dL)	2.4
Blood gases (mm Hg)	$Paco_2$ 20, Pao_2 45
ESR (mm/hr)	60

Blood pressure fell to 90/60 mm Hg. Cultures were obtained, and the empirical antibiotic therapy was started. Blood and urine cultures subsequently revealed the etiologic agent, *Escherichia coli.*

Questions

1. What are the most likely etiologic agents?
2. The clinical findings and laboratory findings suggest developing organ dysfunction in which organ systems?

Discussion

1. Urinary tract infection with subsequent blood stream infection (urosepsis) in males is most commonly associated with a variety of gram-negative bacilli. Enteric organisms are most common, but in a patient compromised by an indwelling catheter, nonfermenters such as *Pseudomonas aeruginosa* can occur. Empirical coverage would likely include consideration of either organism with a broad-spectrum β-lactam antibiotic plus an aminoglycoside given.
2. The abnormal results in this patient are suggestive of early development of MODS. The early lethargy suggests central nervous system (CNS) involvement, and the decreasing BP indicates cardiovascular collapse and worsening of sepsis. Thrombocytopenia suggests evolution of coagulation deficits, and hypoxemia suggests evolution of respiratory failure. In addition, hyperbilirubinemia indicates development of hepatic dysfunction, and elevated creatinine levels indicate development of renal failure.

References

1. Centers for Disease Control: Increase in national hospital discharge survey rates for septicemia—United States, 1979–1987. MMWR 39:31, 1990.
2. Bone R, Balk R, Cerra F, et al: Definitions for sepsis and organ failure and guidelines for the use of innovative therapies in sepsis. Chest 101:1644, 1992.
3. Bone R: The pathogenesis of sepsis. Ann Int Med 115:457, 1991.
4. Manthous C, Hall J, Samsel R: Endotoxin in human disease. Part 1: Biochemistry, assay, and possible role in diverse disease states. Chest 104:1572, 1993.
5. Bone R: Gram-negative sepsis: A dilemma of modern medicine. Clin Microbiol Rev 6:57, 1993.
6. Danner R, Elin R, Hosseini J, et al: Endotoxemia in human septic shock. Chest 99:169, 1993.
7. Parrillo J: Pathogenetic mechanisms of septic shock. N Engl J Med 328:1471, 1993.
8. Christman J, Holden E, Blackwell T: Strategies for blocking the systemic effects of cytokines in the sepsis syndrome. Crit Care Med 23:955, 1995.
9. Thomas L: The Medusa and the Snail: More Notes of a Biology Watcher. New York, Bantam Books, 1979, p 77.
10. Barriere S, Lowry S: An overview of mortality risk prediction in sepsis. Crit Care Med 23:376, 1995.
11. Giroir B: Mediators of septic shock: New approaches for interrupting the endogenous inflammatory cascade. Crit Care Med 21:780, 1993.
12. Goldie A, Fearon K, Ross J, et al: Natural cytokine antagonists and endogenous antiendotoxin core antibodies in sepsis syndrome. JAMA 274:172, 1995.
13. Thijs L, deBoer J, de Groot M, et al: Coagulation disorders in septic shock. Int Care Med 19:S8, 1993.
14. Bone R: Sepsis syndrome, the diagnostic challenge. J Crit Illness 6:525, 1991.
15. Beal A, Cerra F: Multiple organ failure syndrome in the 1990's: Systemic inflammatory response and organ function. JAMA 271:226, 1994.
16. Rangel-Frausto M, Pittet D, Costigan M, et al: The natural history of the systemic inflammatory response syndrome (SIRS): A prospective study. JAMA 273:117, 1995.
17. Cobb J, Danner R: Nitric oxide and septic shock. JAMA 275:1192, 1996.
18. Bick R: Disseminated intravascular coagulation: Objective laboratory diagnostic criteria and guidelines for management. Clin Lab Med 14:729, 1994.
19. Jensen R, Ens G: Septicemia and hemostasis. Clin Hemost Rev 4:10, 1990.
20. Marshall J, Cook D, Christou N, et al: Multiple organ dysfunction score: A reliable descriptor of a complex clinical outcome. Crit Care Med 23:1638, 1995.
21. Pollack M, Getson PL: Pediatric critical care cost containment: Combined actuarial and clinical program. Crit Care Med 19:12, 1991.
22. Meduri G, Mauldin G, Wunderink R, et al: Causes of fever and pulmonary densities in patients with clinical manifestations of ventilator-associated pneumonia. Chest 106:221, 1994.
23. Washington J: Collection, transport, and processing of blood cultures. Clin Lab Med 14:59, 1994.
24. Leong D, Greisen K: PCR detection of bacteria found in cerebrospinal fluid. *In* Persing DH, Smith TH, Tenover FC, White TJ (eds): Diagnostic Molecular Microbiology: Principles and Applications, Washington, DC, American Society for Microbiology, 1993, p 300.
25. Bernard G: Sepsis trials. Intersection of investigation, regulation, funding, and practice. Am J Respir Crit Care Med 152:4, 1995.
26. Luce J: Introduction of new technology into critical care practice: A history of HA-1A human monoclonal antibody against endotoxin. Crit Care Med 21:1233, 1993.
27. Cronin L, Cook D, Carlet J, et al: Corticosteroid treatment for sepsis: A critical appraisal and meta-analysis of the literature. Crit Care Med 23:1430, 1995.
28. Abraham E, Wunderink R, Silverman H, et al: Efficacy and safety of monoclonal antibody to human tumor necrosis factor in patients with sepsis syndrome. JAMA 273:934, 1995.
29. Wenzel R, Pinsky M, Ulevitch R, et al: Current understanding of sepsis. Clin Infect Dis 22:407, 1996.

Chapter 55

Nosocomial Infections

Peggy Prinz Luebbert

The term *nosocomial* derives from the Greek words *nosos,* meaning "disease," and *komeo,* meaning "to care" for; therefore, nosocomial infections are those infections that develop within a health care setting or are produced by microorganisms acquired while a patient is receiving care in this setting. Traditionally, the term has been used to describe infections in hospital settings, but it may also apply in long-term care facilities, home health care settings, psychiatric facilities, and so on. Nosocomial infections may involve not only patients but also anyone else who has contact with the facility, including members of the staff, volunteers, and visitors. The majority of nosocomial infections become clinically apparent while the patients are still in the facility; however, the onset of disease can occur after a patient has been discharged. As many as 25% of postoperative wound infections, for example, become symptomatic after the patient has been discharged.

INFECTIOUS PROCESSES

Infections incubating at the time of the patient's admission to a facility are not nosocomial and are considered community acquired. These infections are significant, however, because they may serve as a ready source of infection for other patients or personnel and must be considered in the total scope of facility-related infections.

Organisms that cause nosocomial infections come from either *endogenous* (autogenous) or *exogenous* sources. Endogenous infections are caused by the patient's own flora. Exogenous infections result from transmission of organisms from a source other than the patient. Endogenous organisms are either brought into the hospital by a patient (colonization outside the hospital) or colonize the patient after he or she is admitted to the hospital. In either instance, the organisms colonizing the patient may subsequently cause a nosocomial infection. The organisms most commonly responsible for endogenous nosocomial infections are *Escherichia coli, Klebsiella, Proteus,* and group D enterocci in the intestine; *Staphylococcus aureus* in the nares; and *S. epidermidis* on the skin. In exogenous infections, the causative organisms are not part of the patient's normal flora, but spread from the external environment. For example, *Pseudomonas* may originate from water or equipment, and *Mycobacterium tuberculosis* may spread from visitors or patients with pulmonary tuberculosis.

Nosocomial infectious diseases may persist at a relatively constant level in a facility (*endemic*) or can be characterized by the number of existing cases in a population (*prevalence*), the number of new cases in a population (*incidence*), and the risk of transmission (*contagiousness*). A *sporadic* infection is one that occurs occasionally and irregularly, without any specific pattern. An *epidemic* is a definite increase in the incidence of a disease above its expected endemic occurrence. The term *outbreak* is used interchangeably with epidemic; however, some infection control practitioners (ICPs) use the term "outbreak" to mean a higher rate of occurrence but not at levels as serious as an epidemic.

Nosocomial infections involve diverse anatomic sites, but the risk of these various types of infections, and consequently their relative frequency, appear to be very similar in most acute care hospitals. Table 55–1 lists the estimated nationwide infection rates and relative frequency of the most common sites found in Centers for Disease Control and Prevention (CDC) National Nosocomial Infections Surveillance (NNIS) reports.[1] Note that urinary tract infections make up one-fourth of all nosocomial infections. Surgical wound infections constitute almost 19%, followed by pneumonias and bacteremias. The NNIS system, which was started in 1970, consists of the aggregation of surveillance

Table 55–1. Frequency Distribution of Major Sites of Nosocomial Infections, by Bedsize and Teaching Affiliation, Hospital-wide Component, January 1993 to April 1995

Major Site	Nonteaching Hospitals <200 beds	Nonteaching Hospitals ≥200 beds	Teaching Hospitals <500 beds	Teaching Hospitals ≥500 beds	All Hospitals
Urinary tract infection	504 (36.0%)	1560 (33.6%)	3045 (28.2%)	2267 (22.1%)	7376 (27.2%)
Surgical site infection	198 (14.1%)	903 (19.5%)	1934 (17.9%)	2023 (19.7%)	5058 (18.7%)
Pneumonia	261 (18.6%)	779 (16.8%)	1822 (16.9%)	1811 (17.7%)	4673 (17.3%)
Primary blood stream infection	146 (10.4%)	443 (9.5%)	1647 (15.2%)	2051 (20.0%)	4287 (15.8%)
Other	292 (20.8%)	958 (20.6%)	2356 (21.8%)	2094 (20.4%)	5700 (21.0%)
All infections	1401 (5.2%)	4643 (17.1%)	10,804 (39.9%)	10,246 (37.8%)	27,094 (100%)

Do not use the data in this table for interhospital comparison, because the frequencies are not adjusted for risk of infection or intensity of surveillance. The data should be used as a general guide for determining the relative frequency of infection at the major sites.

From National Nosocomial Infections Surveillance (NNIS): Semiannual Report, May 1995, Special Communications. Am J Infect Control 23:377, 1995.

data in a national database from approximately 200 acute care facilities in the U.S.

Data from the hospital-wide component of the NNIS System in the period 1986–1990 indicated that *E. coli* is the most commonly isolated pathogen from all nosocomial infections, regardless of site.[2] This is primarily because of its substantial role in urinary tract infections. *S. aureus* is the second most common, because of its frequent involvement in many types and sites of infections. The third leading pathogen, enterococci, has engendered growing concern owing to its ability to develop resistance patterns. *Pseudomonas* and coagulase-negative staphylococci are fourth and fifth, respectively, as commonly isolated pathogens.

The average infection incidence rates of hospitals participating in the NNIS System were reported to vary from 1.7% in small community hospitals to more than 11% in chronic disease hospitals.[3] Patient risk factors, average length of stay, completeness of diagnostic evaluation for infection, and seasonal trends are intrinsic factors adding to the individuality of the incidence rates of a specific hospital.

CHAIN OF INFECTION

A nosocomial infection results from the interaction between an infectious agent and a susceptible host. This interaction, or transmission, occurs by means of contact between the agent and the host. Three factors, the agent, transmission, and the host, are necessary for an infection to occur, and this triad is often described as the *chain of infection.*

Causative Agent

The first link in the chain of infection is the causative agent. The majority of nosocomial infections are caused most often by bacteria and viruses, occasionally by fungi, and rarely by parasites. All organisms have a reservoir and a source. The *reservoir* is the place where the organism maintains its presence, metabolizes, and replicates. Viruses and gram-positive cocci (e.g., *S. aureus* in nares), survive better in human reservoirs, whereas gram-negative bacteria often prefer an inanimate reservoir (e.g., *Pseudomonas* in water). The *source* is the place from which the infectious agent passes to the host through a vehicle of transmission.

For example, a reservoir for *S. aureus* organisms may be a health care worker's nares, but the source from which it is transmitted to the patient may be the worker's hands. Even though most nosocomial outbreaks are associated with person-to-person spread of an organism, the role of fomites in transmitting infection has also been emphasized. A *fomite* is an inanimate object that may be contaminated with microorganisms and serve in their transmission. Potable water, sinks, urine measuring devices, food, flowers, air filters, suction apparatus, ice machines, and water baths have all been incriminated as fomites associated with water. Medical equipment such as endoscopes, prosthetic devices, cataract lens implants, prosthetic heart valves, bandages, thermometers, and stethoscopes can also function as fomites.

The effectiveness of an organism as an infectious agent also depends on its pathogenicity, or the ability of the organism to induce disease. Pathogenicity is determined by many factors, including virulence, dose, invasiveness, antigenic makeup, and ability to develop resistant strains.

Transmission

Transmission, the second link in the chain of infection, is the movement of organisms from the source to the host. Transmission may occur through one or more of four different routes: contact, common-vehicle, airborne, and vector-borne.[4] In *contact* transmission of disease, the patient has contact with the source through either direct or indirect means or by droplets. *Direct contact* occurs when there is actual physical contact between the source and patient; *indirect contact* refers to transmission from the source to the patient through an intermediate object, which is usually inanimate (e.g., endoscopes). *Droplet spread* is the brief passage of an agent through the air when the source and patient are within several feet of each other.

In *common-vehicle transmission,* a contaminated inanimate vehicle serves as the transmission of the agent to multiple persons. Common vehicles are shared items such as ingested food, blood products, and intravenously administered fluids.

Airborne transmission occurs with organisms that have a true airborne phase in their route of dissemination and usually involves a distance of more than several feet between the source and the patient.

Vector-borne nosocomial infections have not been reported in the United States.

The Host

The third link in the chain of infection is the host or victim. Resistance among persons to infection varies greatly. Some people may be immune to infection or may be able to resist colonization by an infectious agent. Others exposed to the same agent may form a commensal relationship with the infecting organism and become asymptomatic carriers, and still others may develop clinical disease.

PREVENTION OF NOSOCOMIAL INFECTIONS

In any attempt to control nosocomial infections, an attack on the chain of infection at its weakest link is generally the most effective procedure. Efforts should be directed at optimizing the resistance of the patient to infection, controlling the reservoir of infection, and limiting the transmission of infectious agents.

Optimizing Resistance

Optimizing resistance begins with treatment of underlying illnesses. For example, patients with poorly controlled diabetes mellitus have a higher incidence of urinary tract, respiratory tract, and skin infections. Overuse or improper use of medications may also decrease a patient's resistance. Antibiotics, for example, may disturb normal flora and facilitate colonization of the pharynx by gram-negative bacilli. Anticholinergics may predispose to urinary retention, raising the risk of urinary tract infection. Antacids reduce gastric acid, an important antibacterial defense mechanism. Improving local defenses also raises the body's resistance. Proper skin care programs to avoid ulcers and skin breakdown are useful. Avoiding the use of such devices as indwelling bladder catheters, and intravascular cannulae aid in limiting exposure to the risk of colonization.

Controlling Reservoirs

Providing a clean and sanitary facility and equipment is the cornerstone of the infection control program. Proper plumbing and sewer systems limit the spread of organisms such as *Pseudomonas* and *Klebsiella*. Well-maintained ventilation systems assist in limiting the spread of airborne infections. Even though infections associated with linen are quite rare in health care facilities, soiled linens may potentially become a reservoir for microbes and should be handled and washed for effective decontamination.

The disinfection of environmental surfaces is probably the most useful tool in decreasing the rate of day-to-day transmission of diseases in the environment. Disinfectants are chemicals formulated to destroy or inactivate microorganisms on inanimate surfaces. It is important, therefore, that body fluids be removed from equipment and instruments prior to use of the chemical. The Association of Practitioners in Infection Control and Epidemiology (APIC) has developed guidelines that can assist in selecting the proper disinfectant for a specific area or equipment.[5] In general, disinfectants are classified according to their level of effectiveness and the type of equipment appropriate for their use.[6]

Low-level disinfectants are chemicals that destroy most bacteria, viruses, and fungi, but not *M. tuberculosis* or bacterial spores. They are labeled as "hospital disinfectants" by the United States Environmental Protection Agency (EPA) but bear no label claim for tuberculocidal activity. Low-level disinfectants, such as quaternary ammonium products, are excellent cleaners and can be used for routine housekeeping or soil removal (in the absence of visible body fluid contamination) on noncritical surfaces such as floors and countertops.

Intermediate-level disinfectants are more effective, in that they destroy *M. tuberculosis* and most bacteria, viruses, and fungi, but not bacterial spores. Labeled as "hospital disinfectants" by the EPA with a label claim for tuberculocidal activity, intermediate-level disinfectants are often used to disinfect noncritical surfaces (tourniquets, stethoscopes, blood pressure cuffs, laboratory work surfaces) that come in contact with intact skin and potentially are contaminated with body fluids. As with all disinfectants, visible body fluids should be removed from surfaces before the germicidal chemical is applied. Examples of intermediate-level disinfectants are the 1:10 and 1:100 dilutions of common household bleaches, phenolics, and formulated alcohol.

High-level disinfectants remove all forms of microbial life except bacterial spores present in high numbers. Reusable semicritical items that come in contact with mucous membranes or nonintact skin but do not enter tissue or vascular systems (oral thermometers, respiratory equipment, endoscopes) are usually immersed in the product for a specific time as directed by the manufacturer. Two percent (2%) glutaraldehydes and paracetic acid are common high-level disinfectants often used in surgical areas of the hospital.

The most effective disinfectants sterilize or destroy all viruses, bacteria, fungi, and their spores on inanimate surfaces. *Sterilants* are used on critical items that will enter tissue, vascular systems, or blood (needles, surgical equipment, catheters). Steam under pressure (autoclave), gas (ethylene oxide), dry heat, and liquid sterilants such as 2%-glutaraldehyde–based formulations, 6% stabilized hydrogen peroxide, peracetic acid, and demand-release chlorine dioxide are all considered sterilants when they are used under the conditions set by the manufacturer.

Limiting Transmission

Handwashing

Handwashing has been recognized for more than a century as the primary method to prevent the spread of infectious agents. Many guidelines for cleansing the skin have been published in recent years to support this practice.[7-9] Guidelines now indicate that plain soaps are probably sufficient for the routine 10-second handwashing procedure in health care settings, such as after performance of a routine phlebotomy; however, antiseptics are still recommended for certain high-risk situations, such as handling of newborns and immunosuppressed patients and in the clinical laboratory setting. Antiseptics—chemical agents formulated to be used on skin or tissue—are not used to decontaminate inanimate objects or surfaces. Besides handwashing, antiseptics are often used for skin preparation prior to phebotomy procedures, surgical procedures, and skin testing. Common antiseptics used in health care facilities are as follows.

Ethyl or isopropyl alcohols, in 70% to 90% concentrations, degerm the skin quickly by dehydration and coagulation; they are used to decontaminate the skin prior to routine phlebotomy. They are also found in rinses and foams for hand cleaning whenever running water and towels are not available.

Iodophores, which have excellent and fairly rapid antimicrobial activity, eliminate bacteria by oxidation. Although iodophores are often used as surgical preps and as skin preparation for phlebotomy for alcohol testing, this type of antiseptic is harsh on skin and stains skin and clothing.

Chlorohexidine gluconate (CHG) products contain an antimicrobial agent that is effective when used over time. This antiseptic does not act as quickly as alcohol but is milder and leaves a residual action on the skin, making it a common component of health care handwashing soaps.

The *parachlorometaxylenol* (PCMX) antiseptic products are also commonly used in handwashing soaps, particularly surgical scrubs. PCMX decontaminates by cell wall destruction and leaves good residual activity between washings with slight skin irritation.

In sites where adequate handwashing facilities are not available, antiseptic foams, which can be used without water, are excellent substitutes. More important than the agent used to clean hands, however, has been the issue of motivating health care workers to actually perform the procedure. Unfortunately, educational efforts to improve handwashing behavior have had only a minimal effect.

Isolation Guidelines

In 1996, the CDC released new isolation guidelines to minimize the transmission of microorganisms in health care facilities.[4] These guidelines combined the philosophies of "universal precautions" (designed to reduce the risk of transmission of blood-borne pathogens) and "body substance isolation" (designed to reduce the risk of transmission of pathogens from moist body substances). This two-tiered approach consists of "standard precautions" and three transmission-based categories: airborne, droplet, and contact.

Table 55–2 lists various clinical situations and the isolation practices recommended for them by the CDC.

STANDARD PRECAUTIONS

Standard precautions apply to blood, all body fluids (except sweat), secretions, nonintact skin, mucous membranes, and excretions regardless of whether or not they contain visible blood and regardless of the diagnosis of the patient. These precautions are designed to reduce the risk of transmission of microorganisms from both recognized and unrecognized sources of infection. The basic principles of standard precautions are as follows:

- Washing hands, even when gloves are worn, to avoid transfer of microorganisms to other patients or environments.
- Wearing gloves, masks, eye protection, and gowns when contact with any body fluids, tissues, or contaminated items is expected.
- Using mouthpieces and resuscitation devices for cardiopulmonary resuscitation.
- Handling contaminated items, such as linens, in a way to prevent further transfer of microorganisms.

TRANSMISSION-BASED CATEGORIES

The second level of transmission-based precautions is designed for patients documented or suspected to be infected with highly transmissible or epidemiologically important pathogens and for which additional precautions are needed. The following measures should be used to supplement standard precautions.

Airborne Precautions. These precautions are necessary for patients known or suspected to be infected with microorganisms transmitted by airborne droplet nuclei. The etiologic agents of measles, varicella, and tuberculosis can remain suspended in the air and can be widely dispersed by air currents within a room over a long distance.

With airborne precautions, the patient is placed in a private room that has monitored negative air pressure in relation to the surrounding areas. Air must either be discharged outdoors or, if air is circulated to other areas of the facility, through monitored high-efficiency filtration. The door should remain closed, and the patient should remain in the room. Cohorting of patients is acceptable. Respiratory protection, such as an N95 respirator approved by the National Institute for Occupational Safety and Health (NIOSH), should be worn by anyone entering the room. Susceptible employees should not enter rooms of patients known or suspected to have measles or varicella. Movement and transporting of the patient from the room should also be minimized. If necessary, the patient should wear a surgical mask when outside the room.

Droplet Precautions. In addition to standard precautions, droplet precautions should be used for patients known or suspected to be infected with microorganisms transmitted by large-particle droplets (i.e. pertussis, influenza) that can be generated by the patient during coughing, sneezing, or talking or by the performance of procedures. Ideally the patient is also placed in a private room but may be cohorted. Such a patient may even share a room with noninfected patients as long as a distance of at least 3 feet is maintained between the infected patient and other patients. Personnel should wear a mask, not a respirator, when working within 3 feet of the patient. Also, the patient's movement outside the room should be limited; the patient should wear a mask when outside the room.

Contact Precautions. In addition to standard precautions, contact precautions should be used for specified patients known or suspected to be infected or colonized with epidemiologically important microorganisms that can be transmitted by direct contact. Organisms of current

Table 55–2. Clinical Syndromes or Conditions Warranting Additional Empiric Precautions*

Clinical Syndrome or Condition†	Potential Pathogens‡	Empiric Precautions
Diarrhea		
Acute diarrhea with a likely infectious cause in an incontinent or diapered patient	Enteric pathogens§	Contact
Diarrhea in an adult with a history of recent antibiotic use	*Clostridium difficile*	Contact
Meningitis	*Neisseria meningitidis*	Droplet
Rash or exanthems, generalized, etiology unknown		
Petechial/ecchymotic with fever	*Neisseria meningitidis*	Droplet
Vesicular	Varicella	Airborne and contact
Maculopapular with coryza and fever	Rubeola (measles)	Airborne
Respiratory infections		
Cough/fever/upper lobe pulmonary infiltrate in an HIV-negative patient or a patient at low risk for HIV infection	*Mycobacterium tuberculosis*	Airborne
Cough/fever/pulmonary infiltrate in any lung location in an HIV-infected patient or a patient at high risk for HIV infection	*Mycobacterium tuberculosis*	Airborne
Paroxysmal or severe persistent cough during periods of pertussis activity	*Bordetella pertussis*	Droplet
Respiratory infections, particularly bronchiolitis and croup, in infants and young children	Respiratory syncytial or parainfluenza virus	Contact
Risk of multidrug-resistant microorganisms		
History of infection or colonization with multidrug-resistant organisms‖	Resistant bacteria	Contact
Skin, wound, or urinary tract infection in a patient with a recent hospital or nursing home stay in a facility where multidrug-resistant organisms are prevalent	Resistant bacteria	Contact
Skin or wound infection		
Abscess or draining wound that cannot be covered	*Staphylococcus aureus,* Group A streptococcus	Contact

*Such precautions aid in the prevention of transmission of epidemiologically important pathogens pending confirmation of diagnosis. Infection control professionals are encouraged to modify or adapt this table according to local conditions. To ensure that appropriate empiric precautions are implemented always, hospitals must have systems in place to evaluate patients routinely according to these criteria as part of their preadmission and admission care.

†Patients with the syndromes or conditions listed below may present with atypical signs or symptoms (e.g., pertussis in neonates and adults may not have paroxysmal or severe cough). The clinician's index of suspicion should be guided by the prevalence of specific conditions in the community, as well as clinical judgment.

‡The organisms listed in the column "Potential Pathogens" are not intended to represent the complete, or even most likely, diagnoses, but rather possible etiologic agents that require additional precautions beyond standard precautions until they can be ruled out.

§These pathogens include enterohemorrhagic *Escherichia coli* O157:H7, *Shigella*, hepatitis A, and rotavirus.

‖Resistant bacteria judged by the infection control program, the basis of current state, regional, or national recommendations, to be of special clinical or epidemiologic significance.

From Garner JS: The Hospital Infection Control Practices Advisory Committee: Guidelines for isolation precautions in hospitals. Infect Control Hosp Epidemiol 17:53, 1996.

concern include multidrug-resistant bacteria, *Clostridium difficile, E. coli* O157:H7, and rotavirus. Contact consists of hand or skin-to-skin contact during patient care activities that require touching the patient's dry skin; indirect contact is touching environmental surfaces or patient care items in the patient's environment. In general, these precautions expand standard precautions from using protection when coming in contact not only with body fluids but also with the body itself or environment contaminated by the body. Personnel should wear gloves when entering the patient's room and should change when they are contaminated or when leaving the room. When body contact with the patient or the contaminated environment is expected, clean, nonsterile gowns should be worn. Movement and transportation of the patient should be limited to essential services. Patient care items, bedside equipment, and frequently touched surfaces should receive daily cleaning. If possible, noncritical patient care items such as tourniquets should be dedicated to a specific patient. If use of common equipment or items is unavoidable, the items should be adequately cleaned and disinfected between patient uses.

SURVEILLANCE AND EPIDEMIOLOGIC INVESTIGATION

In the health care setting, surveillance is used to identify nosocomial infections and other adverse events that may be prevented.[10] At the First International Conference on Nosocomial Infections, the CDC implemented initial recommendations for a national surveillance program of nosocomial infections in patients. In the 1980s, this surveillance was expanded to include assessment of risk to the hospital employee as well. To validate the effectiveness of a surveillance program, the CDC established the Study on the Efficacy of Nosocomial Infection Control (SENIC) project.[11] The SENIC study involved a representative sample of U.S. hospitals from 1976 to 1985.[12] In 1985, using data from the SENIC project, Haley and colleagues[13] projected an overall rate of nosocomial infections at 5.7 per 100 admissions or at least 2.1 million nosocomial infections occurring annually in hospitals at an estimated nationwide cost of $3.8 billion. This cost included extra charges for antibiotics, prolonged hospital stays, and further medical interventions. On the basis of the initial SENIC study findings, it was determined that one-third of these infections could be avoided with the establishment of an intensive surveillance program.

The overriding objective for a surveillance program is to provide data for improvement of patient care outcomes and processes. The basic elements of nosocomial surveillance programs among institutions are as follows:

- Defining categories of infection
- Systematically finding and collecting data

- Tabulating data
- Analyzing and interpreting data
- Reporting relevant infection surveillance
- Implementing appropriate actions

A simple set of definitions developed by the CDC for surveillance was piloted by hospitals participating in the National Nosocomial Infection Survey (NNIS) in 1987 and has now been integrated into most hospital surveillance programs.[14] For example, for a facility to classify an infection as a blood infection, a positive culture must be documented from the laboratory with contaminant possibility ruled out.

Types of Surveillance

Traditional or "whole-house" surveillance systems have been used successfully for years. In this system, all infections from all patients or populations are included. This method can give a "big picture" of the types of infections encountered and help to establish baseline data. It is, however, very costly and time consuming. Many facilities have now moved to targeted surveillance programs to maximize resources and to generate meaningful data in a few specific areas, such as surgical wound infections or intravenous catheter sites.[15] In targeted surveillance, only patients with the targeted concern are included in the study.

Another useful and often used surveillance system is known as "surveillance by objective," or SOB. This system uses quantitative objectives to study priority, problem-oriented processes, procedures, or case types. For example, SOB might be used to calculate incidence rates occurring with coronary arterial bypass grafts in a large teaching medical center.

Sources of Infection Data

A wide variety of sources of infection information, from both within and outside the hospital, must be utilized to ensure a complete picture. Concurrent case findings are strongly preferred to retrospective reviews. Concurrent reviews tend to be more complete and provide the ICP the opportunity to gain first-hand knowledge of the infection while interacting with the staff at the time of the concern.

Typical sources of data for most facilities include review of laboratory reports, chart reviews, antibiotic monitoring, radiology reports, ward rounds, discharge summaries, and post-discharge follow-up. Examination of laboratory data should include culture results and antimicrobial susceptibility patterns. Clusters of organisms according to unit, site, and antimicrobial susceptibility patterns should also be monitored. Unit-specific surveillance of antimicrobial susceptibilities may demonstrate changes in susceptibility patterns that may correlate with antimicrobial use.

Data Documentation

When an infection meets the established criteria for a nosocomial infection, the pertinent data that should be documented are any information that will be useful in determining the infection and its causes. Typically, these data will include patient's name, age, sex, hospital number, ward, and service, the admission and infection onset dates, and the organism and antimicrobial susceptibility patterns. Information regarding culture results, clinical features including the presence of fever, and pertinent physical findings and laboratory data, such as chest x-ray and white blood cell count, are also recorded. Predisposing factors, such as surgery, chemotherapy, antibiotics, steroids, and underlying disease, as well as exposure factors, such as urinary or intravenous catheters, are also important to record. These data do not become part of the patient's medical record, but rather are tools to assist the ICP.

Data Analysis and Reporting

Each nosocomial infection becomes one entity in a statistical review. The most common statistic reported is the *incidence rate*—the proportion of new cases of a disease occurring in a population in relation to the number of persons at risk for developing the disease.[16] Most acute care facilities calculate incidence rates as infections per 100 discharges or infections per 1,000 patient days. Because the number of resident discharges from a long-term care facility is usually low, the average census per month or the number of resident-days is often used to calculate incidence rates for these facilities.

The attack rate is a type of incidence rate used to describe clusters or outbreaks. It is appropriate when the population is at risk for a limited period only and the study period incorporates the entire epidemic. *Attack rate* is the proportion of persons who develop an illness in relation to the total number exposed.

Another important epidemiologic rate is the *prevalence rate*. This is the number of persons with a disease at any given time relative to the total number of persons in a group. Such a rate is usually determined with data accumulated over a single 24-hour period. Prevalence rates can often assist in testing the validity of monthly incidence rates; they also may identify hidden trends.

Caution should be used in comparing statistics such as these from several other facilities, to avoid erroneous conclusions. Each facility has its own acuity level and individualized methods of gathering, identifying, and calculating rates. These data should be used only for internal comparison, in order to change the behavior of persons or environmental factors, with the ultimate goal to minimize incidence rates. This information should, however, be shared as a "progress report" with administration, physicians, and staff as appropriate.

EPIDEMICS

Infected sites involved in outbreaks tend to differ from the usual endemic situations. In epidemics, blood stream infections predominate, followed by surgical wound infection, pneumonia, gastrointestinal infection, and meningitis. Similarly, the pathogens vary markedly from those seen in endemic infections. For example, from 1956 to 1990, the CDC investigated more than 381 hospital outbreaks. The problems most commonly noted by investigators were epidemics due to gastrointestinal *Salmonella* species and *E. coli* as well as *S. aureus* infections in newborn nurseries. Later investigators found gram-negative pathogens, bacteremias, surgical wound infections, and problems related to intensive care units, newly introduced medical devices, and invasive procedures. Outbreaks of hepatitis A and B, necrotizing enterocolitis in nurseries, sternal wound infections following open-heart surgery, and nosocomial legionnaires' disease are currently being reported. The emergence of microorganisms resistant to multiple antimicrobials, particularly vancomycin-resistant enterococcus (VRE), methicillin-resistant *S. aureus* (MRSA), and multidrug-resistant *M. tuberculosis* are also of concern in current outbreak situations.[2]

Even though infection control programs have greatly reduced nosocomial infections, outbreaks still occur. In general, outbreaks are considered preventable and should always be investigated. Once a facility's established threshold of concern has been surpassed, the investigation begins with a preliminary case review to evaluate clinical severity. Pseudoepidemics, generally caused by surveillance artifact or laboratory errors, must also be ruled out. If the outbreak is similar to any that have previously occurred, usual effective infection prevention and control measures should be implemented. A major investigation is necessary, however, if the problem is unusual, complex, or of substantial scientific importance or when the basic investigation has been unsuccessful.[17]

Today's health care facility cannot afford to investigate every nosocomial infection that occurs. Infection control programs should focus efforts and time on preventable infections rather than evaluating issues that cannot be affected by changes in practices. In fact, the Joint Commission for the Accreditation of Healthcare Organizations (JCAHO) now evaluates infection control programs on the basis of outcomes rather than the extent of their programs.

ROLE OF THE LABORATORY

The clinical laboratory is essential in efforts to recognize and control nosocomial infections. The isolation and identification of pathogens are the first steps in any surveillance and control program. Species identification is especially important for coagulase-negative staphylococci (CNS), the enterococci, and mycobacteria, as are the antimicrobial susceptibility patterns of these organisms, because resistance to therapeutic agents continues to grow. When an unusually resistant organism or otherwise suspected nosocomial organism is encountered by the laboratory, both the clinician and the ICP should be contacted, so that therapeutic or control procedures can be implemented. In many instances, the laboratory is the first to recognize a possible problem. With respect to unusual antimicrobial resistance, ongoing monitoring and tabulation of antimicrobial susceptibility patterns in the hospital are extremely important, so that deviations from the norm can be recognized and evaluated in a timely manner.

When the ICP undertakes an epidemiologic investigation, the laboratory should be prepared to save isolates associated with the cases being analyzed in case further testing is necessary. The laboratory may also be called upon to assist in identifying possible reservoirs and to undertake typing procedures to further elucidate the etiology of outbreaks in the hospital. Participation in educational efforts for hospital or facility staff is also an important contribution of laboratory practitioners.

The challenge for the clinical laboratory and the clinical laboratory scientist is to provide timely, effective assistance and yet maintain a cost-effective response. This balance requires careful collaboration with the ICP so that overutilization or inappropriate testing can be avoided. In addition to biotyping, antimicrobial susceptibility testing, and serotyping, methods utilized to determine whether isolates represent a single strain of the suspected organism are bacteriophage and bacteriocin typing, various electrophoretic protein typing techniques, and gene typing techniques. Although many of the more sophisticated techniques are not feasible for the routine laboratory, the standard typing (biotyping and antimicrobial susceptibility testing) should be available. More esoteric typing should be obtained from reference laboratories with this expertise, so that the epidemiologic investigation can be complete.[18–20]

Case Study 1

One floor of an acute care hospital reported an unusual number of urinary tract infections and bacteremias associated with *Serratia marcescens* during a short period. Upon chart review by the infection control practitioner, it was noted that all patients in question had orders for urine specific gravity determinations. Procedure for this diagnostic test included the patient's saving the urine to be tested by the nurse on the floor. A common urine collection device was used for all patients.

Questions

1. What is the most likely source of the outbreak?
2. What steps should be taken to minimize the recurrence?
3. What is the role of the laboratory in controlling such nosocomial outbreaks?

Discussion

1. The most likely source and reservoir are the urine collection containers and the specific gravity devices. No documented routine disinfection was noted by procedure or in staff interviews for either piece of equipment. Cultures from both yielded *S. marcescens*. Transmission was most likely through contaminated hand contact.
2. After control measures are established and documented, the infection control practitioner, epidemiologist, or clinical laboratory scientist should conduct a nursing in-service program to explain how organisms are transmitted from patient to patient on hands and that standing reservoirs of urine can actually increase the quantities of the organisms. Nurses should be instructed to use new collection containers for each patient, to disinfect the specific gravity devices after each use, and to wash their hands after handling each patient sample. To illustrate the point, sample culture plates of *S. marcescens* with colony counts could be demonstrated and explained.

The infection control practitioner should continue to monitor for reappearance of the organism and for recurrence of problematic nursing practices. Additional in-service programs should be conducted if previous practices recur.

3. The role of the laboratory consists of reporting all isolates to the infection control department; devising optimized culture techniques to detect the agent in question; providing guidance on the selection of sites to be cultured; assisting in teaching about the organism and its transmission; and continuing monitoring for the agent in the future.

Case Study 2

A series of *S. aureus* isolates from cerebrospinal fluid (CSF) was noted on one nursing unit within a few days. Initial investigation noted that no single physician or assistant was involved in all cases. Even though two different types of lumbar puncture trays were utilized, a common multi-dose bottle of antiseptic was observed to be used for all the skin preparations. The bottle was removed, along with others of the same lot number, examined, and cultured. Although no etiologic agents were cultured from the skin preparation agent, removal of the bottles coincided with the end of the outbreak.

Questions

1. What appears to be the source of the outbreak?

2. What steps should the laboratory take to increase the possibility of isolating an organism from this source?

3. What other explanations might account for the end of the outbreak?

Discussion

1. The common bottle of antiseptic solution used for skin preparation is the most likely source.

2. The skin preparation should be filtered to concentrate the organisms, and its antibacterial activity should be neutralized prior to culture.

3. If the antiseptic bottle was not the source, some other unidentified nursing practice was altered during the investigation, resulting in the end of the outbreak.

References

1. National Nosocomial Infections Surveillance (NNIS) Semiannual Report, May 1995, Special Communications. Am J Infect Control 23:377, 1995.
2. Marone WJ, Jarvis WR, Culver DH, Haley RW: Incidence and nature of endemic and epidemic nosocomial infections. *In* Bennent JV, Brachman PS (eds): Hospital Infections, ed 3. Boston, Little, Brown 1992.
3. Bennett JV, Scheckler WE, Make DG, Brachman PS: Current national patterns: United States. *In* Proceedings of the International Conference on Nosocomial Infections, August 3–6, 1970. Chicago, American Hospital Association. 1971.
4. Garner JS: The Hospital Infection Control Practices Advisory Committee: Guidelines for Isolation Precautions in Hospitals. Infect Control Hosp Epidemiol 17:53, 1996.
5. Rutalla WA: Draft APIC guidelines for selection and use of disinfectants. Am J Infect Control 23:35A, 1995.
6. Spaulding EH: Chemical disinfection of medical and surgical materials. *In* Lawrence CA, Block SS (eds): Disinfection, Sterilization and Preservation. Philadelphia, Lea & Febiger, 1968.
7. Larson EL, and the 1992, 1993 and 1994 APIC Guidelines Committees: Draft APIC guideline for handwashing and hand antisepsis in health care settings. Am J Infect Control 22:25A, 1994.
8. Larson E: Guidelines for use of topical antimicrobial agents. Am J Infect Control 16:253–266, 1988.
9. Association of Operating Room Nurses: Standards and Recommended Practices for Perioperative Nursing: Recommended Practices for Surgical Scrub III. Denver, Colo, The Association of Operating Room Nurses, 1990.
10. Wenzel RP: Is there infection control without surveillance? Chemotherapy 34:548–552, 1988.
11. Haley RW, Quade D, Freeman HE, Bennett JV; The CDC SENIC Planning Committee: The SENIC project; study of the efficacy of nosocomial infection control; summary of study design. Am J Epidemiol 111:472–485, 1980.
12. Quade D, Culver DH, Haley RW, et al: The SENIC sampling process—design for choosing hospitals and patients and results of sample selection. Am J Epidemiol 111:486–502, 1980.
13. Haley RW, Culver DH, White JW, et al: The nationwide nosocomial infection rate: A new need for vital statistics. Am J Epidemiol 121:159–167, 1985.
14. Garner JS, Jarvis WR, Emori TG, et al: CDC definitions for nosocomial infections, 1988. Am J Infect Control 16:128–140, 1988.
15. Perl TM: Surveillance, reporting and the use of computers. *In* Wenzel RP (ed): Prevention and Control of Nosocomial Infections, ed 2. Baltimore, William & Wilkins, 1993.
16. Rusnak PE, Horning LA: Surveillance in the long term care facility. *In* Smith PW (ed): Infection Control in Long Term Care Facilities, ed 2. Albany, NY, Delmar Publishers, 1994.
17. Dixon RE: Investigation of endemic and epidemic nosocomial infections. *In* Bennett JV, Brachman PS (eds): Hospital Infections, ed 3. Boston, Little, Brown, 1992.
18. Herwaldt LA, Wenzel RP: Dynamics of hospital acquired infection. *In* Murray PR, Baron EJ, Pfaller MA et al (eds): Manual of Clinical Microbiology. Washington, DC, ASM Press, 1995.
19. McGowan, JE Jr, Metchock B: Infection control epidemiology and clinical microbiology. *In* Murray PR, Baron EJ, Pfaller MA, et al (eds): Manual of Clinical Microbiology. Washington, DC, ASM Press, 1995.
20. Arbeit RD: Laboratory procedures for the epidemiologic analysis of microorganisms. *In* Murray PR, Baron EJ, Pfaller MA, et al (eds): Manual of Clinical Microbiology. Washington, DC, ASM Press, 1995.

Chapter 56

Infections in the Immunocompromised Host

Linda L. Ross

The *immunocompromised host* is an individual without normal host defense mechanisms. Organisms that do not cause disease in individuals with normal immune systems often act as *opportunists,* causing diseases known as *opportunistic infections* in these persons.[1] Infectious complications in the immunocompromised host have higher morbidity and mortality, often supplanting the primary disease as the cause of death. From 1980 to 1992, the rate of death due to infectious agents rose from 41 to 65 deaths per 100,000 population in the United States, an increase of 58%.[2] Infectious diseases are currently the third leading cause of death, preceded only by heart disease and cancer.[3]

Organ transplantation, intensive radiation and chemotherapy, treatment with corticosteriods, extensive prophylactic and therapeutic administration of antibiotics, use of intravascular catheters, and the increase in the population of patients with human immunodeficiency virus (HIV) are contributing to the dramatic increase in the numbers of immunocompromised patients. The number and nature of opportunistic microorganisms are also changing. This change is due to improved culturing techniques, better recognition of organisms by the clinical laboratory, and identification of new agents of disease, such as *Bartonella henselae,* the cause of bacillary angiomatosis.[4] Therefore, the definition of immunocompromised host depends on the type and extent of the deficiency of normal defense mechanisms and the pathogenicity of the organism.[1]

HOST DEFENSE MECHANISMS

A number of distinct yet interactive mechanisms protect the host from invasion of foreign microorganisms. They are physical and motility barriers, chemical antagonism, action of the phagocytic cells, and humoral and cell-mediated immunity[1] (Box 56–1). The skin and mucous membranes act as physical barriers and are the host's first line of defense. The antimicrobial activity of fatty acids in the skin, lysozyme and lactoferrin in the saliva, ciliated cells of the lungs, coughing, the flushing action of tears, the acidity, mucus, and peristalic action of the gastrointestinal tract, and regular urine voiding act locally to remove or kill microorganisms.[5] The female genital tract secretes glycogen, which is fermented by vaginal normal flora, in turn producing an acidic milieu that inhibits potential pathogens.

The phagocytic system encompasses the polymorphonuclear neutrophils (PMNs) and eosinophils that act systemically, monocytes in the blood, and tissue macrophage cells. The first phagocytes to reach an infected area are the PMNs, which can nonspecifically phagocytize some organisms. Eosinophils seem to be essential in the removal of immune complexes. Alveolar macrophages remove microbes that enter the lungs and tissue macrophages act similarly as the Kupffer's cells of the liver and as histiocytes in other tissues eliminating circulating particles and microorganisms.

The fourth element in host defense systems is the hu-

Box 56–1. Host Defense Mechanisms

Anatomic barriers
  Skin
  Mucous membranes
Chemical and motility barriers
  Skin—fatty acids and normal flora
  Conjunctiva—tears for flushing, lactoferrin, and lysozyme
  Respiratory tract
    Filtration (nasal hairs and ciliated tissues)
    Coughing
    Mucus
    Lysozyme
  Mouth, stomach, and GI tract
    Normal flora and saliva (mucus, lysozyme, and lactoferrin)
    Stomach acidity and mucus
    Peristaltic action of the GI tract
  Urinary tract—normal voiding of urine
  Female genital tract—glycogen, normal flora, acidic milieu
Phagocytic defenses
  Granulocytes
  Monocytes
  Tissue macrophages
Humoral immunity
  Complement
  Immunoglobulins
  Cytokines
Cell-mediated immunity
  T lymphocytes
    Cytotoxic T cells
    Natural killer T cells
    T-suppressor cells
  B lymphocytes

moral immunity, consisting of soluble and circulating specific and nonspecific effectors. The classical pathway of the complement system acts to lyse microbial cell membranes and release inflammation-enhancing substances. Triggered by a specific antigen-antibody complex, the complement schema cannot be considered nonspecific, although complement effector proteins act nonspecifically. Polysaccharides in the cell walls of bacteria and fungi, including the lipid A of endotoxin, can initiate an alternative pathway leading to cell lysis and release of protein fragments that act as chemotactic factors, promoting release of histamines. They also act as opsonins.[6] Fibronectin and tuftsin are serum factors that enhance the activity of phagocytosis and promote clearance of particles by the reticuloendothelial system.[5] Immunoglobulins (Igs) have long been recognized as specific factors that activate and bind complement, neutralize and agglutinate antigens, prevent attachment of microbes to the endothelium, and promote endocytosis. For example, secretory IgA, present in nonvascular fluids, binds to infectious agents such as respiratory pathogens and viruses and prevents their attachment. IgM initiates the complement cascade and aids in phagocytosis. Serum IgG, which can cross the placenta, inactivates some bacterial

toxins, prevents viruses from entering host cells, and, when bound to antigen, initiates the complement cascade. Produced by monocytes, macrophages, and T lymphocytes, the cytokines (lymphokines, interleukins, monokines, and colony-stimulating factors), which include a variety of polypeptides, have been recognized as critical to successful immune response by the host. Understanding of the role of cytokines in the immunologic cascade is increasing as advancements are made in understanding of the molecular biology of these substances.[5]

Much overlap and interaction exist between the humoral and cell-mediated defense systems. T-helper lymphocytes promote maturation of B lymphocytes and enhance antibody production in these cells. Stimulated by the binding of T-cell–independent antigens, such as lipopolysaccharide (LPS) and the flagella of some microbes, B lymphocytes produce specific antibodies, primarily IgM. T-suppressor cells regulate immune responses by preventing activation of T-helper cells. Cytotoxic T lymphocytes kill virus-infected host cells. The dynamic interplay among the host's defense mechanisms acts cumulatively to protect against the invading organism.

ENDOGENOUS MICROORGANISMS

The lifelong connection between humans and microorganisms is established at birth, when infants are colonized with organisms from the mother and from the surrounding environment. The surface of the skin of normal hosts is composed of a transient population of coagulase-negative staphylococci (CNS), *Corynebacterium, Propionibacterium* species, spore-forming gram-positive bacilli from the soil, and contaminating organisms from the intestinal tract. The mouth and upper respiratory tract are colonized with streptococci of the viridans group, coagulase-negative staphylococci, corynebacteria, nonpathogenic *Neisseria* and *Mycoplasma* species, yeasts, spirochetes, and anaerobes such as *Fusobacterium* species and *Prevotella melaninogenica.* Present also are organisms that, under other conditions, may be pathogenic, such as *Staphylococcus aureus, Neisseria meningitidis, Haemophilus influenzae, Streptococcus pneumoniae, S. pyogenes,* and members of the Enterobacteriaceae. Anaerobes predominate in the gastrointestinal (GI) tract including *Bacteroides fragilis* group, *Clostridium* species, *Eubacterium* species, and *Veillonella* species. Members of the Family Enterobacteriaceae, enterococci, and fungi also exist in the GI tract in large numbers. Male and female genital tracts are colonized with microorganisms. The predominant resident microbial flora of the female genital tract are *Lactobacillus,* but yeasts, the streptococcus viridans group, CNS, members of the Enterobacteriaceae family, and anaerobes also reside there.

Certain organisms, once acquired, are present, but long dormant in host macrophage cells. Fungi such as *Cryptococcus neoformans, Histoplasma capsulatum,* and *Pneumocystis carinii,* the *Mycobacterium* species, and viruses such as cytomegalovirus (CMV), Epstein-Barr virus (EBV), herpes simplex virus (HSV), and varicella-zoster virus (VZV) remain inactive.[7] Initial acquisition of these organisms may not result in serious infection but in the immune-depressed state, the host may succumb to systemic infection.[8, 9]

The normal flora of the host represent a dynamic, changing population. "New" flora are acquired by the host from the environment and from foods and water. New flora are influenced by the environment from which they come (community vs. hospital setting). Hospitalized patients become colonized with microorganisms in the hospital environment such as *Pseudomonas,* antibiotic-resistant strains of the Enterobacteriaceae, staphylococci, and enterococci. Antibiotic treatment, whether prophylactic or therapeutic, alters the host's normal flora, thus removing its protective effects and allowing for selection of resistant strains. Therapy with cytotoxic drugs and corticosteroids and empiric use of broad-spectrum antibiotics may result in depletion of normal flora, allowing *Candida* species to flourish.[10]

An understanding of the relationship between organism colonization and pathogenicity is critical to the understanding of the origins of an infection in the immunocompromised host[5] (Fig. 56-1). The immunocompromised host is as susceptible as persons with a functioning immune system to microbes with primary virulence factors. Poorly understood, however, are the complex factors that change a microbe into an invasive, opportunistic microorganism. Breaks in the integrity of the mucosal surfaces following cytotoxic therapy may predispose endogenous microbes, which colonize the oropharynx and gastrointestinal tract, to entry into the blood stream and lungs, resulting in infection.[11]

TYPES OF IMMUNOCOMPROMISED CONDITIONS

Many diseases and conditions that hinder the normal immune response have been identified over the past several decade. In many instances, specific organisms are associated with particular types of immunosuppression, as outlined in Table 56-1. Some children are born with inherited immune disorders, including congenital deficiencies in the production of components in the complement complex, defects in immunoglobulin synthesis, congenital disorders that result in defects in cell-mediated immunity (e.g., DiGeorge's syndrome), and severe combined immunodeficiency disease, which affects both cell-mediated and humoral immunity. Persons with antibody deficiencies are at risk for developing infections with encapsulated bacteria such as *S. pneumoniae, N. meningitidis,* and *H. influenzae.* Chronic granulomatous disease of childhood, a disease

of defects in the polymorphonuclear neutrophils (PMNs), predisposes children to infections with gram-negative bacteria and *Staphylococcus.*

The immune system may be also be depressed owing to a number of underlying conditions. Patients may have a decrease in the absolute number of leukocytes or may have a normal number of defective leukocytes. A critical factor in determining the risk of granulocytopenic patients with neoplastic conditions or organ transplantation is the number of circulating leukocytes, particularly PMNs. When the number of PMNs decreases to less than 0.5×10^9/L, particularly to less than 0.1×10^9/L, there is risk of severe infection.[12]

Cytotoxic drugs used to treat neoplasms, such as methotrexate and cyclophosphamides, depress bone marrow production of white blood cells. Radiation therapy can lead to granulocytopenia and damage to the skin and mucous membranes, allowing infective organisms a portal of entry. Suppression of the host inflammatory defense system is a complicating factor of therapy with prednisone and other corticosteroids used to treat rheumatoid arthritis and other autoimmune diseases. Successful treatment of the primary disease by the transplant physician, hematologist, oncologist, and rheumatologist has afforded individuals with neoplasms and HIV the chance for longer, productive lives, but the price paid for such success is the danger of life-threatening infections.

Neoplastic Conditions

The most common group of vulnerable hosts are those with neoplasms. The nature of the malignancy, the treatment protocol, or both may evoke immunosuppression. A direct consequence of the successful chemotherapy and radiation protocol is the higher risk of serious infections.[3, 7]

Hematologic Malignancies

Intensive chemotherapy protocols are administered to leukemic patients with the intent to induce remission. A granulocyte count of less than 1.0×10^9/L predisposes these patients to infection.[11] Bacterial pathogens are most commonly isolated from patients with leukemia and other granulocytopenic conditions. Infections caused by gram-negative organisms in the families Enterobacteriaceae and Pseudomonadaceae as well as those caused by staphylococci are common. α-Hemolytic streptococci have been recognized as pathogens in granulocytopenic persons after dental extraction or mucositis.[11] Pneumonia and bacteremia are common infections at the time of therapy. Patients receiving treatment for leukemia and myelodysplastic disorders are also at higher risk for developing invasive fungal infections.[10, 13] Disseminated candidiasis and pulmonary aspergillosis are two of the more common life-threatening fungal infections in these patients. Seen with increasing frequency are opportunistic fungi from the environment, such as *Fusarium* species, *Trichosporon* species, the phaeophyomycetes (dematiaceous fungi), *Scedosporium* species, and the zygomycetes.[10, 14] As the granulocyte count rebounds, the danger of infection persists. Impairments in cell-mediated immunity increase the risk of infection by fungi such as *Cryptococcus* species, *Nocardia* species, and

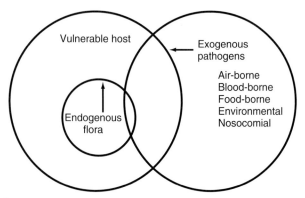

Figure 56-1. Relationship between the immunocompromised host and opportunistic pathogens.

Table 56–1. Relationship Between Host Immunodeficiencies and Specific Infection

Conditions of Immunosuppression	Defective Host Defense	Organisms Associated with Infection

Cytotoxic chemotherapy, myeloproliferative disorders, congenital disorders	Decrease in the number of functioning granulocytes	Bacteria
		  Enterobacteriaceae
		  Pseudomonas species
		  S. aureus
		  Coagulase-negative staphylococci
		Fungi
		  Candida species
		  Aspergillus species
		  Environmental fungi

AIDS, transplantation, long-term corticosteroid therapy, lymphoma, congenital disorders	Impaired cell-mediated immunity	Bacteria
		  Mycobacterium species
		  Legionella species
		  L. monocytogenes
		Fungi
		  Nocardia species
		  Cryptococcus species
		  P. carinii
		Parasites
		  T. gondii
		  Strongyloides stercoralis
		Viruses
		  Cytomegalovirus
		  Varicella-zoster virus
		  Herpes simplex virus
		  Epstein-Barr virus
		  Measles

AIDS, B cell malignancies, congenital and acquired hypoglobulinemia	Defects in antibody production	Bacteria
		  S. pneumoniae
		  H. influenzae type b
		  N. meningitidis

Congenital and acquired hypocomplementemic states	Defects in complement system	Bacteria
		  S. pneumoniae
		  H. influenzae type b
		  N. meningitidis
		Virus
		  Enterovirus

P. carinii, bacteria such as *Listeria monocytogenes* and *Legionella* species, and viruses in the herpes family.[7]

Patients with Hodgkin's disease, although not granulocytopenic, have defects in cell-mediated immunity, putting them at risk for developing infections characterized by granuloma formation, such as those due to *Mycobacterium* species, and those characterized by persistence in monocytes and macrophages, such as those due to *Salmonella* and *L. monocytogenes*.[11] There is risk of developing infection with encapsulated bacteria such as *S. pneumoniae* following splenectomy in patients with Hodgkin's disease.

Patients with a diagnosis of non-Hodgkin's lymphoma are predisposed to infections with aerobic bacteria because of aggressive treatment with cytotoxic drugs, radiation therapy, and breach of anatomic barriers by indwelling urinary and intravenous catheters. Urinary tract infections, pneumonia, and bacteremia are seen in individuals with lymphomas. Bacterial infections of the skin are observed in cutaneous lymphomas, illustrating the importance of the anatomic location of the primary disease.

Solid Tumors

Treatment of solid tumors may increase a host's susceptibility to infection, because patients treated with corticosteroids, cytotoxic therapies, and radiation may demonstrate neutropenia, and damage to the skin or mucous membranes. Infections with staphylococci, streptococci, and both aerobic and anaerobic gram-negative bacilli are observed in patients with solid tumors. Observed less commonly are infections due to *Aspergillus* species and other environmental fungi.[14]

Other Leukopenic Conditions

Treatment strategies for malignant neoplasms are not the only reasons for leukopenia. A small number of persons have congenital abnormalities in the structure and function of neutrophils, such as chronic granulomatous disease, Chédiak-Higashi syndrome, myeloperoxidase deficiency, and other rare conditions. A larger number of persons are leukopenic because of HIV infection.

Acquired Immunodeficiency Syndrome

Patients with acquired immunodeficiency syndrome (AIDS) due to HIV infection have mixed defects in the normal immune response to invading organisms. Opportunistic infections diminish the quality and duration of life for the approximately 1 million individuals who have HIV infection.[15] Impairments in the cell-mediated immune system, due to decreases in the population of T helper lymphocytes, make them vulnerable to infections with *Mycobacterium* species, especially *M. avium* complex (MAC), *L. monocytogenes,* and the *Legionella* species. Cryptosporidiosis, microsporidosis, and toxoplasmic encephalitis are parasitic infections to which the HIV patient is susceptible. Fungal infections in HIV patients individuals include those due to *Candida* species as well as *C. neoformans, Nocardia* species, and *P. carinii. P. carinii* pneumonia (PCP) is a common finding in persons with AIDS. Infections with viruses in the herpes family (e.g., CMV, HSV, and VZV) can cause serious complications in these severely immunocompromised patients.[14, 15]

Nonleukopenic Conditions

Patients with autoimmune disorders, such as systemic lupus erythematosus and rheumatoid arthritis, although not leukopenic, are treated with corticosteroids, which impair cell-mediated immunity. The neonate and elderly patient represent more subtle examples of the vulnerable host. The growing population of elderly persons has led to recognition of age as a factor in the pathogenesis of infection. Age-related dysfunction in cell-mediated immunity is known to predispose the elderly to bacterial and systemic fungal infections, including bacterial endocarditis.[16] Nutritional status of the host, breach in anatomic barriers such as occurs with use of intravascular and urinary catheters, and drug abuse are thought to be factors that alter immune status (Box 56–2).

Organ Transplantation

Transplant recipients are at risk for infection by a myriad of microorganisms from both endogenous and exoge-

nous sources. Use of immunosuppressive drugs such as cyclosporine to prevent rejection of the graft results in nonspecific immunosuppression, especially cell-mediated immunity. A relationship between the time following renal transplant and the causative agent involved in infection was identified by Rubin and Ferraro[7] and has application to infections following transplantation of bone marrow, liver, heart, lung, and other organs (Fig. 56–2). This timetable approach is useful to the physician and laboratorian as an infection control tool and as aid in the differential diagnosis of a specific patient who presents with signs of an infectious process.[7]

CLINICAL MANIFESTATIONS

Fever and Bacteremia

Unexplained fever in the immunocompromised patient starts the search for an etiologic agent. Sources of blood stream infection include respiratory tract infections, central nervous system infections, breaks in the integrity of the gut mucosa or other mucocutaneous surfaces, urinary tract infections, and intravascular catheters. Rapidly fatal septic shock may result from infections with gram-negative bacteria such as the Enterobacteriaceae and *Pseudomonas* species as well as staphylococci, streptococci, yeasts, and anaerobes.[17] Culture-negative sepsis often responds to a course of antimicrobial therapy (see Chapter 54).

Pneumonia

Conventional bacterial pneumonias are the most common cause of pulmonary infection in the vulnerable host and are a chief cause of death.[2] Pulmonary infiltrates may be absent in patients with active pneumonia; therefore, the presence of fever may be the only indication of developing infection.[12] Fever and cough may not be accompanied by

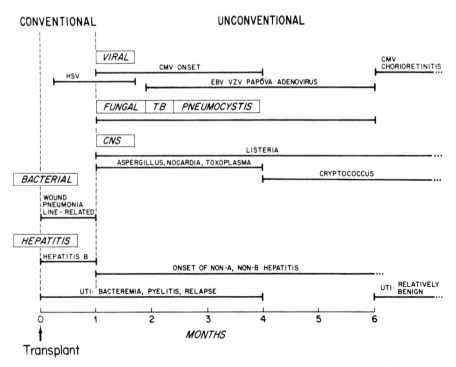

Figure 56–2. Timetable for occurrence of infection in the organ transplant recipient. Abbreviations: CMV, cytomegalovirus; HSV, herpes simplex virus; UTI, urinary tract infection; VZV, varicella zoster virus; EBV, Epstein-Barr virus; TB, tuberculosis; CNS, central nervous system. (Reprinted with permission from Rubin RH, Ferraro MJ: Understanding and diagnosing infectious complications in the immunocompromised host. Hematol Oncol Clin North Am 7:799, 1993.)

Nonleukopenic Conditions Resulting in Immunosuppression

Breach in anatomic barriers
  Surgical procedures
  Burns
  Severe trauma
  Intravascular and urinary tract catheters
Organ transplantation
  Kidney
  Bone marrow
  Liver
  Heart
  Lung
  Pancreas
Age
  Neonate
  Elderly
Metabolic abnormalities
  Malnutrition
  Alcoholism
  Drug abuse
  Diabetes mellitus
  Pregnancy
Autoimmune diseases
  Rheumatoid arthritis
  Systemic lupus erythematosus

patients may show a rapidly progressive fungal infection due to organisms such as *Curvularia, Bipolaris,* and other dematiaceous organisms (phaeohyphomycosis), which travel to the brain from the nasal passages or palatal region.[18]

Urinary Tract Infection

The vulnerable host is at no greater risk for developing urinary tract infections than the immunocompetent host, and the presence of a urinary catheter predisposes any person to the possibility of infection. Gastrointestinal flora, including members of the Enterobacteriaceae and the *Enterococcus* species, are common isolates from urine specimens. Isolation of *Candida* species from urine samples in granulocytopenic patients is significant as an indication of disseminated candidiasis.[10] Removal of the indwelling Foley catheter from patients with urinary tract infections is warranted whenever possible.

Other Infections

Gastrointestinal tract infections include esophagitis due to *Candida* species and herpes simplex virus, intra-abdominal infections, and perirectal cellulitis caused by a variety of anaerobes and *Enterococcus* species. Use of cytotoxic drugs and antibiotic therapy may permit overgrowth of the toxin-producing *Clostridium difficile,* resulting in pseudomembranous colitis.

production of sputum in the neutropenic patient, and radiologic changes may not be especially useful because of the wide array of potential pathogens presenting diverse patterns of infiltration of the lung. Bacterial pneumonia may be evident as consolidation and cavitation, whereas fungal infection may be indicated by a nodular pulmonary infiltrate. *P. carinii* and cytomegalovirus generally produce an interstitial pneumonia. Initial lung injury due to bacterial pathogens is often followed by secondary infection by unusual fungi (phaeohyphomycetes) and other opportunistic pathogens (Box 56–3).

Central Nervous System Infection

Central nervous system infections in the compromised host include meningitis, meningoencephalitis, and brain abscesses. Fever, stiff neck, headache, mental confusion, and other typical symptoms of infection may be slight. Meningitis may be due to encapsulated bacteria in patients with defects in antibody production. *L. monocytogenes* and *C. neoformans* can be isolated from patients with impaired cell-mediated immunity. Ventricular shunts provide skin flora, including coagulase-negative staphylococci, *Corynebacterium* species, and streptococci of the viridans group, with a portal of entry into the central nervous system. Chronic meningitis due to *Mycobacterium, Candida,* and *Nocardia* species as well as other fungal, bacterial, and parasitic agents may occur in immunocompromised patients. Meningoencephalitis may be caused by reactivation of viruses or *Toxoplasma gondii* in patients with AIDS and other cell-mediated immune defects. Immunosuppressed

Organisms Causing Pulmonary Infection in the Vulnerable Host

Bacteria
  Enterobacteriaceae
  Pseudomonas and related species
  S. aureus
  Legionella species
  Mycobacteria (tuberculosis and nontuberculosis)
Fungi
  Candida species
  Cryptococcus species
  Nocardia species
  Hyalohyphomycetes
  Aspergillus species
  Fusarium species
  Scedosporium species
Zygomycetes
  Mucor species
  Rhizopus species
Endemic mycoses
  H. capsulatum
  C. immitis
Parasites
  P. carinii
  Strongyloides stercoralis
Viruses
  Cytomegalovirus
  Herpes simplex virus

Infections of the skin are often seen in the vulnerable host. Lesions on the skin may indicate disseminated infection with organisms such as *Candida* species. Disseminated varicella-zoster virus is problematic in leukemic children, whereas, shingles, a reactivation of VZV, has commonly been observed in adults with impaired cell-mediated immunity.

LABORATORY ANALYSES AND DIAGNOSIS

For the most part, diagnosis of infectious diseases in the vulnerable host is handled in the laboratory just for the normal host; however, standard methods for cultivation of infectious agents may require modification. In addition to routine collection of blood and body fluids for culture, invasive procedures, including fine-needle aspiration, computed tomography (CT)–guided biopsies, and bronchoalveolar lavage (BAL) using fiberoptic bronchoscopy may be necessary to obtain fluids and tissue.[1, 19] Histologic analysis is important, because some organisms may be demonstrated only histologically or may be nonculturable.

Direct examination of the specimen in the microbiology laboratory aids in rapid determination of the infecting organism. Conventional Gram stains of specimens for visualization of bacteria may not be sufficient in the case of the immunocompromised patient. In addition to Gram stain, fluorescent stains such as acridine orange, to visualize low numbers of bacteria and cell-wall damaged organisms; calcofluor white, for *P. carinii* and fungi; and auramine rhodamine, for mycobacteria, are prepared from appropriate specimens and examined.[20] Immunofluorescent stains for *Legionella* species, cytomegalovirus, and herpes simplex virus are useful. Rapid reporting of direct smear results to the physician is important, because the immunocompromised patient must be started on empiric therapy without delay. Cultures for bacterial pathogens in the immunocompromised patient should be screened as they are for the normal host. Antimicrobial susceptibility testing should be performed on usual and unusual suspected pathogens.

Fever and Bacteremia

The clinical laboratory scientist must be mindful that unusual bacterial agents are commonly recovered from blood of the compromised host (Box 56–4). Intravascular catheters are often used in these patients, and although it is tempting to draw blood for culture from these devices, doing so must be avoided. Several studies have demonstrated positive blood cultures from specimens drawn through the cannula tip despite negative cultures from peripheral blood and the absence of sepsis.[16] Catheter-related sepsis due to coagulase-negative staphylococci and *Candida* species is a common cause of nosocomial infection in these patients, however, so culture of the intravascular catheter tip may be indicated when infection is suspected.[10, 21] Special attention should be given to skin preparation prior to collection of blood for culture, because isolation of coagulase-negative staphylococci, *P. acnes*, *Corynebacterium jeikeium,* or streptococci of the *viridans* group may indicate infection if these organisms can be

---

Box 56–4. Unusual Organisms Causing Bacteremia in the Vulnerable Host Bacteria

Bacteria
  Gram-positive
    Coagulase-negative staphylococci
    Streptococcus viridans group
    Enterococcus faecalis
    C. jeikeium
    L. monocytogenes
    Bacillus species
    P. acnes
  Gram-negative
    Salmonella species
    Shigella flexneri
    B. henselae
    Capnocytophaga species
    Campylobacter species and related organisms
  Mycobacteria
    M. tuberculosis
    M. avium complex (MAC)
    Mycobacterium other than tuberculosis (MOTTs)
Fungi
  Candida species
  Trichosporon species
  Rhodotorula species
  Malassezia furfur
  H. capsulatum
  Blastomyces dermatitidis
  Scedosporium species
  Fusarium species
Viruses
  Cytomegalovirus
  Human immunodeficiency virus

---

discounted as contaminants only (see Chapter 54). Isolation of these organisms from multiple blood culture bottles is indicative of bacteremia, and speciation of the bacteria helps the physician determine their significance.

Recovery of mycobacteria from blood was uncommon until the increase in recovery from individuals with AIDS; however, recovery of mycobacteria species other than tuberculosis (MOTTs) has been reported in patients with non-Hodgkin's lymphoma and hairy cell leukemia, increasing the need for blood culture techniques for mycobacteria.[8] Fungal blood cultures may also require special culturing techniques, such as [lysis-centrifugation] for isolation of *Candida, Trichosporon, Rhodotorula,* and other yeasts from the blood of the immunocompromised host.[21] Viral blood cultures for cytomegalovirus by shell vial assay are appropriate in both HIV-infected persons and transplant recipients.

Pneumonia

Respiratory specimens are often screened microscopically by laboratory personnel to determine the quality of the specimen (Q score) submitted for culture. Criteria for acceptance of sputa must be flexible enough to accommodate samples from immunocompromised patients with absence or low numbers of PMNs. Sputum collected from long hospitalized patients may be colonized with a number of bacterial species, making it difficult to determine which microbe is causing infection. Culture of BAL fluids and catheter-protected brushes has supplanted transtrachial aspiration as a means to avoid normal oropharyngeal flora.[19] Open pulmonary biopsy was utilized extensively in the 1970s and 1980s and was associated with a high rate of nonhealing because of the debilitative state of patients undergoing cytotoxic and steroid therapy. Ultrasonic or CT-guided transtracheal pulmonary aspiration or biopsy of peripheral lung lesions is currently in use.[1] These invasive procedures are not without risk in patients in whom hemorrage is possible. When pneumonia is suspected, blood specimens should also be collected for culture.

Central Nervous System Infection

Microorganisms responsible for meningitis are usually recovered from cerebrospinal (CSF) and ventricular fluid and may be observed from cytocentrifuged smears of fluid stained with Gram's stain, acridine orange stain, and others. Although the capsule of *C. neoformans* may be visualized with India ink stain, cryptococcal antigen testing by latex agglutination has greater sensitivity and specificity. Blood cultures specimens usually accompany CSF specimens, because the patient may be septic. The etiologic agent of brain abscesses is not often demonstrated in CSF; therefore, a biopsy specimen collected with the aid of radiologic or CT imaging for culture and histologic examination is indicated. As in other specimens from the vulnerable host, the presence of unusual pathogens should be suspected.

Urinary Tract Infection

Clean-catch midstream urine is the specimen of choice for diagnosis of urinary tract infections in both immunocompetent and compromised patients without urinary catheters. Urines may be screened for the presence of white blood cells using leukocyte esterase test strips. Quantitative cultures are performed, and bacterial counts of less than 10^5 colony-forming units (CFUs) per milliliter are considered significant.

Other Infections

Punch biopsy of the skin may be performed for histologic examination and culture of bacterial, fungal, and viral pathogens. Skin scrapings should be collected at the edges of obvious lesions. Observation of multinulceated giant cells in vesicular skin lesions following staining with Wright's, Giemsa's, Papanicolaou's or other available stains (Tzanck's smear) is useful to identify infection with varicella zoster virus in the compromised host.[22]

Patients with suspected esophagitis should be screened for the presence of *Candida* and herpes simples viruses by collection of scrapings for stain and cultures of these agents, because both may be present.[12] Stool specimens should be submitted for culture in cases of gastroenteritis and diarrhea. In addition to common enteric pathogens such as *Salmonella*, *Shigella*, and *Campylobacter*, the vul-

nerable host is susceptible to a number of unusual pathogens, including *Helicobacter cineadi* and *H. fennelliae*, which have been isolated from patients with AIDS.[23] Patients receiving long-term antibiotic and chemotherapy should be tested for the presence of *C. difficile* toxin if diarrhea occurs. Stool from patients with AIDS should be examined for the presence of *Cryptosporidium* and *Microsporidium* species.

Serologic testing for the diagnosis of infection has been disappointing in immunocompromised patients. Detection of antifungal antibodies is neither sensitive nor specific enough to be useful in establishing a diagnosis of fungal infection. Determination of viral infection using antiviral antibodies requires paired serum samples obtained at least 1 or 2 weeks apart in order to demonstrate a rise in titer. The mere presence of the IgM antibody is not sufficient to prove that cytomegalovirus is causing the disease syndrome under investigation; however, the presence of cryptococcal antigen in cerebrospinal fluid of patients suspected of having meningitis is diagnostic.

Traditional cultural approaches to identify infecting organisms from tissues and body fluids will continue to be utilized, augmented with non–culture-dependent technologies such as DNA probe and amplification techniques and specific monoclonal antibodies, to detect low numbers of microoganisms in clinical specimens in the immunosuppressed patient.

Other Laboratory Tests

Assessment of the hematologic state of the immunocompromised host is crucial to determine anemia, severity of neutropenia, thrombocytopenia, and coagulopathic changes. Other laboratory analyses, such as blood chemistry analysis, are performed when indicated to determine organ dysfunction. The level of immunosuppression at which opportunistic infection is most likely to occur is monitored in HIV-infected patients by measurement of CD4+ T lymphocyte counts.[24] Patients considered severely immunosuppressed have a CD4+ T lymphocyte count of less than 200 cells/µL.

PREVENTION AND TREATMENT STRATEGIES

Emphasis is placed on prevention of exposure to opportunistic pathogens and early detection of infection to permit directed treatment. Environmental exposure to opportunists during diverse activities, such as gardening, gathering wood, playing with pets in the home, using tobacco products, consuming raw foods, and traveling to foreign countries, may endanger immunocompromised persons.

Recommendations have been suggested for prevention of infection by 17 opportunistic agents for persons infected with HIV. These recommendations serve as guidelines for prevention of (1) exposure to opportunistic pathogens, (2) the first episode of infection by vaccination or chemoprophylaxis, and (3) disease recurrences through long-term maintenance antimicrobial therapy.[24] Factors considered in developing these recommendations are as follows:

- Level of immunosuppression at which opportunistic infection is most likely to occur

- Incidence of disease
- Severity of disease in terms of cost of care, morbidity and mortality
- Feasibility, efficacy, and cost of the preventive measure
- Impact of preventive measures on quality of life
- Drug toxicity, interaction, and potential for development of drug resistance[24]

Recommendations have similarly been made for immunization of bone marrow transplant recipients to include diphtheria and tetanus toxoid, inactivated killed polio vaccine, the polysaccharide vaccines (pneumococcus, meningococcus, and *H. influenzae* type B), measles, mumps, and rubella (MMR), and the influenza vaccine.[25] Vaccination against diphtheria, pertussis, and tetanus (DPT) and varicella zoster is recommended for patients with cancer or undergoing chemotherapy, especially the asplenic patient, in addition to those previously mentioned.[25]

Antibiotic therapy is guided by the specific offending organism isolated (see Chapter 58). Response to therapy is measured from the clearing of cultures of the opportunistic pathogen. Antimicrobial resistance has developed in immunocompromised hosts because of the extensive use of empiric therapy with antibacterial and antifungal drugs, which select for resistant organisms, further complicating treatment.[14, 26] During the course of antimicrobial therapy with the aminoglycosides, serum drug levels should be monitored to ensure that the therapeutic window of treatment is maintained without reaching toxicity. Serum bacteriostatic and bactericidal levels (Schlichter's test) may be requested for patients with severe infection.

Innovative therapies for treatment of infections in the compromised host that are currently under investigation include the use of biologic agents that can stimulate or modulate immunohematologic deficiencies.[27, 28] Referred to as interleukins, lymphokines, colony-stimulating factors, and cytokines, these proteins can stimulate the production and differentiation of myeloid progenitor cells as well as the function of mature phagocytes. Reports of their effectiveness are conflicting, and the future role of these innovative therapies remains to be defined. Issues that remain unanswered are whether the addition of cytokines to the treatment of infections improves survival rates and whether the use of cytokines is cost-effective. It is possible that cytokines will be utilized with antimicrobials to further improve the outcome of infectious complications in immunocompromised patients.

Case Study 1

A 63-year-old man, a resident of a small town, is admitted to a tertiary care hospital with fever (102 °F) of sudden onset and mental confusion. The patient has been taking 40 to 60 mg prednisone daily for the past 4 years for rheumatoid arthritis. Blood culture specimens were drawn, cerebrospinal fluid was collected, and he was started on erythromycin and ceftriaxone pending culture confimation of infection. When evidence of pulmonary and gastrointestinal bleeding was detected, bronchoscopy was performed. Thirty-four hours after specimen collection, Gram stain of the positive blood

cultures demonstrated a tiny gram-positive bacillus suspected of being *L. monocytogenes*. Biochemical tests confirmed the identity of the organism in both blood and CSF cultures. Antibiotic susceptibility tests showed the organisms to be resistant to clindamycin and erythromycin and sensitive to vancomycin.

Questions

1. What predisposed this particular patient to infection?
2. What is the most likely source of the infection?

Discussion

1. The patient was predisposed to infection because of treatment with corticosteroids, which impair cellular immunity.
2. *L. monocytogenes* can be found in the bowel as normal flora and can cause bacteremia in pregnant females and immunocompromised patients for reasons that remain unknown. The portal of entry is the gastrointestinal tract. Contaminated dairy and meat products can lead to outbreaks of systemic infection, because the organism can replicate at refrigeration temperatures (2 to 8 °C). Although any portion of the brain may be infected in CNS involvement, *Listeria* has a predilection for the brain stem.

Case Study 2

A 29-year-old female was admitted to the hospital for severe community-acquired pneumonia, which remained unresponsive to erythromycin therapy. Other than a case of "shingles" 3 months earlier, she had been in good health until 2 weeks prior, when she developed low-grade fever, shortness of breath, and tachycardia. Chest x-ray revealed bilateral interstitial infiltrates, and she was treated for bronchospasm. Gram stain of material obtained by bronchoscopy demonstrated what the clinical laboratory scientist described as "foamy, organized trash." Calcofluor white stain revealed organisms with a "double-parentheses"–like appearance resembling *P. carinii*. Subsequent testing revealed the patient to be HIV positive.

Questions

1. Following observation of the Gram stain, why was the clinical laboratory scientist suspicious that *P. carinii* might be the etiologic agent?
2. What course of treatment should be initiated for this infection?
3. What other laboratory tests would be useful in determination of the extent of immunosuppression in this patient?

Discussion

1. *P. carinii* stains faintly with Gram stain. The observation of a thick clump of precysts and cysts with

numbers of intracystic bodies and trophic forms overlying each other prompted initial suspicion. Stained with calcofluor white, the cyst walls and thickenings (double-parentheses–like) are highly fluorescent.

The increased incidence of HIV in the heterosexual population has resulted in recovery of unsuspected opportunistic pathogens from heretofore immunocompetent persons. Patients with infections that are unresponsive to treatment with conventional antimicrobials should be suspected of having infection with unusual microbes. Shingles, a reactivation of latent varicella zoster virus infection, has also been commonly observed in adults with impaired cell-mediated immunity.

2. USPHS (United States Public Health Service)/IDSA (Infectious Disease Society of America) Guidelines for prevention of opportunistic infections in persons infected with HIV recommend trimethoprim-sulfamethoxazole (TMP-SMZ) for treatment of PCP and to prevent recurrence of infection. Dapsone alone or in combination with other agents can be used if TMP-SMZ cannot be tolerated.

3. CD4+ T lymphocyte counts are recommended for determination of extent of immunosuppression. For example, the threshold for prophylaxis against disseminated infection with *M. avium* complex is a CD4+ T lymphocyte count less than 75 cells/μL in a HIV-infected adult.

References

1. Howard RJ: Infections in the immunocompromised patient. Surg Clin North Am 74:609–620, 1994.
2. Pinner RW, Teutsch SM, Simonsen L, et al: Trends in infectious diseases mortality in the United States. JAMA 275:189–193, 1996.
3. National Center for Health Statistics: Annual summary of births, marriages, divorces, and deaths: United States, 1993. Monthly Vital Statistics Report 42:13, 1994.
4. Armstrong D: History of opportunistic infection in the immunocompromised host. Clin Infect Dis 17(Suppl 2):S318–S321, 1993.
5. Hathorn JW: Critical appraisal of antimicrobials for prevention of infection in immunocompromised hosts. Hematol Oncol Clin North Am 7:1051–1099, 1993.
6. Miller JN, Baron EJ: Host-parasite interactions. *In* Baron EJ, Chang RS, Howard DH, et al (eds): Medical Microbiology: A Short Course. New York, Wiley-Liss, 1994.
7. Rubin RH, Ferraro MJ: Understanding and diagnosing infectious complications in the immunocompromised host. Hematol Oncol Clin North Am 7:795–812, 1993.
8. Young LS: Mycobacterial diseases and the compromised host. Clin Infect Dis 17(Suppl 2):SS436–S441, 1993.
9. Koll BS, Brown AE: Changing patterns of infections in the immunocompromised patient with cancer. Hematol Oncol Clin North Am 7:753–769, 1993.
10. Walsh TJ: Management of immunocompromised patients with evidence of an invasive mycosis. Hemotol Oncol Clin North Am 7:1003–1026, 1993.
11. Chanock S: Evolving risk factors for infectious complications of cancer therapy. Hematol Oncol Clin North Am 7:771–793, 1993.
12. Lee AW, Pizzo PA: Management of the cancer patient with fever and prolonged neutropenia. Hematol Oncol Clin North Am 7:937–959, 1993.
13. Walsh TJ, Hiemenz J, Pizzo PA: Evolving risk factors for invasive fungal infection: All neutropenic patients are not the same. Clin Infect Dis 18:793–798, 1994.
14. Vartivarian SE, Anaissie EJ, Bodey GP: Emerging fungal pathogens in immunocompromised patients: Classification, diagnosis, and management. Clin Infect Dis 17(Suppl 2):S487–S491, 1993.
15. Centers for Disease Control: Estimates of HIV prevalence and projected AIDS cases: Summary of a workshop, October 31–November 1, 1989. MMWR Morbid Mortal Wkly Rep 39:110–112, 1990.
16. Stratton CW: Blood cultures and immunocompromised patients. Clin Lab Med 14:31–49, 1994.
17. Sundaresan R, Sheagren JN: Current understanding and treatment of sepsis. Infect Med 12:261–268, 1994.
18. Saubolle MA, Sutton J: The dematiaceous fungal genus *Bipolaris* and its role in human disease. Clin Microbiol News 18:1–6, 1996.
19. Baselski VS, Wunderink MD: Bronchoscopic disgnosis of pneumonia. Clin Microbiol Rev 7:533–558, 1994.
20. Baselski VS, Robison MK, Pifer LW, Woods DR: Rapid detection of *Pneumocystis carinii* in bronchoalveolar lavage samples using calcofluor staining. J Clin Microbiol 28:393–394, 1990.
21. Jarvis WR: Epidemiology of nosomical fungal infections, with emphasis on *Candida* species. Clin Infect Dis 20:1526–1530, 1995.
22. Solomon AR: New diagnostic tests for herpes simplex and varicella zoster infections. J Am Acad Dermatol 18:218–221, 1988.
23. Allos BM, Lastovica AJ, Blaser MJ: Atypical campylobacters and related organisms. *In* Blaser MJ, Ravdin JI, Smith PD, et al (eds): Infections of the Gastrointestinal Tract. New York, Raven Press, 1995.
24. Center for Disease Control and Prevention: USPHS/IDSA Guidelines for the prevention of opportunistic infections in persons infected with human immunodiffency virus: a summary. MMWR Morbid Mortal Wkly Rep 44(No. RR-8):1–34, 1995.
25. Ambrosino DM, Molrine DC: Critical appraisal of immunizations stategies for prevention of infection in the compromised host. Hematol Oncol Clin North Am 7:1027–1049, 1993.
26. Shlaes DM, Binczewski B, Rice LB: Emerging antimicrobial resistance and the immunocompromised host. Clin Infect Dis 17(Suppl 2):S527–S536, 1993.
27. Roilides A, Pizzo PA: Modulation of host defenses by cytokines: Evolving adjuncts in prevention and treatment of serious infection in immunocompromised hosts. Clin Infect Dis 15:508–524, 1992.
28. Roilides A, Pizzo PA: Biologicals and hematopoietic cytokines in prevention or treatment of infections in immunocompromised hosts. Hematol Oncol Clin North Am 7:841–857, 1993.

Chapter 57

Osteomyelitis

Louis B. Caruana

Osteomyelitis is an infection of the bone and bone marrow that may be acute or chronic. The infection is usually caused by gram-positive cocci such as *Staphylococcus aureus*, but a variety of gram-negative bacteria, fungi, rickettsiae, and viruses may be implicated as etiologic agents. The number of unusual organisms that have been found to cause osteomyelitis is expanding; however, *Staphylococcus* is the most commonly isolated infectious agent in pyogenic osteomyelitis. The acute infection occurs more often in children than in adults. The most common sites in children are the distal end of the femur and the proximal ends of the tibia, humerus, and radius. In adults, the acute infection occurs most frequently in the pelvis and vertebrae.

Osteomyelitis is considered a surgical disease and as such requires the attention of the orthopedic surgeon and the clinician.[1-3] Prolonged antimicrobial therapy, selected on the basis of culture and susceptibility data and often administered in conjunction with drainage and debridement, is critical to the successful treatment of osteomyelitis.[4] With prompt treatment, the prognosis of acute osteomyelitis is good, but the prognosis is poor for the chronic form. If not diagnosed during the acute state or if inadequately treated, the infection may persist to become chronic.[4]

ETIOLOGY AND PATHOPHYSIOLOGY

Osteomyelitis may affect any age group and either sex, but the disease is usually found in children and adolescents in whom bone is still growing. It is more common in boys than in girls. Pyogenic vertebral osteomyelitis is uncommon in children younger than 10 years, but from ages 10 to 19 years, there is increased frequency in this form of the disease. The majority of cases, however, occur in males older than 50 years. Diabetics, as well as other compromised hosts such as heroin addicts, appear to have a predilection for vertebral osteomyelitis. Infections of the bones are usually the result of blood-borne (hematogenous) spread to the infected site but may also result from trauma with secondary infection. Osteomyelitis may also arise by spread of infection from a contiguous abscess; however, involvement of the bone in addition to subcutaneous or surrounding tissues must be confirmed.[5] Increasingly common forms of this disease are vertebral osteomyelitis, seen in immunocompromised adults,[6-8] and clavicular osteomyelitis, a complication of the use of subclavian catheters.[9] Osteomyelitis of the pubis has been reported after surgical procedures such as prostatectomy, bladder resection, and urethral suspension.[10] Osteomyelitis of the skull bones has been reported but is a relatively rare disease.[11] Today, acute osteomyelitis occurs less commonly than in the past because of effective antimicrobial treatment; however, if treatment is not adequate in amount or duration, chronic osteomyelitis will result.[12]

The onset of acute osteomyelitis is usually abrupt but can be insidious. If the infected bone or bones are left untreated or inadequately treated, chronic osteomyelitis leads to avascular necrosis of the affected site. No specific criteria separate acute from chronic osteomyelitis. Clinically, newly diagnosed bone infection is considered acute, whereas recurrent infection, characterized by the presence of a large area of dead bone (sequestrum), is considered the chronic stage of the disease. The high frequency of infection of the metaphyses of the bone suggests that this site is susceptible to bacterial infection. It is possible that the decreased blood flow with subsequent decreased numbers of phagocytes favors the growth of organisms at this site and, consequently, their spread to the entire bone. Because children with rich red-marrowed bones are affected more commonly than adults, it has been suggested that bones rich in red marrow favor bacterial colonization.

Etiologic agents responsible for osteomyelitis reach the bones through one of three routes: (1) hematogenous spread, (2) extension from a contiguous site of infection, and (3) direct penetration through the overlaying skin as a result of trauma or surgery.

Hematogenous Causes

The bone marrow may be seeded with an organism following a blood-borne systemic disease, such as bacterial endocarditis, brucellosis, mycosis, typhoid fever, or tuberculosis, to produce a latent source for subsequent infection. *S. aureus* causes 60% to 90% of acute hematogenous bone infections in children younger than 12 years, although adults can be affected as well.[13–15] *S. aureus* is often found to be penicillin-resistant in cases of osteomyelitis. *S. aureus* osteomyelitis has been reported in adult males with human immunodeficiency virus (HIV)[15] Acute hematogenous osteomyelitis in children commonly localizes in the diaphyseal ends of the long bones, especially the femur and tibia. The infection originates in the metaphyseal sinusoidal veins, where blood flow is diminished and the lack of phagocytic leukocytes favors the growth of infectious organisms. *Streptococcus pyogenes* and *Staphylococcus* species other than *aureus*, as well as gram negative bacilli, may be implicated.

The number of unusual organisms found to cause osteomyelitis is expanding, possibly owing to better isolation and identification methods. In a recent case study report, the authors confirmed *Corynebacterium jeikeium* as the causative bacterium of osteomyelitis of the fifth metatarsal bone.[16] Gram negative bacilli are responsible for vertebral infections in adults, whereas Group B streptococci are emerging as agents commonly found in neonatal osteomyelitis.[12]

Osteomyelitis is a well-recognized complication of sickle cell disease, and although the etiologic agent is usually *Salmonella*, it may also be caused by other gram-negative organisms, such as *Escherichia coli* and *Haemophilus influenzae*.[12–14, 17–19] Anaerobes such as *Bacteroides* species or *Actinomyces* species have also been reported.[20]

A single microbic organism is usually responsible for the infection in hematogenous osteomyelitis. Polymicrobic hematogenous osteomyelitis is rare.

Contiguous Focus

Bone infections from a contiguous abscess, often associated with diabetic foot ulcers, can have a wide range of etiologic agents and, according to some reports, may even be polymicrobic. *S. aureus* is the organism isolated most commonly in these cases, but a variety of gram-negative organisms may be implicated, especially in the immunocompromised patient.[21] Novel routes of bone infection should not be overlooked. For example, sneakers were found to be a source of *Pseudomonas aeruginosa* in children with osteomyelitis of the foot following puncture wounds.[22, 23] Human bites, if deep enough, may result in osteomyelitis due to indigenous anaerobic mouth flora. The pathogen most commonly isolated from wounds inflicted by domestic animal bites is *Pasteurella multocida*, but other species, such as *P. pneumotropica, P. ureae, P. haemolytica*, and *Eikenella corrodens*, may be isolated in cases of contiguous focus etiology.[24, 25] Because the infection develops as a direct extension of the local infection, multiple aerobic and anaerobic bacteria may be isolated from the infected bone.

Direct Penetration via Trauma or Surgery

Penetrating trauma or surgery, in which local infection gains access to traumatized bone, offers another focus route

of infection. Insertion of prostheses in or adjacent to the bone and other surgical procedures for nontraumatic bone or joint disorders offer additional routes of infection. The likely organism implicated is *S. aureus*, but aerobic gram-negative bacilli may be the causative agent as well.[26]

CLINICAL MANIFESTATIONS

Acute Osteomyelitis

Acute osteomyelitis should be suspected in febrile patients with localized bone pain. Generally, it is characterized by local pain, fever, swelling, and tenderness to palpitation over the affected site. Infections usually occur in the hip, vertebrae, sacroiliac joints, or other deep-seated bones.[27, 28] The clinician should suspect osteomyelitis in cases of rheumatic fever, rheumatoid arthritis, septic arthritis, cellulitis, and tumor. Hematogenous infection of a long bone in children or of vertebrae in adults may be more easily overlooked than an infected peripheral joint.

The abrupt onset of pain of increasing severity and fever are the cardinal signs of osteomyelitis. Irritability, nausea, lethargy, and often dehydration are present as well. The symptoms are both local and general, depending on the bones affected. The local symptoms are pain and tenderness at the end of a long bone, with acute inflammation. Back pain may be a diagnostic clue to vertebral osteomyelitis if other causes of the pain are ruled out.[8] Because vertebral osteomyelitis manifests as very common symptoms such as back and neck pain, the clinician should be aware of the possibility of osteomyelitis and take necessary steps to establish a definitive diagnosis.[29]

Back and neck pain, with or without rigidity, is a common complaint, and is seen in at least 90% of cases. Atypical symptoms include occipital, arm, chest, abdominal, or leg pains.[29]

Pubic bone pain or tenderness should alert the clinician to possible osteomyelitis of the pubis. This is a rare but serious infection resulting from bacteremia following pelvic surgery or trauma.[10]

Chronic Osteomyelitis

Chronic osteomyelitis is usually seen in adults and is associated with underlying predisposing factors, such as vascular disease, history of postoperative infection, heroin addiction, hemodialysis, and hemoglobinopathy. Some patients tolerate chronic osteomyelitis well, with symptoms that are nonspecific but may include local swelling and pain in the affected bone. Sequestrum formation is common, and sinuses may develop that drain the bone abscess to the surface. Draining sinuses is a deep-seated infection sequela and is often caused by chronic osteomyelitis.

Organisms associated with chronic osteomyelitis are *S. aureus*, gram-negative bacilli such as *E. coli, P. aeruginosa*, anaerobic gram negative bacilli, anaerobic gram positive cocci as well as other anaerobic organisms, mycobacteria, and fungi. Long-term antimicrobial treatment is necessary for chronic osteomyelitis. Surgical drainage is also essential for cure.[1, 2]

LABORATORY ANALYSES AND DIAGNOSIS

Although radiographic or radionuclide studies may be helpful, definitive diagnosis of osteomyelitis rests on the isolation and identification of the etiologic agent from blood cultures or from a biopsy of the bone lesion itself. *S. aureus* is the leading pathogen, but other microbes may also be identified. *Mycobacterium tuberculosis*, for example, can produce a chronic vertebral osteomyelitis. Blood cultures should include both aerobic and anaerobic phases as well as methods to isolate unusual etiologic organisms, such as *Aspergillus, Candida,* and *Rhizopus.* Multiple blood cultures may be necessary to isolate and identify the etiologic agent; however, if they are negative, bone biopsy material should be cultured to establish the diagnosis.[27, 30] Immediate Gram staining of biopsy material is recommended; however, a negative result should not rule out the presence of osteomyelitis. Culture of sinus tract drainage is not reliable and is not recommended.[26]

Bone scanning often shows positive results before radiographic findings appear; however, bone scans may give false-negative results, especially in neonates.[31] Magnetic resonance imaging provides a means for presumptive diagnosis in the evaluation of musculoskeletal infections when the causative agent is not recovered by cultural techniques.[32] Bone biopsy remains the procedure of choice for establishing a definitive diagnosis in patients in whom osteomyelitis is suspected clinically but who have negative radiographic or bone scan findings.[28, 33]

Often the erythrocyte sedimentation rate (ESR) is elevated in pyogenic vertebral osteomyelitis, and this feature may be of value in both diagnosis and follow-up studies.[34, 35] The ESR may or may not be elevated in other sites of infection and, therefore, has limited diagnostic value in these cases. Levels of acute-phase reactants, for example, C-reactive protein, may also be elevated.[23, 35] Routine blood counts are frequently of no value, but leukocytosis is often present in children with acute osteomyelitis. Serologic tests, such as teichoic acid antibody, have been evaluated for *S. aureus* osteomyelitis and found to be useful diagnostic tools.[36]

TREATMENT

Antimicrobial susceptibility studies should be performed on all organisms isolated from specimens appropriately collected from legitimate sites of the bone or from blood cultures. Precise bacteriologic identification is fundamental for appropriate antimicrobial therapy.[37] Four to 8 weeks of antimicrobial therapy and surgical debridement and drainage of the affected site are essential for complete recovery and to prevent the development of chronic osteomyelitis. Acute hematogenous osteomyelitis is often a life-threatening disease in children, and early treatment with antibiotics is necessary to avoid surgery.[13] Surgical debridement must be performed if radiologic evidence of bone destruction is present or if there is soft tissue fluctuance, indicating abscess formation.

Treatment may be difficult, because the identity of the etiologic organism may be unresolved. If the causative agent cannot be determined in a patient with clinical symptoms, empiric antimicrobial therapy should be instituted. The agent's spectrum of activity should include *S. aureus* as well as gram-negative bacilli and anaerobes. Clindamycin, oxacillin, or penicillin G, depending on β-lactamase test results, afluoroquinolone, and tobramycin may be an effective battery; however, results of susceptibility studies should be considered first.[10, 12, 38] Currently, there are both public and private economic incentives to reduce the length of hospital stays; thus, outpatient treatment for some cases of osteomyelitis may be indicated.[39]

Prophylactic use of antimicrobial agents might be useful in cases of contiguous infection. Osteomyelitis associated with a prosthesis generally requires the removal of the appliance and the initiation of appropriate antimicrobial therapy.

Case Study

A 2-week-old newborn girl was referred to the hospital by a visiting nurse because the baby disliked passive movement of the left arm. The mother reported that the patient had been feverish and was not feeding well. Radiographic films of the left shoulder excluded a fracture, and a consultant pediatrician diagnosed Erb's palsy. One week later, the physical therapist, at an outpatient session, noticed that the girl cried when her left arm was moved. Repeat x-rays revealed an osteolytic lesion of the humerus with a periosteal reaction. A bone scan was normal, however.

Questions

1. What organism is a likely cause of osteomyelitis in this age group?
2. What steps should be taken, and how often will this condition be encountered?

Discussion

1. *Streptococcus agalactiae,* grown in pus from the shoulder joint, is a likely cause of the osteomyelitis.
2. The patient should be started on specific antimicrobial treatment until symptoms clear. Neonatal osteomyelitis is rare, and early diagnosis is essential for effective treatment. Neonatal osteomyelitis should be considered in the differential diagnosis of neonates presenting postnatally with limb palsy. Group B streptococcus and *S. aureus* are two of the microbes commonly isolated in these cases.[40]

References

1. Calhoun JH, Cobos JA, Mader JT: Does hyperbaric oxygen have a place in the treatment of osteomyelitis? Orthop Clin North Am 22:467, 1991.
2. Cierny G: Classification and treatment of adult osteomyelitis. *In* Evarts CM (ed): Surgery of the Musculoskeletal System. New York, Churchill Livingstone, 1990.
3. Graham GD, Lundy MM, Frederick RJ, et al: Predicting the cure of osteomyelitis under treatment: Concise communication. J Nucl Med 24:110, 1983.
4. Stiefeld SM, Graziani AL, MacGregor RR: Toxicities of antimicrobial

agents used to treat osteomyelitis. Orthop Clin North Am 22:439, 1991.

5. Schmid FR: Infections: Arthritis and osteomyelitis. Prim Care 2:295, 1984.

6. Modic MT, Feiglin DH, Piraino DW, et al: Vertebral osteomyelitis: Assessment using MR. Radiology 157:157, 1985.

7. Holzgang J, Wehrli R, von Graevenitz A, et al: Adult vertebral osteomyelitis caused by *Haemophilus influenzae*. Clin Microbiol 3:261, 1984.

8. William MR, Berry PH: Pseudomonas vertebral osteomyelitis following open heart surgery: Case report. Texas Med 80:47, 1984.

9. Joklik WK, Willett HP, Amons DB (eds): Zinsser Microbiology, ed 18. Norwalk, Conn., Appleton-Century-Crofts, 1984.

10. Hoyme UB, Tamimi HK, Eschenbach DA, et al: Osteomyelitis pubis after radial gynecologic operations. Obstet Gynecol 63(Suppl):475, 1984.

11. Balm AJ, Tiwari RM, deRiyeke TB: Osteomyelitis in the head and neck. J Laryngol Otol 99:1059, 1985.

12. Waldvogel FA, Vasey H: Osteomyelitis: The past decade. N Engl J Med 303:360, 1980.

13. Morrey BF, Peterson HA: Hematogenous pyogenic osteomyelitis in children. Orthop Clin North Am 6:935, 1975.

14. Mollan RAB, Piggot J: Acute osteomyelitis in children. J Bone Joint Surg (Br) 59:2, 1977.

15. Turck M, Counts GW: Staphylococcal infections. *In* Isselbacher KJ, Braunwald E, Wilson JD, et al (eds): Harrison's Principles of Internal Medicine, ed 10. New York, McGraw-Hill, 1983.

16. Boc SF, Martone JD: Osteomyelitis caused by *Corynebacterium jeikeium*. J Am Podiatr Med Am Assoc 85:338, 1995.

17. Barter SJ, Hennessy O: Actinomycetes as the causative organism of osteomyelitis in sickle cell disease. Skeletal Radiol 111:271, 1984.

18. Mallouh A, Talab Y: Bone and joint infection in patients with sickle cell disease. J Pediatr Orthop 5:158, 1985.

19. Ebony WW: Septic arthritis in patients with sickle-cell disease. Br J Rheumatol 26:99, 1987.

20. Vichinsky EP, Lubin BH: Sickle cell anemia and related hemoglobinopathies. Pediatr Clin North Am 27:429, 1980.

21. Fierer J: The fetid foot: Lower extremity infections in patients with diabetes mellitus. Rev Infect Dis 1:210, 1979.

22. Fisher MC, Goldsmith JF, Gilligan PH: Sneakers as a source of *Pseudomonas aeruginosa* in children with osteomyelitis following puncture wounds. J Pediatr 106:607, 1985.

23. Crosby LA, Powell DA: The potential value of the sedimentation rate in monitoring treatment outcome in puncture-wound-related *Pseudomonas* osteomyelitis. Clin Orthop 188:168, 1984.

24. Gadberry JL, Zipper R, Taylor JA: *Pasteurella pneumotropica* isolated from bone and joint infections. J Clin Microbiol 19:926, 1984.

25. Shimizu K, Away G, Matsuda F, et al: *Eikenella corrodens* stenosynovitis and osteomyelitis of the hand: A case report. Arch Jpn Chir 53:800, 1984.

26. Andreoli TE, Carpenter CCJ, Plum F, et al (eds): Osteomyelitis. Philadelphia, WB Saunders, 1986.

27. Norden CW: Osteomyelitis. *In* Stein JH (ed): Internal Medicine. Boston, Little, Brown, 1983.

28. Wheat J: Diagnostic strategies in osteomyelitis. Am J Med 78:218, 1985.

29. Strausbaugh LJ: Vertebral osteomyelitis: How to differentiate it from other causes of back and neck pain. Postgrad Med 97:147, 1995.

30. Dich VQ, Nelson JD, Haltalin KC: Osteomyelitis in infants and children: A review of 163 cases. Am J Dis Child 129:1273, 1975.

31. Longmaid HE 3rd, Kruskal JB: Imaging infections in diabetic patients. Infect Dis Clin North Am 9:163, 1995.

32. Totty WG: Radiographic evaluation of osteomyelitis using magnetic resonance imaging. Orthop Rev 18:587, 1989.

33. Fletcher BD, Scoles PV, Nelson AD: Osteomyelitis in children: Detection by magnetic resonance. Pediatr Radiol 150:57, 1984.

34. Kern RZ, Houpt JB: Pyogenic vertebral osteomyelitis: Diagnosis and management. Can Med Assoc J 130:1025, 1984.

35. Selker RG, Wilder BL: The erythrocyte sedimentation rate: An interface between science and the law. Surg Neurol 43:290, 1995.

36. Wheat LJ, White AC, Norden C: Serological diagnosis of *Staphylococcus aureus* osteomyelitis. J Clin Microbiol 21:764, 1985.

37. Ray CG: Bone and joint infections. *In* Ryan KJ (ed): Sherris Medical Microbiology: An Introduction to Infectious Diseases, ed 3. Norwalk, Conn., Appleton & Lange, 1994.

38. Marguise JH: Osteomyelitis and infections of prosthetic joints. *In* Isselbacher KJ, Braunwald E, Wilson JD, et al (eds): Harrison's Principles of Internal Medicine. New York, McGraw-Hill, 1994.

39. Tomczak RL: Outpatient treatment of osteomyelitis. J Am Podiatr Med Assoc 75:261, 1985.

40. Isaacs D, Bower DB, Moxon ER: Neonatal osteomyelitis presenting as nerve palsy. Br Med J 292:1071, 1986.

Chapter 58

Antimicrobial Therapy and Sensitivity Testing

Vickie S. Baselski and Theodore H. Morton

Antimicrobial agents can prevent or cure many diseases and have contributed significantly to the advancement of modern medicine. The clinical laboratory provides much of the information essential to optimizing anti-infective therapy. Understanding the clinical use of antimicrobials facilitates the efficient selection and interpretation of diagnostic tests. This chapter describes the fundamental principles of anti-infective therapy, the clinical use of common agents, and the role of the laboratory in guiding therapy.

GENERAL PRINCIPLES OF ANTI-INFECTIVE THERAPY

All medications act by binding a receptor or target that produces a desired therapeutic effect; for antibiotics, this effect is the inhibition or killing of pathogenic organisms. It is important, therefore, to target a receptor that is not found in human cells; otherwise, the medication would be too toxic. For the antibiotic to be effective, a specified minimum amount must be present at the site of infection. In the laboratory, in vitro susceptibility testing can establish a minimum inhibitory concentration (MIC) for that organism. If the MIC is greater than the concentrations that can safely be achieved in a patient, the organism is considered resistant. Most antibiotics have maximal effect as long as the in vivo concentration is always above the MIC. Two important exceptions, the aminoglycosides and the quinolones, have dose-dependent killing. Their maximal effect is seen when peak concentrations are at least 10 times the MIC. This fact changes the dosing strategy toward single large doses as opposed to frequent small doses or continuous infusion.

Antibiotics that kill bacteria are considered bactericidal. They can be used to treat life-threatening infections of the central nervous system (meningitis) and heart (endocarditis) as well as blood stream infections in many patients without an immune system (febrile neutropenia). Other agents are bacteriostatic, and merely inhibit the organism so the patient's immune system can eradicate them. Some combinations of antibiotics work better than others. Using two agents with different mechanisms of action often yields a net killing effect that is greater than expected (*synergy*). Combinations of drugs with duplicative mechanisms can actually be less effective than the individual drugs, because they compete for the same receptors (*antagonism*). In vitro testing can be used to clarify the effect of drug combinations on a specific organism.[1, 2]

Pharmacokinetics

The blood stream serves to deliver the drug to the infection, and there are two major ways to get a medication into the blood. The first is parenteral, which can be either intravenous (IV) or intramuscular (IM). Parenteral administration usually achieves the highest bood concentrations, but not all medications can be given by this route because of their biochemistry. The second most common route is oral administration (PO), which requires a drug to be absorbed from the gastrointestinal (GI) tract into the circulation. This route is not appropriate for many drugs, because they are broken down by acid in the stomach or cannot be absorbed from the GI tract. Blood levels achieved with oral administration tend to be lower than with parenteral administration, because of limited absorption (termed *bioavailability*), but oral administration is more convenient and less expensive than parenteral administration. It is also important to consider an agent's ability to penetrate into sites that are naturally protected by physical and biochemical barriers, such as the lung or central nervous system. Higher doses can be effective in reaching these sites but are also more toxic. Alternative routes of administration sometimes used to overcome this problem are intrathecal administration and aerosolization to maximize lung secretion levels.[3]

Adverse Effects

All medications have the potential to produce undesired effects. They are generally divided into side effects and toxicity. *Side effects* can occur at usual therapeutic doses and include a number of physiologic alterations as well as allergic reactions. *Toxicity* refers to negative cellular effects that increase with use of higher doses. Both types of adverse effects can limit the clinical usefulness of an antibiotic if the adverse effects are greater than the drug's beneficial effects, especially compared with other agents. It is also important to consider whether the antibiotic adversely interacts with other medications the patient is taking.[1, 2]

Types of Therapy

There are essentially three uses of antibiotics: prophylactic, empiric, and definitive. A patient with a known risk of developing an infection may be given *prophylactic* antimicrobics if the benefit of preventing the infection outweighs the risk and cost of using the drug. Risk includes the chance for individual adverse events from the drug, and cost includes the actual cost of the drug; but risk also includes the potential of promoting the development of resistant organisms. *Empiric* treatment is used when a patient presents with signs and symptoms of infection, but the specific causative organism is not known. This therapeutic strategy uses agents active against the organisms that are likely to be causing the presenting illness. Local trends in antibiotic susceptibility can vary and should be carefully considered in the selection of empiric therapy. When a specific organism has been identified and its in vitro susceptibility to antibiotics has been established, the patient should receive *definitive* treatment. This means giving the most specific, least toxic, and most cost-effective agent for that organism. That agent is most often referred to as the "drug of choice" for that organism.[1, 2]

Resistance

For every mechanism by which an antibiotic acts against a bacterium, there are several ways for the organism to resist it. The first is for the bacteria to destroy or inactivate the antibiotic.[4] For example, some bacteria have β-lactamases, enzymes designed to break apart molecules like penicillin. The second method is to prevent the antibiotic from getting to the target.[5] This can involve a change in permeability of the outer membrane of the organism or even active removal of the drug from the periplasmic space.

The last method is for the bacteria to alter the targeted receptor, thereby preventing the antibiotic from working even if it manages to reach the target.[6]

Some organisms are intrinsically resistant to a specific antibiotic. Others may acquire resistance through transfer of genetic determinants on chromosomal or plasmid DNA from resistant organisms. Expression of resistance may be continuous (constitutive) or may require pre-exposure to initiate the process (inducible). Knowledge of operative mechanisms is commonly important in determining an effective in vitro test strategy for detection of the organism and for prediction of susceptibility to related agents.[1, 2, 7]

OVERVIEW OF MAJOR THERAPEUTIC AGENTS

A basic understanding of the pharmacology, mode of action, and spectrum of activity of antimicrobial agents is key to the implementation of appropriate antimicrobial susceptibility test methods. Agents may be divided into broad classes relating to the organism category they are effective against (e.g., antibacterial, antifungal, antiviral), and into more specific classes on the basis of their mode of action. In general, an antimicrobial susceptibility testing panel is designed for testing a specific group of organisms, and represents all antimicrobial classes potentially of benefit for that organism group (Table 58–1).

Antibacterials

Cell Wall Active Agents

VANCOMYCIN

This cell wall active agent acts by inhibiting transport of precursor molecules. It is active against gram-positive organisms, and it is the only drug with reliable activity against methicillin-resistant *Staphylococcus aureus* (MRSA) as well as *Streptococcus pneumoniae* that is resistant to penicillins and cephalosporins.

Vancomycin is given IV and has difficulty penetrating the central nervous system. It may be infused into the cerebrospinal fluid (CSF) for life-threatening infection. It

Table 58–1. Classes of Antibacterial Agents

Target in Bacteria	Class of Antibiotic (Examples)
Cell wall	Glycopeptides: vancomycin, teicoplanin
	β-lactams: penicillins, cephalosporins, others
Ribosomes	Aminoglycosides: gentamicin, tobramycin, amikacin
	Macrolides: erythromycin, clarithromycin, azithromycin, clindamycin
	Tetracyclines: tetracycline, doxycycline, minocycline
Metabolic pathways and enzymes	
DNA gyrase	Quinolones: ciprofloxacin, ofloxacin
Folic acid synthesis	Sulfonamides, sulfones: sulfamethoxazole, sulfisoxazole, dapsone
	Dihydrofolate reductase inhibitors: trimethoprim, pyrimethamine
Other	Metronidazole, rifampin, nitrofurantoin

can be given PO to treat diarrhea caused by *Clostridium difficile* that has not responded to metronidazole. There is great concern over the indiscriminate use of vancomycin because of fear of developing vancomycin-resistant strains of *S. aureus* and *S. pneumoniae*.[8]

β-LACTAMS

The β-lactams are the largest group of antibacterials. They have a common chemical structure called a β-lactam ring. This ring binds to penicillin-binding proteins (PBPs) on the cell walls of gram-positive and gram-negative organisms. Binding to the PBP disrupts cell wall synthesis and results in cell death. These agents are bactericidal and exert maximal killing as long as concentrations are maintained that are 3 to 4 times above the MIC at the site of infection. There are three mechanisms by which bacteria are, or become, resistant to a β-lactam: the agent's inability to penetrate the outer membrane of gram-negative bacteria to reach the PBP; destruction of the agent by bacterial enzymes (β-lactamases); and inability of the agent to bind the PBP. There are four major classes of β-lactams: penicillins, cephalosporins, carbapenems, and monobactams (Table 58–2). Various side chains on the β-lactam ring determine each agent's antibacterial spectrum, pharmacokinetics, and toxicities. These factors in turn determine clinical utility.

PENICILLINS

The first β-lactam was penicillin. Modifications of the core penicillin molecule were made in an effort to improve its spectrum and pharmacokinetics. This attempt led to the discovery of many agents that we now classify by their antibiotic spectra. The current classes are natural, extended-spectrum, antistaphylococcal, and antipseudomonal penicillins. In addition, some penicillins have been combined with β-lactamase inhibitors to further increase their spectra. Despite the common mechanism of action, there are significant differences in their clinical use.[9, 10]

Natural Penicillins. The antibiotic spectrum of penicillin is very limited, but it remains essential in the definitive treatment of many infections. It is active against most streptococci, although resistance is now being seen in up to 60% of *S. pneumoniae* and half of the viridans group. It is active against almost all *Neisseria meningitidis* and is the drug of choice for syphilis. This spectrum makes penicillin useful, combined with an antistaphylococcal penicillin, as part of empiric treatment for endocarditis, although the latter is generally used with an aminoglycoside for this purpose. Penicillin should not be used empirically for community-acquired meningitis or pneumonia but is the drug of choice if a susceptible strain of *N. meningitidis* or *S. pneumoniae* is the identified pathogen.

There is both a parenteral and oral form of penicillin, and an intramuscular slow-release formulation (benzathine penicillin) can be used for streptococcal pharyngitis in children or if patient compliance with oral penicillin therapy is questionable.

Extended-Spectrum (Amino) Penicillins. Ampicillin and amoxicillin have better activity than penicillin against some gram-positive organisms and are considered the drugs of choice for *Listeria* and *Enterococcus*. The gram-negative spectrum includes up to 70% of *Escherichia coli* and most *Proteus mirabilis*, as well as up to 75% of *Haemophilus influenzae*. Only ampicillin is available parenterally. For oral administration, amoxicillin has superior bioavailability.

For meningitis in infants and the elderly, ampicillin is included with ceftriaxone or cefotaxime (third-generation cephalosporins) to provide coverage for *Listeria*. Ampicillin is also included in regimens for intra-abdominal infections to cover enterococci. Enterococcal urinary tract infections (UTIs) can be treated with ampicillin or amoxicillin alone, but outside the urinary tract, ampicillin is often combined with gentamicin for effective killing. Amoxicillin can be used for many other uncomplicated UTIs, and ampicillin can be combined with gentamicin for treating pyelonephritis. Because of its low cost, good tolerability, and activity against many strains of *S. pneumoniae* as well as *H. influenzae*, amoxicillin is recommended as first-line treatment of otitis media in pediatric patients and of bronchitis or sinusitis in adults.

Antistaphylococcal Penicillins. This class was developed to treat penicillinase-producing strains of *S. aureus* but is otherwise limited in clinical use. Methicillin was the first of this class, and although this agent is not used clinically, the term "methicillin-susceptible or methicillin resistant *S. aureus*" (MSSA/MRSA) is still widely used. In clinical practice, nafcillin and oxacillin are the parenteral agents, and dicloxocillin is used orally. This class is often used for cellulitis and is combined with penicillin or an aminoglycoside for empiric treatment of endocarditis. The antistaphylococcal penicillins are the drugs of choice for

Table 58–2. Categories of β-Lactam and Related Antibiotics

Class	Subtype	Examples
Penicillins	Natural penicillins	Penicillin
		Pen VK (PO)
	Extended-spectrum (amino) penicillins	Ampicillin (IV/PO)
		Amoxicillin (PO)
	Antistaphylococcal penicillins	Oxacillin, Nafcillin
		Dicloxacillin (PO)
	Antipseudomonal penicillins	Piperacillin, mezlocillin, azlocillin
		Ticarcillin, carbenicillin
	Penicillins with β-lactamase inhibitors	Amoxicillin/clavulanic acid
		Ampicillin/sulbactam
		Ticarcillin/clavulanate
		Piperacillin/tazobactam
Cephalosporins	First-generation	Cefazolin, cephalexin (PO)
	Second-generation	Cefuroxime (IV/PO), cefamandole
	Second-generation with anaerobic	Cefoxitin, Cefotetan
	Third-generation	Ceftriaxone, Cefotaxime, Ceftizoxime
	Third-generation with antipseudomonal activity	Ceftazidime
Other	Monobactam	Aztreonam
	Carbapenems	Imipenem, meropenem

MSSA and may be combined with gentamicin for synergy in treatment of staphylococcal endocarditis or pneumonia. Resistance to the agents is now common, with up to 50% of staphylococci resistant due to an altered PBP.

Antipseudomonal Penicillins. The antipseudomonal penicillins have an antibiotic spectrum similar to that of ampicillin, with very good additional activity against enteric–gram negative organisms and *P. aeruginosa*. They are not active against penicillinase-producing organisms and should not be used for serious streptococcal infections. Their use is usually reserved for nosocomial pneumonias and UTIs as well as febrile neutropenia because of their broad antibiotic spectrum. Most antipseudomonal agents are parenteral and include ticarcillin, piperacillin mezlocillin, and azlocillin. Ticarcillin may be active against slightly fewer strains of *Pseudomonas*. Against *P. aeruginosa*, these agents should be combined with an aminoglycoside to provide synergistic killing and prevent resistance. Orally, carbenicillin can be used for urinary tract infection but may have unpleasant sensory side effects.

Penicillins With β-Lactamase Inhibitors. Many significant pathogens, including MSSA, *H. influenzae*, anaerobes, and some enteric gram-negative organisms, are resistant to penicillins because of the production of β-lactamases, which degrade the penicillins before they are able to bind to the bacteria's PBPs. Combining a β-lactamase inhibitor with a penicillin expands the spectrum to include these otherwise resistant pathogens. Ampicillin combined with sulbactam (Unasyn) is available parenterally, and amoxicillin with clavulanate (Augmentin) is available orally. Both drugs are useful for community acquired infections. Unasyn is often used for intra-abdominal infections to cover enterococci, enteric gram-negative organisms, and anaerobes. Augmentin is often used for amoxacillin failure in otitis or bronchitis to cover β-lactamase–producing strains of *H. influenzae*. It is also the drug of choice for some bite wounds.

Two commercially available products include an inhibitor with an antipseudomonal penicillin. Ticarcillin with clavulanic acid (Timentin) is useful for nosocomial sepsis, pneumonia, and other life-threatening mixed infections in which *Pseudomonas* is a probable pathogen. Piperacillin with tazobactam (Zosyn) is similar in spectrum and use to Timentin. None of these products has improved activity against organisms with resistance due to altered PBP, and they should not be used for central nervous system (CNS) infection, because they do not reliably cross the blood-brain barrier.

CEPHALOSPORINS

This group of β-lactams shares some characteristics with penicillins. They are usually subdivided into "generations" on the basis of their relative activity against *Staphylococcus* and gram-negative bacilli. First-generation cephalosporins have the most activity against *S. aureus* and about 90% of enterics, whereas third-generation cephalosporins have less staphylococcal activity but cover up to 99% of enterics and almost all *H. influenzae*, and some have antipseudomonal activity. Some second-generation cepha-

losporins are active against anaerobes. Differences in pharmacokinetics and side effects also determine the clinical utility of each agent. Only agents that adequately cross the blood-brain barrier can be used for CNS infections, and those with an *N*-methylthiotetrazole (MTT) side chain on the core cephalosporin molecule can cause bleeding and vomiting.[11, 12]

First-Generation Cephalosporins. These agents have activity against MSSA and most streptococci. They are active against common enteric gram-negative bacilli but do not have significant activity against *Enterococcus, H. influenzae, Pseudomonas*, or anaerobes. Given this spectrum, they are often used IV to prevent surgical wound infections, with cefazolin being preferred because its slow elimination allows the use of a single dose prior to the incision. Cefazolin is also commonly used for cellulitis and for non-CNS infections with susceptible gram-negative organisms. The most commonly used oral agent is cephalexin, which is useful for cellulitis as well as uncomplicated UTI. The use of first-generation cephalosporins in otitis and bronchitis is limited by lack of activity against *H. influenzae* and *S. pneumoniae*.

Second-Generation Cephalosporins. A diverse group of antibiotics, the second-generation cephalosporins are best subdivided according to antibiotic spectrum. Cefoxitin (IV) and cefotetan (IV) both have significant anaerobic activity and can be used for moderate mixed infections, including pelvic inflammatory disease (PID). Cefotetan's long half-life allows for less frequent dosing (twice a day compared with 4 times a day for cefoxitin), but it has an MTT side chain. Cefuroxime (IV, PO) does not have anaerobic activity but has good activity against *H. influenzae* and *S. pneumoniae*, and it can be used for community-acquired pneumonia. Oral second-generation cephalosporins, including cefuroxime (Ceftin) and cefaclor (Ceclor), can be used for bronchitis and otitis.

Third-Generation Cephalosporins. This group of cephalosporins is commonly used in hospitals. Ceftazidime (IV) and cefoperazone are notable for antipseudomonal activity and are also active against almost all enteric gram-negative organisms and *H. influenzae*. They have poor activity against staphylococci and streptococci and should not be used for community-acquired pneumonia or meningitis. They can be used in the same settings as antipseudomonal penicillins, and should also be combined with an aminoglycoside for *Pseudomonas*.

Of the other available agents, ceftriaxone (Rocephin, IV) and cefotaxime (Claforan, IV) are most commonly used. Ceftriaxone is eliminated mostly by the liver and can be given once a day, compared with an average of 3 times a day for cefotaxime. These two agents are so similar in spectrum and clinical use that most institutions do not carry both; however, the latter may be preferred in patients with liver disease. They have excellent activity against *S. pneumoniae* and most nonpseudomonal gram-negative organisms. They are drugs of choice for adult community-acquired pneumonia, meningitis, and pyelonephritis. Ceftriaxone is also used for uncomplicated and disseminated *N. gonorrhoeae*.

Cefixime is an oral third-generation cephalosporin that can be used for mild gram-negative (nonpseudomonal) respiratory and urinary tract infections. Cefipime is a new "extended-spectrum" cephalosporin that has gram-negative coverage comparable to that of ceftazidime as well as significant gram-positive coverage, except for MRSA and *Enterococcus*.

Other β-Lactam–Like Agents

Carbapenems. Imipenem and meropenem are the two carbapenems. Their spectra are similar and are so broad that these agents are usually described in terms of the organisms they do *not* cover. Gram-positive bacteria the carbapenems are not active against include MRSA and some enterococci. Although they are active against most gram-negative organisms, suprainfection with *Stenotrophomonas maltophilia* and *Burkholderia cepacia* is not uncommon, and resistance may occur in *P. aeruginosa* and *Acinetobacter* infections. Most pathogenic anaerobes are susceptible. *Mycoplasma*, *Chlamydia*, and *Legionella* are resistant. Given this spectrum, the carbapenems are used in infections that fail to respond to multiple-antibiotic combinations, and for cephalosporin-resistant gram-negative pathogens such as *Acinetobacter* and *Enterobacter*. Imipenem is used combined with cilisatin (Primaxin, IV). It is not used for CNS infections, because it can cause seizures. These drugs are very expensive and should be used judiciously to preserve their role as the last line of defense against several multidrug-resistant gram-negative pathogens.[13]

Monobactams. The only commercially available agent in the monobactams is Aztreonam (Azactam, IV). It has a spectrum similar to that of ceftazidime but is less active against *Pseudomonas*. The chemical structure is such that aztreonam can be used safely in patients allergic to penicillins and cephalosporins. Thus, it is usually only used for an allergic patient who would otherwise be treated with an extended-spectrum penicillin or cephalosporin.[13]

Ribosome-Targeting Agents

Aminoglycosides

The aminoglycoside class of antibiotics is bactericidal and acts on 30 and 50S bacterial ribosomes. These agents are bactericidal against many gram-negative organisms, including *P. aeruginosa*, and provide synergistic killing of certain gram-positive organisms when combined with a penicillin or vancomycin. The aminoglycosides lack clinical activity against *H. influenza*, *S. pneumoniae*, and *Neisseria* species. This lack limits their role in community-acquired meningitis and pneumonia. They do not reliably penetrate the CNS and are not active in oxygen-poor environments (abscesses) or against anaerobes. The most clinically useful aminoglycosides are gentamicin, tobramycin, and amikacin. Their spectra of activity and relative cost are compared in Box 58–1. Netilmicin is used uncommonly, and streptomycin is generally reserved for serious enterococcal infections and mycobacterial disease. The aminoglycosides' potential for nephrotoxicity and ototoxicity demands careful use, particularly in patients with compromised renal function.[14]

Macrolides

Literally named "big molecules," macrolides are most notable for their activity against streptococci and atypical bacteria like *Chlamydia*, *Mycoplasma*, and *Legionella*. They can be bactericidal, and they act by binding and inhibiting the 30S bacterial ribosomal subunit.

Erythromycin, which is available both orally and parenterally, is the prototype. It is a useful alternative to penicillin for mild streptococcal infections in β-lactam–allergic patients. For otherwise healthy young outpatients, erythromycin is the drug of choice for community-acquired pneumonia and is often given IV in high doses to patients requiring hospitalization in whom *Legionella* is suspected.

Erythromycin's clinical utility is limited by its frequent dosing (four times a day), common gastrointestinal side effects, and lack of activity against significant respiratory pathogens such as *H. influenzae*. This situation has led to development of extended-spectrum agents clarithromycin (Biaxin) and azithromycin (Zithromax). These agents are better tolerated than erythromycin and have better *H. influenzae* activity. Clarithromycin is notable for its significant activity in preventing and treating *Mycobacterium avium* complex infections. Azithromycin can be used for single-dose treatment of *Chlamydia trachomatis*, and an abbreviated (5-day) course is effective for many upper respiratory infections. Both clarithromycin and azithromycin are available in oral formulations only and cost up to $75 for a course of therapy (compared with $10 for oral erythromycin). Side effects are mild, but drug interactions

---

Box 58–1. **Cost and Antimicrobial Spectra of Common Aminoglycosides**

Gentamicin $7/day	>95% enteric gram-negative bacilli*
	85% *P. aeruginosa* (use combination therapy†)
	MSSA: Synergistic with oxacillin
	Enterococci: Synergistic with ampicillin or vancomycin
Tobramycin $28/day	>95% enteric gram-negative bacilli*
	97% *P. aeruginosa* (use combination therapy†)
Amikacin $55/day	Reserve for documented gentamicin- and tobramycin-resistant gram-negative bacilli
	Some *Mycobacterium* (TB, MAC)

*Common enteric gram-negative bacilli are *E. coli*, *Proteus*, *Klebsiella*.
†For synergy, add an antipseudomonal β-lactam (piperacillin, ceftazidime).

with theophylline, nonsedating antihistamines, and cyclosporin can be problematic.[15]

CLINDAMYCIN

Clindamycin is active against many gram-positive and anaerobic bacteria but not against aerobic gram-negative organisms. It is also inactive against enterococci, most MRSA, *S. pneumoniae*, and *C. difficile*. Bacteriostatic, clindamycin acts by binding the 50S bacterial ribosomal subunit. Combination with gentamicin is the treatment standard for mixed aerobic and anaerobic infections such as intra-abdominal sepsis, PID, and diabetic foot infection. In outpatient therapy, it can be combined with a quinolone for oral treatment of milder infections. It is used with penicillin for necrotizing fasciitis caused by *S. pyogenes* and is an alternative for patients with cellulitis who are allergic to β-lactams. As monotherapy, clindamycin is the drug of choice for aspiration pneumonia. It has additional use in high doses with pyrimethamine in treating toxoplasmosis. Clindamycin is available in IV and PO forms and is generally well tolerated. Diarrhea and subsequent colitis with *C. difficile* are an uncommon but serious adverse effect of clindamycin.[15]

TETRACYCLINES

Tetracyclines, which are bactericidal, act by binding and inhibiting the 30S bacterial ribosomal subunit. Despite activity against select gram-positive and gram-negative pathogens, they are usually third-line treatment, after the more effective and better-tolerated β-lactams. They are invaluable in the treatment of many unusual or rare pathogens, as well as the more common *C. trachomatis*. Tetracycline (PO) is usually reserved for treatment of acne and must be given 4 times a day. Doxycycline (IV or PO) is the most useful agent in this class because of its spectrum, twice-daily dosing, and lower incidence of side effects. It is the drug of choice for the following important pathogens: *Borrelia*, *Brucella*, *Chlamydia* species, *Erhlichia*, *Rickettsia*, and *Vibrio cholerae*. It also may be useful for select methicillin-resistant staphylococci. Minocycline is more ototoxic and expensive than doxycycline, but may be more active against staphylococci.[16]

Metabolic Pathways and Enzymes

QUINOLONES

The quinolones are notable for their activity against gram-negative organisms (including *P. aeruginosa* and *H. influenzae*) and their excellent oral bioavailability. Gram-positive organisms have quickly become resistant to these agents, and resistance has been increasing among *P. aeruginosa* and *N. gonorrhoeae*. The quinolones are bactericidal and act by binding and inhibiting bacterial DNA gyrase. They can be used for some β-lactam–resistant organisms, and to provide gram-negative coverage in β-lactam–allergic patients. When an aminoglycoside is contraindicated, a quinolone may be used, although it has only additive, not synergistic, effect with β-lactams. The quinolones are not the drugs of choice for *P. aeruginosa*, but their oral administration makes them useful for outpatient

treatment of mild or resolving pseudomonal infections. Ciprofloxacin has the best antipseudomonal and antimycobacterial activity. Ofloxacin can also be used for 7 days to treat *C. trachomatis*.[17, 18]

FOLIC ACID SYNTHESIS INHIBITORS

Trimethoprim-Sulfamethoxazole. This product (co-trimoxazole; Bactrim, Septra) combines two synergistic inhibitors of folic acid synthesis in a fixed 1:5 ratio of trimethoprim to sulfamethoxazole. This combination is active against most gram-positive organisms except enterococci and some MRSA, and against most gram-negatives except *P. aeruginosa*. It is also the drug of choice for *Nocardia*, for prevention and treatment of *Pneumocystis carinii* pneumonia (PCP) in patients infected with human immunodeficiency virus (HIV), and for some unusual gram-negative bacilli *(S. maltophilia)*. Trimethoprim-sulfamethoxazole is commonly used for urinary tract infections as well as for otitis, bronchitis, and sinusitis. It is inexpensive and generally well tolerated, although hematologic toxicity and rash are seen, particularly with concurrent HIV infection.[19]

Others. Sulfisoxazole inhibits folic acid synthesis and can be used for prevention and treatment of UTIs and otitis media. It is a second-line agent for chlamydial infection in pregnant patients.[19] Dapsone, which also inhibits folic acid synthesis, is useful for treatment of leprosy *(M. leprae)* and is a second-line agent for prevention of PCP in HIV-infected patients.[19]

Miscellaneous Antibacterials

METRONIDAZOLE

A unique antibiotic, metronidazole is active against anaerobes and select protozoa. For treatment of mixed infections, it must be combined with an agent such as cefazolin or ceftriaxone to cover gram-positive and negative pathogens. Metronidazole is the drug of choice of for *C. difficile* colitis as well as giardiasis and amebiasis. A single large dose is effective treatment for trichomoniasis. It is available in IV and PO forms and generally well tolerated. Disulfuram-like reactions (severe nausea and vomiting when metronidazole is combined with alcohol) are significant side effects.[20]

RIFAMPIN

Rifampin inhibits bacterial RNA synthesis and is used in combination treatment of tuberculosis. It can be added to vancomycin for use against MRSA and used to treat nasal carriage of *N. meningitidis*. Rifampin should not be used as monotherapy, however, because of development of resistance. This agent has many adverse effects, including staining of all body fluids red, causing liver damage, and interacting with practically all drugs metabolized by the liver.

NITROFURANTOIN

A urinary antiseptic, nitrofurantoin acts by an unknown mechanism to kill common urinary tract pathogens, including enterococci, but is not active against *Pseudomonas, Klebsiella,* or *Proteus.* It can also cause toxicity of the lungs.

Antimycobacterials

The acid-fast bacilli continue to be major pathogens, and few agents are effective against them. Infections should be treated with at least three drugs to prevent emergence of resistance, and therapy must be continued for more than 6 months to be effective. Against *M. tuberculosis,* the most active agents are isoniazid (INH) and rifampin, which are usually combined with pyrazinamide (PZA) for the first 2 months of treatment of a patient with active disease. INH can be used alone in recently infected patients who do not have clinical disease, to prevent the development of active disease. All these agents are hepatotoxic (particularly INH), can cause malaise, and interact with many drugs. Noncompliance with a full course of treatment is common and has led to the development of tuberculosis (TB) strains that are resistant to primary agents, termed multidrug-resistant TB (MDR-TB). Treatment of MDR-TB requires the use of at least four agents other than INH and rifampin, including ciprofloxacin, ethambutol, and amikacin. Prognosis in MDR-TB is especially grim for patients co-infected with HIV.[21]

Antifungals

Amphotericin B is the drug of choice for life-threatening systemic mycoses, including aspergillosis, cryptococcal meningitis, disseminated histoplasmosis, and disseminated candidiasis. Use of this agent in less severe infections is limited by its nephrotoxicity and the need for parenteral administration. The azoles—fluconazole (IV, PO), itraconazole (PO), and ketoconazole (PO)—can be useful in the treatment of select moderate fungal diseases. Fluconazole is active against most *C. albicans* and can be used to treat disseminated and localized infection. It is also used in HIV-infected patients to prevent recurrence of cryptococcosis after treatment with amphotericin B. Itraconazole has poor activity against *Candida* species but is very useful in histoplasmosis, blastomycosis, and with some dermatophytes. Fluconazole and itraconazole are well tolerated but expensive, and interact with some other hepatically metabolized drugs. Ketoconazole is second- or third-line treatment for many systemic mycoses, but compared with the other oral azoles, it is not as well tolerated and is more likely to interact with other drugs.

Clotrimazole and nystatin are topical antifungals that can be used for oral, dermatologic, or vaginal fungal infections. Griseofulvin, an oral antifungal, is used for mild dermatophytic infections and onychomycosis. Fluorocytosine (5-FC) is used with amphotericin B for cryptococcal meningitis, but at serum concentrations above 100 μg/mL, it is extremely toxic to the bone marrow.[22, 23]

P. carini, now considered a fungus, causes pneumonia in patients with HIV. Agents effective against PCP include trimethoprim-sulfamethoxazole, pentamidine, atovaquone, and dapsone. Trimethoprim-sulfamethoxazole is the drug of choice for treatment and also prevention of PCP in patients at risk. Pentamidine (IV), which acts by an un-

known mechanism, is a second choice for treatment and a third choice (as inhalation) for prevention but is very toxic. Atovaquone, which also acts by an unknown mechanism, is indicated for treatment of mild PCP in patients who cannot tolerate co-trimoxazole, and dapsone is a second choice for prevention of PCP. The mechanism of these agents' activities against PCP is generally unknown. True resistance to these drugs is rare.[24]

Antivirals

Human Immunodeficiency Virus

Currently, two classes of drugs can delay the progression of HIV infection: the reverse transcriptase inhibitors and the protease inhibitors. There is no cure, but life-threatening opportunistic infections can be delayed by use of these agents, especially in combination. The most effective therapy at this time appears to be one or two reverse transcriptase inhibitors combined with a protease inhibitor[24, 25] (Table 58–3).

Herpes Viruses

Acyclovir, valaciclovir, and famciclovir are agents activated within herpes-infected cells to a form that inhibits DNA polymerase. They are used for herpes simplex virus (HSV) and varicella-zoster virus (VZV) infection, in which they may reduce the severity of oral, genital, and skin lesions, but cannot effect a cure. Acyclovir can be used at high doses IV for herpetic infections of the central nervous system. Resistance has been detected in vitro and may be clinically significant.[26]

Ganciclovir is similar in activity to acyclovir but much more active in cytomegalovirus (CMV)–infected cells. It can be used IV to treat CMV and orally to maintain remission or prevent CMV in patients at risk, but it has bone marrow toxicity. Foscarnet is more toxic (renal) than ganciclovir and must be given IV, but it may be effective against ganciclovir-resistant strains of CMV.[24]

Respiratory Viruses

Infection with influenza virus is best prevented with vaccination, but after exposure, amantidine and rimantidine can be used to prevent infection and reduce the severity of disease for influenza A only. For treatment, these agents reduce the severity of illness in children and the elderly only if started within 48 hours of onset of symptoms. For

Table 58–3. Antivirals for HIV Infection

Class	Abbreviation	Generic Name	Brand Name
Reverse transcriptase inhibitors	AZT	Zidovudine	Retrovir
	ddC	Zalcitabine	Hivid
	ddI	Didanosine	Videx
	d4T	Stavudine	Zerit
	3TC	Lamivudine	Epivir
Protease inhibitors	SQV	Saquinavir	Invirase
		Ritonavir	Norvir
		Indinavir	Crixivan

patients at risk for complications of respiratory syncytial virus (RSV) infection (primarily children), ribivarin is available as an aerosol treatment to decrease signs and symptoms, but it is very expensive.[26]

Antiparasitics

Pathogenic parasites are divided into multicellular helminths and unicellular protozoa (see also Chapter 53). Anthelmintics are available only for oral administration. Mebendazole is most useful, being active against intestinal nematodes (other than *Strongyloides*). Pyrantel pamoate is an alternative to mebendazole for ascarias, enterobiasis, and hookworm. Ivermectin and albendazole are investigational drugs that have potential for indication similar to those of mebendazole. For strongyloidiasis, thiabendazole is the drug of choice, but ivermectin may also be effective. The trematodes and cestodes may respond to praziquantel.

Among intestinal protozoa, giardiasis is usually treated with metronidazole (an antianaerobic antibiotic with antiparasitic activity), and albendazole has also been effective. Cyclosporiasis and isosporiasis can be treated with trimethoprim-sulfamethoxazole. Lastly, cryptosporidial diarrhea in HIV-infected patients is usually treated with fluids and electrolyte support, but paromomycin (an aminoglycoside) has been effective in select patients.

For blood and tissue protozoa, several agents are used. Malaria may be treated with chloroquine, primaquine (for some species), and quinine if chloroquine resistance is likely. Toxoplasmosis in a normal host may be treated with a combination of pyrimethamine and sulfisoxazole, but this infection is notoriously difficult to treat in HIV-infected patients. Anti-infective agents are also available for other significant protozoa *(Leishmania, Trypanosoma)*.[27, 28]

LABORATORY ASPECTS

Increasing antimicrobial resistance and the threat of newly emerging resistance mechanisms[29] have placed the clinical laboratory in a central role in the recognition, surveillance, and control of the problem.[30] The purposes of antimicrobial susceptibility testing (AST) can be seen as twofold. First is the appropriate, accurate, and reliable detection of resistance. It must be appreciated at the outset that susceptibility cannot be guaranteed. Many pharmacokinetic factors (e.g., protein binding, bioavailability) and innate host defense mechanisms (or lack thereof) influence in vivo effectiveness. In vitro susceptibility testing assesses only the interaction of a microorganism and an antimicrobial agent. It is not possible to include the many complex and variable host factors that contribute to a successful therapeutic outcome. However, it is possible to detect the inability of an antimicrobial to inhibit an organism to an extent that clinical failure is likely. The second major purpose is effective communication of results for both individual patient therapy and surveillance. In defined populations, surveillance reports indicating prevailing susceptibility patterns are essential for logical selection of empiric therapy for presumed infection. Periodic surveillance of isolates for newly recognized or potentially emergent resistance may have even broader implications for patient care or public health. Effective reporting of results in a manner

that will encourage appropriate utilization of antimicrobial agents will facilitate control efforts to reduce or at least restrict emerging resistance rates and ultimately control costs.

To accomplish these goals, it is imperative that the laboratory work closely with other members of the health care team. Communication with requesting physicians regarding issues of specimen collection, suspected etiologic agents, and appropriate antimicrobial agents to test is essential for optimal patient results. Interaction with infection control personnel is essential in matters pertaining to surveillance. Finally, interaction with the pharmacy is desired in promoting choices of cost-effective and pharmacologically appropriate agents for testing.

Test Variables

The primary concept behind AST is simple. Clinically significant microbial isolates are placed in the presence of pharmacologically appropriate concentrations of antimicrobial agents, and the impact upon growth is measured. An organism is considered sensitive if growth is inhibited by a therapeutically achievable concentration, and, conversely, resistant if growth occurs. The major variables in the test system, therefore, are the organisms, the antimicrobials and their concentrations, and the method used to assess growth.[31]

Selection of Organisms

Three categories of organisms can be identified.[32] The first category is organisms for which AST need not be routinely performed because there are clear-cut drugs of choice, and no clinically significant resistance to those agents has been demonstrated. This does not preclude periodic surveillance of recent isolates to detect emerging resistance. This list is decreasing steadily, but most β-hemolytic streptococci belong in this category. Also included in this category are isolates from mixed infections contiguous to a mucous membrane surface. Here, empiric therapy aimed at predominant species is as likely to be successful as attempts to find a single antimicrobial or combination to which all isolates are sensitive. The same holds for other mixed infections in which contamination or colonization is likely and an etiologic agent cannot be presumed (e.g., by predominance) from the culture results.

The second category of organisms is that for which limited testing for select resistance is indicated. These are isolates for which significant levels of resistance have been noted to agents that are otherwise clearly cost-effective drugs of choice. Examples are penicillin and third-generation cephalosporin testing against *S. pneumoniae* or *N. meningitidis*; ampicillin, high-level aminoglycoside, and vancomycin testing against enterococci; penicillin, tetracycline, and quinolone testing against *N. gonorrhoeae*; and β-lactamase testing of a variety of organisms, including *H. influenzae*, *N. gonorrhoeae*, and significant anaerobe species to detect penicillin or cephalosporin resistance.

The third category of organisms are those that require extensive testing against a variety of agents. These organisms, when encountered as significant etiologic agents, have resistance to multiple types of antimicrobials in varying percentages, so that there are no clear-cut drugs of choice designated for a given clinical situation. Staphylococci, enterics, nonfermenting gram-negative bacilli such as *Pseudomonas and Acinetobacter*, and others belong in this category. For these organisms, close collaboration with physician-users and pharmacist-consultants is essential to select an appropriate antibiotic test panel.

Selection of Antimicrobials

A number of criteria are considered in the selection of antimicrobics for testing and reporting. The criteria pertain to type of organism, antimicrobial characteristics, host factors, institutional needs, and practical issues. With regard to organism type, the discussion of antimicrobials and modes of action has already demonstrated that each antimicrobial has an expected spectrum of activity. Drawing upon this concept, the National Committee for Clinical Laboratory Standards (NCCLS) Guidelines for susceptibility testing have suggested groupings of antimicrobial agents that should be considered for routine testing and reporting by clinical microbiology laboratories.[33–36] These groupings are as follows:

- Nonfastidious gram-positive cocci in the genera *Staphylococcus, Enterococcus*, or nonpneumococcal *Streptococcus*
- Nonfastidious gram-negative bacilli in the family Enterobacteriaceae or in the genera *Pseudomonas, Stenotrophomonas, Burkholderia*, and *Acinetobacter*
- Fastidious genera *Haemophilus, Neisseria* (particularly *N. gonorrhoeae*), *S. pneumoniae*, and anaerobes

For other organism types, each laboratory must use published clinical guidelines[37, 38] to determine which agents may be appropriate.

With regard to antimicrobial characteristics, several factors must be considered, all of which pertain to the utility of the data generated. First, within a given class of agents, only a single agent needs to be tested unless there are significant differences in antibiotic spectrum. Examples are selection of a single first-generation cephalosporin based on utilization patterns for testing gram-positive or -negative organisms, and selection of oxacillin, because of its greater in vitro stability, to represent all semisynthetic antistaphylococcal penicillins. Second, agents may be grouped in primary panels for testing against all organisms of a given type, with secondary or supplemental panels used for testing and/or reporting only when resistance to primary agents occurs or in select clinical circumstances (e.g., testing with urinary isolates only, testing in an inpatient setting for IV use vs. outpatient setting for PO use). For this situation, NCCLS documents provide suggested groupings to consider. Finally, agents may be chosen for testing because of their proven ability to detect specific resistance mechanisms of clinical importance. They are termed "predictor panels."[39] Examples are use of high-level gentamicin with *Enterococcus* species to predict resistance to aminoglycosides other than streptomycin, and selection of ceftazidime to detect extended-spectrum β-lactamase activity in certain enterics, most notably *Klebsiella pneumoniae*.

Certain host factors must also be included in the antibiotic test selection process. Of particular note is the site of infection, which can be presumed from the specimen source. Examples are testing of urinary infection agents only on urine isolates, selection of agents with good central nervous system penetrability for CSF isolates, and testing of topical ophthalmic compounds on ocular isolates. Other host factors to be considered are age, pregnancy, renal or hepatic function, and state of immunocompetency, because specific inclusion or exclusion criteria for use may apply (Table 58–4).

Table 58–4. Drug(s) of Choice for Common Pathogenic Bacteria

Organisms		Usual Drug of Choice
Gram-positive		
S. aureus	Methicillin-sensitive	Oxacillin, nafcillin, dicloxacillin (PO)
Coagulase-negative staphylococci		Cefazolin
	Methicillin-resistant	Vancomycin
S. pneumoniae	Penicillin-sensitive	Penicillin
	Penicillin-resistant, cephalosporin-sensitive	Cefotaxime, ceftriaxone
	Penicillin- and cephalosporin-resistant	Vancomycin
Streptococcus species		Penicillin, macrolides, cephalosporins, etc.
Enterococcus		Ampicillin or vancomycin *with* gentamicin or streptomycin
Gram-negative		
Enteric	*E. coli, Proteus, Klebsiella*	First- to third-generation cephalosporin
		Trimethoprim-sulfamethoxazole, quinolone
		Aminoglycoside
	Serratia, Enterobacter	Imipenem *or* Piperacillin + aminoglycoside
		Ciprofloxacin
Nosocomial	*P. aeruginosa*	Piperacillin or ceftazidime *with* aminoglycoside
		Ciprofloxacin, imipenem, aztreonam
	Acinetobacter	Imipenem + amikacin
Respiratory	*H. influenzae, Moraxella (Branhamella) catarrhalis*	Third-generation cephalosporin for life-threatening disease
		Amoxicillin-clavulanate, ampicillin-sulbactam, oral cephalosporin, trimethoprim-sulfamethoxazole
Anaerobic		
Mouth/lungs	*Peptostreptococcus, Clostridium*	Clindamycin
Lower GI tract	*Bacteroides fragilis*	Metronidazole, clindamycin, cefoxitin/cefotetan, imipenem

Of key emerging importance in the antimicrobial selection process are factors relating to cost,[40] in addition to considerations of clinical efficacy and low toxicity. To ensure cost-effective utilization of antimicrobials, most health care organizations employ a formulary that either suggests or specifies agents to use in given clinical situations. Clearly, the laboratory must design its testing battery to be compatible with the approved formulary. When a formulary does not exist, or if the client base is more diverse, the laboratory should include prevailing utilization patterns as a factor in the design of appropriate test batteries.

Finally, all laboratories should be flexible enough to recognize that special circumstances may dictate that antibiotics not usually tested need to be considered upon specific physician request. Factors such as host allergies, unusual sites of infection, and multidrug resistance may all be indications for additional testing.

Test Methods for Bacteria

A number of variables should be considered in determining which test methods to employ in a routine clinical laboratory setting. Factors relating to the type of data generated (e.g., qualitative vs. quantitative, bacteriostatic vs. bactericidal), specific organism considerations (particularly pertaining to detection of emerging resistance), and a variety of practical considerations enter into such decisions.[41] For a full appreciation of these factors, it is worthwhile to briefly describe the types of test formats available.

Qualitative Tests

Qualitative tests provide data that are categorical and separate organisms into "sensitive," "resistant," and, in some cases, "intermediate" groups. The most obvious examples are tests for specific enzymes that inactivate antibiotics and confer clinical resistance. These tests rely on visual detection of the action of the enzymes on antimicrobial substrates. The most widely used enzyme test is detection of β-lactamase activity in a variety of organisms, including *Staphylococcus, Haemophilus, N. gonorrhoeae,* and some anaerobes, to predict resistance to penicillins. Another enzyme test, used primarily for *Haemophilus,* is that for chloramphenicol acetyltransferase, which is indicative of chloramphenicol resistance. Although rapid, easy, and specific, these tests have rather limited clinical utility.[42]

Also available are a limited number of growth-dependent screening tests that employ single critical concentrations of antimicrobials to classify organisms as sensitive or resistant. Examples are screening for MRSA (including one rapid-test format) and screening for *Enterococcus* with resistance to vancomycin or high-level resistance to aminoglycosides.[42]

On the horizon are tests employing molecular probes to detect specific nucleic acid target sequences. To improve sensitivity, these tests may depend on amplification (e.g., polymerase chain reaction). Although none is yet commercially available, several such tests, including one for the *mec* gene responsible for "methicillin" resistance in *S. aureus,* one for the *van* genes responsible for vancomycin resistance in *Enterococcus,* and one for the genes responsible for primary drug resistance in *M. tuberculosis,* have proved both accurate and reliable.[30]

Disk Diffusion (Kirby-Bauer) Testing

The disk diffusion method constitutes one of the most widely used qualitative susceptibility test procedures. The test indicates resistance to antimicrobial agents by the reduction of a zone of growth inhibition around an antimicrobial disk. Zone size values are established by regression analysis of populations of isolates chosen through consideration of several factors—pharmacologic factors, particularly relating to the peak attainable therapeutic levels one can achieve using the most common dosage regimens; microbiologic factors, primarily relating to the distribution of isolates with known susceptibility and resistance patterns; and clinical factors, relating to clinical response of isolates to therapy. It is of note that if an isolate's resistance has not been previously recognized, false-susceptible results may occur until an appropriate analysis has been done.

The disk diffusion test offers a relatively easy and flexible format, with highly reproducible results, when performed in strict accordance with NCCLS guidelines.[33] However, the test is indicated only for rapidly growing aerobic organisms, such as staphylococci, most streptococci, enterococci, enterics, and common nonfermenting gram-negative bacilli. With appropriate media and incubation modifications, the disk diffusion test may also be applied to *S. pneumoniae, H. influenzae, N. gonorrhoeae,* and *N. meningitidis.* This test method has not been standardized for other organisms. Alternative methods should be employed, or if disk diffusion testing is attempted, results should be reported as nonstandard or investigational. It is also of note that in medically urgent situations, early readings (6–12 hours) can be made and are generally consistent with overnight readings. Despite primary use of the disk diffusion test to provide qualitative data, one company has developed a software package (BioMic; Giles Scientific) that relates zone size to antimicrobic concentration, thereby potentially providing quantitative data. It is also recommended that data be recorded as inhibition zone size in order to detect significant trends that may be overlooked if only interpretive data (e.g., sensitive or resistant) are recorded.[30]

Quantitative Tests

In contrast to qualitative tests, quantitative tests generate actual numeric data that are reported in addition to an interpretive category. The most common such assay generates a value termed the MIC (minimal inhibitory concentration). In an MIC assay, varying concentrations of antimicrobials, generally comprising serial twofold dilutions within a broad biologic and therapeutic range, are tested for their ability to inhibit growth of organisms. Standard methods are described by the NCCLS.[34] The MIC value is reported as the smallest amount of antimicrobial tested that will completely inhibit growth of an organism. Categorical interpretations are made by comparison of MIC values with NCCLS tables, which establish break points similar to a process for disk tests (Fig. 58–1).

The major advantage of an MIC test is the ability to

A. Relative peak achievable levels

(μg/mL)

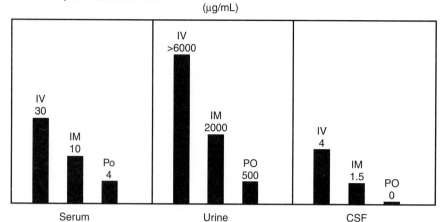

B. MIC Break point by organism type

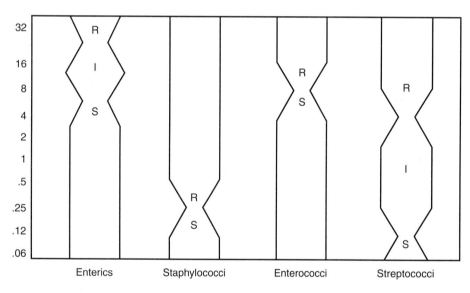

Figure 58–1. Relationship of *(A)* achievable levels by varying routes of administration and *(B)* break point interpretation for ampicillin. Abbreviations: IV, intravenously; IM, intramuscularly; PO, orally; CSF, cerebrospinal fluid; R, resistant; S, sensitive; I, intermediate.

perform site-specific categorical interpretation. As shown schematically in Figure 58–1, one can see the influence of both route and anatomic site on the achievable drug levels. In general, it is desirable to have the peak attainable level at the site of infection at least several-fold (i.e., twofold to fourfold) higher than the MIC to account for the "peaks and troughs" in drug concentration that occur during interval dosing. For any isolate with a given MIC, predicted efficacy may vary widely according to pharmacologic parameters. It has been proposed that an "inhibitory quotient" (peak drug level divided by the MIC) be determined to facilitate interpretation of results.[43] For serious infection in compromised patients, such an approach may be very helpful.

Like disk tests, MIC tests have been highly standardized by NCCLS and are reproducible for the same organism groups. In addition, agar dilution has been recommended as a standard test for anaerobic bacteria.[35] In fact, MIC results may be generated for virtually any organism group

that can be grown in vitro. However, one must be cautious in applying categorical interpretations when such organisms have not been evaluated and included in the NCCLS documents. The major disadvantage to MIC tests is that they can be labor intensive and expensive, particularly if the dilution panels are prepared by the laboratory. This disadvantage can be overcome by using commercially available, prepared panels from a number of sources. Many of the commercial systems also have automated readers, which can improve reliability and reduce labor, and come in "combo" forms with computer-based biochemical identification systems.

RAPID, AUTOMATED MIC SYSTEMS

In addition to the automation and convenient miniaturized packaging available through commercial MIC test systems, several systems are available with the capability to generate rapid, "same-day" results for both MICs and identification of many rapidly growing aerobic or facultative organisms. The concept that generation of rapid results may positively affect patient care by reducing overall costs has been reaffirmed.[44] The reduced costs are primarily related to more timely institution of appropriate and cost-effective antimicrobial therapy. The instruments that are commercially available either rely on rapid (2–4 hour) endpoint analysis using colorimetric, turbidometric, or fluorometric detection, or employ complex assessment of growth coefficients to extrapolate MIC values. The two major suppliers at present are Dade-Microscan, employing the former method, and BioMerieux Vitek Systems, using the latter.[45]

On a performance basis, the two systems are comparable. One cautionary note for both, however, is that the combination of microvolumes (i.e., low absolute organism numbers) and rapid readout may render false-susceptible results for specific organism-antibiotic combinations when resistance is inducible.[39]

E Test

A relative newcomer to the susceptibility test market is the E test strip (AB BioDisk). This product employs a continuous gradient antibiotic strip that is placed on an inoculated agar surface. The MIC is determined by assessing where the growth edge intersects the strip markings. Thus, the test combines the ease of the disk diffusion method with the quantitative data potential of an MIC method. This test has been widely accepted for use with many fastidious organism groups, including drug-resistant *S. pneumoniae*, vancomycin-resistant *Enterococcus* species, anaerobes, rapidly growing mycobacteria, and some yeasts. The major disadvantages are its high cost for individual strips and lack of U.S. Food and Drug Administration (FDA) clearance for all published applications.[31]

Special Organism Considerations

The continued emergence of novel antimicrobial resistance mechanisms frequently necessitates the implementation of special methods to facilitate detection. A number of examples of unique organism test strategies have been developed.

Gram-Positive Cocci

The earliest example of an organism requiring specific test strategies was methicillin-resistant *S. aureus* (MRSA).[46] Resistance is due to the presence of altered penicillin-binding proteins. Optimal detection of MRSA and resistant coagulase-negative species (MRCNS) requires manipulation of test conditions to promote expression of heterotypic resistance.[30, 33] Because MRSA and MRCNS are commonly multidrug-resistant, a high index of suspicion must be maintained when multidrug resistance is noted. In addition, both MRSA and MRCNS should be reported as resistant to all other β-lactam type antimicrobials, because clinical failure is likely regardless of the in vitro test result.

Enterococcus species have also emerged that require special testing.[30, 42] Penicillin and ampicillin resistance due to altered penicillin-binding proteins may be detected by standard tests. However, detection of β-lactamase–producing strains requires an enzyme method. Either type of resistance may result in failure to respond to synergistic penicillin and aminoglycoside therapy. Because β-lactamase production remains uncommon and occurs primarily in high-level aminoglycoside–resistant strains, a selective test strategy may be employed.

High-level aminoglycoside–resistant *Enterococcus* species carry plasmids with enzymatic resistance genes and also fail to respond to synergistic therapy. For their detection, screening agar or broth with gentamicin (500 μg/mL) or streptomycin (1000 μg/mL in broth, 2000 μg/mL in agar) should be used. Testing of other aminoglycosides is unnecessary, because gentamicin resistance predicts resistance to the other agents. Finally, vancomycin-resistant enterococci (VRE) have also emerged to a level at which routine testing is indicated.[47] For optimal detection, a 6 μg/mL screening agar is recommended, with MIC verification. Multiple mechanisms are responsible, with the basis still incompletely understood. However, three resistance genes (termed *van* A, *van* B, and *van* C) are known, which may be surmised from MIC level and teicoplanin cross-resistance and may be confirmed by molecular testing. VRE is of particular concern for its potential to transmit resistance to MRSA.[48]

Drug-resistant *S. pneumoniae* (DRSP) similarly requires special attention.[49] In the last few years, rapid increases in resistance to penicillin and cephalosporins (including third-generation agents) has been noted. Resistance occurs through chromosomal alteration of PBPs in a stepwise fashion. Although an oxacillin screening disk test strongly suggests an elevated MIC, a specific MIC test should be performed to verify level of resistance. Special interpretive guidelines apply to the two agents. Whereas serious infection with moderately susceptible strains may respond to therapy, absolute resistance usually predicts clinical failure, especially in meningitis. DRSP is also commonly multidrug-resistant, so testing against alternate agents is appropriate.

Gram-Negative Bacilli

Aerobic and facultative gram-negative bacilli, particularly the Enterobacteriaceae and common nonfermenters (e.g., *Pseudomonas, Acinetobacter, Burkholderia, Stenotrophomonas*) have built an extensive armamentarium of resistances to virtually every antimicrobial class. Although most clinically significant resistances are reliably detected by standard methods, resistance to β-lactam–type agents remains problematic.[39, 50] Resistance due to activation (derepression) of a chromosomally mediated β-lactamase may be problematic, because the resistance is inducible. A small proportion of stably expressing mutants may fail to be detected initially, but through selective therapeutic pressure, they emerge as predominant in a setting of clinical failure. Tests using low concentrations of inocula or short incubation times are especially prone to generate false-susceptible results. Because certain genera characteristically carry such enzyme activity (i.e., *Enterobacter, Serratia, Citrobacter, Pseudomonas*), correct identification is a key to recognition of resistance. A second problem area is the detection of strains with extended-spectrum, plasmid-mediated β-lactamases (ESBLs), which have emerged through mutations in common plasmid-borne genes. These resistant organisms are more reliably detected with ceftazidime and aztreonam than other β-lactams but are clinically resistant to all. ESBLs can be demonstrated by the potentiation of β-lactam activity with the β-lactamase inhibitor, clavulanic acid. Again, awareness of the primary organisms involved (i.e., *K. pneumoniae, E. coli*) is a key to their recognition.

Anaerobes

Like other bacteria, anaerobic species may also express a diverse array of antimicrobial resistance. There is general agreement that isolates from serious infections with possible significant resistances should be tested with antibiotics appropriate for anaerobic therapy.[51] The problem lies in selection of a test method.[52] The NCCLS-approved method uses a tedious agar dilution approach that is not practical for most laboratories.[35] Commercial MIC panels and E tests offer possible solutions, and β-lactamase tests may be useful for some isolates.

Other Bacteria

It is now clear that virtually every clinically significant bacterial species has the potential to develop resistance to agents considered drugs of choice. Therefore, the laboratory must be vigilant in detection, and flexible in adapting new methods as appropriate. Penicillin-resistant *N. meningitidis*, quinolone-resistant *Campylobacter*, and quinolone-resistant *N. gonorrhoeae* all represent contemporary concerns.[53] On the horizon are other concerns, for example, vancomycin-resistant *S. aureus* and penicillin-resistant *S. pyogenes*.

Testing of Other Microorganism Groups

Although most clinical microbiology laboratories perform bacterial AST, testing of other groups of organisms is generally confined to regional specialty laboratories. That is not to say that antimicrobial resistance is not a concern, but rather that the techniques employed require special expertise and a sufficient volume for the costs to be justified.

Mycobacterial Testing

Multidrug-resistant *M. tuberculosis* (MDR-TB) has become a major concern, particularly in high-risk patients, including the HIV infected, the homeless, recent immigrants, and cohort groups such as prison populations. The Centers for Disease Control and Prevention (CDC) guidelines encourage routine testing of primary drugs for new isolates, and retesting if emergence of new resistance is likely.[54] In addition, second-line agents should be tested when primary resistance is encountered. Traditional test methods employ a "proportion of resistance" approach, in which clinical resistance can be inferred when 1% or more of a test population shows growth on selected test concentrations of antimicrobials.[55] Alternatively, a more rapid test

method employing the radiometric Bactec 460 system of Becton Dickinson is commercially available. This method assesses the ability of 1% or more of a test population to grow in broth with antibiotics at least as well as in a 100% control suspension.[56] New methods employing nucleic acid probe and amplification techniques[30] and a novel mycobacterial phage-luciferase reporter technique[57] may further shorten laboratory turnaround times in the future, thereby facilitating institution of appropriate therapy.

For mycobacteria other than tuberculosis (MOTTs), susceptibility testing may also be indicated. Rapid-growing *M. fortuitum-chelonae* complex isolates may be tested in a nonstandard fashion with disk diffusion or E test.[42] Other MOTTs, particularly those encountered in HIV-infected patients (e.g., *M. avium-intracellulare* complex, *M. kansasii*), may be tested with an agar method similar to that used for *M. tuberculosis*, with appropriate antimicrobials.[55]

Fungal Testing

Although the array of antifungals available is limited, fungal resistance has also been noted, particularly in immunocompromised patients on prophylactic therapy.[58] For some isolates, resistance is intrinsic and may be presumed from a correct identification (e.g., amphotericin resistance in *Pseudoallescheria boydii* or *C. lusitanae*). Particularly for *Candida* species, however, emergence of resistance has been noted, and in vitro testing may be indicated. An NCCLS broth microdilution or macrodilution method has been proposed[59] but is not practically possible for many laboratories. However, an alternative convenient investigational approach employs the E test method.[58] For all fungi, break point interpretation and standardization remain concerns.

Viral Testing

The battery of antimicrobials used to treat viral infections is still quite limited, yet viral resistance has already been noted. Although testing strategies and even clinical significance of in vitro resistance have not been clearly established, testing may be appropriate for some infections. Of particular note are resistance of HSV to acyclovir and of CMV to gancyclovir. Testing relies on either cell culture–based replication inhibition or molecular methods. In addition, for HIV, viral nucleic acid quantification using amplification on blood samples is used to assess the therapeutic efficacy of combination anti-HIV therapy.[60]

Protozoal Infections

Resistance has been documented for a few clinically significant protozoal infections. Testing is rarely performed except in highly specialized centers, but requests may occasionally be made. Examples are the emergence of metronidazole resistance in *Trichomonas vaginalis*, and of chloroquine resistance in *Plasmodium falciparum*. Detection relies on growth inhibition or molecular methods.

Special Categories of Tests

Occasionally, methods other than those previously described may be employed for in vitro assessment of potential therapeutic efficacy. These tests are used primarily for serious bacterial infections in compromised hosts but may occasionally be requested in mycobacterial or fungal infection.

MBC (Minimal Bactericidal Concentration)

Derived from the MIC procedure, the MBC test assesses the ability of an antimicrobial to kill bacteria (or other organism types) rather than simply inhibit growth. Following completion of a broth MIC procedure using a known inoculum concentration, measured amounts of broth from dilutions showing apparent inhibition are inoculated to agar media to detect remaining viable organisms. By convention, one generally evaluates the concentration where 99.9% killing (i.e., a 3 log_{10}-reduction) occurred. Although an NCCLS-proposed standard exists,[61] the procedure is wrought with technical variables and interpretive problems, particularly for testing of β-lactam antimicrobials. However, when killing activity is essential because of a patient's immunocompromised state (e.g., in neutropenia), or in situations with poor antibiotic access (e.g., meningitis, endocarditis), MBC results may help in selecting the "best" agent to use.[62]

Serum Bactericidal (Schlichter's) Test

Serum bactericidal tests (SBTs) are used in circumstances similar to the MBC test and are performed in a similar manner. However, instead of preparation of dilutions of known concentrations of antimicrobial agents, dilutions of a patient's serum are inoculated with the patient's own infecting organism. Typically, both peak and trough serum samples are obtained for testing. The dilutions are examined at 24 hours for growth inhibition, and at 48 hours for 99.9% killing activity. In general, it is desirable to demonstrate a peak killing titer of 1:8 or higher, with some residual trough activity. An NCCLS-proposed document exists,[63] but as for MBC tests, the performance of the SBT is subject to many technical variables. Nevertheless, in serious infections, the SBT may be useful in maximizing the pharmacodynamic effects of one or more antimicrobial agents.[62] The test may be modified for organisms other than bacteria. Collection of samples may be problematic when multiple antimicrobials are being delivered on variable dosage schedules.

Synergy Testing

Occasionally, testing may be performed to assess interactions between a combination of two agents. The interactions observed may be synergistic (indicating greater activity than expected), indifferent (indicating expected combined activity), or antagonistic (indicating less activity than expected). Most assays are technically difficult, not standardized, and only rarely indicated. There are four main assay approaches, as described by Eliopoulos and Moellering.[64] Few laboratories perform such assays, although they may provide valuable assistance in optimizing therapy in difficult infections involving multidrug-resistant pathogens (e.g., pulmonary infections in patients with cystic fibrosis, multidrug-resistant mycobacterial infections).

Antibiotic Levels

In situations in which there is a narrow toxic-to-therapeutic ratio, assays for antimicrobial levels in serum or other body fluids may be necessary to avoid a potential adverse outcome. Although historically bioassays were performed using sensitive indicator organisms, current methods rely primarily on automated immunoassays. Agents for which monitoring is typically performed include aminoglycosides and vancomycin.[41]

Other Techniques

As the number and types of immunocompromising or otherwise compromising medical interventions increase, the need for implementation of convenient assays to maximize therapy of resultant infections will also grow. Attention has been focused on rapid "-cidal" assays employing instrumentation. One such approach uses flow cytometry with organisms tagged by differential viability dyes.[65]

CONSIDERATIONS IN SELECTION OF LABORATORY TESTS

Table 58–5 summarizes the laboratory methods available to assist clinicians in selection of appropriate anti-infective therapy. The various AST formats evaluate interactions between organisms and antimicrobials, antibiotic assays evaluate attainable levels in a given host, and the SBT attempts to evaluate the interaction of all components—organism, antimicrobial, and host. As previously discussed, each has a specific role in directing anti-infective therapy.[41]

Of these tests, the one showing the greatest diversity in available formats is the in vitro antimicrobial susceptibility test. There is variability not only in methods but also in commercial suppliers. Each laboratory must therefore evaluate a number of factors in selecting a test system for use.[45, 66] Foremost are the patient care needs of the institution. A tertiary care center with complex or compromised patients at risk for infection with drug-resistant organisms will of necessity make quantitative and killing activity assays available. Other centers may need only qualitative data.

In considering which specific commercial (or perhaps

Table 58–5. Summary of Laboratory Tests Used to Guide Antimicrobial Therapy

Test	Purpose
Antimicrobial susceptibility tests	Measure in vitro sensitivity or resistance to antimicrobics
Disk diffusion	Measures inhibition qualitatively
MIC	Measures inhibition quantitatively
MBC	Measures killing quantitatively
Synergy	Measures combination effects
Enzyme assays	Detect inactivating enzymes
Antibiotic levels	Measure amount in blood to assess toxic-therapeutic levels
Serum bactericidal test	Measures how much a patient's serum can inhibit and kill an infecting organism to predict therapeutic efficacy

in-house) system to use, one must next consider a number of performance issues. Through literature review and internal validation, one must be comfortable that the accuracy and reliability of the test system are adequate. Practical performance issues, such as space requirements, workflow adaptability, organism and antibiotic flexibility, quality control requirements, aesthetic aspects (particularly ergonomics, noise considerations, and waste disposal), and equipment maintenance requirements and downtime frequency must also be given significant consideration. Most laboratories will need to have more than one approach available to address all of these issues.

Reporting issues are equally important. The necessity for and potential effectiveness of a rapid turnaround system, compared with a standard overnight system, must be determined. Reporting format utility and flexibility must be established. Finally, all data management aspects, including laboratory and hospital information system interface capabilities, must be evaluated. Of particular note is the availability of epidemiology and pharmacy management software for several automated systems that must be considered.

Finally, as with all decisions in contemporary health care, a complete cost analysis that takes into consideration all of the aforementioned issues must be performed. The laboratory must assume a rightful and knowledgeable role in this process.

EFFECTIVE COMMUNICATION OF RESULTS

It is imperative that the susceptibility and resistance data generated by the microbiology laboratory be presented in a manner that facilitates a desired patient care outcome. That is, the data must allow physicians and clinical pharmacists to formulate therapeutic strategies that meet the goals of clinical efficacy, low toxicity, and cost-effectiveness.

For individual patient reports, there are a number of goals to strive for. Reports should be both timely and accurate.[30] The data should be presented with an interpretive category as defined by NCCLS. Conditional reporting should selectively display results for organisms and agents determined to meet patient care goals, with rule-supported editing, suppression, and release mechanisms. The chart versions should be annotated with additional information to support appropriate use (e.g., costs, toxicity, common dosage, attainable levels). Finally, a system for *STAT* broadcasting of highly significant resistant organisms should be established. These results may serve as a laboratory alert to the possibility of a novel or incorrect finding (e.g., vancomycin-resistant *S. aureus*). Alternatively, the results may signal an alert to a health care provider that an infection control risk exists (e.g., MRSA, VRE). Finally, innovative and sophisticated interactions between pharmacy and laboratory information systems may actually be programmed to flag the use of an inappropriate antimicrobial agent for an etiologically confirmed infection and/or to recommend change to a more appropriate agent.[40]

In addition to individual patient reports, the laboratory has an obligation to provide periodic summary data for specific organisms, antimicrobial agents, anatomic sites of infection, and/or physical locations or specific population.

Such surveillance data are essential to selection of empiric therapy for specific infection types in defined patient groups.[67] Surveillance data may also serve a sentinel function in the recognition of significant emerging trends in resistance. Periodic reports should be given to appropriate health care organization committees and distributed to health care providers as part of the quality assurance or performance improvement program for the laboratory.[68]

Case Study 1

A 57-year-old white man from a southern state was picked up in a midtown entertainment district for "acting crazy" and was taken to an area hospital psychiatric unit. On admission, he was noted to be febrile (100.8 °F) with blood pressure of 121/70 mm Hg and a pulse of 92 beats/min. A peripheral white blood cell count was 19.2×10^9/L with significant neutrophilia. A lumbar puncture was performed with a CSF count of 9750 cells µL (100% polymorphonuclear leukocytes); a gram-positive coccobacillus was visualized microscopically and presumptively identified by CSF latex agglutination. A diagnosis of meningitis was made, and the patient was started on IV ceftriaxone. Of note is that the patient had been taking amoxicillin for the previous week for treatment of computed tomography–confirmed sinusitis. Blood cultures were negative, but on CSF culture, 5 colonies of an α-hemolytic, catalase-negative, gram-positive coccus in chains was noted in the second streak area of the primary plates (blood agar, chocolate agar). The organism was identified as *S. pneumoniae* by latex agglutination. Susceptibility testing by disk diffusion revealed resistance to oxacillin, erythromycin, trimethoprim-sulfamethoxazole, and chloramphenicol. Subsequent E tests revealed a penicillin MIC of 4 µg/mL and a ceftriaxone MIC of 3 µg/mL. With the addition of vancomycin and rifampin, the patient improved and was discharged without sequelae.

Questions

1. Are the therapeutic strategies used in treating this patient appropriate for the clinical scenario described?

2. This case illustrates a number of laboratory features that are unusual for *S. pneumoniae* meningitis. What are these unusual aspects?

3. The MIC values for both penicillin and ceftriaxone demonstrate resistance in accordance with NCCLS guidelines. Why would clinical failure be associated with these values in a case of meningitis?

Discussion

1. The clinical signs and symptoms and the laboratory findings are consistent with bacterial meningitis. In a normal, otherwise healthy adult, the primary etiologic agent to be considered is *S. pneumoniae*, with *N. meningitidis* and *H. influenzae* being secondary con-

siderations. Because of significant emerging penicillin resistance in *S. pneumoniae*, a third-generation cephalosporin is the drug of choice in many regions for empiric therapy of community-acquired meningitis. This agent would also be appropriate for coverage for β-lactamase–producing *H. influenzae* and moderately penicillin-resistant *N. meningitidis*. Because penicillin resistance in the southern United States may be as high as 30%, the empiric choice of ceftriaxone is appropriate. It should also be remembered that third-generation cephalosporins have good CSF penetrability.

2. The most notable unusual observation in this case is the history of development of meningitis secondary to sinusitis despite prior therapy with amoxicillin and, subsequently, ceftriaxone. This finding suggests than an organism resistant to these β-lactam agents may be involved. Cephalosporin-resistant *S. pneumoniae* has been reported, so depending on the prevailing community resistance rates, it may be appropriate to add other antimicrobial agents to cover this possibility. In select pediatric groups in which resistant isolates have been documented, it has become community practice to add vancomycin and perhaps rifampin until a definitive susceptible etiologic agent has been documented. It can be seen that the laboratory has a very important role in monitoring community resistance rates to facilitate adequate empiric use of antibiotics.

Second, the microscopic and culture features are also unusual and probably also relate to the recent antibiotic history. The morphology on direct Gram stain was atypical for *S. pneumoniae*, that is, coccobacilli rather than diplococci. β-Lactam agents commonly alter morphology of both susceptible and resistant organisms. On culture, the antibiotics present in the specimen also probably reduced the quantity of growth expected given the positive Gram stain, with only a few colonies detected in a nonprimary streak area, where the antibiotics were diluted by the streaking process. It is also possible that the normal inflammatory milieu of the specimen contributed to the scant growth denoted by inhibiting or killing the bacteria present. It is well accepted that *S. pneumoniae* is a fastidious organism that may be difficult to recover from clinical specimens, particularly when antecedent therapy has been given.

3. Because an organism is considered to be clinically susceptible to an antibiotic when the peak achievable level at the site of infection exceeds the MIC by several-fold, one can look at both values to predict therapeutic success. In this case, the NCCLS interpretations for *S. pneumoniae* and penicillin or ceftriaxone are as follows:

MIC (µg/mL)

Interpretation	Penicillin	Ceftriaxone
Sensitive	≤.06	≤0.25
Intermediate	>.06–<2	>.25–<2
Resistant	≥2.0	≥2.0

The approximate attainable levels for these agents at several possible sites of infection are as follows:

		Peak Level (µg/mL)	
Site	**Route**	*Penicillin*	*Ceftriaxone*
Serum	IV	1.0	128
CSF	IV	0.5	5–10
Sputum	IV	0.2	4
Ear fluid	PO	2	
Sinus fluid	PO	0.5	

With the patient isolate MICs of 4 µg/mL for penicillin and 3 µg/mL for ceftriaxone, it is readily obvious that the attainable levels would fail to predictably eradicate the organism in the settings of meningitis, pneumonia, otitis media, or sinusitis.

Case Study 2

The Pharmacy and Therapeutics (P&T) Committee of an academic medical center tertiary care hospital performed a medication utilization evaluation of ciprofloxacin, which was added to the formulary in 1992. The data presented to the committee were as follows:

			Findings	
Justification of Use	**Standard (%)**	**Threshold (%)**	*Year*	*Compliance (%)*
IV ciprofloxacin was used for the following indications:				
Culture and sensitivity documented resistance of other formulary alternatives	100	80	1993	43
			1994	57
			1995	66
Suspected or proven osteomyelitis	100	80	1993	40
			1994	36
			1995	55

The data indicated that the agent was commonly being used for indications other than those approved. Review of the outliers indicated that most inappropriate use was in the surgical ICU (SICU) settings and for treatment of suspected ventilator-associated pneumonia.

Questions

1. The microbiology laboratory was asked for assistance in evaluating the impact of the unapproved usage. What kind of data would be useful to the P&T Committee?

2. In a related matter, the P&T Committee was also investigating whether ofloxacin could be used as a more cost-effective alternative to ciprofloxacin, and requested that the laboratory assist. What kind of data would be useful to the P&T Committee for this issue?

Discussion

1. Antibiotics have been categorized as being the only medications given to patients that may have an ad-

verse outcome on other patients. That is, if use of an antibiotic results in increased resistance of microorganisms to that agent, then infection with the antibiotic-resistant organisms may be transmitted to another patient. In this situation, the unapproved utilization could be targeted in specific hospital locations and for a specific infectious process. Thus, the laboratory could review antibiotic resistance patterns by both parameters and look for evidence of increased resistance. The data provided by the laboratory were as follows:

Indicator Organisms	Hospital Location	% Resistant to Ciprofloxacin			
		1992	1993	1994	1995
S. aureus	ER	46	39	42	37
Enterococcus sp.		3	8	15	20
E. coli		0	0	1	0
E. cloacae		20	23	18	22
P. aeruginosa		6	11	9	13
Acinetobacter		20	25	27	29
S. aureus	MICU	52	50	48	50
Enterococcus sp.		4	10	12	15
E. coli		0	2	3	0
E. cloacae		30	28	25	30
P. aeruginosa		12	15	17	15
Acinetobacter		30	35	40	35
S. aureus	SICU	46	48	55	60
Enterococcus sp.		8	12	20	25
E. coli		0	2	5	8
E. cloacae		30	32	35	40
P. aeruginosa		8	15	20	25
Acinetobacter		30	56	68	78

The data demonstrated that isolates from community-based infections seen in the emergency room showed little increase in resistance except for Enterococcus, which could be attributed to increasing quinolone use for urinary tract infection in elderly patients.

Similarly, for a nonsurgical ICU, although resistance rates were higher than in the community (presumably due to increased exposure to antibiotics), there was no unexpected increased ciprofloxacin resistance.

However, for the SICU identified as a site of misappropriate utilization, increasing resistance was documented for a number of clinically significant organisms.

Additional specimen-specific data for the SICU were as follows:

Organisms	Specimen	% Resistant to Ciprofloxacin			
		1992	1993	1994	1995
S. aureus	Urine	43	45	45	50
P. aeruginosa		8	12	15	15
Acinetobacter		20	22	25	40
S. aureus	Sputum	43	45	50	65
P. aeruginosa		10	15	22	30
Acinetobacter		32	55	70	80
S. aureus	Blood	42	48	55	64
P. aeruginosa		8	14	18	25
Acinetobacter		34	55	70	76

These data suggested that use of the quinolone for treatment of respiratory infections was associated with increasing resistance in specimens from that site, with resistance also documented in secondary bacteremias. In contrast, resistance was less marked in urinary tract infections.

Taken together, these data supported the emergence of ciprofloxacin resistance secondary to greater utilization of the agent in a setting for which it is not accepted as appropriate. On the basis of these data, an intervention strategy was designed to reduce utilization in the SICU.

2. When more than one antimicrobial agent is commercially available within a given class, a number of factors are considered in the decision as to which to use. Efficacy in treatment is given first priority, followed by low toxicity, and the cost issues. In the assessment of efficacy, both clinical performance data and in vitro susceptibility data are considered. Therefore, the laboratory is often asked to provide data on organisms derived from within the patient groups served. In this case, a variety of organisms from significant infections were tested by a disk diffusion procedure, which generated the following results:

Organism	% Ciprofloxacin			% Ofloxacin		
	Resistant	Intermediate	Susceptible	Resistant	Intermediate	Susceptible
S. aureus	45	16	39	48	14	38
Staphylococcus sp.	55	16	29	56	17	27
Enterococcus sp.	18	4	78	20	5	75
Acinetobacter sp.	44	10	46	47	12	41
C. koseri	0	0	100	0	0	100
E. cloacae	2	6	92	1	8	91
E. coli	1	0	99	1	1	98
K. pneumoniae	0	1	99	1	0	99
P. mirabilis	0	0	100	0	0	100
P. aeruginosa	8	9	83	18	12	70

The only organism tested for which a significant difference in resistance rate was noted was P. aeruginosa. The data suggested that ofloxacin antimicrobial inhibitory levels might be greater than ciprofloxacin levels. Therefore, this organism was selected for further MIC testing using E tests to determine whether the difference might be clinically significant.

The following data were obtained for P. aeruginosa:

	Ciprofloxacin	Ofloxacin
Average MIC ($\bar{x}$)	0.19	1.14
"S" breakpoint	1.0	2.0
Breakpoint/MIC $\bar{x}$	5.3	1.7
PO peak level	2.3	4.4

PO peak/MIC $\bar{x}$	12.43	3.85
IV peak level	4.6	4.25
IV peak/MIC $\bar{x}$	24.86	3.72

In addition to increased resistance, among sensitive *P. aeruginosa* isolates, the average MICs for ciprofloxacin were sixfold lower than those for ofloxacin. When compared with peak serum levels by either intravenous (IV) or oral (PO) dosing, the ratio of attainable level to MIC is significantly higher with ciprofloxacin. Particularly if monotherapy is being considered, this increased "inhibitory quotient" is desirable to ensure therapeutic efficacy. On the basis of these data, a decision was made to keep ciprofloxacin on the medical center's formulary.

In summary, this case illustrates how data from antimicrobial susceptibility testing may have an impact on the care of patient's care beyond those from whom the data was derived.

References

1. Moellering RC: Principles of anti-infective therapy. *In* Mandell GL, Bennett JE, Dolin R (eds): Mandell, Douglas and Bennett's Principles and Practice of Infectious Diseases, ed 4, vol 1. New York, Churchill Livingstone, 1995.
2. Wilkowske CJ: General principles of antimicrobial therapy. Mayo Clin Proc 66:931, 1991.
3. Drusano GL: Pharmacology of anti-infective agents. *In* Mandell GL, Bennett JE, Dolin R (eds): Mandell, Douglas and Bennett's Principles and Practice of Infectious Diseases, ed 4, vol 1. New York, Churchill Livingstone, 1995.
4. Davis J: Inactivation of antibiotics and the dissemination of resistance genes. Science 264:375, 1994.
5. Nikaido H: Prevention of drug access to bacterial targets: Permeability barriers and active efflux. Science 264:382, 1994.
6. Spratt BG: Resistance to antibiotics medicated by target alterations. Science 264:388, 1994.
7. Mayer KH, Opal SM, Medeiros AA: Mechanisms of antibiotic resistance. *In* Mandell GL, Bennett JE, Dolin R (eds): Mandell, Douglas and Bennett's Principles and Practice of Infectious Diseases, ed 4, vol 1. New York, Churchill Livingstone, 1995.
8. Ffekety R: Vancomycin and teicoplanin. *In* Mandell GL, Bennett JE, Dolin R (eds): Mandell, Douglas and Bennett's Principles and Practice of Infectious Diseases, ed 4, vol 1. New York, Churchill Livingstone, 1995.
9. Wright AJ, Wilkowske CJ: The penicillins. Mayo Clin Proc 66:1047, 1991.
10. Chambers HF, Neu HC: Penicillins. *In* Mandell GL, Bennett JE, Dolin R (eds): Mandell, Douglas and Bennett's Principles and Practice of Infectious Diseases, ed 4, vol 1. New York, Churchill Livingstone, 1995.
11. Gustaferro CA, Steckelberg JM: Cephalosporin antimicrobial agents and related compounds. Mayo Clin Proc 66:1064, 1991.
12. Karchmer AW: Cephalosporins. *In* Mandell GL, Bennett JE, Dolin R (eds): Mandell, Douglas and Bennett's Principles and Practice of Infectious Diseases, ed 4, vol 1. New York, Churchill Livingstone, 1995.
13. Chambers HF, Neu HC: Other β-lactam antibiotics. *In* Mandell GL, Bennett JE, Dolin R (eds): Mandell, Douglas and Bennett's Principles and Practice of Infectious Diseases, ed 4, vol 1. New York, Churchill Livingstone, 1995.
14. Gilbert DN: Aminoglycosides. *In* Mandell GL, Bennett JE, Dolin R (eds): Mandell, Douglas and Bennett's Principles and Practice of Infectious Diseases, ed 4, vol 1. New York, Churchill Livingstone, 1995.
15. Steigbigel NH: Macrolides and clindamycin. *In* Mandell GL, Bennett JE, Dolin R (eds): Mandell, Douglas and Bennett's Principles and Practice of Infectious Diseases, ed 4, vol 1. New York, Churchill Livingstone, 1995.
16. Standiford HC: Tetracyclines and chloramphenicol. *In* Mandell GL, Bennett JE, Dolin R (eds): Mandell, Douglas and Bennett's Principles and Practice of Infectious Diseases, ed 4, vol 1. New York, Churchill Livingstone, 1995.
17. Hooper DC, Wolfson JS: Fluoroquinolone antimicrobial agents. N Engl J Med 324:384, 1991.
18. Hooper DC: Quinolones. *In* Mandell GL, Bennett JE, Dolin R (eds): Mandell, Douglas and Bennett's Principles and Practice of Infectious Diseases, ed 4, vol 1. New York, Churchill Livingstone, 1995.
19. Zinner SH, Mayer KH: Sulfonamides and trimethoprim. *In* Mandell GL, Bennett JE, Dolin R (eds): Mandell, Douglas and Bennett's Principles and Practice of Infectious Diseases, ed 4, vol 1. New York, Churchill Livingstone, 1995.
20. Finegold SM, Mathisen GE: Metronidazole. *In* Mandell GL, Bennett JE, Dolin R (eds): Mandell, Douglas and Bennett's Principles and Practice of Infectious Diseases, ed 4, vol 1. New York, Churchill Livingstone, 1995.
21. Drugs for tuberculosis. Med Lett Drug Ther 37:67, 1995.
22. Systemic antifungal drugs. Med Lett Drug Ther 38:10, 1996.
23. Georgopapadakous NH, Walsh TJ: Antifungal agents: Chemotherapeutic targets and immunologic studies. Antimicrob Agents Chemother 40:279, 1996.
24. Drugs for AIDS and associated infections. Med Lett Drug Ther 37:87, 1995.
25. The new drugs for HIV infection. Med Lett Drug Ther 38:35, 1996.
26. Drugs for non-HIV viral infections. Med Lett Drug Ther 36:27, 1994.
27. Drugs for parasitic infections. Med Lett Drug Ther 37:99, 1995.
28. Liu LX, Weller PF: Drug therapy: Antiparasitic drugs. N Engl J Med 334:1178, 1996.
29. American Society for Microbiology: Report of the ASM Task Force on Antibiotic Resistance. Public and Scientific Affairs Board. Washington, DC, American Society for Microbiology, 1995.
30. Sahm DF: The role of clinical microbiology in the control and surveillance of antimicrobial resistance. ASM News 62:25, 1996.
31. Sahm DF, Newman MA, Thornsberry C, et al: Current concepts and approaches to antimicrobial agent susceptibility testing. (Cumitech 25.) Washington, DC, American Society for Microbiology, 1988.
32. Jorgensen JH: Antimicrobial susceptibility testing of bacteria that grow aerobically. Infect Dis Clin North Amer 7:393, 1993.
33. National Committee for Clinical Laboratory Standards: Performance Standards for Antimicrobial Disk Susceptibility. (NCCLS Document M2-A5.) Villanova, Pa., NCCLS, 1993.
34. National Committee for Clinical Laboratory Standards: Methods for Dilution Antimicrobial Susceptibility Tests for Bacteria that Grow Aerobically. (NCCLS Document M7-A3.) Villanova, Pa., NCCLS, 1993.
35. National Committee for Clinical Laboratory Standards: Methods for Antimicrobial Susceptibility Testing of Anaerobic Bacteria. (NCCLS Document M11-A3.) Villanova, Pa., NCCLS, 1993.
36. National Committee for Clinical Laboratory Standards: Supplemental Tables for M2-AS, M7-A3, and M11-A3. (NCCLS Document M100-55.) Villanova, Pa., NCCLS, 1993.
37. The choice of antibacterial drugs. Med Lett Drug Ther 38:25, 1996.
38. Amsden GW, Shentag JJ: Tables of antimicrobial agent pharmacotherapy. *In* Mandell GL, Bennett JE, Dolin R (eds): Mandell, Douglas and Bennett's Principles and Practice of Infectious Diseases, ed 4, vol 1. New York, Churchill Livingstone, 1995.
39. Sanders CC, Thomson KS, Bradford PA: Problems with detection of β-lactam resistance among nonfastidious gram-negative bacilli. Infect Dis Clin North Amer 7:411, 1993.
40. Schentag JJ, Ballow CH, Fritz AL, et al: Changes in antimicrobial agent usage resulting from interactions among clinical pharmacy, the infectious disease division, and the microbiology laboratory. Diagn Microbiol Infect Dis 16:255, 1993.
41. Rosenblatt JE: Laboratory tests used to guide antimicrobial therapy. Mayo Clin Proc 66:942, 1991.
42. Neumann MA, Sahm DF, Thornsberry C, et al: New developments in antimicrobial susceptibility testing: A practical guide. (Cumitech GA.) Washington, DC, American Society for Microbiology, 1991.
43. Ellner PD, New HC: The inhibitory quotient: A method for interpreting minimum inhibitory concentration data. JAMA 246:1575, 1981.
44. Doern GV, Vautour R, Gaudet M, et al: Clinical impact of rapid in vitro susceptibility testing and bacterial identification. J Clin Microbiol 32:1757, 1994.

45. Hindler JA: Antimicrobial susceptibility testing of gram-negative bacteria: Meeting the challenge of increasing resistance and decreasing budgets. Clin Microbiol Newsl 17:77, 1995.

46. Chambers HF: Detection of methicillin-resistant staphylococci. Infect Dis Clin North Am 7:425, 1993.

47. Woodford N, Johnson AP, Morrison D, et al: Current perspectives on glycopeptide resistance. Clin Microbiol Rev 8:585, 1995.

48. Edmond MB, Wenzel RP, Pasculle AW: Vancomycin-resistant *Staphylococcus aureus*: Prospective measures needed for control. Ann Intern Med 124:329, 1996.

49. Defining the public health impact of drug-resistant *Streptococcus pneumoniae*: Report of a working group. MMWR CDC Surveill Summ 45:1, 1996.

50. Livermore DM: β-Lactamases in laboratory and clinical resistance. Clin Microbiol Rev 8:557, 1995.

51. Rosenblatt JE, Brook I: Clinical relevance of susceptibility testing of anaerobic bacteria. Clin Infect Dis 16:S446, 1993.

52. Wexler H: Anaerobic susceptibility testing: Where are we and where do we go from here? Clin Microbiol Newsl 18:41, 1996.

53. Neu HC: The crisis in antibiotic resistance. Science 257:1064, 1992.

54. Tenover FC, Crawford JT, Huebner RE, et al: The resurgence of tuberculosis: Is your laboratory ready? J Clin Microbiol 31:767, 1993.

55. National Committee for Clinical Laboratory Standards: Antimycobacterial Susceptibility Testing: Proposed Standard. (NCCLS Document M24-P.) Villanova, Pa., NCCLS, 1990.

56. Siddiqui SH, Liborati JP, Middlebrook G: Evaluation of a rapid radiometric method for drug susceptibility testing of *Mycobacterium tuberculosis*. J Clin Microbiol 13:908, 1981.

57. Jacobs WR Jr, Barletta RG, Udani R, et al: Rapid assessment of drug susceptibilities of *Mycobacterium tuberculosis* by means of luciferase reporter phages. Science 260:819, 1993.

58. Pfaller MA, Rinaldi MG: Antifungal susceptibility testing: Current state of technology, limitations, and standardization. Infect Dis Clin North Amer 7:435, 1993.

59. National Committee for Clinical Laboratory Standards: Reference Method for Broth Dilution Antifungal Susceptibility Testing of Yeasts: Proposed Standard. (NCCLS Document M-27P.) Villanova, Pa., NCCLS, 1992.

60. Keating MR: Antiviral agents. Mayo Clin Proc 67:160, 1992.

61. National Committee for Clinical Laboratory Standards: Methods for Determining Bactericidal Activity of Antimicrobial Agents: Tentative Proposal. (NCCLS Document M26-T.) Villanova, Pa., NCCLS, 1992.

62. Stratton CW: Bactericidal testing. Infect Dis Clin North Amer 7:445, 1993.

63. National Committee for Clinical Laboratory Standards: Methodology for the Serum Bactericidal Test. (NCCLS Document M21-T.) Villanova, Pa., NCCLS, 1992.

64. Eliopoulos GM, Moellering RC Jr: Antimicrobial combinations. *In* Lorian V (ed): Antibiotics in Laboratory Medicine, ed 3. Baltimore, Williams & Wilkins, 1991.

65. Mason DJ, Power EGM, Talsania H, et al: Antibacterial action of ciprofloxacin. Antimicrob Agents Chemother 39:2752, 1995.

66. Jorgensen JH, Doern GV: Practical guidelines for in vitro susceptibility testing of selected gram-positive bacteria. Clin Microbiol News 17:81, 1995.

67. Evans RS, Classen DC, Pestotnik SL, et al: Improving empiric antibiotic selection using computer decision support. Arch Intern Med 154:878, 1994.

68. McGowan JE Jr: Antibiotic-resistant bacteria and healthcare systems: Four steps for effective response. Infect Control Hosp Epidemiol 16:67, 1995.

Nutritional and Metabolic Disorders

Chapter **59**

Major Aminoaciduria

Jesse Guiles and Felicia A. Czekaj

ETIOLOGY AND PATHOPHYSIOLOGY
General Categories

Aminoaciduria (AAU) refers to high levels of amino acids in the urine. Generally, the cause of AAU is either a malfunction in the manufacture of these compounds by the liver or a malfunction in the transport or reabsorption of them by the kidney. AAUs can be grouped into four categories. The first three categories are collectively known as *primary aminoacidurias.* They are caused by a genetic defect resulting in the nonmanufacture or defective manufacture of an enzyme necessary for synthesis, metabolism, or tubular reabsorption of a specific amino acid. These genetic defects are also known as *inborn errors of metabolism.* The four AAU categories and their descriptions are as follows:

1. *Overflow AAU* is caused by an enzyme defect that leads to overproduction of one or more amino acids by the liver. This results in the amino acid(s) exceeding its renal threshold, therefore spilling into the urine. Both serum and urine amino acid levels are increased in these diseases.
2. *Renal transport AAU* is caused by a congenital defect in the reabsorption of an amino acid by the kidney tubules. Serum levels for one or more amino acids are normal or decreased, whereas urine levels are high.
3. *No-threshold AAU* is caused by an inherited enzyme defect in the biochemical processing of an amino acid, which leads to an accumulation in the urine of an intermediate amino acid not normally seen in the urine.

It should be noted that these AAUs are not due to a congenital defect in the tubules but to a normal lack of a physiologic mechanism for the reabsorption of the intermediate metabolites by the tubules.

4. *Secondary AAU* is caused by other diseases or toxins resulting in liver necrosis or destruction of tubular function. Many or all amino acids are usually increased in these diseases.

A list of AAUs can be seen in Tables 59–1 and 59–2. Although this table lists the major AAUs found today, more than 50 hereditary diseases of amino acid metabolism have been identified. Fortunately, as can be seen from the table, the incidence of these diseases is low and identification of those AAUs with a relatively high frequency can easily be accomplished through screening tests.

Primary Overflow Aminoaciduria

PHENYLKETONURIA

Phenylketonuria (PKU) results from a block in phenylalanine (Phe) metabolism due to a congenital lack of the enzyme phenylalanine hydroxylase (PAH), which causes a buildup of Phe in blood and urine (Fig. 59–1). This PAH enzyme deficiency is an autosomal recessive trait. PKU is the prototype for overflow AAU, and as shown in Table 59–1, it is the most common type. Variant forms exist, some of which are caused by partial PAH deficiencies; others are caused by defects in the metabolism of biopterin, a cofactor of PAH.[1]

MATERNAL PHENYLKETONURIA

Mass screening and treatment of PKU has existed in many states and countries for almost 30 years, resulting in a new problem, maternal PKU. The number of mothers who had been diagnosed and treated for PKU as infants but subsequently taken off treatment is increasing. In pregnancies of such women, the infant is at greater risk of mental retardation, microcephaly, and congenital heart disease. These increased risks correlate with the blood Phe levels of the mothers.[2, 3] Several studies have reported that any degree of hyperphenylalaninemia in the mother can cause harm to the fetus.[2] Infants are at a lesser risk when such mothers follow dietary therapy before conception and throughout the pregnancy.[4] In many treatment centers, patients with PKU are receiving continued follow-up and counseling regarding treatment and prevention of maternal PKU.[2]

TYROSINEMIA

The genetically controlled lack of enzyme activity causing tyrosinemia (formerly referred to as *tyrosinosis*) is shown in Figure 59–1. Blockage leads to an alternate route for tyrosine metabolism, with a concurrent rise in urinary tyrosine dihydroxyphenylalanine (DOPA), and other metabolites. Variant forms of the disease exist, depending on the specific enzyme affected and whether the genetic defect causes a partial or total loss of enzymatic activity. A milder, transient form of neonatal tyrosinemia is seen relatively frequently, caused by the decreased ability of the premature infant's liver to synthesize enzymes. This is a temporary, self-correcting condition, although recent study has indicated that infants afflicted with this condition may have some diminished mental abilities.[5] In transient neonatal tyrosinemia, Phe also accumulates because of an accompanying PAH deficiency. The clinical laboratory scientist must be aware of this possibility when PKU testing is performed to avoid an erroneous diagnosis. Although the neonatal form of tyrosinemia is the most common, it must be distinguished from the more severe forms of the disease to ensure proper treatment.

ALKAPTONURIA

Alkaptonuria results from an abnormality along the same metabolic pathway as PKU and tyrosinemia (see Fig. 59–1). Deficiency of homogentisic acid (HGA) oxidase leads to a buildup of HGA.

MAPLE SYRUP URINE DISEASE

Maple syrup urine disease (MSUD) or branched-chain ketoaciduria (BCKA) is caused by an inborn error in the catabolism of the branched-chain amino acids (BCAAS)—leucine, isoleucine, and valine. The affected enzyme catalyzes the decarboxylation of intermediate BCAA metabolites to α-ketoacids (see Fig. 59–2). The enzyme is nonspecific, resulting in an increase of all three amino acids in serum and urine.

Variant forms of MSUD exist and have been identified by biochemical markers and clinical signs. In the intermittent form, enzymatic activity is sufficient during periods of relative health; however, in times of stress (e.g., infections, surgery, vaccinations), children may show symptoms identical to the classic MSUD. In milder forms, BCAAs are increased in urine, but clinical symptoms are less severe.

Primary Renal Transport Aminoaciduria

Cystinuria is the classic example of renal transport AAU. It is caused by the defective reabsorption of cystine by the renal tubular epithelial cells and is transmitted as an autosomal recessive trait.

Primary No-Threshold Aminoaciduria

No-threshold AAU is characterized by the abnormal presence of an amino acid in the serum and urine (see Table 59–1). No-threshold AAU is due to a blockage of an intermediate metabolic step of an amino acid, causing the metabolite to be filtered into the urine. No physiologic mechanism allows for tubular reabsorption of these intermediates; consequently, they are excreted by the kidneys.

Secondary Aminoaciduria

Causes of secondary AAU are listed in Table 59–1. The AAU can be an overflow type (fulminant hepatic failure) or a renal type (Fanconi's syndrome). Certain diseases, such as galactosuria, result in the accumulation of intermediate products of metabolism, which in turn can cause renal toxicity. Other causes of secondary AAU include poisons,

Table 59–1. Primary Aminoacidurias

Disease	Prevalence	Deficient Enzyme	Amino Acid Increase	Clinical Features	Treatment
Primary Overflow AAUs (Autosomal Recessive)					
Phenylketonuria (PKU) with variants (I–V)	1:10,000	L-Phenylalanine hydroxylase	Phenylalanine and metabolites	Mental retardation Seizures	Diet low in Phe
Tyrosinemia (variants) (neonatal)	1:100,000	Fumarylacetoacetate hydrolase, tyrosine amino transferase (neonatal = liver immaturity)	Tyrosine, methionine, and metabolites (Phe in neonatal)	Hepatic cirrhosis Renal damage Tyrosine needles	Diet low in tyrosine, Phe, and methionine
Alkaptonuria	1:250,000	Homogentisic acid oxidase	Homogentisic acid	Degenerative arthritis	None known
Maple Syrup Urine Disease (MSUD) or Branched Chain Ketoaciduria (BCKA)	1:200,000	Branched chain ketoacid decarboyxlase	Valine, leucine, isoleucine (ketoacids)	Spasticity Severe acidosis Convulsions Respiratory failure Mental retardation Leucine crystals Early death	Diet low in leucine, valine, and isoleucine
Histidinemia	1:20,000	Histidase	Histidine, alanine, and metabolites	Speech defects Motor deficiencies Mental retardation (to no symptoms)	Diet low in histidine
Citrullinemia	Rare	Argininosuccinate synthetase	Citrulline, alanine (ammonia)	Seizures Vomiting Mental retardation	Low protein diet
Primary No-Threshold AAUs (Autosomal Recessive)					
Homocystinuria (and variants)	1:200,000	Cystathionine β-Synthase (and variants)	Homocystine, methionine (normal in variants)	Vascular thrombosis Ocular dislocation Skeletal deformity Mental retardation	Diet low in methionine Vitamin B6, B12 therapy
Cystathioninuria	1:70,000	Cystathionase	Cystathionine and metabolites	Benign to mild mental retardation	Vitamin B12 therapy
Primary Renal AAUs (Autosomal Recessive)					
Cystinuria (and variants)	1:7,000	Tubular dysfunction	Lysine, ornithine, arginine	Cystine crystals Renal calculi Renal damage	Hydration Alkaline urine D-penicillamine
Hartnup Disease	1:18,000	Tubular dysfunction	13 Neutral amino acids	Normal to pellagra-like rash Retarded growth Mental retardation Neurologic symptoms	Adequate protein diet Nicotinamide therapy
Iminoglycinuria	1:15,000	Tubular dysfunction	Glycine Proline, hydroxyproline	Renal tubular defect in reabsorption of iminoacids and glycine	None known

Table 59–2. Causes of Secondary Aminoacidurias

Fulminant hepatic failure
Acute massive necrosis of liver
Acute yellow atrophy of liver
Acute tubular necrosis
Fanconi syndrome
Galactosemia
Wilson's disease
Wasting/starvation
Poisons (lead, mercury)
Acetaminophen overdose

From Guiles HJ: Aminoaciduria. *In* Davis BG, Bishop ML, Mass DM (eds): Clinical Laboratory Science. Philadelphia, JB Lippincott, 1989.

wasting (from starvation), acute tubular necrosis, and acetaminophen overdose.

Secondary causes can result in the abnormal excretion of one or usually more amino acids. In addition to increases in amino acids, other substances, such as glucose, protein, phosphate, and galactose, can be, and usually are, increased in the urine.

CLINICAL MANIFESTATIONS

General Clinical Signs

As can be seen in Table 59–1, clinical manifestations are similar in many of these diseases. They appear very early in life, beginning within a few days after birth and continuing through infancy into childhood and adulthood.

The following clinical signs in infants and children[6, 7] should alert the clinician to the possibility of AAU:

- Mental retardation
- Deterioration of motor skills or language
- Profound developmental delay
- Corneal clouding
- Abnormalities in urine color or odor
- Sparse, short, brittle hair
- A family history of AAU or of siblings who died young

Very young infants who appear healthy at birth but begin manifesting signs of life-threatening illness (anorexia, vomiting, difficulty in breathing, coma) after the onset of feeding, should be evaluated immediately for aminoacidopathy. The disease progression is very rapid once the first symptoms appear.

Primary Overflow Aminoaciduria

PHENYLKETONURIA

Neonates with PKU appear normal at birth. After the onset of feeding, symptoms such as feeding difficulties, vomiting, and delayed development begin to appear. Brain injury occurs between the second and third weeks of life and becomes maximal at 8 to 9 months. Untreated patients have significantly lower intelligence quotients (IQs) than treated patients.[8] Other symptoms include hypopigmentation, skin lesions, eczema, and urine with a characteristic "mousy" odor.

TYROSINEMIA

Clinical symptoms of tyrosinemia include jaundice, failure to thrive, hepatosplenomegaly, ascites, edema, and bleeding. Symptoms usually begin in infancy and vary according to the severity of the disease (partial vs. total enzyme deficiency). Patients with partial enzymatic defects develop cirrhosis. Death due to hepatocarcinoma and liver failure is the usual result in patients with a complete defect.[9]

ALKAPTONURIA

In infancy and childhood, the only symptom of alkaptonuria is darkening of the urine when exposed to air or alkaline pH. The disease can be detected in neonates if dark stains in diapers are noticed and investigated. Clinical symptoms begin in adulthood and include degenerative arthritis and dark pigmentation of cartilage, which is caused by the binding of HGA and its metabolites to collagen in the cartilage and connective tissue.

MAPLE SYRUP URINE DISEASE

The incidence of MSUD is rare (see Table 59–1). Although the neonate is normal at birth, symptoms such as listlessness, refusal to eat, and vomiting appear within the first 5 days of life. These symptoms rapidly progress to include loss of reflexes, alternating hypotonicity and hypertonicity, lethargy, episodes of acute ketoacidosis (often triggered by recurrent infections), irregular respiration, convulsions, and coma. Unless the disease is diagnosed properly and promptly, the infant will die of respiratory insufficiency. Those who survive the acute neonatal period show severe retardation and cerebral palsy.[6, 7] Morbidity is minimal if the diagnosis is made and treatment is initiated within 24 hours of the initial symptoms. Prognosis is unpredictable if there is a delay of 3 to 14 days; it is inevitably grave if delayed beyond 14 days.[6, 7]

Primary No-Threshold Aminoaciduria

The clinical symptoms listed in Table 59–1 are the major reason for laboratory screening of suspected no-threshold AAU. Symptoms may develop later in life or not at all.

Secondary Aminoaciduria

Clinical symptoms of secondary AAU are consistent with the primary condition that is responsible for the liver or kidney malfunction that has caused the AAU.

LABORATORY ANALYSES AND DIAGNOSIS

Screening Tests for Aminoaciduria

Specimens for laboratory analysis come either from patients who exhibit AAU symptoms or from participants of massive screening programs. Blood analyses on infants for AAU, especially PKU, are mandatory in most states.[10]

Screening tests are designed to call attention to suspi-

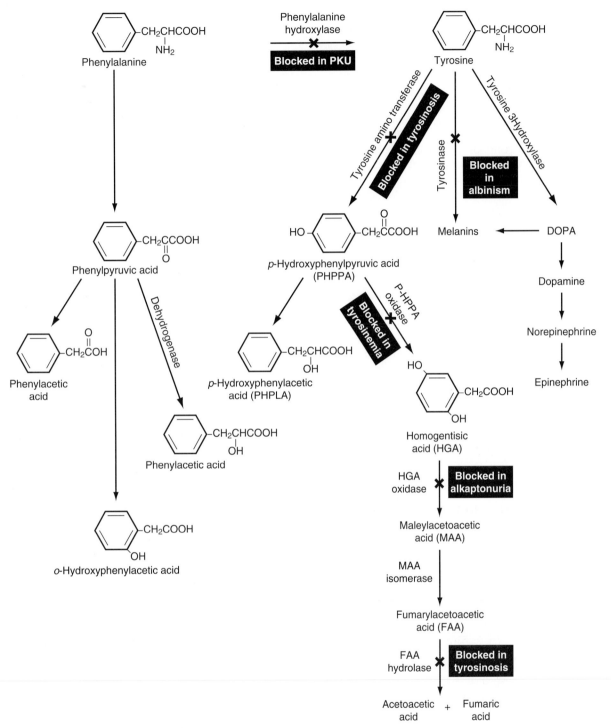

Figure 59–1. Metabolism of phenylalanine and tyrosine.

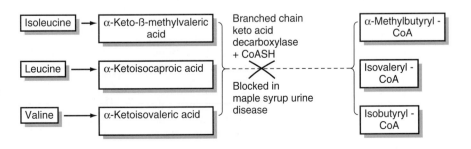

Figure 59–2. Catabolism of branched chain amino acids. Abbreviations: CoA SH, uncombined coenzyme A; CoA, coenzyme A. (Adapted from Efron ML: Aminoaciduria. N Engl J Med 272:1058–1066, 1965. Massachusetts Medical Society. All rights reserved.)

cious cases; therefore, confirmatory testing is always necessary. These preliminary tests have "high sensitivity" that is, patients with the disease will be positive for the test. However, to obtain high sensitivity, some clinical specificity is sacrificed, resulting in a concurrent high rate of false-positive results. In some screening programs, only 1 in 40 infants testing positive will actually have the disease. This sacrifice of specificity for sensitivity is insignificant because treatment, consisting of a prescribed dietary regimen, can begin on all screen-positive infants without any ill effects. However, prompt initiation of treatment is necessary to prevent permanent impairment of an affected infant.

The first, and still utilized, highly sensitive mass screening test is the Guthrie test system,[12] which has been adapted for screening other types of AAU in addition to PKU. Any positive result must be followed with confirmatory testing. It should be noted that a potential for false-negative results using Guthrie's test exists. The clinical laboratory scientist should be certain that the specimen is collected from an infant whose age is at *least* 24 hours. This ensures that sufficient time has elapsed, allowing for a rise in concentration of the amino acid in question to detectable levels.[12]

Although state law may prescribe mandatory screening of neonates for one or more amino acids, infants and children up to several years of age may also present with symptoms of AAU. These individuals may have been missed in the screening program or may have a defect not tested for in the initial screen. The next level of testing calls for urine and serum screening by qualitative chemical colorimetric methods, chromatography, or high-voltage electrophoresis (HVE).

Chemical Screening Tests

Simple chemical screening tests are available and are quick and easy to perform. They can be used *with* thin-layer chromatography (TLC) but never alone as a screen. Drawbacks include being positive for a number of other metabolic disorders and drugs and being negative in the presence of many interfering substances, resulting in poor sensitivity and specificity. These tests are described in standard texts on urinalysis.

Thin-Layer Chromatography Screens

One- and two-dimensional TLC is the preferred methodology for screening suspected AAU urine and blood samples (Fig. 59–3). HVE can also be used. Principles of result interpretation are similar for both methods.

TLC gives a qualitative measurement of the amino acids that are present. Screen interpretation requires great skill and experience. For this reason, reference laboratories experienced in the interpretation of test results are typically utilized. Generally, a positive result should be reported with caution because this test is a screening test, and positive results can occur for a wide variety of reasons. Clinical laboratory scientists should be aware of the following limitations before making an interpretation of the chromatograph:

1. A *fresh* urine sample is crucial for best results using this technique. Bacterial contamination can be an important source of false-positive or false-negative results. Bacte-

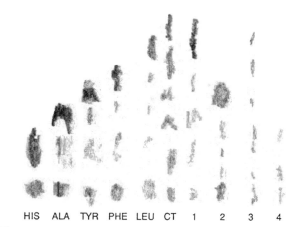

HIS ALA TYR PHE LEU CT 1   2   3   4

Figure 59–3. Thin-layer chromatography (TLC) amino acid screen.

ria utilize amino acids and produce metabolites that can cause interference with TLC. Laboratories must insist that only "clean catch random urine" samples brought to the laboratory as soon as possible are tested.[13]

2. Administration of medication (especially penicillins) or dietary therapy can cause results resembling AAU.[12]

3. Oliguria, with resulting concentration of metabolites, can cause false-positive results. To rule out this possibility, suspected urine samples must be tested for specific gravity.

4. Inadequate metabolic development or enzymatic maturation in the infant can cause false-negative results.

The TLC screen, like the Guthrie screen, is designed for high sensitivity, and its specificity is limited. The laboratory requires patient information such as diagnosis, medication, and diet to help in the interpretation of the test.[13]

Quantitation of Amino Acids

When a screening test is positive, a quantitative determination is the next course of action. Quantitative results can be obtained using high-pressure liquid chromatography (HPLC) with an appropriate ion exchange column and a fluorescent detection system. Interpretation of testing must be made with the same precautions noted for qualitative examinations. Should a delay occur in the reporting of the confirmatory (quantitative) results, it is advisable that a preliminary report indicating the probability of an AAU be issued so that appropriate therapy can be initiated promptly. Possible causes for false-positive results should be ruled out after a thorough review of the patient's status and the laboratory protocol as it relates to the specimen. An algorithm for handling specimens of suspected AAU is presented in Figure 59–4. DNA sequencing analysis for suspected PKU is now possible, as is measurement of gene product catalytic protein and enzyme activity in cultured cells from amniocentesis.[14] These techniques are currently available.

Primary Overflow Aminoaciduria

TYROSINEMIA

A Guthrie system for tyrosinemia is currently available, and mass screening of infants is done in most states. Urine

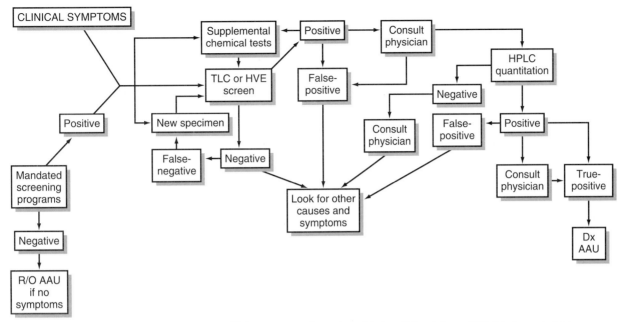

Figure 59–4. Use and interpretation of laboratory tests for aminoacidurias. Abbreviations: TLC, thin-layer chromatography; HVE, high-voltage electrophoresis; HPLC, high-pressure liquid chromatography; R/O, rule out; AAU, aminociduria; Dx, diagnosis.

samples can be used for qualitative screening, but serum must be used for final quantitation by chromatography. Urine contains interfering compounds in high enough concentrations to give poor specificity. An enzymatic method is also available, which gives better sensitivity and specificity for tyrosine. *p*-Hydroxyphenylpyruvic acid (PHPPA) can also be detected by chromatography, which is considered one of the most reliable ways of diagnosing tyrosinemia because urinary excretion of PHPPA can reach up to 25 times the normal amount.[15]

Hepatobiliary test result values are elevated with tyrosinemia, especially as the disease progresses. Patients who exhibit characteristic symptoms along with increased levels of hepatic enzymes and bilirubin should have further testing for tyrosinemia.

Tyrosine crystals may be seen in the urine of patients affected with any form of tyrosinosis. The urine also has a cabbage-like odor. The crystals must be distinguished from similar-looking crystals, such as sulfonamide or X-ray dye crystals. Solubility tests help to distinguish them. The discovery of tyrosine crystals in urine should always be considered a significant finding. The clinical laboratory scientist should check the age, symptoms, and suspected diagnosis of the patient to see if the the diagnostic profile of tyrosinemia fits. Tyrosine crystals can also be seen in patients with severe liver disease due to oasthouse urine disease or to other etiologies.

ALKAPTONURIA

The darkening of urine over a 12- to 24-hour period when exposed to air or sunlight is a presumptive indication of alkaptonuria. A similar darkening of urine may be caused by other substances, such as phenols, melanin, and metabolites of salicylate and tryptophan. These substances must be ruled out by chemical testing. Furthermore, high

levels of vitamin C, sometimes used to treat alkaptonuria, reduce HGA levels and produce a false-negative result.

A combination of positive screening tests and darkening of urine left standing should lead to the performance of qualitative and quantitative chromatography procedures to confirm the presence of HGA. The chromatography results should correlate with symptoms in adults only, since infants are symptomless.

MAPLE SYRUP URINE DISEASE

The breath, skin, earwax, and urine of patients with MSUD have a characteristic burnt sugar or maple syrup odor, from which the disease derives its name.[15] The odor is believed to be caused by the increase of α-keto-β-methylvaleric acid, a metabolite of isoleucine in the urine.[16] The urine will test positive for this amino acid in chemical analyses but must be screened by TLC or HVE, which will show increases in all three amino acids.

Prompt diagnosis after appearance of the first clinical symptoms is the single most important factor in determining the outcome of treatment. Within 24 hours after birth, newborns with classic MSUD can have a diagnostically relevant plasma leucine concentration, regardless of feeding.[7] The infant may rapidly progress into acidotic episodes; therefore, it is imperative that clinical symptoms and urine amino acid results be correlated with other laboratory tests, particularly electrolyte and blood gas studies.

Leucine crystals may be found in the urine sediment of MSUD patients. They are identified by their appearance and solubility characteristics. The finding of leucine crystals in urine is always abnormal and should initiate a protocol similar to the one described earlier when finding tyrosine crystals.

The incidence of MSUD is very low; however, some states mandate neonatal mass screenings. MSUD can also be diagnosed by characterization of the MSUD enzyme phenotype in cultured skin fibroblasts. Measurement of chorionic villi enzyme activity has been reported as a means of prenatal diagnosis.[17]

Primary No-Threshold Aminoaciduria

Chemical tests can be useful for the detection of no-threshold AAUs, but, again, these tests are nonspecific (Table 59–3). Qualitative and quantitative assays are best performed by chromatography, in which the intermediate metabolites can be visualized. Both urine and serum samples should be analyzed because a no-threshold AAU may show a positive result in the urine and a normal result in the serum.

Secondary Aminoaciduria

Clinical symptoms, laboratory data, and patient history should be utilized in the diagnosis of secondary AAU. Supporting laboratory data can include markedly increased liver enzyme and bilirubin levels, drug or toxin levels, electrophoretic abnormalities, and a positive hepatitis profile.

TREATMENT

Primary Overflow Aminoaciduria

PHENYLKETONURIA

Treatment consists of a dietary regimen low in Phe. Over-restriction of Phe, however, can lead to impaired growth or brain damage. At the beginning of treatment, Phe measurements should be performed every 1 to 2 days until the level drops below 10 mg/dL. Thereafter, weekly measurements for 1 or 2 months, followed by monthly measurements, are recommended.[7]

Infants are placed on a Phe-free formula. Commercial formulas are hydrolysates of protein and contain other amino acids and nutrients required for growth and development. Phe is also essential for growth, it is added to the diet in accordance with the patient's individual tolerance. The additional Phe can be added as cow milk–based formula or breast milk.[18] Breast milk is preferred because it is lower in both Phe and total protein content than infant formula. Breast milk also contains immunoglobulins, which are beneficial for any infant.

After infancy, conventional foods are added to slowly replace breast milk or commercial formula. High protein foods such as meat, eggs, milk, and cheese are highly restricted or forbidden. Most other conventional foods, especially fruits and vegetables, are acceptable and are selected with consideration of the patient's needs in terms of age, weight, and development. The composition of conventional foods is readily found in standard tables of food composition, which can be utilized by the clinician and nutritionist to select foods that meet the patient's requirements and provide a varied and palatable diet.

Dietary control, along with Phe monitoring, should continue indefinitely. Physical examination, motor skills tests, and neuropsychologic tests should be performed periodically. Additionally, hemoglobin levels and bone age adequacy should be monitored.[7] Data have shown that changes in cerebral function have occurred in children who, after several years of dietary compliance, have discontinued their Phe-restricted diet.[19]

TYROSINEMIA

Treatment of hereditary tyrosinemia includes dietary restriction of tyrosine, Phe, and methionine. Dietary treatment does not reverse liver damage or prevent progression to hepatocarcinoma and liver failure. However, it can correct biochemical abnormalities, including tubular complications.[8] Liver transplant has been tried with some success.[9] The number of infants with transient neonatal tyrosinemia has reportedly decreased with the increase in breast-feeding and lowered protein concentration in commercial formulas.[20]

Treatment and laboratory protocol for monitoring tyrosinemia parallels that described for PKU. As disease progresses, hepatic function worsens and should be monitored for life. Renal complications can be demonstrated via routine urinalysis.

ALKAPTONURIA

There is no completely satisfactory treatment for alkaptonuria. If detected early, dietary restriction of tyrosine and Phe may be beneficial. Vitamin C therapy has also been tried. Monitoring of HGA concentration should continue once a diagnosis is made, to follow the progression of disease and the effectiveness of therapy.

MAPLE SYRUP URINE DISEASE

Treatment of MSUD, consisting of a diet low in BCAA, should be initiated within the first week of life but no later than the second week, if permanent neurologic damage is to be prevented. Commercial formula products that are devoid of one or more BCAA are available. The formulas contain other essential nutrients (e.g., fat-soluble vitamins, minerals, and caloric sources) that provide a complete diet for infants with MSUD. Older children can receive appropriately balanced mixtures of natural foods of known composition in accordance with the National Academy of Science report on recommended dietary allowances (RDA) to meet nutritional requirements.[21]

In the variant forms of MSUD, levels of BCAA can frequently be maintained within normal limits by limiting daily protein intake without the need for special amino acid mixtures or by requiring a restricted diet only at times of acute stress. One variant form of MSUD is responsive to a regimen of thiamine at 10 times the normal daily requirement.

Measurement of serum concentrations of BCAA may be necessary on a daily basis early in life or whenever an acidotic crisis occurs. Daily analysis of urine for ketoacids should continue throughout life. This can be done at home, using dinitrophenylhydrazine strips. As long as the urine is negative or contains only trace amounts of ketoacids, measuring serum amino acids at monthly intervals along with a simple chemistry screen, is usually sufficient.[6]

Table 59–3. Some Diseases Detectable by Inborn Error Screening Tests

	Ferric Chloride (FeCl₃)	Reducing Substance	Cetyltrimethyl Ammonium Bromide (CTAB)	Dinitrophenylhydrazine (DNPH)	Sodium Cyanide (NaCN−) Sodium Nitroprusside	Nitrosonaphthol	Ninhydrin (4)	Amino Acid Chromatography
Phenylketonuria	Green	±	−	+	−	−	±	+
Tyrosinemia	Quick-fading green	±	−	+	−	+	+	+
Galactosemia	−	+	−	−	−	±	+	−
Histidinemia	Olive	−	−	±	−	−	±	+
Maple syrup urine disease	Greenish gray	±	−	+	−	−	+	+
Lowe's syndrome	−	−	−	−?	−	−	+	+
Hartnup's disease	−	−	−	−	−	−	+	+
Wilson's disease	−	−	−	−?	−	−	+	+
Arginosuccinicaciduria	−	−	−	+	−	−	±	+
Hyperglycinemia	Green	−	−	−	±	−	±	+
Citrullinuria	−	−	−	−	−	−	±	+
Homocystinuria	−	−	−	+	+	−	±	+
Cystinuria	−	−	−	−	+	−	+	+
Hyperlysinemia	−	−	−	+	−	−	±	+
Cystathionuria	−	−	−	±?	−	−	±	+
Fructosuria	−	+	−	−	−	±?	−	−
Alkaptonuria	Transient blue-green	+	−	−	−	−	−	−
Hurler's syndrome	−	−	+	−	−	−	−	−
Morquio-Ullrich syndrome	−	−	+	−	−	−	−	−
Marfan's syndrome	−	−	±	−	−	−	−	−

Primary No-Threshold Aminoaciduria

Treatment for no-threshold AAUs usually consists of diets low in intermediate metabolites supplemented with amino acids required for growth and development. Vitamin therapy is sometimes recommended.

Secondary Aminoaciduria

Treatment of secondary AAUs involves resolution of the underlying disease. Laboratory follow-up should continue during the course of the treatment.

Case Study

A positive result on a Guthrie screen for PKU is reported on a premature 5-day-old infant. A ferric chloride screen on the same patient shows a green color that fades quickly. A diet low in Phe is initiated, and serum and urine samples for TLC are ordered. In the interim, the patient develops symptoms leading to a "failure to thrive" diagnosis, and additional tests are ordered. A sweat test is negative, and liver enzymes (aspartate aminotransferase [AST] and alanine aminotransferase [ALT]) appear in the high reference range. Glucose, creatinine, blood urea nitrogen (BUN), and protein levels are normal. Bilirubin concentration fell from 15.6 mg/dL on day 1 to 8.9 mg/dL on day 5 (reference range, 1–12 mg/dL). The TLC plate showed "an elevation in the reference areas of phenylalanine and tyrosine."

Questions

1. What is the most likely diagnosis?
2. What tests correlate with this diagnosis?
3. Why would a dietary regimen low in Phe not improve the patient's condition?
4. What additional therapy is now indicated?
5. What additional tests are needed?
6. What are the advantages and limitations of the Guthrie test as it applies to this patient?

Discussion

1. Transient neonatal tyrosinemia is the most likely diagnosis.
2. The FeCl₃ test turns green, Phe and tyrosine are detected on TLC, and chemistry test results (e.g., ALT, bilirubin) are a normal level.
3. The problem was not PKU, but overall enzymatic deficiencies due to underdeveloped liver function.
4. Dietary restriction of tyrosine, Phe, and total protein are indicated.
5. HPLC quantitative testing for Phe and tyrosine should be done, in addition to laboratory follow-up of the patient in the next few weeks.

6. Guthrie's test for PKU is sensitive but not specific. It is designed to bring a possible abnormality to the attention of the clinician, but it is not diagnostic. Further testing is always indicated with a positive Guthrie test. In this case, it correctly identified an increase in Phe in the blood, but this was not due to PKU.

References

1. Dhondt JL: Strategy for the screening of tetrahydrobiopterin deficiency among hyperphenylalaninaemic patients: 15 years experience. J Inherit Metab Dis 13:641–650, 1991.
2. Koch R, Hanley W, Levy H, et al: A preliminary report of the collaborative study of maternal phenylketonuria in the US and Canada. J Inherit Metab Dis 13:641–650, 1990.
3. Matalon R, Michals K, Azen C, et al: Maternal PKU collaborative study: pregnancy outcome and prenatal head growth. J Inherit Metab Dis 17:353–355, 1994.
4. Smith I, Glossop J, Beasley M, et al: Fetal damage due to maternal phenylketonuria: effects of dietary treatment and maternal phenylalanine concentrations around the time of conception. J Inherit Metab Dis 13:651–657, 1990.
5. Rice DN, Houston IB, Lyon IC, et al: Transient neonatal tyrosinaemia. J Inherit Metab Dis 12:13–22, 1989.
6. Waber L: Inborn errors of metabolism. Pediatr Ann 19:105–118, 1990.
7. Burton BK: Inborn errors of metabolism: The clinical diagnosis in early infancy. Pediatrics 79:359, 1987.
8. Waisbren SE, Mahon BE, Schnell RR, et al: Predictors of intelligence quotient and intelligence quotient change in persons treated for PKU early in life. Pediatrics 79:351, 1987.
9. Kvittingen EA: Tyrosinemia type I—an update. J Inherit Metab Dis 14:554–562, 1991.
10. Schuett VE: National Survey of Treatment Programs for PKU and Selected Other Inherited Metabolic Diseases. U.S. Department of Health and Human Services Office of Maternal and Child Health. DHHS Publication Number HRS-M-OH-89-5, 1990.
11. Buist NRM: Laboratory aspects of newborn screening for metabolic disorders. Lab Med 19:145–150, 1988.
12. Doherty LB, Rohr FJ, Levy HL: Detection of PKU in the very early newborn specimen. Pediatrics 87:240–244, 1991.
13. Edwards MA, Grant S, Green A: A practical approach to the investigation of amino acid disorders. Ann Clin Biochem 25:129–141, 1988.
14. Woo SLO: Molecular basis and population genetics of phenylketonuria. Biochemistry 28:1–7, 1989.
15. Danner DJ, Elsas U II: Disorders of branched chain amino acid and keto acid metabolism. In Scriver CR, Stanbury JB, Wyngaarden DS, et al (eds), The Metabolic Basis of Inherited Disease, ed 6. New York, McGraw-Hill, 1989.
16. Chalmers RA: Disorders of organic acid metabolism. In Holton JB (ed): The Inherited Metabolic Diseases, ed 2. Edinburgh, Churchill Livingstone, 1994, p 129.
17. Kleijer WJ, Horsman D, Mancini GM, et al: First trimester diagnosis of maple syrup urine disease on intact chorionic villi. N Engl J Med 333:1608, 1985.
18. McCabe L, Ernest AE, Neifert MR, et al: The management of breast feeding among infants with phenylketonuria. J Inherit Metab Dis 12:467–474, 1989.
19. Thompson A, Smith I, Brenton D, et al: Neurological deterioration in young adults with phenylketonuria. Lancet 336:602–605, 1990.
20. Pollitt RJ: Amino acid disorders. In Holton JB (ed): The Inherited Metabolic Diseases, ed 2. Edinburgh, Churchill Livingstone, 1994, p 80.
21. Subcommittee on the Tenth Board of the Recommended Dietary Allowances, Food and Nutrition Board, Commission on Life Sciences, National Research Council: Recommended Dietary Allowances, ed 10. Washington DC, National Academy Press, 1989.

Chapter 60

Malnutrition, Eating Disorders, and Starvation

Deborah T. Firestone and Craig A. Lehmann

Public interest in nutrition has been increasing throughout the years, as people have become better informed about the short- and long-term effects of the food that they eat. This increased attention has led a number of investigators to study the nutritional status of various populations and to identify those that are malnourished. Such studies have drawn attention to the prevalence of malnourished patients in hospitals and nursing homes.[1, 2]

Malnutrition describes a condition of poor nourishment. Prolonged intake of a nutritionally deficient diet or an abrupt or gradual withdrawal of food can lead to starvation. The identification of patients who are malnourished or of those at risk of becoming malnourished is important because studies have shown that these patients have an increased rate of morbidity and mortality.[3, 4] A nutritional assessment of the patient is the first step in identifying malnutrition and starvation. The clinical laboratory plays a central role in this evaluative process.

ETIOLOGY AND PATHOPHYSIOLOGY OF NUTRITIONAL DEFICIENCIES

Nutritional deficiencies can develop over a short or long period of time and may involve one or, more commonly, many nutrients. The way in which the body adapts to these changes depends on (1) whether reserves of the nutrient are available in the body, (2) the difference between the amount of intake of the nutrient and the amount needed by the body, and (3) the amount of time during which the reduced intake of the nutrient continues.

The physiologic response of the body to nutritional deficiency occurs in three stages. In stage 1, the body responds to the insufficient intake of nutrients by utilizing reserves of the nutrient, if any. Stage 2 results if deficient intake of the nutrient continues. It is characterized by altered serum and/or urine concentrations of the nutrient or of its metabolites. In this stage, although the patient may be asymptomatic, nutritional deficiency may be detected using appropriate laboratory tests. The final physiologic response of the body, the development of stage 3, is determined by the available stores of fat in the body. When the available stores of lipid are depleted, protein in the body is used as a last source of energy, which ultimately leads to the death of the patient. In stage 3, the patient is symptomatic, and nutritional deficiency can be detected by using a number of laboratory tests.

Vitamin deficiencies can be either primary, due to inadequate vitamin intake, or secondary, as the result of various disease processes. Vitamins can be divided into two groups, fat-soluble (vitamins A, D, E, and K) and water-soluble (vitamins C and B-complex). They perform a variety of physiologic functions, for example, as cofactors in numerous enzymatic reactions. The body's adaptation to vitamin deficiency is diverse, and it depends on the particular function that is being compromised.

Minerals are necessary for many normal functions within the body, for example, cellular and humoral immunity. Although the body is able to compensate over a period of time for deficiencies in the mineral content of the diet, if the deficiency continues for a prolonged period, compensatory mechanisms are no longer adequate, and serious diseases such as iron-deficiency anemia or osteomalacia can result.

Studies of hospitalized patients in the United States have shown that nutritional deficiency is associated with compromised immunity and may be a significant contributor to severe infections.[4, 5] In undernourished children and adults, lymphoid tissues, such as the tonsils, spleen, and thymus, atrophy in response to nutritional deprivation. There is a decrease in the number of T lymphocytes, an impairment in delayed hypersensitivity skin reactions to various antigens, and a decrease in the serum concentration of many complement components. The primary antibody response to most antigens is depressed, although the secondary antibody response is usually unaffected. The bactericidal activity of polymorphonuclear leukocytes (PMNs) is reduced, and breaks in the integrity of the mucocutaneous junction may be caused by deficiencies in specific vitamins and minerals, thus making the patient more susceptible to infections.

CLINICAL SYNDROMES

Acute malnutrition, due to any one of many clinical syndromes, may lead to a state of starvation in the patient. Patients with *anorexia nervosa*, an eating disorder most often seen in teenage girls, suffer from a distorted body image that makes them preoccupied with losing weight and being thin. Weight loss is accomplished by either fasting or eating small amounts of food and may be accompanied by self-induced vomiting. Anorexia nervosa may be life-threatening because of the medical complications of starvation. Patients with *bulimia* show poor control of their food intake. These patients indulge in binge eating, or the ingestion of large quantities of food, followed by induced vomiting to avoid a gain in weight. The compulsive overeating that occurs in bulimia may also occur to varying degrees in other clinical conditions. Patients may also be classified as *bulimic anorexics*, persons who normally fast or ingest small quantities of food but periodically gorge themselves and then vomit to maintain their low weight.

Cancer patients often experience a condition of acute malnutrition, as a result of the disease process itself or as a result of treatment modalities such as chemotherapy and radiation. In fact, one of the first symptoms of cancer in a patient may be an unexplained weight loss.

Conditions of protein-calorie malnutrition (PCM) can also lead to a state of starvation. PCM in children is most prevalent in areas of the world that are underdeveloped. The two most common classifications of PCM are marasmus and kwashiorkor. *Marasmus*, generally being more severe in nature, is characterized by a diet that is deficient in protein and calories. This results in a depletion of the adipose tissue and skeletal muscle (somatic) protein, which leads to a general wasting. *Kwashiorkor*, however, can vary from mild to severe and is characterized by a diet that is low in protein, with carbohydrates as the major source of calories. In kwashiorkor, the somatic protein stores are generally maintained, whereas the visceral protein stores are depleted. Patients with *marasmic kwashiorkor* exhibit symptoms of both conditions.

There are syndromes in which chronic malnutrition, over a period of time, may lead to starvation. This may occur in drug addicts and alcoholics due to prolonged ingestion of diets rich in "empty calories," such as ethanol. These individuals may have an unbalanced diet to begin with, and the presence of drugs and/or alcohol can compound the problem by interfering with the normal absorption and utilization of ingested nutrients. Chronic malnutrition with eventual starvation may also be present in cancer patients, as well as in patients who fail to eat well-balanced meals because of inadequate or inferior nutrients supplied

from the environment or from a self-imposed weight loss diet.

Patient populations may be suffering from acute or chronic malnutrition that does not progress to conditions of starvation. This population includes the increasing number of elderly patients, who for financial, emotional, or physical reasons do not consume foods that supply the proper nutritional requirements. Patients with malabsorption syndromes or diets deficient in a specific nutrient or metabolite may exhibit clinical signs and symptoms indicative of acute or chronic malnutrition. These patients, although they are malnourished, do not have deficiencies in their diets that are severe enough to lead to starvation.

CLINICAL MANIFESTATIONS

Although the syndromes of malnutrition and starvation are complex in their etiology, so too are the clinical signs and symptoms of these disorders. The clinical picture of afflicted patients is variable and depends on the degree, type, and duration of the eating disorder. On the one hand, a patient may present with symptoms that are specific enough to suggest a possible deficiency in a class of nutrients, such as bleeding tendencies (vitamin K deficiency) or hypochromic anemia (iron deficiency). On the other hand, symptoms may reflect a combination of nutritional deficiencies, including bradycardia, hypotension, hypothermia, dry skin, amenorrhea, hyperactivity, abdominal pain, lethargy, weight loss, wasting, muscle weakness, anorexia, growth retardation, desquamation and pigmentation of the skin, diarrhea, and hepatomegaly.

Clinical assessment of patients with nutritional disorders can be made using a combination of history-taking, evaluation of signs and symptoms, and anthropometric measurements (measurements of the size, weight, and proportions of the human body). A nutritional history should include questions that establish whether there have been any recent weight losses or gains, illnesses, changes in dietary habits, and medications taken. An assessment of food intake, which can be obtained through either the patient's recall of food eaten or a diary of food intake over a period of time, can at best provide only an estimate of the nutritional status of the patient, due to the variability in methods.

Anthropometric measurements, if interpreted correctly, can be used to monitor the nutritional status of a patient. Changes in body weight, as well as rapidity of weight loss, can be an accurate indicator of a change in the nutritional status of nonedematous patients. Height measurements can be a more sensitive indicator of malnutrition in children than in adults, because children frequently exhibit a retardation in growth in response to malnutrition. Triceps skinfold (TSF) measurements are frequently used to estimate body fat. In cases of severe malnutrition, subcutaneous body fat disappears. Midarm circumference (MAC) measurements of the nondominant arm have been used to evaluate changes in skeletal muscle mass. TSF and MAC measurements are useful tools in the identification of severe malnutrition, but values must be interpreted carefully when distinguishing mild to moderately malnourished patients from lean, healthy individuals.

LABORATORY ANALYSES AND DIAGNOSIS
Routine Laboratory Tests for Assessing Nutritional Status

Laboratory tests used as part of the initial nutritional evaluation of a patient vary, depending on the patient population under study.

Anemia, leukopenia, and decreased hemoglobin and hematocrit associated with malnutrition can be detected by a complete blood cell count (CBC). Total lymphocyte counts are decreased and cell-mediated immunity, as determined by delayed hypersensitivity responses, is frequently abnormal because the immune defenses of undernourished children and adults are impaired. Studies have shown a correlation between the degree of anergy and the severity of nutritional deficiency in a patient. The degree of anergy has also been used as an indicator of prognosis, sepsis, and mortality.[2-4]

Triglyceride and cholesterol determinations can be used to determine whether fat content of the diet is appropriate and whether fat is being absorbed properly.

Albumin is one of the biochemical markers most frequently used in assessing the protein status of an individual. However, the long half-life of albumin (18 days) and the equilibration of extravascular albumin with the intravascular stores[6] limit its usefulness as a marker of recent protein changes in the diet.[7] Although it is not a sensitive indicator of short-term nutrition deprivation, albumin has been identified as a predictor of postoperative complications.[3] A detailed discussion of nutrition in the hospitalized patient may be found in Chapter 62.

Measuring individual levels of minerals is of little value, unless a patient history dictates otherwise. A decrease in sodium, potassium, chloride, bicarbonate, calcium, phosphate, and magnesium levels could corroborate a diagnosis of malnutrition in the absence of other disease.

Blood urea nitrogen (BUN) levels are increased, reflecting the breakdown of protein in the body. A 24-hour urine creatinine test can be used to measure the somatic protein status (muscle mass) of a patient. Creatinine, a breakdown product of skeletal muscle, is excreted into the urine in decreasing amounts as the degree of malnutrition becomes more severe.[7] An accurate determination of urinary creatinine is dependent on proper sample collection. The creatinine height index (CHI) is obtained by dividing the 24-hour creatinine excretion of a patient by the 24-hour creatinine excretion of a control matched by height and weight.[8] The CHI is affected by changes in creatinine excretion caused by age and variability in the standards and therefore must be interpreted carefully when evaluating cases of PCM.

The total iron-binding capacity (TIBC), an indirect measurement of transferrin, can serve as an overall indicator of protein nutrition. Interpretation of TIBC values, however, must take into consideration limiting factors, such as iron stores of the patient, which can affect TIBC results.

Nonroutine Tests for Assessing Nutritional Status

The determination of rapid-turnover visceral proteins, such as thyroxine-binding prealbumin (2-day half-life) and retinol-binding protein (10-hour half-life), has proved to be particularly useful in evaluating the short-term effect of nutritional therapy with respect to protein. In addition, these proteins are the first of the visceral proteins to respond to total parenteral nutrition (see Chapter 62). The plasma levels of these proteins are low during periods of protein depletion and increase rapidly when nutritional deficiency is corrected.[9] Inflammatory conditions can also have a direct effect on levels of thyroxine-binding prealbumin and retinol-binding protein.[10]

Transferrin determinations can also be used as an indicator of visceral protein depletion. Transferrin has a half-life of approximately 8 days, and the levels of this protein correlate with short-term changes in protein deficiency. Transferrin levels have also been shown to accurately predict which patients will develop postoperative complications.[3]

The serum concentration of many of the complement components is decreased in conditions of PCM. The decrease may be due to a reduced rate of synthesis and to an increased rate of consumption in antigen-antibody reactions (e.g., infections). The extent to which C3 levels are reduced correlates with morbidity.[5]

Leukocyte terminal deoxynucleotidyl transferase (TdT) is present in large amounts in immature thymocytes, and levels of the enzyme decrease as T cells mature. In PCM, a decreased activity of thymic hormone results in defects in the normal maturational sequence of T lymphocytes.[11] This results in an increase in "null" cells, which may be immature T cells.[12] Determination of TdT can, therefore, be used as an indirect measurement of nutritional deficiency and of defects in the maturational sequence of T lymphocytes.

Deficiencies in the essential fatty acids (EFAs) are most often a result of side effects of treatment modalities, such as fat-free parenteral feeding, or of certain disease processes, such as fat malabsorption in Crohn's disease. Total lipid analysis can be performed to assess the EFA status of a patient; however, this test does not separate the classes of lipids. The performance of more sophisticated procedures, such as 5,8,11-eicosantrienoic acid levels and the eicosantrienoic acid/arachidonic acid ratio (the triene/tetrane ratio) can be used to accomplish such classification.[13]

The reasons for nutritional deficiencies in vitamins and trace elements are varied. They include inadequate dietary intake and impaired absorption, metabolism, or excretion due to disease, medical treatments, or increased nutritional demands (e.g., pregnancy, surgery). Indications for the measurement of a specific vitamin or trace element most commonly are based on information obtained from a patient's dietary history or presenting clinical symptoms, for example, xerophthalmia due to vitamin A deficiency.

Factors Influencing Laboratory Analyses

The laboratory test used as part of a nutrition profile can be affected by a patient's diet and intake of drugs. It is, therefore, imperative that laboratory scientists become familiar with the various factors that can influence the interpretation of a particular laboratory analysis. Drugs can reduce food intake and digestibility, impair absorption, increase excretion, inhibit synthesis, and interfere with the utilization of nutrients. These interactions can result in mineral and electrolyte imbalances and affect the levels of vitamins in laboratory assays. Clinical laboratory scientists must evaluate test results in the light of these interfering factors to avoid reporting erroneous or misleading results.

TREATMENT

Treatment of patients with nutritional deficiencies can be accomplished by change in diet, oral supplementation, enteral feeding, or parenteral feeding. Patients requiring nutritional support can be separated into three categories: (1) those who have decreased oral intake (anorexia), (2) those with increased nutritional losses (diarrhea), and (3) those who have increased nutrient requirements (burns). Assessment of treatment is based on dietary history, physical examination, laboratory test results, and anthropometric measurements. If the body weight has decreased by 5% or less and the problem has been present for less than 7 days, nutritional intervention may not be warranted. However, if the body weight has decreased more than 5% and the illness has been present for more than 7 days, forced enteral or parenteral nutrition may be required. Forced enteral feeding is a common procedure for anorexia. Parenteral nutrition is necessary when the gastrointestinal tract is not properly functioning or when the patient cannot take anything by mouth. The laboratory plays a critical role in the monitoring of patients on enteral and parenteral feedings, and the laboratory scientist should be aware of complications that may develop. These include fluid and electrolyte imbalance, acid-base imbalance, glycosuria, hyperglycemia, and hepatic and hematologic abnormalities. Prolonged use of total parenteral nutrition may result in vitamin (folic acid, vitamins A and E, biotin) and mineral (zinc) deficiencies.[14]

Case Study 1

A 17-year-old girl was seen by her physician at her mother's request. The mother reported that the girl was chronically tired and had trouble concentrating in school. She had previously been on a diet and had lost 30 lb but appeared to be eating well now.

A physical examination was performed and a detailed medical history was taken. Both proved to be unremarkable.

After an overnight fast, blood was drawn for a routine 20 chemistry profile and a CBC.

The CBC was within normal limits, and the only abnormalities on the 20 chemistry profile were an elevated bicarbonate level and decreased plasma potassium and chloride concentrations. Based on these results, the patient appeared to be in metabolic alkalosis and was both hypokalemic and hypochloremic. Because no finding pointed to a diagnosis, the patient was seen on a follow-up visit.

On further investigation, the patient revealed that she felt tremendous social pressure from her peers at school. All of her friends were very fashion-conscious and

placed great emphasis on being thin. She felt particular pressure because of a previous weight problem, and she was afraid of gaining back the weight she had lost.

When questioned about how she was keeping her weight off, the patient reluctantly revealed that although she enjoyed eating and therefore ate whatever she liked, she was vomiting and taking laxatives at least once a day to avoid a gain in weight.

Questions

1. Given this patient's history, what disorder is probable?
2. Are the reported laboratory findings consistent with this diagnosis?
3. What next step is warranted in the treatment of this patient?

Discussion

1. Bulimia is the probable disorder in this case.
2. Many disorders can cause hypochloremia (e.g., renal disorders, prolonged vomiting), hypokalemia (e.g., chronic starvation, gastrointestinal loss), and metabolic alkalosis (e.g., prolonged diuretic use, loss of hydrochloric acid [HCl] from the stomach). Using a combination of the patient's medical history, physical examination, and laboratory results, it is possible to rule out some of the causes and thereby limit the number of possibilities.

   The most common laboratory findings in bulimia are metabolic alkalosis, hypokalemia, and hypochloremia. In cases that involve dehydration, BUN and serum amylase levels may be elevated when gastric dilatation is present.

3. At this point, the patient should be referred to an eating disorders center.

Case Study 2

A 19-year-old female freshman demonstrated weakness and dizziness. Clinical examination demonstrated that she was 5 ft 6 in. in height and weighed 170 lb. She revealed that she has been on a new diet for 2 weeks that would assure her of a major weight loss. The diet consisted of a grapefruit in the morning, salad for lunch and salad with a slice of whole wheat bread for dinner. The diet also recommended drinking at least ten glasses of water a day. The patient was placed under observation and blood was drawn for a routine chemistry profile and a CBC. The chemistry profile only revealed a decreased level of potassium. On further investigation the patient revealed that she had read about this diet in a magazine that she found in the dorm, and had lost 18 lb in 2 weeks.

Questions

1. Given the condition of the patient, what do you believe to be her problem?

2. Do you think, knowing the clinical signs, that the clinician ordered the appropriate tests?

3. What would be your recommendation to the patient in reference to her diet?

Discussion

1. The patient was not providing sufficient nourishment to her body and was essentially starving herself.

2. If the clinician was attempting to assess the patient's nutritional status, a routine albumin found in most routine chemistry profiles would not be appropriate. The patient has only been on the diet for 2 weeks and albumin has a half-life of 18 days. A more appropriate test would be prealbumin (half-life, 2 days) or transferrin (half-life, 8 days).

3. All diets should be nutritionally sound and should be planned in conjunction with a clinician.

References

1. Bistrian BR, Blackburn GL, Vitale J, et al: Prevalence of malnutrition in general medical patients. JAMA 15:1567, 1976.
2. Shaver HJ, Loper JA, Lutes RA: Nutritional status of nursing home patients. J Parenter Enteral Nutr 4:367–370, 1980.
3. Mullen JL, Gertner MH, Buzby GP, et al: Implications of malnutrition in the surgical patient. Arch Surg 114:121–125, 1979.
4. Harvey KB, Ruggiero JA, Regan CS, et al: Hospital morbidity and mortality risk factors using nutritional assessment. Clin Res 26:581A, 1978.
5. Chandra RK: Serum complement and immunoconglutinin in malnutrition. Arch Dis Child 50:225–229, 1975.
6. Hoffenberg R, Black E, Brock JF: Albumin and γ-globulin tracer studies in protein depletion states. J Clin Invest 45:143–151, 1966.
7. Forbes GB, Bruining GJ: Urinary creatinine excretion and lean body mass. Am J Clin Nutr 29:1359–1366, 1976.
8. Viteri FE, Alvarado J: The creatinine height index: Its use in the estimation of the degree of protein depletion and repletion in protein-calorie-malnourished children. Pediatrics 46:696–706, 1970.
9. Shetty PS, Watrasiewicz KE, Jung RT, et al: Rapid-turnover transport proteins: An index of subclinical protein-energy malnutrition. Lancet 2:230–232, 1979.
10. Ramsden DB, Prince HP, Burr WA, et al: The interrelationship of thyroid hormones, vitamin A, and their binding proteins following acute stress. Clin Endocrinol 8:109–122, 1978.
11. Chandra RK: Serum thymic hormone activity in protein-energy malnutrition. Clin Exp Immunol 38:228–230, 1979.
12. Chandra RK: T- and B-lymphocyte subpopulations and leukocyte terminal deoxynucleotidyl-transferase in energy-protein undermalnutrition. Acta Paediatr Scand 68:841–845, 1979.
13. Holman RT: The ratio of trienoic:tetranoic acids in tissue lipids as a measure of essential fatty acid requirement. J Nutr 70:405, 1960.
14. Howard L, Bigaonette J, Chu R, et al: Water-soluble vitamin requirements in home parenteral nutrition patients. Am J Clin Nutr 37:421–428, 1983.

Bibliography

Burritt MF, Anderson CF: Laboratory assessment of nutritional status. Hum Pathol 15:130–133, 1984.

Carpentier YA, Barthel J, Bruyns J: Plasma protein concentration in nutritional assessment. Proc Nutr Soc 41:405–417, 1982.

Durnin JVGA, Fidanza F: Evaluation of nutritional status. Bibl Nutr Dieta 35:20–30, 1985.

Groer ME, Shekleton ME: Basic Pathophysiology: A Conceptual Approach. St Louis, CV Mosby, 1979.

Labbe RF: Symposium on laboratory assessment of nutritional status. Clin Lab Med 1:605–796, 1981.

Mitchell JE: Anorexia Nervosa and Bulimia: Diagnosis and Treatment. Minneapolis, University of Minnesota Press, 1985, pp 48–77.

Tomaiolo PP: Malnutrition in the elderly: Its recognition and treatment. Compr Ther 11:54–58, 1985.

Truswell AS: Malnutrition in the third world. Br Med J 291:525–528, 1985.

Woods HF: Biochemical methods in nutritional assessment. Proc Nutr Soc 41:419–424, 1982.

Chapter 61

Disorders of Carbohydrate Metabolism

H. Elise Galloway

SIMPLE SUGARS

Lactose, galactose, fructose, and pentose are reducing sugars classified as simple sugars. Although other sugars may present problems, the incidence is extremely low. See Chapter 32 for a discussion of impaired glucose metabolism.

The inability of the body to use monosaccharides and disaccharides can be attributed to the lack of a specific enzyme. This results in either a malabsorption problem or an increase in the amount of precursors of the affected metabolic pathway. Malabsorption is addressed elsewhere (see Chapter 24) and is discussed only briefly here.

Etiology and Pathophysiology

Lactose, or milk sugar, is a disaccharide composed of galactose and glucose. Lactase, an enzyme produced in the brush borders of the intestinal mucosa, splits lactose into its two monosaccharides. As mammals mature, the ingestion of lactose normally decreases, paralleling a decrease in the production of lactase. Adults normally have a low level or absence of lactase.[1] In some individuals, this condition may produce an acquired intolerance to milk products.

The more serious dysfunctions of sugar metabolism are due to the lack of specific enzymes involved in metabolic pathways. These disorders affect the metabolism of fructose, galactose, and the pentose sugar, xylulose. Occasion-ally, infants are not able to manufacture lactase, resulting in a congenital lactose intolerance. All of these disorders are autosomal recessive defects, and the incidence of occurrence is low (Table 61–1).

Fructose intolerance can result from the lack of three different enzymes: fructokinase, fructose 1-phosphate aldolase, and fructose-1,6-diphosphatase.[2] Galactosemia is most often due to the lack of galactose 1-phosphate uridyltransferase. This deficiency results in the accumulation of galactose 1-phosphate and galactitol, the metabolite implicated in the development of cataracts. Two other enzymes also involved in galactose metabolism have been associated with intolerance. They are galactokinase and (very rarely) uridine diphosphate galactose 4-epimerase.[3] Pentosuria is a relatively benign autosomal recessive defect of the glucuronic acid oxidation pathway resulting from a decrease in the activity of L-xylulose reductase.[4] It is found primarily in people of Jewish extraction. Congenital lactose intolerance, first described in 1959 by Hoezal,[5] results from the absence of lactase in infants. It is a rare condition that can prove fatal if not diagnosed and treated.

Clinical Manifestations

Sugar intolerance disorders manifest as similar clinical symptoms. Diarrhea or loose stools after eating, abdominal pain, cramps or distention, and failure to thrive are all relatively nonspecific signals pointing to either malabsorption or an enzyme deficiency. It is also possible for a patient to have no clinical signs initially.

Children who present with cataracts should be considered for galactose intolerance, because galactokinase-deficient patients have no aversion to milk and are asymptomatic except for the development of cataracts. Uridyltransferase-deficient patients, however, present with vomiting, hepatomegaly, diarrhea, edema, and lethargy, symptoms that commonly do not appear until several days after milk feeding begins. Cataracts may also be observed within a few days of milk ingestion.[3]

Fructokinase deficiencies are relatively benign and may be undetected. Hereditary fructose intolerance (HFI or aldolase B deficiency) is manifested when sucrose or fructose, in fruits, for instance, becomes part of the diet. It can appear as a severe acute reaction with vomiting, convul-

Table 61-1. **Summary of Simple Sugar Disorders***

Disorder	Substrate	Incidence	Presumptive Diagnosis	Definitive Diagnosis
Lactose intolerance				
Acquired: no lactase	Lactose → galactose and glucose	Low in whites; high in blacks and East Asians	Lactose tolerance test or hydrogen breath test	Biopsy of mucosal cells of intestine
Congenital: no lactase		Low	Thin-layer chromatography (TLC)	
Fructose intolerance				
Fructokinase	Fructose → fructose 1-phosphate	1/130,000	Fructose tolerance test TLC	Demonstration of block or decrease in activity of affected cells (liver, intestine)
Fructose 1-phosphate aldolase B	Fructose 1-phosphate → glyceraldehyde and dihydroxyacetone phosphate	1/20,000 (Switzerland)		
Fructose 1,6-diphosphatase	Key enzyme in gluconeogenesis	85 known cases reported		
Galactose intolerance				
Galactose 1-phosphate uridyltransferase	Galactose 1-phosphate → UDP galactose	1/40,000	Inhibition test or enzyme activity detection by fluorescent technique TLC	Demonstration of decrease in enzyme activity in red cells or amniotic fluid cells
Galactokinase	Galactose → galactose 1-phosphate	< 1/100,000		
Uridine diphosphate galactose 4-epimerase		1/23,000 (Japan)		
Pentosuria				
L-Xylulose reductase		1/50,000	TLC	

*Screening test for all these intolerances is detection of reducing substances in urine.

sions, and coma, or in a milder, chronic form with failure to thrive, vomiting, hepatomegaly, and jaundice.[2] Fructose-1,6-diphosphatase deficiency can be life threatening and should be suspected in full-term newborns of normal weight who begin to hyperventilate and go into convulsions or coma after eating a fortified diet.

Laboratory Analyses and Diagnosis

Several simple screening tests yield presumptive evidence of these defects (see Table 61–1). Because glucose is the primary circulating carbohydrate, it is the one generally seen in the urine when the renal threshold is exceeded. The presence of a reducing substance that is not glucose is preliminary evidence of some other sugar defect. Galactose, fructose, xylulose, and lactose are all reducing substances that will give a positive result with a test for reducing substances such as Benedict's test. At the same time, the specific test for glucose with an enzyme method such as glucose oxidase (dipstick method) is negative. All newborns should be checked with this procedure and should be followed for several days, because the sugar may not be present initially. In any child with clinical symptoms, especially jaundice, reducing sugar levels should be checked.

In infants, the presence of reducing substances in feces and an acid pH of the stool suggests a congenital lactose deficiency;[6] however, this is not a useful screening procedure for the acquired lactose intolerance seen in adults. Acquired lactose intolerance may be more common than has been previously thought. Medical record reviews and interviews with elderly people have revealed that many people start self-limiting diets by removing milk products or by using lactase pills to relieve symptoms of diarrhea and abdominal discomfort.

Changes in blood analytes can also be helpful in diagnosis of some of these intolerances. In HFI, there may be a pronounced hypoglycemia and decrease in phosphate levels owing to the accumulation of fructose 1-phosphate in the liver.[2] Levels of methionine and tyrosine may be increased in the blood. Fructose 1,6-diphosphate deficiency may manifest as hypoglycemia and ketoacidosis. Increased levels of lactate, ketones, alanine, and uric acid are seen in the blood and appear in the urine. Galactosemia due to the transferase defect commonly manifests as a decrease in blood glucose. In many states, infant screening procedures for galactosemia are now mandatory.[7-9] They usually consist of direct fluorescent measurement of galactose-1-phosphate uridyltransferase activity or an inhibition test.

Presumptive tests include chromatography, which can be used to identify the specific sugar present in the urine or blood.[10] Tolerance tests for fructose and lactose are also used to assess the patient's ability to metabolize these substances. The hydrogen breath test for lactose intolerance has been used with success and is considered by some to be the diagnostic method of choice when used in combination with clinical findings.[11] Others believe that it is of no greater value than the tolerance test.[1]

Definitive tests to confirm lactose and fructose intolerance require an intestinal mucosal biopsy to determine the exact defect in enzyme activity. Galactose enzyme defects, however, are present in the red blood cell and can be determined from enzyme activity of red cell hemolysates. Cultured cells from amniotic fluid can also be used to detect the defect. A gas-liquid chromatograph method for the detection of galactitol in amniotic fluid has been reported to correlate well with cell culture results.[12] It is a more rapid method for prenatal diagnosis, because it eliminates the time needed for cell culture growth.

Treatment

In all of these defects, diet is the best therapy. Absence of the sugar from the diet results in complete recovery in most instances and emphasizes the need for early detection. Compliance with dietary restrictions can be confirmed by monitoring the patient with a urine test for reducing substances.

In HFI, removal of all food containing sucrose and fructose can result in complete recovery. It is sometimes necessary to provide supportive measures, such as infusion of fresh plasma or exchange transfusions. The prognosis is good, however, if the sugar is removed, and affected patients generally adopt self-imposed diets that avoid foods containing sucrose and fructose. With fructose 1,6-diphosphatase deficiency, removal of the two sugars fructose and sucrose usually proves effective. It may be necessary to correct for hypoglycemia and acidosis with intravenous measures, depending on the severity of symptoms.

Recognizing classic galactosemia early and immediately withdrawing galactose from the diet can prevent serious complications.[9] Failure to do so can result in liver damage and death. Although this disorder is not as severe as phenylketonuria (PKU), both mental retardation and cataracts are consequences of galactosemia.

In galactokinase deficiency, removal of galactose from the diet usually results in complete recovery, and cataracts, if present, will regress.

Lactose intolerance can be managed by removal of lactose from the diet. A study of people who self-reported severe lactose intolerance suggested that people who identify themselves as lactose intolerant may mistakenly attribute other abdominal symptoms to lactose intolerance.[13] When these subjects' lactose intake was limited to less than 240 mL a day, their symptoms were negligible, and lactose-digestive aids were not needed.

Genetics

Genetic counseling and prenatal diagnosis are important in galactosemia. This disorder can be assessed prior to birth.[8] Mothers who have fetuses with the defect should avoid consuming lactose. Prior knowledge of the condition also provides information necessary for proper management of the neonate.

GLYCOGEN STORAGE DISEASES

Glycogen storage diseases are disorders resulting from a specific enzyme deficiency. In most cases, the clinical laboratory plays a minor role in diagnosis. There are at least nine types, whose associated enzyme defects and incidences are listed in Table 61–2. All are autosomal recessive enzyme defects with the possible exception of type IX.[14] With some of the types, there are variants that manifest a different clinical picture.[15] The overall incidence of hepatic glycogen storage diseases is about 1 in 60,000 live births.[16] In general, these diseases affect primarily either the liver or the muscle, and the symptoms result from the enzyme defect in those tissues.

Clinical Manifestations

Type I glycogen storage disease manifests as hepatomegaly, xanthomas, and renal enlargement. There may be bleeding due to impaired platelet function, and diarrhea may be present.

Type II, which is a lysosomal defect, may be seen in three forms, depending on the age of the patient.[17] The classic case is seen in the infant who presents with hypotonia, muscle weakness, and congestive heart failure. The symptoms appear within 6 months after birth, and average life expectancy is 1 year. The disease may not manifest until childhood, when symptoms of muscle weakness and hypotonia appear. Death is frequently due to pneumonia and respiratory failure. In adults, the primary symptom is muscle weakness. Hypoglycemia, increased lipid levels, and mild cirrhosis are common.

Type III glycogen storage disease has a presentation like that of type I, but the clinical course is milder.

Type IV should be suspected in infants who fail to thrive and have little weight gain. There is an increase in the size of the liver and spleen, and cirrhosis with early death is not uncommon.

People with type V commonly are normal, well-developed individuals who have no problems at rest but have a limited ability to perform strenuous exercise. This defect usually manifests later in life, typically between 20 and 40 years of age.

Type VI glycogen storage disease is difficult to diagnose clinically, as there may be few symptoms. It is a milder form of type I.

Type VII manifests like type V, because it is primarily a muscle glycogen storage problem.

Type VIII has been excluded, because as yet, no enzyme deficiency has been demonstrated.[16]

Type IX, which is sex linked, may be more common than previously suspected, because the phosphorylase kinase defect is often asymptomatic.

Table 61–2. Types of Glycogen Storage Disease

Type	Name of Disease	Enzyme Deficiency	Incidence
0	Lewis's	Glycogen synthetase	3 documented cases
I	Von Gierke's	Glucose 6-phosphase, type Ia	1/200,000
II	Pompe's	Lysosomal α-1,4-glucosidase (acid maltase)	1/100,000
III	Cori's	Amylo-1,6-glucosidase	1/100,000
IV	Andersen's	Amylo 1,4 1,6-transglucosidase	1/500,000
V	McArdle's	Muscle phosphorylase	1/500,000
VI	Hers's	Liver phosphorylase	1/200,000
VII	Tarui's	Muscle phosphofructokinase	1/500,000
IX	—	Phosphorylase kinase	1/100,000

Type 0, which is a deficiency of glycogen synthetase, is very rare. To date, three cases have been documented. Children may present with ketosis and hypoglycemic convulsions after fasting.

Laboratory Analyses and Diagnosis

The definitive diagnosis of type I glycogen storage disease is made by liver biopsy. Patients with type I have a pronounced hypoglycemia after fasting,[18] and hyperlipidemia, increased uric acid, and increased lactic acid are commonly found. An oral glucose tolerance test demonstrates a diabetic-type response.

In type II, a muscle biopsy shows an increase in the concentration of glycogen and a decrease in enzyme activity. Activity may also be assayed in leukocytes, and fibroblast culture allows for prenatal diagnosis.[19]

Type III manifests as hypoglycemia and an increase in cholesterol levels. Lactate levels are generally normal, a feature that may help to distinguish this type from type I. Amylo 1,6-glucosidase levels in white cells can be determined, and the glycogen content of red cells is also elevated.

In type IV, the glucose tolerance test is normal, and serum transaminase levels are increased. Fibroblasts can be cultured for prenatal diagnosis, but the prognosis is poor.

Types V and VII occasionally result in myoglobin in the urine. Lactic acid levels are not elevated after exercise. Diagnosis can be made by measuring lactic acid levels both before and after ischemic exercise. Under normal conditions, there should be a two to three-fold increase over basal levels. In patients with both type V and type VII diseases, this increase does not occur.

Type VI glycogen storage disease is difficult to diagnose. True deficiencies of liver phosphorylase are rare. It is difficult to distinguish these cases from others that present with hypoglycemia, and liver biopsy is necessary.

Type IX, phosphorylase kinase deficiency, can be detected by measurement of this enzyme's activity in red blood cells.

Treatment

In those types of glycogen storage disease that can be treated, diet has proven effective. In types I and III, nocturnal nutrient infusions with an enteral feeding pump along with a high-starch meal every 3 hours during the day have been successful.[14] In type I, once growth potential is achieved, cornstarch feedings can be used in place of nocturnal infusion in most patients.

Types III and V[20] have been more successfully managed with a high-protein intake. It has been reported that type II was managed successfully with a protein diet high in branched-chain amino acids.[14] Successful therapy in the past has not been demonstrated. Absence of strenuous exercise is helpful in types V and VII.

Genetics

Genetic counseling can be very helpful with the glycogen storage diseases. Heterozygous screening is available for types II, III, IV, VI, and VII. Prenatal diagnosis is possible with types II and IV.[8]

Case Study

A 65-year-old white woman was admitted with a tentative diagnosis of irritable bowel syndrome manifested as episodic diarrhea and chronic upper quadrant abdominal pain. She had a long history of abdominal complaints, having had watery bowel movements at various times since age 18 years. Approximately 2 years prior to admission, she had recurrent diarrhea and abdominal pain with weight loss. She was seen by a gastroenterologist, who found no organic etiology for either symptom. Her diarrhea is currently controlled with Metamucil, paregoric, and other similar agents.

Routine laboratory findings were normal except for an elevated bicarbonate level (32 mEq/L). A lactose tolerance test was performed, using 50 grams of lactose given orally. This resulted in five or six loose, watery bowel movements within 2 hours of ingestion. Glucose levels remained close to the fasting result of 69 mg/dL. With a 100-gram-fat, high-residue diet, the patient's weight stabilized, and stool studies were normal.

Questions

1. For what two conditions was this patient evaluated?
2. What condition is suggested by the laboratory findings?
3. What treatment is likely to be effective?

Discussion

1. The patient was evaluated for malabsorption and lactose intolerance.
2. The laboratory findings suggest lactose intolerance, because the ability to metabolize lactose is apparently absent.
3. Diet modifications to eliminate lactose should be effective treatment. The patient should be instructed regarding a lactose-free diet and told to try a high-carbohydrate, high-residue, lactose-free diet with several small feedings per day.

References

1. Taylor RH: Clinical tests for hypolactasia, lactose malabsorption, and lactose tolerance. Lancet 2:766, 1982.
2. Gitzelmann R, Steinmann B, von den Bughe G: Disorders of fructose metabolism. *In* Scriver CR, Stanbury J, Wyngaarden JB, et al: The Metabolic Basis of Inherited Disease, ed 6. New York, McGraw-Hill, 1989.
3. Segal S: Disorders of galactose metabolism. *In* Scriver CR, Stanbury J, Wyngaarden JB, et al: The Metabolic Basis of Inherited Disease, ed 6. New York, McGraw-Hill, 1989.
4. Hiott H: Pentosuria. *In* Scriver CR, Stanbury J, Wyngaarden JB, et al: The Metabolic Basis of Inherited Disease, ed 6. New York, McGraw-Hill, 1989.
5. Editorial: When does lactose malabsorption matter in adults? Br Med J 2:351, 1975.
6. Savilatiti E, Lauviola K, Kiutunen P: Congenial lactose deficiency: A clinical study on sixteen patients. Arch Dis Child 58:246–252, 1983.
7. Lyson M, Russo PJ: Normal initial blood galactose levels in a newborn with galactosemia. Am J Dis Child 136:747–748, 1982.
8. McCormack MK: Screening for genetic traits and diseases. Am Fam Physician 24:153–166, 1981.

9. Lewis V, Welch F, Cherry F, et al: Galactosemia: Clinical features, diagnosis and management. J Louisiana State Med Soc 147:262–265, 1995.
10. Bhatti T, Clamp J: Identification and estimation of monosaccharides and disaccharides in urine by GLC. Clin Chim Acta 22:563–567, 1968.
11. Rings EH, Grand RJ, Buller HA: Lactose intolerance and lactase deficiency in children. Curr Opin Pediatr 6:562–567, 1994.
12. Allen J, Holton J, Gilets M: Gas-liquid chromatographic determination of galactitol in amniotic fluid for possible use in prenatal diagnosis of galactosemia. Clin Chim Acta 110:59–63, 1981.
13. Suarez FL, Savaiano DA, Levitt MD: A comparison of symptoms after the consumption of milk or lactose-hydrolyzed milk by people with self-reported severe lactose intolerance. N Engl J Med 333:1–4, 1995.
14. Hers HG, Van Hof F, deBarry T: Glycogen storage diseases. *In* Scriver CR, Stanbury J, Wyngaarden JB, et al: The Metabolic Basis of Inherited Disease, ed 6. New York, McGraw-Hill, 1989.
15. Cornblath M, Schwartz R: Disorders of Carbohydrate Metabolism in Infancy, ed 3. Boston, Blackwell Scientific, 1991.
16. Dunger DB, Holton JB: Disorders of carbohydrate metabolism. *In* Holton JB: The Inherited Metabolic Diseases, ed 2. Edinburgh, Churchill Livingstone, 1994.
17. Matsusiki T, Yoshino M, Terasawa K, et al: Childhood acid maltase deficiency. Arch Neurol 41:47–52, 1984.
18. Maire I, Baussan C, Moatti N, et al: Biochemical diagnosis of hepatic glycogen storage disease: 20 years French experience. Clin Biochem 24:169–178, 1991.
19. Midorihawa K, Okada T, Kato T, et al: Diagnosis of Pompe's disease using pyridylaminomaltosligosaccharides as substrates of 1,4 glucosidase. Clin Chim Acta 147:97–102, 1985.
20. Slovim AE, Goan PJ: Myopathy in McArdle's syndrome: Improvement with a high protein diet. N Engl J Med 312:355–359, 1985.

Chapter 62

Nutrition in the Hospitalized Patient

Elia Mears

During the past three decades, numerous studies have documented the prevalence of malnutrition among hospitalized patients.[1-4] Malnourished patients are at higher risk of developing nutrition-related complications while being treated for other conditions. These complications include higher morbidity and mortality, infections, and impaired wound healing. Malnutrition can also have an adverse impact on length of hospital stay.[5] Reilly and colleagues[5] and Robinson and associates[6] demonstrated that malnourished medical and surgical patients stay in the hospital longer and they also incur twice the hospital charges and costs compared with similar well-nourished patients. In addition, Reilly and colleagues[5] found an average delay of 4 to 5 days in identifying patients with possible malnutrition.

Malnutrition can be defined as a state induced by altered dietary intake or nutrient utilization resulting in impaired subcellular, cellular, or organ function. Malnutrition occurs in patients either as a part of their primary disease or because the procedures they undergo for treatment of the primary disease prevent them from receiving appropriate nutritional intake for prolonged periods. Although it is difficult to determine the presence of subclinical nutritional deficiencies, it is important to do so in order to assess the possible benefits of aggressive nutrition therapy and to provide timely and appropriate treatment for those patients found to be malnourished or at risk for developing malnutrition.

PROTEIN MALNUTRITION

In the human body, proteins are essential for structural and regulatory function. In addition, proteins act as specific carriers and mediators of the immune response. Humans have no dispensable protein stores, and loss of body protein stores results in loss of essential structural elements and impaired function. Most of the body's protein is found in the skeletal muscle and in the visceral protein pool. There are three classifications of overt protein calorie/energy malnutrition. *Marasmus* is a chronic condition resulting from a deficiency in total energy intake in which reserves of protein and energy are depleted. There is wasting of skeletal muscle and adipose tissue stores, but visceral protein production is preserved. The relative weight loss threshold is 85% of ideal body weight. This form of malnutrition is most commonly encountered in developing countries and results from a prolonged reduction of food intake; however, it may occur in hospital patients with chronic illnesses or from prolonged use of clear fluid diets.

Kwashiorkor, another form of protein malnutrition, also occurs in certain regions of developing countries as well as in hospitalized patients. In the latter, it tends to occur as a result of inadequate intake of dietary protein but with adequate calorie intake, concomitant with acute protein losses induced by stress, hypermetabolism, or some other catabolic state. There is depletion of visceral protein pools with relative preservation of adipose tissue. Kwashiorkor is classically characterized by hypoalbuminemia and edema. *Mixed kwashiorkor/marasmus* is a form of severe protein malnutrition in chronically ill, starved patients who are undergoing hypermetabolic stress. It manifests as reduced visceral protein synthesis superimposed on wasting of somatic protein and energy stores. Immunity is lowered, incidence of infection is increased, and there is poor wound healing.[6-8]

NITROGEN BALANCE

Nitrogen balance, the difference between nitrogen intake and nitrogen excretion, is one of the most widely used indicators of protein change. In the healthy individual, anabolic and catabolic rates are in equilibrium, and thus the nitrogen balance is essentially zero.[6, 8] During trauma or stress, such as burns, nutritional intake decreases, and nitrogen loss may be greater than intake, putting the patient in a state of negative nitrogen balance. During recovery, nitrogen balance should become positive with nutrition support. Nitrogen balance studies provide the best information about meeting the patient's current metabolic nitrogen requirements. Total urinary nitrogen excretion provides information on the amount of nitrogen being lost from stress-related proteolysis. The hypermetabolic response that occurs in stressed states differs from nutritional depletion and is characterized by an increase in overall metabolic expenditure, accelerating the loss of lean body mass. For the hypermetabolic patient in a state of catabolism, the principal objective of nutrition support is to minimize loss of lean body mass.

CHOLESTEROL AND OTHER NUTRIENTS

The use of cholesterol as a nutritional assessment marker may be more important than previously believed. A cholesterol level below 130mg/dL is medically significant, and concentrations below 90mg/dL may be indicative of severe malnutrition and predictive of a poor clinical outcome.[8]

Trace metals, vitamins, minerals, and other nutrients can also be individually assessed when necessary in order to ensure that the patient's needs are being met. Because a deficiency of trace metals or minerals usually occurs in a generally malnourished individual, assessment methods should include consideration of these deficiencies. The following factors may increase the risk of trace metal deficiencies:[8]

- A vegetarian diet, especially one high in fibers and phytates that bind metals
- Alcohol consumption
- Drug treatment
- Increased losses secondary to malabsorption
- Intravenous nutrition for longer than two weeks without added trace metals

When a trace element deficiency is identified, the likelihood of the presence of a deficiency of more than one element increases. Clinical indicators warranting an in-depth evaluation are (1) keilosis and skin disorders, (2) anemia, (3) malabsorption syndromes, and (4) poor wound healing and infection.[8] The trace metals of most concern in nutrition are zinc, copper, selenium, chromium, manganese, and molybdenum. Clinical signs and symptoms of trace metal deficiency, except for zinc, are usually nonspecific, and their measurement in body fluids has not been proven to be a reliable predictor of overall trace metal adequacy. Consequently, routine screening for trace metals is not cost-effective or necessary. If any sign or symptom associated with a trace metal deficiency is found, justification exists to measure that metal.

As for trace metals deficiencies, the signs and symptoms of vitamin deficiencies may be nonspecific. The more common vitamins of concern are detailed in Box 62–1. Vitamins are routinely provided with parenteral and enteral nutrition support; therefore, hospitalized patients are at low risk of developing vitamin deficiencies and do not require routine monitoring of vitamin levels. Those who have clinical signs of a deficiency, however, should be assessed for the particular vitamin. Patients on long-term intravenous nutrition support should undergo periodic assessments of vitamin concentrations.[8]

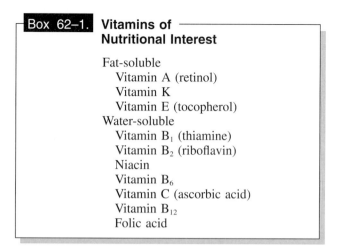

Box 62–1. **Vitamins of Nutritional Interest**

Fat-soluble
    Vitamin A (retinol)
    Vitamin K
    Vitamin E (tocopherol)
Water-soluble
    Vitamin B_1 (thiamine)
    Vitamin B_2 (riboflavin)
    Niacin
    Vitamin B_6
    Vitamin C (ascorbic acid)
    Vitamin B_{12}
    Folic acid

NUTRITIONAL ASSESSMENT

Nutritional assessment has become an essential component of the care of the hospitalized patient, and the Joint Commission for the Accreditation of Health Organizations (JCAHO) now requires compliance with certain nutrition care standards.[9] The objectives of these assessments are (1) to accurately define the nutritional status of the patient, (2) to define clinically relevant malnutrition, and (3) to monitor changes in nutritional status and follow the response of the patient during nutrition support. Nutritional assessments use a variety of methods, based on dietary, laboratory, anthropometric, and clinical measurements, that may be used alone but are most effective as a "system." Protein-energy/calorie malnutrition is the type of malnutrition most prevalent in hospital patients at present; thus, greater attention has been given to the selection of tests and criteria to assess and identify patients at risk.

The primary stage of nutritional deficiency is identified by dietary assessment methods. In this stage, inappropriate dietary intake of one or more nutrients occurs, as a result of either a primary deficiency or a secondary deficiency. Primary deficiency results from low levels in the diet. A secondary deficiency may be due to interference by certain drugs or disease states with the ingestion, absorption, transport, excretion, or utilization of nutrients.[6]

Certain stages in the development of nutritional deficiencies can be identified by laboratory methods. In primary or secondary deficiencies, tissue stores gradually become depleted of nutrients. The resulting reduction in the levels of the nutrients or their metabolic products in the body fluids and tissues can be detected by biochemical tests or protein markers.

Anthropometric methods use measurements of the physical dimensions and gross composition of the body, which vary with age and level of nutrition. There are certain advantages in using such methods. These procedures use simple, safe, and noninvasive measurements that can be performed at the bedside, and are applicable to large sample sizes. The required equipment is inexpensive and portable, and the information is generated on past, long-term nutritional history. Despite the advantages, however, anthropometry has important limitations: First, it is relatively insensitive and cannot detect short-term nutritional status or identify specific nutrient deficiencies. Second, it cannot distinguish disturbances induced by nutrient deficiencies from those caused by imbalances in protein and energy intake. Third, clinical conditions such as edema, obesity, and loss of skin elasticity and turgor prevent accurate measurements in patients. In addition, the equipment used, scales and skinfold calipers, must be calibrated regularly and kept in good condition.

Clinical assessment methods consist of a routine medical history and a physical examination to detect signs and symptoms associated with malnutrition. These signs and symptoms usually develop during the advanced stages of nutritional depletion, when overt disease is present. Clinical assessments, therefore, miss the marginally malnourished states or the preclinical stage of malnutrition. The medical history can be obtained by an interview with the patient and from the medical record. It generally consists of a description of the patient and relevant social, environmental, and family factors. This information is used to establish whether a nutrient deficiency is primary, as from inadequate dietary intake, or secondary in origin.

The physical examination detects changes that can be seen or felt in superficial epithelial tissue and is usually performed by a physician. This technique has the following limitations: (1) nonspecificity of the physical signs, (2) multiple physical signs confusing the diagnosis, (3) occurrence of some signs during malnutrition as well as during treatment, and (4) examiner inconsistencies depending on experience. In addition, there is variation in the pattern of physical signs because of genetic factors, activity level, environment, dietary pattern, age, and the duration and severity of malnutrition.

LABORATORY TESTS FOR NUTRITION ASSESSMENT

It is preferable and cost-effective to detect marginal nutrient deficiencies before a clinical syndrome develops, and laboratory methods should be included in the assessment process to confirm the existence of specific nutrient deficiencies. In primary or secondary deficiencies, tissue stores become gradually depleted of the nutrients, resulting in the reduction of the levels of nutrients or their metabolic products in certain body fluids. Laboratory assessment provides an objective means of assessing nutritional status.

Biochemical tests for nutritional assessment have been classified into two main categories, measurement of a nutrient in serum and measurement of the urinary excretion rate of the nutrient. Plasma/serum carries newly absorbed nutrients as well as those being transported throughout the body; thus, plasma/serum levels reflect recent dietary intake, providing present rather than long-term nutrient status. If the patient's renal function is normal, urine specimens can be used for the biochemical assessment of some minerals, vitamins, and proteins. Urinary excretion assessment methods primarily reflect recent dietary intake rather than long-term status. These methods depend on the presence of a renal conservation system that reduces the urinary excretion of the nutrient or metabolite when body stores of the nutrient are depleted.[6]

Serum Protein Markers

Biochemical assessment of the visceral protein component involves measurement of serum proteins. The main site of synthesis for most of these is the liver, one of the first organs to be affected by protein malnutrition. The serum proteins used as indices in the assessment of nutritional status are albumin, transferrin, retinol-binding protein, prealbumin, and, to a lesser extent, somatomedin C and fibronectin (Table 62–1). All of these proteins have transport functions separate from their use in nutrition assessment. The ideal marker for measuring short-term changes in protein status is one that has a small body pool and a rapid rate of synthesis, responds specifically to protein deprivation, has a short biologic half-life, and is not affected by nonnutritional factors.

Albumin is considered the first biochemical marker of malnutrition and has long been used in the assessment of hospitalized patients. There is a relatively large body pool of albumin, more than half of which is found outside the vascular space. Serum albumin reflects changes occurring within the intravascular space. Redistribution of albumin from the extravascular space to the intravascular space also occurs. Owing to its long half-life of 21 days, albumin is not a sensitive indicator of short-term nutrition deprivation, or of the efficacy of nutrition support. It does help identify patients with chronic protein deficiency, under conditions of adequate non–protein calorie intake, leading to marked hypoalbuminemia. It is known that low levels of albumin (less than or equal to 3.5g/dL) on admission to the hospital correlate with poor surgical outcome, poor diagnosis, higher costs, and prolonged length of stay.[10] Albumin can be affected by liver or kidney disease and by the hydration state of the patient. Age can also influence serum albumin, which declines in the elderly, probably because of a decreased rate of albumin synthesis.

Serum transferrin is a β-globulin protein but, unlike

Table 62–1. Serum Proteins Used in Nutrition Assessment

Protein	Half-Life	Reference Range*	Site(s) of Synthesis
Albumin	21 days	3.6–5.0 g/dL	Liver
Transferrin	8 days	200–400 mg/dL	Liver
Prealbumin	2 days	16–35 mg/dL	Liver
Somatomedin C	24 hr	0.10–0.40 mg/L	Primarily liver†
Fibronectin	15 hr	22.0–40.0 mg/dL	Endothelial cells, fibroblasts, macrophages, and liver
Retinol-binding protein	12 hr	3.0–6.0 mg/dL	Liver

*May vary with age and methodology.
†Also in tissue to lesser extent.

albumin, is found almost completely in the intravascular space, where it serves as the iron transport protein. It also has a bacteriostatic role, binding with free iron to prevent the growth of bacteria, which require iron for growth. Transferrin has a shorter half-life (8 days) and smaller body pool than albumin, making it a potentially better marker of protein status. Unfortunately, transferrin concentrations are affected by iron deficiency, pregnancy, gastrointestinal, renal, and liver disease, oral contraceptives, high-dose antibiotic therapy, and neoplastic disease.[6, 11, 12]

Retinol-binding protein (RBP) is a protein of low molecular weight that functions as a carrier for retinol. The complex RBP and retinol circulate together with one molecule of thyroxine-binding prealbumin, forming a trimolecular complex. Thus, loss of retinol during filtration at the kidney glomerulus is avoided. RBP has a very short half-life (approximately 12 hours) and a small body pool, so RBP concentrations tend to fall rapidly in response to protein and calorie deprivation and to respond quickly to dietary treatment.[6, 11, 12] Unfortunately, RBP concentrations can decrease in liver disease, vitamin A deficiency, acute catabolic states, after surgery, and in hyperthyroidism.

Thyroxine-binding prealbumin serves as a transport protein for thyroxine and as a carrier protein for RBP. Prealbumin (PAB), or transthyretin, has a half-life of 2 days and a slightly larger body pool than RBP, and the sensitivities of both proteins to protein deprivation and treatment are similar. Serum levels of prealbumin are higher than RBP, however, and are easier to measure. Patients with acute renal failure may have increased serum prealbumin values because of the role of the kidneys in prealbumin catabolism. Prealbumin levels decrease in patients with acute phase reactions. Ingenbleek[13] has recommended the combined measurements of prealbumin and an acute-phase reactant, such as C-reactive protein, to discriminate between the effects of inflammation and nutritional status in acutely or chronically ill patients receiving nutritional therapy.[13] PAB measurements are very useful at the initiation of nutrition therapy and to monitor response to the therapy. A serum transthyretin concentration greater than 11mg/dL is an entropy value that should be obtained for any patient in transition from parenteral to enteral to oral feeding. The serum concentration of the protein increases when more than 55% of the assessed protein and energy needs are met. When levels do not increase or when they remain below 11mg/dL, and nutritional support is being provided, the mode of feeding, amount of nutrients, and presence of disease, must be reexamined.[11]

Retinol-binding protein and prealbumin have been reported to be sensitive indicators of changes in nutritional status. Carpentier and associates[14] found a definite increase in the concentrations of RBP and prealbumin in protein-depleted, nonstressed patients receiving total parenteral nutrition (TPN). Prealbumin was the most sensitive indicator of nutritional status in cancer patients receiving total parenteral nutrition.[15] Winkler and colleagues[16] studied the use of RBP and prealbumin in monitoring response to nutritional therapy during the transition of total parenteral to oral or enteral feeding. They showed a significant improvement in the concentration of the proteins during the transitional feeding period. Their data demonstrate that plasma concentration of RBP and prealbumin rise at a time when other plasma proteins, albumin and transferrin in particular, do not change. These changes are persistent over time, and the rise in levels is maintained during the entire transitional period from TPN to oral or enteral feeding.

Both fibronectin and somatomedin C have been used in nutrition assessment and as markers of response to nutrition support. Fibronectin is a glycoprotein found in the lymph, blood, basement membranes, and many cell surfaces with structural functions as well as host defense functions. Levels have been found to increase significantly after 1 to 4 days of adequate enteral/parenteral feeding. Fibronectin is useful in nutritional panels, because it is one of the few nutritional markers that is not exclusively synthesized in the liver. Somatomedin C (insulin-like growth factor 1) is a growth-hormone dependent factor produced by the liver. It has a proinsulin-like structure and broad anabolic properties. Somatomedin C circulates bound to carrier proteins and has a half-life of several hours. Because of its short half-life and sensitivity to nutrient intake, somatomedin C may be more specific and sensitive as a marker of nutritional status. Reductions in levels occur in patients who have hypothyroidism and with estrogen administration.[6, 11, 12] Although both fibronectin and somatomedin C measurements appear to have potential uses in nutrition assessment, they are not easily performed in the laboratory and may be too costly to justify their routine use at this time.

Nitrogen Balance

In the assessment of nitrogen balance and excretion, there are two ways of measuring urinary nitrogen losses: Measuring urinary urea nitrogen and estimating total nitrogen, or directly measuring total urinary nitrogen (TUN). Direct measurement is preferred and recommended and is most significant for the unstable critically ill patient. For measurement, it is essential to collect a clean, properly preserved urine sample over a complete 24-hour period. There is significant day-to-day variation in nitrogen excretion; therefore, multiple samples may be needed. TUN may need to be measured every other day during the initial, most catabolic stage of an illness, and then weekly thereafter. Total urea nitrogen is important in determining the success of a nutrition treatment plan.[17]

Lymphocyte count is also a marker of nutritional deprivation. Total lymphocyte count (TLC) is a quick and inexpensive test that may be a useful indicator of nutritional status and outcome. In protein calorie malnutrition, the lymphocyte count is often below 2.5×10^9/L. Blackburn and colleagues[18] have suggested that a count of 0.8 to 1.2 $\times 10^9$/L indicates a moderate nutritional deficit and a value below 0.8×10^9/L represents a severe nutritional deficit. Marked lymphopenia in the absence of other primary causes, such as immunodeficiency or a viral infection, may suggest the presence of malnutrition.

Laboratory Approach to Nutritional Testing

Development of protocols, panels, or standardized orders can ensure consistent nutritional monitoring of patients and quality patient care. Individual tests can be performed, but offering clinicians various nutrition test panels can aid in specific clinical situations. There are several advantages to grouping nutrition tests into panels. Most important to the patient is the consolidation of blood sampling and fewer specimen requirements. It is easier for the physician to order medically necessary nutrition panels to assess a patient's status instead of listing the individual test. Panels also ensure selection of the best available and most cost-effective tests. The laboratory benefits by reduction in costs and a more predictable workload.

Global testing is the use of one or more laboratory tests individually or as a panel to screen an entire hospital population or subpopulation. It is often applied to surgical and medical patients, particularly upon admission. Prealbumin level is an example of a test that can be used to screen subpopulations such as medical and surgical patients, patients in intensive care, and the elderly. The test offers information pertaining to the nutritional status of the patient, and it is inexpensive to perform with present-day automation. In addition, it is sensitive for identifying nutritional depletion early, and allows the implementation of nutrition support early in the hospital stay. Prealbumin testing can be completed within 24 to 36 hours of admission.

Reflexive testing is the serial performance of a test on the basis of the outcome of another test or condition. An application of this principle is performance of a prealbumin test on a patient who meets certain clinical criteria, such as age greater than 65 years. Another use of reflexive testing is to monitor the nutrition support of a patient every 3 days with prealbumin measurements. Yet another application of reflexive testing is the use of C-reactive protein (CRP) measurement. The concentrations of several proteins increase dramatically during the inflammatory response; these are called acute-phase reactants, and of these, CRP is the most sensitive, with a half-life of 8 hours. The

serum concentration of CRP can be used to help interpret changes in PAB or RBP. If the level of CRP is normal, low level of the nutrition marker is most likely to be associated with protein malnutrition. The inverse, increased CRP and low PAB, may show the nutrition marker to be falsely decreased, because prealbumin is a negative acute-phase reactant. During monitoring, patients with decreasing levels of CRP and increasing levels of PAB are more likely to have improving protein energy status. Once the CRP value returns to normal, PAB can once again help define the nutrition status of the patient. Optimally, the CRP level should be measured on the same specimen used to assay the prealbumin. Figure 62–1 shows how prealbumin can be used as a part of a program for effective monitoring of patients. Implementation of such a program can be used to monitor the effectiveness of the nutritional care a patient is receiving, improve quality of care, and reduce costs.

NUTRITION SUPPORT

Nutrition support can be provided by either the enteral or the parenteral route, depending on whether the gastrointestinal tract is functioning. Nutrients can be administered enterally through a feeding tube. Enteral feeding is always preferable and less costly than total parenteral nutrition. *Total parenteral nutrition* (TPN) is defined as the intravenous provision of all the essential nutrients to the patient. These nutrients, including protein hydrolysates or amino acids in addition to glucose, are administered through a central venous catheter in amounts sufficient to meet the normal calorie and nitrogen needs of a patient. *Hyperalimentation* is the provision through a central venous catheter of calories in excess of normal requirements.[19, 20] Because it is part of therapy for many diseases and conditions, TPN is used in a variety of clinical settings and by many differ-

Figure 62–1. Prealbumin flow chart for positive patient outcome. Abbreviation: CRP, C-reactive protein.

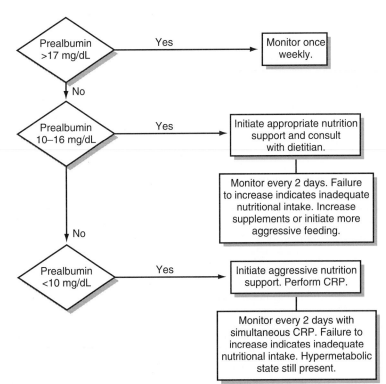

Table 62–2. **Laboratory Results to Monitor During Parenteral and Tube Feeding**

Analyte(s)	Rationale
Glucose	To determine whether the insulin release in response to the glucose in the formula is stimulating cellular glucose uptake
Electrolytes BUN Serum creatinine Ionized calcium	To monitor imbalance in those who have not been eating or who suffer from diarrhea or fluid losses, or who are being treated with medications *Note:* Calcium may tend to precipitate in TPN solutions, limiting its availability.
Phosphorus Magnesium	Severely malnourished patients are susceptible to rapid vascular depletion during refeeding Phosphate deficiency can also interfere with protein and ATP synthesis.
Liver enzymes Bilirubin	Indicative of TPN-induced liver complications, including impaired bile flow
Triglycerides	Evaluation of tolerance to intravenous lipid emulsions
Nitrogen balance	To ensure that adequate protein is available to compensate for normal amino acid turnover and to cover the extra demands of wound healing and stress.
Osmolality	Indicative of hydration status
Prealbumin	Best analyte available reflecting short-term protein/energy balance
Albumin	Prognostic indicator of hydration, and visceral protein status
Vitamin C Zinc Vitamin A	Important for optimal wound healing and immunocompetence
Zinc protoporphyrin	Indicator of subclinical iron deficiency
Copper	Required for activity of a number of oxidases
Selenium	Crucial in maintaining the body's antioxidation protection

ent medical specialties. The following are some situations in which TPN should be considered:

- Dysfunctional gastrointestinal tract
- Necessity to minimize intestinal activity
- Malnutrition in a patient who cannot meet conventional nutritional requirements owing to organ failure, stress, trauma, and malignancies.

There are two types of TPN, peripheral (PPN) and central. Peripheral parenteral nutrition is usually limited to 5 to 7 days. Central TPN allows the administration of 25% glucose, amino acids, and 10% to 20% lipids through a subclavian venous catheter. PPN uses a 10% glucose solution with amino acids and lipids. Although PPN is administered through a peripheral line, it has the same daily costs as central TPN, but it cannot deliver the same amount of calories. Nevertheless, PPN is commonly used because of the reluctance to place a central line.[21]

Although TPN is widely used, serious clinical considerations are issues involved in its administration, as follows:

- Prevention and management of complications such as infections, as well as metabolic complications
- Determination of nutritional requirements to support anabolism/positive nitrogen balance
- Choice of techniques and materials to ensure successful TPN administration, such as vein catheter selection and dressing maintenance
- Monitoring objectively to assess metabolic function and adequacy of protein and calories
- Management of the psychological ramifications associated with long-term oral deprivation

Risks in the use of TPN include complications such as hyperglycemia, vitamin or mineral deficiencies, pneumothorax, and infection at the catheter site. Knowledge of the potential complications of TPN can reduce occurrence. Multidisciplinary nutrition support teams can be formed to establish policies and monitor the administration of TPN. These individuals set basic practice standards and techniques, remain alert to potential problems, and intervene rapidly to minimize the morbidity associated with these complications.

TPN is expensive to administer, a fact that needs to be examined in view of the current efforts in health care to contain costs. The costs of providing nutrition support involve costs associated with formulary (TPN or enteral formulations), administration sets (lines or feeding tubes, and pumps and controllers), labor (nurses, dietitians, and pharmacists), and laboratory and radiology monitoring.[21]

Table 62–2 lists the laboratory results that should be monitored during parenteral and tube feeding nutrition support. Monitoring intervals depend on whether TPN is initial, stable, or long term and whether tube feeding is to be short or long term.

Transitional feeding—the gradual weaning of nutritional support from TPN to oral or enteral feeding—is an important element of the nutrition care plan. The smooth progression from one form of nutrition support to another must be carefully implemented and monitored in order to prevent deterioration of the patient's nutritional status. A combination of oral or enteral feeding methods may be used simultaneously while parenteral solutions are decreased.

Case Study

A 68-year-old male visited an emergency department with the complaint of voiding difficulty and decreased urinary output. Upon his admission to the hospital, laboratory findings revealed elevated BUN and creatinine, and an electrolyte imbalance. Urinalysis demonstrated proteinuria, and many RBC casts were present on microscopic examination. Hematologic studies showed a normochromic, normocytic anemia of moderate severity. In addition, the patient's urine output was measured as less than 400mL/24 hours. The patient also had a serum albumin of 2.5 g/dL and a serum prealbumin of 56 mg/dL. Nutritional history included improper eating for the past 2 months and a 10-lb weight loss.

Questions

1. What is the primary diagnosis for this patient?
2. How should the serum prealbumin value be interpreted by the physician and dietitian, and what form of nutrition support should the patient receive?
3. How should the patient's nutritional progress be monitored in this type of situation?

Discussion

1. The laboratory data in this case study suggest that the patient may be suffering from acute renal failure. Nutritional history indicates that the patient has been suffering from chronic malnutrition, although the prealbumin value is not decreased. The albumin is below the reference range; however, albumin is affected by so many other factors that it cannot be used to assess the patient's nutritional status.

2. The prealbumin value of this patient is above the reference range. In renal failure, prealbumin concentration increases; however, of all the markers available, it is the least affected by this condition. From the nutritional history and weight loss problem, it is evident the patient is experiencing protein depletion and is in a state of malnutrition. The dietitian must take all conditions into account and start the patient on a nutrition support program appropriate for renal disorders.

3. In these situations, the patient is started on appropriate nutrition support and can be monitored with prealbumin levels every 3 days. Any changes are likely to reflect alterations in nutritional status and nitrogen balance. Urinary nitrogen studies can also be performed, which can indicate when the patient has entered an anabolic state. Albumin should not be used for monitoring, because it is affected by so many other factors.

References

1. Bristrian BR, Blackburn GL, Hallowell E, et al: Protein status of general surgical patients. JAMA 230:858–860, 1974.
2. Bristian BR, Blackburn GL, Vitale J, et al: Prevalence of malnutrition in general medical patients. JAMA 235:1567–1570, 1976.
3. Baker JP, Detsky AS, Wesson DE, et al: Nutrition assessment: A comparison of clinical judgment and objective measurements. N Engl J Med 306:969–972, 1982.
4. Detsky AS, Baker JP, O'Rourke K, et al: Predicting nutrition-associated complications for patients undergoing gastrointestinal surgery. J Paren Ent Nutr 11:440–446, 1987.
5. Reilly JJ, Hull S, Albert N, et al: Economic impact of malnutrition: A model system for hospitalized patients. J Parent Ent Nutr 12:371–376, 1988.
6. Gibson R: Principles of Nutritional Assessment. New York, Oxford University Press, 1990.
7. Baumgartner T: Clinical Guide to Parenteral Micronutrition, ed 2. Deerfield, Ill, Lymphomed, Division of Fugisawa, 1991.
8. Kaplan L (ed): National Academy Clinical Biochemistry: Standards of Laboratory Practice—Consensus Guidelines. Cincinnati, Pesce Kaplan Publishers, 1994.
9. Dougherty D, Bankhead R, Kushner R, et al: Nutrition care given new importance in JACHO standards. Nutr Clin Pra 10:26–31, 1995.
10. Mullen JL, Buzby GP, Walman MT, et al: Prediction of operative morbidity and mortality by preoperative nutritional assessment. Surg Forum 30:80–82, 1979.
11. Spiekerman M: Proteins used in nutritional assessment. Clin Lab Med 13:353–369, 1993.
12. Charney P: Nutrition assessment in the 90's: Where are we now? Nutr Clin Pract 10:131–139, 1995.
13. Ingenbleek Y: Usefulness of prealbumin as nutritional indicator. In Allen RC, Bienvenu J, Laurent P, Suskind RM (eds): Marker Proteins in Inflammation. New York, Walter de Gruyter, 1982.
14. Carpentier YA, Barthel J, Bruyns J: Plasma protein concentration in nutritional assessment. Proc Nutr Soc 4:405, 1982.
15. Bourry J, Milano G, Caldani C, et al: Assessment of nutritional proteins during parenteral nutrition of cancer patients. Ann Clin Lab Sci 12:158, 1982.
16. Winkler MF, Gerrior S, Pomp A, et al: Use of retinol-binding protein and prealbumin as indicators of the response to nutrition therapy. Journal of Am Diet Assoc 89:5:684–687, 1989.
17. Konstantinides FN: Nitrogen balance studies in clinical nutrition. Clin Pract 7:231–238, 1992.
18. Blackburn GL, Bistrian BR, Maini BS, et al: Nutritional and metabolic assessment of the hospitalized patient. Parent Ent Nutr 1:11, 1977.
19. Perry S, Pillar B, Radany M: The appropriate use of high-cost, high-risk technologies: The case of total parenteral nutrition. Technology Assessment and Practice Guidelines Forum. Washington DC, Georgetown University School of Medicine, 1990.
20. Morsi ML: Total Parenteral Nutrition. In Davis BG, Bishop ML, Mass D: Clinical Laboratory Science: Strategies for Practice. Philadelphia, JB Lippincott, 1989, pp 854–862.
21. Bernstein L, Shaw-Stiffel T, Schorow M, et al: Financial implications of malnutrition. Clin Lab Med 13:491–507, 1993.

Chapter 63

Hyperlipoproteinemias

Craig A. Lehmann

Hyperlipoproteinemias were first classified in 1965 by Fredrickson and Lees,[1] who separated them into five major categories. Since then, laboratory methodologies and research have provided a better understanding of these disorders and have shown that the term *hyperlipoproteinemia* is not fully representative. The term *dyslipoproteinemia* better describes these abnormalities, because it accounts for decreases in some lipoproteins that occur and for physiologic variations in the phenotype.

Fredrickson's classification accounts for all variations of hyperlipoproteinemias except for hyperalphalipoproteinemia, which is usually primary (familial) and involves autosomal dominant inheritance.[2, 3] Patients have increased concentrations of plasma high-density lipoproteins (HDLs). Because increased HDLs have not been shown to have harmful effects on health, no further discussion of them will be presented here, except to say that research has shown that high levels of HDLs appear to be related to lower risk of coronary artery disease.

The primary clinical interest in hyperlipoproteinemias centers on their association with increased risk of coronary artery disease and pancreatitis. This association requires that an accurate distinction be made between primary disorders, which are familial, and secondary disorders, which are associated with other disease processes, so that the proper treatment may be administered. This distinction can be made only through careful evaluation of patient and family history and of the clinical signs and symptoms, use of appropriate sampling methods, and proper utilization, interpretation, and correlation of laboratory tests.

ETIOLOGY AND PATHOPHYSIOLOGY
Type I

Type I hyperlipoproteinemia is very rare, almost exclusively primary, and acquired by autosomal recessive inheritance. The abnormality is manifested as an inability to clear chylomicrons. This is due to decreased activity of lipoprotein lipase (LPL) or a deficiency in apolipoprotein C-II.[4, 5] The presence of plasma chylomicrons results in increases in triglyceride levels that are among the highest within the hyperlipoproteinemias. These high concentrations inflame the pancreas and result in recurring episodes of pancreatitis. For these reasons, a diagnosis is generally made early in life.

Although most primary disorders are diagnosed early in life, secondary conditions must be ruled out, especially in the adult. Conditions that can cause lipid abnormalities resembling type I hyperlipoproteinemia are systemic lupus erythematosus, pancreatitis, dysglobulinemia, oral contraceptive therapy, hypothyroidism, and uncontrolled diabetes mellitus.

Type II

Fredrickson's type II, a common hyperlipoproteinemia, has been divided into two subclasses, IIa and IIb. Type IIa is primary heterozygous and acquired by autosomal dominant inheritance. It leads to hypercholesterolemia and increased low-density lipoproteins (LDLs). Type IIb is almost always primary, with a possibility of being either inherited as an autosomal dominant trait or derived from a combination of genetic causes that leads to a combined hyperlipoproteinemia of very-low-density lipoproteins (VLDLs) and low-density lipoproteins (LDLs). Type IIb is almost exclusively heterozygous and rarely appears in the homozygous state.

Patients with type IIa hyperlipoproteinemia may lack sufficient LDL receptors or may have a defect either in the receptors or in LDL metabolism within the cell.[6] Homozygous patients demonstrate much higher levels of LDL cholesterol than heterozygous patients. Patients with type IIb familial combined hyperlipoproteinemia have high plasma levels of LDLs and VLDLs. The exact defect has not yet been resolved. The increase in VLDLs may be polygenic or may involve a variety of secondary conditions. Family studies usually reveal other family members with type IIa or IV hyperlipoproteinemia.

Lipid elevations that resemble primary type II patterns are seen in patients who have diabetes mellitus, myxedema, hypothyroidism, nephritic syndrome, hepatic disease, anorexia nervosa, or stress, consume high-cholesterol, high-fat diets, or are undergoing treatment for another disease with numerous drugs.

Type III

Type III hyperlipoproteinemia is very rare, almost exclusively primary, and acquired by autosomal recessive inheritance. The primary condition is due to dysbetalipoproteinemia, resulting in plasma increases of VLDLs that are high in cholesterol. Type III hyperlipoproteinemias are apolipoprotein E^2 homozygotes. Normal individuals possess the apolipoprotein in the E^3 genotype form. Other variations have been reported that involve apolipoprotein E.[7-9]

A primary role of apolipoprotein E is to clear chylomicron remnants and intermediate-density lipoproteins (IDLs). The site of its involvement is the liver receptors, where chylomicron remnants and IDLs are taken up. The apolipoprotein E^2 homozygote appears to lack the ability to bind the remnants to the receptors.

Although most dysbetalipoproteinemias are primary, secondary disorders can cause lipid abnormalities resembling those in type III hyperlipoproteinemia. These include hypothyroidism, diabetes mellitus, myxedema, biliary cirrhosis, systemic lupus erythematosus, and gout.

Type IV

Type IV is a very common hyperlipoproteinemia, sometimes referred to as endogenously induced hyperlipoproteinemia, that may be primary by autosomal dominant inheritance. The precise biochemical defect involved in type IV is not known. The lipid increase appears to be caused by a decrease in VLDL catabolism, an increase in the synthesis of VLDLs, or both. Patients can present with either a familial hypertriglyceridemia or a familial combined hyperlipoproteinemia. Research has demonstrated an association between apolipoprotein A-I and C-III genes for hypertriglyceridemia.[10]

Often, moderate alcohol ingestion may cause a lipoprotein pattern consistent with type IV hyperlipoproteinemia. Other conditions that may cause lipid abnormalities resembling those of type IV hyperlipoproteinemia are stress, diet, use of estrogens, oral contraceptives, diet, thiazides, or β-adrenergic blockers, diabetes mellitus, and lipid storage diseases (*e.g.,* Gaucher's disease, Niemann-Pick disease).

Type V

Type V hyperlipoproteinemia is a rare form of mixed familial hypertriglyceridemia that appears to be heterozygous or homozygous for an uncommon apolipoprotein $E^{4,11}$ and/or may have elevations in sialylated apolipoprotein C-III2.[11,12] These defects produce elevations in VLDLs and chylomicrons, which in turn cause inflammation of the pancreas.

As with type IV, secondary forms of hypertriglyceridemia are numerous and common, and a careful effort must be made to distinguish them from the primary form. Common conditions causing hypertriglyceridemia are alcoholism, myeloma, pancreatitis, diabetes mellitus, obesity, use of estrogens, and hyperuricemia.

CLINICAL MANIFESTATIONS

Early and frequent occurrence of abdominal pain and pancreatitis are key factors in making a diagnosis of type I hyperlipoproteinemia. Patients who consistently have triglyceride levels greater than 1500 mg/dL may also exhibit eruptive xanthomas, lipemia retinalis, splenomegaly, and hepatomegaly. Patients generally complain of abdominal pain after the intake of a fatty meal, which is due to the increase in chylomicrons and their effect on the pancreas. The episodes of pancreatitis are the most serious complications of type I hyperlipoproteinemia for the patient, because this type is not associated with a higher risk of coronary artery disease.

Type II hyperlipoproteinemias are associated with a high incidence of coronary artery disease. Heterozygotes tend to develop coronary artery disease as early as the third decade of life. Type IIa generally results in higher cholesterol levels than the familial combined type IIb. Homozygotes tend to have very high plasma cholesterol levels and to develop coronary artery disease before the second decade of life. Planar and tuberous xanthomas are usually present on the patient's elbows, knees, and hands. Patients with type IIb tend to be overweight and have elevated plasma VLDLs in addition to their LDLs. It is very rare for type IIb to cause xanthomas.

Patients with dysbetalipoproteinemia (type III) present unique tubero-eruptive and palmar xanthomas (*xanthoma striatum palmare*). These xanthomas appear in various hues of yellow and orange. Many patients have glucose intolerance and are obese. Coronary artery disease, ischemic vascular disease, and peripheral vascular diseases are prevalent. Clinical signs and symptoms vary with age, sex, and, secondary disease, with the related primary disorder.

Most patients with type IV hyperlipoproteinemia are obese and have no xanthomas. They are generally adults and may have an additional disorder, such as hypertension, diabetes mellitus, or hyperuricemia. Familial hypertriglyceridemia seems to have little correlation with coronary artery disease, unlike combined hyperlipoproteinemia.[13]

Patients with type V disease are generally obese and describe dryness of eyes and mouth along with numbness of distal extremities. Patients usually present with pancreatitis and eruptive xanthomas, but not as early in life as in type I, because type V hyperlipoproteinemia usually occurs in adults.

LABORATORY ANALYSES AND DIAGNOSIS

Patient history is very important for proper interpretation of laboratory results. Patients should be questioned about a family history of hyperlipoproteinemia and coronary heart disease. They should also be asked about alcohol consumption, because of its association with hypertriglyceridemia.

Other circumstances may affect the results of laboratory tests used to assist in the diagnosis of hyperlipoproteinemia, such as recent surgery or myocardial infarction within the previous month. Recent illness, current drug therapy, such as contraceptives, or alteration of dietary habits within the previous 2 weeks may also interfere with the interpretation of test results.

Blood samples for the analysis of LDL and triglycerides must be collected from fasting patients, and analysis should not be delayed. For total and HDL cholesterol, patients need not be fasting. For very short delays (2 to 4 hours), samples should be stored at 4°C. For electrophoresis, samples can be stored at 4°C with ethylenediaminetetraacetic acid (EDTA) up to 5 days.[14] Samples for cholesterol, triglyceride and/or HDL cholesterol measurements can be either serum or plasma; however, levels measured in samples from EDTA plasma need to be multiplied by 1.03.

Although cholesterol and triglyceride analyses still remain the primary tests for screening hyperlipoproteinemias, many physicians automatically include HDL cholesterol. A variation of the methods used to quantitate HDL cholesterol involving precipitation of VLDL and LDL may prove to be helpful, especially in the screening of large populations.[15, 16] Once cholesterol and triglycerides have been estimated and one or both are demonstrated to be elevated in at least two samples on different occasions, preliminary phenotype classification should be established by the 18-hour 4 °C plasma observation test, as shown in Figure 63–1. After preliminary classification has been made and secondary factors have been ruled out, additional information for phenotyping and risk of coronary artery disease can be obtained by the series of tests shown in Figure 63–1.

Although there is debate about the relevance of lipoprotein electrophoresis as a routine clinical tool, it is useful in detecting the presence of chylomicrons in type I and type V hyperlipoproteinemia and of a lipoprotein X band, a marker of obstructive jaundice. Electrophoresis also helps to distinguish between types III and IV by revealing the presence of a broad band of β-lipoprotein, present in type III; therefore, electrophoresis for selected samples is still appropriate. On a routine basis, many laboratories measure HDL, LDL, and VLDL cholesterol tests as a lipid profile. The LDL and VLDL cholesterol levels are generally calculated from relationships among total cholesterol, triglycer-

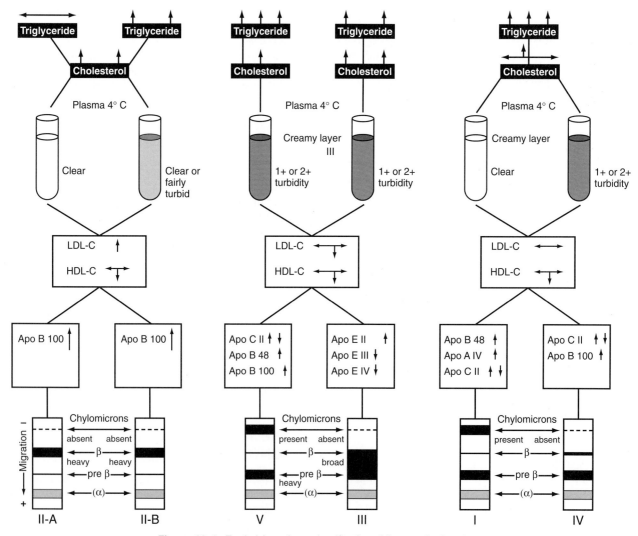

Figure 63–1. Frederickson-Levy classification of lipoprotein disorders.

ides, and HDL cholesterol values. Direct LDL testing can be performed if triglycerides are too high to use the calculation method.

Apolipoproteins are becoming part of the diagnostic testing requests for many clinicians, especially requests for apo A-I and apo B. Although methodologies have improved, there are still problems associated with these assays, primarily in the area of standardization. Apolipoproteins are being used to help identify hyperlipoproteinemias and help predict risk of coronary artery disease. Apolipoproteins play a major role in lipoprotein metabolism. Apolipoproteins A-I and A-II are the major proteins of HDL. Apo A-I is involved in removing free cholesterol from peripheral tissue through the activation of lecithin-cholesterol acyltransferase (LCAT), and A-II's function is to inhibit LCAT. Apolipoprotein B is the major apolipoprotein in all other lipoproteins and occurs in two forms, B-100 and B-48. Apo B is involved with transporting and clearing lipids in circulation. As demonstrated in Figure 63–1, apolipoprotein assays can yield additional information for identifying specific phenotypes, although many clinical laboratories are not performing apolipoprotein analyses at this time.

Most hyperlipoproteinemias can be classified by the tests previously described; however, other measurements and measurement ratios have been helpful in their classification or in predicting risk of coronary artery disease. The ratios most widely used for this purpose are cholesterol-triglycerides, LDL cholesterol–HDL cholesterol, and VLDL cholesterol–triglycerides. For example, type III hyperlipoproteinemia demonstrates a ratio of VLDL cholesterol–triglycerides greater than 0.30. A more involved procedure, useful in separating phenotype I from phenotype V, is post–heparin lipase activity (PHLA); lipoprotein lipase levels in type I do not rise following the infusion of heparin.

Laboratory analyses that are helpful in assessing secondary conditions include those for glucose intolerance and hepatic, renal, and endocrine function, which are discussed elsewhere in this text.

TREATMENT

Type I

Currently, there is no effective drug for type I hyperlipoproteinemia; however, changing the diet works well in controlling the condition and in preventing the occurrence of pancreatitis, a major objective of the therapy. The diets should consist of less than 20 g of fat per day. In addition to diet changes, patients are counseled to restrict alcohol and to supplement their diet with fat-soluble vitamins.

Type II

Both subclasses of type II hyperlipoproteinemia respond well to diet alterations. The diet should include low-fat and low-cholesterol intake. Type IIb responds well to niacin and gemfibrozil, whereas type IIa responds best to niacin and colestipol. It should be noted that homozygous familial hypercholesterolemia is far more difficult to treat, as it responds poorly to diet and drugs. When patients cannot

Table 63–1. Drug Therapy for Hyperlipoproteinemias

Drug (Mechanism)	Phenotype(s)	Effect(s)	Adverse Effect(s)	Laboratory Monitoring
Nicotinic acid (niacin) (Mechanism for lipid reduction unknown)	II, III, IV	↓ Triglyceride ↓ VLDL cholesterol ↓ LDL cholesterol ↑ HDL cholesterol	Hepatic Peptic ulcers	HDL cholesterol, liver function tests, glucose, cholesterol, triglyceride, LDL cholesterol, uric acid
Cholestyramine and colestipol (anion-exchange resin that binds intestinal bile acids)	IIa	↓ LDL cholesterol	Constipation Nausea Hypoprothrombinemia (<vitamin K)	Cholesterol, triglyceride, prothrombin time, LDL cholesterol, HDL cholesterol
Clofibrate (mechanism not yet clear)	III, IV	↓ Triglyceride ↓ VLDL cholesterol ↓ LDL cholesterol ↑ HDL cholesterol	Myositis Hepatic Gastrointestinal Many additional effects	HDL cholesterol, cholesterol, triglycerides, liver function tests, complete blood count, protein, creatine kinase
Gemfibrozil (mechanism not yet clear; research has demonstrated that the drug inhibits peripheral lipolysis and decreases hepatic extraction of free fatty acids)	IIa, IIb, III IV, V	↓ VLDL ↓ LDL ↑ HDL	Myositis Hepatic Many additional effects	Cholesterol, triglyceride, potassium levels, complete blood count, HDL cholesterol, LDL cholesterol, liver function tests
Probucol (increased rate of fractional catabolism of LDL also inhibits cholesterol synthesis)	II	↓ LDL ↓ HDL	Hepatic Diarrhea Nausea	Cholesterol, triglyceride, HDL cholesterol, liver function tests, glucose, urea nitrogen, uric acid, LDL cholesterol
Fluvastatin sodium (HMG CoA reductase inhibitor)	IIa IIb	↓ Total cholesterol ↓ LDL cholesterol	Digestive	Liver function tests, creatine kinase, total cholesterol, LDL cholesterol
Lovastatin (HMG CoA reductase inhibitor)	IIa IIB	↓ Total cholesterol ↓ LDL cholesterol	Central nervous system Gastrointestinal hypersensitivity CK, AST, ALT	Creatine kinase, AST, total cholesterol, LDL cholesterol, VLDL cholesterol

tolerate standard drugs, probucol is an effective alternative.[17]

Type III

Type III disease responds well to cholesterol and caloric restrictions. Generally, to normalize lipid levels, drug intervention is also required. The drug most widely prescribed is niacin, but for patients who cannot tolerate this drug, gemfibrozil and clofibrate are excellent alternatives.[17]

Type IV

Most cases of type IV hyperlipoproteinemia respond well to diets that restrict fats, cholesterol, and calories. The avoidance of certain drugs as well as of alcohol is imperative. If drugs become necessary, niacin, gemfibrozil, and clofibrate are recommended.[17]

Type V

Type V disease responds to diets in which intake of both fat and cholesterol is low. Restriction of alcohol and exogenous estrogens is imperative. For patients whose disease does not respond well to dietary changes, the drug gemfibrozil is effective (Table 63–1).[17]

Case Study 1

A routine physical examination of a 45-year-old male accountant revealed that the patient was overweight for his height and frame size. In addition, the patient's blood pressure was elevated (165/90 mm Hg). Fasting blood samples were drawn for a 20-test chemistry profile, complete blood count, and urinalysis. The laboratory results were all normal except for a moderate elevation in cholesterol and a major elevation in triglycerides.

During a follow-up visit to his physician, the patient was questioned about a family history of hyperlipoproteinemia and coronary heart disease. To rule out secondary complications, the patient was also questioned about dietary habits, drug therapy, recent illness, and alcohol consumption. All responses were negative, so these factors were considered noncontributory to the lipid elevations.

Laboratory tests performed at this time were measurements of cholesterol, triglycerides, HDL cholesterol, LDL cholesterol, as well as 18-hour, 4°C refrigeration observation. The laboratory was also directed to hold an additional sample for possible lipoprotein electrophoresis.

The cholesterol and triglyceride analyses were consistent with the previous data, moderately elevated cholesterol and extremely elevated triglycerides. The HDL and LDL cholesterol levels were normal. The 18-hour, 4°C refrigeration observation showed a 2+ turbidity. There was no creamy layer at the surface of the sample.

Questions

1. What hyperlipoproteinemia types can be eliminated in light of the initial laboratory test results?

2. Considering the additional laboratory findings, what hyperlipoproteinemia type is most likely?

3. What treatment is most effective for this type?

Discussion

1. Hyperlipoproteinemia types IIa and IIb can be ruled out immediately, because they involve extremely elevated cholesterol levels and normal to slightly elevated triglycerides, as demonstrated in Figure 63–1.

2. The absence of a creamy layer at the surface of the sample after refrigeration rules out phenotypes I and V, as indicated in Figure 63–1. This leaves two possibilities, phenotypes III and IV. Of these two, the laboratory data present more supportive evidence for phenotype IV, because the LDL cholesterol level is normal, as it would not be for phenotype III (see Fig. 63–1). The slight elevation in cholesterol with phenotype IV is due to the increased cholesterol found in the higher VLDL fraction and not in the LDL fraction; this can be confirmed by electrophoresis. The electrophoretic pattern should reveal no broad band of β-lipoproteins, as seen in phenotype III, but a heavy band of pre-β lipoproteins that is consistent with phenotype IV.

3. The patient should be started on dietary restrictions of fats, cholesterol, and calories, because most cases of phenotype IV respond well to this regimen; however, if drug therapy becomes necessary, tests other than cholesterol and triglyceride measurements should be included as part of the monitoring process. Drug therapy can cause such adverse side effects as hepatic and gastrointestinal problems and peptic ulcers, as seen in Table 63–1.

Case Study 2

An initial lipid screen performed for a 55-year-old man revealed a triglyceride level of 600 mg/dL and a total cholesterol level of 220 mg/dL. Complete blood count (CBC) demonstrated macrocytosis. The clinician ordered another lipid screen plus HDL cholesterol, CBC, and a general blood chemistry profile. The results revealed the following elevated results: triglycerides, 580 mg/dL; total cholesterol, 210 mg/dL; red blood cell macrocytosis; and slight elevation of aspartate aminotransferase (AST).

Questions

1. On the basis of the laboratory findings, should this patient undergo phenotyping?

2. On the basis of the laboratory findings, would you order any additional tests? If so what would they be, and why?

Discussion

1. It is far too early to phenotype the patient. Cholesterol and triglyceride levels should be measured in

at least three fasting blood samples taken at separate times with at least several weeks between samplings. This routine should be accompanied by tests that could possibly rule out secondary disorders in question.

2. On the basis of the elevated AST and the presence of macrocytosis, one should be suspicious of a secondary disorder. AST is located in the microsomal and mitochondrial segment of the hepatic cell as well as other areas of the body. When AST becomes elevated and exceeds alanine aminotransferase (ALT), inflammation and necrosis of the liver are generally indicated. This finding, along with macrocytosis and elevated triglycerides, should prompt further investigation of a secondary hepatic condition. The clinician should be advised to order additional liver function tests to evaluate possible liver disease and a vitamin B_{12}–folate assay to address macrocytosis. It is very important to rule out secondary conditions before putting the patient through the unnecessary procedures and costs associated with phenotyping. Once the secondary condition is treated, lipid assays should again be checked, because the patient may still have a primary hyperlipoproteinemia.

References

1. Fredrickson DS, Lees RS: A system for phenotyping hyperlipoproteinemina (editorial). Circulation 31:312–327, 1965.
2. Glueck CJ, Fallat RW, Millet F, et al: Familial hyperalphalipoproteinemia. Metabolism 24:1243, 1975.
3. Fredrickson DS, Levy RI: Familial hyperlipoproteinemias. *In* Wyngaarden JB, Fredrickson DS (eds): The Metabolic Basis of Inherited Disease, ed 3. New York, McGraw-Hill, 1972.
4. Fredrickson DS, Levy RI, Lees RS: Fat transport in lipoproteins—an integrated approach to mechanisms and disorders. N Engl J Med 276:148–156, 1967.
5. Breckenridge WC, Little JA, Steiner G, et al: Hypertriglyceridemia associated with the deficiency of apolipoprotein C-11. N Engl J Med 298:1265–1273, 1978.
6. Tolleshaug H, Hobgood KK, Brown MS, et al: The LDL receptor focus in familial hypercholesterolemia: Multiple mutations disrupt transport and processing of a membrane receptor. Cell 32:941–951, 1983.
7. Rall SC Jr, Weisgraber KH, Innerarity TL: Identification of new structural variant of human apolipoprotein E, E2 (Lys 146 Gln) in a type III hyperlipoproteinemic subject with E3/2 phenotype. J Clin Invest 72:1288–1297, 1983.
8. Gregg RE, Ghiselli G, Brewer HB Jr: Apolipoprotein E bethesda: A new variant of apolipoprotein E associated with type III hyperlipoproteinemia. J Clin Endocrinol Metab 57:969–974, 1983.
9. Havel RJ, Kotite L, Kane JP, et al: Atypical familial dys-β-lipoproteinemia associated with apolipoprotein phenotype E3/3. J Clin Invest 72:379–387, 1983.
10. Karathansis SK, McPherson J, Zannis VI, et al: Linkage of human apolipoproteins Al and C-111 Gene. Nature 304:371–373, 1983.
11. Ghiselli G, Schaffer EJ, Zech LA, et al: Increased prevalence of apolipoprotein E4 in type V hyperlipoproteinemia. J Clin Invest 70:474–477, 1982.
12. Holdsworth G, Stocks J, Dodson P, et al: An abnormal triglyceride-rich lipoprotein containing excess sialyated apolipoprotein C-III. J Clin Invest 69:932–939, 1982.
13. Sniderman AD, Wolfson C, Teng B, et al: Association of hyperapobetalipoproteinemia with endogenous hypertriglyceridemia and atherosclerosis. Ann Intern Med 97:833–839, 1982.
14. Ballantyne CF: Role of the clinical biochemistry laboratory in the assessment of dyslipoproteinemias. Ann Clin Biochem 21:166–175, 1984.
15. Lehmann CA, Rosenfeld MH, Danielson LA: A rapid, reliable screening method for hyperlipidemia. Lab Med 14:782–784, 1983.
16. Lehmann CA, Treanor WJ, Malchiodi L: Efficacy of a simplified screening procedure for hyperlipoproteinemias. J Med Technol 2:174–176, 1985.
17. Physicians' Desk Reference, ed 40. Oradell, NJ, Medical Economics Books, 1986.

Bibliography

Brensike JF, Levy RI, Kelsey SF, et al: Effects of therapy with cholestyramine on progression of coronary arteriosclerosis: Results of the NHLBI Type II Coronary Intervention Study. Circulation 69:313–324, 1984.

Coronary Drug Project Research Group: Clofibrate and niacin in coronary heart disease. JAMA 231:360–381, 1975.

Ghiselli G, Schaefer EJ, Gascon P, et al: Type III hyperlipoproteinemia associated with apolipoprotein E deficiency. Science 214:1239–1241, 1981.

Glueck CJ, Levy RI, Glueck HI, et al: Acquired type I hyperlipoproteinemia with systemic lupus erythematosus, dysglobulinemia, and heparin resistance. Am J Med 47:318–325, 1969.

Goldstein JL, Schrott HG, Hazzard WR, et al: Hyperlipidemia in coronary heart disease. II: Genetic analysis of lipid levels in 176 families and delineation of a new inherited disorder, hyperlipidemia. J Clin Invest 52:1544–1568, 1973.

Grundy SM: AHA special report: Recommendations for the treatment of hyperlipidemia in adults—a joint statement of the Nutrition Committee and the Council on Arteriosclerosis of the American Heart Association. Arteriosclerosis 4:445A–468A, 1984.

Holdsworth G, Stocks J, Donson P, et al: An abnormal triglyceride-rich lipoprotein containing excess sialylated apolipoprotein CIII. J Clin Invest 69:932–939, 1982.

Kashyap ML, Hynd BA, Robinson K, et al: Abnormal preponderance of sialylated apolipoprotein CIII in triglyceride-rich lipoproteins in the type V hyperlipoproteinemia. Metabolism 30:111–118, 1981.

Levy RI: Drugs used in the treatment of hyperlipoproteinemia. *In* Goodman AS, Goodman LS, Gilman A (eds): The Pharmacological Basis of Therapeutics, ed 6. New York, Macmillan, 1980.

Levy RI, Fredrickson DS, Shulman R, et al: Dietary and drug treatment of primary hyperlipoproteinemia. Ann Intern Med 77:267–294, 1972.

Mellies MJ, Gartside PS, Glotfelter L, et al: Effects of probucol on plasma cholesterol, high-and low-density lipoprotein cholesterol, and apolipoproteins A1 and A2 in adults with primary familial hypercholesterolemia. Metabolism 29:956–964, 1980.

Norum RA, Lakier JB, Goldstein S, et al: Familial deficiency of apolipoproteins A1 and C-III and precocious coronary artery disease. N Engl J Med 306:1513–1519, 1982.

Schaefer EJ: Dietary and drug treatment. Ann Intern Med 98:623–640, 1983.

Specher DS, Schaefer EJ, Kent KM, et al: Cardiovascular features of homozygous familial hypercholesterolemia: Analysis of 16 patients. Am J Cardiol 54:20–30, 1984.

WHO cooperative trial on primary prevention of ischemic heart disease using clofibrate to lower serum cholesterol: Mortality followup. Report of the Committee of Principal Investigators. Lancet 2:379–385, 1980.

Zannis VI, Breslow JL: Characterization of a unique human apolipoprotein E variant associated with type III hyperlipoproteinemia. J Biol Chem 255:1759–1762, 1980.

Toxicology and Drug Monitoring

Chapter 64

Toxicology and Drug Monitoring

Thomas Spillman and Brian D. Andresen

Toxicology is the science of the adverse effects of chemicals on living organisms.[1] Toxicologists seek to describe how and why chemicals are toxic, ascertain overall risk of exposure, and provide information to aid in the implementation of regulations governing exposure limits. Forensic toxicologists consider medicolegal questions aimed at the characterization of all toxic agents and the determination of toxin levels and possible route of administration.

EMERGENCY TOXICOLOGY AND DRUG MONITORING

Drug analyses can provide the physician with immediate and valuable insight into planning emergency treatment for the toxic patient. Treatment of the unconscious or obtunded (dull or confused) patient with an unknown, inaccurate, or incomplete history requires differentiation among almost unlimited possibilities of toxic exposures and disease states. Even when the history or symptoms indicate the presence of a particular drug, the detection of other unsuspected substances may require special measurement techniques or may alter management of the patient.

The Comatose or Convulsing Patient

Emergency room guidelines are well established for the immediate treatment of the comatose or convulsing patient, addressing a critical condition if it exists, but introducing minimal risk if it does not.[2, 3] Specifically, glucose (for hypoglycemic coma), thiamine (for alcoholic or dietary chronic deficiency crisis), and naloxone (for opiate toxicity) are administered routinely. Respiratory support guidelines consist of intubation, maintenance of blood pressure with pressor drugs, control of seizures with anticonvulsants, and correction of acidosis by alkalinization with intravenous bicarbonate.

Minimizing Absorption of the Toxic Oral Drug Dose

Following initial stabilization of the patient, oral ingestion of a toxic drug may warrant emesis if the patient is awake. Emesis is accomplished by the administration of syrup of ipecac, the extract of the root of an alkaloid-containing South American plant, *Ipecacuanhae radix*. Alternatively, gastric lavage may be used if the patient is comatose or having seizures and is at risk of aspirating the gastric contents after emesis. Activated charcoal is often given orally after emesis to adsorb the remaining traces of the drug. Charcoal adsorption is effective for most drugs, both acidic and basic, but not for organic liquids such as alcohols. Once the lavage is completed, absorption of drug remaining in the intestinal tract is sometimes further decreased by administration of cathartics such as magnesium sulfate.

Identification of the Toxic Drug(s)

Identification of the toxin is required for selection of an appropriate antidote or a method to enhance its removal from the body. A broad, all-purpose drug screen, if immediately available, may provide identification of the toxic agent. Patient history, clinical symptoms upon admission to the hospital, and routine laboratory tests may narrow the possibilities if sophisticated analytical toxicology instrumentation is not available. Opiates, barbiturates, alcohol, methaqualone, and benzodiazepines, for example, tend to produce slowed respiration, hypotension, drowsiness, or coma. Stimulants such as amphetamines, theophylline, and cocaine produce agitation, convulsions, hypertension, and rapid respiration. Additional specific clinical characteristics may provide more specific information; for example, pinpoint pupils are often seen with opiate use.[3]

Once the toxin is identified, blood level monitoring may be useful in determining the need for special rescue procedures. Nomograms have been developed to predict the risk of delayed toxicity from specific blood levels of aspirin and acetaminophen at known periods after ingestion. The relationship of circulating levels to the known risk of immediate reaction is available in reference sources for other drugs with pronounced toxicities. Although a urine specimen is the medium of choice for detecting accumulated drugs and metabolites, drug quantitation is meaningful only when performed on blood. For drugs of habitual use, interpretation of blood levels is sometimes complicated by an individual's tolerance to the toxic agent. Behavioral tolerance to barbiturates, opiates, and alcohol is well known, although lethal thresholds do not increase appreciably in parallel with behavioral response. It should be noted that interpretation of blood levels requires knowledge of the state of absorption and distribution of the drug at the time of sampling.

Other Laboratory Analyses

A variety of sophisticated tools are available to the analytical toxicologist to identify and measure massive overdose amounts as well as ultratrace levels of drugs and metabolites in all body fluids and tissues.[4, 5] Antibody screening can identify a group of drugs during a routine drug screen. Thin-layer chromatography (TLC) in conjunction with specific color tests allows large numbers of samples to be analyzed simultaneously for different classes of drugs or toxins. New solid-phase extraction cartridges and solid-phase microextraction (SPME) fibers allow samples to be prepared easily within minutes for gas chromatography (GC), mass spectrometry (MS), and computer guided GC-MS. High-performance liquid chromatography (HPLC) can allow for quantitative analyses of drug and toxin levels during the recovery phase of treatment. Inductively coupled plasma MS (ICP/MS), flame photometric, and atomic absorption spectrometry procedures allow for rapid and highly reliable identification of inorganic toxic substances at parts-per-billion concentrations. Many analytical toxicology tests can be performed in less than 30 minutes.

Additional important clinical laboratory tests involved in a rapid assessment of the patient's condition are measurements of electrolytes and blood gases, which will reveal an anion gap and metabolic acidosis in the presence of several toxins, including ethanol, methanol, ethylene glycol, and salicylates. Alcohol toxicity generates an osmolal gap, which can also be measured easily.

Treatment to Reduce Drug Levels

The net result of the processes of absorption, distribution, and clearance of a drug is an increase and subsequent decline in circulating drug levels in a complex but reasonably predictable pattern. Levels first rise during absorption of the drug from the site of administration and its distribution into the circulation. Following this rise, blood levels decline as the drug begins to be partitioned into any tissue spaces in addition to the blood and then cleared from the blood by metabolism or excretion. During a simple excretion phase of decline, the circulating level decreases by half of the existing level during each fixed period, called the *circulating half-life*.

A steady-state level can be established if a second dose of the drug is administered before the first dose is completely eliminated from the body. The result is a new level, higher than that seen after the initial dose, because the new dose is superimposed on the old one. When the total level is higher, the absolute amount cleared during the same period is also greater. This sequence of increasing peak concentration followed by increasing rate of elimination continues until the two effects offset each other (after 5 to 6 cycles), and a steady state is reached in which peak and trough levels, respectively, are the same after each dose. Whenever this process achieves steady-state levels too slowly for the clinical need, a loading dose may be given intravenously, followed by smaller regular maintenance doses. The time required for a toxic drug level to subside to safety may be calculated from the known half-life, although the patient's hepatic and renal integrity, use of other drugs, and possible saturation of the normal pathways of drug clearance must be considered.

If life-threatening levels of toxic drugs are not cleared quickly enough for the clinical need by physiologic means, invasive measures may be useful. All such measures focus on the toxin existing largely in the blood rather than in other tissue compartments.

The simplest invasive procedure is *peritoneal dialysis,* in which volumes of dialysis fluid are introduced through an incision into the peritoneal cavity and left for 1 to 2 hours before draining.[6] *Hemodialysis* is a higher-risk procedure involving continuous-flow removal of blood from the body, incubation of the blood with dialysis fluid across a semipermeable membrane, and ultimate return of the blood to the body.[7] The procedure introduces a volume of fluid equal to the volume of the dialysis apparatus, which must be filled initially with fluid to prevent decrease of blood volume on initiation of treatment. Hemodialysis and also *hemoperfusion,* in which the blood flows through a column filled with charcoal or ion-exchange resin, require the patient to be treated with heparin to prevent coagulation of the blood in the apparatus, and both reduce platelet counts. *Plasmapheresis* is a similar process that separates the blood cells from the plasma and returns them to the body suspended in a buffered electrolyte solution.[8] Drugs located in the blood but bound to protein are not removed by dialysis, but may be removed by hemoperfusion owing to competition for binding by the charcoal or resin, and they will be removed efficiently by plasmapheresis or the more radical measure of exchange transfusion.

Examples of drugs for which overdose may justify invasive removal are digoxin, with cardiotoxic action and a long circulating half-life, and phenytoin, which can induce lethal seizures, particularly when its clearance by the liver has been oversaturated. Invasive measures may also be used for phenobarbital, salicylates, and theophylline. Even

if removed from the circulation by invasive measures, most drugs will rebound as the portion compartmentalization in the extracellular fluid, tissues, or membranes reequilibrates with the blood. Repeated cycles of treatment may be necessary to bring about a successful detoxification.

Few specific antidotes are available for treatment of toxic patients. Naloxone, a specific antagonist (blocker), is available for opiates; *N*-acetylcysteine can be given to reduce toxicity of acetaminophen overdose; deferoxamine chelates and promotes renal excretion of toxic levels of iron; and controlled ethanol administration competitively reduces the metabolism and subsequent toxicity of methanol and ethylene glycol.[9]

GENERAL PATHOPHYSIOLOGY OF DRUG ABSORPTION, DISTRIBUTION, AND CLEARANCE

Absorption

The absorption of a drug and its distribution through the tissues and body fluids are highly dependent on many factors (Fig. 64–1), including its physiochemical properties, protein binding or solubility in body fluids, metabolism, and diffusion through biologic membranes under prevailing local conditions. The distribution of the active form of the drug is also strongly influenced by the pH-dependent state of ionization, which often determines which route of administration, oral or parenteral, is the more effective with respect to drug absorption. The maximum biologic impact of drugs or toxins is most always seen as drugs pass cellular membranes in the un-ionized form. The passage of drugs through biologic membranes can also have a profound impact on the developing fetus.[10]

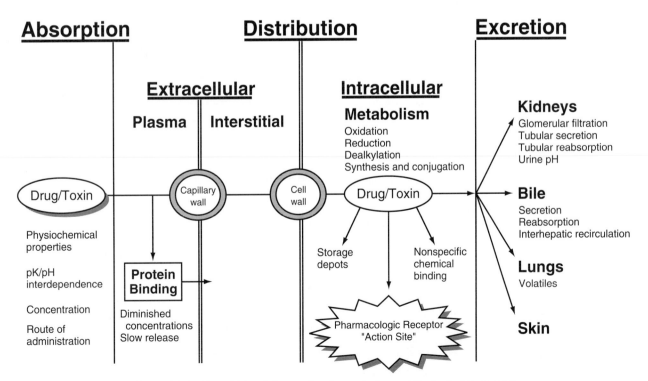

Figure 64–1. Many factors influence the drug or toxin reaching the target receptor.

The pK of a drug indicates the relationship between pH and the amount of ionization of the drug in an aqueous environment. Most important, when the pH equals the pK of the drug, half of a population of the drug molecules is ionized. At 1 pH unit on either side of the pK, the distribution of the ionized form is 1:9 or 9:1, and at 2 pH units from the pK, the ratio is 1:99 or 99:1. A basic drug with a pK of 4.3 would be more than 99% ionized in the stomach at a pH 1.0, but would be only 10% ionized in the duodenum at pH 5.3, and thus would be more rapidly absorbed as the drug is carried out of the stomach. Morphine, for example, exhibits a basic ionization with a pK (pKb) of 6.1, so that in the stomach it is more than 99% ionized in the acid environment, and in the duodenum somewhat less than 90% ionized; therefore, a delayed toxicity can be observed as an overdose of morphine leaves the stomach and is absorbed in the duodenum. The low pH and consequently inadequate gastrointestinal absorption for most drugs can be overcome by parenteral administration, either by intramuscular or by intravenous route.

Rapid hepatic metabolism of a drug is another process limiting the potency of orally administered drugs.[11] Because the blood flow from the intestinal tract passes through the liver before reaching the central venous system, drugs that are metabolized efficiently reach the peripheral circulation in reduced concentrations. An example is cocaine, which is extremely ineffective if taken by mouth owing to rapid first-pass liver metabolism as well as extensive hydrolysis in the blood before it reaches the brain. In contrast, smoking cocaine elicits a faster high, because the drug is carried directly to the brain with little or no delayed absorption or metabolism.

Distribution

Gastrointestinal absorption or direct introduction of a drug into the circulation is followed by distribution of the substance throughout the body. The pattern of distribution of a drug is determined by its chemical properties, and information is available regarding these patterns for each drug. Whereas some substances are highly water-soluble and are distributed through the vascular and extracellular spaces, others tend to accumulate in body lipids or bind to circulating protein, especially albumin. The protein-bound portion of a drug is a temporarily inactive reservoir, with only the unbound or free portion exerting biologic activity. For highly toxic drugs such as phenytoin, which may be more than 90% protein-bound, fluctuations in drug binding by protein as seen in uremia may profoundly alter the biologically active levels without changing total blood levels, so that determination of the amount of *free* or *unbound* drug in the blood is more diagnostic.

The *volume of distribution* is the apparent volume into which a drug is distributed, based on calculations from blood levels. If the drug is accumulated in tissues outside the blood, the appearance will be that of distribution into a large volume, sometimes larger than the entire body volume. When drugs undergo such distribution into theoretic compartments in the body other than the blood, clearance from the body will be slow.

Clearance

Clearance of drugs from the circulation usually occurs by metabolism in the liver, followed by excretion of metabolites in the urine, although some drugs are excreted without being metabolized extensively. Many chemical modifications occur in the hepatic microsomal system, including oxidation, hydroxylation, deamination, methylation, acetylation, and conjugation with glycine, sulfate, and glucuronic acid.[11] These reactions most often reduce the biologic activity and increase the solubility of the parent drug, although a few metabolites are known to be biologically active or toxic.

The capacity of these metabolic pathways is stimulated or *induced* by the presence of many substances on which they act, and it is usually adequate to process circulating levels of drugs at a constant percentage of the total each hour (first-order kinetics). Aspirin, theophylline, and phenytoin, however, are three important exceptions for which hepatic metabolic pathways become saturated at high concentration, resulting in a leveling-off of metabolism at a maximal rate, despite increasing blood levels.

In cases in which excretion of the parent drug in the urine is a significant pathway for elimination, enhancement of that process will improve the rate of patient recovery. Tubular reabsorption of a drug involves passage across biologic membranes and is blocked by ionization of the drug. For acidic drugs with pKs between 3.0 and 7.5, or for basic drugs with pKs between 7.5 and 10.5, appropriate adjustment of urine pH can enhance the ionization and excretion of drugs in the urine. Within these ranges, the pK is close enough to the typical urine pH that the drug is not already fully ionized but is still within the range in which attainable changes of urine pH will increase the degree of ionization.[7] Commonly encountered drugs for which ion trapping after the administration of either sodium bicarbonate or ammonium chloride effectively enhances elimination are amphetamines, imipramine, phencyclidine, and quinidine in acidic urine, and barbiturates and salicylates in alkaline urine.

MAJOR CLASSES OF SPECIFIC PHARMACOLOGICALLY ACTIVE AGENTS ASSAYED IN THE LABORATORY

Nonnarcotic Analgesics

Aspirin

Aspirin is the acetate ester of salicylic acid, the parent compound of the salicylates, a family of analgesic, antiinflammatory, and antipyretic compounds. Therapeutic levels of these drugs act primarily by inhibiting prostaglandin synthesis, which is directly involved in generation of inflammation, fever, and pain. Aspirin is the least toxic and most commonly used of the salicylates.[12] After oral ingestion, aspirin is absorbed from the stomach and small intestine, and levels peak in the blood in 2 hours. Metabolism occurs mainly in the liver, with excretion of the metabolites and a small amount of the unmetabolized drug in the urine.

The circulating half-life of aspirin is only 15 minutes, but two important mechanisms may prolong the action of the drug. First, salicylic acid, a major metabolite of aspirin, is also biologically active and has a longer circulating half-life (2 to 3 hours). Second, the enzyme pathways for liver metabolism of aspirin are easily saturable, and with increasing doses, the circulating lifetime of aspirin itself becomes much greater. Long-term aspirin use may lead to serious salicylate poisoning, particularly in children, by gradually overburdening the metabolic capacity of the liver. Symptoms of aspirin toxicity are nausea, vomiting, tinnitus, hyperpnea, coma, and convulsions. Direct stimulation of the central nervous system (CNS) causes hyperventilation and respiratory alkalosis. Uncoupling of oxidative phosphorylation causes a compensatory increase in glycolysis, which may lead to hypoglycemia and greater production of lactic and pyruvic acids. Direct inhibition of Krebs' cycle enzymes by salicylate prevents normal metabolism of these acids and can lead to severe metabolic acidosis, requiring clinical intervention.[13]

When acute aspirin poisoning is suspected, a rapid semi-quantitative test for aspirin may be performed in the laboratory. Ferric nitrate reacts with salicylic acid to generate a deep red complex. Solvent extraction and TLC analysis generate fluorescent spots in an ammonia-filled atmosphere. If aspirin toxicity is confirmed, standard measures are taken to minimize uptake of the drug remaining in the gastrointestinal tract, followed by 6 hours of observation and medical support. Quantitative salicylate measurements utilizing HPLC in serum can then be performed for prediction of the ultimate severity of the poisoning. The nomogram constructed by Done[13] (Fig. 64–2) predicts the ultimate toxicity on the basis of circulating levels at a specific time after salicylate ingestion.

Acetaminophen

Acetaminophen (Tylenol) is an *N*-acetylated para-aminophenol with analgesic and antipyretic action similar to that of the salicylates, although its anti-inflammatory activity is minor. The drug is absorbed from the gastrointestinal tract more rapidly than aspirin, and peak blood levels occur within 1 hour. Elimination occurs by hepatic metabolism to a number of conjugates and hydroxylated forms, and the serum half-life is 1 to 4 hours.

As with aspirin, laboratory analysis is typically performed only for suspected acute toxic overdose. The initial symptoms of acetaminophen toxicity are nonspecific, consisting of nausea, vomiting, and sweating. Following this initial toxic phase, the symptoms resolve; however, potentially fatal liver injury may have already occurred. The hepatotoxicity results from accumulation of a highly toxic metabolite of acetaminophen, para-aminoquinone, that binds with liver proteins. In low concentration, this toxic acetaminophen metabolite is normally inactivated by liver stores of glutathione. In overdose, the metabolite may deplete glutathione reserves and injure the liver. As with testing for aspirin, a rapid spot test, which generates a colored product with α-naphthol and sodium nitrite, may be performed to confirm the presence of acetaminophen.

The chemical reducing potential in the body may be reestablished by administration of *N*-acetylcysteine within the first 16 hours after ingestion of a toxic overdose of acetaminophen and at 4-hour intervals for 3 days. As with the Done[13] nomogram for salicylates, the Rumack nomogram for acetaminophen toxicity (Fig. 64–3) predicts hepatotoxicity and indicates the need for *N*-acetylcysteine therapy and hospitalization on the basis of serum levels determined 4 hours or more after ingestion.[14] Serum bilirubin and enzyme level measurements will reflect hepatotoxicity. Typically, aspartate aminotransferase (AST) levels peak 72 hours after ingestion.[15]

Opiates (Narcotics)

Opiates are drugs and analogues of drugs obtained from the opium poppy. The major natural opiates are morphine and codeine. Heroin is a synthetic, acetylated derivative of morphine that is about 3 times more potent owing to increased lipid solubility and ease of passage into the CNS. Other important synthetic opiate-like drugs are meperidine (Demerol), methadone, and the opiate blocker naloxone (Narcan). The major clinical uses of the opiates are for pain relief, cough suppression, and diarrhea control.[16] They act on the CNS to suppress pain impulses and the cough stimulatory mechanism, and to induce hypertonic contrac-

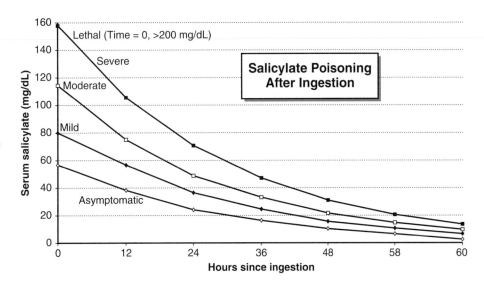

Figure 64–2. Salicylate poisoning after ingestion.

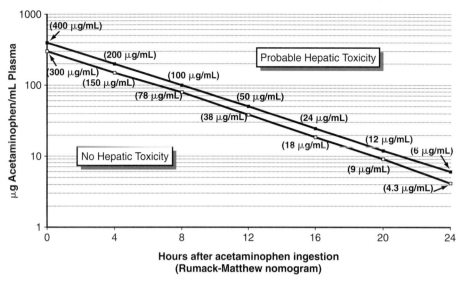

Figure 64–3. Rumack-Matthew nomogram.

tion of the intestinal walls and reduce peristalsis. With the exception of methadone, the uptake of opiates in the gastrointestinal tract is slow, incomplete, and variable, so that for analgesia or recreational use, they are commonly smoked or administered by injection. Opiates can be vaporized by heat, so smoking provides an efficient route of administration that rapidly produces high circulating levels of the drugs.

The opiates are cleared mainly by hepatic metabolism and renal excretion of the metabolites, largely as the glucuronides, with a duration of action of 4 to 5 hours. Opiate overdose leads to potentially lethal respiratory depression. Miosis (contraction of the pupils) is usually noted after opiate use, a reaction sometimes useful in recognizing opiate intoxication, although respiratory depression itself may cause dilation of the pupils.[17] Regular use of opiates leads to tolerance, which is due both to induction of liver microsomal enzyme levels and to decreased response of the CNS to the drug.

The withdrawal syndrome following opiate addiction is a clinically important state in itself. Symptoms include elevation of heart rate and blood pressure, sweating, severe aching, diarrhea, anxiety, respiratory stimulation, vomiting, fever, and chills. A spectrum of withdrawal symptoms develops within 8 to 12 hours after circulating blood levels of morphine diminish and requires several days for resolution.

Opiates are often detected with a urine screen to identify the source of a toxic overdose. In acute toxicity with respiratory depression, the inactive synthetic analogue of the opiates, naloxone (Narcan), may be administered to block the opiate receptor. Naloxone is capable of inducing rapid and severe opiate withdrawal symptoms in the addict. To lessen these withdrawal symptoms, a second opiate, methadone, may be required. Methadone itself is capable of producing physical addiction, respiratory depression at toxic doses, and withdrawal symptoms when discontinued, although these effects are milder than those for morphine.[18]

In long-term drug rehabilitation programs, methadone is substituted for other recreational opiates to provide a transitional substance from which later withdrawal will be more easily accomplished. In these programs, the labora-

tory may be used to verify the presence of urinary methadone and its major metabolite to ensure compliance. The metabolite will not be present if the methadone tablet was dissolved directly in the urine specimen.

Behavioral Depressants

The sedative-hypnotics, most notably the barbiturates, alcohol, methaqualone, glutethimide, and methyprylon, depress the CNS, an effect that differs according to the dosage. At low doses, these agents depress anxiety and inhibition and generate a euphoria, giving the impression of CNS stimulation. As the dosage is increased, however, they progressively produce sedation, hypnosis (sleep), general anesthesia, coma, and death from respiratory depression.[19]

Barbiturates

Barbiturates are the derivatives of barbituric acid. They are used mainly as sedatives or hypnotics, although the sleep they produce is an abnormal state in which rapid-eye-movement (REM) sleep is reduced. In contrast to the opiates, the barbiturates produce sedation without relief of pain. Certain rapidly cleared barbiturate derivatives are also used as anesthetics, and phenobarbital is used as an anticonvulsant at subsedative concentrations. Recreational use of the barbiturates is mainly directed at the low-dose euphoria.[20]

Barbiturates are acidic, highly lipophilic, and easily absorbed from the gastrointestinal tract, so that unlike with opiates, their oral administration is effective and common. The barbiturates are rapidly distributed to the brain and cross the blood-brain barrier easily. As the drug equilibrates with more remote body lipids, however, it is shifted rapidly out of the brain. The nature of side-chain lipid characteristics determines the distribution and action of the barbiturates, which are classified as ultrashort-acting (thiopental), short-acting (secobarbital, pentobarbital), intermediate-acting (amobarbital), or long-acting (phenobarbital). Clearance of barbiturates from the blood occurs through metabolism by microsomal liver enzymes, production of which is increased by barbiturate exposure.

Barbiturate toxicity includes loss of judgment and significantly reduced motor coordination, followed by respiratory failure at high doses. The depressant effects of alcohol are additive to the barbiturates, and toxicity may occur with amounts of the two combined that would not be toxic for either if taken alone. As with opiate tolerance, barbiturate tolerance develops with consistent use, and increasing dosages are required to attain constant effects.

Serious physical dependence, characteristic of chronic depressant abuse, also develops. Withdrawal symptoms develop over about a day and, like those for the opiates, run their course in several days to a week. Barbiturate withdrawal produces hypotension, weakness, tremors, and, in extreme cases, convulsions. A state of delirium may develop, leading to exhaustion, cardiovascular collapse, and death.[14] This state and the similar state seen with alcohol withdrawal are often treated with the benzodiazepines, such as chlordiazepoxide (Librium) and diazepam (Valium).

Laboratory analysis of the barbiturates is generally aimed at either the detection of barbiturates in suspected abuse or addiction or in quantitation of levels of phenobarbital when it is used as an anticonvulsant. GC-MS analysis of serum extracts can provide accurate quantitative data of both the parent drug and metabolites in serum. Currently, no specific antidote or blocker, analogous to naloxone for the opiates, is available for the barbiturates.

Alcohol

The mechanism of action of ethanol on the CNS is not known, although nonphysiologic concentrations have been shown to inhibit ion pumps responsible for generation of electrical nerve impulses. Ethanol, as well as methanol and ethylene glycol, the other alcohols that are often ingested, is readily absorbed from the stomach and the small intestine owing to its small molecular dimensions and lipid solubility. Although alcohols other than ethanol possibly have direct CNS effects, their toxicities are predominantly due to their metabolic products.[21]

Withdrawal from ethanol addiction is a potentially fatal state similar to that of barbiturate withdrawal, although seizures are somewhat less common. The patient experiences agitation, increasing for 1 to 2 days to a state known as delirium tremens (the DTs). The agitation may be counteracted by phenothiazines, particularly chlorpromazine (Thorazine), but reversal of the syndrome is better accomplished with benzodiazepines, especially chlordiazepoxide.[14]

Metabolism of ethanol is mostly by oxidation in the liver to acetyl coenzyme A (CoA), which is normally oxidized to carbon dioxide and water. The first two metabolic reactions for ethanol, however, consume the enzyme cofactor nicotinamide adenine dinucleotide (NAD). The eventual shortage of NAD blocks aerobic metabolism and limits the progression of metabolism of carbohydrates and amino acids to the final product of glycolysis, lactic acid. Lactic acid accumulates in the blood, creating metabolic acidosis. Methanol and ethylene glycol both share the metabolic pathway of ethanol and also induce anion-gap metabolic acidosis, although the actual metabolic products of these alcohols are different.[22] These metabolites are considerably more toxic than the alcohols themselves. For this reason, ethanol may be given therapeutically to compete for the metabolic processes of the liver and allow the usually minor pathways of renal or respiratory clearance to remove these alcohols instead.

Whereas metabolic acidosis has many nontoxicologic causes, the existence of an osmolal gap specifically indicates large amounts of non-ionized substances such as alcohol in the blood. The *osmolal gap* is the difference in the measured and calculated serum osmolalities. Serum osmolality is measured by determination of its freezing point. Normally, the osmolality value obtained by this process corresponds to that calculated from the serum sodium, glucose, and blood urea nitrogen (BUN) concentrations (the major contributors to the ionic content or osmolality of the serum) by means of the following formula:

$$\text{Osmolality} = 2 \times [\text{Na}] + \frac{[\text{Glucose}]}{18} + \frac{[\text{BUN}]}{2.8}$$

When any of the alcohols is present in intoxicating concentrations, this calculated result is different from the measured value. For example, for each 10 mg/dL (2.17 mmol/L) of ethanol, the osmolal gap increases by 2.2 mOsm/kg.[23] When direct assays of alcohols are not available, this approximation is useful, although it does not identify the non-ionized substance specifically. However, all alcohols are easily analyzed by gas chromatography, and complex mixtures of solvents and alcohols can be characterized easily by GC-MS analysis when there is a need for an exact identification of the toxic substances.

Methaqualone

A nonbarbiturate sedative-hypnotic, methaqualone (Quaalude) is popularly abused for a barbiturate-like euphoria with less drowsiness. Administered orally, the drug is completely absorbed in 2 hours. Clearance is by hepatic metabolism, with excretion of most metabolites in the urine and a minor portion in the bile. Toxic effects include delirium, convulsions, and coma, with cardiovascular and respiratory depression only slightly less severe than those caused by the barbiturates.[24] The effects are additive with those of the barbiturates and alcohol. Methaqualone detection in screening is used to confirm the source of toxicity. The parent drug can easily be detected by antibody screen, thin-layer chromatography and color spot test, and by GC-MS.

Psychedelic Anesthetics/Sedatives

Phencyclidine

Phencyclidine (PCP) was developed as an anesthetic, but its clinical use was discontinued as a result of its hallucinogenic properties. These properties and PCP's low cost have in turn popularized its illicit use. PCP creates an unresponsive state characterized by a blank stare, in which the subject can communicate and appears to be awake but is detached and unresponsive to pain. PCP may be injected, smoked, inhaled, or ingested and is often taken inadvertently with other drugs that have been diluted with inactive fillers, to which it has been added to create the impression of potency. PCP is easily detected in the urine for identification of the cause of drug-induced delirium. PCP is also hydroxylated in the liver before excretion of the metabolites in the urine. The parent drug can be easily detected by urine subsequent to solvent extraction and TLC screening (with iodoplantinate over spray). Hydroxylated PCP metabolites are also easily detected by GC-MS in both the serum and urine.

Toxic reaction to PCP consists mainly of several hours of aberrant behavior in which the most common cause of death is violent or delusional acts.[25] Myoglobinuria may also be pronounced in the overdose victim, owing to intense muscle contractions, even in the absence of seizures. This is important, because acidification of the urine is often used to enhance PCP excretion by ion-trapping and may cause serious renal damage by precipitating the myoglobin.[26] Diazepam and chlorpromazine are often used to treat the PCP-induced elevated state of agitation.

Cannabinoids (Marijuana)

The psychoactive agent in the marijuana plant is Δ-9-tetrahydrocannabinol (THC), which may be smoked or ingested directly or used as a concentrated extract called *hashish.* This primarily recreational drug is a mild sedative-hypnotic at low levels, at which anxiety and inhibitions are relieved. Higher doses, however, result not in coma or death but rather in hallucinogenic effects.[27] The role of the laboratory in its detection is generally for evaluation of behavioral influences. The parent drug can be screened with antibody tests and easily quantitated in urine utilizing GC-MS analysis. Metabolism of THC occurs primarily in the liver, after which the metabolites are excreted in the urine and in the feces, over a period of a several days. Because of apparent distribution of small amounts of the parent drug or its lipophilic metabolites into body tissues, low levels of the urinary metabolites have been reported for weeks after cessation of heavy marijuana use by chronic abusers.[28]

Antianxiety Drugs (Minor Tranquilizers)

Benzodiazepines constitute a family of commonly used sedatives with effects similar to those of the barbiturates and alcohol. Three of the most common are chlordiazepoxide (Librium), diazepam (Valium), and oxazepam (Serax). The ability of the benzodiazepines to suppress anxiety is much stronger than their induction of sleep, and they depress respiration much less than the barbiturates.[29] Although they are commonly used in suicide attempts, overdose with benzodiazepines alone is rarely fatal. The effects are additive with alcohol and barbiturates, and such combinations in overdose may be lethal.

Absorption of benzodiazepines is slow at the acid pH of the stomach and occurs mainly in the small intestine, with maximum blood levels occurring 8 to 24 hours after ingestion. This slow absorption may cause quantitation to lead to underestimation of the actual dose if obtained too soon after a toxic ingestion. In addition to contributing to benzodiazepine-induced CNS depression, ethanol increases the rate of benzodiazepine absorption. Clearance of the

benzodiazepines from the blood takes place by oxidation and conjugation in the liver, followed by renal excretion. This metabolism occurs in a nonsaturable mode, so that unlike with aspirin or phenytoin, even massive overdoses of benzodiazepines are cleared rapidly by natural processes.

Toxicity may manifest as minor respiratory depression, hypotension, and coma. Hemoperfusion is rarely useful in the comatose patient, unless there is suspicion of concomitant barbiturate ingestion. A benzodiazepine receptor antagonist, flumazenil, is now available as an antidote.

Anticonvulsant/Antiepileptic Drugs

Anticonvulsant/antiepileptic drugs reduce seizure activity in a wide range of epileptic disorders, although each is most effective with a certain type of seizure.[29] The major drugs for treatment of seizure disorders have some limited structural similarity. Phenytoin (Dilantin), primidone (Mysoline), phenobarbital, ethosuximide (Zarontin), and carbamazepine (Tegretol) reflect structural similarity, whereas valproate sodium (Depakene) does not.

Phenytoin, primidone, phenobarbital, and carbamazepine are all effective to variable degrees in both simple and complex partial as well as general tonic-clonic seizures, and are used individually or in combination.[29] These drugs are much less effective in the absence of myoclonic types of general seizures, for which ethosuximide and valproic acid are selectively effective and most often used.

With the exception of acute seizure emergency (status epilepticus) and neonatal seizure control, the antipeleptics are generally administered as oral preparations. Peaks of circulating drug typically occur 1 to 8 hours after oral administration, with phenobarbital and phenytoin being absorbed more slowly and peaking as late as 18 to 24 hours after ingestion. Dosage intervals are typically 8 hours for drugs in this group, circulating half-lives of which range from 20 to 40 hours. Exceptions are phenobarbital, with a longer half-life of 4 days, and valproic acid, with a shorter half-life of 8 to 15 hours that requires slightly shorter dosing intervals.

Clearance of these drugs is mainly by hepatic metabolism. The metabolic pathway for phenytoin is particularly sensitive to saturation at high levels, and intestinal reabsorption (enterohepatic recirculation) of the binary excretion products slows its excretion. A third of carbamazepine excretion takes place directly into the stool without hepatic metabolism, and half of phenobarbital and a third of ethosuximide are excreted in the urine without metabolism. Otherwise, clearance of hepatic metabolites in the urine is the final mechanism of disposition.

Antipsychotic/Neuroleptic Drugs (Major Tranquilizers)

Psychosis refers to a mental state of dissociation from reality and lack of the ability to communicate with one's surroundings, as contrasted with simple feelings of anxiety, tension, depression, or frustration. The sedatives or minor tranquilizers previously discussed are used to treat these latter conditions, whereas the antipsychotics or neuroleptics are used to manage psychotic behavior.

Phenothiazines

Phenothiazines are the largest group of antipsychotic drugs, including chlorpromazine (Thorazine), fluphenazine (Prolixin), and promethazine (Phenergan). The mechanism of action of this group is thought to be blockage of dopamine receptors in the brain.[30] The phenothiazines are usually administered orally and absorbed slowly. The drugs are metabolized by the liver, and the metabolites excreted in the urine. Clearance of these drugs is among the slowest of any group, with metabolites reported in the urine a year after discontinuation of the drug. Side effects, in addition to sexual dysfunction, include muscular tremor and twitching, increased heart rate, dry mouth, blurred vision, constipation, and hepatotoxicity.

These side effects may discourage patient compliance with therapy, so monitoring of serum drug levels serves both to adjust the dose and to verify compliance. Overdose of phenothiazines is also common, owing to their use in a patient population with a high tendency for suicide attempts. Urine screening for metabolites may be useful in identification in toxic overdose. TLC analysis of solvent extracts of urine samples often generate highly colored TLC bands following heating, which reflect the many metabolites generated from the phenothiazines. The usual expression of phenothiazine overdose is a state of lethargy or sedation compounded by episodes of restlessness, tremors, or spasms. Coma is encountered mostly in accidental overdose in children.

Haloperidol

A butyrophenone, haloperidol (Haldol) is structurally different from the phenothioazines but pharmacologically similar.[30] Haloperidol differs in being less hepatotoxic but more apt to cause involuntary muscle tremors. It is metabolized more rapidly than the phenothiazines. Determination of serum levels of the drug serves the same purpose as for the phenothiazines.

Clinical Antidepressants (Tricyclics and Lithium)

Tricyclic Antidepressants

The major tricyclic antidepressants are amitriptyline (Elavil), nortriptyline (Pamelor), imipramine (Tofranil), desipramine (Norpramin), doxepin (Sinequan), and protriptyline (Vivactyl). These drugs are used in the control of depression, both for autonomous forms, in which no specific external events trigger the state, and for conditions such as terminal illness.[31] Standard oral doses are increased in slow stepwise fashion, guided by blood levels and observed clinical response, which is maximal after a delay of 2 to 3 weeks. Oral administration is used for convenience, although extensive first-pass clearance by the liver impairs absorption from the intestine into the peripheral circulation. Peak levels are obtained in 4 to 8 hours. Side effects include dry mouth, urinary retention, blurred vision, hypotension, and constipation (anticholinergic action). At toxic levels, confusion, agitation, irritability, difficulty in speaking, respiratory depression, coma, convulsions, and cardiac arrhythmias can occur. Physostigmine is used for reversal of the anticholinergic effects.

Lithium

The mechanism of action of lithium salts in stabilizing mood is unknown. There is no known role of lithium in normal physiology, and therapeutic levels of the substance do not alter the mood of the normal individual.[32] Its close chemical relationship to potassium and sodium ions has led to experimentation, suggesting a possible influence on membrane polarization in neurologic transmission. Lithium carbonate is administered orally for the treatment of mood disorders, particularly manic-depressive states.

The salt is readily absorbed from the gastrointestinal tract, with peak blood levels occurring in 2 to 4 hours. One-third to two-thirds of the dose is excreted in the urine in the first 6 to 12 hours, after which excretion continues slowly for 10 to 14 days. Toxicity in overdose consists of nausea and vomiting, ataxia, seizures, coma, and cardiac arrhythmias. Renal clearance of lithium is reduced by sodium depletion. A reuptake and increase in lithium levels may quickly create toxicity; therefore, regular monitoring of blood levels is important in maintaining the drug in the therapeutic range. The concentration of lithium in plasma, urine, or other body fluids can be determined with either flame emissions photometry or atomic absorption spectrometry.

Behavioral Stimulants

Behavioral stimulants act on the nervous system to alter chemical transmission of nerve impulses in complex and only partially understood ways. For some drugs, such as cocaine, the best-understood influences are secondary to the main purpose of the drug. The distinction among the types of chemical nerve transmitters involved is important to understanding what is known about the actions of these drugs.

Transmission of nerve impulses at adrenergic synapses between nerve cells is generally accomplished by the release of either catecholamines (epinephrine, norepinephrine) or acetylcholine.[33] After release, catecholamines are reabsorbed by the transmitting nerve cell, to return the synapse to the resting state. Because large amounts of catecholamines are produced by the adrenals, epinephrine is also known as *adrenaline*, and these catecholamine-reactive nerve endings are known as *adrenergic synapses*. The skeletal muscle (somatic) system and part of the visceral (autonomic) nervous system are equipped with nerves using acetylcholine rather than norepinephrine as neurotransmitters. That portion of the autonomic nervous system using only acetylcholine is known as the *parasympathetic* system, whereas the other portion, which uses catecholamine transmission, is the *sympathetic* nervous system. Drugs stimulating catecholamine synapses or mimicking the action of norepinephrine are thus known as *sympathomimetic amines*. The effects of stimulation of norepinephrine synapses include general vasoconstriction, higher heart rate, sweating, raised body temperature, increased mental activity, dilation of the pupils, and reduced intestinal peristalsis.

Amphetamines/Sympathomimetic Amines

Amphetamines/sympathomimetic amines constitute a family of analogues of norepinephrine, of which the prototype drug of abuse is amphetamine. Amphetamine is thought both to stimulate the release of norepinephrine into the adrenergic synapse and to have a direct effect on the postsynaptic receptor.[34] The effect of amphetamine is to stimulate a physiologic response like that to norepinephrine, and it has found clinical applications in the treatment of absence seizures and hyperactivity in children. An amphetamine analogue, methylphenidate (Ritalin), has also been used in hyperactivity, although its mode of action is not understood. The widest uses of sympathomimetic amines are as weight control drugs, decongestants (due to their vasoconstrictive properties), inducers of wakefulness and alertness, and euphoriants.

Sympathomimetic amines are taken orally to obtain the moderate-dose stimulatory effects, which in addition to increased alertness, energy, and sense of well-being include undesired side effects such as sweating, dry mouth, increased blood pressure, and increased respiration. Intravenous use induces an intensely pleasurable sensation or "rush" that in high concentrations is associated with a manic paranoia. The high lipid solubility of the sympathomimetic amines promotes their ready absorption across nasal, lung, and gastrointestinal membranes. Blood levels peak within 3 hours of oral ingestion, and the half-life in the blood is 7 to 34 hours. Hepatic metabolism consists of hydroxylation, dealkylation, deamination, and oxidation, before excretion of these metabolites into the urine.

Acute toxicity is associated with nausea, vomiting, headache, palpitations, confusion, dizziness, and even seizures and coma. Pupils are dilated but reactive. Hypertension and ventricular tachyarrhythmias are of particular concern, because cerebral vascular and cardiac events are often responsible for death in amphetamine toxicity.

Cocaine

A naturally occurring alkaloid from the South American plant *Erythroxylon coca*, cocaine has limited medical application but widespread social use.[35] Cocaine exerts many of the same effects as sympathomimetic amines, not by acting directly on the norepinephrine receptor, but by inhibiting the uptake of norepinephrine from the synapse once it is secreted. The accumulation of norepinephrine leads to sympathetic stimulation. This effect is responsible for the increased heart rate and blood pressure experienced with cocaine use.

The euphoria created by cocaine, however, is a result not of the sympathetic stimulation but rather of the interaction with dopamine receptors in the brain. Additionally, cocaine acts as a local anesthetic at the area of membrane absorption, leading to its medical application as a local anesthetic for ophthalmologic procedures. Rapid hydrolysis in the blood and liver minimizes the effect of orally administered cocaine. The highly hydrophobic nature of the drug promotes its passage across membranes in the oral, nasal, and bronchial passages, thus enabling it to gain access to a shorter circulatory pathway to the brain. The hydrochloride salt is often snorted, and the non-ionized or free-base form, also known as "crack," is vaporized by smoking

and absorbed directly through the lungs. Although the vasoconstrictive activity of cocaine progressively reduces absorption through the nasal passages, sympathetic stimulation actually opens bronchial passages for better absorption and passage to the brain.

Cocaine toxicity proceeds through a biphasic process of increasing CNS stimulation followed by CNS depression. Symptoms similar to those of amphetamine toxicity, including nausea, vomiting, and seizures with increased blood pressure and respiration rate, later give way to paralysis, respiratory failure, circulatory failure, and loss of vital functions. Cocaine is eliminated rapidly, having a short half-life of 75 minutes, and the pleasurable effects last for a shorter time. Cocaine is metabolized rapidly in the blood by pseudocholinesterase and liver enzymes before being excreted in the urine. The parent drug is excreted only when high levels are present. Laboratory testing consists of detection of the cocaine or metabolites, particularly benzoylecgonine, in the urine to monitor cocaine use or to confirm the etiology of a toxic crisis. The metabolites are easily detected with antibody screening reagents or solvent extraction of the urine and TLC analysis.

Cardiac Drugs

Neurologic stimulation of the heartbeat occurs by means of nerve impulses, the timing of which is normally controlled by the design and arrangement of the conduction pathways.[36] The sinoatrial (S-A) node at the junction of the venous sinus and the atrium transmits a natural rhythmic pulse throughout the atrial walls. A second nerve bundle at the junction of the atria and ventricles, the A-V node, passes the impulse to the ventricles. At the A-V node, the impulse is delayed to allow the ventricles to fill before the impulse is finally transmitted throughout the ventricles, leading to an abrupt contraction and ejection of the blood out of the heart.

Much of the heart is subject to self-excitation and is capable of initiating uncoordinated heartbeats. The S-A node normally controls the heartbeat because it discharges more frequently than the rest of the pathway, and each impulse from the S-A node depolarizes the nerves, overriding their tendencies to self-excitation. An abnormal site of impulse initiation may develop owing to increased excitability of the heart, which can result from local lack of blood flow (ischemia), lack of sleep, anxiety, or overuse of stimulants such as caffeine.

Quenching of the excitation of each heartbeat once it has been completed is accomplished by the existence of a refractory period, in which the nerves cannot be stimulated. All nerves are stimulated during the contraction and then enter the refractory period at once, so that the nerve impulse dies. If the refractory period is shortened, as in response to an increase of epinephrine, some pathways may recover their excitability before the previous impulse has been terminated, and a continuous cycle of contraction may begin to move around the heart (circus movements), resulting in flutter or fibrillation in which the heart no longer functions as a pump.

Flutter or fibrillation in the atria is much less serious than that in the ventricles, because the movement of the blood is primarily driven by the ventricular beats. Despite atrial fibrillation, transmission of impulses from the atria to the ventricles is still controlled by the A-V node, which causes stimulation to pass to the ventricles only periodically and along the proper pathways. Ventricular fibrillation, in contrast, causes immediate cessation of blood flow throughout the body. Once initiated, flutter or fibrillation may be terminated by application of an intense electric current through the heart to cause all the nerves to become refractory at once. Otherwise, within 60 to 90 seconds, the heart muscle itself is so weak from lack of perfusion that correction of the nerve impulse pattern alone can no longer reinitiate the heartbeat. Cardiac massage in conjunction with recoordination of nerve impulses is required for resuscitation.

Antiarrhythmic Drugs

Quinidine, procainamide/N-acetyl procainamide, and *disopyramide* act to slow the high-velocity conduction rates and prolong the refractory period of the high-velocity pathways throughout the heart, ensuring the complete termination of each impulse.[37] These agents are favored for use in atrial flutter, fibrillation, and tachycardia. The drugs are cardiotoxic in overdose, resulting in depression of nodular conduction. They are absorbed rapidly from the gastrointestinal tract, with peak blood levels occurring at 1 to 2 hours after administration. Clearance is by hepatic metabolism and renal clearance, with half-lives of 3 to 6 hours. Laboratory monitoring is used to adjust the dosage to maintain therapeutic levels. One major metabolite of procainamide, *N*-acetyl procainamide, is biologically active and requires quantitation in procainamide therapy.

Lidocaine and *phenytoin (Dilantin)* both reduce abnormal initiation of nerve impulses, particularly in the ventricles, and depress high-velocity conduction, altering the kinetics of nerve fiber voltage development.[37] First-pass inactivation by the liver renders oral administration of lidocaine ineffective. When administered intravenously, lidocaine is cleared by the liver, with a half-life of 1 to 2 hours. Lidocaine overdose results in convulsions, coma, and respiratory arrest. Phenytoin, an established anticonvulsant, has similar electrophysiologic actions and is particularly useful in counteracting digoxin toxicity.

β-BLOCKERS

Propranolol and other β-adrenergic blockers specifically counteract the increased excitability and spontaneous discharges promoted by epinephrine (adrenaline), and act to slow conduction and prolong the refractory period at the A-V node.[34] Clearance is hepatic, with a circulating half-life of 3 to 6 hours. Toxicity may include A-V node block and circulatory collapse.

DIGITALIS FAMILY

The *digitalis* family of drugs, including digoxin, digitoxin, and ouabain, slows the heart rate by influencing vagal nerve activity, slowing conduction and prolonging the refractory period of the A-V node.[37] These drugs are particularly useful for ventricular control in atrial tachyarrhythmias. Whereas the majority of digoxin and ouabain is excreted by the kidneys, digitoxin is eliminated nearly entirely by hepatic metabolism. The circulating half-lives of these drugs are long—2 to 5 days. A narrow therapeutic index requires periodic monitoring of blood levels. Toxic effects are premature ventricular beats, ventricular tachycardia, and even ventricular fibrillation, which may be counteracted by lidocaine and phenytoin. Accidental overdose occurs most often with children, and the long half-life of the digitalis family requires aggressive intervention. Digoxin-specific antibody treatments that bind and inactivate the circulating drug are available but are very expensive. Charcoal hemoperfusion is also effective.

Antibiotics

Aminoglycosides

The aminoglycoside antibiotics, which include gentamicin, tobramycin, amikacin, kanamycin, streptomycin, and neomycin, exert their biologic activity by binding directly to the ribosomes of gram-negative bacteria and inhibiting protein synthesis.[38] Their highly polar nature limits passage across biologic membranes, and absorption from the gastrointestinal tract is minimal. Administration is parenteral, either intramuscular or intravenous, with peak blood levels occurring in 30 to 90 minutes. Clearance is almost totally renal, with a half-life of 2 to 3 hours, and 50% to 60% of the dose is excreted in 24 hours. Toxicity consists of permanent ototoxicity (loss of hearing) and reversible nephrotoxicity, primarily acute tubular necrosis, due to high concentrations of the drug in the urine. Clearance of the drugs varies 10-fold with renal status, so that regular monitoring of drug levels is important in limiting the incidence and severity of renal damage.

Vancomycin

Vancomycin is a complex glycopeptide not structurally related to the aminoglycosides but similar in many respects. The drug is active mainly against gram-positive bacteria and acts by inhibiting cell wall synthesis.[39] Like the aminoglycosides, vancomycin is poorly absorbed from the gastrointestinal tract and is therefore administered intravenously. Excretion is mainly renal, with ototoxicity and nephrotoxicity similar to and additive to that of the aminoglycosides. Therapeutic drug monitoring serves to minimize renal damage.

Chloramphenicol

Chloramphenicol is a bacteriostatic agent that inhibits growth of a fairly broad spectrum of organisms, including many strains of gram-negative bacteria and all anaerobic species.[40] The drug is lipophilic and readily crosses biologic membranes, including the blood-brain barrier, but is only slightly soluble in water. Oral absorption is consequently rapid, with peak concentrations 1 to 2 hours after dosing. The limited solubility of chloramphenicol causes it to be 50% bound to blood proteins. Intravenous administration is in the form of an inactive but highly water-soluble succinate ester, which is hydrolyzed to the active drug. Metabolism occurs mainly by glucuronidation in the liver, followed by renal excretion of the glucuronide, with a half-life in the normal adult of 1.5 to 3.5 hours.

Chloramphenicol has induced aplastic anemia in rare

cases of long-term use, although this phenomenon is not related to dose. More importantly, potentially fatal acute toxicity can develop in overdose or accumulation because of inadequate hepatic metabolism, a particular risk with neonates (gray baby syndrome).[41] In humans, the drug inactivates the bacterial-like mitochondrial ribosomes and causes circulatory collapse. Circulating levels require frequent monitoring to avoid accumulation.

Other Drugs and Toxins

Theophylline

Theophylline is a xanthine, chemically related to caffeine and theobromine, which are consumed in large amounts in coffee, tea, and chocolate. The xanthines stimulate respiration, heart rate, and, to some extent, mental alertness, while relaxing certain smooth muscle and systemic blood vessels. Theophylline has found clinical application in stimulating respiration in apnea of the newborn and relaxation of the bronchi in chronic asthma.[42] Absorption after oral dosage is rapid, with maximal blood levels attained within 2 hours. Elimination is primarily by hepatic metabolism, followed by urinary excretion of the metabolites. The circulating half-life in children is 3.5 hours, and in adults, 8 to 9 hours. Toxic reaction consists of headache, palpitation, dizziness, nausea, hypotension, tachycardia, and seizures. Clearance of theophylline, like that of salicylates and phenytoin, is saturable at high circulating levels and, because of the drug's toxicity, may require hemoperfusion while seizure control is exerted with diazepam. Quantitation of blood levels in the laboratory is useful in adjusting dosage and evaluating suspected or documented toxicity.

Organophosphorous Compounds

Organophosphorous compounds are used widely as insecticides, including home aerosol products. They are also a highly toxic class of chemical warfare agents and have been used in the treatment of glaucoma, myasthenia gravis, nerve blocking, and smooth muscle inhibition. Their mechanism of both insect and human toxicity is tight binding to and inhibition of cholinesterase, the enzyme that destroys acetylcholine in the synapse after each discharge of a cholinergic neuron. The consequence of this inhibition is interruption of the conduction of normal nerve impulses.[43] The organophosphorus compounds may be inadvertently inhaled, ingested, or absorbed through the skin, especially by children. The onset of the symptoms, known as a cholinergic crisis, is rapid, and includes a syndrome with the acronym SLUDGE: salivation, lacrimation, urination, defecation, gastrointestinal cramping, and emesis. Respiratory or cardiac arrest may also be induced.

Organophosphorus toxicity may be inferred from a low serum pseudocholinesterase level. Inhibition of this circulating enzyme to half or less of the normal range indicates serious inhibition of synaptic cholinesterase as well. Organophosphorus poisoning is treated by respiratory support and the administration of the acetylcholine receptor blocker atropine at 10- to 30-minute intervals for 24 to 48 hours. Atropine binds to the muscarinic class of acetylcholine receptors, counteracting the high acetylcholine concentra-

tion and reversing the cardiac and bronchoconstricting effects of the drug. Atropine does not bind to the nicotinic class of acetylcholine receptor to relieve the respiratory depression. A second antidotal substance, pralidoxime (2-PAM), displaces the organophosphorus compound from the cholinesterase and gradually reverses the poisoning. Plasma pseudocholinesterase levels may not return to normal for 1 to 4 weeks after recovery.

Iron

Iron is another toxin commonly encountered in accidental overdose in children.[44] The regulation of uptake of iron in the intestine normally prevents dietary iron overload, but in extreme overdose, the iron induces hemorrhagic gastroenteritis, and damage to the gastric mucosa is so severe that absorption can no longer be controlled. In turn, the iron-binding capacity of the blood is overloaded, and toxic circulating levels of free iron develop. Intestinal damage occurs within 2 hours, but other symptoms do not appear for several more hours. After that period, hypotension, metabolic acidosis, pulmonary edema, and liver and kidney failure develop, with a high incidence of death in the absence of treatment.

Laboratory evaluation of the serum iron and total iron-binding capacity (TIBC) are important in determining the severity of the excess of free iron. An iron chelator, deferoxamine, is given to complex the iron and allow it to be excreted into the urine, where it creates a pink coloration that is useful in monitoring the course of therapy.

Case Study 1

A 30-year-old white woman was found by her husband, obtunded, at 9 PM. A nearby bottle that had contained 40 to 50 100-mg tablets of phenobarbital was empty. She was taken to a local community hospital, where gastric lavage was performed and pill fragments were recovered. Lavage was followed by instillation of activated charcoal, but the patient's condition continued to deteriorate, and she was nearly comatose.

Following a failed attempt at endotracheal intubation for respiratory support, the patient was transported by helicopter to a tertiary care trauma center, where she arrived at midnight, comatose, and was successfully intubated. Gastric lavage was repeated. Tachycardia was noted (110–115 beats/min) in compensatory reaction to falling blood pressure, which was maintained at 130/80 mm Hg. Pupils were sluggishly reactive, indicating the absence of midbrain injury. A stat. urine drug screen was performed, which revealed only phenobarbital. At 2:30 AM, the serum phenobarbital was 106 μg/mL (toxic levels, >30 μg/mL). Blood ethanol was 225 mg/dL (toxic level, >100 mg/dL).

The patient was heparinized, and charcoal hemoperfusion was initiated at 3:30 AM. Within 30 minutes, the patient was noted to be more alert. Perfusion was continued for a total of 2 hours. Seventy-five minutes after the completion of the treatment, the phenobarbital level was 51 μg/mL. The patient was observed for the next 24 hours, and psychiatric consultation was requested.

Questions

1. The first serum measurement of phenobarbital was obtained more than 2 hours after the patient's arrival at the trauma center. Should it have been obtained sooner?

2. If the urine drug screen had shown the presence of barbiturates as a class and the identification of phenobarbital had not been known from the history, would differentiation among the barbiturates by the laboratory have been important in determining treatment?

3. What alternative methods of increasing the elimination rate for phenobarbital exist, and why would they be better or worse than the method used?

Discussion

1. There was no need to obtain the serum phenobarbital level sooner. Gastric lavage was performed again upon arrival, and continued absorption of the drug seemed probable. Peak blood levels of phenobarbital normally occur 6 to 18 hours after ingestion, so that deferring the blood testing until the moment of decision for hemoperfusion gave a higher level and better indication of the extent of toxicity to be expected. The maximum blood levels expected from the information available were calculated as 5 g phenobarbital distributed in 0.9 L/kg body weight (standard volume of distribution for phenobarbital) in a 50-kg individual, or 111 μg/mL. This toxic level, confirmed by the blood testing, in conjunction with the additive effects of ethanol was considered to justify the hemoperfusion.

2. Barbiturate differentiation would have been important. Properties of barbiturates vary enormously. The normal serum half-life for phenobarbital is about 3 days and may be increased by the induced hypotension, which impairs kidney function. By contrast, the next most slowly cleared agent, pentobarbital, has a serum half-life of about 30 hours, and the other barbiturates, 12 to 24 hours. Further, short- and ultra-short-acting barbiturates (pentobarbital, secobarbital, and thiopental) are rapidly sequestered in adipose tissue and, although not eliminated from the body, are largely partitioned out of the CNS, where they are no longer dangerous. Thus, phenobarbital overdose requires more aggressive intervention than does overdose of the other barbiturates.

3. Renal clearance of phenobarbital accounts for a significant portion (25%) of the total clearance. Phenobarbital is an acidic drug with a pKa of 7.24, within the range in which alkalinization of the urine enhances excretion. Ion-trapping is effective for phenobarbital, although less so than hemoperfusion. Like hemoperfusion, ion-trapping would not enhance ethanol removal. Hemodialysis would be better for the removal of alcohol but is of limited use with drugs

as highly protein bound as phenobarbital, which is 50% protein bound. Plasmapheresis or exchange transfusion would be ideal for removal of both the protein-bound drug and the alcohol, although hemoperfusion is simpler and was effective in this case.

Case Study 2

A 1100-g premature female infant whose delivery was associated with foul-smelling amniotic fluid developed a fever of 102 °F with a white blood cell count on the fifth day of life (DOL) of 6.7×10^9/L (reference range $10-30 \times 10^9$/L at birth). A lumbar puncture (LP) was performed; the cerebrospinal fluid (CSF) protein was determined to be 324 mg/dL (reference range, $\leq$ 150 mg/dL during the first month of life), and CSF glucose 34 mg/dL (reference range, 45–70 mg/dL). CSF cultures were initiated, and ampicillin and gentamicin were administered empirically.

On DOL 7, the white cell count was 58×10^9/L and the infant developed seizure activity, which was controlled with phenobarbital. LP was performed again. CSF protein was 452 mg/dL; CSF glucose was 5 mg/dL; and CSF cell count was 903/mm³, indicating persistent bacterial infection. *Gardnerella vaginalis* was isolated from the earlier CSF specimen, and chloramphenicol therapy was initiated on DOL 9. Daily blood levels of chloramphenicol were 23, 32, and 16 μg/mL on the next 3 days, respectively (therapeutic range, 10–20 μg/mL). Total bilirubin had peaked on DOL 4 at 7.2 mg/dL (reference range, <1.0 mg/dL), and even with discontinuation of phototherapy, it was only 2.3 μg/mL on the day before chloramphenicol was initiated.

On the fourth day of chloramphenicol therapy (DOL 13), the infant developed a pallor described as dusky or cyanotic, and blood pressure began to decline. Metabolic acidosis developed, with a CO_2 level of 12 mEq/L (reference range, 24–32 mEq/L). A chloramphenicol level, measured in blood drawn at 7:25 AM, was 120 μg/mL. Stat. analysis of a second specimen drawn at 10:30 AM was 223 μg/mL.

The apparently misformulated chloramphenicol solution was stopped immediately, and dopamine was administered to improve tissue perfusion. One hour after a complete exchange transfusion, the chloramphenicol level was 149 μg/mL. Seven hours later, a second transfusion was performed. Two hours after that transfusion, the drug level was 114 μg/mL. Two hours after a third complete exchange transfusion, the blood chloramphenicol level was 83 μg/mL. On the fifth and sixth days of therapy (DOLs 14 and 15), chloramphenicol levels were 33 and 14 μg/mL, respectively. Further CSF cultures were negative, and the infant recovered without apparent secondary effects.

Questions

1. Why did a complete exchange transfusion not remove the chloramphenicol altogether?

2. Should drug levels be measured more than once a day?

Discussion

1. This case illustrates the "rebound" phenomenon seen with lipid-soluble drugs, which are distributed extensively into the tissues of the body and diffuse back into the blood over time. Although chloramphenicol is administered as a highly water-soluble ester, it is hydrolyzed rapidly in the blood to the poorly soluble active form. The water insolubility reflects a lipophilic nature that allows free passage across the blood-brain barrier, promoting effectiveness in the CSF but also causing a pronounced rebound effect. The determination of blood levels of the drug was delayed for 1 to 2 hours after each transfusion to allow some reequilibration and to avoid overestimation of the benefit of the transfusion.

2. In adults, chloramphenicol levels do not usually need to be measured more than once a day. The particular need for aggressive chloramphenicol monitoring in neonates is due to the importance of a diminished hepatic enzyme, which normally allows elimination of the drug through the kidneys by converting it into the water-soluble glucuronide. This enzyme also conjugates bilirubin, so that neonatal jaundice parallels and reflects the limitation of the liver's capacity to eliminate the drug. The usual reason for chloramphenicol toxicity in the neonate, which typically develops on the fourth day of treatment, is gradual accumulation of unmetabolized drug, so that daily monitoring is usually adequate. In this case, bilirubin metabolism had already developed, and chloramphenicol metabolism was probably not a critical factor. Misformulation is a rare, unforeseeable event that first became evident in the characteristic gray pallor (gray baby syndrome) that was recognized by the alert medical staff. Blood chloramphenicol measurements served to confirm the situation and monitor therapy.

References

1. Klaassen CD: Principles of Toxicology. *In* Gilman AG, Rall TW, Niles AS, Taylor P (eds): Goodman and Gilman's The Pharmacological Basis of Therapeutics, ed 9. New York, McGraw-Hill, 1996.
2. Hanenson IB: General principles in the management of acute poisoning. *In* Hanenson IB (ed): Quick Reference to Clinical Toxicology. Philadelphia, JB Lippincott, 1980.
3. Shuckit MA: Overview of treatment—goals of treatment. *In* Galanter M, Kleber HD (eds): The American Psychiatric Press Textbook of Substance Abuse Treatment. Washington, DC, American Psychiatric Press, 1994.
4. McCarron MM: The use of toxicology tests in emergency room diagnosis. J Anal Toxicol 7:131, 1983.
5. Mills T, Roberson CJ, Mcurdy HH, Wall WH: Instrumental Data for Drug Analysis (IDDA), vol 1–5. Boca Raton, Fla, CRC Press, 1993.
6. Wanke LA, Bennett WM: Enhancement of elimination: Diuresis, peritoneal dialysis, hemodialysis, and hemoperfusion. *In* Bayer NU, Rumack BH, Wanke LA (eds): Toxicologic Emergencies. Bowie, Md, PJ Brady, 1984.
7. Rosenbaum JL, Kramer MS, Raja RM, et al: Current status of the hemoperfusion in toxicology. Clin Toxicol 17:493, 1980.
8. Jones JS, Dougherty J: Current status of plasmapheresis in toxicology. Ann Emerg Med 15:474, 1986.
9. Getman CJR, Conner CS: Rational use of antidotes in toxicology. *In* Bayer MJ, Rumack BH, Wanke LA (eds): Toxicologic Emergencies. Bowie, Md, RJ Brady, 1984.
10. Rayburn WF, Andresen BA: Principles of perinatal pharmacology. *In* Rayburn WF, Zuspan FP (eds): Drug Therapy in Obstetrics and Gynecology. Norwalk, Conn, Appleton-Century-Crofts, 1986.
11. Gram TE: Metabolism of drugs. *In* Craig CR, Stitzel RE (eds): Modern Pharmacology. Boston, Little, Brown, 1982.
12. Gossel TA, Bricker JD: Nonnarcotic analgesics. *In* Principles of Clinical Toxicology. New York, Raven Press, 1984.
13. Done AK: Salicylate intoxication: Significance of measurements of salicylate in blood in cases of acute ingestion. Pediatrics 26:800, 1960.
14. Rumack BH, Matthew H: Acetaminophen poisoning and toxicity. Pediatrics 55:871, 1975.
15. Rumack BH, Kulig K: Acetaminophen overdose. *In* Bayer NU, Rumack BH, Walke LA (eds): Toxicologic Emergencies. Bowie, Md, RJ Brady, 1984.
16. Wald PH, Weisman RS, Goldfrank L: Opioids. Top Emerg Med 7:9, 1985.
17. Jaffe JH, Martin WR: Opioid analgesics and antagonists. *In* Gilman AG, Rall TW, Niles AS, Taylor P (eds): Goodman and Gilman's The Pharmacological Basis of Therapeutics, ed 9. New York, McGraw-Hill, 1996.
18. Jaffe JH: Drug addiction and drug abuse. *In* Gilman AG, Rall TW, Niles AS, Taylor P (eds): Goodman and Gilman's The Pharmacological Basis of Therapeutics, ed 9. New York, McGraw-Hill, 1996.
19. Julien RM: Sedative-hypnotic compounds. *In* A Primer of Drug Action. New York, WH Freeman, 1985.
20. Battarowich LL: Barbiturates. Top Emerg Med 7:46, 1985.
21. Kuling K, Duffy JP, Linden CH, et al: Toxic effects of methanol, ethylene glycol, and isopropyl alcohol. Top Emerg Med 7:14, 1985.
22. Wanke LA: Methanol and ethylene glycol poisoning. *In* Bayer MJ, Rumack BH, Wanke LA (eds): Toxicologic Emergencies. Bowie, Md, RJ Brady, 1984.
23. Glasser L, Stemglanz PD, Combie J, et al: Serum osmolality and its applicability to drug overdose. Am J Clin Pathol 60:695, 1973.
24. Rall TW: Hypnotics and sedatives: Ethanol. *In* Gilman AG, Rall TW, Niles AS, Taylor P (eds): Goodman and Gilman's The Pharmacological Basis of Therapeutics, ed 9. New York, McGraw-Hill, 1996.
25. Hartness CC, Buchan JE, Bayer MJ: Phencyclidine. Top Emerg Med 7:33, 1985.
26. Rowland LP, Penn AS: Myoglobinuria. Med Clin North Am 56:1233, 1972.
27. Julien RM: Marijuana: The ancient drug of cannabis. *In* A Primer of Drug Action. New York, WH Freeman, 1985.
28. Dackis CA, Pottash ALC, Annitto W, et al: Persistence of urinary marijuana levels after supervised abstinence. Am J Psychiatry 139:9, 1982.
29. Gerson B: Antiepileptic agents. *In* Gerson B (ed): Essentials of Therapeutic Drug Monitoring. New York, Igaku-Shoin, 1983.
30. Gosset TA, Bricker JD: Antipsychotic agents. *In* Principles of Clinical Toxicology. New York, Raven Press, 1994.
31. Gerson B: Tricyclic and tetracyclic antidepressants. *In* Gerson B (ed): Essentials of Therapeutic Drug Monitoring. New York, Igaku-Shoin, 1983.
32. Baldessarini RJ: Drugs and the treatment of psychiatric disorders. *In* Gilman AG, Goodman LS, Gilnan A (eds): The Pharmacological Basis of Therapeutics, ed 6. New York, Macmillan, 1980.
33. Julien RM: Synaptic transmission and transmitters. *In* A Primer of Drug Action. New York, WH Freeman, 1985.
34. Linden CH, Kulig KW, Rumack BH: Amphetamines. Top Emerg Med 7:18, 1985.
35. Grinspoon L, Bakalar JB: Cocaine: A Drug and Its Social Evolution. New York, Basic Books, 1976.
36. Guyton AC: Rhythmic excitation of the heart. *In* Textbook of Medical Physiology. Philadelphia, WB Saunders, 1991.
37. Bump TE: Clinical pharmacology of conventional and newer antiarrhythmic drugs. *In* Das Gupta DS (ed): Principles and Practice of Acute Cardiac Care. Chicago, Year Book Medical, 1984.
38. Frame P: Antibiotics. *In* Hanenson IB (ed): Quick Reference to Clinical Toxicology. Philadelphia, JB Lippincott, 1980.

39. Sande MA, Kapusnik-Uner JE, Mandell GL: Antimicrobial agents: Miscellaneous antibacterial agents; antifungal and antiviral agents. *In* Gilman AG, Rall TW, Niles AS, Taylor P (eds): Goodman and Gilman's The Pharmacological Basis of Therapeutics, ed 9. New York, McGraw-Hill, 1996.

40. Sande MA, Mandell GL: Antimicrobial agents: Tetracyclines and chloramphernicol, erythromycin, and miscellaneous antibacterial agents. *In* Gilman AG, Rall TW, Niles AS, Taylor P (eds): Goodman and Gilman's The Pharmacological Basis of Therapeutics, ed 9. New York, McGraw-Hill, 1996.

41. Burns LE, Hodgman JE, Cass AB: Fatal circulatory collapse in premature infants receiving chloramphenicol. N Engl J Med 261:1318, 1959.

42. Rall TW: Drugs used in the treatment of asthma: The methylxanthines, cromolyn sodium and other agents. *In* Gilman AG, Rall TW, Niles AS, Taylor P (eds): Goodman and Gilman's The Pharmacological Basis of Therapeutics, ed 9. New York, McGraw-Hill, 1996.

43. Gossel TA, Bricker JD: Pesticides. *In* Principles of Clinical Toxicology. New York, Raven Press, 1984.

44. Banner W, Tong TG: Iron poisoning. Pediatr Clin North Am 33:393, 1986.

The Neonate

Chapter **65**

Laboratory Results in the Newborn

Michael L. Bishop

Laboratory Values
Hematology
Coagulation
Clinical Chemistry
Summary

Pediatric patients are classified together in medicine but in reality are a group of rapidly changing individuals. Two pediatric patients with the same chronologic age may often be as different from each other as they are from adult or geriatric patients. These patients can be divided into subgroups on the basis of the physiologic changes occurring. A patient who is 6 hours old will differ physiologically from one who is 36 hours old.[1]

Nonetheless, various classification schemes have been developed for biologic age groups. Typically, the biologic age groups used are the newborn (less than 1 month old), the infant (1 month to 5 years), the prepubescent child (6 to 10 years), the pubescent child (10 to 14 years), the adolescent (15 to 18 years), the adult (older than 18 years), and the geriatric population. The one common factor in these classification schemes is the fact that chronologic age and biologic age are not equivalent throughout the population.[1] Regardless of the classification scheme, results are referenced as an age-related effect as compared with the values attained during adulthood.

All pediatric patients, whatever their health status, are involved in a dynamic growth process, which is reflected in a different rate of development for each child. Moreover, the biologic processes occurring in a newborn are reflected in very different laboratory results from those obtained from a 1-year-old. Similarly, the results of both will vary markedly from those of a 14-year-old, and no two 13-year-olds are at the same developmental stage. Laboratory results, therefore, must often be evaluated according to developmental level to avoid false interpretation of results.[2] The focus of this discussion is on those changing laboratory parameters of the neonatal period that reflect normal physiologic processes. Abnormal conditions found in neonates are discussed elsewhere in this text, and the reader is referred to the appropriate chapters of interest.

Immediately after birth, an adaptation to extrauterine life begins. The infant begins active respiration and begins eating. Kidney function increases, and closure of the patent ductus arteriosus of the heart occurs. The process of birth alters analyte and fluid volume in the circulatory system, in interstitial fluid, and at intracellular levels; therefore, laboratory results for some analytes will change each hour for the first few days after birth. Infants experience weight loss owing to the loss of insensible water, which is offset by weight gain from caloric intake.

Organ systems undergo dynamic changes throughout the first year of life. In many newborns, the liver is less than completely developed at birth, resulting in abnormal liver function enzyme and protein tests. Generally, protein and enzyme levels are lower in the neonate than in the adult. Mature liver function is accomplished at approximately 2 months of age. By the end of the first year, kidney function approaches adult levels. The shift from fetal to adult hemoglobin in the first 90 days of life may result in increased bilirubin levels. The fairly rapid metabolic rate of the neonate and associated rapid changes often make it difficult to interpret laboratory results and identify the significant changes.

The stages of development of the immune system in the neonate are also reflected in laboratory findings. From 2

635

Table 65–1. Red Blood Cell Values for Term Infants During the First 12 Weeks of Life (All ± Standard Deviation)

Age	Hemoglobin (g/dL)	Red Blood Cell Count (×10¹²/L)	Hematocrit (%)	MCV (fL)	MCHC	Reticulocyte Count (%)
Days						
1	19.3 ± 2.2	5.14 ± 0.7	61 ± 7.4	119 ± 9.4	31.6 ± 1.9	3.2 ± 1.4
2	19.0 ± 1.9	5.15 ± 0.8	60 ± 6.4	115 ± 7.0	31.6 ± 1.4	3.2 ± 1.3
3	18.8 ± 2.0	5.11 ± 0.7	62 ± 9.3	116 ± 5.3	31.1 ± 2.8	2.8 ± 1.7
4	18.6 ± 2.1	5.00 ± 0.6	57 ± 8.1	114 ± 7.5	32.6 ± 1.5	1.8 ± 1.1
5	17.6 ± 1.1	4.97 ± 0.4	57 ± 7.3	114 ± 8.9	30.9 ± 2.2	1.2 ± 0.2
6	17.4 ± 2.2	5.00 ± 0.7	54 ± 7.2	113 ± 10.0	32.2 ± 1.6	0.6 ± 0.2
7	17.9 ± 2.2	4.86 ± 0.6	56 ± 9.4	118 ± 11.2	32.0 ± 1.6	0.5 ± 0.4
Weeks						
1–2	17.3 ± 2.3	4.80 ± 0.8	54 ± 8.3	112 ± 19.0	32.1 ± 2.9	0.5 ± 0.3
4–5	12.7 ± 1.6	3.60 ± 0.4	36 ± 4.8	101 ± 8.1	34.9 ± 1.6	0.9 ± 0.8
8–9	10.7 ± 0.9	3.40 ± 0.5	31 ± 2.5	93 ± 12.0	34.1 ± 2.2	1.8 ± 1.0
11–12	11.3 ± 0.9	3.70 ± 0.3	33 ± 3.3	88 ± 7.9	34.8 ± 2.2	0.7 ± 0.3

Abbreviations: MCV, mean corpuscular volume; MCHC, mean corpuscular hemoglobin concentration.
Adapted from Segel GB: Hematology of the newborn. *In* Beutler E, Lichtman MA, Coller BS, et al (eds): Williams Hematology, ed 5. New York, McGraw-Hill, 1995.

years of age to puberty, growth spurts have a profound effect on laboratory results for a number of chemistry analytes. Prior to puberty, endocrine changes will result in changes in chemistry values for proteins, lipids, and analytes transported by proteins.

Once stabilization has occurred after birth, the change of the cellular and chemical composition of venous blood is gradual, and any significant shifts are usually due to underlying physiological conditions. The ability of clinical laboratory scientists to identify significant changes, therefore, is directly related to his or her understanding of the dynamic nature of the neonatal period.[1, 3]

LABORATORY VALUES

Laboratory testing for the newborn has historically been performed in specialized pediatric laboratories with procedures and instruments designed to handle the small volumes of plasma, serum, and blood available. Advancements in technology that utilize smaller sample volumes no longer require such specialized methods. In the past, different reference intervals were necessitated partially by the differences in test methodologies. With the advances in technol-

ogy that allow the utilization of small volumes for all laboratory procedures, different reference intervals now reflect true physiologic differences, although reference intervals that are age indexed are still required for some analytes.

Hematology

Hematologic changes occur as the newborn adapts to extrauterine life. These changes are significant and differ for full-term and premature infants. Fluctuations in cell counts reflect shifts and changes in total body water. As fluid moves from extracellular to intracellular compartments, the count of the cells per unit volume increases. The laboratory scientist must determine whether an observed change is due to a relative change (dilutional effect) or an absolute change (increased or decreased production). Tables 65–1 and 65–2 show the changes in hematologic parameters of healthy, term infants over time.

Coagulation

The newborn coagulation factors have different maturation rates, but most approach adult levels by 6 months of

Table 65–2. The White Cell Count and the Differential Count During the First 2 Weeks of Life*

Age	Leukocytes	Neutrophils			Eosinophils	Basophils	Lymphocytes	Monocytes
		Total	Segmented	Band				
Birth								
Mean	18.0	11.0	9.4	1.6	.40	.10	5.5	1.05
Mean %		61	52	9	2.2	0.6	31	5.8
7 Days								
Mean	12.2	5.5	4.7	0.83	0.50	0.05	5.0	1.1
Mean %		45	39	6	4.1	0.4	41	9.1
14 Days								
Mean	11.4	4.5	3.9	0.63	0.35	0.05	5.5	1.0
Mean %		40	34	5.5	3.1	0.4	48	8.8

*All white cell counts are expressed as cells × 10⁹/L.
Adapted from Segel GB: Hematology of the newborn. *In* Beutler E, Lichtman MA, Coller BS, et al (eds): Williams Hematology, ed 5. New York, McGraw-Hill, 1995.

Table 65–3. Coagulation Factors in Newborn and Premature Infants in Relationship to Adult Levels

Coagulation Factor	Ratio of Plasma-Clotting Factor Concentration	
	Newborn/Adult	*Premature/Adult*
Fibrinogen	0.90	0.80
Prothrombin	0.50	0.30
Factor V	0.90	0.80
Factor VII	0.55	0.35
Factor VIII	1.00	0.75
Factor IX	0.40	0.25
Factor X	0.40	0.35
Factor XI	0.35	0.20
Factor XII	0.50	0.20
Factor XIII	0.70	
Plasminogen	0.50	0.25
Antithrombin III	0.60	0.25

Adapted from Segel GB: Hematology of the newborn. *In* Beutler E, Lichtman MA, Coller BS, et al (eds): Williams Hematology, ed 5. New York, McGraw-Hill, 1995.

Table 65–5. Reference Ranges for Arterial pH and Blood Gas Parameters in the Newborn

Test	Reference Values	Alert Values
pH	7.27–7.74	<7.10 >7.55
$Paco_2$ (mm Hg)	27–40	>80
Pao_2 (mm Hg)	65–80	<40 >250
Bicarbonate (mmol/L)	16–23	

Adapted from Sherwin JE, Sobenes JR: Pediatric clinical chemistry. *In* Bishop ML, Duben-Engelkirk, Fody EP, et al (eds): Clinical Chemistry: Principles, Procedures, Correlations, ed 3. Philadelphia, Lippincott-Raven, 1996.

age.[5] Newborn plasma levels of some coagulation factors are reduced, but other coagulation proteins are similar to those of adults. Relative levels of coagulation factors are shown in Table 65–3.[4] Coagulation status is normally assessed by several screening tests, whose reference intervals are summarized in Table 65–4.

Prothrombin and factors VII, IX, and X require vitamin K for the final step in their synthesis. These vitamin K–dependent factors decrease in the first 3 to 4 days of life, possibly resulting in hemorrhagic disease of the newborn. Administration of vitamin K usually prevents this condition.[6]

Clinical Chemistry

Acid-Base Balance

The trauma of labor and delivery results in a significant asphyxia in the infant, which may cause an acidosis. Within 1 hour of delivery, however, the pH should return to normal (Table 65–5). Infants who remain acidotic and clinically depressed several hours after birth require additional evaluation. Premature infants with respiratory distress syndrome usually become rapidly acidotic and exhibit an elevated arterial carbon dioxide tension ($Paco_2$). In many cases, the only treatment required is oxygenation. Owing to the rapidly changing environment of the newborn, transcutaneous monitoring is recommended. The use of this technology in infants with acid-base imbalances has greatly reduced the need for more invasive blood gas analyses in the newborn.[3]

Electrolyte Composition and Body Fluid Levels

Rapid changes in electrolyte composition occur in the newborn and often correlate with the shift or loss of body water, which accounts for approximately 80% of the infant's weight. This water is 55% intracellular and 45% extracellular (20% plasma water, 80% interstitial fluid). The volume of interstitial fluid decreases during the first month to a level such that the total body water is 60%. The normal neonate has immature renal function with a glomerular filtration rate only 25% of that in the adult (Table 65–6), and the maximal concentrating rate of the kidney is only about 68%. Levels of the major electrolytes (sodium, potassium, chloride, and bicarbonate) in the newborn approximate the adult levels (Table 65–7). Fluctuation

Table 65–4. Normal Values for Coagulation Screening Tests

Test	Older Child and Adult	Full-Term Newborn Infants Who Received Prophylactic Vitamin K	Normal Thriving Premature Infants Who Received Prophylactic Vitamin K
Prothrombin time (seconds)	10–13	11–15	11–16
Activated partial thromboplastin time (seconds)	25–35	30–40	35–80
Fibrinogen (mg/dL)	175–400	175–350	150–325
Fibrin split products (μg/mL)	<10	<10	<10

Adapted from Segel GB: Hematology of the newborn. *In* Beutler E, Lichtman MA, Coller BS, et al (eds): Williams Hematology, ed 5. New York, McGraw-Hill, 1995.

Table 65–6. Glomerular Filtration Rates of Infants and Adults

Age	Glomerular Filtration Rate (mL/min/1.73 m²)	
	Mean	*Range*
1 day	24	3–38
2–8 days	38	17–60
10–22 days	50	32–69
37–95 days	58	30–86
1.5–2 years	115	95–135
Adult	100	85–115

Adapted from Sherwin JE, Sobenes JR: Pediatric clinical chemistry. *In* Bishop ML, Duben-Engelkirk, Fody EP, et al (eds): Clinical Chemistry: Principles, Procedures, Correlations, ed 3. Philadelphia, Lippincott-Raven, 1996.

Table 65–7. Age-Related Reference Intervals for Serum Electrolytes

Analyte	Age	Concentration Range (mmol/L)
Sodium	2–5 days	135–148
	1–12 months	130–145
	Older than 12 months	135–147
Potassium	Newborn to 3 years	3.5–5.1
	3–8 years	3.6–5.0
	8–15 years	3.5–4.9
	Older than 15 years	3.5–4.7
Chloride	Newborn to 3 years	100–110
	3–10 years	99–109
	10–19 years	99–107
	Older than 19 years	100–106
Bicarbonate	Infant	19–24
	Child	21–27
	Adult	23–32

Adapted from Sherwin JE, Sobenes JR: Pediatric clinical chemistry. *In* Bishop ML, Duben-Englekirk, Fody EP, et al (eds): Clinical Chemistry: Principles, Procedures, Correlations, ed 3. Philadelphia, Lippincott-Raven, 1996.

Table 65–9. Reference Ranges for Serum Lipids

Age	Cholesterol (mg/dL)	HDL Cholesterol (mg/dL)	LDL Cholesterol (mg/dL)	Triglycerides (mg/dL)
Up to 1 year	90–260			20–120
1–5 years	95–215	35–82	55–160	20–120
5–10 years	95–240	35–65	75–165	20–190
10–20 years	110–230	35–65	50–160	25–270

Adapted from Sherwin JE, Sobenes JR: Pediatric clinical chemistry. *In* Bishop ML, Duben-Englekirk, Fody EP, et al (eds): Clinical Chemistry: Principles, Procedures, Correlations, ed 3. Philadelphia, Lippincott-Raven, 1996.

of these electrolytes is common because of changes or shifts of body water in the newborn, who often is not able to respond physiologically to these changes, requiring appropriate supportive therapy.[3]

Nitrogen Metabolism

The liver is primarily responsible for nitrogen metabolism and the production of metabolic end products, including creatinine, urea, ammonia, and uric acid. The liver is also involved in the conjugation and excretion of bilirubin produced by the breakdown of hemoglobin, which results in the production of 12 mg of bilirubin per hour that must be processed. Because of the immaturity of the liver at birth, the circulating levels of these substances change as the liver function improves (Table 65–8).[3]

Lipid Metabolism

Once the newborn liver matures, the metabolism of lipids is the same as in adults; however, the expected

laboratory results are different. The age-related serum reference ranges are listed in Table 65–9.[3]

Drug Disposition

Drug disposition depends on a variety of factors, such as absorption, distribution, binding, and metabolism. In the neonate, a rapid maturation of body and organ functions affects these factors. Changes in gastric pH, gastric motility, gastric emptying time, protein binding of drugs, body fat, total body water distribution, and renal excretion affect drug disposition. In the pediatric patient, these factors change with every stage of development; therefore, careful monitoring of peak and trough drug levels in infants is extremely important.[7]

SUMMARY

The newborn undergoes dynamic physiologic changes as adaptation to the environment occurs. The laboratory scientist and physician must assess each laboratory result in light of the clinical situation and must determine whether any change is relative or absolute. Once this assessment is made, the determination must be made as to whether the change is due to a normal stage of development or is the result of a disease state. For these reasons, assessment of laboratory results in the newborn requires an especially thorough and frequent review of the patient's status.

Table 65–8. Reference Ranges for Selected Nitrogenous Metabolites and Bilirubin

Age	Ammonia (μmol/L)	Urea (mg/L)	Creatinine (mg/L)	Uric Acid (mg/L)	Total Bilirubin (mg/L)	Conjugated Bilirubin (mg/L)	Δ-Bilirubin (mg/L)
Up to 1 week					1–12	0–12	Not detected
Up to 1 year		60–450	2–10	10–76	2–12	0–5	3–6
Older than 1 year					2–14	0–2	3–6
1–5 years	10–40	50–170	2–10	18–50			
5–19 years	11–35	80–220	4–13	30–60			
Adult male	11–35	100–210	5–12	40–90			
Adult female	11–35	100–210	4–10	30–60			

Adapted from Sherwin JE, Sobenes JR: Pediatric clinical chemistry. *In* Bishop ML, Duben-Englekirk, Fody EP. et al (eds): Clinical Chemistry: Principles, Procedures, Correlations, ed 3. Philadelphia, Lippincott-Raven, 1996.

References

1. McClatchey, Kenneth D (eds): Clinical Laboratory Medicine. Baltimore, Williams & Wilkins, 1994.
2. Randolph V: The neonate. *In* Davis BG, Bishop ML, Mass D (eds): Clinical Laboratory Science: Strategies for Practice. Philadelphia, JB Lippincott, 1989.
3. Sherwin JE, Sobenes JR: Pediatric clinical chemistry. *In* Bishop ML, Duben-Englekirk, Fody EP, et al (eds): Clinical Chemistry: Principles, Procedures, Correlations, ed 3. Philadelphia, Lippincott-Raven, 1996.
4. Segel GB: Hematology of the newborn. *In* Beutler E, Lichtman MA, Coller BS (eds): Williams Hematology, ed 5. New York, McGraw-Hill, 1995.
5. Andrew M, Paes B, Milner B, et al: Development of the human coagulation system in the full term infant. Blood 70:165, 1987.
6. Aballi AJ, de Lamerens S: Coagulation changes in the neonatal period and in early infancy. Pediatr Clin North Am 9:785, 1962.
7. Mondy V: Therapeutic drug monitoring and antibiotics. *In* Tilton RC, Balows A, Hohnadl, DC (eds): Clinical Laboratory Medicine. St Louis, Mosby–Year Book, 1992.

Chapter 66

Screening for Congenital Disorders

Lucy J. Randles

ISSUES IN NEONATAL SCREENING

Cost vs. Benefits

The objectives of neonatal screening are early diagnosis and early treatment when each can improve the long-term outcomes for newborns with congenital disorders. The parameters within which decisions to implement screening programs have been made in the past have been based on the medical consequences of early diagnosis, early intervention, and potential long-term benefits to researchers and families. The current trends toward a health care delivery system that is focused heavily on economic considerations, however, have changed both the parameters within which screening decisions are made and the identity of the decision-makers.

Although cost-benefit ratios of mass screening programs for congenital disorders have long been the subjects of controversy and debate, they have never before been examined so closely. When cost-effectiveness becomes a major criterion for decision-making, the cost considerations for a neonatal screening program go well beyond those of initial testing. Screening tests are intended only to identify neonates who may have a disorder when clinical signs are not apparent, but the costs associated with everything that is done after a positive screening test result must be considered in the total costs of such a program. These include the costs of (1) confirmatory testing to eliminate false-positive results, (2) effective treatment modalities, and (3) long-term social and clinical outcomes. If harmful effects can be reversed after birth and after a later clinical diagnosis, there is no justification to screen for the disorder neonatally.[1] If treatment will not significantly improve the long-term outcome, will not prolong life for more than a few months or even years, or is not made available to all those who are confirmed to have the disorder, screening is not considered appropriate.[2, 3] The issue of costs forces a comparison of the dollars spent on screening large normal populations in which there is no evidence or preindications of disease, with the dollars that might be saved if neonates were tested only when clinical evidence or history suggests the presence of disease, and if treatment begins only after the disorder is confirmed.

A 1991 cost-benefit analysis of a French neonatal screening program for phenylketonuria (PKU) and congenital hypothyroidism (CH) has provided a model for developing an analytic framework that can be applied to any new or existing neonatal screening programs.[4] The study determines the cost-benefit ratio per detected case. The screening costs include laboratory costs, medical costs, and additional costs identified from interviews with families of children diagnosed with PKU and CH. The medical costs are determined from considerations of frequency of disease, life expectancy without early detection of the disease, life expectancy after neonatal screening and proper treatment, and duration of institutionalization without detection of disease (for PKU, between 20 and 30 years, and for CH, variable, according to severity of disease). The costs saved by screening are directly related to the incidence of the disorder in the tested population. A higher incidence of the disorder results in a greater benefit, and a lower incidence results in a lesser benefit. In the French study, PKU was determined to have a positive 6.6 ratio and CH a positive 13.8 ratio.

The benefits of early diagnosis to researchers and to families of diagnosed newborns has also come under severe attack. Some strongly believe that justification for screening can come only from the direct benefit to the infant[5]; therefore, any benefits to a research agenda are not supported if the infant does not also benefit. The benefits to families of early diagnosis and treatment can be significant, in that a disorder can be identified and treated before a child is irreversibly harmed, and genetic testing and counseling can be provided immediately to those parents whose newborn has a confirmed genetic disorder. The negative impact of both confirmed and false-positive results upon parents, however, can also be very significant. Positive screening test results trigger a cascade of emotional, diagnostic, and therapeutic events.[3] The consequences of these events are magnified by delays in repeat or confirmatory testing. Delays can result from parents' refusal of follow-up testing or from an inability to locate a discharged newborn because of inaccuracy of address or other parent information. Other delays in repeat testing or treatment occur because the physician of record in the newborn nursery is not the physician who provides ongoing care, or because the physician is unfamiliar with the disease and fails to refer the newborn to another physician who can provide the necessary follow-up. The latter scenario illustrates the need for all primary care physicians, considered the "gatekeepers" in a managed care environment, to be fully aware of screening tests and associated diseases.[6]

Laboratory Test Performance Criteria

The result of an effective laboratory screening test should yield the most information about clinical condition or diagnosis at the least cost. It must contribute significantly to the diagnosis decision tree and should indicate clearly what should be done next.

The proper selection of laboratory screening tests to achieve these intended outcomes requires careful consideration of test performance characteristics, including analytic sensitivity (ability of a test to detect small concentrations of analyte) and specificity (ability of a test to measure only the analyte that it is intended to measure), predictive value (the percentage of patients who test positive for a disease and are later confirmed to have the disease), specimen requirements, cost, and simplicity of procedure.

Ideally, a laboratory test should be 100% specific and 100% sensitive and should have a predictive value of 100%; however, the limitations of methodologies and cost constraints prevent the availability of such a test for screening purposes. Fortunately, advances in DNA technology have greatly improved both the sensitivity and the specificity of laboratory testing methods. Some are still too costly to be used for screening tests, but others have made screening for new analytes both possible and cost-effective.

The sensitivity differences in laboratory methodologies explain the differences that are reported in the literature regarding the reliability of testing for specific analytes when specimens are drawn from an infant 24 hours old or younger. Several PKU screening studies provide data on the frequency of the problem with false-negative results.[7, 8] One study concluded that all cases of PKU could be detected during the first 48 hours of life.[9] Other studies have reported that the false-negative rate, if testing were done in the first 24 hours of life, could be as low as 2% to 6%[7] or as high as 15% to 16%, with the false-negative rate decreasing to 0.6% to 2% on the second day of life, and to 0.3% on the third day.[10, 11] One solution to the failure to identify newborns who have PKU, but have not had sufficient time or feedings to raise the phenylalanine to a detectable level, is to mandate repeat testing. Studies have suggested, however, that detecting even one case of PKU through repeat testing would require performing from 600,000 to as many as 6,000,000 additional tests, making the cost of repeat testing far exceed the financial benefit.[12]

The "cutoff point" or medical decision level determines the concentration of analyte deemed positive for presumptive presence of the disease and directly affects the predictive value of a test; therefore, both the predictive value and cost-effectiveness of routine screening programs can be improved by adjusting the cutoff points to decrease the numbers of false-positive results,[13] if the risk of increasing the numbers of false-negative results is not too high. The predictive value is also improved when the incidence of the disease in a population is higher, as would be the case if the screened population consisted only of newborns who showed symptoms of the disease. For these reasons, screening is justified only when the frequency of the disease is high enough in the population being tested; therefore, a disease may not be included in a state screening program if the state's population has a very low incidence of the disease, even though consequences of no treatment are severe. Conversely, if a single state or a specific location within a state has a uniquely high incidence of a disease, a screening program for that disease may be mandated in that state or geographic area, as is the case in Pennsylvania, which has a high population of Amish who have a higher incidence of Duchenne's muscular dystrophy.[14]

The overwhelming majority of false-positive results in newborn screening are due to the transient aberrations that can occur postprandially or can occur from antibiotic therapy, prenatal maternal transfer, prematurity, or other situations of a temporary nature.[8] Although these results are usually only mildly abnormal, they cannot be ignored. It becomes important in screening programs that the cutoff point not be set so high as to eliminate mildly abnormal results, even though most of the patients have normal results upon repeat testing.

Erroneous test results contribute to unnecessary expense and anxiety[15] and generally result from improper specimen collection and handling, poor timing of the collection, and performance of the procedure by untrained, unqualified personnel. An Oregon study determined that 58% of newborn screening samples were either improperly collected or mishandled in some way. The most common error resulted from the mislabeling of specimens, but 28% of the errors resulted from the times that the samples were drawn.[16] Because improper collections can produce false-negative and false-positive results, it is important that sample collection follow accepted guidelines, such as those developed by the National Committee for Clinical Laboratory Standards (NCCLS). Screening programs should ensure that usable specimens are obtained from all newborns to minimize unnecessary repeat testing and parent anxiety.

This goal is often difficult now, because of current health care trends and practices, whereby newborns are discharged from the nursery at or before 24 hours of age. Many inborn errors of metabolism are detected only after a newborn has made the transition from placental nutrition to oral feedings, at which time the key metabolites begin to increase. If the specimen is collected too early, the metabolite may not have had sufficient time to reach a detectable level or it may be diluted by the maternal blood that remains in the neonate for a short time. Table 66–1 identifies the neonatal disorders most commonly included in state screening programs and the reliability with which the marker analyte can be screened in newborns less than

Table 66–1. Disorders Included in Newborn Screening Programs

Disorder	Number of States Where Screened (Includes District of Columbia)	Reliably Screened at <24 Hours?
PKU	51	Yes
Galactosemia	44	Yes
Maple syrup urine disease	24	Yes
Homocystinuria	21	No
Biotinidase deficiency	17	Yes
Tyrosinemia	7	Yes
Congenital hypothyroidism	51	Possibly
Cystic fibrosis	3	Possibly
Sickle cell disease	44	Yes
Congenital toxoplasmosis	2	Yes

Data from National Screening Status Report: Infant screening. 17:5, 1994. Adapted from Levy HL, Cornier AS: Current approaches to genetic metabolic screening in newborns. Current Opin Pediatr 6:707–711, 1994.

24 hours of age. Because some disorders require time for the analyte marker to appear, a second specimen should be collected after the newborn has left the hospital but no later than 7 days of age, so that treatment can begin as soon as possible if the result is positive. For infants who have received transfusions, a second screening specimen should be drawn near 2 months of age, when most of the transfused erythrocytes have been replaced by those of the infant. This is very important when the analyte marker for a disorder is contained within the infant's erythrocyte.

Social Issues in Neonatal Screening

Because individual states ultimately decide whether or not routine screening will take place, the rights of states to impose their authority over individual rights becomes an issue. If the state has made a decision to screen all neonates for a treatable disorder, do the parents have a right to refuse testing? Many authorities believe that it is the right of each child to be identified and to receive treatment and that parents should not have the right to refuse testing or treatment.[17] This issue becomes more controversial when genetic disorders are identified, because of concerns that the state may potentially impose genetic counseling or intervene in parental rights of procreation. Further debate ensues when the question regarding "patient rights of confidentiality" is raised. The consequences to families could be potentially catastrophic if insurers, employers, or others had access to screening information. The answers to these questions are obtained by the states on the basis of the projected benefits vs. the perceived risks, the competition for scarce health care dollars, the extent of public pressure, and the amount of influence health care providers and insurers have on public policy.

Screening Criteria

The National Academy of Sciences published genetic screening criteria in 1975.[18] Although they are no longer totally acceptable in today's environment because of the technologic, regulatory, and social changes that have oc-

curred, these criteria still provide valuable guidance for the use of screening tests. The criteria are as follows:

- Neonatal diagnosis and treatment must significantly improve the long-term patient outcome.
- There must be a high incidence of the disorder in its preclinical state.
- The test methodology must yield few false-positive and false-negative results.
- The test must be inexpensive and relatively easy to perform.
- The disease detected must be treatable.
- Parents must be informed and educated regarding the tests that are being conducted and the symptoms to watch for after the baby is discharged from the nursery.
- Protocols must include provisions and procedures for repeat testing on newborns who are discharged from the nursery at 24 hours or less after birth.
- Early treatment, before confirmatory testing is completed, should not cause harm or create potential risk to the patient.
- Screening programs should be evaluated on a regular basis to evaluate the sensitivity and specificity of tests, the effects on long-term patient outcomes, and the effects of false-positive and false-negative results.[18]

Laboratory Screening as a Preventive Service

The long-term outcomes of laboratory screening programs will likely be measured by their success in reducing the costs of care associated with specific disorders, which in turn will determine whether or not mass screening for the disorder will occur. Routine screening must (1) prevent progression of a disorder to irreversible consequences, (2) initiate treatment before secondary manifestations of the disorder appear, (3) ultimately improve the growth and development of the neonate, and (4) result in a savings of health care dollars.

It will no longer be acceptable to assume the benefits of early detection and intervention: they will have to be well documented, as they have been for phenylketonuria and congenital hypothyroidism. Infants who once suffered severe mental retardation from PKU and CH now retain normal cognitive function as a result of routine newborn screening and treatment.[19, 20] Consequently, all 50 states and Washington, DC, mandate screening for PKU and CH (see Table 66–1).

METABOLIC DISORDERS
Inborn Errors of Metabolism

"Inborn errors of metabolism" were first described by Garrod in 1908.[21] They are caused by enzyme deficiencies that block specific metabolic sequences and are inherited as autosomal recessive disorders. Currently, more than 300 human diseases in this category have been recognized. Many of these disorders are not clinically expressed until later in infancy or in childhood, and others may not appear until adulthood. Because newborn screening may be the only way to detect some of these disorders before irreversible complications occur, mandated screening is strongly indicated from a strictly clinical perspective. PKU, homo-cystinuria, tyrosinemia, carnitine deficiencies, and biotini-dase deficiency belong in this category. Other metabolic disorders, such as maple syrup urine disease and galac-tosemia, commonly produce symptoms neonatally but may not always be recognized until irreversible damage has occurred; therefore, neonatal screening is clinically indi-cated for these disorders as well. Those disorders that cause serious medical problems resulting in multiple hospitaliza-tions, institutionalization, or lifelong medical treatment are tremendously costly to society and are also considered strong candidates for neonatal screening for economic rea-sons.

Laboratory Analyses and Diagnosis

Metabolic disorders are identified with laboratory screening tests by the measurement of "analyte markers" that result from an increase of the substrate proximal to the metabolic block, from an absence or reduced amount of the product normally produced by the enzymatic reac-tion, and from the presence of the metabolites of the substrate that are not normally detectable.[8] Routinely, in-fants appear normal during the first 24 hours of life, having experienced full-term delivery, and seemingly are active and alert. Nonspecific signs and symptoms commonly be-gin to appear on the second or third day of life,[22, 23] after the onset of milk feeding, which triggers the presentation of clinical signs in metabolic disorders. Such infants are often misdiagnosed with sepsis, viral infection, respiratory distress syndrome, asphyxia, or liver dysfunction.[24] Presen-tation of metabolic disorders ranges from severe neurologic abnormalities, seizures, hypotonia, and coma to poor feed-ing, persistent vomiting, failure to thrive, and hepatomeg-aly.[25, 26]

Levy and Cornier[27] suggest the following categories for metabolic disorders:

- The "intoxication type," which produces neurologic dis-tress with symptoms such as vomiting, metabolic acido-sis, hypotonia or hypertonia, lethargy, and coma (e.g., organic acid and urea cycle disorders, such as PKU and maple syrup urine disease)
- The "energy-deficient type," with severe hypotonia, car-diomyopathy, seizures, possible congenital malforma-tions, and metabolic acidosis (e.g., fatty acid oxidation disorders such as carnitine deficiency)
- The disorders leading to liver damage (e.g., galactosemia and tyrosinemia).[28]

Although this scheme may be helpful, there is overlap in clinical features among the types of metabolic disorders, making it impossible to diagnose them using only these characteristics. It is important to note that many people perceive that a screening program for neonatal disorders screens for all metabolic disorders. This misinterpretation can lead to an omission of metabolic testing in a clinically abnormal infant who otherwise would be tested, resulting in a delay of diagnosis and appropriate therapy. Also, if clinical symptoms persist, the pediatrician must be careful not to assume that no metabolic disease is present even if the screening test is negative.

The timing of specimen collections is critical to neonatal screening for metabolic disorders. The Maryland Depart-ment of Health and Mental Hygiene (DHMH) implemented an extensive screening program in 1986.[29] It recommends that initial blood specimens be collected from each new-born not sooner than 24 hours after milk feeding begins, but as late as practical before discharge from the hospital. This timing permits reliable results to be obtained from screening that require adequate milk intake or amino acid metabolism—thus enabling the detection of galactosemia, PKU, maple syrup urine disease, homocystinuria, and tyro-sinemia. A second screening sample must be collected no later than 15 days after birth.[30]

Metabolic screening in a neonatal intensive care unit (NICU) population requires a different protocol, because NICUs consist only of critically ill and premature neonates who are being transfused and treated with antibiotics and other medications, and may be receiving parenteral nutri-tion. All of these treatment regimens potentially cause both false-positive and false-negative laboratory screening results. Initial specimens must be drawn prior to transfusion of any blood products or implementation of antibiotic ther-apy, and the grams of amino acids in parenteral solutions must be documented for laboratory interpretation. A second specimen should be obtained on the seventh day of life or after the infant receives milk feedings that provide 75 kcal/kg/day for 72 hours, and a third specimen should be drawn on the 21st day of life, or 2 weeks after the second screening specimen.[30]

Treatment for metabolic disorders generally includes dietary supplements and total or limited dietary restrictions, depending on the metabolic pathway that is interrupted and the enzyme that is deficient. Because the prognosis is, in most cases, excellent when the metabolic error is corrected through dietary treatment, inclusion of inborn errors of metabolism in state screening programs is justified. Gener-ally speaking, the laboratory tests to measure the analyte markers are inexpensive and fairly simple to perform as well; however, the incidence in the general population is very small for some disorders, diminishing the overall cost-benefit ratio of mass neonatal screening for those disorders.

Table 66–2 provides a comprehensive summary of the metabolic problem, incidence, diagnoses, treatments, and prognoses for the most common disorders associated with inborn errors of metabolism.

Congenital Hypothyroidism

Congenital hypothyroidism fits all of the criteria for inclusion in routine neonatal screening and is included in the screening programs of all states and the District of Columbia. It is the most common endocrine disorder of childhood, with a prevalence of 1 in 3000 to 5000 live births and a 2:1 female-to-male ratio.[31] Most children who are diagnosed with CH but who do not receive early treatment develop irreversible mental retardation and a variety of neuropsychological deficits, including cretin-ism.[32] Further, most infants with CH look completely nor-mal at birth, and fewer than 5% are diagnosed clinically before screening test results are known.[33] Once a diagnosis is confirmed, early replacement therapy prevents both the physical and mental retardation that occurs with untreated CH.[34, 35]

Table 66–2. Inborn Errors of Metabolism

Disease	Description	Incidence; Signs and Symptoms	Blood/Urine Analyte Markers; Special Considerations*	Dietary Restrictions/ Supplements; Prognosis
Biotinidase deficiency	Autosomal recessive enzyme deficiency resulting in deficient biotin (vitamin H) recycling and multiple carboxylase deficiency	1 : 70,000; sex ratio: M = F Racial/ethnic variability: no cases known in blacks or Asians: ↑ incidence in Amish and Mennonite populations Seizures, dermatitis, alopecia, ataxia, hearing loss, mental retardation, developmental abnormalities, organic acidemia with acute metabolic decompensation, coma, death	Biotinidase should be present in RBCs† Blood products and sulfonamides can alter results	Biotin supplementation Prognosis excellent with early therapy, variable with late diagnosis
Maple syrup urine disease	Autosomal recessive disorder of branched chain ketoacid decarboxylation resulting in high serum levels of leucine, isoleucine, valine, and other ketoacids	1 : 250,000–300,000; 1 : 70,000 in Amish and Mennonite populations; sex ratio: M = F Racial/ethnic variability: may be more common in blacks and Asians Lethargy, irritability, emesis, failure to thrive, dehydration If untreated: seizures, mental retardation, coma, death from metabolic acidosis, ketosis, hypoglycemia	Serum: ↑ leucine†, isoleucine, and valine (Guthrie test +)† Urine: ↑ ketoacids (ferric chloride test gray-blue color +) (DNPH +), > 4 mg/ dL leucine False negatives: early specimen collection False positives: specimen contains antibiotics Requires 24 hours of milk intake	Lifelong restriction of branched-chain amino acid/ protein intake monitored by daily DNPH testing and monthly amino acid assays Prognosis is lethal if left unrecognized and untreated Age and neurologic symptoms at time of therapy institution affect outcome
Galactosemia	Autosomal recessive disorder of galactose metabolism caused by a deficiency or absence of galactose-1-phosphate uridyltransferase (classic galactosemia), galactokinase, uridine diphosphate galactose-4-epimerase	1 : 20,000; sex ratio M = F Racial/ethnic variability unknown Emesis, diarrhea, failure to thrive, jaundice, metabolic acidosis, hemolytic anemia, excessive bleeding, sepsis, hepatosplenomegaly, cataracts (↑ galactitol in lens), irritability, mental retardation, death	Whole blood: <5 mg/dL galactose (Pagen microbiological assay +),† Gal-1-P assay (Beutler + no fluorescence) Urine: galactose (Clinitest) + with glucose (Dipstick) neg. False positives: other reducing sugars or substances, vitamin C in urine False negatives: EDTA anticoagulant, infusion of blood products, and exposure of specimen to heat and humidity when whole blood used; early specimen collection Requires 24 hours of lactose intake prior to specimen collection	Lifetime galactose and lactose (all milk products) restrictions or elimination dependent on enzyme and extent of deficiency; administration of inositol to counter galactitol Prognosis variable, dependent on enzyme and extent of deficiency If untreated, liver, kidney, eye, and brain damage and death
Homocystinuria	Autosomal recessive disorder in pathway of methionine breakdown resulting in elevated levels of homocystine, methionine, and metabolites of homocystine in the blood and urine Inability to metabolize methionine for protein synthesis	1 : 50,000–150,000; U.S. < 1 : 200,000 by screening; sex ratio: M = F Racial/ethnic variability: more common in Anglo-Saxons Thromboembolism, ectopia lentis, skeletal abnormalities, osteoporosis, seizures, mental retardation, psychiatric disturbances, myopathy	Serum: ↑ methionine > 1 mg/ dL† and homocystine detectable (Guthrie test +) Urine: ↑ methionine and homocystine (cyanide nitroprusside test +)	Methionine restriction, cystine supplementation, pyridoxine (B₆) supplementation valuable in some variants Treatment dependent on underlying cause Prognosis is variable

Most cases of CH are transient and are not associated with permanent thyroid damage. Elevated concentrations of maternal iodide, antithyroid drugs, radioactive iodine, and environmental goitrogens can be transferred and may result in a mild, transient CH. The most common maternally transferred hypothyroidism conditions manifest as endemic goiter or cretinism from an iodine deficiency.[36] Maternally transferred immunoglobulin G antithyroid antibodies have also been demonstrated to cause congenital transient immunoglobulin-mediated hypothyroidism (CTIH). Serum thyroxine (T_4) and thyroid-stimulating hormone (TSH) levels are slightly decreased, and thyroid antibodies are demonstrable in the maternal neonatal sera. Therapy with L-thyroxine should be initiated promptly, and the dosage should be adjusted according to changes in thyroid function tests. TSH levels should be maintained between 0.05 and 5 μU/mL; free T_4 in the upper range; and triiodothyronine (T_3) below 250 μg/dL.[37]

Because the placenta is relatively impermeable to the transfer of T_3, T_4, and TSH, newborn hypothyroidism,

Table 66–2. **Inborn Errors of Metabolism** Continued

Disease	Description	Incidence; Signs and Symptoms	Blood/Urine Analyte Markers; Special Considerations*	Dietary Restrictions/ Supplements; Prognosis
Phenyl-ketonuria	Autosomal recessive aminoacidopathy Most cases due to phenylalanine hydroxylase deficiency (classic) but some due to biopterin cofactor deficiencies (atypical) Transient hyperphenylalaninemia is short term, related to immature liver development, and not considered PKU	1 : 12,000–15,000; sex ratio: M = F Racial/ethnic variability: rare in blacks, varies within geographic regions Neurologic and developmental retardation, decreased pigmentation, eczema, "mousy" odor to urine, neurobehavioral disorders	Blood: phenylalanine >† 2 mg/dL some states, other states 4 mg/dL (Guthrie microbiologic test +)† Atypical PKU <15 mg/dL; classic PKU >20 mg/dL Urine: classic PKU only: ↑ phenylpyruvic acid (PPA) (ferric chloride test dark green-blue green color+) (Phenistix gray-green color+) False positives: many from benign transient hyperphenylalaninemia; increasing cutoff point to 4 mg/dL decreases # false positives False negatives: Guthrie test if specimen contains antibiotics; increasing cutoff point to 4 mg/dL increases # false negatives; early specimen collection PKU infants have normal phenylalanine during first day of life Infants tested in 1st 24 hours of life should be retested the third week of life; requires 24 hours milk intake	Phenylalanine restriction; tyrosine supplementation Prognosis is good to excellent with early treatment Outcome depends on age at which dietary restrictions began
Carnitine deficiency	An autosomal recessive disorder of mitochondrial fatty acid metabolism that is demonstrated in medium-chain Acyl-CoA dehydrogenase deficiency (MCADD) and multiple Acyl-CoA dehydrogenase deficiency (MADD) as secondary carnitine deficiencies; also exists as primary systemic carnitine deficiency	1 : 5,000; 10–15% incidence in SIDS patients Symptoms appear after fasting and include high plasma fatty acids with hypoketosis, hypoglycemia, hyperammonemia, seizures, apnea, bradycardia, hypotension, cardiomyopathies, coma, neurologic deterioration	Serum: ↑ ammonia, ↑ glucose with absence of ketones Whole blood: carnitine† <43 nmol at birth; will normally drop 50% after 7 days of age because of normal decrease in RBCs after birth and high concentration of carnitine in RBCs Urine: absence of ketones Specimen collection should occur after fasting or feedings with soy-based formula that contain no carnitine	Avoid fasting and reduction of dietary fat; high doses of oral carnitine Prognosis is good with early recognition and treatment If treatment does not begin early, cardiorespiratory arrest, reduced liver function and cardiac function may result
Tyrosinemia	Group of autosomal recessive enzyme defects in metabolic pathway of tyrosine. May result in impaired CNS development, hepatic and renal tubular dysfunction (tyrosinemia Type I) or corneal plaques, erosion of skin on palms and soles (tyrosinemia Type II)	1 : 100,000 Type I: listlessness, vomiting, diarrhea, hepatosplenomegaly, hepatoma, abdominal distension, ascites, severe hepatic dysfunction, bleeding disorders, coma, death Type II: ocular manifestations, skin erosions	Serum: >12 mg/dL tyrosine† (Guthrie test +) Urine: type I only: ↑ paraphenylpyruvic acid and tyrosine; type II: ↑ tyrosine False negatives: specimen containing antibiotic	Limit intake of tyrosine, phenylalanine, sometimes methionine, altering CHO source as needed Treatment may include liver transplant (type I) Prognosis varies with cause and management, ranging from remission to death

*All blood specimens are collected in predefined circles on filter paper.
†Identifies the analyte traditionally used in screening tests
Adapted from Strobel SE, Keller CS: Metabolic screening in the NICU population: A proposal for change. Pediatr Nursing 19:114, 1993.

which is characterized by a deficiency in thyroid hormones, results primarily from maldevelopment of the thyroid gland or the hypothalamic pituitary axis and deficiencies in thyroxine-synthesizing enzymes.[38] Permanent hypothyroidism is most often caused by thyroid dysgenesis (1:4500), in which thyroid glands are hypoplastic, absent, or ectopic. The extent of the hormone deficiency in these cases is a function of how much thyroid tissue is present. Thyroid dyshormonogenesis (includes all inborn defects in thyroid hormone synthesis) occurs at an incidence of 1:30,000;

hypothalamic-pituitary (TSH) deficiency at 1:100,000; and transient hypothyroxinemia, found most commonly in premature infants, at 1:200.[39] Family history can be helpful in determining the etiology of CH. If a recurrence is in males, there is strong indication that the basis for CH is an X-linked thyroxine-binding globulin (TBG) deficiency. If thyroid disease has existed throughout the family, an autosomal recessive thyroid hormone synthesis disorder is indicated.

Newborns who are hypothyroid may show clinical signs of thyroid dysfunction at birth that include defective skeletal maturation and length of growth in utero as well as other symptoms[40, 41]; most appear normal, however, having subtle, nonspecific symptoms or absolutely no clinical signs at birth.[33, 42] The most common clinical signs and symptoms are umbilical hernia, rough and dry skin, enlarged tongue, constipation, hypotonia, mottled skin, poor feeding, respiratory problems, and inactivity.[43] Other presentations include failure to thrive, temperature instability, peripheral cyanosis, hoarse cry, prolonged jaundice (> 2 weeks), protuberant abdomen, edema, enlarged posterior fontanelle, a palpable goiter, gestational age greater than 40 weeks, and above-average size. Because premature neonates unaffected by hypothyroidism have many of these same signs, extra caution should be taken in diagnosing neonatal congenital hypothyroidism.[44]

Laboratory Analyses and Diagnosis

The measurement of serum T_4 is still the least expensive and best screening test for congenital hypothyroidism.[45] TSH measurement alone is not recommended as a screening test, because elevated TSH values take longer to appear, although neonates may exhibit a TSH surge within 24 to 48 hours of birth. TSH measurements are not helpful in diagnosing TBG deficiency, and T_3 measurement is not helpful in detecting hypothalamic pituitary hypothyroidism. For these reasons, all North American screening programs utilize T_4 measurements. The American Academy of Pediatrics and the American Thyroid Association recommend a two-tiered system that screens first for decreased T_4 and follows with a TSH measurement.[46] The guidelines further recommend as follows:

1. Specimens should be drawn before discharge at no less than 24 to 48 hours after birth. It is highly desirable to collect a blood specimen 3 to 6 days after birth. For home births, early discharge, and critically ill or premature infants, specimens should be drawn 7 days after birth.
2. The T_4 cutoff may be determined by the individual screening program, but is usually 1.5 to 2 S.D. below the mean of normal range.
3. If the T_4 value is decreased, TSH should be measured immediately. A second specimen should be collected 4 to 6 weeks later from infants who have a decreased serum T_4 level and a TSH level > 40 μU/mL, and these infants should be considered to have primary hypothyroidism until proven otherwise.
4. These newborns should be examined immediately and should undergo confirmatory tests. Treatment with replacement L-thyroxine should begin before results of confirmatory tests are known.

A small number of infants who have transient hypothyroidism from intrauterine exposure to antithyroid drugs, maternal antithyroid antibodies, or endemic iodine deficiency have normal T_4 and TSH levels upon confirmatory testing 4 to 6 weeks later. Both T_4 and TSH levels should be normal in 1 to 3 weeks without treatment, if the mother is receiving antithyroid drugs. Transient hypothyroidism indicated by modest TSH elevations (20 to 100 μU/mL) may result from sex-linked hypothyroidism or an ectopic gland.

The American Academy of Pediatrics–American Thyroid Association[46] guidelines contain information and recommended actions for the following abnormalities:

Decreased T_4 (2 S.D. Below Mean of Normal Range) and Normal TSH. This combination of results occurs in 3% to 5% of neonates and usually is caused by a protein-binding disturbance. The choices the attending physician should consider are as follows:

- Take no further action.
- Follow the patient until T_4 returns to normal.
- Collect a second blood sample and test for TBG and free T_4.
- Perform thyrotropic-releasing hormone test to confirm hypothalamic pituitary hypothyroidism.

In any event, if the patient has a decreased T_4 and a normal TSH, L-thyroxine treatment is not justified and may be harmful.

Decreased T_4 and Delayed TSH Increase. Because there is now proof that infants with CH can be born with decreased T_4 and normal TSH and then exhibit an increase in TSH in the first few weeks of life, it is critical to repeat the testing of any infant who demonstrates clinical signs of hypothyroidism. Some programs rescreen all newborns at 2 to 4 weeks of age, but justification of this policy is difficult because of higher cost, low yield of confirmed cases, diversions of key personnel, and uncertain prognosis.

Decreased T_4 and Increased TSH Levels. The attending physician should:

1. See the infant without delay; a pediatric endocrinologist should evaluate.
2. Obtain a complete history, including parental therapy status, and perform a complete physical examination.
3. Perform serum T_4 and TSH confirmatory testing.
4. *Optional*: Perform ^{123}I-radioiodine uptake and/or thyroid scan to identify functional thyroid tissue. (Treatment should begin immediately, however. Never delay treatment until the scan can be done. Because of controversy regarding the risks of a thyroid scan, the scan can be delayed until the child is old enough to not risk danger to the central nervous system.)

Replacement therapy should be with T_4 and not with triiodothyronine. The T_4 level should be maintained in the upper half of the normal range during the first year of life, because evidence exists that if T_4 decreases to less than 8.0 μg/dL with a TSH higher than 15 μU/mL for a significant time, intelligence quotient values will be lower than in patients whose T_4 was maintained at a higher level.

Follow-up for these patients consists of these actions:

1. Two to 4 weeks after start of treatment, perform a clinical examination and measure serum TSH and T_4 levels.
2. Perform a physical examination and measure serum T_4 and TSH levels after each change in L-thyroxine dosage.
3. Perform a physical examination and measure serum T_4 and TSH levels at 3, 6, 9, 12, and 24 months of age and at each succeeding birth date.

Because most screening programs are not set up to detect high T_4 levels, filter paper should not be used to collect the specimen for this measurement. The specimen must reflect circulating serum T_4.

Missed Diagnosis

Missed diagnoses of congenital hypothyroidism occur because of (1) biologic variants from hypothalamic pituitary hypothyroidosis, (2) delayed TSH rise or mild disease, and (3) errors in sample collection, sample processing, reporting, and treating. It has been reported that, in the United States, 1 of 120 neonates with CH is missed because of a false-negative screening result.[47] False-positive screening results occur at a ratio of 24 to 44 for every confirmed case. Although these patients are easily confirmed as negative with follow-up testing, the anxiety and long-term effects for families are well documented.[48] Because of the potentially severe consequences of undiagnosed CH, it is critical that screening programs and protocol include a comprehensive quality assurance system that addresses all of these sources of error. The monograph *Legal Liability and QA in Newborn Screening* provides guidance.[49]

CYSTIC FIBROSIS

Cystic fibrosis (CF) is an autosomal recessive disorder that results in a defect in cell function. The cells in patients with CF have a faulty transport system between sodium and chloride ions and the outer surfaces of epithelial cell membranes in sweat gland ducts, the pancreas, the gastrointestinal tract, and the airway. Because the movement of water follows the movement of sodium and chloride ions, insufficient water reaches the secretions, which become highly viscous. The increased viscosity causes a buildup of mucous secretions, which in turn causes a number of secondary conditions. These include pancreatic obstruction that results in an inability to transport pancreatic enzymes needed for food digestion to the intestine, frequent infections that cause permanent damage to organs, and bronchial obstructions that produce respiratory complications. Individuals with CF experience chronic and long-term lung problems and digestive disorders that result in multiple hospitalizations, multiple infections requiring bacterial cultures and antibiotic therapy, very frequent visits to primary care physicians, numerous lung radiographs, and significant ambulatory care expenses during the first few years of life. At present, the median longevity/survival of patients with CF is 30 years.[50]

An analysis of the Wisconsin CF screening program that assessed the direct medical costs (considered to be a small portion of the total costs of the disease) associated with screening concluded that neonatal screening contributes a small additional cost to the overall cost of diagnosis and management of CF.[51] Although it is possible that screening may decrease the total cost of the diagnostic process, early identification of CF could lead to short-term higher costs because of the probability of hospitalization for management of respiratory illnesses. If early therapy prevents progressive lung disease, the long-term costs of care and hospitalization could be reduced. Other studies have also suggested that early diagnosis and initiation of treatment for CF significantly reduce hospital admissions in the first 2 years of life.[52, 53] Despite early intervention, however, there is no convincing evidence from controlled studies that age of diagnosis or treatment influences long-term outcomes for patients with CF.[54] Wood[55] has identified the following as unfavorable prognostic indicators:

- Female gender (greater mortality rate in females than in males, especially after adolescence)
- Occurrence of meconium ileus
- Pancreatic insufficiency
- Presence of *Pseudomonas aeruginosa* colonization of the respiratory tract

Other indicators are the extent of "underweight" and presence of established respiratory disease at the time of diagnosis.[56] Patients with CF who also have a pancreatic sufficiency seem to have a better prognosis than those with poor pancreatic function.[57]

Even though 1 in 23,000 American children are born with CF and 12 million Americans (1 in 23) are symptomless carriers of the CF gene,[58] screening for CF is rarely performed (see Table 66–1). CF screening has been and continues to be highly controversial because of the undocumented long-term savings; the lack of convincing evidence that morbidity and mortality are improved with early diagnosis and intervention; the lack of a screening test that is highly specific and highly sensitive and has a high positive predictive value; the many social issues that must be resolved; and the questionable overall cost-benefit ratio. The isolation of the CF gene, the determination of the gene product, CF transmembrane conductance regulator (CFTR) that controls chloride channel activity, and the identification of the major mutation, F508,[59] which causes the disease, have led to an acceptable screening test that is now being used in some screening programs.

Laboratory Analyses and Diagnosis

Screening programs for CF have traditionally used a one-tiered system that uses the immunoreactive trypsinogen test (IRT) assay on dried filter paper blood specimens. Although the sensitivity for IRT is high, false-positive results are estimated at 90%; of every 10 patients found to have increased IRT, only one has CF: therefore, the positive predictive value is an unacceptable 10%. Furthermore, data indicate that there is significant overlap between the CF and non-CF populations when repeat IRT tests are analyzed statistically, strongly suggesting that the IRT test is not specific enough to be used in a "recall" approach that incorporates repeat IRT testing on a new blood specimen. Sweat chloride testing has traditionally been used as the confirmatory test for CF. Although it is relatively inexpensive to quantitate chloride in a sweat specimen, the procedure for collecting the specimen (pilocarpine iontophoresis) is costly, time-consuming, and inconvenient for patients and their families.

The application of DNA technology to laboratory testing has resulted in the development of a highly specific direct gene analysis test that detects delta F508 gene deletions and other gene mutations using dried blood collected onto Guthrie filter paper.[60, 61] A hundred different mutations (e.g., G551 and R553X) of the CF gene have been identified, and the delta 508 mutation has been found in 30% to 80% of CF chromosomes in various populations.[62] With the development of direct gene analysis test, a two-tiered approach to screening that reduces the number of false-positive and false-negative results and sweat testing referrals becomes available.

A two-tiered strategy is currently being used in Australia that uses IRT as the initial screening test and direct gene analysis as the second tier of testing.[63] Direct gene analysis for delta F508 mutation is performed on the dried blood specimens that exhibited increased IRT. There is no need to collect a second specimen if enough blood is collected initially, thereby minimizing the costs of a two-tiered test system. Those patients who are either homozygous or heterozygous for the delta F508 gene mutation are then referred for sweat testing. This insertion of the direct gene analysis between the initial screening IRT test and the confirmatory sweat chloride test reduced the number of patients referred for sweat testing by 50%.

Other molecular genetics tests could reduce the numbers of false-positive results even further. Polymerase chain reaction (PCR) amplification of KM.19 polymorphic DNA marker increases the specificity of CF testing and can diagnose patients with CF by the 15th or 20th day of life.[64] The cost-benefit ratio for using additional molecular genetics tests must demonstrate a savings of health care dollars, or they are not justified for inclusion in screening programs. If only relatively few false-positive results are eliminated by performing more tests on all positive samples, the result will not be cost-effective, and the tests are not likely to be added.

Another two-tiered strategy is suggested by a study of 106,000 neonates in Western Pennsylvania, again using a combination of IRT testing, direct gene analysis, and sweat chloride testing.[65] The strategy is as follows:

1. IRT is quantitated on the initial dried blood spot (DBS) specimen.
2. If the initial IRT is > 140 ng/mL, a direct gene analysis for delta F508 gene deletion is performed using the initial DBS.
3. If the newborn is heterozygous for F508 deletion, tests for G551D and R553X mutations are conducted using the initial DBS.
4. If the newborn is homozygous for F508, G551, or R553X mutations or demonstrates a heterozygote combination, the newborn is confirmed as having CF.
5. If no gene mutation is detected, a second specimen is collected for IRT quantitation prior to 2 months of age.
6. If the IRT is > 100 ng/mL, the patient is referred for sweat testing.
7. If only one gene mutation is present, and the second

IRT is < 100 ng/mL, the patient does not have CF, and sweat testing is not needed.

Even with the clear positive contributions of direct gene analysis, there still is no clearly documented evidence that early diagnosis reduces the morbidity or mortality of CF. The National Cystic Fibrosis Foundation Task Force[66] has recommended on newborn screening that "no mass population screening test for cystic fibrosis be implemented, even if a valid and reliable test is available." The American Academy of Pediatrics Committee on Genetics[67] published the following statement in 1989: "Extensive research is needed to determine value of early treatment, reliability, and validity of screening methods and benefits and/or risks of early detection."

Although the benefits of neonatal screening for CF are unclear, the risks are clearly articulated and well documented as (1) severe psychological stress, stigmatization, and confusion from false-positive screening results; (2) missed diagnoses from laboratory, communication, and procedural errors; (3) inappropriate medical practices because of the misunderstanding of screening test(s); (4) disturbed parent-child relationships; (5) higher costs of care because of screening expenses and unnecessary therapies and hospitalizations; and (6) earlier respiratory colonization by *P. aeruginosa* resulting from continuous oral antibiotic therapy for minor respiratory symptoms.[50, 51, 68]

A number of social and ethical issues must also be resolved before routine screening for CF will occur. Informed consent is currently required for any medical procedure that could potentially result in harm to the patient. Do parents have the right and the knowledge or understanding to make such a decision? The direct gene analysis procedures that are likely to be used in any CF screening program will identify heterozygous CF gene carriers. Should they be identified and counseled, and what will be the impact upon their lives and those of their families? Because the information gained from screening appears to benefit only families and researchers, with no benefit to the infant with CF, are the screening costs justified? The use of gene therapy in infants confirmed to have CF could, unquestionably, result in a direct benefit to the infant, would decrease morbidity and mortality, and would save billions of health care dollars, but the controversies and ethical and moral questions surrounding gene therapy may prevent its application to genetic disorders. Until these social issues and those surrounding the use of gene therapy for genetic disorders are resolved, and the cost-benefit ratio for CF screening is clearly established and documented, it is unlikely that states will implement mass screening programs for CF.

The Cystic Fibrosis Foundation further recommends in its position paper, "Besides considering technical reliability and validity of newborn screening methods, it is crucial that all other aspects of screening (including medical, ethical, psychosocial, and economic aspects) be rigorously examined before implementing mass screening." They further recommended that more research be performed in a comprehensive fashion. The future of CF and its victims will most definitely become a product of evolving technology, social conscience, economic priorities, and public pressure.

OTHER DISORDERS

Other disorders, such as congenital toxoplasmosis, human immunodeficiency virus (HIV), sickle cell anemia and other hemoglobinopathies, and prenatal addiction to drugs and substances of abuse that are currently included in mass or selected population screening programs are discussed in their respective chapters in this text.

Case Study

A newborn of Amish descent showed no symptoms of neonatal disorders at birth. The pregnancy was full term, and the delivery was normal; however, the parents stated that the infant had a mentally retarded sibling who had been diagnosed with phenylketonuria (PKU). The sibling had been delivered at home and was taken to the doctor only after symptoms persisted for several months.

Questions

1. Does a positive Guthrie test on the infant's blood confirm a diagnosis of PKU?
2. If the sibling's mental retardation had resulted from galactosemia instead of PKU, how would the confirmation protocol have differed?
3. What value do screening tests have in situations in which a newborn has a sibling who has an autosomal recessive metabolic disorder or exhibits symptoms of a metabolic disorder?
4. What can be done to alleviate the problem of inadequate neonatal screening in communities where home births are predominant?

Answers

1. No. Guthrie's test is a screening test that will detect increased amounts of all amino acids. It will not differentiate among leucine, isoleucine, methionine, valine, phenylalanine, tyrosine, and homocystine. To differentiate among the metabolic disorders that result in elevated amino acid levels in the blood and urine, it is necessary to identify and quantitate each specific amino acid present. In classic PKU, phenylalanine levels are > 20 mg/dL after 1 week. If the level is < 15 mg/dL, atypical PKU is suggested.

    Also, in classic PKU, both serum levels of phenylalanine and tyrosine are elevated, because tyrosine metabolism is part of the phenylalanine metabolic pathway. The ratio of phenylalanine (P) to tyrosine (T) is normally 1:1, but in classic PKU, the ratio is > 1:1, because phenylalanine levels are substantially higher than those of tyrosine. In tyrosinemia, both phenylalanine and tyrosine are elevated, but they are elevated equally, so that the P/T ratio is still approximately 1:1.

    The P/T ratio is valuable in establishing a presumptive diagnosis early on (after 2 days of feeding), because it could take several months for the phenylal-

anine to reach a significant level, depending on whether the enzyme is deficient or totally absent. If an early presumptive diagnosis can be made, dietary treatment (restriction of phenylalanine intake) should be instituted. The serum phenylalanine level should be kept between 2 and 8 mg/dL to both maintain a quantifiable level and protect the infant from the risks associated with high phenylalanine levels.

2. The screening test, which only identifies an increase in galactose-1-phosphate, is an unnecessary step and delays the diagnosis of galactosemia when a sibling is known to have the disease. Also, challenging an infant suspected of having galactosemia with galactose feedings puts the infant at risk if he or she lacks the enzyme galactose-1-phosphate uridyltransferase, which converts galactose to galactose-1-phosphate.

    Because there is good cause to suspect galactosemia in this newborn, the direct measurement of galactose-1-phosphate uridyl transferase should be done just after birth. If the levels are normal, the parents' anxieties can be quickly relieved, and the infant can begin normal feedings without concerns of limiting galactose intake.

3. Mass population screening tests are primarily useful in identifying disease states when symptoms are not readily observable or present. The costs of screening largely normal populations are high compared with the return of identifying only a few patients with the disease. When selective screening is done with an emphasis on symptomatic patients or patient populations that are likely to have a high incidence of the disease, however, the cost-benefit ratio is much higher.

    The primary benefit of screening tests in symptomatic patients is to rule out certain diseases or conditions that manifest similar symptoms. In the case of neonates who have been born prematurely, it is critical that any metabolic disorders be diagnosed quickly, because of their weakened states and the aggressive treatments that are required in neonatal intensive care units. In addition, because inborn errors of metabolism mimic so many of the conditions routinely found in neonatal intensive care units, it is imperative to rule out metabolic diseases in order to determine and implement the course of treatment that will most benefit the infant.

4. Individual state Departments of Health need to have clearly defined and enforced policies relative to neonatal screening. They must detail specimen requirements, handling, and collection times, as well as follow-up protocol for unacceptable specimens and abnormal results. Communities also need to be educated about the benefits of neonatal screening and the necessity to identify neonatal disorders in the first few days or weeks of life.

References

1. Holtzman NA: What drives neonatal screening programs in every state? N Engl J Med 325:802–807, 1991.

2. Willer PH, West JV: Neonatal screening: Should we or shouldn't we? J R Soc Med 84 (Suppl 18):7–9, 1991.
3. Clayton EW: Comment on issues in state newborn screening programs. Pediatrics 91:853, 1993.
4. Dhondi JL, Farriaux JP, Sailly JC, et al: Economic evaluation of cost-benefit ratio of neonatal screening programs for phenylketonuria and hypothyroidism. J Inherit Metab Dis 14:633–639, 1991.
5. Blood spots in the year 2000: Directions for policy. In Kroppers BM, Losberge CM (eds): Genetic Screening From Newborns to DNA. (International Congress Series No. 901.) Amsterdam, Excerpta Medica, 1990.
6. Listerwick R, Frisone L, Silverman BL: Delayed diagnosis of infants with abnormal neonatal screens. JAMA 267:1095–1099, 1992.
7. Kirkman HN, Carroll CL, Moore EG, et al: Fifteen year experience with screening for phenylketonuria with an automated fluorometric method. Am J Hum Genet 34:743–752, 1982.
8. McCabe ERB, McCabe L, Mosher GA, et al: Newborn screening for PKU: Predictive validity as a function of age. Pediatrics 72:390–398, 1983.
9. Meryash DL, Levy HL, Guthrie R, et al: Prospective study of early neonatal screening for phenylketonuria. N Engl J Med 304:294–296, 1981.
10. Holtzman NA, McCabe ERB, Cunningham GC, et al: Screening for phenylketonuria. N Engl J Med 304:1300, 1981.
11. Schneider AJ: Newborn phenylalanine/tyrosine metabolism: Implications for screening for phenylketonuria. Am J Dis Child 137:427–432, 1983.
12. Sepe SJ, Levy HL, Mount FW: An evaluation of routine follow-up blood screening of infants for phenylketonuria. N Engl J Med 300:606, 1979.
13. Galen RS, Peters T Jr: Analytical goals and clinical relevance of laboratory procedures. In Tietz NW (ed): Fundamentals of Clinical Chemistry, ed 3. Philadelphia, WB Saunders, 1987.
14. National Screening Status Report: Infant screening. 17:5, 1994.
15. Sorensen JR, Levy HL, Mangione TW, et al: Parental response to repeat testing of infants with false positive results in newborn screening programs. Pediatrics 73:183–187, 1984.
16. Tuerck JM, Buist NRM, et al: Computerized surveillance of errors in newborn screening practices. Am J Public Health 77:1528–1531, 1987.
17. Arnold G: Screening for treatable disorders (letter, comment). Pediatrics 90:641–646, 1992.
18. Committee on Screening for Inborn Errors of Metabolism: Genetic Screening Programs: Principles and Research. Washington, DC, National Academy of Sciences, 1975.
19. Williamson ML, Koch R, Azen C, et al: Correlates of intelligence test results in treated phenylketonuric children. Pediatrics 68:161–167, 1981.
20. Hudson FP, Mordaunt VL, Leahy I: Evaluation of treatment begun in first three months of life in 184 cases of phenylketonuria. Arch Dis Child 45:5–12, 1970.
21. Garrod AE: Inborn Errors of Metabolism. Oxford, Oxford University Press, 1963.
22. American Academy of Pediatrics Committee on Genetics: Newborn Screening Fact Sheets. Pediatrics 83:449–464, 1989.
23. Collin J: A practical approach to the diagnosis of metabolic disease in the neonate. Dev Med Child Neurol 32:79–86, 1990.
24. Wright L, Brown A, Davidson-Mundt A: Newborn screening: The miracle and the challenge. J Pediatr Nurs 7:26–41, 1992.
25. Arn PH, Valle DL, Brusilow SW: Inborn errors of metabolism: Not rare, not hopeless. Contemp Pediatr 5:47–63, 1988.
26. Cloherty JP: Inborn errors of metabolism. In Cloherty JP, Stark AR (eds): Manual of Neonatal Care. Boston, Little, Brown, 1991.
27. Levy HL, Cornier AS: Current approaches to genetic screening in newborns. Curr Opin Pediatr 6:707–711, 1994.
28. Saudubray JM, Narcy C, Lyonnet L, et al: Approach to inherited metabolic disorders in neonates. Biol Neonate 58:44–53, 1990.
29. Acosta PB, Yannicelli S, Cameron AM: A Practitioner's Guide to Selected Inborn Errors of Metabolism. Columbus, Ross Laboratories, 1992.
30. Strobel SE, Keller CS: Metabolic screening in the NICU population: A proposal for change. Pediatr Nurs 19:113–117, 1993.
31. Sobel EH, Saenger P: Hypothyroidism in the newborn. Pediatr Review 111:15–20, 1989.
32. Postellon DC, Abdallah A: Congenital hypothyroidism: Diagnosis, treatment, and prognosis. Compr Ther 12:67–71, 1986.
33. Fisher DA: Clinical Review 19: Management of congenital hypothyroidism. J Clin Metab 89:550–552, 1991.
34. New England Congenital Hypothyroidism Collaborative: Hanover, New Hampshire: Elementary school performance of children with congenital hypothyroidism. J Pediatr 116:27–32, 1990.
35. Ilicki A, Larson A: Psychomotor development of children with congenital hypothyroidism diagnosed by neonatal screening. Acta Paediatr Scand 77:142–147, 1988.
36. Foley TP Jr: Maternally transferred thyroid disease in the infant: Recognition and treatment. Adv Exp Med Biol 299:209–226, 1991.
37. Germak JA, Foley TP Jr: Longitudinal assessment of L-thyroxine therapy for congenital hypothyroidism. Pediatrics 117:211–219, 1990.
38. Villee D: Thyroid gland. In Avery M, First LR (eds): Pediatric Medicine. Baltimore, William & Wilkins, 1989.
39. Fisher DA: Effectiveness of newborn screening programs for congenital hypothyroidism: Prevalence of missed cases. Pediatr Clin North Am 34:881–890, 1987.
40. Rovet JF, Ehrlich RM, Sorbara DL: Effect of thyroid hormone temperament in infants with congenital hypothyroidism detected by screening of neonates. J Pediatr 114:63–68, 1989.
41. Virtanen M: Manifestations of congenital hypothyroidism during the first week of life. Eur J Pediatr 147:270–274, 1988.
42. Price DA, Ehrlich RM, Walfish PG: Congenital hypothyroidism: Clinical and laboratory characteristics in infants detected by neonatal screening. Arch Dis Child 56:845–851, 1981.
43. Gravdal JA, Meenan A, Dyson AE: Congenital hypothyroidism. J Fam Pract 29:49, 1989.
44. Miculan J, Turner S, Paes BA: Congenital hypothyroidism: Diagnosis and management. Neonatal Network 12:25–34, 1993.
45. Schultz AL: Thyroid function tests: Selective use for cost containment. Postgrad Med 80:219–228, 1986.
46. Holtzman NA: American Academy of Pediatrics–American Thyroid Association Newborn Screening for Congenital Hypothyroidism: Recommended guidelines. Pediatrics 80:745–749, 1987.
47. Holtzman C, Slazyk WE, Cordero JF, et al: Descriptive epidemiology of missed cases of phenylketonuria and congenital hypothyroidism. Pediatrics 78:553–558, 1986.
48. Fyro K, Bodegard G: Four year follow-up of psychological reactions to false positive screening tests for congenital hypothyroidism. Acta Paediatr Scand 76:107–114, 1987.
49. Andrews LB (ed): Legal Liability and QA in Newborn Screening. Washington, DC, National Center for Education in Maternal and Child Health (Georgetown University, 38th & R Streets NW, 20057), 1985.
50. Farrell PM, Mischler EH, Frost NC, et al: Current issues in neonatal screening for cystic fibrosis and implications of the CF gene discovery. Pediatr Pulmonol Suppl 7:11–18, 1991.
51. Farrell PM, Mischler EH, the Cystic Fibrosis Neonatal Screening Study Group: Newborn screening for cystic fibrosis. Adv Pediatr 39:35–70, 1992.
52. Wiklens B, Chalmers G: Reduced morbidity in patients with CF detected by neonatal screening. Lancet 2:1319–1321, 1985.
53. Chatfield S, Owen G, Ryley HC, et al: Neonatal screening for CF in Wales and the West Midlands: Clinical assessment after 5 years of screening. Arch Dis Child 66:29–33, 1991.
54. Wilford B, Gregg R, Laxova A, et al: Mutation analysis for newborn screening: A two tiered approach. Pediatr Pulmonol Suppl 6:238, 1991.
55. Wood RE: Prognosis. In Verlag GT (ed): Cystic Fibrosis. New York, Thieme-Stratton, 1984.
56. Kraemer R, Hadorn B, Rossi E, et al: Classification at time of diagnosis and subsequent survival in children with cystic fibrosis. Helv Paediatr 32:107–114, 1977.
57. Gaskin K, Gurwitz D, Durie O, et al: Improved respiratory prognosis in patients with cystic fibrosis and normal fat absorption. J Pediatr 100:857–862, 1982.
58. About Cystic Fibrosis and CFRI. CFRI News Fall:15, 1994.
59. Kerem BS, Rommens JM, Buchanan JA, et al: Identification of the cystic fibrosis gene. Genet Anal 245:1073–1080, 1990.
60. Lyonnet S, Caillaud C, Rey F, et al: Guthrie cards for detection of point mutations in phenylketonuria. Lancet 2:507, 1988.
61. McCabe ERB, Zhang YH, Descartes M, et al: Rapid detection of β DNA from Guthrie cards by chromogenic probes. Lancet 1:741, 1989.
62. Worldwide survey of the delta F508 mutation: Report from the Cystic Fibrosis Genetic Analysis Consortium. Am J Hum Genet 47:354–359, 1990.

63. Ranieri E, Ryall RG, Morris CP, et al: Neonatal screening strategy for CF screening using IRT and direct gene analysis. Br Med J 302:1237–1240, 1991.
64. Laroche D, Travert G: The application of PCR amplification and the polymorphic marker KM.19 to dried blood spots: Comparison with deletion 508 for the confirmation of the neonatal screening test for cystic fibrosis. Pediatric Pulmonol Suppl 7:19–22, 1991.
65. Spence WC, Paulus-Thomas J, Orenstein DM, et al: Neonatal screening for cystic fibrosis: Addition of molecular genetics to increase specificity. Biochem Med Metab Biol 49:201–211, 1993.
66. Ad Hoc Committee Task Force on Neonatal Screening, Cystic Fibrosis Foundation: Neonatal screening for cystic fibrosis: Position paper. Pediatrics 72:741–745, 1983.
67. Committee on Genetics, American Academy of Pediatrics: Newborn Screening Fact Sheets. Pediatrics 83:449–464, 1989.
68. Hammond KB, Reardon MC, Accurso FJ, et al: Early detection and follow up of cystic fibrosis in newborns: The Colorado experience. *In* Carter TP, Wiley AM (eds): Genetic Disease: Screening and Management. New York, Alan R. Liss, 1986.

Chapter 67

Hemolytic Disease of the Fetus and Newborn

Diane Wyatt

Hemolytic disease of the fetus and newborn (HDN) is caused by the destruction of fetal or neonatal red cells by maternal antibody directed toward antigens of paternal origin on the red blood cells of the fetus. The severity of the condition varies widely, ranging from death *in utero* to absence of clinical symptoms after a normal delivery. The incidence of severe HDN has shown a marked decrease since the introduction of Rh immune globulin (RhIG) in 1968, and improved methods for diagnosis and treatment have contributed to a higher rate of favorable outcomes for HDN.

ETIOLOGY AND PATHOPHYSIOLOGY

Origin of the Offending Antibodies

Hemolytic disease of the fetus and newborn occurs when the mother mounts a humoral immune response toward foreign antigens of paternal origin on fetal red cells. The mother must have been immunized previously to the antigen, and the antibodies must be of the G immunoglobu-

lin (Ig) class, because other immunoglobulin classes are unable to cross the placenta to sensitize fetal cells.

Categories of HDN are based on the specificity of the offending antibody. The three categories, listed in order of descending severity are:

- Rh hemolytic disease, due to anti-D alone or, less often, in combination with anti-C or anti-E
- "Other" HDN, due to antibodies against other antigens in the Rh system or against antigens in other blood group systems
- ABO HDN, due to anti-A,B in group O mothers, and rarely to anti-A or anti-B

HDN due to antibodies directed toward Rh or "other" antigens rarely occurs in the first pregnancy, because the immunizing event is usually the fetomaternal bleed occurring during delivery of an antigen-positive infant in an earlier pregnancy. It should be noted, however, that maternal immunization can occur during a first pregnancy after invasive procedures such as amniocentesis, cordocentesis, and chorionic villus sampling. Abdominal trauma and previous transfusion also can cause maternal immunization.

HDN due to an ABO incompatibility can occur in a first pregnancy, because ABO antibodies are already present in the mother. It has been noted that the presence of an ABO incompatibility offers a degree of protection against Rh and other categories of HDN, presumably because the ABO antibodies destroy fetal cells before an immune response to the other foreign antigens can be initiated.[1]

Effects of HDN on the Fetus

As maternal IgG antibody crosses the placenta and attaches to fetal cells, accelerated extravascular destruction of the fetal cells occurs. The resulting fetal bilirubin is processed by the maternal liver, posing no threat to the child in utero; however, the loss of red cells stimulates increased hematopoiesis in the fetus, resulting in enlargement of the liver and spleen. If red cell destruction becomes so severe that the fetal hematopoietic system cannot compensate, anemia and loss of oxygen-carrying capacity result. The severely affected fetus develops cardiac failure with generalized edema, and the outcome can be death in utero due to anemia. The primary concern for the HDN affected fetus, therefore, is anemia.

Effects of HDN on the Newborn

The accelerated destruction of red cells continues in the untreated newborn affected with HDN. Although anemia remains a problem in the affected newborn, the accumulation of bilirubin becomes the primary concern, because the newborn liver is unable to conjugate bilirubin adequately. Dangerously high levels of 20 mg/dL or more may permit bilirubin to cross the blood-brain barrier, causing kernicterus.[2]

CLINICAL MANIFESTATIONS

The live-born infant suffering from classic HDN appears anemic and jaundiced and has an enlarged liver and spleen. Depending on the severity of the disorder, the newborn may exhibit edema associated with heart failure.[1]

LABORATORY ANALYSES AND DIAGNOSIS

Prenatal Testing

The goals of prenatal testing and history are to identify women at risk of having a child who could be affected with HDN and to determine the extent of fetal red cell destruction that may exist. Blood for serologic testing should be collected as early as possible during each pregnancy. Appropriate testing consists of ABO grouping, Rh typing, a test for weak D (D^u) if the mother is apparently Rh-negative, and a screening test for unexpected alloantibodies. If the antibody screen is positive, testing to identify the antibody is performed. Decisions for further prenatal testing are based on results of these tests.

ABO grouping is performed only for the purpose of patient identification, in case transfusions become necessary, because it is of no value in predicting ABO HDN. Rh typing is performed to identify Rh-negative women who are candidates for RhIG therapy and who require special attention during pregnancy and at delivery. Women who test positive for weak D are considered Rh-positive, but it should be noted that such testing can be misleading if a significant fetomaternal bleed has occurred. For this reason, it is recommended that tests for weak D should be called positive only if the reaction is reactive at 2+ or greater with a nonreactive control. If unexpected alloantibodies are detected, methods for identification should be directed toward detection of only those IgG, warm-reactive antibodies implicated in HDN.

Antibody screening may be repeated at 28 to 30 weeks of gestation for Rh-negative mothers whose initial antibody screen was negative. When an antibody is identified, it is recommended that antibody titration be performed to determine the necessity for other means of fetal monitoring and intervention. Titration is considered appropriate only if the offending antibody is anti-D, because other antibodies rarely require intervention before delivery. Titers are performed every 2 to 4 weeks after the 20th week of gestation. A titer of 16 or more or a rising titer during the pregnancy are the indicators most used for initiation of more extensive monitoring, such as amniocentesis, ultrasound imaging, or percutaneous umbilical blood sampling (PUBS).[1, 3]

Amniotic fluid analysis is typically initiated at 18 to 20 weeks of gestation to measure bile pigment as an index of fetal red cell destruction. Bilirubin is measured spectrophotometrically and plotted against gestational age on a semilogarithmic (Liley's) graph to predict disease severity and necessity for intervention. Generally, higher bilirubin concentrations indicate more severe disease. The amniotic fluid also can be used to evaluate fetal lung maturity through performance of the lecithin-sphingomyelin ratio (L/S ratio) if decisions regarding early delivery of the fetus become necessary (see Chapter 35).

Factors affecting results of tests on amniotic fluid include turbidity, presence of blood or meconium, and exposure to light. Turbidity can be corrected by high-speed centrifugation to obtain correct bilirubin levels, but the fluid cannot be used for L/S ratio. Samples containing more than 5% red cells are likely to yield invalid results, as are samples containing meconium. The fluid must be protected from exposure to light to avoid rapid degradation of the bilirubin. Other circumstances that may contribute to false results are dilution due to excess amniotic fluid, accidental contamination of the fluid with other body fluids, and failure to withdraw fluid from each sac in a multiple pregnancy.[1]

Percutaneous umbilical blood sampling, or cordocentesis, is a newer technique that involves sampling of fetal blood through ultrasonic guidance of a needle inserted through the mother's abdomen into the fetal umbilical vein. This technique enhances diagnostic efforts by permitting direct testing of fetal blood for ABO, Rh, and other implicated antigens, and performance of a direct antiglobulin test (DAT) and hemoglobin or bilirubin levels. Care must be taken to ensure that the blood collected through PUBS is of fetal rather than maternal origin. Rapid and cost-effective procedures include ABO grouping, Rh typing, and testing with anti-I.[4, 5]

Amniocentesis and PUBS are invasive procedures that carry some risk to the fetus. In addition, these procedures may be complicated by hemorrhage that causes immunization of previously unsensitized mothers.

Postnatal Testing

Immunohematology

When HDN is suspected in a newborn, the cord blood must be tested for ABO group and Rh type, and a DAT performed using anti-IgG reagent. If the DAT is positive, an elution can be performed, and the antibody in the eluate identified; however, elution studies may not be necessary if maternal serum has been thoroughly tested. If no prenatal history is available, testing of the maternal blood is strongly advised; see Box 67-1 for recommended serologic testing. It should be noted that the strength of the DAT reaction does not necessarily correlate with the severity of disease, especially in the case of ABO HDN. If HDN due to ABO incompatibility is suspected, the cord blood serum should be tested with A, B, and O red cells.

Special problems can arise in the typing of cord blood cells. First, the presence of Wharton's jelly in cord blood can cause rouleaux resembling agglutination of the cells; therefore, the cord cells must be washed thoroughly with saline before group and type can be determined. Second, a

---

Box 67–1. Laboratory Studies Recommended for Maternal and Cord Blood in Cases of Suspected HDN

Maternal Blood

ABO group
Rh type
Weak D (D^u), if apparently Rh-negative
Antibody screening test
Identification of antibody, if present

Cord Blood

ABO group
Rh type
Weak D (D^u), if apparently Rh-negative
Direct antiglobulin test
Eluate from red cells, if DAT is positive and clinical circumstances warrant
Identification of antibody in eluate

---

strongly positive DAT reaction can cause false-positive results owing to spontaneous agglutination of the cells in the high-protein media used for typing. Conversely, cells heavily coated with anti-D also may yield a false-negative result in Rh typing, owing to the presence of "blocked D." Laboratories providing cord blood testing must be prepared to take appropriate steps to recognize and solve these technical problems. Figure 67–1 provides an example of how to proceed with serologic testing of cord blood.[1, 3]

Chemistry

The unconjugated bilirubin concentration of the cord blood also serves as a useful guide in determining the severity of the disease and, thus, the need to perform an exchange transfusion. The significance of the unconjugated bilirubin level depends on the weight and age of the infant. Generally, a cord blood unconjugated bilirubin level of 4 to 7 mg/dL or greater indicates that the baby is in danger. A rapidly rising bilirubin in a newborn provides even stronger evidence that an exchange transfusion is indicated; however, it should be noted that various institutions set their own criteria with respect to bilirubin levels as indicators for exchange transfusion. The occurrence of kernic-

terus depends on the level of unconjugated bilirubin, the extent of hypoalbuminemia, the gestational age, and the severity of hypoxia and acidosis. Table 67–1 shows a comparison of results found in infants with ABO and Rh HDN.[6]

It should be emphasized that blood to be analyzed for bilirubin must be delivered to the laboratory as soon as possible after collection. If it cannot be delivered immediately, it must be stored away from light to prevent the deterioration of bilirubin.

Hematology

Although hematologic testing of cord blood is not diagnostic of HDN, the results are helpful in determining the severity of the disease. In cases of severe Rh HDN, numerous nucleated red blood cells (NRBCs) are seen in the infant's peripheral blood. There also may be a macrocytic anemia with reticulocytosis. The cord blood hemoglobin level yields direct information about the severity of the disease. The normal range for cord hemoglobin is approximately 14 to 20 g/dL, but in moderate to severe cases of HDN, the cord hemoglobin may fall as low as 8 g/dL or less. The medical staff may have established criteria regarding the levels of cord hemoglobin and bilirubin to assist in decisions concerning the need for immediate exchange transfusion. In ABO HDN, the cord blood hemoglobin valve is usually mildly decreased, and microspherocytes may be seen on the peripheral blood smear.[6]

TREATMENT OF HDN

Efforts have been made to alleviate the progress of HDN through treatment of the mother, including high-volume plasma exchange and intravenous immunoglobulin, but they have met with limited success. The most effective methods of intervention involve treatment of the baby rather than the mother. Decisions for treatment methods are based on the severity of disease and the maturity of the baby. These factors guide the choice to treat antepartum or postpartum. Early delivery of a sufficiently mature fetus with subsequent postpartum treatment is the most common treatment for HDN.

Antepartum Treatment

If amniocentesis or cordocentesis has indicated that the life of the fetus is in danger but the fetus is too immature to deliver, the decision may be made to perform an intra-uterine transfusion (IUT). The purpose of an IUT is to

---

Table 67–1. Characteristics of the Three Categories of HDN

	Rh	ABO	Other
Most common offending antibody	Anti-D	Anti-A,B	Anti-c or anti-E
Maternal antibody screen	Positive	Negative	Positive
Cord DAT	Positive	Weakly positive or negative	Positive
Anemia	Present	Mild or absent	Present
Jaundice	First 24 hours	24–48 hours	First 24 hours
Bilirubin	Greatly increased	Slightly increased	Increased
Microspherocytes	Absent	Present	Absent
Nucleated red blood cells	Increased	Increased	Increased

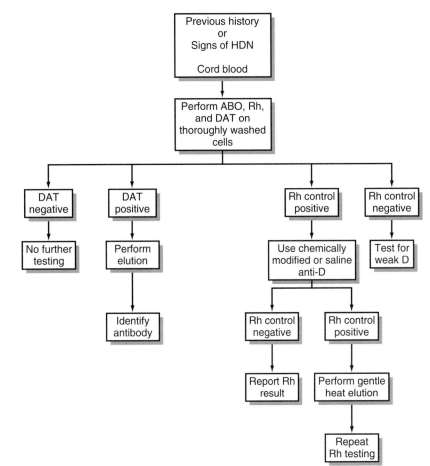

Figure 67–1. Cord blood testing in suspected HDN. Abbreviations: HDN, hemolytic disease of the newborn; Rh, rhesus factor; DAT, differential agglutination titer; D, vitamin D unit.

provide compatible red cells that will correct for the anemia and resulting hypoxia until the baby can be delivered safely. Intrauterine transfusion can be initiated as early as the 20th week of gestation and is repeated at 2-week intervals until delivery.

The standard procedure for IUT involves passage of a needle through the mother's abdominal and uterine walls into the fetal abdominal cavity using ultrasonic guidance. Red blood cells are transfused and enter fetal circulation through lymphatic absorption. A newer technique, described as percutaneous umbilical blood transfusion (PCBT), involves passage of red blood cells directly into the umbilical vein with ultrasonic guidance. It is also possible to perform an exchange transfusion directly through the fetal umbilical vein.

Blood to be used for IUT must be group O and Rh negative and must lack antigens corresponding to any maternal IgG antibodies. The blood should be less than 5 days old to ensure maximum red cell survival. Washed or deglycerolized blood is the product of choice, because it has normal electrolyte levels, provides lower risk for transmission of cytomogalovirus (CMV), and contains minimal amounts of plasma, platelets, anticoagulant, and leukocytes. Depending on the institution, blood that is seronegative for CMV may be required. It is desirable to adjust the hematocrit of the blood to 80% to prevent volume overload, and the blood should be irradiated to prevent graft vs. host disease. The volume transfused depends on fetal age and size.

Problems may occur in ABO grouping and Rh typing of cord cells from a neonate who has been treated with IUT, owing to the presence of transfused cells. In fact, an accurate ABO group and Rh type may not be possible until after the transfused cells have left the circulation. The DAT reaction may be very weak or negative, depending on the volume of transfused cells. In this event, the DAT will not be helpful in assessing the severity of HDN at birth.[1]

Postpartum Treatment

Phototherapy with ultraviolet light is commonly successful in removing the bilirubin from less severely affected infants. Most cases of HDN due to ABO incompatibility are sufficiently mild that phototherapy is all that is needed[2]; however, exchange transfusion may be necessary for the infant born with severe hemolysis. The exchange transfusion accomplishes the following therapeutic objectives:

- Removes excess bilirubin, preventing kernicterus
- Reduces circulating unbound maternal antibody
- Restores albumin and deficient coagulation factors
- Removes antibody-coated cells, preventing further hemolysis
- Provides compatible red cells

The specimen of choice to use in cross-matching for exchange transfusion is the mother's blood, because it contains a high concentration of the offending antibody. If a sample of maternal blood is not available, the second choice is the eluate from cord cells, with the third choice being the infant's serum.

Blood selected for exchange transfusion must be compatible with the maternal ABO group and must lack any other antigens to which the mother has antibody(ies). If the mother and infant have the same ABO group, group-specific cells can be used; however, if they are of different ABO groups, group O blood must be provided. Rh-negative blood is selected for infants affected with HDN due to anti-D, but Rh-positive blood can be given safely to an Rh-positive infant if anti-D is not the cause of the hemolytic process. Protocols vary for selection of components for the exchange transfusion. Recommendations are for CMV-seronegative donor cells that are less than 7 days old and lack hemoglobin S. The cells are reconstituted with compatible fresh-frozen plasma or 5% albumin to adjust the hematocrit to between 40% and 50%. Depending on the size of the infant, enough blood is prepared to provide a two-volume exchange, although this will not remove all the bilirubin, antibody-coated cells, or maternal antibody in the infant's circulation.

When bilirubin is removed from the infant's circulation, bilirubin present in the tissues enters the circulation to reestablish equilibrium. Thus, after the exchange transfusion, the bilirubin in the plasma increases because of this process as well as the continued destruction of newborn red cells that were not removed by the exchange. It is important to monitor bilirubin levels after the exchange transfusion to determine the necessity of performing a second exchange. Additional postexchange laboratory monitoring may include acid-base balance measurement, platelet count, and blood glucose evaluation.[1]

PREVENTION OF HDN DUE TO ANTI-D

The incidence of HDN due to anti-D has decreased dramatically since the development of RhIG, a concentrated solution of IgG anti-D derived from human plasma. The 1-mL full-dose vial, which contains 300 μg of anti-D, will counteract the effects of 15 mL of Rh-positive red cells or 30 mL of fetal whole blood by suppressing formation of anti-D by the maternal immune system. An Rh-negative mother who delivers an ABO-compatible, Rh-positive infant and does not receive RhIG has about a 7% to 8% chance of developing anti-D. This figure drops to approximately 1% if the mother is administered a single dose of RhIG postpartum, and even further, to 0.1%, if RhIG is given both ante- and postnatally.

It should be noted that RhIG also should be provided to susceptible women after abortion, amniocentesis, cordocentesis, ectopic pregnancy, chorionic villus sampling, antepartum hemorrhage, or fetal death, because these events can stimulate immunization. If the pregnancy terminates before 13 weeks, the low-dose vial of 50 μg should be adequate to counteract the effects of the small fetal bleed; otherwise, the standard 300-μg dose is given.

RhIG remains in the circulation for approximately 6 months after administration. It is important that blood bank personnel be advised if the mother has received antepartum RhIG. Otherwise, the blood bank may fail to recommend

administration of postpartum RhIG because of the detection of circulating anti-D in maternal serum.

Testing of Maternal Specimen Prior to Administration of RhIG

Prior to administration of postpartum RhIG to a mother who has delivered an Rh-positive infant, the following tests may be performed on the postpartum maternal specimen:

- ABO group and Rh type, including a test for weak D
- Antibody screen

It should be noted that the American Association of Blood Banks (AABB) Standards also require that the maternal Rh status be determined during admission for delivery, abortion, or invasive obstetric procedures. AABB Standards also require that specimens from all Rh-negative women at risk be tested to detect fetomaternal hemorrhage (FMH) in amount sufficient to require more than a single dose of RhIG. Immunization to the D antigen can occur at delivery despite antepartum administration of RhIG, if the FMH exceeds the 30 mL of whole blood covered by a single dose of RhIG.[1,7]

Methods for Detection and Quantification of Fetomaternal Hemorrhage

The rosette test serves as a practical screening test to detect a large FMH. The technique uses Rh-positive indicator cells that form easily detectable rosettes around fetal Rh-positive red cells in the mother's circulation. A positive rosette test detects the presence of a significant fetal bleed, but it provides qualitative results only. A quantitative procedure must be performed if the rosette test shows positive results.

The Kleihauer-Betke acid elution test is considered the reference method for determining the amount of FMH to use in calculating the number of vials of RhIG to administer. The test is based on the principle that fetal hemoglobin is resistant to elution from the red cell at an acid pH, whereas adult hemoglobin will be eluted. The percentage of fetal cells counted is multiplied by 50 to determine in mL the volume of fetal cells in the maternal circulation. This value is divided by 30 (the amount of fetal blood neutralized by 1 vial of RhIG), and the result is the number of vials of RhIG to administer. Because of the inherent imprecision of this test, it is important to provide a safety margin when calculating RhIG dosage. It is therefore recommended that the calculated dose be rounded to the nearest whole number and that 1 more vial be given.[6,8]

Administration of RhIG

RhIG is administered intramuscularly, usually in the buttocks, within 72 hours of delivery. RhIG is the only type of immune prophylaxis offered to prevent HDN. It must be kept in mind that HDN due to other IgG red cell antibodies can and does occur but is not very common.

A woman who was 33 weeks pregnant fell down a flight of stairs and went into active labor shortly thereafter. She was unconscious at the time of delivery of a girl weighing 1600 g. A detailed history of the mother revealed that she had been transfused with 5 units of packed cells after an automobile accident 3 years earlier. She had delivered her first child 2 years after the accident. Prenatal history revealed the presence of an anti-K, but the first child was delivered with no complications. The Kell genotype of the father was Kk. During this second pregnancy, the anti-K titer rose from 1:8 to 1:64. Amniocentesis was performed at 28 and at 29 weeks to determine the status of the fetus. The change in absorbance was not high enough to warrant any immediate intervention.

A cord blood specimen was taken from the baby girl at birth, and a venous specimen was taken from the mother. Both specimens were sent to the blood bank for testing. DAT reaction was 3+ with polyspecific antihuman globulin (AHG). The cord blood cell typing results were as follows:

Anti-A	0
Anti-B	0
Anti-K	0
Anti-D	4+
Rh Control	3+

The mother was found to be type O-negative with a negative test for weak D. Her blood specimen demonstrated a positive antibody screen at 37 °C and AHG. Anti-K and anti-D were identified. The anti-D reacted 1^{+w} with $R_1 R_2$ cells, and was not enhanced with enzyme-treated cells. The anti-D titer was 1:2. The mother's cells were Kell-negative.

Questions

1. How can Rh typing be determined for the baby?
2. What additional blood tests should be performed on the infant?
3. Explain why the mother's anti-D reacted so weakly.
4. Is this mother a candidate for Rh immune globulin?
5. If blood for an exchange transfusion is needed, what blood type should be selected?

Discussion

1. The original Rh typing was performed with anti-D suspended in a high-protein medium along with the appropriate negative control. Cells that are heavily coated with antibody may spontaneously agglutinate in a high-protein medium. This was probably the case with this baby. The Rh typing should be repeated using a chemically modified or saline-reactive anti-D reagent along with the appropriate negative control. The test for weak D should not be performed when the saline reagent is used, because it is IgM, which cannot react with AHG. It is likely that an accurate test for weak D cannot be performed on these cells, because they are coated with IgG already, which would cause a false-positive result. If, after

testing with chemically modified or saline-reactive anti-D, the Rh control is still positive, a gentle heat elution (45 °C) or elution with chloroquine or ZZAP can be performed to remove the antibody. It should be noted that treatment of the cells with chloroquine may weaken the expression of the D antigen. The Rh testing should then be repeated. In this case, the baby was Rh-positive.

2. It is important to identify the antibody that is causing the positive DAT. In this case, ABO antibodies can be eliminated, because the mother and infant have the same blood group. Although the mother's antibody is known, identification of the antibody coating the infant's cells is still necessary. An elution should be performed on the infant's cells, and the eluate tested against selected panel cells. It is important to save a sample of the saline from the last wash of the cells to test in parallel with the eluate. This saline sample serves as a control to ensure that all unbound antibody was washed free from the cells prior to performance of the elution, providing confidence that any reaction is due to antibody actually eluted from the cells. In this case, anti-K was the only antibody eluted from the baby's cells.

If possible, Kell antigen typing also should be performed on the infant's cells. Because Kell typing requires an indirect antiglobulin technique, any antibody attached to the cells must be removed. ZZAP cannot be used for this purpose, because it has been shown to denature the Kell blood group system antigens. Chloroquine may be used, but it may not render the cells antibody-free, especially if the DAT is strongly reactive. In this case, it seems academic that the infant's cells are Kell-positive, because anti-K was eluted from them and anti-K was identified in the maternal serum. For the sake of completion, however, if Kell typing of the infant's cells is needed, one could wait until the antibody-coated cells are no longer in circulation.

It is also advisable to perform a hemoglobin and bilirubin on the cord blood. In this case, the cord hemoglobin was 12 g/dL, and the total bilirubin was 4 mg/dL.

3. The finding of a very weak anti-D titer should raise suspicions that it may be due to antepartum administration of RhIG. rather than immunologic stimulation. It is very important to explore the mother's history to determine whether this is the case. If the anti-D titer is due to active immunization, then she is not a candidate for RhIG; however, if she did receive RhIG antepartum, she must receive another dose at delivery. In this case, the history revealed that this mother had received RhIG after amniocentesis.

4. This mother meets the criteria for receiving RhIG, because she is Rh-negative, delivered an Rh positive baby, and has no history of active immunization.

5. If blood is needed for an exchange transfusion, the maternal specimen should be used for the crossmatch. In this case, because the mother has anti-D (although it is due to RhIG), group O, Rh-negative, Kell-negative blood must be selected for crossmatch if it is to be compatible with the mother's serum.

Case Study 2

A 24-year-old woman delivered her first child, who appeared healthy at birth. Twenty-four hours later, the baby was observed to be slightly jaundiced. Review of prenatal history revealed the mother to be O-negative with a negative test for weak D. Antibody screens performed in the first and third trimesters were negative. She had no history of prior transfusions or pregnancies, and no invasive procedures had been performed during the gestational period. The neonatalogist immediately ordered a laboratory evaluation of the baby and repeat testing of the mother. The results are as follows:

Baby's Blood

Hemoglobin	15.5 g/dL
Total bilirubin	11 mg/dL
Blood group	A
Rh type	Positive
DAT	Weakly positive with polyspecific AHG

Mother's Blood

Blood group	O
Rh type	Negative
Antibody screen	Negative

Questions

1. What is the most likely cause of the baby's jaundice?
2. What other laboratory studies will be helpful in this case?
3. Is this mother a candidate for RhIG?

Discussion

1. Hemolytic disease of the newborn due to anti-A is the most likely cause of this baby's jaundice, despite the fact that an Rh incompatibility exists. HDN due to anti-D rarely occurs in the first pregnancy, because the immunizing event is usually the fetomaternal bleeding occurring during delivery. A weakly positive DAT is typical of HDN due to ABO antibodies.

2. An elution on the baby's cells should be performed to identify the antibody coating the cells. In this case, the eluate agglutinated A_1 cells but not B cells or O screening cells. These results provide strong evidence that anti-A is causing the baby's jaundice. Bilirubin measurements should be repeated at regular intervals to assess the need for intervention.

3. This mother meets all the criteria for administration of RhIG. She is Rh-negative and weak D-negative with no evidence of immunization to the D antigen, and she delivered an Rh-positive infant less than 72 hours earlier.

References

1. Walker RH (ed): Technical Manual, ed 11. Bethesda, Md, American Association of Blood Banks, 1993.
2. Kennedy MS, Waheed A: Hemolytic disease of the newborn and fetus. *In* Harmening D (ed): Modern Blood Banking and Transfusion Practices. Philadelphia, FA Davis, 1994.
3. Judd, WJ, Luban NLC, Ness PM, et al: Prenatal and perinatal immunohematology: Recommendations for serologic management of the fetus, newborn infant, and obstetric patient. Transfusion 30:175–180, 1990.
4. Strohm, PL: Hemolytic disease of the fetus and newborn. *In* Rudmann SV (ed): Textbook of Blood Banking and Transfusion Medicine. Philadelphia, WB Saunders, 1995.
5. Steiner EA, Judd WJ, Oberman HA, et al: Percutaneous umbilical blood sampling and umbilical vein transfusions: Rapid serologic differentiation of fetal blood from maternal blood. Transfusion 30:104, 1990.
6. Pridgen C: Hemolytic disease of the newborn. In Quinley ED (ed): Immunohematology Principles and Practice, pp 286–290. Philadelphia, JB Lippincott, 1993.
7. Klein HG (ed): Standards for Blood Banks and Transfusion Services, ed 16. Bethesda, Md, American Association of Blood Banks, 1994.
8. Sebring ES, Polesky HF: Fetomaternal hemorrhage: Incidence, risk factors, time of occurrence, and clinical effects. Transfusion 30:344–350, 1990.

Geriatrics

Chapter 68

Geriatric Changes in Laboratory Results

Sharon M. Miller

THEORIES OF AGING
PHYSIOLOGIC AGING
CHANGES IN FUNCTION AND REGULATION
Kidney and Urinary Tract
Glucose Intolerance
Nutritional Status
Anemia
Cardiovascular and Respiratory Systems
Leukocytes and the Immune Response
Hepatic Function
Musculoskeletal System
Thyroid Function
DEFINING REFERENCE RANGES FOR THE ELDERLY

Longevity is commonly described in two ways—life span and life expectancy. *Life span,* usually obtained by averaging the ages of the oldest 5% or 10% of the population, is the maximum age to which an organism can live. For humans, the upper limit of life span seems to be between 110 and 120 years.[1] This maximum attainable age has not been altered substantially by any factors over which we have control. *Life expectancy,* the average number of years a person born in a certain year can anticipate living, has increased steadily since the turn of the century.[2, 3] Improved sanitation, as much as the medical advances of antibiotic therapy and aggressive immunization programs, has reduced deaths from infectious diseases. Better nutri-

tion, sophisticated diagnostics, and advanced therapies have decreased infant mortality as well as reduced adult deaths from acute disease.

Over the last century, there has been a 26-year gain in the average life expectancy. This compares with an estimated 29-year gain from 3000 BC to the end of the 19th century.[2] In 1900, life expectancy at birth was 47 years[4] (Fig. 68–1). Only about 4% of the U.S. population lived long enough to become "elderly," that is, to reach at least 65 years of age. Today, more people are living longer throughout the world.[2]

In the United States, almost 35 million people are 65 years or older, and about 13% of the total population, or 1 in 8 Americans, is elderly.[5, 6] Beginning in 2012, the "baby boomer" generation (individuals born between 1947 and 1957) will begin to swell the ranks of seniors. Projections by the U.S. Census Bureau suggest that in just 20 years, slightly more than 20% of our population (about 52 million people) will be categorized as elderly. By the year 2040, 68 million individuals will be members of this group.[3] In addition to increasing in numbers, our elderly population is getting older. The current mean life expectancy at birth for men is nearly 73 years; for women, it is approaching 80 years.[4] The number of people in the United States aged 85 years or older is expected to reach 8 million by the year 2030, and almost 18 million by 2050.[5, 7] Centenarians will number nearly 110,000 by the year 2000. By 2040, more than 1 million living Americans will have celebrated their 100th birthday.[3]

There are ethnic/racial differences in life expectancy, but it is unclear to what extent these differences are due to socioeconomic factors. In decreasing order, Asians, blacks,

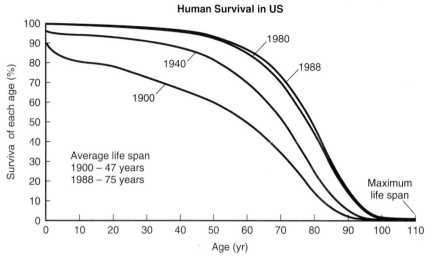

Figure 68–1. Human survival in the United States. (*From* Weindruch R: Caloric restriction and aging. Sci Am 274:46–52, 1996. Copyright © 1996 by Scientific American, Inc. All rights reserved.)

Hispanics, and Native Americans have shorter life expectancies than white Americans.[4] Still, among the elderly, racial and ethnic diversity is increasing steadily. In 1980, 10% of all seniors were members of a minority group. By 2025, that percentage is projected to increase to 15%.[8]

Educational background may also impact health risks and disease. Seniors of the future will be better educated than in the past. Between 1970 and 1990, the percentage of the older population who had completed high school rose from 28% to 55%.[6] With the influx of the baby boomers, the percentage of elderly who have completed 4 or more years of college will rise above the level of about 12% reported in 1990.[6] Multimedia dissemination of information on health and wellness has raised public awareness of the availability of new diagnostic procedures. Interest in the information that laboratory tests can provide and awareness of the personal cost savings derived from disease prevention seem likely to make the better educated seniors of the next century savvy consumers. They will expect to play a key role in all decisions relating to their health and wellness. They will expect substantive answers from their health care providers about the need for and the meaning of laboratory tests. Because women will constitute a greater portion of the elderly in the future, health concerns of seniors will increasingly become women's health issues.

The health care system is increasingly challenged to meet the needs of an aging population. In 1992, persons 65 and older accounted for 35% of all hospital stays and 45% of all days of hospital care in the United States.[4] Few laboratory tests are uniquely required by seniors, but the number of tests necessary to screen, treat, and monitor progress in this segment of the population is typically high. Medication use by seniors raises the potential for drug interference in laboratory analyses. To enhance the diagnostic value of laboratory test results, laboratorians are attempting to compile sufficient data to establish geriatric reference ranges.[9] Although well-publicized national and international efforts are in progress to amass and interpret these data, the task is not easy. Aging is a dynamic, biologic continuum, and chronologic age and physiological age are not synonymous. Individuals advance along this "timeline" at various rates, depending on both intrinsic

(e.g., genetic) and extrinsic (e.g., environmental) factors. The "elderly" as an age grouping exhibit substantially greater heterogeneity than any other chronologically delineated group (e.g., infants, adolescents, perimenopausal women). Laboratory results from studies on older adults are often conflicting. Some parameters show no age-associated change. For others, the magnitude as well as the direction of change reported in studies of the elderly is highly variable. Although confusing, this is not surprising, because different research methodologies are employed in data collection. Most research studies of elderly are cross-sectional rather than longitudinal.

Longitudinal studies follow and reexamine the same individuals over a period of several months or years to determine what changes take place over the life span, and a number of major longitudinal research projects have contributed significantly to a better understanding of the process of aging as distinguished from disease. Three longitudinal research projects are especially well known.[10] The Framingham Study, an epidemiologic investigation of heart disease, was initiated in the town of Framingham, Massachusetts, in 1948 by the U.S. Public Health Service. The original cohort consisted of more than 5000 men and women 29 to 63 years of age. Surviving members of this group have been examined every 2 years to determine the development of cardiovascular disease and to identify risk factors contributing to the disease. The Duke Longitudinal Studies of Aging consisted of three studies focused on noninstitutionalized, healthy elderly. The first study was begun in 1955 and the last continued until 1983. The Baltimore Longitudinal Study of Aging (BLSA), begun in 1958 and sponsored by the National Institute of Aging, is still in progress. The study began by examining certain psychologic and physiologic characteristics of men aged 19 to 96 years living independently in the community. In 1978, women were enrolled in the study. The accumulated data are a great resource of information on the process of aging as distinguished from disease.

Valuable as the data from such major research projects have proved to be, most studies on the elderly are cross-sectional, for reasons of cost and convenience. A problem arising in cross-sectional studies is that some kind of initial matching of different age groups is required.[4] For example, the age groups should be matched on the basis of cultural and socioeconomic factors that may affect results. If this matching is not done, it is difficult to interpret whether the results observed are caused by the aging process per se or by various factors that may translate into lifestyle differences.

Whatever research methodology is employed, it is essential to remember that people age in different ways at different rates. Within a single individual, the aging of specific systems varies according to a complex interaction of inheritance, hormonal and immunologic regulation, and environmental stressors such as drug use, infection, diet, and physical activity. Researchers differ in the criteria they employ to identify "healthy" seniors. There is far less ambiguity in characterizing healthy younger adults. The existence of stable, chronic disease(s) in older adults is common and may be difficult to recognize. Among older adults, the most common chronic conditions are arthritis, hypertension, hearing impairments, and heart disease. Nearly 10% of elderly are diabetics.[4] Whether or not these individuals should be considered healthy for the purposes of establishing geriatric reference ranges is a subject of much discussion. It is easy to understand why differentiating between pathologic changes and age-associated alterations is especially difficult. The laboratorian can provide the physician with a clearer understanding of whether test results reflect age-related changes in healthy elderly or are indicative of disease. This chapter focuses on changes in laboratory values that appear to be associated with aging per se rather than to be the result of illness or use of medications.

THEORIES OF AGING

Aging is the outcome of complex interactions between the individual and the environment. An understanding of factors contributing to the aging process provides a frame of reference for understanding the physiologic and anatomic changes that occur irrespective of disease. Theories of why and how we age may be encompassed by two broad, overlapping concepts. One concept emphasizes the genetic basis of cellular aging; the other, random deterioration due to the accumulation of somatic damage.[1, 11–15]

Cellular aging may be considered to be intrinsic, that is, "genetically programmed," with emphasis placed on the relationship between the cessation of cell growth and aging. DNA is viewed as having a limited capacity to replicate itself: therefore, cell proliferation is also limited. The decline of immune function with age is associated with diminished proliferative capacity.[13] Cytoplasmic accumulation of "senescence factors" or mitotic inhibitors that limit the cell's ability to proliferate has been suggested. Numerous laboratory observations support this paradigm. Aged cells are less sensitive to growth factors; they have a diminished capacity to respond to mitogens. As cells age, they synthesize less of their own growth factors, such as interleukin-2. Additionally, as a cell ages, the pre-DNA synthesis (G_1) phase of its life cycle is lengthened.[1] Accelerated aging syndromes, including progeria, Werner's syndrome, and Down syndrome, are dramatic testimony to the significance of genetic control in the aging process.[15] An additional dimension to genetic involvement in aging is the

existence of genes that confer higher risk for various chronic and degenerative disorders. Many of the diseases encountered among the elderly, such as diabetes, arthritis, heart disease, hypertension, and Alzheimer's disease, have a genetic component.[14]

Aging theories described by the second concept are "injury-based" or stochastic. The environmental factors causing the somatic damage may originate endogenously or exogenously. Aging is regarded as a decreasing ability to adapt to, and thereby survive, stress. Over time, randomly occurring, injurious events are thought to lead to progressive, cumulative damage to macromolecules. In the protein error catastrophe theory, random events in transcription, translation, or post-translational modification result in abnormal proteins that increase to functionally significant levels; the glycation of enzymes and cross-linking of structural proteins are commonly cited examples. Collagen cross-links and nonenzymatic glycation have been suggested as major factors in the aging of connective tissue. The somatic mutation theory of aging proposes that random errors occur during DNA replication and that the DNA repair mechanisms fail to perform adequately. One injury-based theory is currently receiving special attention not only in the scientific and medical communities but also in the public media.

The free-radical theory of cell damage and aging has been enthusiastically embraced, perhaps because it seems to offer a way to manage aging by such relatively simple, low-cost measures as diet and lifestyle modifications. *Free radicals* are atoms or molecules with one or more unpaired electrons in their outer orbitals. They are generated as byproducts of a number of cellular metabolic activities, including mitochondrial electron transport, prostaglandin synthesis, cytochrome P-450 activity, and the oxidative bursts of macrophages and neutrophils.[14, 16] Because they carry an unpaired electron, free radicals can oxidize and thereby damage DNA, lipids, and proteins. Aging may be the result of an accumulation of irreversible oxidative damage to cells and tissues. A variety of defenses prevent or repair molecular damage caused by free radicals. These include scavenging enzymes, such as superoxide dismutase (SOD), glutathione peroxidase and catalase, and antioxidants. The antioxidants attracting special interest are vitamins C, E, and β-carotene (provitamin A).[16, 17] Age-associated decline in levels of scavenging enzymes, due to declining lean body mass, and changes in nutritional status that lower levels of the antioxidant vitamins may be related to numerous changes with age, including diminished immune responsiveness and higher risks for malignant transformation and atherogenesis.[15–17] It seems clear that the structural and functional changes associated with aging are the result of senescence as well as lifestyle factors, such as nutrition and exercise, which can minimize some of the factors that result in cell injury.

PHYSIOLOGIC AGING

The classification of individuals as elderly on their 65th birthday is based on the historical constraints of our retirement and insurance systems. It is an arbitrarily selected cutoff, not a physiologic threshold. There is a gradual decline, even among "healthy" individuals, in many physiologic functions, accompanied by structural changes usually beginning in the late thirties or early forties.[12–14]

In seniors, gradual alterations in structure and function may be academically interesting but have few, if any, clinical consequences. Age-related decline in reserve capacity, however, places the elderly individual closer to the threshold for dysfunction. As long as the body is essentially unstressed, homeostatic mechanisms can adequately cope with minor fluctuations; however, functional impairment and resultant clinical disease are likely to arise in response to stress or challenge. Even in the "oldest-old," reduction in efficiency of function is neither inevitable nor uniform, but the extent of reserves available to adapt to internal and external stressors varies widely.[18]

Cross-sectional and longitudinal studies of community-dwelling adults confirm that physiologic changes occur with age, separate from the effects of disease. Decreases in renal blood flow, cardiac output, lean body mass, glucose tolerance, lung vital capacity, and cellular immunity are most consistently reported[4, 10, 13, 18–22] (Fig. 68–2). The environmental stresses that each individual withstands during an average life span are extremely variable. Furthermore, the specific diseases or disorders that occurred much earlier in life may contribute to compromised regulatory capacity during old age. This variability in personal history also provides an explanation for the wider variation in most laboratory results found in healthy older people compared with younger adults.[18]

Many organs shrink with increasing age, most notably the thymus, spleen, kidney, liver, and brain.[18] Because this change in organ size is widespread, it is probably determined by species inheritance and is only "fine-tuned" by the genes of a specific individual. The varying extent of limitation in the reserve capacity in each organ of the individual then predisposes to the effect of that smaller organ. For example, the liver is well known for its ability to increase its function many-fold and thus is unlikely to

become a limiting factor through loss of size alone. This view is supported by the fact that drug regimens for elderly patients differ from those for young patients mostly on the basis of altered absorption, distribution, and excretion, and not because of limitation of the hepatic detoxification systems arising from the smaller size of the liver. In contrast, the major loss of thymus gland tissue with age overcomes any reserve capacity that it has, and thus, immune functions become limiting in old age both in the absence of external factors (e.g., autoimmune disease, some diabetes mellitus) and in their presence (e.g., infections, some malignancies).[18]

The etiology of some other age-related phenomena apparently relates to regulatory changes without a concurrent change in organ size. Changes in hormone levels that accompany menopause seem to accelerate the aging process. Examples often cited are osteoporosis and atherosclerosis. Although the precise alterations triggering these disorders are not clear, their gradual and irrevocable onset appears to be a failure to resist or recover from the effects of stresses that have existed throughout life. Regulatory alterations that are inherently linked to aging have been suggested for the hypothalamic-pituitary-thyroid axis. Lesions of specific cell types may also depend on the regulation of mitotic capacity. Organs rich in cells with active or potential mitosis are associated with hyperplastic, metaplastic, and neoplastic changes in the elderly.[18] Such organs are the skin, bone marrow, endocrine gland, and liver, and the respiratory, gastrointestinal, and genitourinary tracts.

The combined influence of inheritance, regulation, and exogenous stress on cause of death is reflected in Table 68–1. The major contribution of cardiovascular and renal diseases to shortened life span is most likely due to the limited reserve of functional capacity in these organ systems, whereas malignancies, the class of disease that makes the next greatest contribution, may depend more on altered regulation or exogenous stress.[18]

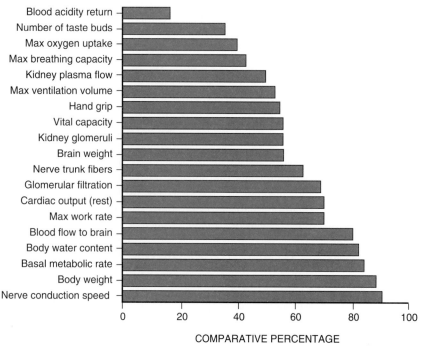

Figure 68–2. Physical characteristics of an average 75-year-old man compared with an average 30-year-old man. (*From* Aiken LR: Aging: An introduction to gerontology. Sage Publications, Thousand Oaks, Cal, 1995.)

Table 68–1. Gain in U.S. Life Expectancy If Selected Causes of Death Were Eliminated

Cause of Death	Years Gained	
	At Birth	*At Age 65*
Major cardiovascular-renal diseases	10.9	10.0
Heart diseases	5.9	4.9
Vascular diseases affecting the central nervous system	1.3	1.2
Malignant neoplasms	2.3	1.2
Accidents (excluding vehicular)	0.6	0.1
Motor vehicle accidents	0.6	0.1
Influenza and pneumonia	0.5	0.2
Other infectious diseases	0.3	0.1
Diabetes mellitus	0.2	0.2

Box 68–1. Functional Changes in the Aging Kidney

Glomerulus
    Decrease in glomerular filtration rate
    Decrease in effective renal plasma flow
Proximal tubule
    Decreased tubular reabsorption of phosphate
    Decreased maximal excretion of glucose and PAH
Distal nephron
    Inability to maximally excrete an acid load
    Impaired diluting ability
    Decreased maximal concentrating ability
    Impaired conservation of sodium

From Sica DA: Renal disease, electrolyte abnormalities, and acid-base imbalance in the elderly. Clin Geriatr Med 10:197–211, 1994.

Whatever etiologies cause the complex of changes referred to as "aging," measurable changes in several laboratory test results occur in elderly people, and many of these changes relate to the functional or regulatory alterations just described.[18]

CHANGES IN FUNCTION AND REGULATION

Kidney and Urinary Tract

Cross-sectional studies of elderly subjects have shown reductions in renal blood flow, glomerular filtration rate, and creatinine clearance.[13, 23] Anatomic abnormalities include progressive loss of renal mass, primarily cortical tissue. The kidneys in an average 40-year-old male that weigh approximately 250 grams are likely to weigh about 200 grams by the time the male is 80 years of age.[24] The total number of functional glomeruli decreases roughly in proportion to changes in renal weight. Histologically, the most important change is the increasing number of sclerotic glomeruli.[25] At 40 years, 5% of glomeruli are sclerotic; by 80 years, 40% have become sclerotic. Factors contributing to these changes may include generalized arteriosclerosis, the higher blood pressure observed in seniors, and damage from lifelong excessive intake of protein[23, 26] (Fig. 68–3).

Glomerular degeneration and reduction in the number of the glomerular capillary tufts or lobes in the cortical nephrons lead to atrophy of afferent and efferent arterioles. There is complete loss of blood flow as the channel is obliterated. As functional glomerular tissue diminishes, the remaining healthy glomeruli are overburdened and are subject to hyperfiltration and hyperperfusion. Over time, these processes are detrimental to glomerular structure and function. Specifically, these changes lead to a decrease in glomerular filtration rate (GFR)—the single most important change in the aging kidney (Box 68–1). In older adults, the GFR seems to remain fairly stable until the mid-30s, then decreases steadily until age 65. After age 65, creatinine clearance decreases markedly.[8] Inulin clearance studies confirm that the alteration is due to a significant change in glomerular filtration rather than in tubular secretion or reabsorption (Fig. 68–4). Cross-sectional studies indicate that the GFR declines about 1% per year after age 40. In a healthy 80-year-old, the GFR may be only ½ to ⅓ the GFR in a young adult.[27]

According to data from longitudinal studies, the GFR declines by about 8 mL/min/1.73 m^2 each decade of life, from a peak at about 30 years. Because muscle creatine is the endogenous source of creatinine, creatinine is excreted into the circulation at a relatively constant rate that is proportional to the individual's muscle mass. Although creatinine clearance declines with advancing age, so does muscle mass. The net effect is that serum creatinine concentrations remain nearly constant even though true GFR

Figure 68–3. The role of increased glomerular pressures and flows in the development of glomerular sclerosis. (*Reprinted from* Anderson S, Brenner B: Effects of aging on the renal glomerulus. Amer J Med 80:435–442, 1986, with permission from Excerpta Medica Inc.)

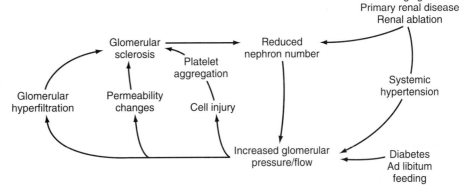

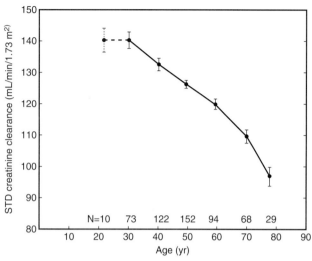

Figure 68–4. The effect of age on creatinine clearance in men. Values plotted indicate standard error of the mean (±1). (*From* Rowe JW: Renal system. *In* Rowe JW, Besdine RW (eds): Geriatric Medicine, ed 2. Boston, Little, Brown & Co, 1988.)

and creatinine clearance decline. Substantial reductions in GFR may be masked by a relatively normal serum creatinine level (Fig. 68–5). For the aged patient, assessment of renal function must never be made solely on the basis of the serum creatinine level. "Correction factors" that take into account the age, weight, and gender of the patient may be applied to the serum creatinine concentration to calculate an estimated glomerular filtration rate,[23] as shown in the following equation:

$$\text{Creatinine clearance (mL/min)} = (140 - \text{age}) \times$$
$$\text{weight (kg)} \div 72 \times \text{serum creatinine (mg/dL)}$$

For women, the result of this equation is multiplied by 0.85.

Physicians must take into account the normal reduction in GFR among seniors when determining the dosage of

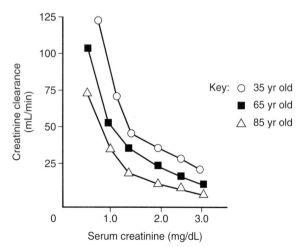

Figure 68–5. Relationship of age and serum creatinine concentration to creatinine clearance (Cockcroft and Gault calculation) in a 50-kilogram man. (*From* Meyer RB: Renal function in aging. J Am Geriatr Soc 37:794, 1989.)

drugs that are eliminated by renal excretion.[28] Drugs commonly monitored in the clinical laboratory that are excreted principally in the urine include aminoglycosides, digoxin, methotrexate, phenobarbital, procainamide, and vancomycin.

Given the wide range of normal values for blood urea nitrogen (BUN), there is disagreement about whether BUN changes with aging. Some investigators have found no difference when the fluid and dietary intakes of the subjects are controlled.[27] Protein catabolic rates (tissue breakdown) also affect BUN. Numerous reports indicate a moderate, steady increase in BUN for individuals between 60 and 90 years of age.[9] Overall, creatinine clearance is the best measure of renal function in the aged.

Although the most dramatic changes in renal function arise as a consequence of modifications in glomerular structure, alterations in tubular structure and function are also noted with advancing age. Reductions in the length and volume of proximal tubules occur and may affect tubular transport. Uric acid is known to be reabsorbed by the renal tubules to a significant extent, and yet its changes with age parallel the change in creatinine at levels at which tubular reabsorption and secretion of creatinine are insignificant. This indicates that glomerular filtration rate, and not renal tubular function, is gradually approaching the limit of compromise over this age span. In seniors, uric acid values have been consistently observed to be higher in men than in women. Similar gender differences have also been reported in younger adults.[9] A reported decrease in mean serum value of uric acid (especially in women) during the eighth decade remains unexplained.[18] It may reflect a larger proportion of reabsorption due to relatively sluggish flow of renal filtrate, or a separate, specific change in uric acid metabolism.[18] Small increases in the amount of albumin or glucose in the urine have been reported in some apparently healthy elderly, but their origin is not clear. Their presence may reflect an unspecified renal tubular reabsorption deficit, or may be the result of the higher rates of subclinical renal disease and glucose intolerance seen in the elderly. It is more common to observe an increase in renal threshold for glucose with aging, thus making the absence of glycosuria an insufficient finding for excluding a diagnosis of diabetes mellitus in an aged patient. Among seniors, the elevation of the renal threshold for glucose may allow blood sugar levels to exceed 300 mg/dL before the appearance of glycosuria.[29]

Inability of the kidney to respond promptly to alterations in fluid and electrolytes is well documented.[30] Impaired handling of water has been noted, especially after seniors have been subjected to several hours of water deprivation. Investigators have calculated an approximately 5% decline in maximum concentrating capacity for each decade after age 50. In addition to impaired ability to maximally concentrate the urine, aging kidneys exhibit a prolonged response time for appropriate adjustment of sodium handling.[27, 30] Despite decreasing renal function in seniors, unless there is significant renal disease, blood pH, PaCO$_2$, and bicarbonate values do not significantly vary from those observed in young adults. Overall, aging decreases the adaptive capacity of the kidneys. Renal response is slower to begin and reduced in magnitude. A summary of mean values for selected renal functions in healthy young and old adults is revealing (Table 68–2).

Table 68–2. Summary of Mean Values for Selected Renal Functions in Normal Young vs. Old Subjects

	Young	Old
Serum creatinine concentration	0.81	0.84
True creatinine (mg/dL)*		
Urinary creatinine excretion (mg/24 h)	1862	1259
Creatinine clearance	140	97
True creatinine (cc/min/1.73 m²)*		
Inulin clearance (mL/min/1.73 m²)†	125	75
PAH clearance (Effective renal plasma flow) (mL/min)	649	289
Concentrating ability	1109	882
Maximum urine osmolality after 12 hours water deprivation (mOsm/kg H₂O)		
Diluting ability	52	92
Minimum urine osmolality after water loading (mOsm/kg H₂O)		
Urine acidification	4.96	4.85
Minimum urine pH after acid loading		

*Total chromogen (autoanalyzer) methodology increases serum creatinine concentrations by 20% to 30% and decreases creatinine clearances by 20% to 30%.

†Estimated means at ages 40 (young) and 80 (old) years.

From Lindeman RD: Assessment of renal function in the old: Special considerations. Clin Lab Med 13:269, 1993.

Altered endocrinologic function also seems to characterize the aging kidney. A well-documented example is the impairment of renal synthesis of the hormone form of vitamin D, that is, 1,25-dihydroxyvitamin D (calcitriol) with age.[31, 32] The significance of this decline for overall calcium homeostasis in the elderly is discussed later in this chapter. In both basal and stimulated states, renin levels decrease with aging. As a result of the changes in renin concentrations, there is an accompanying decline in aldosterone levels.

Painful, frequent, or incomplete urination is a problem for many of the elderly. Stress urinary incontinence (UI) is characterized by loss of urine due to increases in intra-abdominal pressure, such as from coughing, sneezing, and laughing. The origin of the problem may be a general loss of muscle tone in the bladder or urethra. Among women, the most influential factor in lower urinary tract symptoms is the decline in estrogen level. Estrogen retards atrophy of vaginal and urethral tissues.[33] In men, urinary retention may be due to prostatitis or prostatic hypertrophy. Partial obstruction of the urethra is found in 20% to 30% of men over 65 and in 11% to 14% of incontinent women.[34] The consequent stagnation of urine in the bladder predisposes these individuals to an abrupt increase in urinary tract infections after ages 65 to 70.[18] This not only is a source of discomfort but, combined with the decline in immune function that occurs with aging, poses the threat of infection ascending to the kidney.[34]

Glucose Intolerance

Deterioration of glucose tolerance is common among older adults.[13] Reports of the prevalence of diabetes mellitus and impaired glucose tolerance (IGT) have ranged from 20% to 30% and 10% to 35%, respectively, in selected populations of older subjects.[35] Although it has been suggested that fatness, fitness, and fat distribution can account for the decline in glucose tolerance, analysis of glucose tolerance in a community-dwelling population of 742 men and women ranging in age from 17 to 92 years, participants in the BLSA, showed age to be a significant determinant of the further decline in glucose tolerance in healthy old subjects.[36] Elderly subjects tend to have a slightly higher fasting level of serum glucose (FBS) than do younger adults (Fig. 68–6). The elderly also have altered insulin response to a glucose load, which results in diagnostically significant changes in postabsorptive glucose level (Fig. 68–7). The magnitude of the change depends on the challenge; fasting blood glucose levels increase 1 to 2 mg/dL each decade throughout adult life, whereas blood glucose levels 2 hours after a meal increase by as much as 5 to 10 mg/dL each decade.[37] As little as a 50-g oral dose of glucose leads to significant change in the pattern of the glucose tolerance test.[19, 20] This relative intolerance for glucose is a consistent finding even in healthy old people.

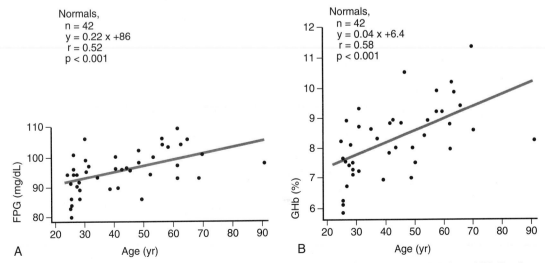

Figure 68–6. Fasting plasma glucose and glycosylated hemoglobin. (*From* Rochman H, Lubrau MM, Bradlaw BA: Clinical Pathology in the Elderly. New York, Karger, 1988. Reproduced with permission of S. Karger AG, Basel.)

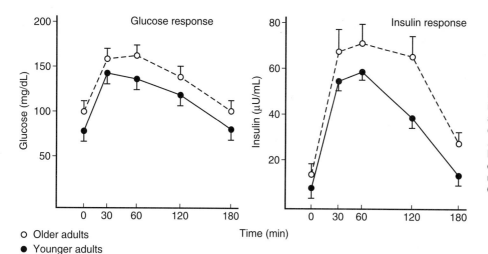

Figure 68–7. Plasma glucose and insulin concentrations over time after a 75 gram oral dose of glucose in older and younger adults. (*With permission from* Reaven GM, Chen N, Hollenbeck C, et al: Effect of age on glucose tolerance and glucose uptake in healthy individuals. J Am Geriatr Soc 37:737, 1989.)

○ Older adults
● Younger adults

In addition, the incidence of type II (maturity-onset) diabetes mellitus is higher among the elderly.[19, 20] The apparent increase in the renal threshold for glucose makes screening, diagnosis, and treatment monitoring for diabetes mellitus more difficult in the elderly.

Long-term monitoring of glycemic control is possible with measurement of glycated hemoglobin (HbA$_{1c}$). However, glycated hemoglobin increases from about 7% in healthy 25-year-olds to more than 9% in healthy people older than age 70 years (see Fig. 68–6). An increase in glycated structural and functional proteins is the basis for one of the stochastic theories of aging and appears to corroborate the belief that impairment of glucose tolerance develops with age, despite dietary restrictions and regular exercise. It has therefore been suggested that glycated hemoglobin measurements in elderly diabetics may be of only limited usefulness, although there is disagreement on this point.[38]

The relatively large changes in glucose levels that follow an oral loading dose, compared with the presumed clinically insignificant changes in FBS, would seem to point toward insulin response as the causative factor. Differences between the young and the elderly have been observed in the plasma concentration of insulin over time, following an oral glucose load.[39, 40] The postabsorptive increase in glucose is properly accompanied by an increase in insulin level. Evidence supports the hypothesis that peripheral tissues or their receptors become less sensitive to the effect of insulin. Thus, a higher insulin level, which results from a higher glucose level, is required for adequate stimulation of peripheral glucose uptake.[38] The postulated change in peripheral receptors for insulin is further supported by data showing that suppression of free fatty acids and stimulation of human growth hormone parallel the changes expected from the alteration in glucose tolerance.[18] Hyperinsulinemia is an independent risk factor for coronary artery disease.[40] The beneficial effect of regular physical exercise and weight control in moderating insulin resistance of peripheral tissues has been documented.[35, 40]

Nutritional Status

Many investigators believe that overwhelming evidence exists to require a modification or adjustment of certain micronutrient recommended dietary allowances (RDAs) for persons aged 50 to 70 years and for those older than 70 years.[41] A significant increase in knowledge of the nutritional and dietary requirements of seniors supports this conclusion. Two large studies that have provided significant amounts of data on this topic are the Boston Nutritional Status Survey, a cross-sectional survey conducted primarily on white elderly subjects older than 60 years, and the New Mexico longitudinal study of nutrition and aging, which examined healthy free-living men and women older than 60 years. Although the physiologic bases of the increased needs for certain specific micronutrients in healthy elderly is not always clear, such observations are well documented.[42] Presumably, age causes differences in metabolism that would increase the RDA above that set on the basis of observing healthy younger adults. Improved immunocompetence in healthy elderly people has been widely reported when the intake of vitamin B$_6$ exceeded the currently established RDA.[43, 44] Other vitamins for which the current RDAs seem to be too low for older adults are vitamin B$_{12}$ and vitamin D.

In the gastrointestinal tract, aging often leads to diminished secretion of gastric acid, with or without accompanying decline in availability of intrinsic factor (IF). The absorptive capacity of the small intestine is also reduced. The outcome is a decline in macronutrient and micronutrient absorption. Calcium is an essential element with key roles in the maintenance of skeletal integrity, regulation of nerve excitability, muscle contraction, and hemostasis. All calcium salts are more soluble in an acidic medium. A reduced ability of older adults to absorb calcium, in part due to a relative achlorhydria, has been suggested.[45]

Krasinski and associates[46] found serologic markers of atrophic gastritis in 32% of patients more than 60 years of age. Impaired digestion of vitamin B$_{12}$–food protein complexes in the stomach may arise from hypochlorhydria, owing to atrophic gastritis. Prevalence of *Helicobacter pylori* increases with age and correlates strongly with the presence of acute and chronic gastritis. The bacterium has been isolated from the stomach in more than 80% of the individuals older than 60 years.[47] Vitamin B$_{12}$ levels decline with advancing age. In 548 surviving members of the Framingham Study cohort, the prevalence of cobalamin deficiency was equal to or greater than 12%.[48] Many of these elderly were found to have serum vitamin B_{12} concentrations within the reference range. However, on the basis of serum concentrations of the metabolites methylmalonic acid and total homocysteine, which are sensitive indicators of tissue status of vitamin B_{12}, these elderly were found to be metabolically deficient in cobalamin. Suboptimal levels of cobalamin may produce neuropsychiatric manifestations without the development of the classic peripheral blood picture of a megaloblastic anemia. Decreased absorption of certain vitamins (B_6) and minerals (zinc and selenium) may contribute to depressed immune responsiveness.

Development of lactose intolerance is age-related. There are conflicting data with regard to calcium absorption in lactase deficiency.[45] However, the avoidance of dairy products, which are rich sources of calcium and vitamin D, jeopardizes the integrity of the individual's bones. With increased age, the concentration in the skin of provitamin D, 7-dehydrocholesterol, declines.[49] This reduces the natural ability of the body to synthesize vitamin D. In the liver, vitamin D is enzymatically hydroxylated to form 25-hydroxyvitamin D (25-OHD). Measurement of serum 25-OHD can help identify elderly at risk of calcium deficiency. Declines in renal cortical tissue restrict the body's ability to maintain calcium homeostasis by limiting the availability of the renal enzyme 1α-hydroxylase, which is responsible for catalyzing the synthesis of the active form of the vitamin, calcitriol. Calcitriol is a potent calciotropic hormone that increases calcium and phosphorus uptake in the small intestine and participates, along with parathyrin (parathyroid hormone, or PTH), in bone mineralization and absorption. There is a great deal of discussion as to what concentrations of the antioxidant vitamins—C, E, and β-carotene (provitamin A)—are appropriate to meet the needs of healthy seniors. Because of the potential relationship of oxidant damage to the aging process, as well as to the development of cancer, cataract, and cardiovascular disease, an extraordinary amount of public and professional interest is focused on the possible health benefits of these micronutrients.

Anemia

The frequency with which the whole blood hemoglobin level is used as a screening test for anemia has prompted many studies investigating this criterion for detecting anemia in the elderly. These studies have focused mainly on factors related to synthesis of hemoglobin and erythrocytes, because there is no evidence for altered erythrocyte destruction in the healthy aged population.[18] There is a slight increase (approximately 4.5 mOsm/kg) of water required for 50% hemolysis in an osmotic fragility test, indicating the presence of spherocytes in the blood of elderly people.[18] On the other hand, there is a gradual tendency toward a slightly increased average cell size as measured by the mean cell volume (MCV). Increased variability in the size of circulating erythrocytes may be indicated by these apparently discrepant findings.[18]

Regional and national surveys have shown that the mean dietary iron intake of elderly men and women meets the RDA of 10 mg/day. However, most investigators report changes in laboratory measures of iron status in the elderly, which perhaps are due to achlorhydria that inhibits ferric iron absorption, or to a marginal status of vitamin C, which enhances intestinal uptake of nonheme iron.[39] Serum iron level decreases with age, and serum ferritin as well as bone marrow iron stores increases, indicating impaired uptake of iron by erythrocyte precursors.[9, 18] In patients with iron deficiency anemia, reduced serum iron usually stimulates a raised serum transferrin level, but transferrin is little changed in the elderly despite their low iron levels.[9, 18] This finding may be due to limited hepatic synthesis of transferrin or to development of a new set point for regulation that perhaps is mediated by altered membrane receptors.[18]

Macrocytic anemia may occur in older adults with marginal or inadequate folate or vitamin B_{12} status. The mean and median concentrations of serum vitamin B_{12} are distinctly lower in aged adults than in younger adults.[9] Serum folate levels decrease between 60 and 90 years of age,[39] but after age 90, values increase and more closely approximate the concentrations found in younger adults.

Bone marrow cellularity decreases 50% during the first 30 years of life, then stabilizes until age 70 years, and subsequently decreases an additional 40% during the following decade.[18] This is thought to reflect an increase in bone marrow fat rather than an absolute decrease in hematopoietic cells, and probably does not reflect any true decrease in potential erythrocyte production rate. Nevertheless, hemoglobin level and erythrocyte count (RBC), which are both constant in men until age 40, gradually decrease until age 70, when a marked decrease parallels the change in bone marrow cellularity. After a rise in values following menopause, women follow the same pattern of change.[18] The significance of these changes is obscured by the fact that there are also increases in the variances of hemoglobin and RBC in older age groups, which result in no change in the average values (per red blood cell) of mean corpuscular hemoglobin (MCH) and mean corpuscular hemoglobin concentration (MCHC).[18] Thus, Htoo and colleagues[50] have rejected the necessity for age-adjusted reference values for erythrocyte parameters in the elderly, on the basis of results of their study of 292 subjects between the ages of 65 and 100 years. Exclusion of only 17 donors from the data pool in this study resulted in identical ranges for RBC, hemoglobin, hematocrit, and red cell indices in the elderly and in younger adults.[50] Dybkaer and associates,[51] in an attempt to reconcile these findings, reviewed 90 publications and derived relative median values of erythrocyte parameters using 30-year-old men as the basis for comparison. These latter researchers confirmed the tendency for age-related decreases in RBC, hemoglobin, hematocrit, iron, and transferrin for men, and for women after menopause.

Cardiovascular and Respiratory Systems

Few tests are available in the routine clinical laboratory that specifically measure pulmonary function; however, blood gas results accurately reflect the decrease in vital capacity that is found in the elderly. Arterial PaO_2 decreases approximately 5% every 15 years starting in the 30s, and $PaCO_2$ increases approximately 2% per decade after age 50.[19] There is also a corresponding, compensating slight increase in bicarbonate with age, such that arterial pH does not change.

Cardiovascular disease (CVD) is the primary cause of death among elderly in the United States. Coronary atherosclerosis, with or without symptoms, occurs in a major proportion of the elderly. Age-related organ changes affecting the cardiovascular system are mostly anatomic and include fibrosis, calcification, and the deposition of lipofuscin, amyloid, and cholesterol in arteries and arterioles and in the heart muscle, its lining and covering, and valves.[18] Intense interest in plasma levels of homocysteine centers on determining whether the amino acid (1) is damaging to the vascular endothelium and directly involved in the pathogenesis of vascular disease, or (2) merely a biochemical marker of increased risk for cardiovascular disease. Levels of total homocysteine (tHcy) are higher in men than in women, though not all studies are in agreement, and increase with age. Sex hormones may play a part in these age and gender differences. Reduced tHcy levels have been reported in postmenopausal women who are receiving estrogen replacement therapy.[52, 53]

Some laboratory tests are used almost exclusively to monitor the pathologic consequences of atherosclerosis, for example, enzyme tests for the diagnosis and prognosis of myocardial and cerebral infarctions. The sequence and predictive value of elevated serum levels of creatine kinase (CK), aspartate aminotransferase (AST), and lactate dehydrogenase (LD) following myocardial infarction are well known, and newer markers, such as Troponin I and T, are being evaluated. Although fewer than 25% of patients with cerebral infarction show elevation of these serum enzymes, levels of CK, AST, and hydroxybutyrate dehydrogenase (a measure of LD isoenzyme 1 [LD-1]) correlate inversely with survival time.[18] Remarkably, there is a weakly positive correlation between the levels of these serum enzymes and the time-to-discharge for survivors of cerebral infarctions.

Because of these findings, it is important to note that serum CK activity in women is 15% to 20% less at all ages than in men. Overall, women show a reduction in enzyme activity of about 2% after 60 years, when lean body mass, total body weight, and physical activity typically decline.[54] CK activity in men falls after age 60 years by about 7%. The drop in CK activity may be due not just to decrease in muscle mass but to a substantial decrease in CK activity in muscle itself.[39] In both sexes, a slight increase in CK activity is noted in patients in their 60s, a decrease after age 70, and a marked decrease after age 90. In populations 90 years and older, the CK-MB isoenzyme has been reported to decrease so dramatically that it may be virtually undetectable by electrophoresis.[39]

Modest increases in AST activity have been reported by some, though not all, researchers for both older men and women, when compared with young adults.[9] Although controversial, it appears that in both men and women older than 60 years, there is a 10% increase in total LD activity.[54] Slight decreases with age have been observed for the LD-5 isoenzyme.[39] Changes in AST and LD levels are insufficient to interfere with their interpretation after either cardiac or cerebral infarction. In frail elderly patients, total CK levels may remain within reference range even in an acute myocardial infarction.

Serum lipid and lipoprotein measurements reflect the propensity for development of atherosclerosis. As in middle-aged adults, an elevated serum cholesterol level in seniors should be interpreted as a risk factor for coronary heart disease.[55] Data from the Framingham Heart Study indicates that in persons 60 to 70 years of age, a 1% increase in serum total cholesterol (TC), although not a direct measurement of the magnitude of arterial plaque formation, produces a 2% increase in incidence of CVD. Age-adjusted reference ranges for serum cholesterol have been advocated by some, and the magnitude of the average increase with age is significant.[18] TC and low-density lipoprotein (LDL) cholesterol have been found to be significantly higher in "old-old" (75 years or older) than in "young-old" (aged 65 to 74 years) persons.[56] A representative study of cholesterol levels in fasting healthy adults between 25 and 79 years of age showed an increase of approximately 40 mg/dL in median serum cholesterol level between ages 60 and 79. A similar increase was observed in a large study of healthy men and women, in the same age range, in which there was no standardization of fasting by the subjects.[18]

High-density lipoprotein (HDL) cholesterol level is inversely related to the risk of CVD. HDL cholesterol has been reported to increase significantly for men aged 60 to 79 years, compared with the levels in men aged 25 to 44 years and 45 to 59 years.[18] HDL cholesterol subfractions may be especially useful in determining cardiovascular health among the elderly. In particular, it may be HDL_2 that is the most "protective" subfraction of HDL cholesterol. Waller and associates[56] found significantly higher levels of HDL cholesterol, HDL_2, HDL_3, and apolipoprotein A-I in a group of older women (mean age about 73 years) than among the male subjects of essentially the same age.[56] The median triglyceride level also shows a tendency to increase with age, although to a lesser extent than the cholesterol level.[57]

The development of methods for fractionating different lipoproteins and for measuring their apolipoproteins has improved the specificity of age-related changes in serum lipid levels. Apolipoproteins may be more sensitive indices of cardiovascular disease than total cholesterol, HDL cholesterol, or triglycerides. A study of 286 men and 289 women aged 27 to 67 years reported that serum apolipoprotein (apo) B and lipoprotein (a) [Lp(a)] concentrations increase with age. There is a substantial correlation of apolipoprotein B with both LDL cholesterol and TC. Individuals with high concentrations of apo B have shown a high prevalence of atherosclerotic disease. Increased atherogenesis and thrombogenesis have been observed in patients with elevated serum Lp(a).[58] Another study of healthy, fasting men between ages 20 and 76 years confirmed the peak in cholesterol and triglyceride values between 40 and 60 years, and the gradual rise with age in HDL cholesterol values. Furthermore, by measuring the apolipoprotein markers of lipoproteins, this study explained that the inverse relationship between very-low-density lipoprotein (VLDL) and HDL is an indicator of successful conversion of VLDL into HDL and, thus, successful metabolism of VLDL triglyceride and VLDL cholesterol. VLDL and HDL, which both contain apolipoproteins C and E, were measured in heparin-magnesium^{+2}–precipitated serum. The amount of cholesterol contained in the precipitated VLDL particles was sharply higher in age-matched patients with angiographically demonstrated cardiovascular disease than in normal donors. The concentrations of apolipoproteins B, C-III, and E followed the same pattern as the concentration of VLDL cholesterol.[59] Clinical testing of these analytes permits identification of high-risk individuals in whom biochemical abnormality predates the occurrence of symptoms of atherosclerotic disease or predicts the presence of arterial plaques or the severity of vascular occlusion. Although higher amounts of total and LDL cholesterol and triglycerides have been reported in elderly subjects, it is not clear whether aging increases LDL oxidizability, enhancing its atherogenicity.[60]

Leukocytes and the Immune Response

The number of total leukocytes and the proportions of monocytes and eosinophils are virtually constant from ages 30 years to 80 years.[18] Neutrophils increase slightly in men and decrease slightly in women during the same age interval, and it is not yet certain whether their function changes with age. The relative constancy of total lymphocyte count with aging belies the significant changes in lymphocyte subsets that occur.

The involution of the thymus during early adulthood and the corresponding decreases in its hormones are well documented. Thymopoietin begins to decline at age 30 years and reaches undetectable levels after age 60.[19] Using monoclonal antibodies to the T3 lymphocyte antigen, several studies have reported conflicting results as to whether total T lymphocytes decrease with age. However, monoclonal antibodies to the CD4 and CD8 surface antigens yield evidence for age-related shifts in the relative numbers of T cells differentiated into the subsets of T-helper lymphocytes (CD4$^+$) and T-suppressor (CD8$^+$) lymphocytes. The ratio of CD4$^+$ to CD8$^+$ T cells increases with advancing age.[61] It is the balance between these T-cell subsets that preserves the normal functioning of the immune response. CD4$^+$ T cells are composed of two major populations, naive T cells and memory T cells. With advancing age, a change within these T-cell subsets occurs. There is a decrease in naive T cells and a concomitant increase in memory T cells. Naive cells mainly produce interleukin-2, which is responsible for T-cell proliferation. Memory cells mainly produce interleukin-4 and interleukin-6, which are responsible for differentiation and proliferation of B cells. It has been suggested that decreased T-cell proliferation in the elderly is related to the decrease in number of naive T cells. Age-related increase in memory T cells could explain the observed rise in the number of antibody-producing cells in tissues and higher serum levels of immunoglobulins (Igs) A and M.[61]

A change in the absolute number of T lymphocytes or fewer mitogen-responsive cells in the T-cell pool may account for the observed decrease in mitogenic responsiveness of T cells with aging. The magnitude of diminished responsiveness, which begins at about age 40, results in only half the proliferative response to mitogens added to T-cell cultures from the 80-year and 90-year age groups as is found in cells from young adult donors. These in vitro findings correlate with an in vivo higher incidence of anergy, that is, a delayed-type hypersensitivity response to antigens, in adults older than 60 years.[62] This lack of differentiation into T-helper and T-suppressor cells also accounts for the decrease seen in sheep red blood cell rosette formation, because this test is a measure of mature T cells.[63, 64]

Circulating levels of natural antibodies, for example, blood group antibodies, begin to decline in young adulthood and reach 50% levels or less at age 80 years.[64] Formation of antibodies to new antigens, such as pneumococcal polysaccharide, parainfluenza virus, and tetanus toxoid, is also impaired in the elderly, contributing to their greater susceptibility to infection.[63, 65] Fortunately, proper booster sequence and strain-matching do result in protective active immunization for the elderly in epidemics.

On the other hand, the incidence of autoantibodies—rheumatoid factor, antinuclear protein, and antithyroglobulin—increases markedly with age.[63] Both the lack of appropriate (natural and acquired) antibodies and the presence of inappropriate (autoimmune) antibodies are thought to reflect lack of T-helper cell and T-suppressor cell influences on B cells, rather than an intrinsic age-related change in B cells.[62]

Nevertheless, serum IgG and IgA levels rise with age, and IgM levels fall.[61] The IgM decrease corresponds to the decrease in blood group antibodies and the relative lack of an initial response to immunogens, whereas the IgG increase may reflect the ability to maintain responsiveness to antigens previously encountered. Total serum globulins in men tend to be slightly higher after age 55 years, whereas values in women tend to increase until menopause and then level off.[18]

Infections are less likely to produce fever in the aged.[18] This condition may be a failure in the leukocyte protection system that prohibits release of pyrogens from invading organisms; such a theory is consistent with depressed neutrophil function, which is implied by their decreased chemiluminescence. However, results of other tests of neutrophil function that measure chemotaxis and phagocytosis, and of the nitroblue-tetrazolium test, have not conclusively shown depression of the inflammatory response in the elderly.[18]

Alternative explanations for lack of fever are depression of the specific hypothalamic response to endogenous pyrogen (interleukin-1) and a generalized suppression of the hypothalamus or the autonomic system.[18] In any case, this suppression is consistent with the inverse relationship between body temperature and infectious morbidity and also contributes to the well-known increase in sensitivity and vulnerability to cold seen in the elderly.

Hepatic Function

Both smaller hepatic mass and reduced organ blood flow are reported with aging, and alterations may affect the clearance of drugs metabolized in the liver.[47] Liver volume declines by about 28%, and hepatic blood flow decreases 25% to 35%, between the ages of 30 and 75 years.[35, 66] Decreased microsomal enzyme activity and diminished response to enzyme-inducing agents have been reported in some studies on animals, but it remains unclear whether hepatic enzyme function degrades with aging in humans.[67] Essentially, clinical assays for hepatic enzymes and tests

Table 68–3. Summary of Enzyme Changes With Aging

Enzyme	Trend over 60	
	Male	*Female*
Acid phosphatase	15%–20% increase due to prostatic component	10% increase from all sources other than prostate
Alanine aminotransferase	Decreases but maintains 10–15 U/L above female value	Decreases but remains less than male value
Alkaline phosphatase	At 60, male values equal female values At 70, male values exceed female values	
Amylase	At 60, P isoenzyme falls to 40% total At 80, P isoenzyme at 20% total	Similar to male trend
Aspartate aminotransferase	Slight increase remaining; higher than female value	Increases but remains 10% lower than male value
Catalase	Slight decrease after 60	Decreases also, but about 5% lower than male value
Creatine kinase	In white males, declines about 7%–10% related to physical condition In black males, also declines, but remains above white activity	Also declines with changes in physical activity and remains 10%–15% less than in males
γ-Glutamyltransferase	About 5%–10% increase	Also increases, but remains 10% less than male value
Glutathione reductase and peroxidase	Unchanged	Unchanged
Lactate dehydrogenase	About 10% increase in total activity	Similar to male trend
Lipase	Slight but gradual increase in total activity	Similar to male trend
Lecithin cholesterol acyltransferase	Remains constant	Similar to male trend

From Griffiths JC: Enzyme changes in healthy older individuals. *In* Faulkner WR, Meites S (eds): Geriatric Clinical Chemistry: Reference Values. Washington, DC, AACC Press, 1994.

of synthetic function do not seem to be substantially affected by aging. However, hepatic conversion of vitamin D to 25-OHD has been reported to decline in older adults.[68]

The synthetic function of the liver is reflected in the concentration of plasma proteins. A gross indicator of plasma protein concentration is the erythrocyte sedimentation rate (ESR), which rises in adults at a rate of 0.22 mm/hr per year because of the corresponding small increases in globulins and fibrinogen.[18] The change in ESR is not related to mortality[18] and has little clinical value because of large interperson variation.[18]

The lower limit, the median, and the mean of the total protein reference range decrease slightly with age.[39] Serum albumin levels decline by 10% to 15% between the ages of 30 and 80 years.[67] Therefore, total serum protein concentration is virtually constant after age 55, because increases in acute phase reactants (e.g., α_1-acid glycoprotein) and globulins are offset by a decrease in albumin.[28, 47] Although this decrease is insufficient to be symptomatic, it may reflect decreasing reserve capacity of the liver and may relate to altered carrier capacity of albumin, for example, protein-bound drugs or calcium. Decreased concentrations of the carrier protein transferrin are seen in the elderly, being lowest in centenarians.[39] Apolipoprotein (apo) A-I concentrations have been reported to be unrelated to age, but apo B and Lp(a) concentrations are age dependent.[58] Decreased albumin level is also a common, nonspecific finding in many illnesses, and the elderly when ill show a decrease to lower levels than younger adults, which may be significant for adjustment of dosages of therapeutic drugs used to treat the illness.[28, 66, 67] Decreased albumin causes an increase in the competition among different drugs for the remaining protein-binding sites, and tends to enlarge the active (non–protein-bound) fraction of a drug. Because

this is coupled with decreases in hepatic blood flow, which reduces the rate of inactivation of a drug, and renal filtration, and with a significantly smaller volume of distribution, therapeutic drug monitoring is especially important in the elderly.[28, 66, 67, 69]

Hepatic enzymes may increase, decrease, or show no change during aging (Table 68–3). Enzyme patterns are highly individualized.[54] The physiologic bases for these changes, when they do occur, are not always clear. Endocrine changes associated with aging or hormone therapy may account for some observed variations in enzyme profiles. AST and LD rise slightly in older women.[9, 19, 54] Although alanine aminotransferase (ALT) declines in both men and women after age 60 years, estrogen preparations increase hepatic ALT.

In older women, alkaline phosphatase (ALP) significantly rises during the years spanning the menopause and shows a 40% increase in activity compared with values in younger women.[18, 39] This increase is commonly attributed to hormonal changes but may also be due to illness such as subclinical osteomalacia associated with secondary hyperparathyroidism. Although women's ALP activity values are lower than for men in all age groups, women's values reached those of men between the ages of 60 and 90 years.[39] ALP activity in elderly men is about 10% greater than in young men.[54] Men show no increase in ALP activity until after 90 years of age.[39] The liver isoenzyme of ALP increases sufficiently to account for this change.

A marked rise in γ-glutamyltranspeptidase (GGT), a more sensitive indicator of hepatobiliary dysfunction, is observed in both men and women between the ages of 60 and 90 years; in men, an increase in ALP activity has been observed only after 90 years of age.[39] On the basis of these findings, it seems prudent that ALP reference ranges should consider the patient's age. Serum bilirubin levels, which also reflect the excretory function of the liver and hepatobiliary integrity, decrease slightly, if at all.[19, 39]

Musculoskeletal System

The volume of muscle is smaller in the elderly. It is important to note, therefore, especially among seniors of slight build, that serum levels of the muscle enzyme creatine kinase may not exceed the enzyme reference range, even in the event of myocardial infarction. Reduced muscle mass, in the absence of overt muscle disease, may also account for minimal change in serum creatinine, even as glomerular filtration declines with aging. In healthy bone, formation and absorption are tightly coupled and bone is lost when an imbalance exists between the rates of these two processes.[70] Bone loss normally accompanies aging,[71] but there is disagreement among researchers as to which factor is of greater importance.[72] Chapter 69 discusses osteoporosis and bone loss in the elderly.

Thyroid Function

Reports on the anatomic effects of aging on the thyroid gland are conflicting. Some, though not all, studies describe a decrease in size. There is agreement that the thyroid becomes more nodular with age. Despite fibrotic changes, decreased colloid, and obliteration of follicles, it is generally accepted that marked changes in serum thyroid hormone levels do not accompany aging[73] (Table 68–4). An abnormal thyroid function test should never be attributed to aging per se.

The incidence of both hypothyroidism and hyperthyroidism rises in the elderly; they present a difficult diagnostic problem because of atypical or more subtle clinical presentation; for instance, skin condition, mental clarity, heat and cold intolerance, and neuromuscular irritability are commonly altered in the elderly population. Postmenopausal women taking thyroid hormone are at risk of developing osteoporosis. However, estrogen therapy reverses the adverse effects of thyroid hormone on bone mineral density.[74]

Table 68–4. Common Age-Related Changes in Thyroid Function Tests

Decreased	No Change	Increased
T$_3$ (maybe)	T$_4$	TSH (in women)
T$_4$ degradation	TSH	
T$_3$ degradation	TSH response to TRH (in women)	
T$_4$ production		
T$_3$ production	Reverse T$_3$	
RAIU		
TSH response to TRH (in men)		
TSH sensitivity to T$_4$		
Circadian TSH variation		

Abbreviations: RAIU, radioactive iodine uptake; T$_3$, triiodothyronine; T$_4$, thyroxine; TRH, thyrotropin-releasing hormone; TSH, thyroid-stimulating hormone.
From Mooradian AP: Normal age-related changes in thyroid hormone economy. Clin Geriatr Med 11:159, 1995.

Table 68–5. Similarities and Dissimilarities Between the Clinical Manifestations of Hypothyroidism and Changes Commonly Seen in Elderly Subjects

	Hypothyroidism	Aging
Slow mentation	Yes	Yes
Delayed relaxation phase of deep tendon reflexes	Yes	Yes
Muscle fatigue	Yes	Yes
Cold intolerance	Yes	Yes
Decreased appetite	Yes	Yes
Depression	Yes	Yes
Constipation	Yes	Yes
Hair loss	Yes	Yes
Dry skin	Yes	Yes
Gynecomastia	Yes	Yes
Decreased libido	Yes	Yes
Bradycardia	Yes	Relatively
Hypertension	Yes	Yes
Osteoporosis	No	Yes
Increased adiposity	No	Yes
Decreased water excretion capacity	Yes	Yes

From Mooradian AD: Normal age-related changes in thyroid hormone economy. Clin Geriatr Med 11:159, 1995.

Although there appear to be a multitude of biologic changes in the hypothalamic-pituitary-thyroid axis, steady-state plasma concentrations of thyroid hormones do not seem to change much with age, unless there are concurrent disease or nutritional problems.[73] Thyroxine (T$_4$) levels may be virtually constant across the age span 30 to 80 years. Serum triiodothyronine (T$_3$) concentrations are modestly reduced, without an increase in serum reverse T$_3$ (rT$_3$). A major portion of T$_3$ normally arises from peripheral deiodination of T$_4$; therefore, some investigators have suggested that a lower T$_3$ level may be secondary to peripheral body changes and would not necessarily indicate a functional change in the thyroid gland itself. The amounts of thyroid-binding globulin (TBG) and T$_3$ resin uptake (T$_3$RU)—an index of plasma protein T$_3$ binding capacity—do not change with age.[39, 73] Some investigators have noted, but others cannot confirm, that thyroid-stimulating hormone (TSH) increases slightly with age.[39] Age-related changes in thyroid hormone action may be due to altered tissue responsiveness to the thyroid hormone. Comparison of the similarities between the classic presentation of hypothyroidism and changes commonly observed in healthy elderly lend support to this belief[73] (Table 68–5). Interestingly, the response to a thyrotropin-releasing hormone stimulation test is suppressed in older men, but not in older women, possibly reflecting a sexual difference in set point, because the T$_4$ level in women is about 10% higher than in men throughout life.[18, 73]

DEFINING REFERENCE RANGES FOR THE ELDERLY

Major problems exist in defining reference ranges for the elderly. On the one hand, most studies are cross-sectional rather than longitudinal, and thus, only survivors are available to be studied at advanced age. This may skew the data toward apparent better health. On the other hand, the occurrence of multiple disorders, many of which have atypical presentation or are clinically silent in the elderly, may contaminate a data collection and skew it toward apparently poorer health. The combination of these two opposing possibilities probably contributes to the wider range of values seen for many laboratory tests performed on the elderly.[18] An additional point of contention is whether it is appropriate to apply reference ranges determined from healthy, ambulatory people to the interpretation of results from sick, hospitalized patients irrespective of their ages.[18] Despite their increasing proportion in the population, it remains difficult to recruit substantial numbers of elderly people for reference studies.

It is also very difficult to define reference sets of donors so that changes in laboratory values that are due to aging can be separated from the changing incidence of a disease that occurs with aging. One approach is to compare the data between groups of people who are known to have different incidences of the relevant disease in the population. Using this approach, Larson and Wilson compared the incidence of glucose intolerance in Australians (in whom it is fairly common in the general population) to its incidence in Eskimos (in whom it is much less common in the general population).[74] Because elderly groups from both populations showed decreased tolerance to glucose, the study concluded that this change is due to age. Although highly advantageous, it is obviously not possible to conduct such comparison studies for all laboratory tests.

All of the arguments about reference ranges apply to the elderly as to the young. This discussion of trends and changes has attempted to point out age-related alterations in laboratory test results that appear to be independent of specific diseases. What may be seen in geriatric values compared with the same analytes in younger adults are that the range, median, and mean of the reference ranges increase along with the age ranges. Combined with the diagnostic criteria cited in other chapters of this book, the wealth of data now becoming available on individuals 65 years of age and older should substantially improve the understanding of laboratory results obtained from the elderly.[18] As the population ages and places even more demands on limited health care resources, it is all the more essential that we better understand the aging process. Our success in differentiating disease from aging will contribute to the prompt identification and management of chronic, degenerative disorders that diminish the quality, if not the quantity, of life.

References

1. Rowe JW, Wang S: The biology and physiology of aging. In Rowe JE, Besdine RW (eds): Geriatric Medicine, ed 2. Boston, Little, Brown, 1988.
2. Cassel CK, Brody JA: Demography, epidemiology, and aging. In Cassel CK, Riesenberg DE, Sorenson LB, et al (eds): Geriatric Medicine, ed 2. New York, Springer-Verlag, 1990.
3. Spencer G: Projections of the Population of the United States by Age, Sex and Race: 1988 to 2080. (Current Population Reports. Series P-25. No. 1018.) Washington, DC, U.S. Bureau of the Census, 1989.
4. Aiken LR: Aging; An Introduction to Gerontology. Thousand Oaks, Cal, Sage Publications, 1995.
5. Taeuber CM: Sixty-five plus in America. (U.S. Bureau of the Census, Current Population Reports, Special Studies, P23-178RV.) Washington, DC, U.S. Government Printing Office, 1993.
6. Fowles D: A Profile of Older Americans. Washington, DC, American Association of Retired Persons, 1991.
7. Garry P: The elderly population in the United States. In Faulkner WR, Meites S (eds): Geriatric Clinical Chemistry: Reference Values. Washington, DC, AACC Press, 1994.
8. Espino DV: Ethnogeriatrics. Clin Geriatr Med 11:1, 1995.
9. Faulkner WR, Meites S (eds): Geriatric Clinical Chemistry: Reference Values. Washington, DC, AACC Press, 1994.
10. Crandall RC: Gerontology: A Behavioral Science Approach, ed 2. New York, McGraw-Hill, 1991.
11. Schneider E, Guralnik J: The aging of America: Impact on health care costs. JAMA 263:2335, 1990.
12. Rusting R: Why do we age? Sci Am 267:131, 1992.
13. Abrass IB: The biology and physiology of aging. West J Med 153:641, 1990.
14. Vijg J, Wei JY: Understanding the biology of aging: The key to prevention and therapy. J Am Geriatr Soc 43:426, 1995.
15. Knight JA: The process and theories of aging. Ann Clin Lab Sci 25:1, 1995.
16. Bendich A: Antioxidant micronutrients and immune responses. Ann N Y Acad Sci 587:168, 1990.
17. Bankson D, Kestin M, Rifai N: Role of free radicals in cancer and atherosclerosis. Clin Lab Med 13:463, 1993.
18. Aldrich J: Geriatric changes in laboratory results. In Davis B, Bishop ML, Mass D (eds): Clinical Laboratory Science: Strategies for Practice. Philadelphia, JB Lippincott, 1989.
19. Timiras PS: Physiological Basis of Geriatrics. New York, Macmillan, 1988.
20. Rochman H: Clinical Pathology in the Elderly: A Textbook of Laboratory Interpretations. Basel, Karger, 1988.
21. Young CH: The chemistry of aging. Lab Manage 26:16, 1988.
22. Gorman LS: Aging: Laboratory testing and theories. Clin Lab Sci 8:24, 1995.
23. Perrone RD, Madias NE, Levey AS: Serum creatinine as an index of renal function: New insights into old concepts. Clin Chem 38:1933, 1992.
24. Sica D: Renal disease, electrolyte abnormalities, and acid-base imbalance in the elderly. Clin Geriatr Med 10:197, 1994.
25. Rowe J: Renal system. In Rowe JW, Besdine RW (eds): Geriatric Medicine, ed 2. Boston, Little, Brown, 1988.
26. Anderson S, Brenner BM: Effects of aging on the renal glomerulus. Am J Med 80:435, 1986.
27. Lindeman RD: Assessment of renal function in the old: Special considerations. Clin Lab Med 13:269, 1993.
28. Annesley TM: Special considerations for geriatric therapeutic drug monitoring. Clin Chem 35:1337, 1989.
29. Mersey JH: Diabetes mellitus in the elderly patient. In Reichel W (ed): Clinical Aspects of Aging, ed 3. Baltimore, Williams & Wilkins, 1989.
30. Meyer BR: Renal function in aging. J Am Geriatr Soc 37:791, 1989.
31. Holick M: McCollum Award Lecture, 1994: Vitamin D—new horizons for the 21st century. Am J Clin Nutr 60:619, 1994.
32. Heaney R: Bone mass, nutrition, and other lifestyle factors. Am J Clin Nutr 95(Suppl):1213S, 1993.
33. Ouslander JG: Geriatric urinary incontinence. Disease-a-Month 38:1, 1992.
34. Fox RA, Horan MA: Genitourinary infection. In Fox RA (ed): Immunology and Infection in the Elderly. New York, Churchill Livingstone, 1984.
35. Broughton DL, Taylor R: A review: Deterioration of glucose tolerance with age: The role of insulin resistance. Age Ageing 20:221, 1991.
36. Shimokata H, Muller DC, Fleg JL, et al: Age as independent determinant of glucose tolerance. Diabetes 40:44, 1991.
37. Riesenberg D. Diabetes mellitus. In Cassel CK, Riesenberg DE, Sorenson LB, et al (eds): Geriatric Medicine, ed 2. New York, Springer-Verlag, 1990.
38. Mulkerrin EC, Arnold JD, Dewar R, et al: Glycosylated haemoglobin in the diagnosis of diabetes mellitus in elderly people. Age Ageing 21:175, 1992.
39. Tietz NW, Shuey DF, Wekstein DR: Laboratory values in fit aging individuals—sexagenarians through centenarians. Clin Chem 38:1167, 1992.
40. Reaven GM, Chen N, Hollenbeck C, et al: Effect of age on glucose tolerance and glucose uptakes in healthy individuals. J Am Geriatr Soc 37:735, 1989.

41. Russell RM, Suter PM: Vitamin requirements of elderly people: An update. Am J Clin Nutr 58:4, 1993.
42. Chandra RK: Effects of vitamin and trace-element supplementation on immune responses and infection in the elderly. Lancet 340:1124, 1992.
43. Meydani SN: Vitamin/mineral supplementation, the aging immune response, and risk of infection. Nutr Rev 51:106, 1993.
44. Talbott MC, Miller LT, Kerkvliet NI: Pyridoxine supplementation: Effect on lymphocyte responses in elderly persons. Am J Clin Nutr 46:659, 1987.
45. Levenson DI, Bockman RS: A review of calcium preparations. Nutr Rev 52:221, 1994.
46. Krasinski SD, Russell RM, Samloff M, et al: Fundic atrophic gastritis in an elderly population: Effect on hemoglobin and several serum nutritional indicators. J Am Geriatr Soc 34:800, 1986.
47. Shamburek RD, Farrar JT: Disorders of the digestive tract in the elderly. N Engl J Med 322:438, 1990.
48. Lindebaum J, Rosenberg IH, Wilson PWF, et al: Prevalence of cobalamin deficiency in the Framingham elderly population. Am J Clin Nutr 60:2, 1994.
49. Holick M: Environmental factors that influence the cutaneous production of vitamin D. Am J Clin Nutr 61(Suppl):638S, 1995.
50. Htoo MSH, Kofkoff RL, Freedman ML: Erythrocyte parameters in the elderly: An argument against new geriatric normal values. J Am Geriatr Soc 27:547, 1979.
51. Dybkaer R, Lauritzen M, Krakauer R: Relative reference values for clinical chemistry and haematologic quantities in "healthy" elderly people. Acta Med Scand 209:1, 1981.
52. Nygard O, Voilset SE, Refsum H, et al: Total plasma homocysteine and cardiovascular risk profile. JAMA 274:1526, 1995.
53. Ubbink JB, Vermaak WJH, van der Merwe A, et al: Vitamin B-12, vitamin B-6, and folate nutritional status in men with hyperhomocysteinemia. Am J Clin Nutr 57:47, 1993.
54. Griffiths JC: Enzyme changes in healthy older adults. *In* Faulkner WR, Meites S (eds): Geriatric Clinical Chemistry: Reference Values. Washington, DC, AACC Press, 1994.
55. Benfante R, Reed D: Is elevated serum cholesterol level a risk factor for coronary heart disease in the elderly? JAMA 263:393, 1990.
56. Waller KV, Ward KM, Rudmann SV: Serum lipids, lipoproteins, and apolipoproteins in the healthy elderly. Lab Med 23:109, 1992.
57. West DW, Ash O: Adult reference intervals for 12 chemistry analyses: Influences of age and sex. Am J Clin Pathol 81:71, 1984.
58. Leino A, Impivaara O, Kaitsaari M, et al: Serum concentrations of apolipoprotein A-1, apolipoprotein B, and lipoprotein(a) in a population sample. Clin Chem 41:1633, 1995.
59. Alaupovic P, Knight C, Downs D: Age-related changes in the plasma apolipoproteins of normolipidemic men and male patients with angiographically documented coronary artery disease. *In* Schneider J, Kaffarnik H (eds): Lipoproteins and Age: International Symposium in Marburg, 1980. New York, Thieme-Stratton, 1982.
60. Schmuck A, Fuller CJ, Devaraj S, et al: Effect of aging on susceptibility of low-density lipoproteins to oxidation. Clin Chem 41:1628, 1995.
61. Hirokawa K: Understanding the mechanism of the age-related decline in immune function. Nutr Rev 50:361, 1992.
62. Burns EA, Goodwin JS: Immunology and infectious disease. *In* Cassel CK, Riesenberg DE, Sorenson LB, et al (eds): Geriatric Medicine, ed 2. New York, Springer-Verlag, 1990.
63. Weksler ME: The senescence of the immune system. Hosp Pract 16:53, 1981.
64. Hallgren HM: Immune response alterations during human aging. J Med Technol 2:685, 1985.
65. Schwab R, Walters CA, Weksler ME: Host defense mechanisms and aging. Semin Oncol 16:20, 1989.
66. Nielsen C: Pharmacologic considerations in critical care of the elderly. Clin Geriatr Med 10:71, 1994.
67. Annesley T: Pharmacokinetic changes in the elderly. Clin Lab Sci 3:100, 1990.
68. Edwards BJ, Perry HM III: Age-related osteoporosis. Clin Geriatr Med 10:575, 1994.
69. Warner A: Therapeutic drug monitoring in the elderly. *In* Faulkner WR, Meites S (eds): Geriatric Clinical Chemistry: Reference Values. Washington, DC, AACC Press, 1994.
70. Marcus R: Understanding osteoporosis. West J Med 155:53, 1991.
71. Gunby MC, Morley JE: Epidemiology of bone loss with aging. Clin Geriatr Med 10:557, 1994.
72. Nordin BEC, Need AG, Horowitz M, et al: Treatment of osteoporosis in the elderly. Clin Geriatr Med 10:625, 1994.
73. Mooradian AD: Normal age-related changes in thyroid hormone economy. Clin Geriatr Med 11:159, 1995.
74. Schneider DL, Barrett-Conner EL, Morton DJ, et al: Thyroid hormone use and bone mineral density in elderly women: Effects of estrogen. JAMA 271:245, 1994.

Chapter 69

Osteoporosis

Donna Spannaus-Martin

ETIOLOGY AND PATHOPHYSIOLOGY

Normal Bone Remodeling

The remodeling of bone is primarily the result of two tightly linked processes, the resorption of old bone by osteoclasts and the formation of new bone by osteoblasts. The rates of these two processes are variable throughout the different stages of life. In childhood and young adulthood, more bone is being formed than is being resorbed, which results in a net increase in bone volume. Peak bone mass is achieved sometime in early adulthood, and, for a period of time, bone mass remains relatively stable, with an equal amount of bone resorption and formation occurring. Eventually, the process of bone resorption occurs more rapidly than the formation of new bone, resulting in a loss of bone mass that gradually diminishes skeletal integrity. When the loss of bone mass is to the extent that enhanced bone fragility and increased risk of fracture occurs, the resulting condition is termed *osteoporosis.*

Bone remodeling occurs in a series of steps, beginning with an initial activation of the bone from a quiescent state to an active state. Activation is achieved by means of enzymes that dissolve an unmineralized layer of organic collagenous material to expose the mineralized portion of the bone. This allows the osteoclasts to attach to the calcified bone surface and to dissolve the mineral portion by acidification and hydrolyze the organic matrix by proteolytic digestion.

The osteoclasts are replaced by preosteoblast cells, which differentiate to form osteoblasts, signaling a reversal from bone resorption to bone formation. Osteoblasts begin the process of new bone formation by laying down a matrix of proteins called the *osteoid.* The primary protein produced by the osteoblast is a precursor to type I collagen. Extracellular processing of the precursor proteins results in the formation of mature, three-chained type I collagen molecules that assemble themselves into a collagen fibril. The individual collagen molecules are connected by pyridinoline cross-links, which are unique to bone.[1] Another protein produced by the osteoblasts is *osteocalcin,* a bone-specific protein characterized by the presence of three γ-carboxy-glutamic acid residues. These residues allow osteocalcin to bind calcium and hydroxyapatite, which results in the mineralization of the protein matrix. In addition to its role in the mineralization of bone, osteocalcin has a chemotactic and mitogenic effect on osteoclast cells.

Osteoporosis may develop when the rate of bone resorption is increased, the rate of bone formation is decreased, or when peak bone mass is inadequate. Peak bone mass is defined as the greatest bone mass achieved as a result of normal growth. A greater peak bone mass provides a larger reserve later in life and decreases the risk of developing osteoporosis.[2] Rates of bone resorption and formation are regulated by several hormones and cytokines, and peak bone mass can be influenced by hormonal, genetic, and lifestyle factors.

Involutional Osteoporosis

The most common form of osteoporosis is *involutional osteoporosis,* which can be further classified as type I or *postmenopausal osteoporosis,* and type II or *senile osteoporosis.* Postmenopausal osteoporosis is the most common of these two forms. It characteristically affects women within 15 to 20 years after menopause and is the result of bone loss due to decreased endogenous estrogen concentrations. Estrogen inhibits the secretion of interleukin-6 (IL-6) by osteoblasts.[3] Upon entering menopause, the reduction in circulating estrogen results in increased IL-6 production, which leads to increased osteoclast activity and bone resorption.[4,5] Increased bone resorption increases plasma ionized calcium activity, suppresses parathyroid hormone

(PTH) secretion, and increases the load of calcium filtered by the kidney. Suppressed PTH concentration decreases renal calcium conservation and renal production of 1,25-dihydroxyvitamin D ($1,25\text{-}(OH)_2D_3$). The major function of $1,25\text{-}(OH)_2D_3$ is to increase calcium absorption in the intestine; in fact a decrease in $1,25\text{-}(OH)_2D_3$ concentration decreases the efficiency of intestinal calcium absorption. The net result is that the amount of calcium lost per day increases from 20 mg in premenopausal women, to 38 mg per day in postmenopausal women.[6] Estrogen may also act by more direct means on bone cells because estrogen receptors have been found on both osteoblastic and osteoclastic cells,[7, 8] but other mechanisms of action have not been elucidated.

Senile osteoporosis is the result of age-related bone loss and is typically seen in men and women after the age of 75. Bone loss is due primarily to age-related changes in calcium metabolism and a decrease in osteoblast function. Serum concentrations of $1,25\text{-}(OH)_2D_3$ decrease with age,[9] and intestinal responsiveness to $1,25\text{-}(OH)_2D_3$ that is present is decreased due to a reduction in the number of $1,25\text{-}(OH)_2D_3$ receptors present on duodenal mucosal cells.[10] Intestinal absorption of both calcium and vitamin D have been shown to decrease with age,[11–13] which may be due in part to a reduction in caloric intake among the elderly.

Although senile osteoporosis occurs in both men and women, it occurs twice as frequently in women. Combined with the effects of postmenopausal osteoporosis, one out of every two women age 65 or older develop osteoporosis-related fractures, whereas only one in five men in the same age group develop these fractures.[14] Each year in the United States, osteoporosis results in 1.5 million fractures involving the hip, distal forearm, spinal vertebrae, and other sites, resulting in an estimated annual cost of $7 to 10 billion.[15] Hip fractures have a mortality rate approaching 20%, and for those patients that survive, mobility is a major problem.[16] The financial consequences of hip fractures are significant. Unfortunately, fractures are often the first clinical sign of osteoporosis. Identification of patients at risk is critical for early diagnosis of the disease, before the occurrence of fractures.

A family history of osteoporosis increases the risk of development of disease. Differences in bone mass have been shown to be associated with differences in the genotype of the vitamin D receptor allele.[17] In addition, hereditary factors also play a role in calcium absorption and serum $1,25(OH_2)D_3$ levels.[18] Although ethnicity has been identified as a risk factor in osteoporosis because white and Asian women have a higher incidence of the disease, it is not clear whether this is due to genetic factors or lifestyle differences.

Calcium intake throughout life can influence the onset of osteoporosis. In the United States, up to one-third of the postmenopausal population surveyed between 1976 and 1980 in the National Health and Nutrition Examination Survey (NHANES II) had intakes under 400 mg and thus likely had calcium insufficiency-related bone loss.[19] The decrease in intestinal absorption of calcium and vitamin D in addition to age compounds the problem.

Underweight individuals are at an increased risk of developing osteoporosis. A comparison of osteoporotic women to healthy postmenopausal women revealed that the osteoporotic women had similar lean body mass, but less fat mass.[20] One proposed mechanism for this is the enhanced peripheral conversion of androstenedione to estrone in fat tissue. This coincides with the observation that bone density also correlates with fat tissue mass in premenopausal women, but no correlation is observed in males.[21] Lack of exercise and immobilization have also been shown to result in the loss of bone.[22, 23] The fact that exercise and mechanical loading stimulate bone formation may be another mechanism in which weight affects disease development.[24, 25]

In women, smoking causes an alteration in the hepatic metabolism of estrogen, converting it to an inactive form.[26] It is likely that other mechanisms of action are also involved because smoking causes decreased bone density in pre- and post-menopausal women, as well as in men.[27–29]

Heavy alcohol use alters the calcium-regulating hormones PTH and $1,25\text{-}(OH)_2D_3$, reduces serum osteocalcin, and reduces the rate of bone formation.[30–32] In addition, alcohol use may also lead to osteopenia because of associated hypogonadism, hypercortisolism, metabolic acidosis, malnutrition, and, in advanced disease, cirrhosis of the liver.[25]

Secondary Osteoporosis

Secondary osteoporosis is the term used to describe bone loss that results from specific conditions, including certain diseases, surgical procedures, and the use of certain drugs. Among the most common contributing factors are hypogonadism in men and women, hyperthyroidism, subtotal gastrectomy, hemiplegia, chronic obstructive lung disease, and the use of glucocorticoid and anticonvulsant drugs.[33] Other syndromes that have been mentioned in association with secondary osteoporosis include hypercortisolism (Cushing's syndrome), hyperparathyroidism, hypopituitarism, insulin-dependent diabetes, rheumatoid arthritis, connective tissue disorders such as homocystinuria and osteogenesis imperfecta, and some malignancies, such as multiple myeloma and myeloproliferative disorders.

Hypogonadism arises from a number of causes, and its occurrence leads to an increased risk of osteoporosis. Hyperprolactinemia in both men[34] and women,[35] idiopathic hypogonadatropic hypogonadism,[36] hypothalamic hypogonadism in female athletes,[37] and anorexia nervosa[38] all result in gonadal insufficiency and decrease in bone mass.

Changes in thyroid gland activity can result in the development of osteoporosis by two possible mechanisms. Hyperthyroidism causes an increase in bone remodeling, but the increase in bone resorption is greater than the increase in bone formation resulting in a net loss of bone.[39] Thyroxine (T_4) and triiodothyronine (T_3) stimulate bone resorption.[40] Thyroidectomy results in the loss of C cells, which produce calcitonin. Calcitonin is a potent inhibitor of osteoclast activity, and some evidence documents that thyroidectomized patients have reduced bone mineral content.[41]

Glucocorticoids, from either hypercortisolism or glucocorticoid therapy, induce secondary osteoporosis by increasing bone resorption and by inhibiting bone formation. Bone resorption occurs due to reduced intestinal absorption and increased renal excretion of calcium, which results in a negative calcium balance.[42, 43] The negative calcium balance, in addition to the direct action of glucocorticoids on the parathyroid gland results in increased PTH secretion, further increasing the calcium loss from the bones.[44] Glucocorticoids inhibit bone formation by inhibiting differentiation of preosteoblasts to form mature osteoblasts,[45] and inhibiting the synthesis of collagen and other noncollagenous proteins.[46, 47]

Idiopathic Osteoporosis

Two forms of primary osteoporosis occur in children and young adults. Idiopathic juvenile osteoporosis is a rare disease affecting children usually between the ages of 8 and 14 years, but it may occasionally occur in children as young as 3 years of age.[48] The disease runs an acute course, usually over 2 to 4 years, and then it undergoes spontaneous remission with the resumption of normal linear and radial bone growth. The etiology for idiopathic juvenile osteoporosis is unknown, although both genetics and hormonal factors have been suggested.[49, 50] Although idiopathic osteoporosis in young adults occurs more frequently than juvenile osteoporosis, it is still a relatively rare disease. It has been called an etiologically heterogeneous disease. Some, but not all, patients have been found to have increased levels of interleukin-1, a potent stimulator of bone resorption.[51] Low levels of insulin-like growth factor-1 (IGF-1), a growth factor that enhances osteoblast number and function, have also been observed in idiopathic osteoporosis.[52]

CLINICAL MANIFESTATIONS
Involutional Osteoporosis

Involutional osteoporosis is often asymptomatic, and the first clinical symptom may be a fracture that occurs essentially with no trauma. Manifestation of acute pain in the mid to lower thorax or high lumbar areas of the spine is probably the earliest symptom. The pain may be intermittent, and, if multiple fractures have occurred, a continuous dull ache may ensue. Postmenopausal osteoporosis is characterized by fractures that occur at sites rich in cancellous bone. These include vertebral compression fractures, Colles' fracture of the distal forearm, and fractures of the ankle. Progressive spinal deformity associated with compression fractures of the thoracic vertebrae leads to loss of height and progressive thoracic kyphosis ("dowager's hump"). Age-related osteoporosis is characterized by fractures at sites containing substantial proportions of both cortical and cancellous bone. The main manifestations are fractures of the hip and vertebral wedge fractures, but fractures of the proximal humerus, proximal tibia, and pelvis are also common.

Secondary Osteoporosis

Clinical manifestations of secondary osteoporosis are similar to those of involutional osteoporosis. Bone pain is often the first clinical symptom, and in patients presenting with fractures, the location of fracture is often characteristic of the disease precipitating the osteoporosis. For example, glucocorticoid-induced osteoporosis manifests itself as a loss of cancellous bone, causing an increased risk of verte-

bral fractures but no increase in risk of hip fracture, whereas gastrectomy patients often present with hip fractures.[33] Hyperthyroidism causes reduced bone mass in the axial skeleton but does not usually result in fractures.[53] Patient history can identify the presence of previously diagnosed conditions known to contribute to bone loss, such as diabetes mellitus or hemiplegia.

Idiopathic Osteoporosis

Patients with idiopathic juvenile osteoporosis present with bone pain, difficulty walking, and fractures of the long bones or vertebrae. Osteopenia is evident by radiograph in most patients. Idiopathic osteoporosis in young adults usually presents with multiple vertebral fractures over a period of 5 to 10 years. Fractures of the ribs and metatarsals are common, and unilateral or bilateral hip fractures may also occur. The severity of idiopathic osteoporosis can range from relatively mild cases, resulting in only one or two crushed vertebrae to severe *kyphoscoliosis,* crippling deformities of the extremities, and even collapse of the rib cage and death from respiratory failure.

LABORATORY ANALYSES AND DIAGNOSIS

The diagnosis of osteoporosis is made primarily from radiographic bone mineral density measurements used to establish the presence of osteopenia. A diagnosis of primary osteoporosis is made primarily by the exclusion of conditions that could result in the development of secondary osteoporosis. The age of the patient is of great importance. Primary osteoporosis is the most common form of osteoporosis in postmenopausal women and in patients older than 65 years. Secondary osteoporosis is more common than primary osteoporosis in juveniles and young adults. A thorough patient history is essential in differentiating between primary and secondary osteoporosis. The patient history includes previous history of fractures, family history, age at the onset of menopause, amenorrhea, and previously diagnosed conditions, along with treatments prescribed. Conditions that have been shown to result in secondary osteoporosis include hypogonadism, hypercortisolism, hyperthyroidism, hyperparathyroidism, diabetes mellitus, various malignancies, gastrectomy, malabsorption, primary biliary cirrhosis, anorexia nervosa, severe malnutrition, osteogenesis imperfecta, Marfan's syndrome, Ehlers-Danlos syndrome, prolonged immobilization, chronic obstructive pulmonary disease, radiation treatment, chronic alcoholism, and rheumatoid arthritis.[14]

Diagnosis in Juvenile and Young Adult Patients

In juvenile patients who exhibit osteopenia, secondary osteoporosis is a more likely cause of the osteopenia than primary osteoporosis. Figure 69–1 shows the suggested order of tests to distinguish between primary and secondary osteoporosis in juveniles and young adults. A diagnosis of idiopathic juvenile osteoporosis can be made only after the exclusion of osteogenesis imperfecta, calcium and vitamin D deficiencies, malabsorption, hyperparathyroidism, hyper-

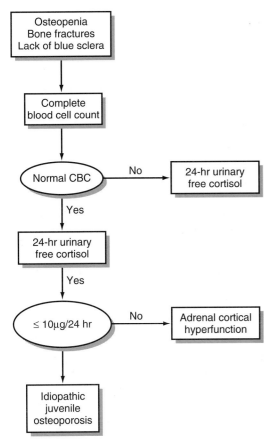

Figure 69–1. Differential diagnosis of osteoporosis in juveniles.

thyroidism, acute leukemias, and Cushing's syndrome. Family and medical history should differentiate between osteoporosis and osteogenesis imperfecta. A patient having osteogenesis imperfecta most likely has a history of fractures of the long bones, a family history of bone disease, and characteristic blue sclera. If it is determined that the patient does not have osteogenesis imperfecta, a 24-hour urinary free cortisol should be done to test for adrenal cortical hyperfunction. If adrenal cortex function is determined to be normal, a complete blood cell count with differential count should be performed for evidence of acute leukemia. Other laboratory tests, such as measurement of serum calcium, phosphate, magnesium, alkaline phosphatase, parathyroid hormone, calcitonin, and 25-hydroxyvitamin D are usually within normal range.[54, 55] Increased urinary calcium excretion has been reported in only 8% of patients at presentation.[56]

Diagnosis in Older Adult Patients

In older patients, primary osteoporosis is much more common than secondary osteoporosis, but secondary causes must still be ruled out before a diagnosis can be made. A suggested ordering of tests can be found in Figure 69–2.

A complete blood cell count should be done to detect the presence of marrow related disorders. Multiple myeloma should be particularly suspect and protein electrophoresis should be considered. Other metastatic malignancies can contribute to the development of secondary osteoporosis, but this is more often related to the treatment

of these cancers, such as therapeutic oophorectomy or adrenalectomy. Chemotherapy can also suppress ovarian function and bone formation, and radiation therapy can produce osteopenia in the radiation field.

A 24-hour urinary free cortisol should be performed on patients who have not been treated with long-term glucocorticoids to rule out adrenal cortical hyperfunction. Serum parathyroid hormone concentration should be used as an indicator of primary or secondary hyperparathyroidism. Secondary hyperparathyroidism is much more common and may be induced by chronic renal disease, anticonvusant medications (especially phenobarbital and diphenylhydantoin), gastrectomy, and malabsorption syndromes. In some adults, an age-related defect in renal hydroxylation of 25-hydroxyvitamin D to the active form

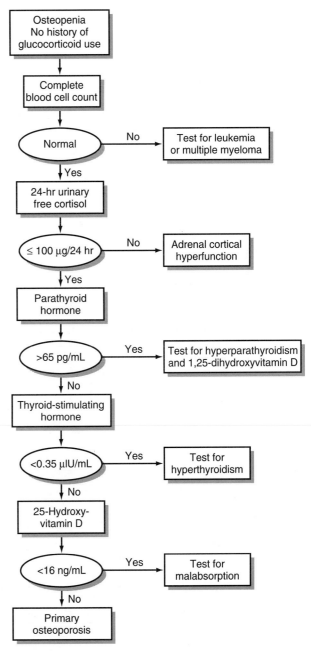

Figure 69–2. Diagnosis of primary osteoporosis in older adults.

of 1,25-(OH)$_2$ D$_3$ can result in elevated PTH concentrations.[15] Laboratory analysis of this form of vitamin D may be beneficial in distinguishing between primary and secondary hyperparathyroidism.

Decreased concentration of thyroid stimulating hormone is an indicator that further thyroid function tests should be done. Accelerated bone loss has been associated with low levels of thyroid-stimulating hormone, which indicates the presence of subclinical hyperthyroidism.[33]

Hypovitaminosis D is relatively common in the elderly. In all older patients being treated for osteopenia, serum 25-hydroxyvitamin D should be determined to assess the adequacy of vitamin D stores and to ascertain if additional tests for malabsorption are necessary.

LABORATORY ANALYSES AND TREATMENT

In cases of primary osteoporosis, the management of the patient involves calcium supplementation that replaces the calcium that has been lost from the bones and prevents further loss. Vitamin D and fluoride supplementation may also be recommended. In the case of secondary osteoporosis, treatment of the condition that resulted in the development of osteoporosis is the main concern, but calcium supplementation would also be initiated. Laboratory tests for monitoring patients are performed primarily for the purpose of monitoring the rates of bone formation and bone resorption.

Bone Resorption Tests

Several markers have been used to monitor rates of bone resorption. The least expensive of these tests is the 24-hour urinary calcium. It is useful to detect a marked increase in bone resorption, but it lacks specificity. Values are influenced by renal handling of calcium and by estrogens.

Urinary excretion of hydroxyproline is the standard measure of collagen breakdown and bone resorption; however, it is not a very sensitive marker of bone resorption. Hydroxyproline represents about 13% of the amino acid content of collagen and approximately 50% of the body's collagen is found in bone. The C1q fraction of complement also contains significant amounts of hydroxyproline. Urinary excretion of hydroxyproline increases following the activation of complement, and it is also affected by liver metabolism and dietary intake of hydroxyproline.

Two pyridium crosslinks, pyridinoline and deoxypyridinoline, are present in the mature form of collagen found in bone. These crosslinks are the result of post-translational modification of collagen molecules and cannot be reutilized for the synthesis of new collagen molecules. As a result, when collagen is degraded during bone resorption, pyridinoline and deoxypyridinoline are released and excreted in the urine. Their concentration can be measured in either serum or urine as a measure of bone resorption. Related to these tests are immunoassays for the peptides containing N-telopeptide and C-telopeptide crosslinks. Deoxypyridinoline is more specific to bone collagen, but both crosslinks and related peptides appear to provide sensitive and specific markers for bone resorption. Pyridinoline and deoxypyridinoline excretion exhibit circadian rhythm with a peak during the night and a nadir during the afternoon, a pattern similar to that of osteocalcin that probably reflects a nocturnal increase of bone turnover and resorption.[57] Pyridinoline and deoxypyridinoline are not absorbed by the intestine, so their concentration is not influenced by diet.

Tartrate-resistant acid phosphatase (TRAP) has been used as a marker for osteoclast activity. Plasma acid phosphatase should be measured rather than serum levels due to the release of platelet phosphatase activity during clotting and the presence of enzyme inhibitors in serum.[57] TRAP is elevated after oophorectomy and is relatively unstable.

Bone Formation Tests

Three biochemical markers can be used to monitor bone formation. These include bone-specific alkaline phosphatase, serum osteocalcin, and procollagen I extension peptides. Serum total alkaline phosphatase activity is the most commonly used marker of bone formation, but it is a test of low specificity and sensitivity for osteoporosis. Levels are usually normal in osteoporosis patients, although they may be elevated after a fracture.

Bone-specific alkaline phosphatase is used to enhance the specificity and sensitivity of alkaline phosphatase activity in monitoring bone formation. The bone, hepatic, and kidney isoenzyme forms are all encoded by a single gene and differ only in post-translational modifications. However, this modification is sufficient to allow for their separation by electrophoresis, and the bone isoenzyme can be precipitated by wheat-germ lectin.[58] The expression of the bone isoenzyme is enhanced by a variety of factors, including parathyroid hormone, calcitriol, glucocorticoids and other steroid hormones, and growth factors.[59]

Osteocalcin, also called *bone GLA protein* or BGP, is very specific for bone tissue and dentin. It is synthesized by the osteoblasts and the majority is incorporated into the extracellular matrix of bone. A small portion is released into the plasma where it can be quantified by radioimmunoassay. Sensitivity of the assay is dependent on the specificity of the antibody. After a few hours at room temperature, a significant fraction of plasma-intact osteocalcin is rapidly converted into the large N-midfragment, resulting in a significant loss of immunoreactivity with most polyclonal antibodies that recognize the C-terminal end of the molecule.[57] The half-life of osteocalcin in plasma is short (minutes), and it is excreted in the urine. Serum levels of osteocalcin demonstrate a circadian rhythm and may also fluctuate during the menstrual cycle.[15] The expression of osteocalcin is enhanced by calcitriol, vitamin K, thyroid hormones, glucocorticoids, insulin, and estrogen. Impaired renal function may also result in an increase in the level of serum osteocalcin.[59]

About 80% of the protein found in bone is type I collagen. Type I collagen is synthesized as a propeptide and processed by cleaving the amino terminal (PINP) and the carboxy terminal (PICP) extension peptides. Serum PICP levels have been found to weakly correlate with bone formation rates, but this test lacks sensitivity.[57] Serum PINP levels did not correlate well with increased bone turnover.[60] PICP has a molecular weight of approximately 100 kD, so it is not affected by glomerular filtration rate. It is believed to be cleared through the liver.

Case Study 1

A 66-year-old white woman was admitted to the hospital after sustaining a fall at home. Initial assessment disclosed facial lacerations and multiple contusions on the arms, legs, thighs, hips, and upper chest. Vital signs showed a temperature of 98.5° F, pulse 65, respirations 15, and blood pressure 115/78 mm Hg. X-rays obtained on admission revealed a simple fracture of the intertrochanteric area of the right proximal femur, and a lateral radiograph of the thoracic and lumbar spine showed visible loss of bone density. Personal and medical history reveal that the patient is a widow with two children and four grandchildren. She resides alone and has had relatively good health, with no history of chronic illness. The patient reported a simple fracture of the left distal radius 5 years prior to this admission.

The laboratory results (with reference ranges) are as follows:

Analyte	Admission Result	Postoperative Result	Reference Range
WBC ($\times 10^9$/L)	5.6	6.0	4.8–10.8
RBC ($\times 10^{12}$/L)	4.0	3.8	4.2–5.4
Hgb (g/dL)	11.8	11.5	12–16
Hct (%)	36	34	37–47
Glucose (mg/dL)	100	115	70–105
Ca (mEq/L)	4.7	4.6	4.3–5.3
PO_4 (mg/dL)	3.7	3.6	2.8–4.1
Mg (mEq/L)	1.7	1.7	1.3–2.1
Alkaline Phosphatase (U/L)	145	150	30–120

Questions

1. What is the most likely diagnosis? Why?
2. What tests would confirm the diagnosis?
3. Do the laboratory findings support this diagnosis?

Discussion

1. Uncomplicated postmenopausal osteoporosis is the most likely diagnosis because it is most commonly found in white females of this age group. The type of fracture sustained by this patient and her history support this diagnosis.

2. Radiologic procedures for the detection of osteopenia would confirm the diagnosis of osteoporosis. A diagnosis of primary postmenopausal osteoporosis can be made after laboratory tests have ruled out causes of secondary osteoporosis.

3. The laboratory findings support this diagnosis. Except for alkaline phosphatase, which is expected to be elevated after a fracture, laboratory findings in uncomplicated postmenopausal osteoporosis are usually normal, even when bone loss has been extensive. Slightly elevated glucose is associated with postoperative IV infusion of 5% dextrose in water.

Case Study 2

During a routine physical, a 46-year-old white male presented with mild dorsal kyphosis and a loss of 1¼ inches in height over the past 12 years. Vital signs showed a temperature of 98.6° F, pulse 100, respirations 17, and blood pressure 120/70. Radiologic findings revealed a decrease in vertebral bone density, but no compression fractures. The patient did not report any back pain. Personal and medical history indicated that the patient is married with two children. He has congenital adrenal hyperplasia and had been taking 30 mg of hydrocortisone daily. He has felt well and is active physically, including a hobby of rollerskating. He did not report any previous fractures.

The laboratory results (with reference ranges) are as follows:

Analyte	Results	Reference Range
Calcium (mEq/L)	4.6	4.3–5.3
Ionized Calcium (mg/dL) at pH 7.4, 37° C	5.25	4.5–5.3
Urinary Calcium (mg/24hr)	261	100–250
Phosphorus (mg/dL)	4.0	2.5–4.5
Albumin (g/dL)	4.2	3.5–5.2
Alkaline Phosphatase (U/L)	80	30–120
Bone Specific Alkaline Phosphatase (U/mL)	10.3	2.8–12.0
Parathyroid Hormone (pg/mL)	25	10–65
25-OH Vitamin D (ng/mL)	30	16–74
1,25-$(OH)_2$ Vitamin D (pg/mL)	56	15–60
Total T_3 (ng/mL)	0.9	0.6–1.8
TSH (μIU/mL)	1.19	0.35–5.5
T_3 Uptake (%)	33.9	24–37
T_4 (μg/dL)	6.6	4.5–12.0
Free Thyroxine (ng/dL)	2.2	1.1–4.4
Urinary Pyridinoline (pmol/μmol Creatinine)	73.1	22–90
Urinary Deoxypyridinoline (pmol/μmol Creatinine)	26.7	4–21

Questions

1. What is the most likely diagnosis? Why?
2. Do the laboratory findings support this diagnosis?

Discussion

1. Glucocorticoid-induced osteoporosis is the most likely diagnosis due to the patient's long-term use of hydrocortisone.

2. Yes. Increased levels of calcium and deoxypyridino-line suggest increased rates of bone resorption. All other laboratory tests are within normal range, which indicates no other cause for secondary osteoporosis other than long-term glucocorticoid use.

References

1. Jilka RL, Manolagas SC: The cellular and biochemical basis of bone remodeling. *In* Marcus R (ed): Osteoporosis. Boston, Blackwell Scientific Publications, 1994, pp 17–48.

2. Heaney RP, Matkovic V: Inadequate peak bone mass. *In* Riggs BL, Melton LJ III (eds): Osteoporosis: Etiology, Diagnosis, and Management. Philadelphia, Lippincott-Raven Publishers, 1995, pp 115–131.

3. Pottratz ST, Bellido T, Mocharla H, et al: 17β-Estradiol inhibits expression of human interleukin-6 promoter-reporter constructs by a receptor-dependent mechanism. J Clin Invest 93:944–950, 1994.

4. Ishimi Y, Miyaura C, Jin CH, et al: IL-6 is produced by osteoblasts and induces bone resorption. J Immunol 145:3297–3303, 1990.

5. Lowik CWGM, van der Pluijm G, Bloys H, et al: Parathyroid hormone (PTH) and PTH-like protein (PLP) stimulate interleukin-6 production by osteogenic cells: A possible role of interleukin-6 in osteoclastogenesis. Biochem Biophys Res Commun 162:1546–1552, 1989.

6. Heaney RP, Recker RR, Saville PD: Menopausal changes in calcium balance performance. J Lab Clin Med 92:953–963, 1978.

7. Eriksen EF, Colvard DS, Berg NJ, et al: Evidence of estrogen receptors in normal human osteoblast-like cells. Science 241:84–86, 1988.

8. Oursler MJ, Pederson L, Fitzpatrick L: Human giant cell tumors of the bone (osteoclastomas) are estrogen target cells. J Bone Min Res 7:S111, 1992.

9. Aksnes L, Rodland O, Odegaard OR, et al: Serum levels of vitamin-D metabolites in the elderly. Acta Endocrinol 121:27–33, 1989.

10. Ebeling PR, Sandgren ME, Dimagno EP, et al: Evidence of an age-related decrease in intestinal responsiveness to vitamin D: Relationship between serum 1,25 dihydroxyvitamin D_3 and intestinal vitamin D receptor concentrations in normal women. J Clin Endocrinol Metab 75:176–182, 1992.

11. Bullamore JR, Gallagher JC, Williams A, et al: Effect of age on calcium absorption. Lancet ii:535–537, 1970.

12. Nordin BEC, Wilkinson R, Marshall DH, et al: Calcium absorption in the elderly. Calcif Tissue Res 21 (suppl):442–451, 1976.

13. Clemens TL, Zhou XY, Myles M, et al: Serum vitamin D_2 and vitamin D_3 metabolite concentrations and absorption of vitamin D_2 in elderly subjects. J Clin Endocrinol Metab 63:656–660, 1986.

14. Gamble CL: Osteoporosis: Making the diagnosis in patients at risk for fracture. Geriatrics 50:24–33, 1995.

15. Mitlak BH, Nussbaum SR: Diagnosis and treatment of osteoporosis. Ann Rev Med 44:265–277, 1993.

16. Cummings SR, Kelsey JL, Nevitt MC, et al: Epidemiology of osteoporosis and osteoporotic fractures. Epidemiol Rev 7:178–208, 1985.

17. Morrison NA, Qi JC, Tokita A, et al: Prediction of bone density from vitamin D receptor alleles. Nature 367:284–287, 1994.

18. Peacock M, Johnston CC, Christian J: Inheritance of calcium-regulating hormones, calcium absorption and bone turnover. J Bone Miner Res 7(Suppl 1):937 (abstr), 1992.

19. Abraham S, Carroll MD, Dresser CM, et al: Dietary intake findings, United States 1976–1980. Hyattsville, MD: Department of Health and Human Services (DHHS publication no. (PHS) 83-1681).

20. Hassager C, Christianson C: Influence of soft tissue body composition on bone mass and metabolism. Bone 10:415–419, 1989.

21. Reid IR, Plank LD, Evans MC: Fat mass is an important determinant of whole body bone density in premenopausal women but not in men. J Clin Endocrinol Metab 75:779–782, 1992.

22. Dalsky G, Stocke K, Ehsani A, et al: Weight-bearing exercise training and lumbar bone mineral content in postmenopausal women. Ann Intern Med 108:824–828, 1988.

23. Donaldson C, Hulley S, Vogel J, et al: Effects of prolonged bed rest on bone mineral. Metabolism 19:1071–1084, 1970.

24. Pead MJ, Skerry TM, Lanyon LE: Direct transformation from quiescence to bone formation in the adult periosteum following a single brief period of bone loading. J Bone Miner Res 3:647–656, 1988.

25. Dawson-Hughes B: Prevention. *In* Riggs BL, Melton LJ III (eds): Osteoporosis: Etiology, Diagnosis, and Management. Philadelphia, Lippincott-Raven Publishers, 1995, pp 335–350.

26. Michnovicz JJ, Hershcopf RJ, Naganuma H, et al: Increased 2-hydroxylation of estradiol as a possible mechanism for the anti-estrogenic effect of cigarette smoking. N Engl J Med 315:1305–1309, 1986.

27. Sparrow D, Beausoleil NI, Garvey AJ, et al: The influence of cigarette smoking and age on bone loss in men. Arch Environ Health 37:246–249, 1982.

28. Krall EA, Dawson-Hughes B: Smoking and bone loss among post-menopausal women. J Bone Miner Res 6:331–337, 1991.

29. Slemenda CW, Hui SL, Longcope C, et al: Cigarette smoking, obesity, and bone mass. J Bone Miner Res 4:737–741, 1989.

30. Labib M, Abdel-Kader M, Ranganath L, et al: Bone disease in chronic alcoholism: The value of plasma osteocalcin measurement. Alcohol 24:141–144, 1989.

31. Bikle DD, Genant HK, Cann C, et al: Bone disease in alcohol abuse. Ann Intern Med 103:42–48, 1985.

32. Diamond T, Stiel D, Lunzer M, et al: Ethanol reduces bone formation and may cause osteoporosis. Am J Med 86:282–288, 1989.

33. Khosla S, Melton LJ III: Secondary osteoporosis. *In* Riggs BL, Melton LJ III (eds): Osteoporosis: Etiology, Diagnosis, and Management. Philadelphia, Lippincott-Raven Publishers, 1995, pp 183–204.

34. Biller BMK, Baum HBA, Rosenthal DI, et al: Progressive trabecular osteopenia in women with hyperprolactinemic amenorrhea. J Clin Endocrinol Metab 75:692–697, 1992.

35. Schlechte J, Walkner L, Kathol M: A longtitudinal analysis of pre-menopausal bone loss in healthy women and women with hyperprolactinemia. J Clin Endocrinol Metab 75:698–703, 1992.

36. Finkelstein JS, Klibanski A, Neer RM, et al: Osteoporosis in men with idiopathic hypogonadotropic hypogonadism. Ann Intern Med 106:354–361, 1987.

37. Drinkwater BL, Bruemner B, Chesnut CH III: Menstrual history as a determinant of current bone density in young athletes. JAMA 263:545–548, 1990.

38. Herzog W, Minne H, Deter C, et al: Outcome of bone mineral density in anorexia nervosa patients 11.7 years after first admission. J Bone Miner Res 8:597–605, 1993.

39. Eriksen EF, Mosekilde L, Melsen F: Trabecular bone remodeling and bone balance in hyperthyroidism. Bone 6:421–428, 1985.

40. Mundy GR, Shapiro JL, Bandelin JG, et al: Direct stimulation of bone resorption by thyroid hormones. J Clin Invest 58:529–534, 1976.

41. McDermott MT, Kidd GS, Blue P, et al: Reduced bone mineral content in totally thyroidectomized patients: possible effect of calcitonin deficiency. J Clin Endocrinol Metab 56:936–939, 1983.

42. Caniggia A, Nuti R, Loré F, et al: Pathophysiology of the adverse effects of glucoactive corticosteroids on calcium metabolism in man. J Steroid Biochem 15:153–161, 1981.

43. Morris HA, Need AG, O'Loughlin PD, et al: Malabsorption of calcium in corticosteroid-induced osteoporosis. Calcif Tissue Int 46:305–308, 1990.

44. Fucik RF, Kukreja SC, Hargis GK, et al: Effect of glucocorticoids on function of the parathyroid glands in man. J Clin Endocrinol Metab 40:152–155, 1975.

45. Chyun YS, Kream BE, Raisz LG: Cortisol decreases bone formation by inhibiting periosteal cell proliferation. Endocrinology 114:477–480, 1984.

46. Canalis EM: Effect of cortisol on periosteal and non-periosteal collagen and DNA synthesis in cultured rat calvariae. Calcif Tissue Int 36:158–166, 1984.

47. Subramaniam M, Colvard D, Keeting P, et al: Glucocorticoid regulation of alkaline phosphatase, osteocalcin and protooncogenes in normal human osteoblast-like cells. J Cell Biochem 50:411–424, 1992.

48. Exner GU, Prader A, Elsasser U, et al: Idiopathic osteoporosis in a three-year-old girl: Follow-up over a period of 6 years by computed tomography bone densitometry (CT). Helv Paediatr Acta 39:517–528, 1984.

49. Treves R, Harang H, Bertin P, et al: Adolescent osteoporosis disclosing familial osteopenia. Clin Rheumatol 11:558–561, 1992.

50. Dent CE: Osteoporosis in childhood. Postgrad Med J 53:450–456, 1977.

51. Pacifici R, Rifas L, Teitelbaum S, et al: Spontaneous release of interleukin-1 from human blood monocytes reflects bone formation in idiopathic osteoporosis. Proc Natl Acad Sci USA 84:4616–4620, 1987.

52. McCarthy TL, Centrella M, Canalis E: Insulin-like growth factor (IGF) and bone. Connect Tissue Res 20:277–282, 1989.

53. Solomon BL, Wartofsky L, Burman KD: Prevalence of fractures in postmenopausal women with thyroid disease. Thyroid 3:17–23, 1993.

54. Saggese G, Bertelloni S, Baroncelli GI, et al: Mineral metabolism and calcitriol therapy in idiopathic juvenile osteoporosis. Am J Dis Child 145:457–462, 1991.

55. Zerwekh JE, Sakhaee K, Breslau NA, et al: Impaired bone formation in male idiopathic osteoporosis: Further reduction in the presence of concomitant hypercalciuria. Osteoporosis Int 2:128–134, 1992.

56. Khosla S, Lufkin EG, Hodgson SF, et al: Epidemiology and clinical features of osteoporosis in young individuals. Bone 15:551–555, 1994.

57. Delmas PD: Biochemical markers of bone turnover I: Theoretical considerations and clinical use in osteoporosis. Am J Med 95 (Suppl 5A):11S–16S, 1993.

58. Rosalki SB, Foo AY: Two new methods for separating and quantifying bone and liver alkaline phosphatase isoenzymes in plasma. Clin Chem 30:1182–1186, 1984.

59. Price CP, Thompson PW: The role of biochemical tests in the screening and monitoring of osteoporosis. Ann Clin Biochem 32:244–260, 1995.

60. Ebeling PR, Peterson JM, Riggs BL: Utility of type I procollagen propeptide assays for assessing abnormalities in metabolic bone diseases. J Bone Miner Res 7:1243–1250, 1992.

Index

Note: Page numbers in *italics* indicate figures; those followed by t indicate tables; those followed by b indicate boxed material.

T

ISBN 0-7216-6934-4